TEXTBOOK of

Diagnostic Ultrasonography

volume **TWO**

TEXTBOOK of

Diagnostic Ultrasonography

sixth edition

Sandra L. **Hagen-Ansert, MS, RDMS, RDCS**

Cardiology Department

Scripps Clinic — Torrey Pines

Former Office Manager and Clinical Cardiac Sonographer

University Cardiology Associates, Medical University of South Carolina

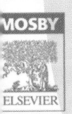

MOSBY

ELSEVIER

with 3217 illustrations

volume **TWO**

11830 Westline Industrial Drive
St. Louis, Missouri 63146

TEXTBOOK OF DIAGNOSTIC ULTRASONOGRAPHY
Copyright © 2006, 2001, 1995, 1989, 1983, 1978 by Mosby, Inc., an affiliate of Elsevier Inc.

ISBN 13: 978-0-323-02803-5
ISBN 10: 0-323-02803-9

ISBN 13: 978-0-323-02803-5
ISBN 10: 0-323-02803-9

Publisher: Andrew Allen
Executive Editor: Jeanne Wilke
Developmental Editor: Linda Woodard
Publishing Services Manager: Pat Joiner
Project Manager: Gena Magouirk
Design Direction: Kathi Gosche

Printed in Canada

Last digit is the print number: 9 8 7 6 5 4 3 2 1

Contributors

DARLEEN CIOFFI-RAGAN, BS, RDMS
Instructor
Obstetrics and Gynecology
University of Colorado Health Sciences Center
Denver, Colorado

M. ROBERT De JONG, RDMS, RDCS, RVT
Radiology Technical Manager, Ultrasound
The Russell H. Morgan Department of Radiology and Radiological
    Science
The Johns Hopkins Hospital
Baltimore, Maryland

TERRY J. DuBOSE, MS, RDMS, FSDMS, FAIUM
Associate Professor and Director
Diagnostic Medical Sonography Program
University of Arkansas for Medical Sciences
Little Rock, Arkansas

M. ELIZABETH GLENN, MD
Women's Health Center at Baptist East
Memphis, Tennessee

CHARLOTTE G. HENNINGSEN, MS, RT, RDMS, RVT
Chair and Professor
Diagnostic Medical Sonography Department
Florida Hospital College of Health Sciences
Orlando, Florida

MIRA L. KATZ, PhD, MPH
Assistant Professor
Division of Health Behavior and Health Promotion
School of Public Health
The Ohio State University
Columbus, Ohio

VALJEAN MacMILLAN, RDMS, RDSC
Sonographer
Shared Imaging Services
Madison, Wisconsin

DANIEL A. MERTON, BS, RDMS
Technical Coordinator of Research
Department of Radiology
The Jefferson Ultrasound Research and Education Institute
Thomas Jefferson University
Philadelphia, Pennsylvania

CAROL MITCHELL, PhD, RDMS, RDCS, RVT, RT(R)
Program Director
School of Diagnostic Medical Sonography
University of Wisconsin Hospitals & Clinics
Madison, Wisconsin

CINDY A. OWEN, RT, RDMS, RVT
Ultrasound Consultant
Diagnostic Ultrasound Services
Memphis, Tennessee

SUSAN RAATZ STEPHENSON, MEd, BSRT-U, RDMS, RT(R)(C)
Clinical Product Specialist
Philips Ultrasound
Bothell, Washington

TAMARA L. SALSGIVER, RT(R), RDMS, RVT
Program Director
Diagnostic Medical Sonography
Kaiser Permanente School of Allied Health Sciences
Richmond, California

JEAN LEA SPITZ, MPH, RDMS, FSDMS, FAIUM
Professor
College of Allied Health
University of Oklahoma Health Sciences Center
Oklahoma City, Oklahoma

DENISE SPRADLEY, BSRT, RDMS, RDCS, RVT
Lead Sonographer
Perinatal Center of Oklahoma
Oklahoma City, Oklahoma

DIANA M. STRICKLAND, BSBA, RDMS, RDCS
Clinical Assistant Professor and Co-Director
Ultrasound Program
Department of Obstetrics and Gynecology
Brody School of Medicine
East Carolina University
Greenville, North Carolina

BARBARA TRAMPE, RN, RDMS
Chief Sonographer
Meriter/University of Wisconsin Perinatal Ultrasound
Madison, Wisconsin

BARBARA J. VANDER WERFF, RDMS, RDCS, RVT
Chief Sonographer
University of Wisconsin-Madison Hospitals and Clinics
Madison, Wisconsin

KERRY WEINBERG, RDMS, RDCS
Director
Diagnostic Medical Sonography Program
New York University
New York, New York

BETH ANDERHUB, MEd, RDMS, RSDMS
Program Director
Diagnostic Medical Sonography
St. Louis Community College
St. Louis, Missouri

GINA M. AUGUSTINE, MLS, RT(R)
Director
School of Radiography and Specialty Programs
Jameson Health System
New Castle, Pennsylvania

KEVIN BARRY, MEd, RDMS, RDCS, RT(R)
Department Head
Diagnostic Medical Imaging
New Hampshire Technical Institute
Concord, New Hampshire

KATHI BOROK, BS, RDMS, RDCS
Clinical Coordinator
Diagnostic Medical Sonography Department
Florida Hospital College of Health Sciences
Orlando, Florida

PAMELA BROWER, RVT, RVS, CRT
Department Chair
Diagnostic Medical Sonography
Tyler Junior College
Tyler, Texas

JAN BRYANT, MS, RDMS, RT(R)
Program Director
Ultrasound
El Centro College
Dallas, Texas

ERIC CADIENTE, AS, RDCS, RVT
Diagnostic Medical Sonography Department
Florida Hospital College of Health Sciences
Orlando, Florida

LYNN CARLTON, MS, RDMS, RT(R)(M)
Staff Sonographer
Metropolitan Hospital
Grand Rapids, Michigan

JOAN M. CLASBY, BvE, RDMS, RT, RDCS
Professor and Director
Diagnostic Medical Sonography Program
Orange Coast College
Costa Mesa, California

**JANICE DIANE DOLK, MA, RT(R), RDMS
(abdomen, ob/gyn, breast)**
Director of Allied Health Education
University of Maryland—Baltimore County
UMBC Training Enterprises
Baltimore, Maryland

KEVIN EVANS, PhD, RT(R)(M)(BD), RDMS, RVT
Assistant Professor and Director
Ohio State University
Columbus, Ohio

JANET M. FELDMEIER, BSRT, RDMS
Staff Ultrasonographer
Cardinal Glennon Children's Hospital
St. Louis, Missouri

THOMAS J. GERVAISE, BS, RT, RDMS
Ultrasound Division Director
Modern Division Director
Anaheim, California

TIM S. GIBBS, RT(R,F), RDMS, RVT, CTNM
Senior Sonographer
West Anaheim Medical Center
Anaheim, California

CHARLOTTE G. HENNINGSEN, MS, RT, RDMS, RVT
Chair and Professor
Diagnostic Medical Sonography Department
Florida Hospital College of Health Sciences
Orlando, Florida

FELICIA JONES, MSEd, RDMS, RCDS, RVT
Director
Diagnostic Medical Sonography
Tidewater Community College
Virginia Beach, Virginia

RUBEN MARTINEZ, BS, RDCS, RVT
Cardiovascular Ultrasound Instructor
Florida Hospital College of Health Sciences
Orlando, Florida

CAROL MITCHELL, PhD, RDMS, RDCS, RVT, RT(R)
Program Director
School of Diagnostic Medical Sonography
University of Wisconsin Hospitals & Clinics
Madison, Wisconsin

JOSEPH B. MORTON III, MBA, RT(R), RDMS
Sonographer/Clinical Instructor
Columbia—St. Mary's Hospitals
Milwaukee, Wisconsin

KATHLEEN MURPHY, MBA, RDMS, RT
Program Director
Diagnostic Ultrasound
Gateway Community College
Phoenix, Arizona

SUSANNA OVEL, RDMS, RVT
Senior Sonographer/Trainer
Radiological Associates of Sacramento (RAS)
Sacramento, California

CRAIG PENOFF, BSAS, RDMS, RVT
Assistant Professor and Program Director
Diagnostic Medical Sonography
Lorain County Community College
Elyria, Ohio

CYNTHIA REBER-BONHALL, BS, RDMS, RVT
Clinical Faculty
Orange Coast College
Costa Mesa, California

DANA SALMONS, BS, RT, RDMS
Sonographer
Florida Hospital
Orlando, Florida

LISA STROHL, BS, RT(R), RDMS, RVT
Marketing Manager
Jefferson Center City Imaging
Thomas Jefferson University
Philadelphia, Pennsylvania

REGINA SWEARENGIN, BS, RDMS (AB, OB, NE)
Sonography Department Chair
Austin Community College
Austin, Texas

ELLEN T. TUCHINSKY, BA, RDMS, RDCS
Clinical Education Coordinator
Diagnostic Medical Sonography Program
School of Continuing Professional Studies
New York University
New York, New York

CHERYL L. ZELINSKY, MM, ARRT(R), RDMS
Associate Professor and Director
Diagnostic Medical Sonography
Oregon Institute of Technology
Klamath Falls, Oregon

To our own little sonic boomers:
Rebecca, Alyssa, and **Katrina,**
who are growing up to make their own waves

Preface

A LOOK BACK

Medicine has always fascinated me. I had my first introduction to this field of study in 1963 when Dr. Charles Henkelmann provided me the opportunity to learn radiography while I was still in high school. Although radiographic technology was interesting, it did not provide the opportunity to evaluate patient history or to follow through on more complex cases, which seemed to be the most intriguing aspect of medicine and my primary concern.

Shortly after I finished my radiographic training in 1968 at UCSD Medical Center, I was assigned to the radiation therapy department. I was introduced to a very quiet, young, dedicated radiologist, whom I would later grow to admire and respect as one of the foremost authorities in diagnostic ultrasound. Convincing Dr. George Leopold that he needed another hand to assist him was difficult in the beginning, and it was through the efforts of his resident, Dr. Dan MacDonald, that I was able to learn what eventually developed into an exciting new medical modality.

Using high-frequency sound waves, diagnostic ultrasound provides a unique method for the visualization of soft tissue anatomic structures. Identifying such structures and correlating the results with clinical symptoms and patient data presents an ongoing challenge to the sonographer. The art of sonography demands expertise in scanning techniques and maneuvers to demonstrate the anatomic structures, for without high-quality images, limited diagnostic sonographic information is available to the physician.

At UCSD, our initial experience in ultrasound took us through the era of A-mode techniques, identifying aortic aneurysms through pulsatile reflections, trying to separate splenic reflections from upper-pole left renal masses, and, in general, attempting to echo every patient with a probable abdominal or pelvic mass. Of course, the one-dimensional A-mode techniques were difficult for me to conceptualize, let alone trust. However, with repeated success and the experience gained from mistakes, I began to believe in this method. The conviction that Dr. Leopold had about this technique was a strong indicator of its success in our laboratory.

In 1969, when our first 2-D ultrasound unit arrived in the laboratory, the "skeptics" started to believe a little more in this modality. I must admit that those early images looked like weather maps to me for several months. The repeated times I asked, "What is that?" were enough to try anyone's patience.

I can recall when Siemens installed our first real-time unit and we saw our first obstetrical case. It was such a thrill for us to see the fetus move, wave his hands, and show us fetal heart pulsations!

We scouted the clinics and various departments in the hospital for interesting cases to scan. With our success rate surpassing our failures, the caseload increased, and soon we were involved in all aspects of ultrasound. There was not enough material for us to read to learn about new developments. It was for this reason that excitement in clinical research soared, attracting young physicians throughout the country to develop techniques in diagnostic ultrasound.

Because Dr. Leopold was so intensely interested in ultrasound, it became the diagnostic method of choice for our patients. It was not long before conferences were incomplete without the mention of the technique. Later, local medical meetings and eventually national meetings grew to include discussion of this new modality. A number of visitors were attracted to our laboratory to learn the technique, and thus we became swamped with a continual flow of new physicians, some eager to work with ultrasound and others skeptical at first, but believers in the end.

In 1970, the beginning of ultrasound education progressed slowly, with many laboratories offering a one-on-one teaching experience. Commercial companies thought the only way to push the field was to develop their own national training programs, and thus several of the leading manufacturers were the first to put forth a dedicated effort in the development of ultrasound education.

The combined efforts of our laboratory and the commercial interests precipitated my involvement in furthering ultrasound education. Seminars, weekly sessions, local and national meetings, and consultations became a vital part of the growth of ultrasound.

As ultrasound grew in popularity, more intense training was desperately needed to maintain the quality that the pioneers strove for. Working with one of the commercial ultrasound companies conducting national short-term training programs, I became acquainted with Dr. Barry Goldberg and his enthusiasm for quality education in ultrasound. His organizational efforts and pioneer spirit led me to the East Coast to further develop more intensive educational programs in ultrasound. The challenge grew in establishing new programs and continuing education in diagnostic medical sonography as we ventured across the United States and Canada in the years to follow.

There are very few moments in life when one is in the right place at the right time, but this was one of those moments for me. I had the opportunity to begin when the field was in its infancy and to work with some of the stellar ultrasound scholars along the way. This textbook is a culmination of knowledge gained throughout the years as I have taught students in sonography.

INTRODUCING THE NEW SIXTH EDITION

The sixth edition of the *Textbook of Diagnostic Ultrasonography* continues the tradition of excellence begun when the first edition was published in the 1978. Each new edition brings impressive updates and vital reorganization. The field of diagnostic ultrasound has changed dramatically over the past 50 years, reflecting the changing approaches to many procedures. Phenomenal strides in transducer design, instrumentation, color flow Doppler, tissue harmonics, contrast applications, and 3-D imaging continue to provide increased resolution in the ultrasound image.

The primary goal of this textbook is to serve as an in-depth resource for students studying sonography, as well as for practitioners in hospitals, clinics, and private radiology, cardiology, and obstetric settings. This sixth edition strives to keep abreast of the rapid advancements, providing students and practitioners with the most complete and up-to-date information in the field of medical sonography.

ORGANIZATION

The *Textbook of Diagnostic Ultrasonography* remains divided into two volumes to compensate for its expanded coverage and to make the book more convenient to use. The content has been critically reviewed, reorganized, and improved to provide a better flow for the reader. Volume One covers general ultrasound applications, techniques, and scan protocols and introduces abdominal anatomy and physiology and the general health history analysis. Sonography of the abdomen, superficial structures, and pediatrics are also found in Volume One. Volume Two focuses on cardiovascular applications and obstetrics and gynecologic sonography. A comprehensive glossary is found at the end of each volume, and a reference of common medical and ultrasound abbreviations is located on the inside covers of each volume.

Each chapter begins with *learning objectives*, a *chapter outline*, and *key terms* and *definitions* to aid the reader. Sonographic concepts are presented in a logical and consistent manner in each chapter. To help the student and the sonographer understand the patient's total clinical picture before the sonographic examination, discussions on anatomy, physiology, laboratory data, clinical signs and symptoms, pathology, and sonographic findings are found within each chapter. The sonographic evaluation of the organ (to include normal measurements) is included in the chapters. Each chapter also offers discussion of the pathology of the organ, including clinical symptoms, gross pathology, ultrasound findings, and differential considerations. Tables throughout the text summarize the pathology discussed in each chapter and break the information

down into Clinical Findings, Sonographic Findings, and Differential Considerations. Key points are also pulled out into numerous boxes in the chapters, making it easy to find important information quickly. References and a Selected Bibliography are found at the ends of the chapters, as relevant. The review questions have been moved into the Instructor's Manual that accompanies the textbook

ILLUSTRATIONS AND VISUALS

Hundreds of beautifully drawn full-color illustrations highlight anatomical information important when performing the different ultrasound examinations presented. Color Doppler illustrations are also included in relevant chapters. Tables and boxes continue to highlight important areas of knowledge throughout both volumes.

One-third of the more than 3000 illustrations in this edition are new. Almost 800 new images have been incorporated, including color Doppler, 3-D, and contrast images. The anatomic illustrations—almost 200 of which are new—clearly add to the understanding of each of the organ structures discussed throughout the textbook. Gross pathology images have also been added to help the reader visually image the particular type of pathology presented.

Sonographic findings for particular pathologic conditions are preceded by the following special heading:

Sonographic Findings. This icon makes it very easy for students and practicing sonographers to find this information.

NEW TO THE SIXTH EDITION

This edition has been completely revised and expanded to offer student and practicing sonographers a comprehensive textbook of general ultrasound.

Chapter 1, *Foundations of Sonography,* was revised to provide more background information for students just entering the field of ultrasound. New to this chapter is the section "Medical Terms for the Sonographer," which introduces students to common medical terms they will encounter in their field. This chapter also introduces key physical principles of sonography.

Chapter 2, *Introduction to Physical Findings, Physiology, and Laboratory Data of the Abdomen,* exposes the student to the clinical assessment that the patient experiences prior to arriving in the ultrasound department. Although in many busy labs the student does not have an opportunity to perform such a thorough evaluation of the patient, an understanding of which questions may be appropriate for specific complaints can be invaluable during the ultrasound examination. Also included in this chapter is an introduction to laboratory tests relevant to various disease processes.

Chapter 14, *Abdominal Applications of Ultrasound Contrast Agents,* by Daniel Merton, provides an excellent introduction to the clinical applications of contrast in ultrasound. This chapter lists and discusses the various types of contrast that are available and includes illustrated examples of how contrast has aided in the diagnostic accuracy of the ultrasound examination.

Chapter 15, *Ultrasound-Guided Interventional Techniques,* by Robert DeJong, offers an excellent step-by-step analysis of how to perform invasive procedures with ultrasound guidance. DeJong has exquisitely illustrated the different types of needles, transducer devices, and protocols for performing the procedure. Guidelines for finding the needle tip for the biopsy procedures are clearly outlined.

Chapter 16, *Emergent Abdominal Ultrasound Procedures,* is a new chapter that focuses on the FAST scan technique used in Emergency Departments throughout the country. A few of the more common "STAT" ultrasound procedures are also included in this chapter for easy reference in an on-call situation.

Chapter 17, *The Breast,* was completely rewritten and updated to provide the student and sonographer with a solid foundation of the applications of ultrasound of the breast.

Chapter 19, *The Scrotum,* by Cindy Owen, is a new chapter that includes many images of normal scrotal anatomy as well as scrotal pathology. This chapter also offers practical tips on scanning techniques as well as discussion of Doppler principles as they relate to scrotal imaging.

Chapter 20, *The Musculoskeletal System,* by Susan Raatz Stephenson, is a new chapter with exquisite images and anatomical drawings. The author shares her practical experience in ultrasound imaging of the musculoskeletal system with excellent descriptions and protocols for performing multiple examinations. Because this is a new area for most sonographers, readers may encounter some new terminology. I recommend reviewing the drawings and images before reading through the text material.

Part IV, Pediatric Applications, was updated with the addition of three new introductory chapters that focus on the basic anatomy and common pathology that sonographers may encounter: Chapter 22, *The Pediatric Abdomen: Jaundice and Common Surgical Conditions;* Chapter 25, *The Neonatal Hip;* and Chapter 26, *The Neonatal Spine.*

Part V, Cardiology, contains four chapters that provide readers with a basic foundation of hemodynamics with an introduction to echocardiography. The subject of fetal echocardiography is now divided into two chapters: Chapter 29, *Introduction to Fetal Echocardiography,* and Chapter 30, *Fetal Echocardiography: Congenital Heart Disease.*

Part VI, Vascular, offers four chapters that help students understand vascular applications within a general ultrasound department.

Part VII, Gynecology, was completely rewritten and reorganized. Tami Salsgiver opens this part of the textbook with the excellent, illustrated Chapter 35, *Normal Anatomy and Physiology of the Female Pelvis.* Barb Vander Werff rewrote and updated four chapters in Part VII. Finally, Carol Mitchell and Valjean MacMillan added an excellent new chapter called *The Role of Ultrasound in Evaluating Female Infertility.*

Several additions have been made to Part VIII, Foundations of Obstetric Sonography. Jean Lea Spitz rewrote Chapter 41, *The Role of Ultrasound in Obstetrics;* Chapter 42, *Clinical Ethics for Obstetric Sonography;* and Chapter 45, *Sonography of the Second and Third Trimesters.* Terry DuBose reevaluated Chapter 46, *Obstetric Measurements and Gestational Age.* Chapter 48, *Ultrasound and High-Risk Pregnancy,* was rewritten by Carol Mitchell and Barbara Trampe. A brief introduction to the clinical applications of 3D ultrasound was contributed by Darleen Cioffi-Ragan (Chapter 50). Chapter 54, *The Fetal Face and Neck,* is beautifully illustrated and rewritten by Diana Strickland.

Each of these chapters was reviewed by numerous sonographers currently working in various areas of ultrasound. Their comments, critiques, and suggestions for change have been incorporated into this edition in an effort to make this textbook practical in a clinical setting and useful for both the student and the practicing sonographer. It continues to be my hope that this textbook will not only introduce the reader to the field of ultrasound but also allow readers to go a step beyond to what I have found to be the very stimulating and challenging experience of diagnostic patient care.

Also Available. *Workbook for Textbook of Diagnostic Ultrasonography* is available for separate purchase and has been created to provide the learner with ample opportunities to practice and apply the information presented in the text. Each workbook chapter covers all the material presented in the textbook. Each chapter includes exercises and activities on image identification, anatomy identification, key term definition, and sonographic technique. Case reviews and self tests are also included at the end of the workbook.

For the Instructor. An *Instructor's Electronic Resource (IER)* has also been created to assist instructors in preparing classroom lectures and activities. This resource consists of:

- Instructor's Manual, which includes detailed chapter outlines, chapter objectives, in-depth lecture notes, and critical thinking questions and exercises.
- Test Bank, which includes 1500 multiple-choice questions in Examview and Word format.
- Electronic Image Collection, which includes all of the images from the text in PowerPoint and jpeg formats.

The IER is also posted on Evolve, which also includes a Course Management system for instructors and WebLinks for students.

Evolve Online Course Management. Evolve is an interactive learning environment designed to work in coordination with *Textbook of Diagnostic Ultrasonography.* Instructors may use Evolve to provide an Internet-based course component that reinforces and expands on the concepts delivered in class. Evolve may be used to publish the class syllabus, outlines, and lecture notes; set up "virtual office hours" and email communication; share important dates and information through the online class Calendar; and encourage student participation through Chat Rooms and Discussion Boards. Evolve allows instructors to post exams and manage their grade books online. An online version of the Instructor's Resource Manual is also available on Evolve. For more information, visit http://www.evolve.elsevier.com/HagenAnsert/diagnostic/ or contact an Elsevier sales representative.

Sandra L. Hagen-Ansert, MS, RDMS, RDCS

Acknowledgments

I would like to express my gratitude and appreciation to a number of individuals who have served as mentors and guides throughout my years in ultrasound. Of course it all began with Dr. George Leopold at UCSD Medical Center. His quest for knowledge and his perseverance for excellence have been the mainstay of my career in ultrasound. I would also like to recognize Drs. Dolores Pretorius, Nancy Budorick, Wanda Miller-Hance, and David Sahn for their encouragement throughout the years at the UCSD Medical Center in both Radiology and Pediatric Cardiology.

I would also like to acknowledge Dr. Barry Goldberg for the opportunity he gave me to develop countless numbers of educational programs in ultrasound in an independent fashion and for his encouragement to pursue advancement. I would also like to thank Dr. Daniel Yellon for his early-hour anatomy dissection and instruction; Dr. Carson Schneck, for his excellent instruction in gross anatomy and sections of "Geraldine;" and Dr. Jacob Zutuchni, for his enthusiasm for the field of cardiology.

I am grateful to Dr. Harry Rakowski for his continued support in teaching fellows and students while I was at the Toronto Hospital.

Dr. William Zwiebel encouraged me to continue writing and teaching while I was at the University of Wisconsin Medical Center, and I appreciate his knowledge, which found its way into the liver physiology section of this textbook.

I would like to acknowledge the feedback from several individuals as I contemplated changes for this edition: Kerry Weinberg, Jean Lea Spitz, and Tami Salsgiver. I would also like to extend gratitude to Misty Johnson and Charlene Fessler from MUSC Medical Center.

My good fortune in learning about and understanding the *total patient* must be attributed to a very dedicated cardiologist, James Glenn, with whom I had the pleasure of working while I was at MUSC in Charleston, South Carolina. It was through his compassion and knowledge that I grew to appreciate the total patient beyond the transducer, and for this I am grateful.

For their continual support, feedback, and challenges, I would like to thank and recognize all the students I have taught in the various Diagnostic Medical Sonography programs: Episcopal Hospital, Thomas Jefferson University Medical Center, University of Wisconsin-Madison Medical Center, UCSD Medical Center, Baptist College of Health Science, and Trident Technical College. These students continually work toward the development of quality ultrasound techniques and protocols and have given back to the ultrasound community tenfold.

I would like to thank the very supportive and capable staff at Elsevier who have guided me though yet another edition of this textbook. Jeanne Wilke and her excellent staff are to be commended on their perseverance to make this an outstanding textbook. Linda Woodard was a constant reminder to me to stay on task and was there to offer assistance when needed. Gena Magouirk, Project Manager, has done an excellent job with the manuscript. She is to be commended on her eye for detail. Also, Jennifer Moorhead has been a tremendous aid in working with this project. Finally, Luke Held, Editorial Assistant, worked on the test bank questions for the Instructor's Manual.

I would like to thank my family, Art, Becca, Aly, and Kati, for their patience and understanding, as I thought this edition would never come to an end.

I think that you will find the 6th Edition of the *Textbook of Diagnostic Ultrasonography* reflects the contribution of so many individuals with attention to detail and a dedication to excellence. I hope you will find this educational experience in ultrasound as rewarding as I have.

Contents

TEXTBOOK of

Diagnostic
Ultrasonography

volume **TWO**

PART V

Cardiology

CHAPTER 27

Anatomic and Physiologic Relationships within the Thoracic Cavity

Sandra L. Hagen-Ansert

OBJECTIVES

- Describe the landmarks of the thoracic cavity
- Define the relational landmarks of the heart
- Discuss the function of the pericardial sac
- Differentiate the three layers of the heart wall
- Describe the anatomic landmarks of the cardiac chambers, valves, and interventricular septum

THE THORAX AND THE THORACIC CAVITY

THE HEART AND GREAT VESSELS

PERICARDIAL SAC
LININGS OF THE HEART WALL
RIGHT ATRIUM AND INTERATRIAL SEPTUM
TRICUSPID VALVE
RIGHT VENTRICLE
PULMONARY VALVE AND TRUNK
LEFT ATRIUM
MITRAL VALVE
LEFT VENTRICLE
INTERVENTRICULAR SEPTUM
AORTIC VALVE
AORTIC ARCH AND BRANCHES

THE CARDIAC CYCLE

THE ELECTRICAL CONDUCTION SYSTEM

BUNDLE OF HIS
CARDIAC NERVES

THE MECHANICAL CONDUCTION SYSTEM

ELECTROCARDIOGRAPHY

P WAVE
QRS COMPLEX
P-R INTERVAL
T WAVE

AUSCULTATION OF THE HEART VALVES

PRINCIPLES OF BLOOD FLOW

VENTRICULAR EJECTION
CORONARY CIRCULATION

KEY TERMS

atrioventricular valves – valves located between the atria and ventricle
continuous murmur – the murmur begins in systole and continues without interruption through the time of the second heart sound into all or part of diastole
depolarization – describes the electrical activity that triggers contraction of the heart muscle
diastolic murmur – the diastolic murmur begins with or after the time of the second heart sound and ends at or before the time of the first heart sound
electrocardiography – method of recording the electrical activity generated by the heart muscle
endocardium – inner layer of the heart wall
epicardium – outer layer of the heart wall
frequency – the predominant frequency band of the murmur varies from high to low as determined by auscultation
intensity – (murmurs) both systolic and diastolic, vary from grade 1 to grade 6. A grade 1 murmur is very faint with progression to a grade 6 murmur that is exceptionally loud and heard with the stethoscope.
murmur – a murmur is a relatively prolonged series of auditory vibrations of varying intensity (loudness), frequency (pitch), quality, configuration, and duration. The murmur is produced by structural changes and/or hemodynamic events in the heart or blood vessels.
myocardium – thickest muscle in the heart wall
pericardium – sac surrounding the heart, reflecting off the great arteries

repolarization – begins just before the relaxation phase of cardiac muscle activity

semilunar valves – valves located in the aortic or pulmonic artery

systolic murmur – the systolic murmur begins with or after the time of the first heart sound and ends at or before the time of the second heart sound

EXTERNAL LANDMARKS OF THE THORAX

costal margin – lower boundary of the thorax, formed by the cartilages of the seventh through tenth ribs and the ends of the eleventh and twelfth cartilages

midaxillary line – runs vertically from a point midway between the anterior and posterior axillary folds

midclavicular line – vertical line from the midpoint of the clavicle

midsternal line – lies in the median plane over the sternum

sternal angle – angle between the manubrium and the body of the sternum; also known as the angle of Louis

suprasternal notch – superior margin of the manubrium sterni; lies opposite the lower border of the body of the second thoracic vertebra

xiphisternal joint – junction between the xiphoid and the sternum

xiphoid – lowest point of the sternum

The cardiovascular system delivers oxygenated blood to tissues in the body and removes waste products from these tissues. The heart pumps blood to all the organs and tissues of the body. The autonomic nervous system controls how the heart pumps, whereas the vascular network (arteries and veins) carries blood throughout the body, keeps the heart filled with blood, and maintains blood pressure.

THE THORAX AND THE THORACIC CAVITY

The thorax constitutes the upper part of the body. (See Figure 27-1 and Key Terms for external landmarks of the thorax.) The thoracic cavity lies within the thorax and is separated from the abdominal cavity by the diaphragm. The diaphragm reaches upward as high as the midaxillary level of the seventh rib. The mediastinum is the medial portion of the thorax, and the pleurae and lungs are the lateral components (Figure 27-2).

Superiorly the upper thoracic cavity gives access to the root of the neck. It is bounded by the upper part of the sternum, the first ribs, and the body of the first thoracic vertebra.

Anteriorly the sternum consists of the manubrium, the corpus sterni (body), and the xiphoid process. The junction between the manubrium and the body of the sternum is a prominent ridge; together they form the angle of Louis. This palpable landmark is important in locating the superior mediastinum or the second rib cartilages, which articulate with the sternum at this point.

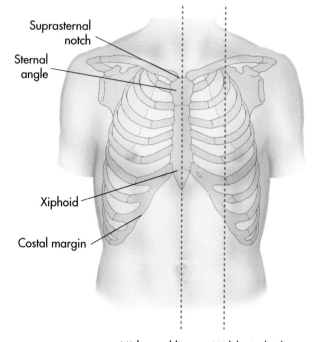

Figure 27-1   External landmarks of the thorax.

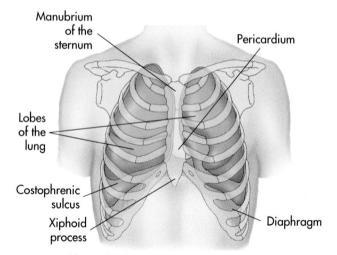

Figure 27-2   Anterior view of the thorax.

The greater part of the thoracic cavity is occupied by the two lungs, which are enclosed by the pleural sac. To understand the pleural sac, imagine a deflated plastic bag covering your fist. Your fist should be enveloped by both sides of the bag to simulate the pleural sac. The internal layer, or visceral pleura, is adherent to each lobe of the lung. The external layer, or parietal pleura, is adherent to the inner surface of the chest wall (costal pleura), diaphragm (diaphragmatic pleura), and mediastinum (mediastinal pleura). The two layers become continuous with each other by a "cuff" of pleura that surrounds the structures at the hilum of the lung.

The costophrenic sinus is the pleural reflection between the costal and diaphragmatic portions of the parietal pleura. This space lies lower than the edge of the lung and, in most cases, is never occupied by the lung. When pleural fluid accumulates, its most common location is in the costophrenic sinus. On a radiographic examination, the costophrenic angle is blunted by the presence of pleural effusion.

The mediastinum is the median partition of the thoracic cavity. The mediastinum is a movable, thick structure and extends superiorly to the thoracic inlet and the root of the neck and inferiorly to the diaphragm. It extends anteriorly to the sternum and posteriorly to the twelfth thoracic vertebra. Within the mediastinum are found the remains of the thymus, the heart and great vessels, the trachea and esophagus, the thoracic duct and lymph nodes, the vagus and phrenic nerves, and the sympathetic trunks.

The mediastinum may be divided into a superior and inferior mediastinum by an imaginary plane from the sternal angle to the lower body of the fourth thoracic vertebra (Box 27-1). The inferior mediastinum is subdivided into three parts: (1) middle, which contains the pericardium and the heart; (2) anterior, which is a space between the pericardium and sternum; and (3) posterior, which lies between the pericardium and vertebral column.

THE HEART AND GREAT VESSELS

The heart lies obliquely in the chest, posterior to the sternum, with the greater portion of its muscular mass lying slightly to the left of midline. The heart is protected within the chest by the sternum and rib cage anteriorly and the vertebral column and rib cage posteriorly. The other structures within the thoracic cavity in close approximation to the heart are the lungs, esophagus, and descending thoracic aorta.

Contrary to most simplified anatomic illustrations, the heart is not situated with its right chambers lying to the right and its left chambers to the left. It may be better considered as an anteroposterior structure, with its right-side chambers located more anterior than its left-side chambers. As we look

---

BOX 27-1   MAJOR MEDIASTINAL STRUCTURES FROM ANTERIOR TO POSTERIOR

SUPERIOR MEDIASTINUM
- Thymus
- Great veins
- Great arteries
- Trachea
- Esophagus and thoracic duct
- Sympathetic trunks

INFERIOR MEDIASTINUM
- Thymus
- Heart within the pericardium with the phrenic nerves on either side
- Esophagus and thoracic duct
- Descending aorta
- Sympathetic trunks

---

at the embryologic development, the heart forms as a tubular right-to-left structure. However, as development continues, the right side becomes more ventral and the left side remains dorsal.

In addition, another change in axis causes the apex (or the inferior surface of the heart) to tilt anteriorly. The final development of the heart presents the right atrium anterior to the left atrium and to the right of the sternum, whereas the right ventricle presents anterior to the left ventricle and slightly to the left of the sternum. The left atrium becomes the most posterior chamber to the left of the sternum, whereas the left ventricle swings its posterior axis slightly toward the anterior chest wall.

The heart has three surfaces: sternocostal (anterior), diaphragmatic (inferior or apex), and base (posterior) (Figure 27-3). The right atrium forms the right border of the heart to the right of the sternum. The vertical atrioventricular groove separates these two structures.

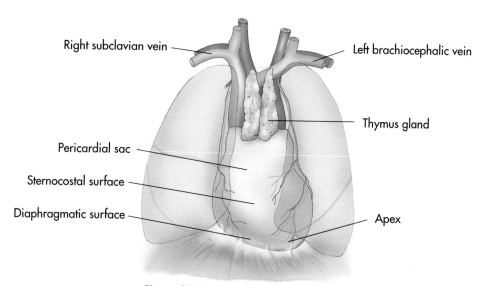

Right subclavian vein

Left brachiocephalic vein

Thymus gland

Pericardial sac

Sternocostal surface

Diaphragmatic surface

Apex

Figure 27-3   The heart and great vessels.

The left border is formed by the left ventricle and left atrial appendage. The right and left ventricles are separated by the anterior interventricular groove. The diaphragmatic surface of the heart is formed principally by the right and left ventricles, separated by the posterior interventricular groove (Figure 27-4). A small part of the inferior surface of the right atrium also forms this surface.

The base of the heart is formed by the left atrium, into which the four pulmonary veins enter from the lungs. The right atrium contributes a small part to this posterior surface (Figure 27-5). The left ventricle forms the apex of the heart, which can be palpated at the level of the fifth intercostal space, about 9 cm from the midline.

PERICARDIAL SAC

The heart and roots of the great vessels lie within the pericardial sac (see Figure 27-3). Like the pleura of the lungs, the **peri-**

cardium is a double sac. The fibrous pericardium limits the movement of the heart by attaching to the central tendon of the diaphragm below and the outer coat of the great vessels above. The sternopericardial ligaments attach to it in the front. The serous pericardium is divided into parietal and visceral layers. The parietal layer lines the fibrous pericardium and is reflected around the roots of the great vessels to become continuous with the visceral layer of serous pericardium. The visceral layer is very closely applied to the heart and is often called the **epicardium.** The slit between the parietal and visceral layers is the pericardial cavity. This cavity normally contains a very small amount of fluid that lubricates the heart as it moves.

The pericardial sac protects the heart against friction. If the serous pericardium becomes inflamed, pericarditis will develop, or if too much pericardial fluid, fibrin, or pus develops in the pericardial space, the visceral and parietal layers may adhere to one another.

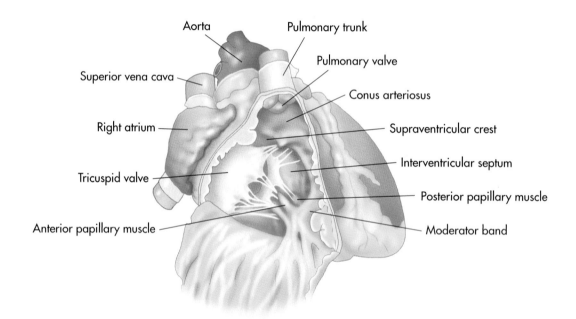

Figure 27-4   Anterior view of the right ventricle.

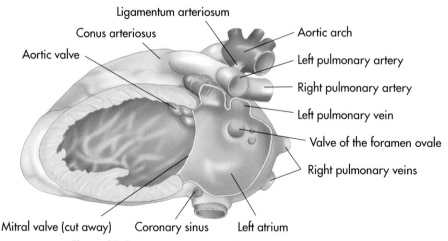

Figure 27-5   Posterolateral view of the left atrium and ventricle.

The pericardial sac does not totally encompass the heart. On the posterior left atrial surface of the heart, the reflection of serous pericardium around the pulmonary veins forms the recess of the oblique sinus. This may be an important landmark in the echocardiographic separation of pericardial effusion from pleural effusion. The transverse sinus lies between the reflection of serous pericardium around the aorta and pulmonary arteries and between the reflection around the pulmonary veins.

LININGS OF THE HEART WALL

The chambers of the heart are lined by the endocardium, myocardium, and epicardium.

The **endocardium** is the intimal lining of the heart and is continuous with the intima of the vessels connecting to it. The endocardium is very similar to the intima of blood vessels. It also forms the valves that lie between the filling (atria) and pumping (ventricle) chambers of the heart and along each base of the two great arterial trunks leaving the heart (the aorta and pulmonary artery).

The muscular part of the heart, the **myocardium,** is a special type of muscle found only in the heart and great vessels. This cardiac muscle is equivalent to the media of a blood vessel. The cardiac muscle is very complex compared with other muscular fibers. Although it is striated like voluntary muscle, the fibers of the cardiac muscle branch and anastomose so that it is impossible to determine the limits of a fiber. The myocardium of both ventricles is one continuous muscle mass, as is the myocardium of both atria. Because of this continuity, an impulse for contraction originating in the atrium can spread throughout the atrial musculature; similarly an impulse originating in a ventricle can spread throughout the ventricular musculature. A special bundle of fibers connects the atria to the ventricles. The unique feature of cardiac muscle is the ability to possess intrinsic rhythmic contractility. It is this rhythmicity that keeps the heart contracting, with nerve impulses modifying rather than initiating the heart beat.

Because the atria work at very low pressures, the musculature of the atria is very thin compared with the ventricular wall mass. The primary purpose of the atria is to act as filling chambers that drive the blood into the relaxed ventricular cavity. In contrast the myocardium of the ventricles is much thicker than that of the atria. The left ventricle has the greatest muscle mass, because it must pump blood to all of the body, whereas the right ventricle needs only enough pressure to pump the blood to the lungs.

The outside layer of the heart is the epicardium, or the visceral layer of the serous pericardium. The outer surface of the epicardium is a single layer of mesothelial cells continuous with the serous (inner) surface of the pericardium.

RIGHT ATRIUM AND INTERATRIAL SEPTUM

The right atrium forms the right border of the heart (Figure 27-6). The superior vena cava enters the upper posterior border, and the inferior vena cava enters the lower posterolateral border. The posterior wall of the right atrium is directly related to the pulmonary veins (which flow from the lungs to empty into the left atrium). The medial wall of the right atrium is formed by the interatrial septum. The septum angles slightly posterior and to the patient's right, so the atrium lies in front and to the right of the left atrium. The central ovale portion of the septum is thin and fibrous. Just superior and in front of the opening of the inferior vena cava lies a shallow depression, the fossa ovalis. Its borders are the limbus fossae ovalis and the primitive septum primum. The foramen ovale lies under the most superior part of the limbus fossae. The limbus fossae ovalis is the remainder of the atrial septum and forms a ridge around the fossa ovalis.

The atrioventricular part of the membranous septum separates the right atrium and left ventricle. Atrial septal defects can occur in this area, causing blood to flow from the high-pressured left ventricle into the right atrial cavity.

The anterior and lateral walls of the right atrium are ridged by the pectinate muscles. The superior portion of the right

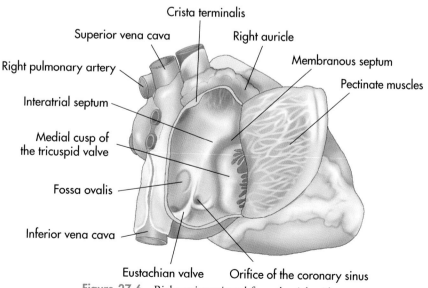

Figure 27-6   Right atrium viewed from the right side.

atrium, the right atrial appendage, contains the most prominent pectinate muscles. The posterior and medial walls are smooth, probably because of the continual flow of blood from the inferior and superior vena cavas and coronary sinus.

The inferior vena cava is guarded by a fold of tissue called the Eustachian valve, and the coronary sinus is guarded by the Thebesian valve.

The coronary sinus drains the blood supply from the heart wall. It is bordered by the fossa ovalis and the tricuspid valve.

TRICUSPID VALVE

The tricuspid valve separates the right atrium from the right ventricle. It has three leaflets: anterior, septal, and inferior (or mural) (Figure 27-7). The septal leaflet may be maldeveloped in association with such conditions as ostium primum defect or ventricular septal defect. The leaflets are attached by their base to the fibrous atrioventricular ring. The chordae tendineae attach the leaflets to the papillary muscles. As these muscles contract with ventricular contraction, the leaflets are pulled together to prevent their being pulled into the atrial cavity. The septal and anterior leaflets are connected to the same papillary muscle, which helps in this process.

RIGHT VENTRICLE

The base of the right ventricle lies on the diaphragm, and the roof is occupied by the crista supraventricularis, which lies between the tricuspid and pulmonary orifices. The right ventricle is essentially divided into two parts—the posteroinferior inflow portion (containing the tricuspid valve) and the anterosuperior outflow portion (containing the origin of the pulmonary trunk). The demarcation between these two parts is several prominent bands—the parietal band, supraventricular crest, septal band, and moderator band (see Figure 27-4). Together these bands form an almost circular orifice that normally is wide and forms no impediment to flow.

The inflow tract of the right ventricle is short and heavily trabeculated. It extends from the tricuspid valve and merges into the trabecular zone. This zone is the body of the right ventricle. The trabeculae carneae enclose an elongated ovoid opening. The inflow tract unites with the outflow tract, which extends to the pulmonary valve. The outflow portion of the right ventricle, or infundibulum, is smooth-walled and contains few trabeculae.

The right ventricle has two walls, an anterior wall (corresponding to the sternocostal surface) and a posterior wall (formed by the ventricular septum).

PULMONARY VALVE AND TRUNK

The pulmonary valve lies at the upper anterior aspect of the right ventricle. It has three cusps: anterior, right, and left (Figure 27-8). The wall of the pulmonary artery bulges out adjacent to each cusp to form pockets known as the pulmonary sinuses of Valsalva.

The pulmonary trunk passes posterior and slightly upward from the right ventricle. It bifurcates into the right and left pulmonary arteries just after leaving the pericardial cavity. The ligamentum arteriosum connects the upper aspect of the bifurcation to the anterior surface of the aortic arch. (The ligamentum arteriosum is a remnant of the fetal ductus arteriosus.)

LEFT ATRIUM

The left atrium is a smooth-walled, circular sac that lies posterior in the base of the heart. Two pulmonary veins enter posteriorly on either side of the cavity (see Figure 27-5). Occasionally, these veins unite before entering the atrium, and sometimes there are more than two veins on either side. The veins may also be congenitally defective and enter the right atrium or other areas in the thoracic cavity. This absence of pulmonary veins entering the left atrial cavity is known as *total anomalous pulmonary venous return.*

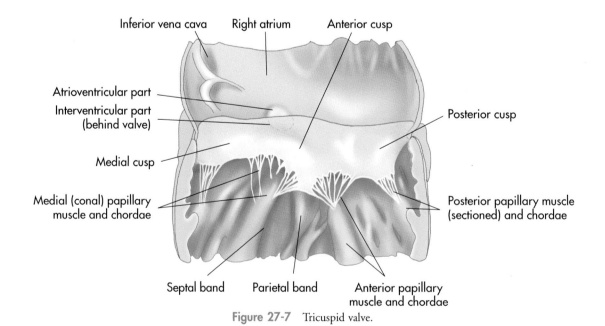

Figure 27-7　Tricuspid valve.

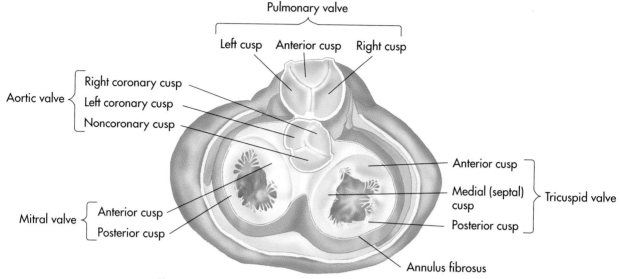

Figure 27-8   Heart viewed from the base with the atria removed.

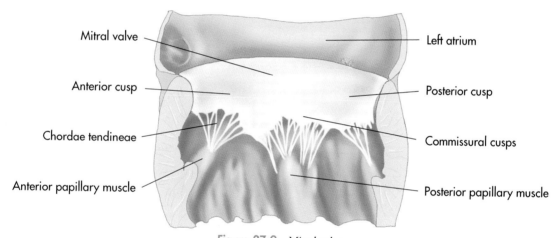

Figure 27-9   Mitral valve.

The septal surface of the atrium is fairly smooth. A somewhat irregular area indicates the position of the fetal valve of the foramen ovale. The left auricle, or left atrial appendage, is a continuation of the left upper anterior part of the left atrium. Small pectinate muscles are located within its lumen.

MITRAL VALVE

The mitral valve separates the left atrium from the left ventricle. It consists of two large principal leaflets (anterior and posterior) and two small commissural cusps (which usually merge with the posterior leaflet). The anterior leaflet is much longer and larger than the posterior leaflet. It projects downward into the left ventricular cavity. The leaflets are thick membranes that are trapezoidal with fine irregular edges (Figure 27-9). They originate from the anulus fibrosus and are attached to the papillary muscles by chordae tendineae. The functions of the chordae tendineae are to prevent the opposing borders of the leaflets from inverting into the atrial cavity, to act as mainstays

of the valves, and to form bands or foldlike structures that may contain muscle.

LEFT VENTRICLE

The left ventricle is conical or egg shaped. The smaller end of the ventricle represents the apex of the heart, and the larger end, near the orifice of the mitral valve, is near the base of the heart (Figure 27-10). The left ventricle has a short inflow tract from the mitral valve to the trabecular zone that merges with the outflow tract extending to the aortic valve. Unlike the right side of the heart (where there is no continuity between the tricuspid and pulmonary valves), the anterior leaflet of the mitral valve is continuous with the posterior aortic wall, and the left side of the interventricular septum is continuous with the anterior aortic wall.

The left ventricle has several wall segments that can be recognized in relation to their surrounding structures. The medial wall is formed by the ventricular septum. The lateral wall,

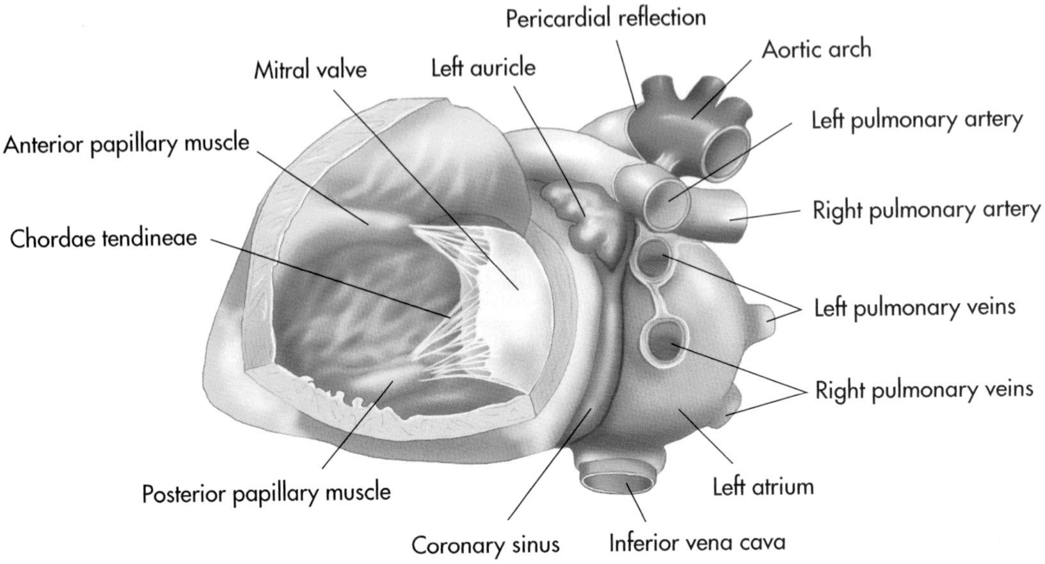

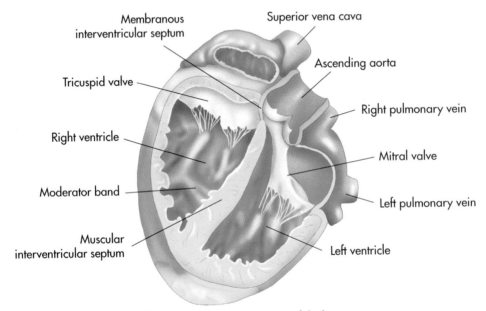

Figure 27-10   Posterolateral view of the left ventricle.

Figure 27-11   Long-axis view of the heart.

posterior wall, posterior-basal wall, and apex are all formed by their relative locations in the heart. The lateral wall is covered with trabeculae, which are finer and more numerous than those found in the right ventricle.

As mentioned previously, the wall of the ventricle consists of the endocardium, the myocardium, and the epicardium. This wall thickness is two to three times thicker than the right ventricular wall because it must handle the increased pressures in the left ventricular cavity.

INTERVENTRICULAR SEPTUM

The septum is somewhat triangular in shape, with its apex corresponding to the apex of the heart and its base fusing posteriorly and superiorly with the atrial septum. The ven-

tricular septum is formed of membranous, inflow, trabecular, and infundibular parts. These parts arise from the endocardial cushions, the primitive ventricle, and the bulbus cordis. The membranous septum varies in size and shape. It merges into the tissue at the aortic root and infundibular septum, but is sharply demarcated from the muscular portion of the septum.

Most of the interventricular septum is muscular and thicker than the membranous portion of the septum (Figure 27-11). The muscular septum makes up about two thirds of the septal length, with the membranous septum located just inferior to the aortic root in the area of the left ventricular outflow tract. Most interventricular septal defects occur in this thin, membranous part of the septum.

The muscular septum consists of two layers: a thin layer on the right side and a thicker layer on the left side. The major septal arteries run between these layers. The muscular portion of the septum has approximately the same thickness as the left ventricular wall.

AORTIC VALVE

The aortic valve lies at the root of the aorta and has right, left, and posterior (or noncoronary) cusps (Figure 27-12). The wall of the aorta bulges slightly at each cusp to form the sinus of Valsalva. The main coronary arteries arise from the right and left coronary cusps. At the center of each cusp is a small fibrous nodule, Arantius' nodule, which aids in preventing leakage of blood from the left ventricle when the aortic cusps are closed.

Often it becomes the site of calcification in patients in whom arteriosclerosis develops.

AORTIC ARCH AND BRANCHES

The aortic arch is a continuation of the ascending aorta (Figure 27-13). The arch lies behind the manubrium sterni and runs upward, backward, and to the left in front of the trachea. It then passes downward to the left of the trachea to become continuous with the descending aorta at the sternal angle.

The brachiocephalic artery arises from the convex surface of the arch. It passes upward and to the right of the trachea and divides into the right subclavian and common carotid arteries. The left common carotid artery arises from the aortic arch on the left side of the brachiocephalic artery. It runs

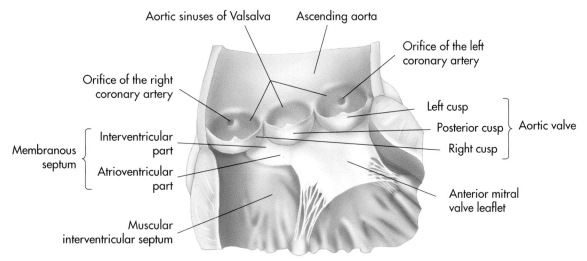

Figure 27-12   Aortic valve.

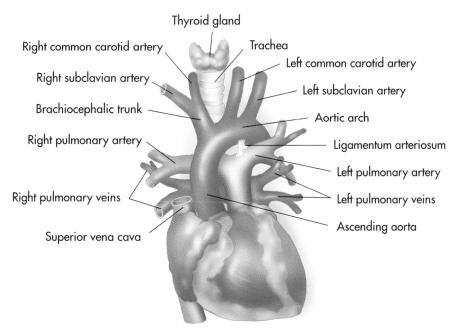

Figure 27-13   Aortic arch and branches.

upward and to the left of the trachea and enters the neck behind the left sternoclavicular joint.

The left subclavian artery arises from the arch behind the left common carotid artery. It runs upward along the right side of the trachea and the esophagus to enter the root of the neck.

THE CARDIAC CYCLE

The heart is a muscular pump that propels blood to all parts of the body. It is able to act in definite strokes, or beats, and in the normal adult usually beats in sinus rhythm at 70 times per minute. The cardiac cycle is the series of changes that the heart undergoes as it fills with blood and empties (Box 27-2). Rhythmic contraction of the heart causes blood to be pumped through the chambers of the heart and out through the great vessels. The forceful contraction of the cardiac chambers is "systole," and the relaxed phase of the cycle is "diastole."

During diastole the venous blood enters the right atrium from the superior and inferior vena cavas. At the same time, the oxygenated blood returns from the lungs through the pulmonary veins to enter the left atrium. At this point the **atrioventricular valves** (tricuspid and mitral) between the atria and ventricles are open so that the blood may flow from the atria into the ventricles. The next phase allows atrial contraction to squeeze the remaining blood from the atria into the ventricles. The combination of atrial contraction and increased

pressure of the full atrial cavities ultimately drains the atrial blood into the ventricles.

Shortly after this phase, the ventricles contract (ventricular systole). The rising pressure in the ventricular cavity closes the atrioventricular valves. As the pressure increases in the ventricles, the **semilunar valves** (pulmonary and aortic) open so that blood can be forced into the lungs and body, respectively.

The ventricles relax when contraction is completed (ventricular diastole). The blood in the aorta is under very high pressure, and the decreased pressure in the ventricles would cause it to flow backward into the ventricle. However, the semilunar valves prevent this reverse flow. The blood fills the sinuses of Valsalva and forces the valves to close. During ventricular contraction, the atria relax and the venous blood starts to fill them again. When the ventricles are completely relaxed, the atrioventricular valves open and blood flows into the ventricles to begin the next cardiac cycle.

THE ELECTRICAL CONDUCTION SYSTEM

The heart consists of a syncytium of striated muscle cells held together with fibrous tissue. The specialized muscle cells with a high degree of inherent rhythmicity are present in conduction tissue in the areas concerned with the generation and propagation of excitatory electrical activity.

The electrical conduction system of the heart consists of specialized cardiac muscle in the sinoatrial node, atrioventricular node, atrioventricular bundle and its right and left terminal branches, and subendocardial plexus of Purkinje fibers (Figure 27-14). The sinoatrial node initiates the normal cardiac impulse and is often called the pacemaker of the heart. It is situated on the lateral wall of the right atrium, at the upper part of the sulcus terminalis just to the right of the opening of the superior vena cava. Once activated, the cardiac impulse spreads through the atrial myocardium to reach the atrioventricular node. The atrioventricular node is located in the right posterior portion of the interatrial septum. It lies subendocardially in the medial wall of the right atrium to the left of the ostium of the coronary sinus and immediately posterior to the basal attachment of the septal cusp of the tricuspid valve.

BUNDLE OF HIS

The atrioventricular node is continuous with the bundle of His, which forms the common bundle that passes along the posterior edge of the membranous septum. The bundle branches include the common bundle, and right and left branches. The common bundle divides into the right and left bundle branch and extends subendocardially along both septal surfaces. The left branch divides into anterior and posterior branches that run along the left interventricular septal surface into the Purkinje fibers, which spread to all parts of the ventricular myocardium.

CARDIAC NERVES

The heart is innervated by cholinergic fibers from the vagus nerve and by adrenergic fibers arising from the thoracolumbar

---

BOX 27-2   PHASES OF THE CARDIAC CYCLE (ELECTRO-MECHANICAL EVENTS)

1. PASSIVE FILLING PHASE (VENTRICULAR DIASTOLE)
   - Early diastole, blood enters ventricles through AV valves
   - Venous blood continues to enter atria during this phase
   - Ventricles expand and pressure slowly rises as ventricular volume increases
   - Inflow volume diminishes in middiastole

2. ATRIAL SYSTOLE (P WAVE ON EKG, LATE DIASTOLE)
   - Active contraction of atria stops venous inflow
   - Rapid push of blood into ventricles
   - Causes pressure rise in both atria and ventricles (a wave)

3. ISOVOLUMETRIC CONTRACTION
   - Part of preejection period from onset of QRS complex to onset of ventricular ejection
   - Occurs from closure of AV valves to onset of ventricular ejection (opening of semilunar valves)
   - Ventricles contract isovolumetrically:
   A. Pressure rises in ventricles until pressure reaches that of corresponding great vessel
   B. Pulling down of mitral/tricuspid valve ring causes fall in atrial pressure
   C. Rate of change in LV pressure during isometric ventricular contraction is dp/dt

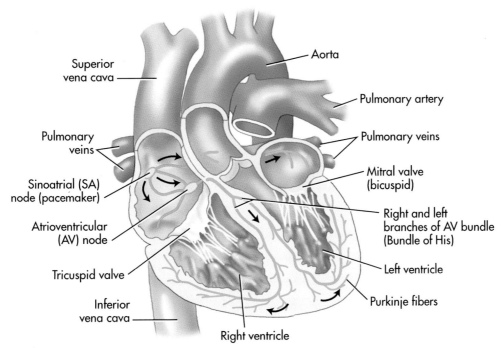

Figure 27-14 Conducting system of the heart. Specialized cardiac muscle cells in the wall of the heart rapidly conduct an electrical impulse through the myocardium. The signal is initiated by the SA node (pacemaker) and spreads to the rest of the atrial myocardium and to the AV node. The AV node then initiates a signal that is conducted through the ventricular myocardium by way of the AV bundle of His and Purkinje fibers.

sympathetic system and passing through the superior, middle, and inferior cervical ganglions.

THE MECHANICAL CONDUCTION SYSTEM

The Frank-Starling law of the heart states that the output of the heart increases in proportion to the degree of diastolic stretch of the muscle fibers. When a sarcomere is maximally shortened, the actin filaments overlap in the middle, covering up and eliminating from cross-linkage a number of active sites. As the sarcomere is stretched, more sites are uncovered and made available for cross-linkage, increasing the force that is developed. The longer the initial resting length of the cardiac muscle (preload), the greater the strength of contraction of the following beat. A further stretch beyond the normal range cuts the amount of overlap and the force of contraction by reducing the number of cross-bridges.

The shortening velocity of cardiac muscle is inversely related to *afterload*, or the force opposing ventricular ejection. The long interval between beats increases the strength of the next cardiac contraction. Tachycardia causes increased strength of contraction. The intracellular calcium ion concentration is probably involved in cellular mechanism.

ELECTROCARDIOGRAPHY

Electrocardiography is a method of recording the heart's electrical activity. It is used to assess cardiac function and disorders of the heart. The contraction of the heart muscle is accompanied by electrical changes, which can be detected by electrodes placed on the skin surface, and they can be recorded as an electrocardiogram on a sheet of graphic paper. On stimulation of a muscle or nerve, the cell membranes are **depolarized**, and on recovery they are **repolarized**. These electrical events are spread throughout the body and can be detected with suitable instruments applied to the skin surface at considerable distances from the sites of origin. There are various standard positions on the front of the chest on which the electrodes are placed to obtain an adequate electrical signal.

The heart's electrical activity is propagated in the following manner:

- Starts with firing of the SA node
- Electrical events precede mechanical events: atrial contraction follows the P wave on EKG and generates the atrial systolic activity (*a wave*). Activation proceeds in an orderly, repetitive fashion as the impulse spreads by several internodal pathways through both atria.

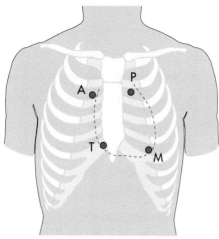

Figure 27-15   The valve opening and closing sounds may be heard best with the least interference at the location of the circles. *A,* Aortic valve; *M,* mitral valve; *P,* pulmonic valve; *T,* tricuspid valve.

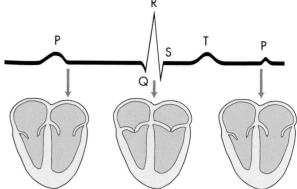

Figure 27-16   Illustration of the ECG components as seen on the real-time image. The P wave represents the depolarization of cardiac muscle tissue in the SA node and atrial walls. Before the QRS complex is observed, the AV node and AV bundle depolarize. The QRS complex occurs as the atrial walls repolarize and the ventricular walls depolarize. The T wave occurs as the ventricular walls repolarize. Depolarization triggers contraction in the affected muscle tissue. Cardiac muscle contraction occurs after depolarization.

- When the impulse reaches the AV node near the tricuspid valve, the cells of the bundle of His are activated and the impulse passes via the right and left bundle branches, the latter splitting into the anterior and posterior divisions.
- The impulse spreads via the Purkinje fibers to activate the ventricles, generating the *Q, R,* and *S* waves of the ECG (*ventricular depolarization*).
- After the ventricles depolarize, they begin to repolarize; this repolarization is demarcated by the T wave on the ECG.

In echocardiography examinations, three ECG lead wires are used for the electrocardiogram (ECG) tracing. Two ECG leads are placed on the patient's right and left shoulders and a ground lead on the right hip. The ECG has three components: P, QRS, and T waves (Figure 27-16).

P Wave

The impulse is initiated by the sinoatrial (SA) node and spreads over the atria. The P wave represents the electrical activity associated with the spread of the impulse over the atria (i.e., the wave of depolarization or activity of the atria).

QRS Complex

The wave of depolarization spreads from the SA node over the bundle branches (bundle of His) and Purkinje system to activate both ventricles simultaneously. The QRS complex is the result of all electrical activity occurring in the ventricles.

P-R Interval

The P-R interval is measured from the beginning of the P wave to the beginning of the QRS complex. It indicates the time that elapses between activation of the SA node and activation of the AV node.

T Wave

The T wave represents ventricular repolarization. The echocardiographic examination is always performed with an ECG.

This allows the cardiac sonographer to assess cardiac events as they occur in systole and diastole.

Excitation Contraction Coupling. The cardiac muscle is a type of striated muscle tissue. The cells are joined by intercalated disks. The calcium ions are stored and released in response to electrical activity.

AUSCULTATION OF THE HEART VALVES

Heart sounds are associated with the initiation of ventricular systole, closing of the atrioventricular valves, and opening of the semilunar valves (see Figure 27-15). The first sound is lower in pitch and longer in duration than the second. Both sounds can be heard over the entire area of the heart, but the first sound, "lubb," is heard most clearly in the region of the apex of the heart.

The second sound, "dupp," is sharper and shorter and has a higher pitch. It is heard best over the second right rib because the aorta approaches nearest to the surface at this point. The second sound is caused mainly by the closing of the semilunar valves during ventricular diastole. Following the second sound, there is a period of silence. Thus the sequence sounds like this: lubb, dupp, silence, lubb, dupp, silence, and so on.

Defects in the valves can cause excessive turbulence or regurgitation of the blood. These are extra abnormal sounds and are called **murmurs** or *clicks*. If the valves fail to close tightly and blood leaks back, a hissing murmur is heard. The hissing sound is heard in the area of the affected valve; thus if the mitral valve is affected, it will be heard in the first sound. Another condition giving rise to an abnormal sound is stenosis or stiffening of a valve orifice. In this case a rumble is heard in the area of the affected valve. A **diastolic murmur** begins with or after the time of the second heart sound and ends at or before the time of the first heart sound. A **systolic murmur** begins with or after the time of the first heart sound and ends at or before the time of the second heart sound. A **continuous murmur** begins in systole and continues without interruption through the time of the second heart sound into all or part of diastole. Murmurs are graded according to **frequency** and **intensity**.

It is beyond the scope of this text to present an in-depth approach to auscultation, and the reader is referred to the Selected Bibliography at the end of this chapter for additional reading on this subject. An understanding of auscultation will help in understanding cardiac physiology and echocardiographic differential considerations.

PRINCIPLES OF BLOOD FLOW

Blood flow may be described in terms of laminar flow or disturbed flow. *Laminar flow* means that blood moves in smooth layers that slide against each other. The blood cells move with similar velocities and directions in an organized manner. *Disturbed flow* means that blood cells move in different directions with varying velocities (disorganized flow). The turbulence denotes the presence of random vortices *(flow eddies).*

The flow dynamics depend on the fluid viscosity and the momentum of molecules in the fluid. The velocity profile indicates two pathways: parabolic flow or flat flow. The *parabolic flow velocity profile* is such that as fluid moves through a tube, fluid layers in the center have a higher velocity than those on outer surfaces. The *flat flow velocity profile* states that as flow accelerates and converges, more fluid travels at velocities closer to peak velocity as layers in the center. This is characteristic of high-velocity flow and at the inlets of the great vessels.

The heart is a pulsatile pump. In systole the ventricles eject blood into the aorta and pulmonary artery. In diastole, the ventricles fill with blood from the atria and flow to the body organs. The damping effect is achieved because of the elasticity of great vessels as they absorb high flow pulsatility of the heart and smooth it out before sending it to the blood downstream. The blood vessels stretch in response to an increase in pressure (compliance). The increase in fluid pressure during systole causes the aorta and pulmonary artery to expand and store some of the ejected blood. Blood is prevented from reentering the ventricles by the closure of the valves. Stored blood is pushed downstream into circulation when the aorta and pulmonary artery begin to return to normal dimensions in diastole. The hardening of the arteries results in loss of vessel compliance. The circulatory impedance occurs because of resistance to flow downstream in small vessels and capillaries. Flow is produced when a pressure gradient exists. The blood flow through a constriction creates a high fluid pressure upstream from constriction. The high fluid pressure forces blood through the constriction in the form of a laminar high-velocity jet. The fluid pressure gradually decreases as it goes downstream. Flow velocity through the constriction is higher than the velocity upstream. The normal resting cardiac output is 5 L/min.

VENTRICULAR EJECTION

Both ventricles eject the same proportion of contents with systole. The normal left ventricular ejection fraction is 67%. The normal stroke volume is 45 +/– 13 ml/m^2. The amount of filling (preload) influences the pressure developed during the next systole via the Frank Starling mechanism. The output of the ventricle depends on resistance encountered by the contracting ventricle when the aortic valve opens during systole (afterload). The most important indicator of cardiac work is the metabolic cost of cardiac activity, which is given by the oxygen consumption of the myocardium.

CORONARY CIRCULATION

The coronary flow is essential to myocardial performance. The right and left coronary arteries arise from the base of the ascending aorta. The left coronary artery flow is mainly diastolic. The right coronary artery flow is more evenly spread through systole and diastole. The flow goes from the epicardium to the endocardium. The diastolic aortic pressure is a major factor in coronary perfusion. Myocardial ischemia may occur in situations in which blood pressure is acutely lowered. The arteries and arterioles anastomose with one another and the small collateral channels increase in number when vessels are occluded.

SELECTED BIBLIOGRAPHY

Adams KF Jr and others: Interrelationships between left ventricular volume and output during exercise in healthy subjects, *J Appl Physiol* 73:2097, 1992.

Anderson PD: *Clinical anatomy and physiology for allied health sciences,* Philadelphia, 1976, WB Saunders.

Clemente CD: *Anatomy: a regional atlas of the human body,* Philadelphia, 1975, Lea & Febiger.

Crafts RC: *A textbook of human anatomy,* New York, 1979, John Wiley & Sons.

DeBakey M, Gotto A: *The living heart,* New York, 1977, Grosset & Dunlap.

Green JH: *Basic clinical physiology,* New York, 1969, Oxford University Press.

Hollinshead WH: *Textbook of anatomy,* Philadelphia, 1985, JB Lippincott.

McMinn RMH, Gaddum-Rosse P, Hutchings RT and others: *McMinn's functional & clinical anatomy,* St Louis, 1995, Mosby.

Northcote RJ and others: The effect of habitual sustained endurance exercise on cardiac structure and function, *Eur Heart J* 11:17, 1990.

Reynolds T: *The echocardiographer's pocket reference,* Phoenix, 2003, Arizona Heart Institute.

Snell RS: *Clinical neuroanatomy for medical students,* Boston, 2003, Little, Brown.

Sokolow M, McIlroy MB: *Clinical cardiology,* Los Altos, CA, 1977, Lange Medical.

Tilkian AG, Conover MB: *Understanding heart sounds and murmurs,* Philadelphia, 1992, WB Saunders.

Wilson DB, Kvacek JL: Echocardiography. Basics for the primary care physician. *Postgrad Med* 87(5):191-193, 196-202, 1990.

Introduction to Echocardiographic Evaluation and Techniques

Sandra L. Hagen-Ansert

KEY TERMS

color flow mapping (CFM) – ability to display blood flow in multiple colors depending on the velocity, direction of flow, and extent of turbulence

continuous wave probe – sound is continuously emitted from one transducer and continuously received by a second transducer

diastole – part of the cardiac cycle in which the ventricles are filling with blood; the tricuspid and mitral valves are open during this time

Doppler frequency – red blood cells move from a lower-frequency sound source at rest toward a higher-frequency sound source; change in frequency is called the Doppler shift in frequency

pulsed wave transducer – single crystal that sends and receives sound intermittently; a pulse of sound is emitted from the transducer, which also receives the returning signal

spectral analysis waveform – graphic display of the flow velocity over time

systole – part of the cardiac cycle in which the ventricles are pumping blood through the outflow tract into the pulmonary artery or the aorta

---

The evaluation of cardiac structures by echocardiography is regarded as an essential diagnostic tool in clinical cardiology. The reason for its widespread use in the evaluation of cardiac disease is its noninvasive, reproducible, and accurate assessment of cardiac structures.

The M-mode technique was limited in that it provided only a one-dimensional or "ice pick" view of the heart. Two-dimensional echocardiography, however, has allowed cardiac structures to be visualized in real-time. Thus, the echocardiographer can assess intracardiac lesions, observe contractility, and estimate valvular function. The combination of real-time, Doppler, and color flow analysis provides an extremely accurate means to evaluate wall thickness, valvular orifice and chamber size, and contractility of the cardiac structures. The introduction of transesophageal echocardiography (TEE) has enabled exquisite visualization of the heart while the transducer is guided through the mouth, into the esophagus, and to the cardiac orifice. Contrast injected into the bloodstream has provided an additional pathway to visualize cardiac perfusion or shunt flow. Exercise echocardiography and dobutamine-injection echocardiography have provided information about the contractility and performance of the left ventricle in a stress situation.

To perform an echocardiographic examination of good diagnostic quality, the sonographer must be aware of anatomic and pathophysiologic parameters of the heart and understand the physical principles of sonography. The purpose of this chapter is to introduce the reader to the basic concepts of echocardiography through two-dimensional, M-mode, Doppler, and color Doppler imaging.

TRANSDUCERS

Several types of transducers are available for echocardiographic techniques. Ideally, one should use as high a frequency as possible to improve the resolution of returning echoes. However, the higher the frequency, the less the penetration; therefore, compromises have to be made to obtain the best possible image. Many echocardiographers working with adults use a 2.5-MHz transducer with a medium focus. A pediatric patient generally requires a 5.0- or 7.5-MHz transducer for improved resolution and near-field definition.

EXAMINATION TECHNIQUES

The patient is generally examined in the left lateral semidecubitus position. This position allows the heart to move away from the sternum and closer to the chest wall, thus allowing a better cardiac window. The cardiac window is found between the third and fifth intercostal spaces, slightly to the left of the sternal border. The cardiac window may be considered that area on the anterior chest where the heart is just beneath the skin surface, free of lung interference.

The cardiac sonographer must keep in mind that different body shapes require variations in transducer position. An obese patient may have a transverse heart, and thus a slight lateral movement from the sternal border may be needed to record cardiac structures. A thin patient may have a long and slender heart, requiring a lower, more medial transducer position. Barrel-chested patients may have echocardiographic difficulties because of the lung absorption interference. It may be necessary to turn these patients completely on their left sides or even prone to eliminate the interference. Sometimes the upright or slightly forward-bent position is useful in forcing the heart closer to the anterior chest wall.

The following techniques are guidelines for the average patient. In the initial echocardiographic study, moving the transducer freely along the left sternal border until all the cardiac structures are easily identified is a better practice than restricting the transducer to one interspace. This procedure saves time and gives the examiner a better understanding of cardiac relationships. If there is difficulty examining the patient in the supine position, a semidecubitus position should be used. If the heart is actually very medial, the best study is performed with the patient completely on his or her left side. If too much lung interference clouds the study, the patient should exhale for as long as possible. This usually gives the examiner enough time to record pieces of valid information.

TWO-DIMENSIONAL ECHOCARDIOGRAPHY

The widespread clinical acceptance of real-time, two-dimensional imaging has tremendously aided the diagnostic results of a typical echocardiographic examination. Improved transducer design, resolution capabilities, focus parameters, gray scale differentiation, gain control factors, cine loop functions, and other computer capabilities have aided the cardiac sonographer in the attempt to record consistent, high-quality images from the multiple scan planes necessary to obtain a composite image of the cardiac structures.

In addition, two-dimensional transducers have the combined function of imaging and performing an M-mode or a Doppler study simultaneously. The addition of color flow Doppler has added a new dimension for the cardiac sonographer in detecting intracardiac shunt flow, mapping regurgitant pathways, and determining obstructive flow pathways. This chapter presents two-dimensional echo with Doppler and color flow Doppler techniques together.

TRANSDUCER LOCATION AND IMAGING PLANES
The Committee on Nomenclature and Standards in Two-Dimensional Echocardiography of the American Society of Echocardiography recommends the following nomenclature and image orientation standards for transducer locations (Figure 28-1):

- **suprasternal**—transducer placed in the suprasternal notch
- **subcostal**—transducer located near the body midline and beneath the costal margin
- **apical**—transducer located over the cardiac apex (at the point of maximal impulse)
- **parasternal**—transducer placed over the area bounded superiorly by the left clavicle, medially by the sternum, and inferiorly by the apical region

The imaging planes are described by the manner in which the two-dimensional transducer transects the heart (Figure 28-2):

- **long axis**—transects the heart perpendicular to the dorsal and ventral surfaces of the body and parallel with the long axis of the heart
- **short axis**—transects the heart perpendicular to the dorsal and ventral surfaces of the body and perpendicular to the long axis of the heart

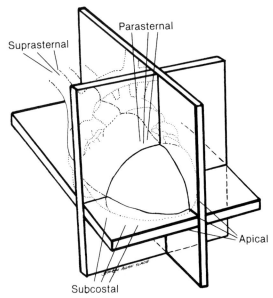

Figure 28-1 Schema of the four transducer positions for the two-dimensional echocardiogram: suprasternal transducer is placed in the suprasternal notch; subcostal transducer is located near the midline and beneath the costal margin; apical transducer is located over the cardiac apex; and parasternal transducer is located in the fourth intercostal space just to the left of midline.

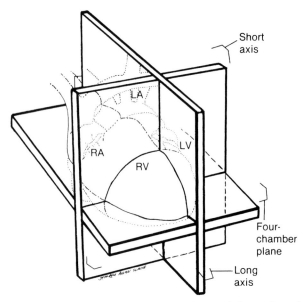

Figure 28-2 Schema of the parasternal long and short axis, and apical four-chamber views of the heart. *LA,* Left atrium; *LV,* left ventricle; *RA,* right atrium; *RV,* right ventricle.

- **four chamber**—transects the heart approximately parallel with the dorsal and ventral surfaces of the body

CARDIAC COLOR FLOW EXAMINATION

The **color flow mapping (CFM)** examination is generally performed along with the conventional two-dimensional examination. The advantage of CFM is its ability to rapidly investigate

BOX 28-1 NORMAL COLOR FLOW MAPPING EXAMINATION AND TECHNIQUES

- The color flow mapping examination is generally performed in the same planes used for conventional Doppler examination.
- Parasternal long-axis view: membranous IVS
- Parasternal short-axis view: AO, PA, RVOT, IAS, TV
- Parasternal short-axis view: MV
- Apical four-chamber plane: MV, TV
- Apical five-chamber plane: LVOT, AV
- Apical long-axis, two-chamber view: LV, LVOT, LA
- Subcostal four-chamber view: IAS, IVS, RV, LV, RA, LA
- Subcostal view: IVC, hepatic veins
- Subcostal view: AO
- Subcostal short-axis view: AO, PA, RVOT
- Suprasternal view (long axis): ascending and descending aorta, SVC
- Suprasternal view (short axis): arch, RPA, LA, SVC
- Right parasternal view: SVC, RA, IVC, LA with pulmonary veins

AO, Aorta; *AV,* aortic valve; *IAS,* interatrial septum; *LA,* left atrium; *LV,* left ventricle; *RA,* right atrium; *RV,* right ventricle; *IVS,* interventricular septum; *LA,* left atrium; *LV,* left ventricle; *LVOT,* left ventricular outflow tract; *MV,* mitral valve; *PA,* pulmonary artery; *RA,* right atrium; *RPA,* right pulmonary artery; *RV,* right ventricle; *RVOT,* right ventricular outflow tract; *SVC,* superior vena cava; *TV,* tricuspid valve.

flow direction and movement within the cardiac chambers (Box 28-1). Flow toward the transducer is recorded in red, and flow away from the transducer is blue (Figure 28-3). As the velocities increase, the flow pattern in the variance mode turns from red to various shades of red, orange, and yellow before it aliases. Likewise flow away from the transducer is recorded in blue; this color turns to various shades of blue, turquoise, and green before it aliases. Depending on the location of the transducer, the flow signals from various structures within the heart appear as different colors. An understanding of cardiac hemodynamics helps the examiner understand the flow patterns.

Although normal cardiac flows are difficult to accurately time during the CFM examination because of its slow frame rate, the use of color M-mode (with a faster frame rate) allows one to precisely determine specific cardiac events in correlation with the ECG. The color M-mode is made in the same manner as a conventional M-mode study (Figure 28-4). The cursor is placed through the area of interest, and the flow is evaluated using an autocorrelation technique. The operator must thoroughly understand the color instrument settings to produce a high-quality image. Familiarity with the color flow maps provided in the software of the equipment is necessary to understand the alias patterns and turbulent flow parameters.

DOPPLER APPLICATIONS AND TECHNIQUE

The Doppler effect, first described by Christian Johann Doppler, is demonstrated on an echocardiogram as red blood cells move from a lower-frequency sound source at rest toward

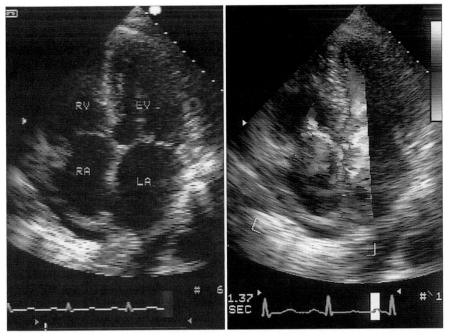

Figure 28-3   Four-chamber view with and without color. The color bar is shown along the right upper margin; yellow and red indicate flow toward the transducer, and blue and turquoise indicate flow away from the transducer. This patient had a small ventricular septal defect *(red flow across the interventricular septum)* and tricuspid insufficiency *(blue flow into the right atrium)*. *LA,* Left atrium; *LV,* left ventricle; *RA,* right atrium; *RV,* right ventricle.

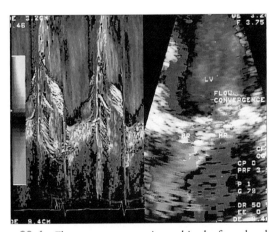

Figure 28-4   Flow convergence as imaged in the four-chamber view and M-mode/color flow mapping image. The red inflow is from the pulmonary veins into the left atrium, the blue is swirling flow within the left atrium, and the multicolored flow at the level of the mitral valve is regurgitant flow. *LV,* Left ventricle; *MR,* mitral regurgitation.

a higher-frequency sound source. The change in frequency is called the Doppler shift in frequency, or the **Doppler frequency** (Figure 28-5).

Doppler echocardiography has emerged as a valuable noninvasive tool in clinical cardiology to provide hemodynamic information about the function of the cardiac valves and chambers of the heart. When combined with conventional two-dimensional and M-mode echocardiography, Doppler techniques may be focused to produce specific information on the flows of a particular area within the heart.

Advances in Doppler technology have made it possible to provide steerable continuous wave and pulsed wave Doppler. The ability to be qualitative and quantitative in evaluating valvular function, intracardiac shunts, dysfunction of a prosthetic valve, and obstruction of a surgically inserted shunt and to record normal cardiac blood flow patterns has contributed to the understanding and diagnostic capability of the Doppler technique in cardiology. However, to record this information, the cardiac sonographer and physician should master cardiac physiology and hemodynamics. In addition, the operator must clearly understand Doppler principles, artifacts, and pitfalls to produce a quality study. Although cardiac instrumentation is fundamentally similar to imaging echocardiography, the approach to Doppler, especially color Doppler, varies considerably from one company to another. A solid understanding of the instrumentation is necessary to produce a valid examination.

This section on the normal Doppler examination is presented so the reader may become familiar with the normal Doppler patterns and the pitfalls in both recording and listening to Doppler signals.

NORMAL CARDIAC DOPPLER FLOW PATTERNS

It is important to understand the relationship between the two-dimensional study and the Doppler flow study. Real-time two-dimensional imaging allows assessment of cardiac anatomy and function. On the other hand, Doppler flow analysis allows examination of blood flow rather than cardiac anatomy. The Doppler principle on which this technique is based involves the backscatter of transmitted ultrasonic waves from circulating red blood cells. The difference in frequency between transmitted and backscattered sound waves (Doppler shift) is used to quantify forward or backward blood flow velocity.

Quality Doppler studies require the patient to be still for several seconds. In adult patients this usually is not difficult, but in pediatric patients it may be a challenge. Therefore, it is necessary that the instrumentation used in pediatrics respond very quickly to changes in the menu or Doppler format. It is essential to be able to change back and forth between the real-time image and the Doppler image or to image the real-time and Doppler images simultaneously. The ability to simultane-

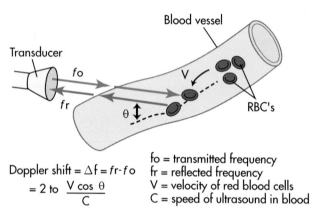

Doppler shift = $\Delta f = fr - fo$

= 2 to $\dfrac{V \cos \theta}{C}$

fo = transmitted frequency
fr = reflected frequency
V = velocity of red blood cells
C = speed of ultrasound in blood

Figure 28-5   Illustration of the Doppler effect. The Doppler shift depends on the transmitted frequency *(fo)*, the velocity of the moving target *(V)*, and the angle *(θ)* between the ultrasound beam and the direction of the moving target.

ously perform the Doppler and two-dimensional study allows the sonographer to image cardiac structures and to place the sample volume in the proper location.

The best-quality Doppler signals are obtained when the sample volume is parallel to the direction of flow. The flow of blood occurs in three-dimensional space, whereas the real-time image is only in two dimensions. Therefore, the two-dimensional image serves as a guide to the operator as small adjustments of the transducer and sample volume are made in the valve orifice to record the optimal Doppler signals. The key is to produce a spectral signal to show a well-defined velocity envelope along with a clearly defined audio tone. The clarity of the audio tone cannot be emphasized enough. Frequently the clarity of tone is used to guide the Doppler cursor into the correct plane to record the maximum velocity.

Blood flow toward the transducer is displayed by a time velocity waveform above the baseline at point zero, or a positive deflection (Figure 28-6). Flow away from the Doppler signal is displayed below the baseline or as a negative deflection. A simultaneous ECG should be displayed to help time the cardiac cycle.

PULSED WAVE DOPPLER

A **pulsed wave transducer** is constructed with a single crystal that sends bursts of ultrasound at a rate called the *pulsed repetition frequency*. Sound waves backscattered from moving red blood cells are received by the transducer during a limited time between transmitted pulses. A time gating device is then used to select the precise depth from which the returning signal has originated because the signals return from the heart at different times.

The particular area of interest undergoing Doppler evaluation is referred to as the *sample volume*. The sample volume and directional line placement of the beam are moved by use of the trackball. The exact size and location of the sample

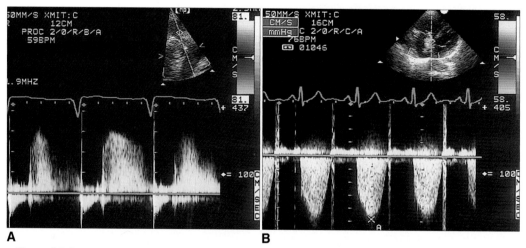

A   B

Figure 28-6   **A,** Flow above the baseline represents forward flow (as seen in this patient with pulmonic insufficiency). **B,** Flow below the baseline represents flow moving away from the transducer (as seen in this patient with tricuspid regurgitation).

volume can be adjusted at the area of interest. Some instruments have a fixed sample volume size. Others allow the operator to select the size appropriate for the particular study.

Velocities under 2 m/sec are recorded without an alias pattern (Figure 28-7). However, pulsed Doppler is limited in its ability to record high-velocity patterns. The maximum frequency shift that can be measured by a pulsed Doppler system is called the Nyquist limit, and is one half the pulsed repetition frequency. Velocities that exceed this limit are known to produce an aliasing pattern (Figure 28-8). Normal cardiac structures do not exceed the Nyquist limit and are very easily measured with the pulsed Doppler system.

CONTINUOUS WAVE DOPPLER

The **continuous wave probe** differs from the pulsed wave probe in that it requires two crystals (Figure 28-9). One crystal continuously emits sound; the other receives sound as it is backscattered to the transducer. This probe may be part of a

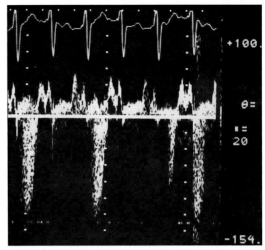

Figure 28-7   Pulsed wave flow pattern at the mitral valve level in a patient with mild mitral regurgitation *(negative flow from the baseline).*

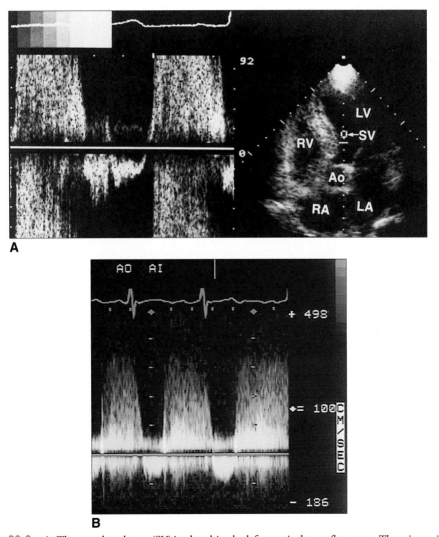

Figure 28-8   **A,** The sample volume *(SV)* is placed in the left ventricular outflow tract. There is aortic insufficiency that exceeds the Nyquist limit of the pulsed wave Doppler (flow is seen above and below the baseline). When the continuous wave transducer is used **(B),** the velocity measures 3.5 m/sec. *Ao,* Aorta; *LA,* left atrium; *LV,* left ventricle; *RA,* right atrium; *RV,* right ventricle.

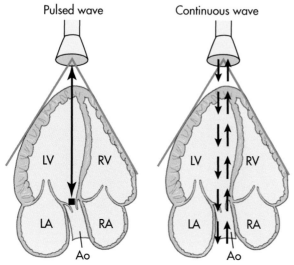

Figure 28-9   Drawing of pulsed-wave and continuous-wave Doppler echocardiography with the transducer placed in the PMI at the apex of the heart.

phased or annular array imaging probe or may be a stand-alone independent probe. If it is part of a two-dimensional imaging transducer, the sample direction can sometimes be steered by use of the trackball. This method has many advantages in the Doppler study; it is quicker and more efficient to be able to image a structure and then move the Doppler cursor to obtain the best audio and spectral signals.

Some instruments have a fixed continuous wave sample direction, which means that the area of interest must be aligned with a stationary line on the screen to obtain the best signal. This method is very tedious and difficult to maintain for a good tracing.

The independent continuous wave probe is smaller than the imaging probe and thus has advantages in obtaining a good Doppler study. Because the diameter of the probe is smaller, it allows greater flexibility to reach in between small rib interspaces or to obtain signals from the suprasternal notch. Many patients will allow the small independent probe to be angled within their suprasternal notch but not the bulky imaging probe. The independent probe is often more sensitive and therefore produces better Doppler signals. The audio portion of the Doppler examination becomes a critical factor in this study because there is no two-dimensional image to guide in the transducer location.

It is often beneficial to use both probes to perform the study. Once the proper transducer position is found with the imaging transducer, the angulation and window are marked for proper placement of the continuous wave transducer (see Figure 28-8). The audio sound and spectral wave pattern are then used to guide the correction angulation of the beam for maximum-velocity recordings. There is not a particular sample volume site within the continuous wave beam. Velocities are recorded from several points along the linear beam. This technique has the ability to record maximum velocities without alias patterns. The recording ability is especially useful for very high-velocity patterns.

AUDIO SIGNALS AND SPECTRAL DISPLAY OF DOPPLER SIGNALS

It is known that the best Doppler signals are obtained when the ultrasound beam is parallel or nearly parallel to the flow of blood. Therefore the best windows used to record the two-dimensional images may not be the best windows to record Doppler flow patterns. The technique for recording quality Doppler signals from the inflow and outflow tracts through the cardiac valves is discussed in this section.

Audio Signals. The audio signal from the frequency shift, as recorded in the Doppler study, is in the audible range, which is conveyed through a headphone or through dual speakers. (Dual speakers allow the operator to differentiate forward and reverse flow.) The recognition of Doppler signals does take experience. The signal from the arterial flow is very different from that of the venous flow; likewise, mitral and tricuspid patterns differ from the aortic and pulmonary valve patterns. The blood flow velocity determines the pitch or frequency of the audio signal. As the velocity becomes higher, the pitch becomes higher; as the velocity decreases, so does the pitch.

Normal blood flow across the cardiac valves demonstrates a narrow range of velocity with a very smooth and even Doppler audio signal. When the flow becomes disturbed, as occurs distal to an obstruction or regurgitation of the valve, the tone becomes harsh. Very high-velocity flows produce a very-high-frequency signal with a sharp "whistling-hissing" tone. This signal may be found in obstruction and regurgitant lesions.

Other movements within the cardiac chambers produce audio signals, but these signals are not as well defined. The valve opening and closure can be heard as a discrete click when the Doppler window is located too close to the valve. The normal cardiac function causes the valve to move in and out of the Doppler beam, producing a lower-frequency signal. Therefore, careful angulation along with the audio signal helps the operator observe the dynamics of the cardiac cycle for correct beam placement to obtain the best quality Doppler signal.

To record accurate velocity measurements, the ideal position of the Doppler beam is along a line of sight in which the angle of the beam is parallel to the transducer. As the angle decreases, the clarity of the audio signal increases, indicating that a quality signal is being recorded.

Spectral Analysis. The **spectral analysis waveform** allows the operator to print a graphic display of what the audio signal is recording because it provides a representation of blood flow velocities over time. The velocity on the vertical axis is measured in centimeters per second or meters per second, whereas time is shown on the horizontal axis. Therefore, the direction and velocity of flow may be measured very accurately when the beam is parallel to the flow. Flow toward the transducer is above the baseline. Flow away from the transducer is below the baseline. Multiple velocity measurements are used to quantify valvular function, stroke volume, and intracardiac shunts and pressures.

TABLE 28-1 **MAXIMAL VELOCITIES RECORDED WITH DOPPLER IN NORMAL INDIVIDUALS**		
	Children (cm/sec)	Adults (cm/sec)
Mitral flow	80-130	60-130
Tricuspid flow	50-80	30-70
Pulmonary artery	70-110	60-90
Left ventricle	70-120	70-110
Aorta	120-180	100-170

A normal spectral display pattern has a very typical appearance. In normal blood flow, the cells generally have a uniform direction with similar velocities. The spectral tracing appears as a smooth mitral velocity pattern bordered by a narrow band of velocities. As the velocity increases, so does the turbulence within the border of the narrow-band velocities, producing a filling of the velocity curve. As the cardiac structure moves in and out of the beam, the Doppler frequency shift is recorded as tall artifact spikes.

Gray scale imaging is used to display the amplitude of the velocity signal, with the highest velocities appearing as the darkest shade (if a black-on-white spectral analysis is used) or white (if a white-on-black spectral analysis is used).

DOPPLER QUANTITATION

Quantitation of the Doppler signal to obtain hemodynamic information is derived from the measurement of blood flow velocity (Table 28-1). As explained previously, it is critical that the angle of the Doppler signal be as parallel to flow as possible. The Doppler equation is based on the principle that the velocity of blood flow is directly proportional to the Doppler frequency shift and the speed of sound in tissue, and is inversely related to twice the frequency of transmitted ultrasound and the cosine of the angle of incidence between the ultrasound beam and the direction of blood flow. Therefore, the relationship between the angle and its cosine becomes significant and can be a source of error if ignored. If the angle is less than 20 degrees, the cosine is quite close to 1 and can be ignored. If the angle increases beyond 20 degrees, the cosine becomes less than 1 and may produce an underestimation of velocity.

DOPPLER EXAMINATION

The Doppler examination is also performed along with the two-dimensional study of the cardiac structures. During this conventional study the sonographer notes structures that may need special attention during the Doppler examination (e.g., a redundant mitral valve leaflet may indicate the need to search for mitral regurgitation). Throughout the Doppler study, various patient positions and transducer rotations are necessary to place the sample volume parallel to blood flow (Box 28-2). There are basically five transducer positions used to record quality Doppler flow patterns: the apical four chamber, left parasternal, subcostal, suprasternal, and the right parasternal.

BOX 28-2 DOPPLER WINDOWS

APICAL WINDOW
Mitral valve, tricuspid valve, left ventricular outflow tract, aortic valve, pulmonary vein inflow, superior vena cava inflow, interventricular septum

PARASTERNAL SHORT-AXIS WINDOW
Pulmonary valve, main pulmonary artery, right and left branches, patent ductus arteriosus flow, tricuspid valve

SUPRASTERNAL NOTCH WINDOW
Ascending aorta, descending aorta, patent ductus arteriosus flow, right pulmonary artery

SUBCOSTAL WINDOW
Interatrial septum, interventricular septum, inferior vena cava flow, superior vena cava flow

PARASTERNAL LONG-AXIS WINDOW
Mitral regurgitation, tricuspid regurgitation, aortic regurgitation

RIGHT PARASTERNAL WINDOW
Ascending aorta

The patient should be forewarned about the audio sounds produced by the Doppler signal because some find the sound alarming if the volume is set too high.

THE ECHOCARDIOGRAPHIC EXAMINATION

The protocol for the evaluation cardiac structures begins with the parasternal long- and short-axis views, followed by the apical four-chamber, long-axis, and two-chamber views. The subcostal and suprasternal views complete the study (Box 28-3).

PARASTERNAL VIEWS

Parasternal Long-Axis Two-Dimensional View. The parasternal long-axis view is the initial image in the echographic examination (Figure 28-10). An attempt should be made to record as many of the cardiac structures as possible (from the base of the heart to the apex). Generally, this is accomplished by placing the long axis of the transducer slightly to the left of the sternum in about the fourth intercostal space. When the bright echo reflection of the pericardium is noted, the transducer is gradually rotated until a long-axis view of the heart is obtained. If it is not possible to record the entire long axis on a single scan, the transducer should be gently rocked cephalad to caudad in an "ice pick" fashion to record all the information from the base to the apex of the heart (Figure 28-11).

The cardiac sonographer should observe the following structures and functions in the parasternal long-axis view:

1. Composite size of the cardiac chambers
2. Contractility of the right and left ventricles

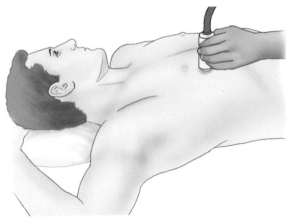

Figure 28-10   Parasternal long-axis view of the heart with the transducer placed along the left sternal border at the fourth intercostal space.

BOX 28-3   TRANSDUCER POSITION AND CARDIAC PROTOCOL

PARASTERNAL
Long-axis view: LV in sagittal plane
    RV inflow
    LV outflow
Short-axis view: LV apex
    Papillary muscles (midlevel)
    Mitral valve (basal level)
    Aortic valve—RV outflow tract
    Pulmonary trunk bifurcation

APICAL
Four-chamber view
Five-chamber view (including aorta)
Two-chamber view

SUBCOSTAL WINDOW
Inferior vena cava
Hepatic veins
RV and LV inflow
LV aorta
RV outflow

SUPRASTERNAL NOTCH WINDOW
Ascending aorta
Descending aorta
Right pulmonary artery
Left atrium

RIGHT PARASTERNAL WINDOW
Ascending aorta

---

3. Thickness of the right ventricular wall
4. Continuity of the interventricular septum with the anterior wall of the aorta
5. Pliability of the atrioventricular and semilunar valves
6. Coaptation of the atrioventricular valves
7. Presence of increased echoes on the atrioventricular and semilunar valves
8. Systolic clearance of the aortic cusps

9. Presence of abnormal echo collections in the chambers or attached to the valve orifice
10. Presence and movement of chordal-papillary muscle structure
11. Thickness of the septum and posterior wall of the left ventricle
12. Uniform texture of the endocardium and myocardium
13. Size of the aortic root and left atrium

Parasternal Long-Axis View for Color Flow Mapping. In **diastole,** the parasternal long-axis view shows the left atrium filled with various shades of red as the pulmonary venous flow enters the atrial cavity from the right and left branches. While the blood is pushed toward the mitral leaflets, some turbulence is shown when the flow enters into the left ventricle.

During **systole,** the mitral leaflets close and the ventricle contracts to push the blood through the left ventricular outflow tract through the open aortic cusps. The blood is now flowing toward the transducer and is shown as a shade of red with some yellow highlights as it approaches the aortic root. Aliasing can occur when the Nyquist limit is lower than the maximum velocity of the flow. No color flow is seen to cross at the level of the membranous septum in the normal patient.

If mitral regurgitation is present, a turquoise flow arising from the mitral valve is seen in the left atrial cavity during systole (Figure 28-12). If aortic insufficiency is present, a yellowish mosaic flow pattern is seen during diastole (this generally hugs the left side of the interventricular septum, but the amount of calcification or thickening present in the aortic cusps determines which direction the regurgitant jet takes) (Figure 28-13).

Left Parasternal Window for Doppler. The parasternal long-axis view with the patient rolled in a left lateral decubitus position has limited applications with Doppler. The transducer is more perpendicular to the cardiac structures than parallel, so the maximum velocity is difficult to record. However, disturbances in flow, especially mitral, aortic, and tricuspid (with the transducer angled medial) regurgitation, may be recorded in some patients with this view. Thickened cusps may direct the regurgitant flow in a pathway not typically seen as well on the apical view as on the parasternal long-axis view (Figure 28-14). A ventricular septal defect may be visualized on this view because the flow of blood is more parallel to the beam. Both muscular and membranous defects may be imaged from this view along with the apical and subcostal views.

Right Parasternal View for Color Flow Mapping. The right parasternal view is performed after the patient has been rolled into a steep right decubitus position. The transducer is placed along the right sternal border in the second intercostal space. This view may be useful for visualization of the entrance of the superior vena cava into the right atrium. The caval flow appears red as it enters the right atrium. This view also provides another window to image the entrance of the pulmonary veins into the left atrium. Flow patterns from the veins may be seen, whereas the actual veins are difficult to image on the two-dimensional study.

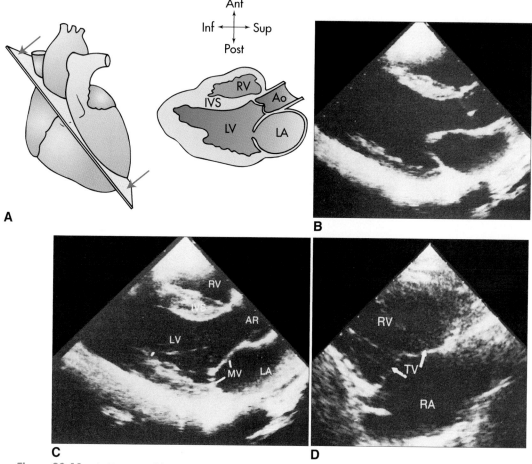

Figure 28-11   **A,** Parasternal long-axis view. The two-dimensional parasternal long-axis view of the heart in early diastole **(B)** and end-systole **(C).** *AR,* Aortic root; *IVS,* interventricular septum; *LA,* left atrium; *LV,* left ventricle; *MV,* mitral valve; *RV,* right ventricle. **D,** Parasternal long-axis view of the tricuspid valve *(TV)* as it separates the right ventricle *(RV)* from the right atrium *(RA).*

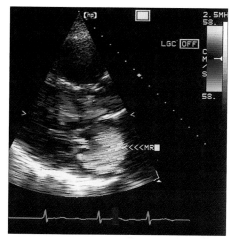

Figure 28-12   Parasternal long-axis view showing disturbed blue and yellow flow representing severe mitral regurgitation in the left atrial cavity.

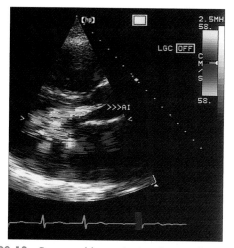

Figure 28-13   Parasternal long-axis view showing flow reversal through the aortic leaflets during ventricular diastole in a patient with aortic insufficiency.

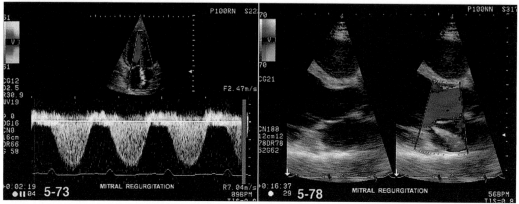

Figure 28-14 Parasternal long-axis view in a patient with mitral regurgitation (blue flow in the left atrium). The continuous wave flow is recorded in the apical position to measure 5 m/sec.

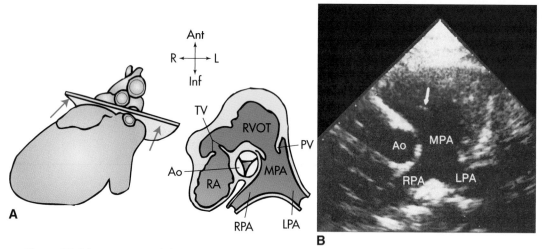

Figure 28-15 **A,** Parasternal short-axis view. *Ao,* Aorta; *LPA,* left pulmonary artery; *MPA,* main pulmonary artery; *PV,* pulmonary valve; *RA,* right atrium; *RPA,* right pulmonary artery; *RVOT,* right ventricular outflow tract; *TV,* tricuspid valve. **B,** High parasternal short-axis view of the aorta pulmonary cusp *(arrow),* main pulmonary artery *(MPA),* right pulmonary artery *(RPA),* and left pulmonary artery *(LPA).*

Right Parasternal Window for Doppler. The right parasternal position is most useful in the difficult-to-image adult or older pediatric patient after surgery who has a jet of aortic stenosis directed more to the right. The patient is rolled into a steep right decubitus position and the transducer placed in the first, second, or third intercostal space to the right of the sternum. Often the independent probe is easier to position in this patient, with the audible sound as the guide to the maximal velocity jet.

Parasternal Short-Axis Two-Dimensional View. The transducer should be rotated 90 degrees from the parasternal long-axis view to obtain multiple transverse short-axis views of the heart, particularly at the following four levels:

1. High parasternal short-axis view to demonstrate the pulmonary valve, right ventricular outflow tract, and aorta (Figure 28-15):

   a. Typical sausage-shaped right ventricular outflow tract and pulmonary artery draped anterior to circular aorta
   b. Semilunar cusp thickness and mobility
   c. Presence of calcification, extraneous echoes, or both in right ventricle or valve areas
   d. Pulmonary valve mobility and thickness

2. Moderate to high parasternal short-axis view to demonstrate the right ventricle, tricuspid valve, aortic cusps, coronary arteries, right and left atria (Figure 28-16):

   a. Size of right ventricle and left atrium
   b. Presence of mass lesions in right or left atrium
   c. Mobility and thickness of tricuspid and aortic valves
   d. Continuity of interatrial septum
   e. Right ventricular wall thickness
   f. Presence of trileaflet aortic valve

3. Mid parasternal short-axis view to demonstrate the right ventricle, left ventricular outflow tract, and anterior and posterior leaflets of the mitral valve (Figure 28-17):

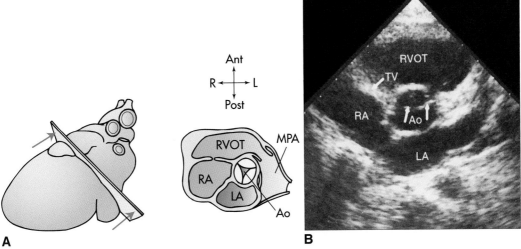

Figure 28-16   **A,** Parasternal short-axis view. *Ao,* Aorta; *LA,* left atrium; *MPA,* main pulmonary artery; *RA,* right atrium; *RVOT,* right ventricular outflow tract. **B,** High midparasternal short-axis view of the right ventricular outflow tract *(RVOT),* tricuspid valve *(TV),* right atrium *(RA),* aorta *(Ao),* aortic cusp *(arrows),* and left atrium *(LA).*

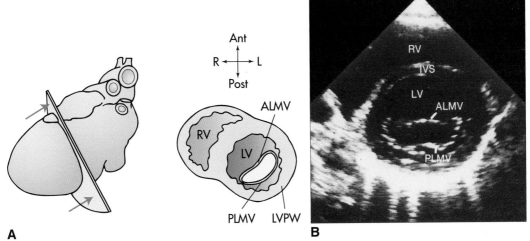

Figure 28-17   **A,** Parasternal short-axis view. *ALMV,* Anterior leaflet mitral valve; *LV,* left ventricle; *LVPW,* left ventricular posterior wall; *PLMV,* posterior leaflet mitral valve; *RV,* right ventricle. **B,** Midparasternal short-axis view of the right ventricle *(RV),* interventricular septum *(IVS),* anterior leaflet mitral valve *(ALMV),* posterior leaflet mitral valve *(PLMV),* and left ventricle *(LV).*

a. Size of the left ventricular outflow tract
b. Size of the septum and posterior wall
c. Presence of mass lesions in left or right ventricle
d. Mobility and thickness of the mitral valve
e. Presence of a flutter on the septum or anterior leaflet of the mitral valve or both
f. Systolic apposition of mitral valve leaflets
g. Contractility of septum and posterior wall

4. Low parasternal short-axis view should demonstrate the right ventricle, left ventricle, and papillary muscles (chordal echoes may also be seen) (Figure 28-18):
a. Contractility of the septum and posterior wall of the left ventricle
b. Thickness of the septum and posterior wall

c. Size of the left ventricle
d. Presence or absence of mural thrombus or other mass
e. Presence or absence of pericardial fluid, constriction, or restriction
f. Presence of increased echo density in posterior wall
g. Number of papillary muscles and their location within the left ventricular cavity

Parasternal Short-Axis View for Color Flow Mapping.
At the level of the aortic valve, the blood flow appears as a red signal moving toward the transducer from the right atrium into the right ventricle through the open tricuspid valve in diastole (Figure 28-19). Flow into the coronary arteries is sometimes seen in the right coronary, left main coronary, and circumflex

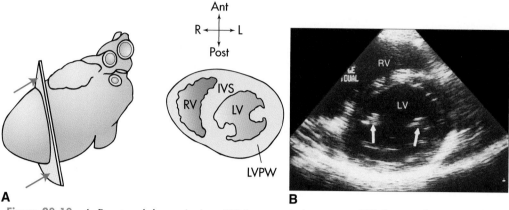

Figure 28-18   A, Parasternal short-axis view. *IVS,* Interventricular septum; *LV,* left ventricle; *LVPW,* left ventricular posterior wall; *RV,* right ventricle. **B,** Low parasternal short-axis view of the right ventricle *(RV),* left ventricle *(LV),* and posterior papillary muscle *(arrows).*

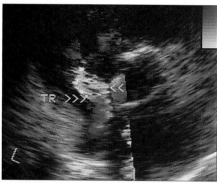

Figure 28-19   Parasternal short-axis view of tricuspid regurgitation *(TR, arrowheads, yellow and blue)* as it leaks into the right atrial cavity.

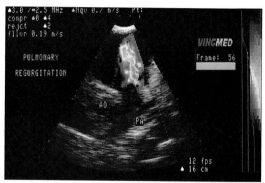

Figure 28-20   Parasternal short-axis view of pulmonic insufficiency *(yellow and blue)* as it leaks into the right ventricular outflow tract. *AO,* Aorta; *PA,* pulmonary artery.

and proximal left anterior descending arteries. Depending on the orientation of the coronary arteries, the blood flow appears yellow-red or bluish.

With slight angulation of the transducer, flow from the inferior vena cava can be seen while it flows into the right atrium. This flow appears red. When atrial systole occurs, blue signals can be seen moving from the right atrium into the inferior vena cava. Blue signals can also be seen as blood leaves the right ventricular outflow tract to enter the pulmonary valve and main pulmonary artery in systole. While the transducer is angled slightly, the flow from the main pulmonary artery is seen to move into the bifurcation of the right and left pulmonary arteries. This flow is still primarily blue while it moves away from the transducer.

Pulmonary insufficiency is shown easily with CFM as a yellow and red high-velocity flow pattern (Figure 28-20). Pulmonary stenosis would appear as a high-velocity disturbed pattern through the narrowed pulmonic orifice.

A short-axis view at the level of the mitral valve in diastole may show flow signals in the mitral orifice and the right ventricle. When the transducer is angled medially, the right ventricular inflow plane may show flow signals while they arise from the coronary sinus into the right heart during diastole.

Flow reversal (yellow-red pattern) toward the transducer is seen in patients with a high membranous ventricular septal defect (Figure 28-21).

Parasternal Short-Axis Window for Doppler. The parasternal short-axis view is very useful for recording flow from the right ventricular outflow tract and pulmonary artery. The sample volume should be placed distal to the pulmonary cusps to record flow in the main pulmonary artery. The flow pattern is very similar to that obtained from the aortic flow when the transducer is placed in the apical position but with a slightly slower upstroke. The spectral display shows a velocity curve below the baseline with a narrow band of frequencies. Normal pulmonary flow velocities range from 60 to 90 cm/sec in adults and 70 to 110 cm/sec in children. This view is useful for recording pulmonary regurgitation and stenosis, as well as abnormal patent ductus arteriosus flow that may be present in the neonate or child (Figure 28-22).

As the sample volume is positioned closer to the bifurcation of the pulmonary artery, the flow velocity increases slightly. To record velocities in the right ventricular outflow tract, the sample volume is placed just proximal to the pulmonary valve. The flow pattern is similar to the pulmonary

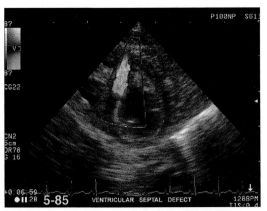

Figure 28-21   Parasternal short-axis view of the right and left ventricle in a patient with a small ventricular septal defect shows flow *(red, yellow, and blue)* flowing across the interventricular septum into the right ventricle.

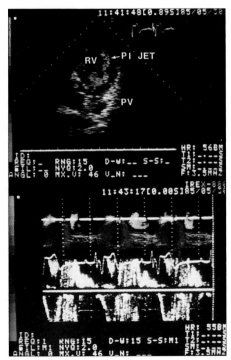

Figure 28-22   Parasternal short-axis view of a patient with pulmonary insufficiency shows flow reversal *(yellow)* through the pulmonary valve into the right ventricle. The spectral Doppler shows the normal forward pulmonary flow and the flow reversal from the insufficiency *(above the baseline)*. *PV,* Pulmonary valve; *RV,* right ventricle.

outflow but has a slightly lower velocity. This view is especially useful for detecting a left-to-right shunt at the membranous ventricular septum, a coronary artery fistula, or a muscle bundle in the right ventricular outflow tract.

Sometimes the parasternal short-axis view with the transducer angled slightly to the right is useful for recording increased flow from tricuspid regurgitation. In this view the sample volume is placed just inferior to the tricuspid leaflets

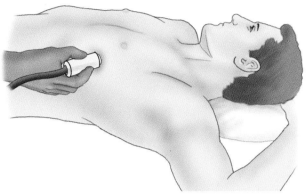

Figure 28-23   The transducer is placed at the PMI for the apical images.

in the right atrial cavity. If the interatrial septum is well seen, the increased flow pattern from a patent ductus arteriosus or atrial septal defect may be recorded.

APICAL VIEWS

Apical Two-Dimensional Views. Two apical views are very useful: the four-chamber view and the apical long-axis view, or two-chamber view. The cardiac sonographer should palpate the patient's chest to detect the point of maximal impulse (PMI) (Figure 28-23). The transducer should then be directed in a transverse plane at the PMI and angled sharply cephalad to record the four chambers of the heart. If there is too much lung interference, then the proper cardiac window has not been found and care should be taken to adjust the patient's position or the transducer position to adequately see all four chambers of the heart. Many laboratories have found it useful to use a very thick mattress in which a large hole has been cut at the level of the apex of the heart. This allows the transducer more flexibility for recording the four-chamber view.

The apical view is excellent for assessing cardiac contractility, size of cardiac chambers, presence of mass lesions, alignment of atrioventricular valves, coaptation of atrioventricular valves, septal or posterior wall hypertrophy, chordal attachments, and the presence of pericardial effusion (Figure 28-24). It is not a good view from which to evaluate the presence of an atrial septal defect because the beam is parallel to the thin foramen ovale and the septum commonly appears as a defect in this view. The subcostal four-chamber view is much better for evaluating the presence of such a defect.

The cardiac sonographer should observe the following structures:

1. Size of the cardiac chambers
2. Contractility of right and left ventricles
3. Septal and posterior wall thickness, contractility, and continuity
4. Coaptation of atrioventricular valves
5. Alignment of atrioventricular valves
6. Presence of increased echoes on valve apparatus
7. Presence of mass or thrombus in cardiac chambers
8. Entrance of pulmonary veins into left atrial cavity

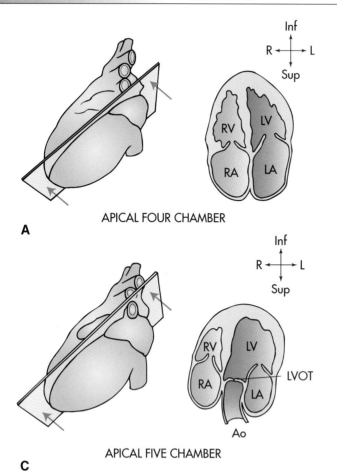

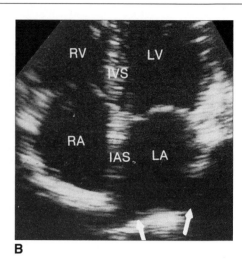

A   APICAL FOUR CHAMBER

C   APICAL FIVE CHAMBER

B

Figure 28-24   A, Apical four-chamber view. The transducer is placed at the posterior maximum impulse (near the midcoronal plane) and angled steeply towards the right shoulder. The patient should be rolled completely on his side for this examination. *LA,* Left atrium; *LV,* left ventricle; *RA,* right atrium; *RV,* right ventricle. **B,** Apical four-chamber view. *Arrows,* Pulmonary veins; *IAS,* interarterial septum; *IVS,* interventricular septum. **C,** Apical five-chamber view (left ventricular outflow tract). Anterior angulation from the four-chamber view will demonstrate the left ventricular outflow tract *(LVOT)* and the ascending aorta *(Ao).*

9. Size of left ventricular outflow tract, signs of obstruction, mobility of aortic cusps, absence of subaortic membrane
10. Entrance of inferior and superior vena cava into the right atrium

The apical long-axis view is very useful for evaluation of the left ventricular cavity and aortic outflow tract (Figure 28-25). Once the apical four-chamber view is obtained, the transducer should be rotated 90 degrees to visualize the left ventricle, left atrium, and aorta with cusps. This view permits the cardiac sonographer to evaluate the wall motion of the posterior basal segment of the left ventricle, the anterior wall, and the apex of the left ventricle. It also permits another view of the left ventricular outflow tract, which may be useful in determining aortic cusp motion or the presence of a subvalvular membrane.

Apical View for Color Flow Mapping. The apical four-chamber view is one of the most useful views in color flow mapping. In the typical four-chamber view, the operator can follow blood flow as it enters the atrial cavities and flows through the atrioventricular valves in diastole to enter the ventricular chambers before it exits through the great arteries.

The right-side events appear slightly earlier as the tricuspid valve opens before the mitral valve. When blood fills the atrial cavities, it appears red as it flows toward the transducer. Pulmonary venous inflow to the left atrial cavity may be seen in this four-chamber view. Flow from the right and left upper veins appears reddish with some yellow, whereas flow from the lower left pulmonary vein appears blue as it moves away from the transducer. Although the transducer is angled more posterior and medial, inflow from the superior vena cava is red when it enters the medial aspect of the right atrium along the border of the interatrial septum.

Diastolic flow through the atrioventricular orifice occurs at a slightly higher velocity, giving rise to changes in colors from red to yellow. The flow returns to red as the inflow chamber of the ventricles fills. When the flow reaches the apex, it begins to swirl toward the ventricular outflow tract and the color changes to blue. Again the velocity increases as the flow moves toward the leaflets of the aorta in systole, changing the color

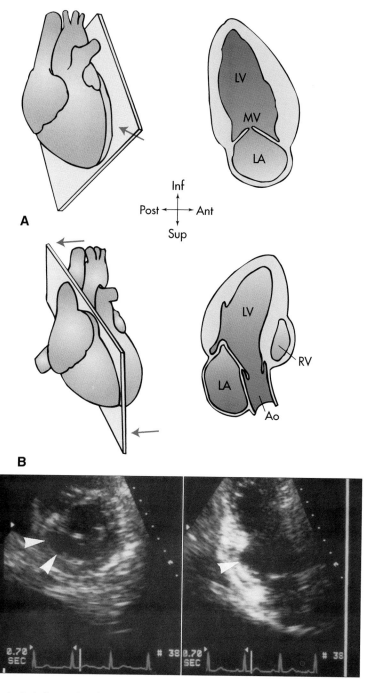

Figure 28-25 **A,** Apical two-chamber view. The transducer is rotated 90 degrees from the apical four-chamber view to show only the left ventricle *(LV)*, mitral valve *(MV)*, and left atrium *(LA)*. **B,** Apical three-chamber view. Medial angulation from the two-chamber view will show the left ventricular outflow tract and aorta *(Ao)*. **C,** Parasternal short-axis and apical two-chamber views are used to show abnormal motion in the posterobasal segment of the left ventricular wall *(arrowheads)*.

into more intense blue shades. Flow in the ascending aorta should be a uniform blue.

Regurgitant flow into the left atrium from the incompetent mitral or tricuspid valve will appear as a blue-green mixed pattern (Figure 28-26).

Apical Window for Doppler. The apical four-chamber position is one of the most widely used for recording multiple

Doppler patterns. The patient lies in the left lateral decubitus position with the transducer placed at the apical impulse and directed toward the patient's right shoulder. This position allows sampling of flow through the mitral, tricuspid, and aortic valves at nearly parallel angles to the beam.

Inflow through the mitral valve leaflets may be recorded by placing the Doppler signal at the level of the tips of the leaflets. The pulsed sample volume may be moved from the tips of the

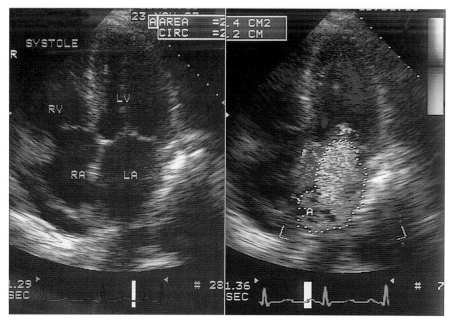

Figure 28-26   Apical four-chamber view is ideal to evaluate the inflow filling patterns of the ventricles and competency of the atrioventricular valves. This patient has severe mitral regurgitation; the left atrium is filled with a mixed blue pattern indicating severe mitral regurgitation. The red indicates inflow from the pulmonary veins into the left atrium and ventricle. *A,* Area; *LA,* left atrium; *LV,* left ventricle; *RA,* right atrium; *RV,* right ventricle.

leaflets to the level of the mitral annulus to obtain a clean recording. The normal mitral flow velocity tracing is similar to that found on an M-mode recording.

The initial peak occurs during the rapid-filling phase of diastole. The smaller second peak occurs late in diastole (with atrial contraction) (Figure 28-27). In patients with decreased left ventricular compliance, the first peak may be lower and the second peak higher. Normal flow velocity across the mitral valve ranges from 60 to 130 cm/sec in adults and similar velocities in children. Mitral regurgitation can be recognized as the sample volume is moved into the left atrial cavity. Careful angulation of the Doppler beam is necessary to sweep across the level of the annulus. An abnormal, high-pitched systolic flow pattern below the baseline represents regurgitation.

The tricuspid valve flow may be recorded in the apical position while the transducer is angled slightly to the right. With the transducer position at the level of the leaflets, a pattern similar to mitral valve flow is recorded with two peaks during diastole. The first occurs during ventricular filling and the second with the onset of atrial contraction. The velocity pattern is much lower in the tricuspid valve, with significant respiratory changes that increase during inspiration and decrease during expiration. The normal velocity range is 30 to 70 cm/sec for adults and is similar for children (Figure 28-28 [see Table 28-1]).

In the apical position, the transducer may be angled slightly anterior or rotated into a long-axis view to record blood flow from the left ventricular outflow tract as it enters the aortic root and ascending aorta. With the pulsed-wave sample volume placed just proximal to the aortic root (in the left ventricular outflow tract), the flow is away from the transducer during systole. The spectral display shows a narrow band of frequencies below the baseline (Figure 28-29).

The normal velocity pattern in the left ventricular outflow tract in the adult is 70 to 110 cm/sec and is similar in children. As the sample volume is moved across the aortic valve, flow can be recorded within the ascending aorta. This velocity pattern is slightly higher and peaks earlier. Normal velocities range from 100 to 170 cm/sec in adults and 120 to 180 cm/sec in children.

SUBCOSTAL VIEWS

Subcostal Two-Dimensional View. The subcostal view also has multiple windows in the four-chamber and short-axis planes (Figure 28-30). Many of the views are only available in the pediatric patient (because of the flexible abdominal muscles). The subcostal four-chamber view is generally a useful view in many adults and may serve as an alternative view if the apical four-chamber view is unobtainable. The transducer should be placed in the subcostal space and, with moderate pressure applied, angled steeply toward the patient's left shoulder. The plane of the transducer is transverse for visualization of the four chambers of the heart (Figure 28-31).

It is usually easy to follow the inferior vena cava into the right atrium of the heart. With careful angulation, the interatrial septum may be visualized between the anterior right atrial chamber and the posterior left atrial chamber. It is usually more difficult to open the right ventricular cavity in this view; therefore, no size assessment should be made. This view is usually

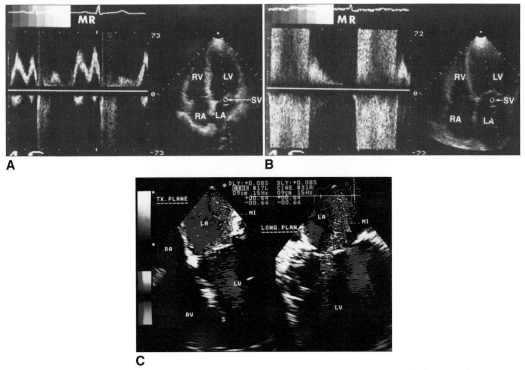

Figure 28-27 **A,** Pulsed wave Doppler of the mitral valve shows the initial valve peak during early diastole; the second peak occurs late in diastole (with atrial contraction). Reversal of flow below the baseline indicates mild mitral regurgitation *(MR)*. *LA,* Left atrium; *LV,* left ventricle; *RA,* right atrium; *RV,* right ventricle; *SV,* sample volume. **B,** The sample volume *(SV)* is placed just below the mitral valve (in the left atrium) to record the high-velocity flow pattern of moderate mitral regurgitation; the aliasing indicates the flow is greater than 2 m/sec with pulsed Doppler. **C,** Transesophageal echocardiography in the transverse and longitudinal plane shows the regurgitant jet pattern of mitral regurgitation in the left atrium. *S,* Septum.

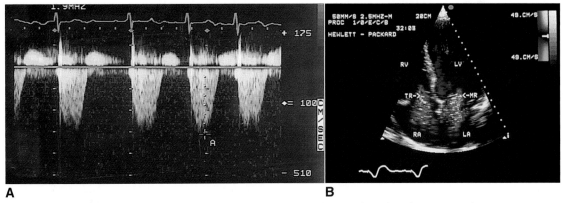

Figure 28-28 **A,** Continuous wave Doppler recorded from the apical window shows tricuspid regurgitation measuring 3.1 m/sec, indicating a right heart pressure of 38.4 mm Hg. **B,** Apical view shows turbulent jets in systole from the mitral and tricuspid valves. *LA,* Left atrium; *LV,* left ventricle; *MR,* mitral regurgitation; *RA,* right atrium; *RV,* right ventricle; *TR,* tricuspid regurgitation.

very good for assessing the presence of pericardial effusion, especially because it surrounds the anterior segment of the right side of the heart (Figure 28-32).

Subcostal View for Color Flow Mapping. The subcostal view is a long-axis view that shows the inferior vena cava inflow pattern as primarily red as it enters the right atrial cavity. The flow from the hepatic veins appears blue when blood enters the inferior vena cava at the level of the diaphragm throughout diastole and systole. During atrial systole, some retrograde flow is seen as it moves from the right atrium into the inferior vena cava and hepatic veins. With the transducer angled slightly to the left, blue pulsatile flow signals through the descending and abdominal aorta may be seen in systole.

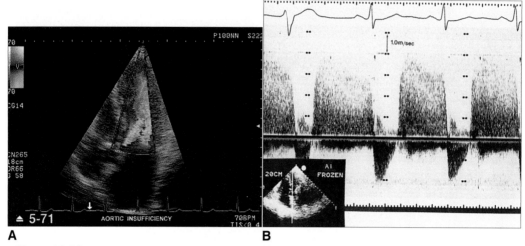

A **B**

Figure 28-29 **A,** Color flow mapping helps to show the direction of the jet from the aortic insufficiency in this apical view. **B,** Correct placement of the sample volume is within the strongest jet to record maximum velocity *(above the baseline)* from the insufficient valve. The aortic outflow is seen below the baseline.

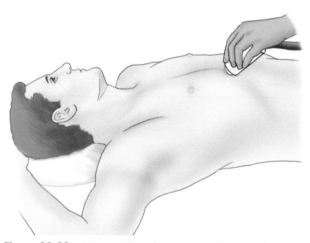

Figure 28-30 Subcostal four-chamber view. The transducer is placed below the costal margin and angled steeply toward the head to record the four-chamber view.

In the subcostal short-axis view, the right ventricular outflow tract and pulmonary artery may be demonstrated. The right ventricular outflow tract appears blue as it leaves the right ventricle to enter through the pulmonary cusps. The velocity increases slightly, causing some color change from blue to turquoise and green before returning to blue when it enters the main pulmonary artery. Some aliasing may be experienced as the flow bounces off the tricuspid leaflets and right ventricular walls. Red and yellow flow can be seen arising from the coronary artery along the posterior wall of the right ventricle. Superior vena cava inflow appears as red and orange flow as it enters the right atrium.

Subcostal Window for Doppler. The subcostal position is especially useful in the neonatal and pediatric population because the transducer is placed in the subcostal region and, with gentle pressure applied, the transducer is angled superi-

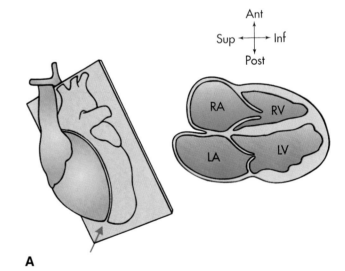

A

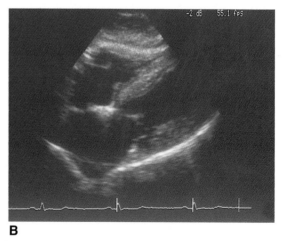

B

Figure 28-31 **A,** Subcostal view shows the four chambers of the heart, interatrial and interventricular septa. *LA,* Left atrium; *LV,* left ventricle; *RA,* right atrium; *RV,* right ventricle. **B,** Ultrasound image of the subcostal four-chamber view.

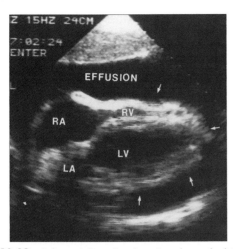

Figure 28-32 Subcostal four-chamber view shows the left lobe of the liver anterior to the large pericardial effusion that surrounds the heart wall *(arrows)*. The right ventricle *(RV)* is collapsed from the increased pressure of the effusion. *LA,* Left atrium; *LV,* left ventricle; *RA,* right atrium.

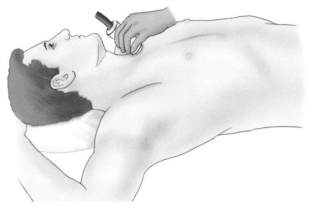

Figure 28-33 Suprasternal view. The transducer is placed in the suprasternal notch and angled steeply toward the arch of the aorta.

orly to record the four chambers of the heart. In adults with pulmonary obstructive disease, this view is very useful because the increased size of the lungs pushes the heart into the view of the transducer without too much pressure on the diaphragm.

In this position the interatrial and interventricular septa are perpendicular to the transducer, so the presence of a left-to-right defect shows positive high-velocity flow from the baseline on the spectral display and the flow is parallel to the beam. A right-to-left flow shows as a negative deflection on the spectral display. This view may also be useful for recording the flow pattern from the pulmonary veins (upper right and left and lower left) when they enter the left atrium.

The superior vena cava flow is shown as a high-pitched, low-velocity, positive deflection from the baseline on the spectral display. The inferior vena cava flow may be recorded as a negative display on the spectral display. A better view of the inferior vena cava flow is made in the subcostal long-axis view through the right lobe of the liver. The inferior vena cava may be well seen as it moves slightly anterior to pierce the diaphragm before it enters the right atrial cavity. This display would project as a low-velocity positive reflection from the baseline.

SUPRASTERNAL VIEWS

Suprasternal Two-Dimensional View. In the suprasternal view, the transducer is directed transversely in the patient's suprasternal notch and angled steeply toward the arch of the aorta (Figure 28-33). This view is only useful if the transducer is small enough to fit well into the suprasternal notch. The patient is best prepared if several towels or a pillow are placed under the shoulders. In this position the patient's neck should flex, avoiding interference with the neck of the transducer and cable. The patient's head should be turned to the right, again to avoid interference with the cable. With careful angulation, the cardiac structures visualized are the aortic arch, brachio-

cephalic vessels, right pulmonary artery, left atrium, and left main bronchus (Figure 28-34). This view is especially useful in determining supravalvular enlargement of the aorta, coarctation of the aorta, or dissection of the aorta.

Suprasternal View for Color Flow Mapping. In the suprasternal long-axis plane of the ascending aorta, arch, and descending aorta, flow signals begin as red in the ascending aorta and turn to blue when flow moves into the arch (some aliasing and reversal of color is seen along this point as the flow bounces off the walls in the arch) (Figure 28-35). When the flow enters the descending aorta, a bright blue color is seen. The atrial and ventricular septa are well seen on this view, and adequate visualization of a possible defect may be made in this imaging plane.

In the short-axis plane the superior vena cava flow is blue when it enters the right atrium. Flow within the aortic arch and right pulmonary artery is also seen. In some patients pulmonary venous inflow may be seen in the suprasternal view.

Suprasternal Window for Doppler. The suprasternal position is used to record velocities in the ascending and descending aorta, right pulmonary artery, superior vena cava inflow, and pulmonary venous return into the left atrium. Initially the patient's shoulders are elevated by a pillow, the neck extended, and the transducer placed in the suprasternal notch with an inferior angulation of the beam (Figure 28-36).

The transducer sample volume is placed in the ascending aorta when the walls of the aorta are as nearly perpendicular to the beam as possible. The flow is then parallel to the pulsed Doppler cursor, and a positive deflection with a narrow band of frequencies is shown above the baseline. Careful sweeping back and forth allows the operator to determine the highest velocity possible. The audio sound helps direct the probe to the maximal jet flow. If high velocities are suspected, the continuous wave probe is used.

The spectral tracing from this probe contains a wider range of frequencies with the same peak velocity measurements as the pulsed wave. As the transducer is angled to the left and posterior, velocity from the descending aorta is recorded. Generally with the pulsed Doppler, the sample volume is placed

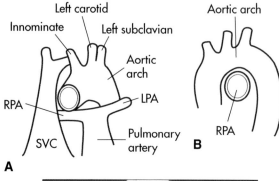

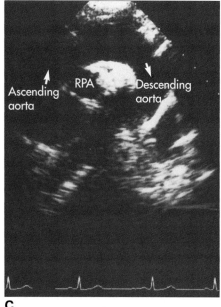

Figure 28-34 **A,** Transverse suprasternal notch view of the superior vena cava *(SVC)* as it lies to the right of the arch of the aorta. The right pulmonary artery *(RPA)* is posterior to the arch of the aorta. *LPA,* Left pulmonary artery. **B,** Longitudinal suprasternal notch view of the ascending aorta and right pulmonary artery. **C,** Suprasternal long view of the ascending, arch, and descending aorta. The right pulmonary artery *(RPA)* is posterior to the arch.

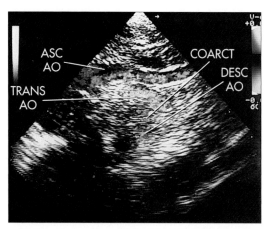

Figure 28-35 Color flow mapping from the suprasternal notch shows turbulence in a neonate with coarctation *(COARCT)* of the aorta *(yellow disturbed flow pattern)*. *ASC AO,* Ascending aorta; *DESC AO,* descending aorta; *TRANS AO,* transverse aorta.

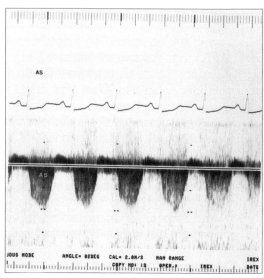

Figure 28-36 Continuous wave Doppler of the descending aortic artery measures 2 m/sec in a patient with aortic stenosis *(AS)*.

near the level of the left subclavian artery to record the maximum flow away from the transducer as it flows down the descending aorta to the abdominal aorta.

The suprasternal notch position is extremely useful for recording abnormal velocities, such as those found in aortic stenosis, coarctation of the aorta, and patent ductus arteriosus. In aortic stenosis, the harsh systolic velocities increase in the ascending and descending aorta. In coarctation of the aorta, the velocity increases slightly proximal to the area of narrowing, and velocity increases dramatically throughout systole as the beam traverses the area of coarctation. In patients with a patent ductus arteriosus, a positive, high-pitched, high-velocity flow will be seen on the spectral display at the level of the subclavian artery.

The flow pattern of the superior vena cava may be recorded from the suprasternal position while the transducer is directed inferiorly and to the right (medial) of the ascending aorta. Flow away from the transducer is recorded with two low-velocity peaks in systole and diastole, which may increase in height during inspiration. This view is useful for recording flow patterns that may be obstructed in the area of the superior vena cava.

The demonstration of the pulmonary veins from the suprasternal notch is more difficult to obtain. With the transducer aligned with the ascending aorta, the beam is angled more posterior to record the dorsal aspect of the left atrial cavity. The right and left upper pulmonary veins appear as a negative flow away from the baseline, whereas the right and left lower veins appear as a positive flow from the baseline. The velocity is low, with changes in respiration and cardiac motion.

M-MODE IMAGING OF THE CARDIAC STRUCTURES

MITRAL VALVE
Echographically, the mitral valve is one of the easiest cardiac structures to recognize. With M-mode, the mitral valve has the greatest amplitude and excursion and can be unquestionably

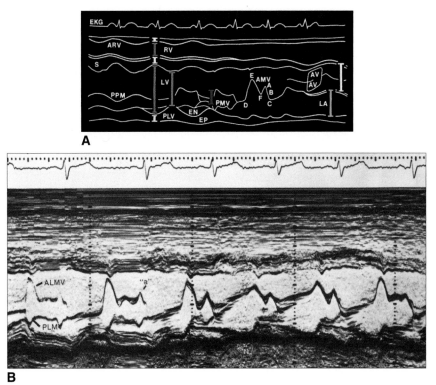

Figure 28-37 **A,** Illustration of the M-mode sweep. *AMV,* Anterior leaflet mitral valve; *ARV,* anterior wall right ventricular wall; *AV,* Aortic cusp; *EN,* endocardium; *EP,* epicardium; *LA,* left atrium; *LV,* left ventricle; *PLV,* posterior wall left ventricle; *PMV,* posterior leaflet mitral valve; *PPM,* posterior papillary muscle; *RV,* right ventricle; *S,* septum. **B,** Both leaflets of the mitral valve are clearly seen in this patient. The systolic segment moves slightly anteriorly until diastole begins, which causes the anterior leaflet *(ALMV)* to sweep anteriorly while the posterior leaflet *(PLMV)* dips posteriorly. Atrial contraction gives rise to the smaller *"a"* kick until the valve closes at end diastole.

recognized by its "double," or biphasic, kick. This kick is caused by the initial opening of the valve in ventricular diastole and the atrial contraction at end diastole (Figure 28-37).

When diastole begins, the anterior mitral leaflet executes a rapid anterior motion, coming to a peak at point *e.* While the ventricle fills rapidly with blood from the left atrium, the valve drifts closed at point *f.* The rate at which this movement takes place represents the rate of left atrial emptying and serves as an important indicator of altered mitral function. As the left atrium contracts, the mitral valve opens in a shorter anterior excursion and terminates at point *a,* which occurs just after the P wave on the electrocardiogram. This motion is followed by a rapid posterior movement from point *b* to point *c,* which coincides with the QRS systolic component on the electrocardiogram produced by the left ventricular contractility closing the valve.

AORTIC VALVE AND LEFT ATRIUM

The echoes recorded from the aortic root on M-mode should be parallel, moving anteriorly in systole and posteriorly in diastole. When the transducer is angled slightly medial, two of the three semilunar cusps can be visualized. The right coronary cusp is shown anterior and the noncoronary cusp posterior (Figure 28-38). When seen, the left coronary cusp is shown in the midline between the other two cusps. The onset of systole

causes the cusps to open to the full extent of the aortic root. The extreme force of blood through this opening causes a fine flutter to occur during systole. As the pressure relents in the ventricle, the cusps begin to drift to a closed position until they are fully closed in diastole.

The chamber posterior to the aortic root is the left atrium, which can be recognized by its immobile posterior wall. As one sweeps from the mitral apparatus medially and superiorly, the left ventricular wall blends into the atrioventricular groove and finally into the left atrial wall (Figure 28-39). Thus the sweep demonstrates good contractility in the left ventricle, with anterior wall motion in systole to the atrioventricular area, where the posterior wall starts to move posteriorly in systole, and then to the left atrium, where there is no movement.

Other structures posterior to the left atrial cavity that may lead to confusion in the identification of the left atrial wall are the left atrial appendage and descending aorta. The left atrial appendage may appear very prominent posterior to the left atrial wall if there is severe enlargement of the left atrial cavity (especially seen in patients with severe mitral valve disease). Real-time evaluation with the transducer in the apical four-chamber position clarifies the atrial appendage as a separate structure. The descending aorta may also be recognized as a parallel, pulsating, tubular structure posterior to the left atrial cavity (Figure 28-40). The aorta is not continuous with the left

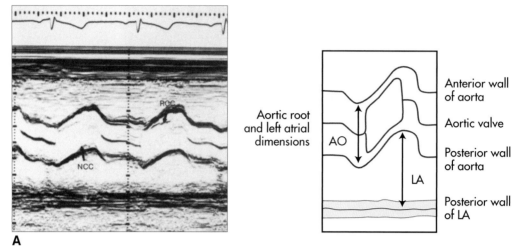

A

Figure 28-38   A, The right coronary cusp *(RCC)* is the most anterior cusp seen in the aortic sweep, and the noncoronary cusp *(NCC)* is the most posterior. The left coronary cusp is sometimes seen in the middle of the other two cusps. **B,** Measurements of the aortic root diameter and size of the left atrium may be made.

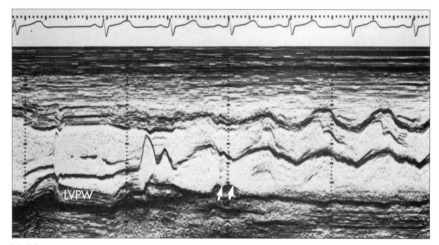

Figure 28-39 M-mode sweep from the left ventricle through the mitral valve to the aorta and left atrium demonstrates the changing movement of the posterior wall of the left ventricle *(LVPW)* as it passes the mitral valve at the atrioventricular junction *(arrows)*. The left atrial wall should be an immobile line contiguous with the posterior heart wall.

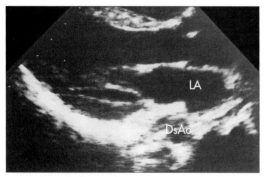

Figure 28-40 The descending aorta *(DsAo)* flows posterior to the left atrial *(LA)* cavity and is shown as a pulsatile tubular structure on the parasternal long-axis view.

ventricular wall, but the left atrial wall is. Thus, the cardiac sonographer should be able to distinguish this echo reflection as normal anatomy.

INTERVENTRICULAR SEPTUM

The septum thickens in systole at the midportion of the ventricular cavity (Figure 28-41). The measurement and evaluation of septal thickness and motion should be made at this point. Normal septal thickness should match that of the posterior left ventricular wall and not exceed 1.2 cm.

LEFT VENTRICLE

Correct identification of the left ventricle may be made when both sides of the septum are seen to contract with the posterior heart wall (Figure 28-41). If the septum is not well defined

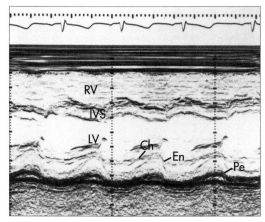

Figure 28-41 M-mode recording in the left ventricular cavity. *Ch,* Chordae; *En,* endocardium; *IVS,* interventricular septum; *LV,* left ventricle; *Pe,* pericardium; *RV,* right ventricle.

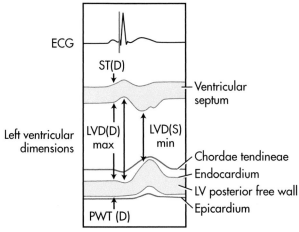

Figure 28-42 Measurements of the interventricular septum, left ventricle in diastole and systole, and the posterior wall are made. M-mode recording in the left ventricular cavity demonstrates the layers of the posterior heart wall: endocardium *(En),* myocardium *(Myo),* epicardium *(Ep),* pericardium *(Pe),* and chordae *(Ch).* The distinction between the endocardium and chordal structures may be made by assessing the velocity of the two structures. The normal endocardial velocity is always much greater than the chordal velocity.

or does not appear to move well, a more medial placement of the transducer along the sternal border with a lateral angulation may permit better visualization of this structure.

The three layers of the posterior heart wall—endocardium (inner layer), myocardium (middle layer), and epicardium (outer layer)—should be identified separately from the pericardium (Figure 28-42). Sometimes it is difficult to separate the epicardium from the pericardium until the gain is reduced. The myocardium usually has a fine scattering of echoes throughout its muscular layer. The endocardium may be a more difficult structure to record because it reflects a very weak echo pattern. The chordae are much denser structures than the endocardium. They generally are shown in the systolic segment along the anterior surface of the endocardium. As the ventricle contracts, the endocardial velocity is greater than the chordae tendineae velocity.

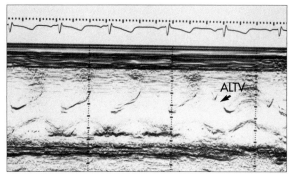

Figure 28-43 M-mode recording of the anterior leaflet of the tricuspid valve *(ALTV).*

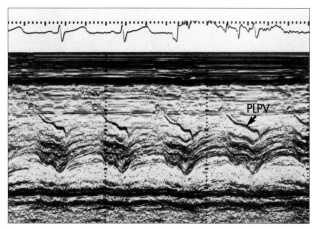

Figure 28-44 M-mode recording of the posterior cusp of the pulmonary valve. The cusp opens in systole and closes in diastole. *PLPV,* Posterior leaflet of the pulmonary valve.

TRICUSPID VALVE

When the transducer has recorded the mitral apparatus, the beam should be angled slightly medially under the sternum to record the tricuspid valve (Figure 28-43). It is fairly easy to identify the whipping motion of the anterior valve in systole and early diastole. However, the complete diastolic period reveals the pathologic changes of stenosis and regurgitation; careful angulation may allow this phase to be recorded.

PULMONARY VALVE

The anterior aortic root forms the posterior boundary of the pulmonary valve area. The appearance of the pulmonic cusp is similar to the aortic cusp and requires very slight angulations of the beam to demonstrate fully (Figure 28-44). With two-dimensional capabilities, the optimal view is generally a high-parasternal short-axis view with a slight angulation of the beam toward the left shoulder.

At the beginning of diastole, the pulmonary valve is displaced downward and is represented anteriorly on the ultrasound recording. The low transducer position with upward beam angulation, together with the vertical inclination of the pulmonary ring, results in the examination of the valve from below. All elevations of the pulmonary valve in the stream of flow are represented as posterior movements on the echo. Likewise, downward movements are represented by anterior cusp positions on the trace.

The pulmonary valve begins to move posteriorly (points *e* to *f*) in a gradual manner as the right ventricle fills in diastole (Figure 28-44). Atrial systole elevates the valve and produces a 3- to 7-mm posterior movement *a (dip)*. The valve completes the opening (points *b* and *c*), and, at the *c* to *d* point, the valve moves upward with ventricular systole.

SELECTED BIBLIOGRAPHY

Davidson WR, Pasquale MJ, Fanelli C: A Doppler echocardiographic examination of the normal aortic valve and left ventricular outflow tract, *Am J Cardiol* 67:547, 1991.

Ding ZP and others: Effect of sample volume location on Doppler-derived transmitral inflow velocity values, *J Am Soc Echocardiogr* 4:451, 1991.

Feigenbaum H. *Echocardiography*, New York, Lippincott Williams & Wilkins; Book & Dvdrm edition, 2004.

Garner CJ and others: Guidelines for cardiac sonographer education, *J Am Soc Echocardiogr* 5:635, 1992.

Hatle L, Anglesen B: *Doppler ultrasound in cardiology*, ed 2, Philadelphia, 1985, Lea & Febiger.

Kremkau FW: *Diagnostic ultrasound: principles and instruments*, ed 6, Philadelphia, 2002, WB Saunders Co.

Labovitz A, Williams G: *Doppler echocardiography*, ed, 2, Philadelphia, 1993, Lea & Febiger.

Oh JK, Seward JB, Tajik AJ: *The echo manual*, ed 2, Philadelphia, 1999, Lippincott Williams & Wilkins.

Otto C: *Valvular heart disease*, ed 2, Philadelphia, 2003, WB Saunders Co.

Otto C: *Textbook of clinical echocardiography*, ed 3, Philadelphia, 2004, WB Saunders Co.

Reynolds T: *The echocardiographer's pocket reference*, Phoenix, 1993, Arizona Heart Institute Foundation.

Reynolds T, Appleton CP: Doppler flow velocity patterns of the superior vena cava, inferior vena cava, hepatic vein, coronary sinus, and atrial septal defect: a guide for the echocardiographer, *J Am Soc Echocardiogr* 4:503, 1991.

Rodevand O and others: Diastolic flow pattern in the normal left ventricle, *J Am Soc Echocardiogr* 12:500, 1999.

St. Vrain JA and others: Multiskilling and multicredentialing of the health professional: role of the cardiac sonographer, *J Am Soc Echocardiogr* 11:1090, 1998.

Tam JW and others: What is the real clinical utility of echocardiography? *J Am Soc Echocardiogr* 12:689, 1999.

Veret C: Cardiovascular applications of the Doppler technique, *J Am Soc Echocardiogr* 12:278, 1999.

Weyman AE. *Principles and practice of echocardiography*, ed 2, New York, 1994, Lippincott Williams & Wilkins.

CHAPTER 29

Introduction to Fetal Echocardiography

Sandra L. Hagen-Ansert

OBJECTIVES

- Learn about the embryology of the fetal heart
- Understand the circulation of the fetal heart
- Discuss how fetal circulation differs from neonatal circulation
- Describe the risk factors that may lead to congenital heart disease
- Identify the type of transducer to use for the fetal echo
- Understand how to evaluate the fetus with two-dimensional, M-mode, pulsed Doppler, and color flow Doppler imaging
- Discuss the sonographic landmarks necessary to obtain before the fetal echo
- Describe the normal anatomy seen in the four-chamber, long-, and short-axis views of the heart
- Discuss the "crisscross" view of the heart
- Describe the relationship of the patent ductus arteriosus to the pulmonary artery and descending aorta

EMBRYOLOGY OF THE CARDIOVASCULAR SYSTEM

DEVELOPMENT OF BLOOD VESSELS
AORTIC ARCHES
DEVELOPMENT OF THE HEART

FETAL CIRCULATION

HEART RATE

RISK FACTORS INDICATING FETAL ECHOCARDIOGRAPHY

FETAL RISK FACTORS
MATERNAL RISK FACTORS
FAMILIAL RISK FACTORS

BEYOND THE FOUR-CHAMBER VIEW

TRANSDUCER REQUIREMENTS
INSTRUMENTATION
MOTION MODE IMAGING
PULSED DOPPLER IMAGING
COLOR FLOW DOPPLER IMAGING
THREE-DIMENSIONAL IMAGING

FETAL ULTRASOUND LANDMARKS

ECHOCARDIOGRAPHIC EVALUATION OF THE FETUS

FOUR-CHAMBER VIEW
LEFT AND RIGHT VENTRICULAR OUTFLOW TRACTS
DUCTAL AND AORTIC ARCH VIEWS: OBLIQUE LONG AXIS

KEY TERMS

atrioventricular node – area of cardiac muscle that receives and conducts the cardiac impulse

bicuspid aortic valve – two leaflets instead of the normal three leaflets with asymmetric cusps

bulbus cordis – primitive chamber that forms the right ventricle

ductus arteriosus – communication between the pulmonary artery and descending aorta that closes after birth

foramen ovale – also termed *fossa ovale;* opening between the free edge of the septum secundum and the dorsal wall of the atrium

fossa ovale – see *foramen ovale*

inferior vena cava – venous return into the right atrium of the heart along the posterior lateral wall

left atrium – filling chamber of the heart

left ventricle – pumping chamber of the heart

main pulmonary artery – main artery that carries blood from the right ventricle to the lungs

mitral valve – atrioventricular valve between the left atrium and left ventricle

patent ductus arteriosus – open communication between the pulmonary artery and descending aorta that does not constrict after birth

pulmonary veins – four pulmonary veins bring blood from the lungs back into the posterior wall of the left atrium; there are two upper (right and left) and two lower (right and left) pulmonary veins

right atrium – filling chamber of the heart

right ventricle – pumping chamber of the heart

septum primum – first part of the atrial septum to grow from the dorsal wall of the primitive atrium; fuses with the endocardial cushions

septum secundum – grows into the atrium to the right of the septum primum

sinoatrial node – forms in the wall of the sinus venosus near its opening into the right atrium

superior vena cava – venous return from the head and upper extremities into the upper posterior medial wall of the right atrium

tricuspid valve – atrioventricular valve found between the right atrium and right ventricle

---

The continued development and improvement of high-resolution, real-time sonography has enabled the sonographer to visualize cardiac activity with endovaginal transducers early in the first trimester. (Detailed visualization of all the anatomic structures of the fetal heart is better imaged in the second and third trimesters.) This ability to visualize cardiac anatomy has aided in the prenatal diagnosis of congenital heart disease. The incidence of congenital heart disease is about 8%, or 30,000 infants/yr in the United States. Ultrasound allows the sonographer and clinician to image the small cardiac structures and obtain hemodynamic information from the fetal heart.

Conditions such as small defects, abnormal size or location of cardiac structures, arrhythmias, or abnormal cardiac function may all be observed with fetal echocardiography. The information obtained about congenital heart defects is usually managed through a team effort, including the pediatric cardiologist, geneticist, cardiovascular surgeon, and imaging specialists, to allow the patient to make educated decisions regarding the opportunities and outcomes for her fetus with a congenital heart defect.

Improvement of high-resolution transducers has permitted good visualization of even the smallest structures within the fetal cardiac chambers. These transducers and dedicated cardiac instrumentation, complete with motion mode (M-mode), two-dimensional, color and Doppler capabilities, enable the sonographer to perform a complete fetal echocardiogram on obstetrical patients in their sixteenth week of pregnancy until the time of delivery. Although fetal heart motion may be seen within the gestational sac as early as 4 to 5 weeks of gestation, structural information is better seen at 14 to 16 weeks of gestation, with more detailed information shown after 18 weeks of gestation.

Fetal echocardiography has been a tremendous clinical aid for the high-risk obstetric patient. The ability to map normal cardiac structures and ventricular function in a patient who has had a previous child with congenital heart disease helps relieve the pregnant patient of worry. Moreover, if a congenital heart condition is found, arrangements may be made to deliver the patient in a facility with the appropriate staff to manage such a neonate.

The addition of Doppler and color flow imaging has aided the diagnosis of congenital heart disease and has helped in the understanding of flow dynamics in the fetus. These two modalities, Doppler and color flow imaging, are used with discretion in the fetus with congenital heart disease. Three-dimensional echocardiography has been introduced in fetal echocardiography to allow more intricate visualization of the cardiac structures. This technique still requires a good axis of the fetal heart to be obtained before adequate interpolation of the data is made.

EMBRYOLOGY OF THE CARDIOVASCULAR SYSTEM

A single major error in the genetic constitution is the basis of congenital malformations. Human teratogens produce or raise the incidence of congenital malformations; 7% are caused by environmental agents or teratogens. A spontaneous abortion usually occurs if the genetic malformation is severe.

The most sensitive period in the first trimester for cardiac development is between $3^{1}/_{2}$ to $6^{1}/_{2}$ weeks. The cardiovascular system is the first organ system to reach a functional state; by the end of the third week, circulation of blood has begun, and in the fifth week, the heart begins to beat.

DEVELOPMENT OF BLOOD VESSELS

The primitive heart is a tubular structure that forms like a large blood vessel from the mesenchymal cells in the cardiogenic area of the embryo. Paired endocardial heart tubes develop before the end of the third week and begin to fuse, thus forming the primitive heart.

The circulation of blood starts by the end of the third week as the tubular heart begins to beat. The embryo obtains sufficient nourishment during the second week of development by diffusion of nutrients from maternal blood flow. The vascular system begins during the third week in the wall of the yolk sac, the connecting stalk, and the chorion. The blood vessels begin to develop 2 days later. Blood islands are formed; cavities develop in the islands to form primitive blood cells and vessels. These primitive vessels form a vascular network in the wall of the yolk sac. Blood vessels form in the mesenchyme associated with the connecting stalk and chorion. Blood vessels also form in the embryo toward the end of the third week and join to form a continuous system of vessels on each side.

Blood vessels from the embryo join those on the yolk sac, connecting stalk, and chorion to form a primitive cardiovascular system (Figure 29-1). The cardinal veins return blood from the embryo, and the vitelline veins return blood from the yolk sac. The umbilical veins return oxygenated blood from the placenta (only one umbilical vein persists). Two dorsal aortas fuse in the caudal half of the embryo to form a single dorsal aorta. Blood formation in the embryo begins at the fifth week.

AORTIC ARCHES

Each branchial arch is supplied by an aortic arch (Figure 29-2). The arteries to the fifth pair are rudimentary or absent. The

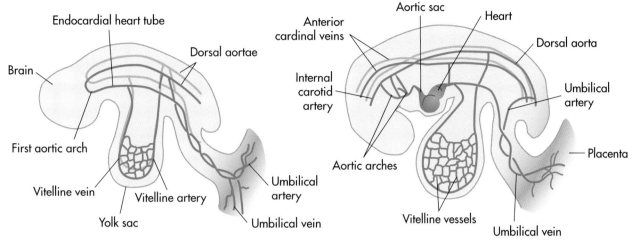

Figure 29-1 Cardiovascular system in a 26-day-old embryo. The two endocardial heart tubes have fused to form a tubular heart ring. The umbilical vein carries oxygenated blood and nutrients to the embryo from the placenta.

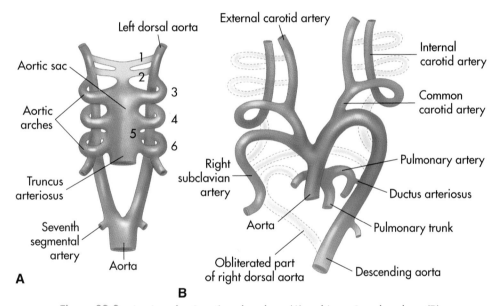

Figure 29-2 Aortic arches in a 6-week embryo (**A**) and in an 8-week embryo (**B**).

third pair of aortic arches becomes the common carotid artery and the proximal parts of the internal carotid arteries. The left fourth arch forms part of the arch of the aorta. The right fourth arch forms the proximal part of the right subclavian artery. The right sixth aortic arch becomes the right pulmonary artery. The left sixth aortic arch forms the left pulmonary artery and the ductus arteriosus (Box 29-1).

DEVELOPMENT OF THE HEART

The heart tube grows rapidly, bending on itself because it is fixed at its cranial and caudal ends. The bending forms a U-shaped bulboventricular loop. The sinus venosus is initially a separate chamber that opens into the **right atrium** (Figure 29-3).

BOX 29-1

CARDIAC DEVELOPMENT

- *Sinus venosus:* The caudal region of the primitive heart, which receives all blood returning to the heart from common cardinal veins, vitelline veins, and umbilical veins
- *Primitive atrium:* Develops into the right and left atria
- *Primitive ventricle:* Develops into the left ventricle
- *Bulbus cordis:* Develops into the right ventricle
- *Truncus arteriosus:* Dilates to form the aortic sac from which the aortic arches arise

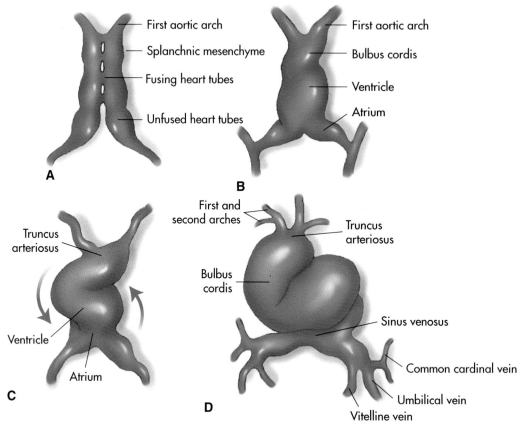

Figure 29-3 The heart during the fourth week of development. The paired endocardial heart tubes (**A**) gradually fuse to form a single tubular heart (**B**). The fusion begins at the cranial end of the tubes and extends caudally until a single tubular heart is formed. As the heart elongates, it bends on itself (**C and D**).

Right Atrium. The left horn of the sinus becomes the coronary sinus. The right horn is incorporated into the wall of the right atrium (forms a smooth portion of the adult right atrial wall). The right half of the primitive atrium persists as the right auricle.

Left Atrium. The **left atrium** is formed by incorporation of the primitive pulmonary vein. As the atrium grows, parts of this vein and its branches are absorbed. Four pulmonary veins eventually enter the left atrium from the lungs. The smooth wall of the left atrium is from the absorbed pulmonary vein. The left auricle is from the primitive heart.

Four-Chambered Heart. During the fourth and fifth weeks of fetal development, the division of the four chambers occurs.

Division of the Atrioventricular Canal. Endocardial cushions develop in the atrioventricular region of the heart. The cushions grow toward each other and fuse to divide the atrioventricular canal into right and left canals.

Division of the Primitive Atrium. The **septum primum** grows from the dorsal wall of the primitive atrium and fuses with the endocardial cushions (Figure 29-4, *A* and *B*). Before the fusion of the septum primum, a communication exists between the right and left halves of the primum atrium through the ostium primum or foramen primum. As the septum primum fuses with the endocardial cushions (obliterating the foramen primum), the superior part of the septum primum breaks down, creating an opening called the *foramen secundum* (see Figure 29-4, *A* and *B*). As this foramen develops, another membranous fold, the **septum secundum,** grows into the atrium to the right of the septum primum. The septum secundum overlaps the foramen secundum and the opening of the septum primum. There is also an opening between the free edge of the septum secundum and the dorsal wall of the atrium called the **foramen ovale** (Figure 29-4, *C*).

Formation of the Ventricles. The **left ventricle** is formed from the primitive vein. The right ventricle is formed from the **bulbus cordis**. The interventricular septum begins as a ridge in the floor of the primitive ventricle and slowly grows toward the endocardial cushions (see Figure 29-4, *B* and *C*). Until the seventh week, the right and left ventricles communicate through a large interventricular foramen. Closure of the interventricular foramen results in formation of the membranous part of the interventricular septum.

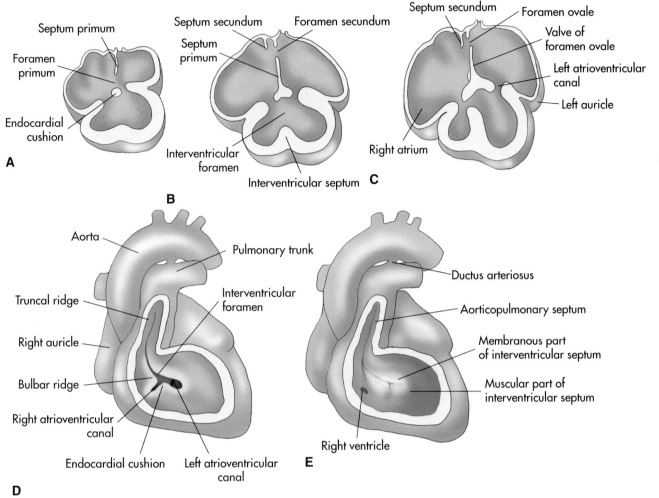

Figure 29-4 The partitioning of the primitive atrioventricular canal, atrium, and ventricle in the developing heart. **A, B,** and **C,** Frontal sections of the embryonic heart during the fourth week. **D,** (5 weeks) and **E,** (7 weeks) show schematic drawings of the heart illustrating closure of the interventricular foramen and formation of the interventricular septum. Note that the interventricular foramen is closed by tissues from three sources.

Partitioning of Bulbus Cordis and Truncus Arteriosus. The division of this part of the heart results from the development and fusions of the truncal ridges and bulbar ridges (Figure 29-4, *D* and *E*). Fused mesenchymal ridges form the aorticopulmonary septum, which divides the **truncus arteriosus** and bulbus cordis into the ascending aorta and pulmonary trunk.

Development of the Conduction System. The **sinoatrial node** forms in the wall of the sinus venosus near its opening into the right atrium; later it is incorporated into the right atrium with the right horn of the sinus venosus. The **atrioventricular node** and bundle are derived from cells in the walls of the sinus venosus and atrioventricular canal.

FETAL CIRCULATION

Blood flow in the fetus varies in two respects from the neonatal stage (Figure 29-5). Communication is open between the right and left sides of the heart through the **fossa ovale,** and

between the aorta and the pulmonary artery via the **ductus arteriosus.** It is useful to know these important communications to appreciate the fetal physiology of the cardiac structures.

Before birth the oxygenated blood is given to the fetus by way of the umbilical vein from the placenta to the heart. Approximately half of the blood passes through the hepatic sinusoids, whereas the remainder bypasses the liver to go through the *ductus venosus* into the inferior vena cava. Blood flows from the **inferior vena cava** and **superior vena cava** and enters the right atrium. Blood in the right atrium is less oxygenated than blood in the umbilical vein.

A small amount of oxygenated blood from the inferior vena cava is diverted by the *crista dividens* and remains in the right atrium to mix with deoxygenated blood from the superior vena cava and *coronary sinus*. Some of the blood from the inferior vena cava is directed by the lower border of the *septum secundum* (the crista dividens) through the *foramen ovale* into the left atrium.

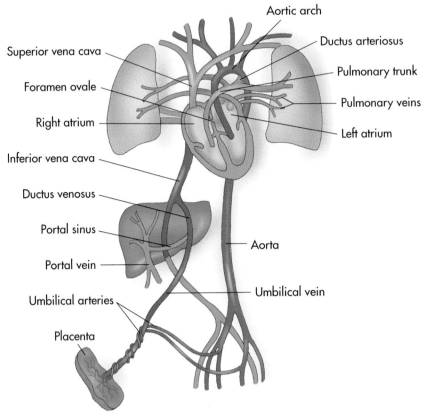

Figure 29-5   Fetal circulation.

The blood in the right atrium flows through the three-leaflet **tricuspid valve** into the **right ventricle** and leaves the right ventricle through the **main pulmonary artery.** This artery bifurcates into right and left pulmonary artery branches that lead to their respective lungs. However, most of this blood passes through the connection of the *ductus arteriosus* into the *descending aorta;* only a very small amount goes to the lungs.

The blood mixes with a small amount of deoxygenated blood as it returns from the lungs via the four **pulmonary veins** into the left atrium. The pulmonary veins enter the posterior of the left atrium. The four veins are named according to their locations: right upper, left upper, right lower, and left lower. The blood then flows from the left atrium into the left ventricle through the bicuspid **mitral valve** and leaves the heart through the *ascending aorta.* The head, neck, and upper torso of the fetus are fed via the three branches off the ascending aorta. These branches are the innominate, left carotid, and left subclavian arteries. The rest of the mixed blood in the descending aorta passes into the umbilical arteries and is returned to the placenta for reoxygenation. The remainder of the blood circulates through the lower part of the body.

After birth, the circulation of the fetal blood through the placenta ceases, and the neonatal lungs begin to function. The fetal cardiac structures no longer necessary are the foramen ovale, the ductus arteriosus, the ductus venosus, and the umbilical vessels (Figure 29-6).

Omission of the placental circulation causes an immediate fall of blood pressure in the newborn's inferior vena cava and

right atrium. As the lungs expand with air, there is a fall in the pulmonary vascular resistance. This causes an increase in pulmonary blood flow and a progressive thinning of the walls of the pulmonary arteries. Thus the pressure in the left atrium becomes higher than that in the right atrium. This causes the foramen ovale to close. With time, complete closure of the foramen occurs from adhesion of the septum primum to the left margin of the septum secundum. The septum primum forms the floor of the fossa ovalis. The lower edge of the septum secundum forms the limbus fossae ovalis, which demarcates the former cranial boundary of the foramen ovale.

The ductus arteriosus usually constricts shortly after birth (usually within 24 to 48 hours) once the left-sided pressures exceed the right-sided pressures. Often there is a small shunt of blood from the aorta to the pulmonary artery until these pressures adjust to neonatal life. The ductus turns into the ligamentum arteriosum in the neonate. If this communication persists, it is called a **patent ductus arteriosus**. This ligament passes from the left pulmonary artery to the arch of the aorta.

The umbilical arteries also constrict after birth to prevent blood loss from the neonate. The umbilical vein may remain patent for some time after birth.

HEART RATE

The normal fetal heart rate is between 120 and 160 beats per minute. In the first trimester of pregnancy, the heart rate begins around 90 beats per minute and increases to 170 beats per minute before returning to a normal rate and sinus rhythm. If

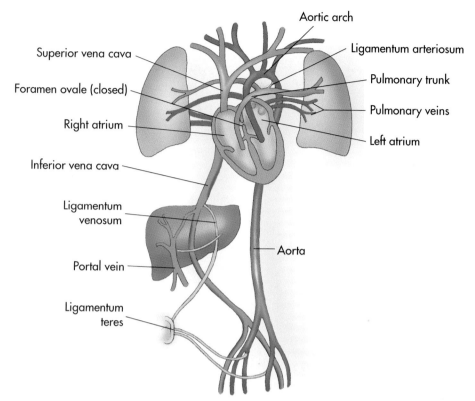

Figure 29-6 Neonatal circulation.

the heart rate is too slow (less than 60 beats per minute), it is called *bradycardia;* a heart rate over 200 beats per minute is termed *tachycardia.*

A very slow fetal heart rate, under 60 beats per minute, places the fetus at high risk of associated heart disease; fetal echocardiography should be performed to rule out the presence of a structural heart defect. The association of complete heart block with structural cardiac defects appears to have a poor prognosis, presumably because of their adverse interaction and the atrioventricular valve regurgitation that commonly complicates the condition. Connective tissue disorder (e.g., systemic lupus erythematosus) is associated with heart block and pericardial effusion.

RISK FACTORS INDICATING FETAL ECHOCARDIOGRAPHY

Specific risk factors indicate that the fetus is at a higher than normal risk for congenital heart disease and warrants a fetal echocardiogram. These may be divided into the following three categories: fetal risk factors, maternal risk factors, and familial risk factors (Box 29-2).[1]

FETAL RISK FACTORS

Fetal risk factors include the presence of intrauterine growth restriction, cardiac arrhythmias, abnormal amniocentesis indicating a trisomy, abnormal amniotic fluid collections, abnormal heart rate, and other anomalies as detected by the sonogram, such as hydrops fetalis.

BOX 29-2 | **INDICATIONS FOR FETAL ECHOCARDIOGRAPHY**

FETAL INDICATIONS
Polyhydramnios (1.5%)
Nonimmune hydrops (7.5%)
Arrhythmias (23%)
Suspected cardiac abnormality on routine ultrasound

FETAL ABNORMALITIES AND DYSMATURITY (11%)
Extracardiac abnormalities
Chromosome abnormalities
Intrauterine growth restriction

The presence of extracardiac abnormalities (e.g., renal anomalies, gastrointestinal anomalies, single umbilical artery, etc.) in the fetus is frequently associated with congenital heart disease. If the abnormality is found in more than one organ system, the incidence of congenital heart disease increases further. Nonimmune hydrops may be cardiac related (heart failure), or may be related to other problems in the fetus.

Cardiac arrhythmias in the fetus may be a common finding if they are simply extrasystoles (premature atrial beats secondary to the immature conducting system). A very small percentage of arrhythmias is associated with significant heart disease. However, a fetus with congenital heart block is usually associated with structural abnormalities in about half of the cases, most commonly atrioventricular septal defect as found in trisomy 21.

MATERNAL RISK FACTORS

Maternal risk factors include the previous occurrence of congenital heart disease in siblings or parents; a maternal disease known to affect the fetus, such as diabetes mellitus or connective tissue disease (e.g., lupus); and maternal use of drugs, such as lithium or alcohol (Box 29-3).[1]

The incidence of congenital heart disease in fetuses whose mothers have uncontrolled diabetes is much higher than when the diabetes is controlled. The most common anomaly is the ventricular septal defect, transposition of the great arteries, and tetralogy of Fallot.

Excessive alcohol during pregnancy has known effects of fetal alcohol syndrome, which includes facial abnormalities, growth restriction, mental retardation, and cardiac abnormalities (ventricular septal defect).

Indomethacin, a nonsteroidal antiinflammatory drug, has been used in the treatment of preterm labor. This drug has an effect on early closure of the patent ductus arteriosus. Evaluation of the fetus may be monitored with ultrasound to measure velocities across the patent ductus to detect if early closure is evident.

FAMILIAL RISK FACTORS

Familial risk factors include genetic syndromes or the presence of congenital heart disease in a previous sibling (Box 29-4). The recurrence risk cited given a sibling with one of the most common cardiovascular abnormalities (ventricular septal defect, atrial septal defect, patent ductus arteriosus, tetralogy of Fallot) varies from 2.5% to 3%.[1] Similar data given one parent with a congenital heart defect suggest that for the common defects listed the recurrence risk ranges from 2.5%

BOX 29-3   **MATERNAL INDICATIONS**

MATERNAL DISEASE AFFECTING THE FETUS (7%)
Diabetes
Lupus erythematosus
Infections during pregnancy

MATERNAL INGESTION OF DRUGS OR TERATOGENS (4.5%)
Alcoholism
Drug exposure during pregnancy

BOX 29-4   **FAMILIAL INDICATIONS**

Familial history of congenital heart disease (44%)

(atrial septal defect) to 4% (ventricular septal defect, patent ductus arteriosus, tetralogy of Fallot).[1]

BEYOND THE FOUR-CHAMBER VIEW

TRANSDUCER REQUIREMENTS

The ideal transducer for fetal echocardiography is a multifrequency transducer that can be quickly and easily changed from a low to a high frequency. This is especially useful when the fetus is located in a position far from the transducer face or when a lower-frequency Doppler signal is necessary to obtain a high-velocity flow profile.

The following guidelines may be used in selecting the proper multihertz transducer for the fetal echocardiogram:

1. A 5.0-MHz transducer or higher with a medium focus is generally ideal for the typical pregnancy in a small to average-size patient in the second trimester.
2. A 3.5-MHz transducer with a medium-to-long focus may be used on patients of average to large build and on patients in the third trimester.
3. A 2.25-MHz transducer with medium-to-long focus is used for the obese patient in the second or third trimester.
4. The higher-frequency endovaginal probe is useful when the fetus is directed in a transverse lie. The probe is placed transabdominally in the mother's umbilicus with gentle pressure and angled toward the fetal heart.
5. The size of the transducer varies. The early second trimester fetus may be adequately imaged with a curved array transducer; however, some laboratories prefer the small-sector, high-frequency probe.

INSTRUMENTATION

Other features useful on the ultrasound equipment include the following: cine-loop feature that allows imaging of the heart in frame-by-frame analysis, videotape or disk recordings for later playback or comparison evaluation, high-power resolution zoom capability, simultaneous M-mode with range expansion (for cardiac arrhythmias), simultaneous Doppler capability with pulsed and continuous wave (to record high-velocity flow), and color Doppler.

MOTION MODE IMAGING

Motion mode (M-mode) is used to evaluate cardiac motion. Once the two-dimensional image is made, a single vertical line of information can be obtained from the face of the transducer through the fetal cardiac structures (Table 29-1). This image is electronically rotated 90 degrees so the depth of the image is along the vertical axis and the time display is shown along the horizontal axis (Figure 29-7). Acquisition of heart wall motion, septal and valve movement, and cavity size may be easily obtained from this technique. Heart rate is measured by counting the number of beats that occur within a specific time frame, usually more than 1 second. If 2.5 beats were shown in a 1-second time period, the heart rate would be 2.5 beats × 60 seconds = 150 beats per minute.

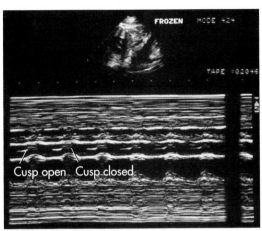

Figure 29-7   M-mode of the aorta and left atrial cavity. Time is depicted along the horizontal axis *(dots along the top of the image)*. The distance between two dots represents 1 second. Distance is located along the vertical axis. The aorta is shown as the two parallel lines moving as a "unit" through systole (pumping) and diastole (resting). The aortic cusps open and remain open during ventricular systole. The left atrial cavity is shown posterior to the aorta. The left atrial wall motion may be seen within the left atrial cavity.

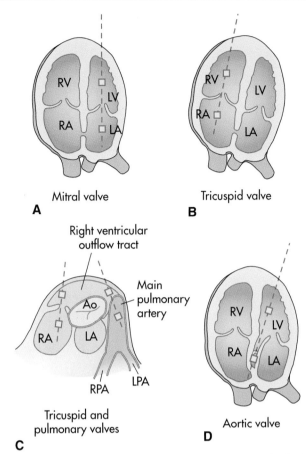

Figure 29-8   Pulsed Doppler sample volume placement for fetal echo. **A** and **B,** The four-chamber view is ideal to sample the velocity flow patterns of the mitral and tricuspid valves. The sample volume is initially placed at the annulus of the valve. To record regurgitation, the volume is moved into the atrial chamber; to record inflow of the valves, the sample volume is moved into the ventricular cavity. *LA,* Left atrium; *LV,* left ventricle; *RA,* right atrium; *RV,* right ventricle. **C,** The high short-axis view is best to obtain velocities from the tricuspid and pulmonary valves. The same procedure is used for the tricuspid valve as described in the four-chamber view. To record flow in the main pulmonary artery, the sample volume is placed at the level of the cusps and then moved back into the right ventricular outflow tract, then into the main pulmonary artery to look for abnormal flow patterns. *AO,* Aorta; *LPA,* left pulmonary artery; *RPA,* right pulmonary artery. **D,** The five-chamber view is good to record velocity flow in the left ventricular outflow tract and the ascending aorta. The sample volume should be placed below the aortic leaflets in the left ventricular outflow tract and then slowly moved through the cusps into the ascending aorta to see flow velocities.

| TABLE 29-1 | NORMAL FETAL M-MODE CARDIAC MEASUREMENTS |

Weeks of Gestation	Cardiac Structure			
	LV/RV	IVS	AO/PA	LA
20	6	1.5	4	5
22	8	1.7	4.8	6
24	9	2	5	6.5
28	10	2.3	6	8
32	12	3	7	10
36	14	3.5	8	11
40	16	3.8	9	12.5

AO, Aorta; *IVS,* interventricular septum; *LA,* left atrium; *LV,* left ventricle; *PA,* pulmonary artery; *RV,* right ventricle.

PULSED DOPPLER IMAGING

Pulsed Doppler demonstrates the direction and characteristics of blood flow within the fetal heart and great vessels and allows the qualitative and quantitative definition of flow disturbances, such as those that occur with valvular stenotic or regurgitant lesions. Doppler uses the principle of the Doppler shift or sound waves reflected from the red blood cells within the fetal heart; if the cells are moving toward the transducer, the pitch increases; if the cells are traveling away, the pitch is decreased. On the spectral display, the flow is displayed above (toward) or below (away) from the baseline. The sample volume may be gated or moved to the area of interest to record the optimum signal as the transducer is parallel to the flow of blood (Figure 29-8).

Higher levels of ultrasound energy are used with Doppler, and although no harmful effects have been reported on the fetal heart, it is recommended by the American Institute of Ultrasound in Medicine (AIUM) to keep the Doppler ultrasonic energy at or below 100 mW/cm^2 spatial peak-temporal average, and Doppler interrogation should be limited to as short a time as possible (Table 29-2).[3]

COLOR FLOW DOPPLER IMAGING

Color flow Doppler may help detect flow disturbances and flow direction (to see if vessels or chambers are patent) and

Table 29-2	Normal Doppler Measurements (Peak Systole)
Mitral valve	40-60-80 cm/sec
Tricuspid valve	45-65-87 cm/sec
Aortic valve	40-60-100 cm/sec
Pulmonic valve	25-55-80 cm/sec
Foramen ovale	20-30 cm/sec
Aortic arch, level of ductal insertion	120-150 cm/sec

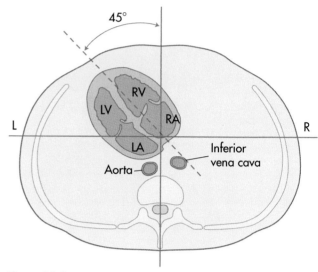

Figure 29-9 Measurement of the cardiac axis from a four-chamber view plane of the fetal chest. *LA,* left atrium; *LV,* left ventricle; *RA,* right atrium; *RV,* right ventricle. The apex of the heart should not exceed a 45-degree angle from the line drawn perpendicular to the fetal spine.

should be integrated into the fetal echocardiogram. Color Doppler flow mapping is a multigated Doppler technique in which sampling along all the scan lines and depths in the field occurs simultaneously. Color displays are usually oriented so that flow toward the transducer is projected in shades of red and orange, and flow away is projected in cool blue colors. Disturbed flow is seen as a mixture of red, orange, and yellow or blues and greens.

THREE-DIMENSIONAL IMAGING

Clinical investigation of three-dimensional echocardiography has been performed both with and without cardiac gating. The gated acquisition showed improved resolution of structures compared with the nongated acquisition. Clarity of images is still the primary problem in this technique: the fetal heart is beating so quickly and the volume is too small to acquire enough data points to display an image better than the current real-time two-dimensional images.

FETAL ULTRASOUND LANDMARKS

In most cases the obstetric patient has had a previous ultrasound and is referred for a dedicated or "target" fetal echocardiographic examination. Generally a dedicated fetal echocardiographic study may take from 30 to more than 60 minutes, depending on the type of pathologic condition present.

The cardiac sonographer must know certain characteristics that will help in the cardiac evaluation. (The reader is referred to Chapter 28 for illustration of these normal structures.)

The fetal survey should demonstrate the following structures before focusing on the fetal heart.

1. The position of the fetus (vertex, breech, transverse)
2. The position of the fetal thorax (spine up or down; determine right side and left side)
3. The position of the fetal stomach (right or left)
4. The location of the apex of the heart (left, right, or midline) (Figure 29-9)
5. The location of the fetal abdominal aorta and inferior vena cava (aorta left, close to spine, inferior vena cava right, and elevated from spine)
6. The position of the fetal placenta (anterior placenta may cause noise that interferes with visualization of the cardiac structures if the thorax is adjacent to the placenta)

7. The biparietal diameter and/or femur length for measurement correlation

Obstacles to obtaining an adequate image include decreased amniotic fluid (oligohydramnios), unusual fetal position (spine up, transverse, or low lie in the maternal pelvis), and maternal obesity. The diabetic mother is generally more difficult to scan; these patients image best in the middle of the second trimester, between 20 and 22 weeks of gestation.

When the fetus is in a difficult-to-image position, the sonographer may ask the mother to get up, use the rest room, walk the hall for a few minutes, or do "toe touches" or jumping jacks to encourage the fetus to change positions. This technique usually works.

ECHOCARDIOGRAPHIC EVALUATION OF THE FETUS

A normal cardiac study should include the following views: four-chamber, outflow tracts, and oblique long-axis view for the aortic arch and ductus arteriosus.

FOUR-CHAMBER VIEW

The four-chamber view is probably one of the easiest views to demonstrate cardiac anatomy (Box 29-5). Remember, the fetal heart lies in a horizontal position within the thorax and the apex of the heart (the left ventricle) is directed toward the left hip (Figure 29-10). The transducer is angled in a cephalic direction through the fetal liver, which serves as a good window to visualize cardiac structures.

The sonographer should note the relative size and function of the atria and inflow ventricular cavities (see Figure 29-10, *D* and *E*). The right heart is slightly larger in utero than the left heart. The right and left sides may be identified by the opening flap of the patent foramen ovale; in utero the foramen opens toward the left atrium; after birth the pressure in the left heart forces the foramen to close. Failure to close results in an atrial septal defect. The moderator band can also be used to identify the right ventricle. It stretches horizontally across the right ventricle near the apex. The right ventricle is also more trabeculated than the left ventricle at the apex.

The position of the mitral and tricuspid leaflets (atrioventricular leaflets) should be assessed. Normally the tricuspid valve is located just slightly inferior to the mitral valve.

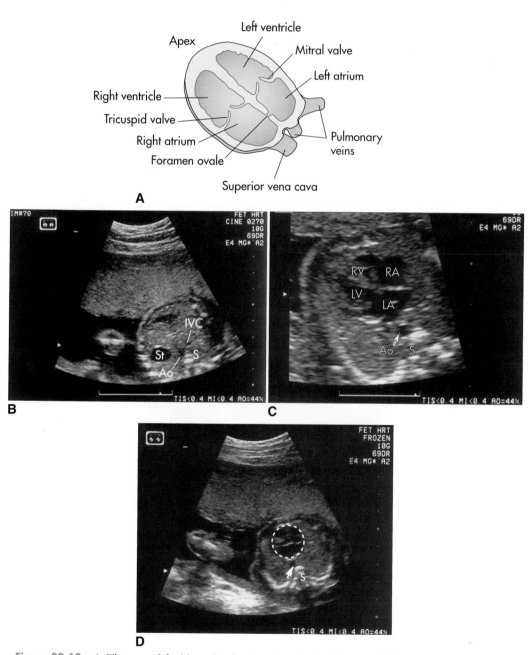

Figure 29-10   A, The normal fetal heart lies horizontal in the fetal thorax, with the apex pointing to the left hip. The four-chamber view shows the superior vena cava as it enters the right atrium. The two upper pulmonary veins enter the left atrium. The foramen ovale opens into the left atrium during fetal life. **B,** Transverse view of the 18-week fetus. The fetus is vertex with the spine *(S)* posterior, aorta *(Ao)* and anterior and inferior vena cavas *(IVC)* anterior and to the right; the stomach *(St)* lies to the left. **C,** As the transducer is angled cephalad, the four-chamber view of the heart is seen within the thorax. The spine *(S)* is posterior with the aorta *(arrow),* anterior to the spine. The left atrium lies directly anterior to the aorta. *LA,* Left atrium; *LV,* left ventricle; *RA,* right atrium; *RV,* right ventricle. **D,** Four-chamber view of the heart with a normal axis.

Continued

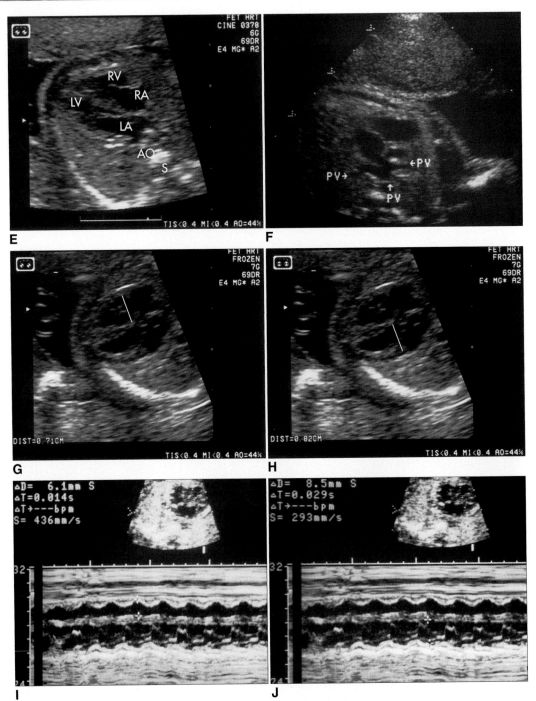

Figure 29-10, cont'd   **E,** *AO,* Aorta; *LA,* left atrium; *LV,* left ventricle; *RA,* right atrium; *RV,* right ventricle; *S,* spine. **F,** Three of the four pulmonary veins *(PV)* enter the left atrial cavity. Measurements of the left ventricle **(G)** and right ventricle **(H)** are made on two-dimensional views at the level of the mitral annulus. **I,** M-mode measurements may also be made at the level of the annulus for the RV and LV **(J).**

The left atrial cavity is generally about the same size as the right atrial cavity and is hypoechoic. The four pulmonic veins enter into the posterior wall of the left atrium. The right upper enters into the medial-posterosuperior wall; the left upper enters into the lateral-posterosuperior wall; the left lower enters lateral inferior wall; and the right lower enters the medial infe-

rior wall (see Figure 29-10, *F*). On the four-chamber view, all the pulmonary veins are imaged except for the right lower vein.

The inferior and superior vena cava may be seen to enter the right atrium. The inferior vena cava enters the posterior wall along the inferior lateral margin; the superior vena cava enters the medial posterosuperior wall.

The right and left ventricular width measurements are performed in the four-chamber view at the level of the atrioventricular annulus. The sonographer should clean up the image as much as possible for this measurement by turning the gain down. The right ventricle is measured from the lateral wall, across the level of the tricuspid annulus, to the midportion of the septum (see Figure 29-10, *G*). The left ventricle is measured from the midportion of the septum, across the level of the mitral annulus, to the endocardial surface of the lateral wall of the ventricle (see Figure 29-10, *H*). Normal values have been established to correspond to appropriate gestational ages. At 18 weeks of gestation, the ventricles should each measure approximately 6 mm.

If any abnormality exists in the atrioventricular valves or if the atria are enlarged, the four-chamber view is excellent to record Doppler tracings of blood flow (Figure 29-11). The transducer should be parallel to the four-chamber view, with the cursor placed at the level of the annulus and slowly moved into the ventricular cavity to record atrioventricular inflow patterns. To record regurgitation of the atrioventricular valves, the cursor is slowly moved into the atrial cavity to map the flow pattern and assess flow dynamics. Normally there is no backward flow through the orifice. The sonographer can assess the atrial size as an additional determinant of the presence of regurgitation.

The atrioventricular valves have a "double peak" of blood flow on the Doppler tracing. The first peak, *e*, is termed the *passive filling phase* (this increases with fetal breathing and with gestational age). This peak is smaller than the second peak because the fetal heart is less compliant than the neonatal heart. The second, taller peak, *a*, is termed the *active atrial phase*. In later pregnancy the *e* point equals or exceeds the *a* point on the Doppler tracing as the pressure on the left side exceeds the right-side pressure. The mean tricuspid valve velocity is 65 cm/sec; the mean mitral valve velocity is 60 cm/sec.[2]

Color flow Doppler (Figure 29-12, *A* and *B*) may be useful in demonstrating the amount and path of regurgitation. A multicolored jet would be present in the atrial cavity posterior to the atrioventricular valve. Remember the pressures in the fetal heart are different than after birth; therefore, the color and Doppler flow patterns will not be truly representative of the velocities obtained after birth.

LEFT AND RIGHT VENTRICULAR OUTFLOW TRACTS

Five-Chamber View. Aortic flow may be recorded in the five-chamber view (Box 29-6); to obtain this view, the transducer should be angled slightly anterior from the four-chamber view to include the left ventricular and aortic outflow tract (Figure 29-13). Doppler flow patterns of the aorta are recorded with the transducer again parallel to flow and the cursor placed first at the level of the aortic cusps and then moved into the ascending aorta. The mean velocity in the aorta is 60 cm/sec.

BOX 29-5   FOUR-CHAMBER VIEW ANATOMY

- Right atrium and ventricle (with moderator band)
- Tricuspid valve
- Left atrium and ventricle
- Mitral valve
- Interventricular septum
- Interatrial septum
- Foramen ovale
- Pulmonary veins as they enter the left atrium

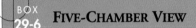

BOX 29-6   FIVE-CHAMBER VIEW

- Left atrium
- Left ventricular outflow tract
- Aortic root
- Right ventricle

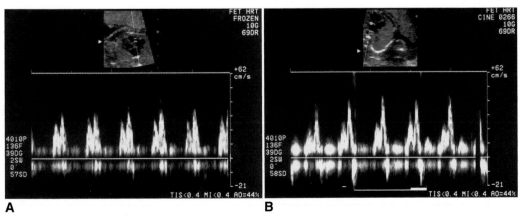

A   **B**

Figure 29-11   Normal Doppler flow patterns made in the four-chamber view of the mitral (**A**) and tricuspid (**B**) leaflets. The smaller first peak is the *e* wave; the second higher peak is the *a* wave.

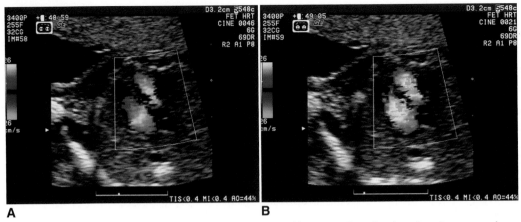

Figure 29-12   Color Doppler inflow patterns of the normal heart in a four-chamber view. **A** corresponds to early diastole at the *e* wave (early inflow filling of the ventricle), and **B** represents the *a* wave.

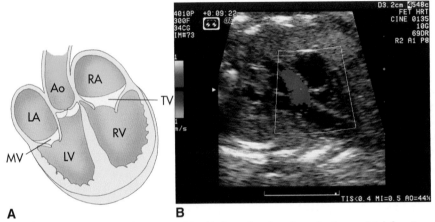

Figure 29-13   Aortic outflow is shown in red in this four-chamber view. *Ao,* Aorta; *LA,* left atrium; *LV,* left ventricle; *MV,* mitral valve; *RA,* right atrium; *RV,* right ventricle; *TV,* tricuspid valve.

Crisscross View.   As the transducer is angled from the aorta slightly to the left, the pulmonary artery may be seen as it arises from the right ventricular outflow tract (Figure 29-14). The pulmonary artery normally is anterior and to the left of the aorta. This "sweep" from the aorta to the pulmonary artery is called the crisscross view and allows the sonographer to see the normal relationship of the great arteries to one another (Box 29-7). Pulmonary flow patterns may be obtained in this view if the cursor is parallel with the flow. The cursor is moved into the main pulmonary artery to record the flow patterns. The mean velocity in the pulmonary artery is 55 cm/sec.

Long-Axis View.   In the long-axis view (Figure 29-15, *A* and *B*), the sizes of the right and left ventricles and the left atrial cavity should be assessed to obtain an overview of cardiac disease and contractility (Box 29-8). The left atrial cavity in this view is generally about the same size as the aorta and is hypoechoic. The crescent-shaped right ventricle is anterior to the left ventricle.

The thickness of the interventricular septum may be assessed from the parasternal long-axis view when the trans-

> **BOX 29-7   CRISSCROSS VIEW OF GREAT ARTERIES**
>
> - Sweep from aorta (located posterior) to pulmonic vessel (located anterior)
> - Left ventricular outflow tract
> - Right ventricular outflow tract

> **BOX 29-8   LONG-AXIS VIEW**
>
> - Right ventricle
> - Interventricular septum
> - Left ventricle
> - Mitral valve leaflets
> - Aorta with aortic cusps
> - Left atrium

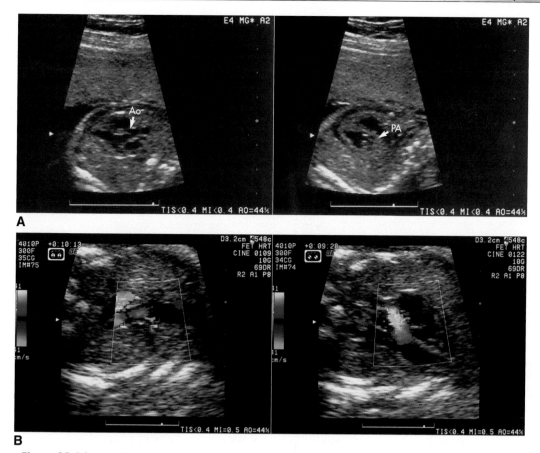

Figure 29-14   **A,** Crisscross view of the heart shows the aorta *(Ao)* posterior in continuity with the ventricular septum. The transducer is angled medial and anterior to image the pulmonic artery *(PA)*. **B,** Color Doppler image of the pulmonary artery outflow is blue as it leaves the right ventricular cavity. The aortic outflow is red as the blood leaves the left ventricle.

ducer is perpendicular to the septum. The septum is divided into membranous and muscular segments. The membranous portion is located just inferior to the aorta. This part of the septum is the last to develop and is very thin and must be examined in several planes to evaluate its inflow and outflow sections. The inflow membranous septum is best seen on the apical four-chamber view at the level of the atrioventricular valves, whereas the outflow may be seen on the long-axis view.

The septum thickens along its muscular component, which makes up the remaining two thirds of the septum. The septum and the posterior left ventricular wall are generally the same thickness at the end of ventricular systole. Normal septal thickness should correspond to the gestational age; a good rule of thumb to remember is that the second-trimester septum should measure about 2 to 2.5 mm and the third-trimester septum should measure under 4 mm. If the septum measures over 5 mm, septal hypertrophy or concentric ventricular hypertrophy should be considered.

On the long-axis view (see Figure 29-15, *C*), the continuity of the right side of the septum with the anterior wall of the aortic root is important to rule out the presence of a membranous ventricular septal defect (VSD), conal truncal abnormality (such as truncus arteriosus), endocardial cushion defect, or tetralogy of Fallot. A very small VSD may not be visualized at this stage, depending on the resolution of the equipment and quality visualization of the fetus. Generally the septal defect must be at least half the size of the aortic diameter to be imaged by ultrasound. Multiple septal defects may be difficult to image in the second trimester.

As the transducer is angled slightly anterior and medial from the aortic root, the right ventricular outflow tract may be imaged (see Figure 29-15, *D*). The pulmonary artery is slightly wider at its origin than the aorta.

The size of the aorta should be assessed. A gestational age of 20 weeks would show a normal aortic measurement of 4 mm. The aortic cusp motion should be assessed on the long- and short-axis views (see Figure 29-15, *E*). Normally the three cusps open in systole to the full extent of the aortic root and close in a midposition in diastole. The cusps do not "flop" into the left ventricular outflow tract, as is sometimes seen to varying degrees with a bicuspid or unicuspid valve. The aortic root should be anechoic from its base throughout the arch and descending aorta. The presence of interluminal echoes with dilation may indicate some degree of aortic

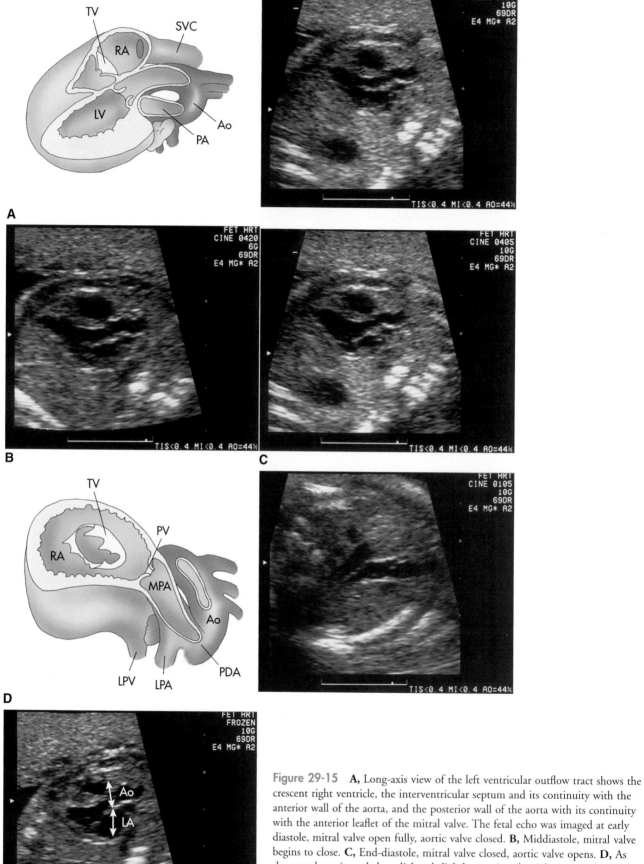

Figure 29-15 **A,** Long-axis view of the left ventricular outflow tract shows the crescent right ventricle, the interventricular septum and its continuity with the anterior wall of the aorta, and the posterior wall of the aorta with its continuity with the anterior leaflet of the mitral valve. The fetal echo was imaged at early diastole, mitral valve open fully, aortic valve closed. **B,** Middiastole, mitral valve begins to close. **C,** End-diastole, mitral valve closed, aortic valve opens. **D,** As the transducer is angled medial and slightly anterior, the right ventricular outflow tract with the pulmonary artery *(PA)* is seen on the fetal echo. *Ao,* Aorta; *LPA,* left pulmonary artery; *LPV,* left pulmonary vein; *MPA,* main pulmonary artery; *PDA,* posterior descending artery; *PV,* pulmonary valve; *TV,* tricuspid valve. **E,** The size of the aorta *(Ao)* and left atrium *(LA)* may be measured in this long-axis view.

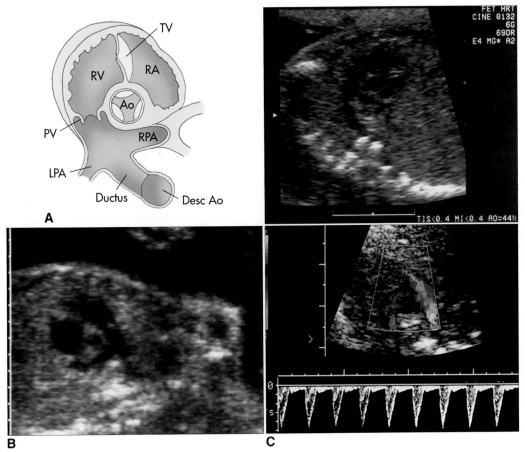

Figure 29-16 A, High, short-axis view of the great vessels. The right ventricular outflow tract wraps anterior to the aorta. The pulmonary artery arises from the right ventricle and bifurcates into right and left branches. The ductal insertion occurs midway between the bifurcation of the pulmonary vessels. Measurement of the great vessel diameters may be made at the level of the cusps. *Ao,* Aorta; *Desc Ao,* descending aorta; *LPA,* left pulmonary artery; *PV,* pulmonary vein; *RA,* right atrium; *RPA,* right pulmonary artery; *RV,* right ventricle; *TV,* tricuspid valve. **B,** Normal relationship of the pulmonary artery (tubular) with the bifurcation into right and left pulmonary arteries as it lies anterior to the aorta. **C,** Color Doppler shows the increased velocity in the main pulmonary artery *(blue)* at the ductal insertion *(yellow). AO,* Aorta; *PA,* pulmonary artery.

> ### BOX 29-9   SHORT-AXIS VIEW
>
> - Right ventricular outflow tract
> - Pulmonary cusps
> - Main pulmonary artery
> - Right and left pulmonary arteries
> - Aorta with cusps
> - Left atrial cavity

stenosis (with poststenotic dilation). The presence of a membrane inferior to the aortic cusps may indicate subvalvular aortic obstruction.

Short-Axis View. Once the long-axis view has been obtained, the transducer is rotated 90 degrees to the transverse or short-axis view. Generally the transducer is angled in a cephalic direction to make this a high parasternal short-axis view (Figure 29-16, *A*). The structures listed in Box 29-9 should be visualized.

The high short-axis is the view we use to measure the diameter of the pulmonary artery and the aorta (see Figure 29-16, *B*). It is also important to visualize the bifurcation of the main pulmonary artery into the right and left pulmonary arteries to demonstrate the normal relationship of the pulmonary artery as it lies anterior and to the left of the aorta. On the short-axis view, normally the right ventricular outflow tract and pulmonary artery "drape" anterior to the circular aorta (see Figure 29-16, *A*). The great vessels are measured two-dimensionally at the level of the semilunar cusps. At 20 weeks of gestation, both arteries should measure approximately 4 mm each.

The trileaflet aortic cusps may be visualized in this short-axis view. A two-leaflet or **bicuspid aortic valve** appears as two

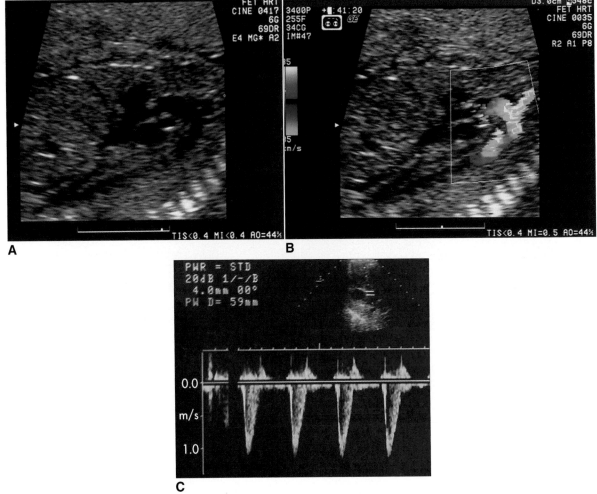

Figure 29-17 Normal gray scale **(A)** and color Doppler **(B)** images of the ascending aorta, arch, and descending aorta. The left subclavian is one of the three vessels that arise from the arch of the aorta and is well seen on the color image. **C**, Normal velocity in the aorta.

cusps with or without eccentric closure, depending on the equal distribution of cusp tissue.

Pulmonic flow patterns are obtained parallel to flow in the high short-axis plane with the Doppler cursor at the level of the pulmonic cusps. The cursor is moved into the main pulmonary artery to map any changes in the flow pattern. The mean velocity in the pulmonary artery ranges from 60 to 80 cm/sec; when the cursor reaches the level of ductal insertion, near the left pulmonary branch artery, the flow dramatically increases to nearly double the velocity in the main pulmonary artery (150 cm/sec) (Figure 29-16, *C*).

DUCTAL AND AORTIC ARCH VIEWS: OBLIQUE LONG AXIS

With careful angulation of the transducer to an oblique longitudinal plane, the root of the aorta, the ascending aorta, the arch, and the descending aorta may be assessed (Figure 29-17). The sonographer may find the fetal spine in the sagittal plane and angle slightly inward toward the left chest to search for the descending aorta and arch. The tubular dimension of this vessel should be somewhat uniform as one follows the aorta from its base into the thorax and abdomen. As the sonographer carefully sweeps back and forth, the inner core should be anechoic. The three head and neck branch arteries (innominate, carotid, and left subclavian) may be seen to arise from the perfect curve of the aortic arch as they ascend into the fetal head. The sonographer should be able to demonstrate the "candy cane" appearance of the ascending aorta, arch, and descending aorta in one image plane.

A second "arch-type" pattern (which appears as large as the aorta) is shown as the transducer is angled inferior from the aortic arch. This represents the patent ductus arteriosus, a communication between the pulmonary artery and the aorta that is patent during fetal life but closes shortly after birth. The ductus is slightly larger than the aortic arch and has a sharper angle ("hockey stick") as it drains into the descending aorta (Figure 29-18). The ductus does not have arterial structures arising from its wall as the aorta does.

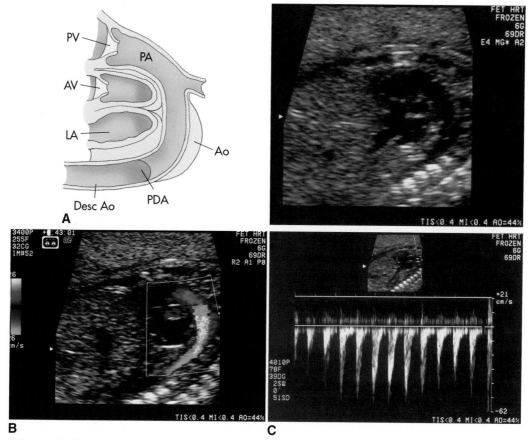

Figure 29-18   The ductal arch is found slightly inferior to the aortic arch. **A,** The short-axis view shows the main pulmonary artery and ductal arch as it empties into the descending aorta. *Ao,* Aorta; *AV,* aortic valve; *Desc Ao,* descending aorta; *LA,* left atrium; *PA,* pulmonary artery; *PDA,* patent ductus arteriosus; *PV,* pulmonary valve. **B,** Color shows the increased velocity *(yellow)* at the level of the ductus. **C,** Pulsed Doppler flow velocity shows the normal pattern of 50 cm/sec in the main pulmonary artery. This velocity may more than double at the level of the ductal insertion.

REFERENCES

1. Allen L: *Manual of fetal echocardiography,* London, 1986, MTP Press Limited.
2. Brand JM, Friedberg DZ: Spontaneous regression of a primary cardiac tumor presenting as fetal tachyarrhythmias, *J Perinatol* 12:48, 1992.
3. Callan NA and others: Fetal echocardiography: indications for referral, prenatal diagnoses, and outcomes, *Am J Perinatol* 8:390, 1991.

SELECTED BIBLIOGRAPHY

Beeby AR and others: Reproducibility of ultrasonic measurement of fetal cardiac haemodynamics, *Br J Obstet Gynaecol* 98:807, 1991.
Bromley B and others: Fetal echocardiography: accuracy and limitations in a population at high and low risk for heart defects, *Am J Obstet Gynecol* 166:1473, 1992.
Bronshtein M, Siegler E, Eshcoli Z and others: Transvaginal ultrasound measurements of the fetal heart at 11 to 17 weeks of gestation, *Am J Perinatol* 9:38, 1992.
Brown DL: Borderline findings in fetal cardiac sonography, *Semin Ultrasound CT MRI* 19(4):329, 1998.
Brown DL and others: The peripheral hypoechoic rim of the fetal heart, *J Ultrasound Med* 8:603, 1989.
Callen PC: *Ultrasonography in obstetrics and gynecology,* ed 3, Philadelphia, 1994, WB Saunders.
Comstock C: Normal fetal heart axis and position, *Obstet Gynecol* 70:2, 1987.
Comstock CH and others: Pulmonary-to-aorta diameter ratio in the normal and abnormal fetal heart, *Am J Obstet Gynecol* 165:1038, 1991.
Copel J, Pilu G, Kleinman CS: Congenital heart disease and extracardiac anomalies: associations and indications for fetal echocardiography, *Am J Obstet Gynecol* 154:1121, 1986.
Copel JA, Hobbins JC, Kleinman CS: Doppler echocardiography and color flow mapping, *Obstet Gynecol Clin North Am* 18:845, 1991.
Cyr D and others: A systematic approach to fetal echocardiography using real-time/two-dimensional sonography, *J Ultrasound Med* 5:343, 1986.
Dolkart LA, Reimers FT: Transvaginal fetal echocardiography in early pregnancy: normative data, *Am J Obstet Gynecol* 165:688, 1991.

Friedman WF: The intrinsic physiologic properties of the developing heart, *Prog Cardiovasc Dis* 15:87-111, 1972.

Haak MC, vanVugt JM: Echocardiography in early pregnancy, *J Ultrasound Med* 21:490-493, 2003.

Hafner E, Schuller T, Metzenbauer M and others: Increased nuchal translucency and congenital heart defects in a low risk population, *Prenatal Diagn* 23:985-989, 2003.

Johnson P, Sharland G, Maxwell D and others: The role of transvaginal sonography in the early detection of congenital heart disease, *Ultrasound Obstet Gynceol* 4:248-251, 1994.

Moore KL: *The developing human,* Philadelphia, 1991, WB Saunders.

Reed KL: Introduction to fetal echocardiography, *Obstet Gynecol Clin North Am* 18:811, 1991.

Reed KL and others: Cardiac Doppler flow velocities in human fetuses, *Circulation* 73:41, 1986.

Respondek M and others: 2D echocardiographic assessment of the fetal heart size in the 2nd and 3rd trimester of uncomplicated pregnancy, *Eur J Obstet Gynecol Reprod Biol* 44:185, 1992.

Rizzo G, Arduini D, Romanini C: Accelerated cardiac growth and abnormal cardiac flow in fetuses of type I diabetic mothers, *Obstet Gynecol* 80:369, 1992.

Romero R and others: *Prenatal diagnosis of congenital anomalies,* East Norwalk, Conn, 1988, Appleton & Lange.

Rychik J, Ayres N, Cueno B and others: American Society of Echocardiography guidelines and standards for performance of the fetal echocardiogram, *J Am Soc Echo* 17:803-810, 2004.

Sahn DJ and others: Quantitative real-time cross sectional echocardiography in the developing normal human fetus and newborn, *Circulation* 62:3, 1980.

Shime J and others: Two-dimensional and M-mode echocardiography in the human fetus, *Am J Obstet Gynecol* 143:178, 1983.

Sklansky M, Tang A, Levy D and others: Maternal psychological impact of fetal echocardiography, *J Am Soc Echo* 15:159-166, 2002.

Sutton MS and others: Assessment of right and left ventricular function in terms of force development with gestational age in the normal human fetus, *Br Heart J* 66:285, 1991.

Tan J and others: Cardiac dimensions determined by cross-sectional echocardiography in the normal human fetus from 18 weeks to term, *Am J Cardiol* 70:1459, 1992.

van der Mooren K, Barendregt LG, Wladimiroff JW: Fetal atrioventricular and outflow tract flow velocity waveforms during normal second half of pregnancy, *Am J Obstet Gynecol* 165:668, 1991.

van der Mooren K, Barendregt LG, Wladimiroff JW: Flow velocity wave forms in the human fetal ductus arteriosus during the normal second half of pregnancy, *Pediatr Res* 30:487, 1991.

Vergani P and others: Screening for congenital heart disease with the four-chamber view of the fetal heart, *Am J Obstet Gynecol* 167:1000, 1992.

Wenink AC: Quantitative morphology of the embryonic heart: an approach to development of the atrioventricular valves, *Anat Rec* 234:129, 1992.

Wilson AD, Rao PS, Aeschlimann S: Normal fetal foramen flap and transatrial Doppler velocity pattern, *J Am Soc Echocardiogr* 3:491, 1990.

Wladimiroff JW and others: Normal fetal cardiac flow velocity waveforms between 11 and 16 weeks of gestation, *Am J Obstet Gynecol* 167:736, 1992.

Wladimiroff JW and others: Normal fetal Doppler inferior vena cava, transtricuspid, and umbilical artery flow velocity waveforms between 11 and 16 weeks' gestation, *Am J Obstet Gynecol* 166:921, 1992.

CHAPTER 30

Fetal Echocardiography: Congenital Heart Disease

Sandra L. Hagen-Ansert

GREAT VESSEL ABNORMALITIES

TRANSPOSITION OF THE GREAT ARTERIES
TRUNCUS ARTERIOSUS
COARCTATION OF THE AORTA
INTERRUPTED AORTIC ARCH
DUCTAL CONSTRICTION

CARDIAC TUMORS

RHABDOMYOMAS

COMPLEX CARDIAC ABNORMALITIES

SINGLE VENTRICLE
COR TRIATRIATUM
CONGENITAL VENA CAVA TO LEFT ATRIAL
   COMMUNICATION
TOTAL ANOMALOUS PULMONARY VENOUS RETURN
CARDIOSPLENIC SYNDROMES
ECTOPIC CORDIS

DYSRHYTHMIAS

ECTOPY
SUPRAVENTRICULAR TACHYARRHYTHMIA
ATRIOVENTRICULAR BLOCK

KEY TERMS

aortic stenosis – abnormal development of the cusps of the aortic valve that results in thickened and domed leaflets

atrial septal defects – defects that provide communication between the left atrium and right atrium. The three most common forms of atrial septal defects are ostium secundum, ostium primum, and sinus venosus.

atrioventricular block – occurs when the transmission of the electrical impulse from the atria to the ventricles is blocked

atrioventricular septal defect (AVSD) – failure of the endocardial cushion to fuse. This defect of the central heart provides communication between the ventricles, between the atria, or between the atria and ventricles. AVSD is subdivided into complete, incomplete, and partial forms.

bicuspid aortic valve – congenital abnormality that causes two of the three aortic leaflets to fuse together, resulting in a two-leaflet valve instead of the normal three-leaflet valve. Usually the cusps are asymmetric in size and position. May be the cause of adult aortic stenosis and/or insufficiency.

cardiomyopathy – disease of the myocardial tissue in the heart. This disease process is caused by several problems, including exposure to a virus-like coxsackie or mumps or a bacterial infection.

coarctation of the aorta – narrowing of the aortic arch (discrete, long-segment, or tubular). Most commonly occurs as a shelflike protrusion in the isthmus of the arch or at the site of the ductal insertion near the left subclavian artery.

corrected transposition of the great arteries – right atrium and left atrium are connected to the morphologic left and right ventricle, respectively, and the great arteries are transposed

cor triatriatum – occurs when the left atrial cavity is partitioned into two components; pulmonary veins drain into an accessory left atrial chamber proximal to the true left atrium

dextrocardia – heart is in the right chest with the apex pointed to the right of the thorax

dextroposition – condition in which the heart is located in the right side of the chest and the cardiac apex points medially or to the left

ductal constriction – occurs when flow is diverted from the ductus secondary to tricuspid or pulmonary atresia or secondary to maternal medications given to stop early contractions

Ebstein's anomaly of the tricuspid valve – abnormal displacement of the septal leaflet of the tricuspid valve toward the apex of the right ventricle. This right ventricle above this leaflet becomes the "atrialized" chamber

hypoplastic left heart syndrome – underdevelopment of the left ventricle with aortic and/or mitral atresia. Left ventricle is extremely thickened compared with the right ventricle.

hypoplastic right heart syndrome – underdevelopment of the right ventricular outflow tract secondary to pulmonary stenosis. Tricuspid atresia is also often found.

levocardia – normal position of the heart in the left chest with the cardiac apex pointed to the left

levoposition – condition in which the heart is displaced further toward the left chest, usually in association with a space-occupying lesion

mesocardia – atypical location of the heart in the middle of the chest with the cardiac apex pointing toward the midline of the chest

mitral atresia – also called *congenital mitral stenosis*. Abnormal development of the mitral leaflet (valve between the left atrium and left ventricle). May lead to development of hypoplastic left ventricle.

mitral regurgitation – occurs when the mitral leaflet is deformed and unable to close properly, allowing blood to leak from the left ventricle into the left atrium during systole

myocarditis – cardiac disease process of necrosis and destruction of myocardial cells, and also an inflammatory infiltrate

partial anomalous pulmonary venous return – condition in which the pulmonary veins do not all enter into the left atrial cavity

pericardial effusion – abnormal collection of fluid surrounding the epicardial layer of the heart

premature atrial contractions (PACs) – benign condition that arises from the electrical impulses generated outside the cardiac pacemaker (sinus node). Immature development of the electrical pacing system causes irregular heart beats scattered throughout the cardiac cycle.

premature ventricular contractions (PVCs) – benign condition that arises from the electrical impulses generated outside the cardiac pacemaker (sinus node). Immature development of the electrical pacing system causes irregular heart beats scattered throughout the cardiac cycle

pulmonary stenosis – abnormal pulmonary valve characterized by thickened, domed leaflets that restrict the amount of blood flowing from the right ventricle to the pulmonary artery to the lungs

single ventricle – a congenital anomaly in which there are two atria but only one ventricular chamber, which receives both the mitral and tricuspid valves

subpulmonic stenosis – occurs when a membrane or muscle bundle obstructs the outflow tract into the pulmonary artery

supravalvular pulmonic stenosis – abnormal narrowing in the main pulmonary artery superior to the valve opening

supraventricular tachyarrhythmias – abnormal cardiac rhythm above 200 beats per minute with a conduction rate of 1:1

tetralogy of Fallot – most common form of cyanotic heart disease characterized by a high, membranous ventricular septal defect; large, anteriorly displaced aorta; pulmonary stenosis; and right ventricular hypertrophy

total anomalous pulmonary venous return (TAPVR) – condition in which the pulmonary veins do not return at all into the left atrial cavity; the veins may return into the right atrial cavity or into a chamber posterior to the left atrial cavity

transposition of the great arteries – abnormal condition that exists when the aorta is connected to the right ventricle and the pulmonary artery is connected to the left ventricle. The atrioventricular valves are normally attached and related.

tricuspid atresia – interruption of the growth of the tricuspid leaflet that begins early in cardiac embryology

truncus arteriosus – congenital heart lesion in which only one great artery arises from the base of the heart. The pulmonary trunk, the systemic arteries, and the coronary arteries arise from this single great artery

ventricular septal defect – defect in the ventricular septum that provides communication between the right and left chambers of the heart; most common congenital lesion in the heart

---

TABLE 30-1	DISTRIBUTION OF TYPES OF CONGENITAL HEART DISEASE AMONG AFFECTED LIVE-BORN INFANTS

Condition	Percentage (%)
Ventricular septal defect	30
Pulmonary stenosis	7
Secundum atrial septal defect	7
Coarctation of the aorta	6
Aortic stenosis	5
Tetralogy of Fallot	5
Transposition of the great arteries	5
Atrioventricular defects	3
Hypoplastic right ventricle	2
Hypoplastic left ventricle	1
Total anomalous pulmonary veins	1
Truncus arteriosus	1
Single ventricle	0.3
Double-outlet right ventricle	0.2
Miscellaneous	17

Data modified from Hoffman C: *Am J Cardiol* 42:641, 1978, with permission from Excerpta Medica, Inc.

This chapter will present the sonographer's approach to evaluating congenital heart disease with examples of many of the more common forms of heart abnormalities. The development of the fetal heart is completed by the eighth week of embryonic life. The presence of congenital heart disease is a result of abnormal cardiac development during this period.

The most common type of congenital heart disease is the ventricular septal defect, followed by atrial septal defects and then **pulmonary stenosis** (Table 30-1). The development of congenital heart disease is multifactorial. Environmental factors, chromosomal factors, and hereditary factors may influence the development of congenital heart disease in the fetus. Fetal echocardiography can help to establish the presence and severity of the cardiac abnormality.

RELATIONSHIP OF GENETICS TO CONGENITAL HEART DISEASE

CHROMOSOMAL ABNORMALITIES

The frequency of chromosomal abnormalities in infants with congenital heart disease is estimated as 5% to 10% from post-natal data. In a control study of 2100 live-born infants with cardiovascular malformations, chromosomal abnormalities were found in 13%.[1] In this study, Down syndrome occurred in more than 10% of the infants, with the other trisomies each comprising the remaining 1%.

The frequency of abnormal karyotypes in fetuses with cardiac defects has been commonly found at 30% to 40%. Of these fetuses, the majority have trisomy 21, followed by trisomy 13, trisomy 18, and Turner's syndrome. The association of congenital heart defects and chromosomal abnormalities is lower in live-born infants than in fetuses because of the high in utero mortality of the fetus with trisomy 18, trisomy 13, and Turner's syndrome (45X).

The occurrence of associated extracardiac abnormalities in fetuses with cardiac defects and chromosomal abnormalities is in the order of 50% to 70%. In the fetus with a single cardiac abnormality, the incidence of chromosomal abnormalities is still increased (15% to 30%). The most common single cardiac abnormality is the **ventricular septal defect.**

Certain cardiac abnormalities are more likely associated with chromosomal defects. In general, malformations of the right side of the heart are rarely associated with karyotypic abnormalities (e.g., pulmonic stenosis and tricuspid atresia). However, abnormalities such as atrioventricular septal defect, perimembranous ventricular septal defect, tetralogy of Fallot, double outlet right ventricle, coarctation of the aorta, and hypoplastic left heart are often associated with chromosomal abnormalities.

The incidence of cardiac defects in the fetus with trisomy is increased, with trisomy 21 showing the highest rate at 40% to 50%, Turner's syndrome (45X) showing 25% to 40%, and more than 90% having cardiac defects with trisomies 13 and 18 (Table 30-2).

TABLE 30-2 CONGENITAL HEART DISEASE AND CHROMOSOMAL ABNORMALITY

Chromosomal Abnormality	Incidence at Live Birth	Associated Cardiac Abnormality	Common Cardiac Abnormalities
Trisomy 21	1:800	40%-50%	Atrioventricular septal defect Ventricular septal defect Cleft mitral valve Heart block
Trisomy 18	1:8000	>90%	Ventricular septal defect Double-outlet right ventricle
Trisomy 13	1:20,000	>80%	Ventricular septal defect Atrial septal defect
Turner's Syndrome (Trisomy 45X)	1:10,000	25%-45%	Coarctation of aorta Bicuspid aortic valve

TABLE 30-3 RECURRENCE RISKS IN CONGENITAL HEART DISEASE

(Normal Parents and One Affected Offspring)

Anomaly	Recurrence Risk
Ventricular septal defect	4.2%
Atrial septal defect	2.9%
Tetralogy of Fallot	3.0%
Pulmonary stenosis	2.7%
Coarctation of aorta	1.8%
Aortic stenosis	2.2%
Transposition of great vessels	1.7%
Atrioventricular septal defect	2.6%
Hypoplastic left heart	2.2%
Tricuspid atresia	1.0%
Ebstein's anomaly	1.0%

Nora JJ, Nora AH: The evolution of specific genetic and environmental counseling in congenital heart diseases, *Circulation* 57:205-213, 1978.

FAMILIAL RISKS OF CONGENITAL HEART DISEASE

The cause of most congenital heart defects has been considered multifactorial, with genetic and environmental factors both playing a role. Only about 10% to 15% of all congenital heart defects have been attributed to known chromosomal abnormalities, genetic syndromes, and teratogenic embryopathies.

The recurrence risk for an isolated congenital cardiovascular malformation is modified for each family based on the number of affected relatives and the severity of the abnormality. In general, a recurrence risk of 1% to 5% is estimated for the majority of congenital cardiac abnormalities (Table 30-3).

Recent studies have noted that the contribution of genetic factors increases the risk of congenital heart disease significantly.[1] For example, a mother who has had a child with a left heart abnormality (mitral atresia or aortic atresia), has a significantly higher risk (13%) of delivering another child with a form of left heart disease. This risk increases significantly with each pregnancy.

INCIDENCE OF CONGENTIAL HEART DISEASE

Congenital heart disease is the most common severe congenital abnormality, with an incidence of 8% in live births. Approximately half of these defects are minor and may be corrected easily with surgery; the remainder are responsible for more than half of the deaths from congenital abnormalities in childhood. Cardiac defects may account for as much as 4% of congenital heart disease in live births. Common cardiac defects include the **bicuspid aortic valve,** patent ductus arteriosus (common in premature infants), and ventricular septal defects. The incidence of the bicuspid aortic valve defect is 10 in 10,000 births; it may lead to cardiac problems in adulthood.

PRENATAL EVALUATION OF CONGENITAL HEART DISEASE

THE FOUR-CHAMBER VIEW

All sonographers should be familiar with the routine four-chamber view that is part of the normal obstetrical examination. This view is easily obtainable after 16 weeks of gestation; however, the anatomy becomes more distinctly imaged with ultrasound at 19 to 20 weeks of gestation. The four-chamber view is normal when the following conditions are seen:

1. The fetal situs is normal. (Heart position is in the left chest and the apex of heart points to the left; stomach is to the left; aorta is anterior and to the left of the spine; and inferior vena cava is anterior and to the right of the spine.)
2. The size of the heart in relation to the chest is normal (Ratio of heart to thorax = 1:3.)
3. The two atria are equal in size and the flap of the foramen ovale is seen to move toward the left atrium. (The atrium should comprise about $1/3$ the size of the heart.)
4. The two ventricles are equal in size and contractility. (The ventricles should comprise about $2/3$ the size of the heart.)
5. The interatrial and interventricular septa are completely formed and normal in thickness.
6. The atrioventricular valves are normal in thickness, position, and opening.

Several cardiac abnormalities may be recognized with the four-chamber view alone (large ventricular septal defect, atrioventricular septal defect, hypoplastic left or right heart, mitral or tricuspid atresia); however, there are many cardiac abnormalities that may be missed with only the four-chamber view. Abnormalities of the cardiac structure (especially the great vessels) that are not located in the four-chamber plane may show a normal four-chamber view, but miss the specific abnormality if a complete study is not conducted (e.g., transposition of the great arteries, truncus arteriosus, coarctation of the aorta, small outlet ventricular septal defect, tetralogy of Fallot, and others). The reader is referred to Chapter 29, which covers the normal fetal echocardiographic examination.

CARDIAC MALPOSITION

When the heart is "out of its normal position," there are several terms that are used to describe the exact position of the heart relative to location and position of the cardiac apex (Figures 30-1 and 30-2). *Dextrocardia* means the heart is in the right chest with the apex pointed to the right of the thorax. Dextrocardia can be associated with a normal visceral situs, situs inversus, or situs ambiguous. *Dextroposition* of the heart refers to a condition in which the heart is located in the right side of the chest and the cardiac apex points medially or to the left. This condition is usually found when extrinsic factors, such as a space-occupying large diaphragmatic hernia or hypoplasia of the right lung, are present.

Levocardia is the term used to denote the normal position of the heart in the left chest (with the cardiac apex pointed to the left) and is often used when visceral situs abnormalities are present. Levocardia can be associated with normal situs (normal anatomy), situs inversus (abdominal organs are located on the opposite side of normal), or situs ambiguous. *Levoposition* of the heart refers to the condition in which the heart is displaced further toward the left chest, usually in association with a space-occupying lesion.

Mesocardia indicates an atypical location of the heart, with the cardiac apex pointing toward the midline of the chest. Usually the heart is located more toward the midline. This may be found with the presence of an extracardiac mass or lung abnormalities.

CARDIAC ENLARGEMENT

CARDIOMYOPATHY

Cardiomyopathy involves a disease of the myocardial tissue in the heart. This disease process is caused by several problems, including exposure to a virus (coxsackie or mumps) or bacteria leading to an infection that causes a cardiomyopathy. Another cause may be errors of metabolism. Endocardial fibroelastosis has also been associated with cardiomyopathies and hypoplastic left-heart syndrome. Asymmetric septal hypertrophy (as seen in patients with hereditary idiopathic subaortic stenosis) and concentric hypertrophy (as seen in some uncontrolled diabetic mothers) have been reported.

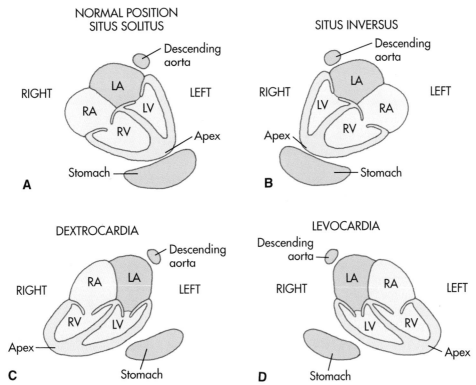

Figure 30-1 The anatomic relationship of the descending aorta, left atrium, apex, and stomach in the four cardiac positions: **A,** Normal position, situs solitus. **B,** Situs inversus. **C,** Dextrocardia; and **D,** Levocardia. *RA,* right atrium; *LV,* left ventricle; *RV,* right ventricle.

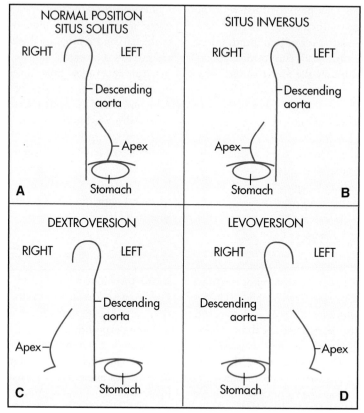

Figure 30-2   The alignment of the descending aorta, apex, and stomach in the four basic cardiac positions from the frontal projection. **A,** In situs solitus, the descending aorta, apex, and stomach are all on the left. **B,** In situs inversus, the descending aorta, apex, and stomach are all on the right. **C,** In dextroversion, the descending aorta and stomach are on the left, but the apex is on the right. **D,** In levoversion, the descending aorta and stomach are on the right, but the apex is on the left.

Myocarditis is characterized by necrosis and destruction of myocardial cells and an inflammatory infiltrate. In a viral cardiomyopathy, all four chambers are dilated, with thinning of the myocardial walls (Figure 30-3). Gross valvular regurgitation may be present, resulting from the stretched mitral and tricuspid anulus. The cardiac function is decreased severely, leading to congestive heart failure with pericardial effusion, bradycardia, and death.

The general prognosis for a fetus with evidence for a cardiomyopathy is very poor. Serial fetal echoes are performed to monitor chamber size, regurgitation, and contractility.

PERICARDIAL EFFUSION

Pericardial effusion is an abnormal collection of fluid surrounding the epicardial layer of the heart. In the four-chamber view, a hypoechoic area in the peripheral part of the epicardial/pericardial interface of 2 mm or less is considered within normal limits and does not represent a pericardial effusion. The separation must be seen on the M-mode to separate both in systole and in diastole and be greater than 2 mm. If the separation surrounds the heart (from the atrioventricular junction around the apex of the heart), it could be associated with hydrops fetalis (Figure 30-4).

With a small pericardial effusion, the separation of the pericardium from the epicardium may localize toward the pos-

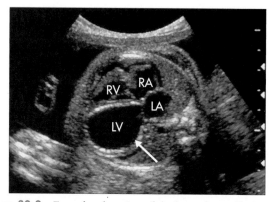

Figure 30-3   Four-chamber view of the heart shows dilation of all four chambers. Regurgitation was present in the mitral and tricuspid valves. Pericardial effusion *(arrow). RV,* right ventricle; *RA,* right atrium; *LV,* left ventricle; *LA,* left atrium.

terolateral and apical walls of the heart. The larger effusion will extend to the atrioventricular groove posteriorly and around the anterior right ventricular wall.

Pericardial effusion may be seen secondary to indomethacin therapy with premature closure of the patent ductus arteriosus. Pericardial effusion has also been associated with coxsack-

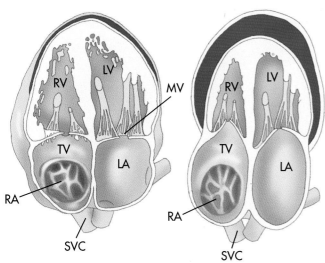

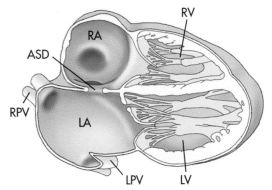

Figure 30-6   Four-chamber view of the heart illustrating the absence of the flap of the foramen ovale. *RV,* right ventricle; *RA,* right atrium; *ASD,* atrial septal defect; *RPV,* right pulmonary vein; *LA,* left atrium; *LPV,* left pulmonary vein; *LV,* left ventricle.

Figure 30-4   **A,** Apical view of a small pericardial effusion. **B,** Apical view of a large pericardial effusion involving the right ventricle, apex, and left ventricle. *RV,* right ventricle; *LV,* left ventricle; *MV,* mitral valve; *LA,* left atrium; *SVC,* superior vena cava; *RA* right atrium; *TV,* tricuspid valve.

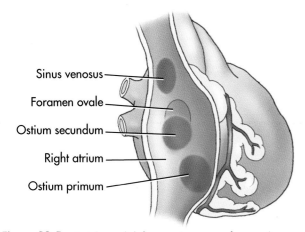

Figure 30-5   Atrial septal defects: ostium secundum, ostium primum, and sinus venosus defects viewed from the right atrium.

ievirus, cytomegalovirus, parvovirus, human immunodeficiency virus, intrauterine growth restriction, and aneuploidy.

SEPTAL DEFECTS

ATRIAL SEPTAL DEFECT

Atrial septal defects provide communication between the left atrium and right atrium. The locations of three common atrial septal defects are shown in Figure 30-5. There are three common forms of atrial septal defects: ostium secundum, ostium primum, and sinus venosus. The ostium secundum defect is the defect in the central atrial septum near the foramen ovale and is the most difficult to see in utero as the flap of the foramen ovale is mobile at this period of development. The ostium primum defect is usually associated with the

chromosomal abnormality of trisomy 21 and often will have a cleft mitral valve and abnormalities of the atrioventricular septum. The least common septal defect is the sinus venosus defect that is seen near the entrance of the superior vena cava into the right atrium. This may be associated with a **partial anomalous pulmonary venous return.**

The atrial septal defect is not always recognized during fetal life unless part of the intraatrial septum is missing. The foramen ovale remains open in the fetal heart until after birth, and the pressures change between the right and left heart to force the foramen to close completely. Failure of the foramen to close may result in atrial septal defect, secundum type. An atrial septal defect provides communication between the right and left atrium. The defect must be quite large in the fetus to be identified by ultrasound.

The area of the foramen ovale is thinner in the fetus than the surrounding atrial tissue; therefore, with echocardiography, the area is prone to signal dropout, particularly in the apical four-chamber view when the transducer is parallel to the septum. Any break in the atrial septum in this view must be confirmed by the short-axis or "subcostal" view (the transducer is inferior to the heart and angled cephalad in a transverse or short-axis plane), in which the septum is more perpendicular to the transducer. Because of beam-width artifacts, the edges of the defect may be slightly blunted and appear brighter than the remaining septum.

In utero the natural flow in the atrium is right to left across the foramen (as the pressures are slightly higher on the right). A small reversal flow may be present. The foramen should flap into the left atrial cavity. The flap should not be so large as to touch the lateral wall of the atrium; when this redundancy of the foramen occurs, the sinoatrial node may become agitated in the right atrium and cause fetal arrhythmias. The sonographer should be sure to sweep inferior to superior along the atrial septum to identify the three parts of the septum: the primum septum, fossa ovalis, and septum secundum.

Ostium Secundum Atrial Septal Defect. The most common atrial defect is the secundum atrial septal defect, which occurs in the area of the fossa ovalis (Figure 30-6).

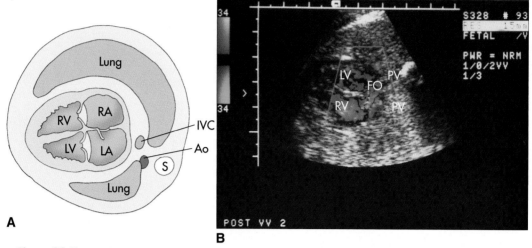

Figure 30-7   A, The most common type of atrial septal defects occur in the area of the fossa ovalis, known as the secundum defect. *Ao,* Aorta; *IVC,* inferior vena cava; *LA,* left atrium; *LV,* left ventricle; *RA,* right atrium; *RV,* right ventricle. **B,** In the fetus, normal flow should occur at the level of the foramen ovale *(FO). PV,* pulmonary vein.

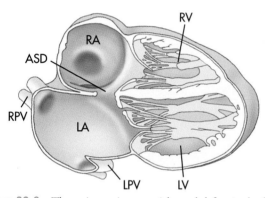

Figure 30-8   The ostium primum atrial septal defect in the four-chamber view. *RV,* right ventricle; *RA,* right atrium; *PRV,* right pulmonary vein; *LA,* left atrium; *LPV,* left pulmonary vein; *LV,* left ventricle; *ASD,* atrial septal defect.

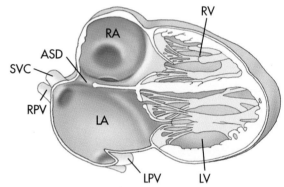

Figure 30-9   The sinus venosus atrial septal defect near the entrance of the superior vena cava and right upper pulmonary vein (RPV). *RV,* right ventricle; *RA,* right atrium; *RPV,* right pulmonary vein; *LA,* left atrium; *LPV,* left pulmonary vein; *LV,* left ventricle; *SVC,* superior vena cava; *ASD,* atrial septal defect.

Usually an absence of the foramen ovale flap is noted, with the fossa ovalis opening larger than normal.

Sonographic Findings. Doppler tracings of the septal defect with the sample volume placed at the site of the defect show a right-to-left flow with a velocity of 20 to 30 cm/sec. Color flow Doppler is performed in the apical four-chamber and subcostal views and may be useful to outline the size and direction of flow as it crosses the foramen ovale (Figure 30-7, *B*). The flow patterns of the mitral and tricuspid valves are slightly increased with the elevated shunt flow.

Ostium Primum Septal Defect.   The primum septal defect is deficient in the lower (inferior) portion of the septum, near the crux of the heart (Figure 30-8). It may be seen in atrioventricular septal defect malformation in which there is malalignment of the atrioventricular valves secondary to the defect. In addition, a cleft of the mitral valve is present, causing mitral regurgitation into the left atrial cavity.

Sonographic Findings. The primum septal defect is best imaged in the four-chamber plane that is parallel to the transducer beam. The gain should be reduced to clearly identify the atrial septum. Look for the flap of the foramen ovale. This defect may be part of an atrioventricular septal defect or be a primary defect with or without a cleft mitral valve.

Sinus Venosus Septal Defect.   The sinus venosus atrial septal defect is technically more difficult to visualize with echocardiography. This defect lies in the superior portion of the atrial septum, close to the inflow pattern of the superior vena cava (Figure 30-9).

Sonographic Findings. Sinus venosus septal defects are best visualized with the subxiphoid four-chamber view. If signs of right ventricular volume overload are present, with no atrial septal defect obvious, care should be taken to study the septum in search of a sinus venosus type of defect. Partial anomalous

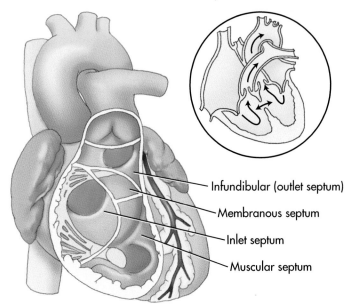

Figure 30-10   Ventricular septal defect. Portions of the ventricular septum showing the infundibular (outlet septum), membranous septum, inlet septum, and muscular septa.

pulmonary venous drainage of the right pulmonary vein is usually associated with this type of defect; thus it is important to identify the entry site of the pulmonary veins into the left atrial cavity. Color flow mapping is useful in this type of problem because it allows the sonographer to actually visualize the venous return to the left atrium and a flow pattern crossing into the right atrial cavity.

VENTRICULAR SEPTAL DEFECT

Ventricular septal defect is the most common congenital lesion of the heart, accounting for 30% of all structural heart defects. The septum is divided into two basic segments: the membranous and muscular areas (Figure 30-10). The septum lies in a curvilinear plane and has different areas of thickness. There are a number of sites where ventricular septal defects may occur within the septum. Muscular defects occur more inferior in the septum, usually are very small, and may be multiple. Often smaller defects will close spontaneously shortly after birth. This type of muscular defect is more difficult to image with echocardiography.

Membranous Septal Defect. The (perimembranous) ventricular septal defect may be classified as membranous, aneurysmal, or supracristal (Figure 30-11). The significant anatomic landmark is the crista supraventricularis ridge. The defect lies either above or below this ridge. Defects that lie above are called *supracristal*. These defects are located just beneath the pulmonary orifice so that the pulmonary valve forms part of the superior margin of the interventricular communication. Defects that lie below the crista are called *infracristal* and may be found in the membranous or muscular part of the septum. These are the most common defects.

Sonographic Findings. The lesion may be partially covered by the tricuspid septal leaflet, and care must be taken to carefully

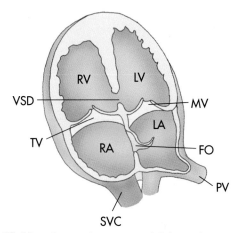

Figure 30-11   The membranous septal defect is shown in this four-chamber view. This is located in the inflow of the ventricles. The muscular defect in this four-chamber view may be large, small, or multiple along the thicker part of the septum. *FO,* Foramen ovale; *LA,* left atrium; *LV,* left ventricle; *MV,* mitral valve; *PV,* pulmonary vein; *RA,* right atrium; *RV,* right ventricle; *SVC,* superior vena cava; *TV,* tricuspid valve; *VSD,* ventricular septal defect.

evaluate this area with Doppler and color flow tracings. The membranous defect is found just below the aortic leaflets; sometimes the aortic leaflet is sucked into this defect (Figure 30-12).

The presence of an isolated ventricular septal defect in utero usually does not change the hemodynamics of the fetus. Defects smaller than 2 mm are not detected by fetal echocardiography. Care must be taken in the four-chamber view to carefully sweep the transducer posterior (to record the inlet part of the septum) to anterior (to record the outlet part of the septum).

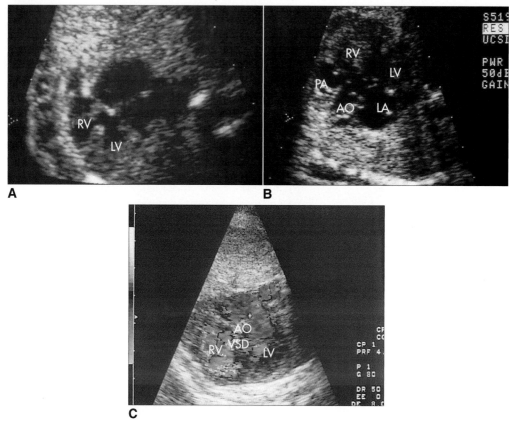

A   B

C

Figure 30-12 Ventricular septal defects. **A,** Large isolated membranous septal defect shown in this four-chamber view. The edges of the defect are slightly brighter than the rest of the septum. *LV,* left ventricle; *RV,* right ventricle. **B,** A patient with trisomy 18 shows a large septal defect involving the membranous and muscular areas. *AO,* Aorta; *PA,* pulmonary artery; *LA,* left atrium. **C,** Color Doppler is helpful when the ventricular septal defect *(VSD)* is large enough to allow crossover of flow from the higher-pressure right side of the heart into the left side of the heart.

Ventricular septal defects may close with the formation of aneurysm tissue, which is commonly found along the right side of the septal defect (Figure 30-13). These aneurysms generally protrude into the right heart in one of the following three directions: (1) above the tricuspid valve and into the right atrium, (2) directly into the septal leaflet of the tricuspid valve, or (3) below the tricuspid leaflets and into the right ventricular cavity. Usually these aneurysms are small, but when they become large, obstruction may occur in the right ventricular outflow tract.

Muscular Defect. A less common infracristal defect is located in the muscular septum. These defects may be large or small, or they may be multiple fenestrated holes (see Figure 30-12, *B* and *C*). The multiple defects are more difficult to repair, and their combination may have the same ventricular overload effect as a single large communication. Small muscular defects are usually found in the neonatal stage and often close spontaneously.

The prognosis is good for a patient with a single ventricular septal defect. However, the association with other cardiac

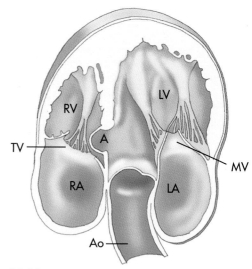

Figure 30-13 Five-chamber view of the heart illustrating the presence of a ventricular septal aneurysm inferior to the aortic cusps near the septal leaflet of the tricuspid valve. *RV,* right ventricle; *LV,* left ventricle; *MV,* mitral valve; *LA,* left atrium; *RA,* right atrium; *A,* atrium; *TV,* tricuspid valve; *Ao,* aorta.

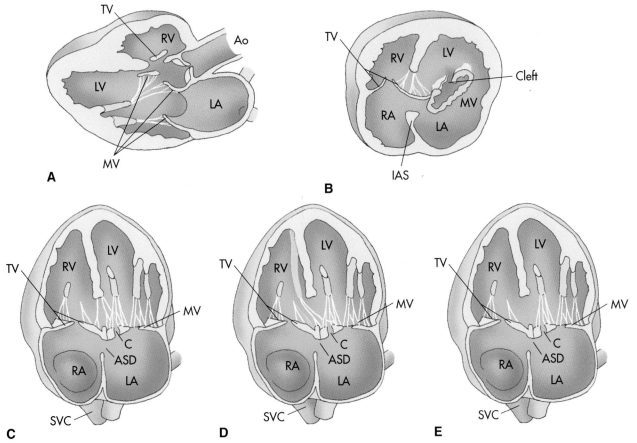

Figure 30-14 Atrioventricular septal defect. **A,** Long-axis view shows the discontinuity of the anterior leaflet of the mitral valve with the posterior wall of the aorta. The membranous septal defect is seen. *Ao,* Aorta; *LA,* left atrium; *LV,* left ventricle; *MV,* mitral valve; *RV,* right ventricle; *TV,* tricuspid valve. **B,** Short-axis through the atrioventricular valves shows the cleft in the anterior leaflet of the mitral valve *(MV).* The primum septal defect is seen. *IAS,* Interarterial septum. **C,** Four-chamber view showing the Rastelli type A large defect in the center (crux) of the heart. The membranous and primum septal defects are seen with the cleft mitral valve. There is a common leaflet from the anterior mitral leaflet to the septal tricuspid leaflet. *ASD,* Atrial septal defect; *SVC,* superior vena cava. **D,** Rastelli type B defect shows the chordal attachments from the medial portion of the cleft mitral leaflet related to the papillary muscle on the right side of the septal defect. **E,** Rastelli type C defect shows a free-floating common atrioventricular leaflet *(C).*

anomalies, such as tetralogy of Fallot, single ventricle, transposition of the great arteries, and endocardial cushion defect, is increased when a ventricular septal defect is found.

One study reported that 40% of ventricular septal defects are closed within 2 years of life and that 60% close by 5 years. The incidence of closure for membranous defects is 25% by 5 years and 65% for muscular defects by 5 years.[3]

Sonographic Findings. The best echocardiographic views to image the septal defect in the outflow tract are the long-axis, short-axis, and five-chamber views. The septal defect in the inflow tract is best seen on the four-chamber view.

Evaluation of shunt flow and direction is made with color flow mapping. Remember that pressures between the right and left heart are almost the same in utero, so a small defect will probably not show a velocity change. If the defect is large, the sample volume should be placed alongside the defect in the left ventricle to see the jet flow.

ATRIOVENTRICULAR SEPTAL DEFECT

The endocardial cushion defect is also called *ostium primum atrial septal defect, atrioventricular canal malformation, endocardial cushion defect,* and **atrioventricular septal defect (AVSD)** (Figure 30-14). These defects are subdivided into complete, incomplete, and partial forms.

Incomplete Atrioventricular Septal Defect. The failure of the endocardial cushion to fuse is termed an incomplete atrioventricular septal defect. This condition results in a membranous ventricular septal defect, abnormal tricuspid valve, primum atrial septal defect, and cleft mitral valve (Figure 30-15). A cleft mitral valve means that the anterior part of the leaflet is divided into two parts (medial and lateral). When the leaflet closes, blood leaks through this hole into the left atrial cavity. The leaflet is usually somewhat malformed, further causing regurgitation into the atrium. In addition, there is a

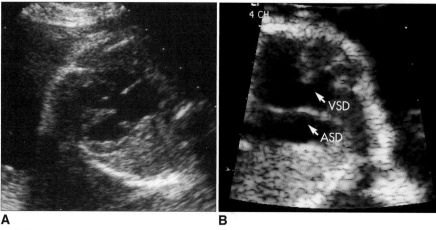

Figure 30-15 Atrioventricular septal defect. **A,** A patient with trisomy 21 had 2:1 heart block secondary to the complete atrioventricular septal defect, which included the membranous and atrial septa. **B,** A patient with trisomy 21 had a huge atrioventricular defect. The membranous and part of the muscular septum is not present *(VSD)*; the primum septum is also absent *(ASD)*.

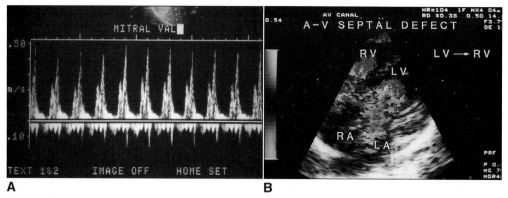

Figure 30-16 Atrioventricular septal defect. **A,** Prominent inflow velocities are seen across the mitral valve. There is a small regurgitant flow into the left atrium seen as flow reversal at the end of diastole below the baseline. **B,** Color flow imaging is helpful to map the flow across the defect and to track regurgitation into the atria. *LA,* Left atrium; *LV,* left ventricle; *RA,* right atrium; *RV,* right ventricle.

communication between the left ventricle and right atrium (left ventricular to right atrial shunt) because of the absent primum atrial septum and membranous interventricular septum. The ventricular septal defect occurs just below the mitral ring and is continuous with the primum atrial septal defect.

Complete Atrioventricular Septal Defect. The endocardial defect may be further classified into Rastelli types A, B, and C. Types A and B are characterized by insertion of the chordae from the cleft mitral and tricuspid valve into the crest of the ventricular septum or a right ventricular papillary muscle (Figure 30-16). Type C is the most primitive form and is called complete atrioventricular septal defect. This defect has a single, undivided, free-floating leaflet stretching across both ventricles. An M-mode sweep from the mitral to the aortic valves would show the anterior mitral leaflet swinging through the ventricular septal defect in continuity with the tricuspid valve. The tricuspid valve is said to cap the mitral valve. The ante-

rior and posterior leaflets are on both sides of the interventricular septum, causing the valve to override or straddle the septum. This is a much more complex abnormality to repair because the defect is larger and the single atrioventricular valve is more difficult to manage clinically, depending on the amount of regurgitation present. Complete AVSDs are frequently associated with malpositions of the heart (mesocardia and dextrocardia) and atrioventricular block (secondary to distortion of the conduction tissues).

AVSDs are frequently associated with other cardiac defects, including truncoconal abnormalities, coarctation of the aorta, and pulmonary stenosis or atresia. There is an increased incidence of Down syndrome (50% of trisomy 21 babies have congenital heart disease) and asplenia and polysplenia syndromes.

Occasionally, complete absence of the interatrial septum is noted in the fetal four-chamber view. With color flow, the entire atria are completely filled throughout systole and diastole. This is termed *common atria.*

With a partial AVSD, the fetus has only some of the above findings, usually an absent primum atrial septum and a cleft mitral valve.

Sonographic Findings. Echocardiographically the ideal views are the long-axis, short-axis (to search for abnormalities in the atrioventricular valves, such as presence of cleft), and four-chamber views (to search for chordal attachment, overriding, or straddling of the valves). The crux of the heart is carefully analyzed by sweeping the transducer anterior to posterior to record the outlet and inlet portions of the membranous septum.

Doppler and color flow techniques are extremely useful in determining the direction and degree of regurgitation present in the atrioventricular valves and the direction of shunt flow (increased right heart pressure causes a right ventricular to left atrial shunt in the fetus).

RIGHT VENTRICULAR INFLOW DISTURBANCE

Abnormalities that affect primarily the right side of the heart are listed as inflow or outflow tract disturbances. Each lesion is presented along with technical advice on how to obtain the ideal fetal cardiac image.

TRICUSPID ATRESIA/STENOSIS

Tricuspid atresia is the interruption of the growth of the tricuspid leaflet that begins early in cardiac embryology. This interruption involves the growth of the tricuspid apparatus, causing the valve to be hypoplastic or atretic.

In tricuspid atresia the inflow portion of the right ventricle has failed to form, and a membrane or dimple in the floor of the right atrium represents the position where the tricuspid valve should have originated (Figure 30-17). A ventricular septal defect may be present to help shunt blood into the

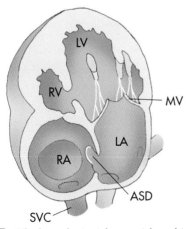

Figure 30-17   The hypoplastic right ventricle and immobile echogenic tricuspid valve apparatus are key factors in the four-chamber view in the patient with tricuspid atresia. The right atrium *(RA)* is enlarged. *ASD,* atrial septal defect; *LA,* left atrium; *LV,* left ventricle; *MV,* mitral valve; *RV,* right ventricle; *SVC,* superior vena cava.

hypertrophied right ventricle. The right ventricular outflow tract and pulmonary artery are generally diminished in size.

Sonographic Findings. Echocardiographically the tricuspid valve is best visualized on the four-chamber view (Figure 30-18). The findings in tricuspid atresia are a large dilated left ventricular cavity with a small, underdeveloped right ventricular cavity. The echogenic tricuspid annulus is seen with no valvular movement. The mitral valve is clearly the dominant atrioventricular valve. On the long- and short-axis views, the right ventricle is seen as a slitlike cavity just anterior to the interventricular septum.

Color flow imaging shows the incoming blood entering the right atrium and crossing over the patent foramen ovale to enter the left heart. If no blood flow passes the tricuspid orifice, then pulmonary stenosis is present. However, if a ventricular septal defect is present, the blood flows from the high-pressure left ventricle across the defect into the hypertrophied right ventricle and out the pulmonary outflow tract.

EBSTEIN'S ANOMALY OF THE TRICUSPID VALVE

Ebstein's anomaly of the tricuspid valve is an abnormal displacement of the septal leaflet of the tricuspid valve toward the apex of the right ventricle (Figure 30-19, *A*). Tricuspid valvular tissue may adhere directly to the ventricular endocardium or may be closely attached to the ventricular wall by multiple, anomalous, short chordae tendineae. The portion of the right ventricle underlying the adherent tricuspid valvular tissue is quite thin and functions as a receiving chamber analogous to the right atrium. This is referred to as the *atrialized chamber* because it registers a right atrial pressure pulse.

The anterior leaflet of the tricuspid valve is the least affected of the three leaflets. The septal and posterior leaflets show the greatest deformity, and the posterior cusp may be rudimentary or entirely absent. The right atrium is usually massively dilated. Often these patients have an incompetent or fenestrated foramen ovale or a secundum atrial septal defect.

The abnormal function of the right heart is related to the following three factors: (1) the malformed tricuspid valve, (2) the "atrialized" portion of the right ventricle, and (3) the reduced capacity of the pumping portion of the right ventricle.

Sonographic Findings. Echocardiographically, there is apical displacement of the septal leaflet of the tricuspid valve with resultant insufficiency (as seen on the apical four-chamber view) (Figure 30-19, *B*). The atrialized right ventricle is well seen. Generally, right ventricular dysfunction is present, which results in an overload pattern of wall motion with paradoxical or anterior septal motion in systole. This right ventricular overload also shows flattening of the septum when viewed in the short-axis plane.

Doppler tracings are useful to record the amount of insufficiency present from the abnormal tricuspid valve. The sample volume should be placed at the annulus of the tricuspid valve and then mapped through the atrialized right ventricle into the right atrial cavity to record the maximum jet of insufficiency. One should note how far the regurgitant jet extends and the width of the jet to determine the degree of insufficiency.

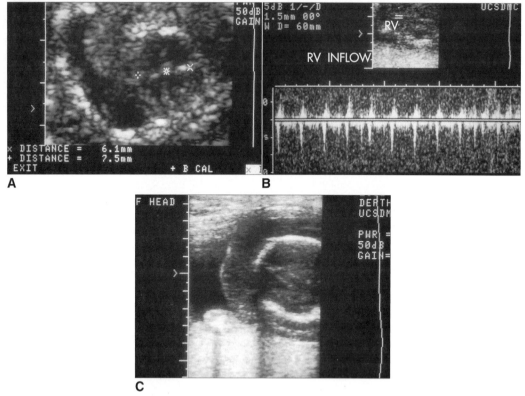

Figure 30-18   Tricuspid atresia. **A,** This patient presented in her 22nd week with the fetus demonstrating asymmetry of the ventricles. The annulus of the tricuspid valve was echogenic and immobile. The right ventricle was smaller than the left ventricle. The right atrium was enlarged. **B,** Pulsed Doppler imaging shows decreased inflow through the immobile tricuspid valve. There is mild to moderate tricuspid regurgitation seen at the end of diastole as flow reversal below the baseline. **C,** The patient developed severe hydrops with edema surrounding the scalp and abdomen, pleural effusion, and ascites.

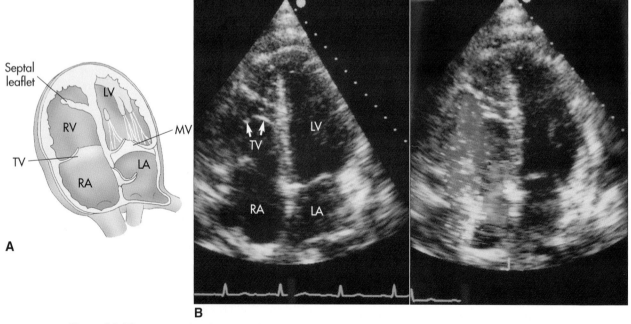

Figure 30-19   **A,** Four-chamber view of Ebstein's anomaly shows the septal leaflet of the tricuspid valve *(TV)* inferiorly displaced from its normal insertion point. The right atrium *(RA)* is markedly enlarged. *LA,* Left atrium; *LV,* left ventricle; *MV,* mitral valve; *RV,* right ventricle. **B,** Inferior displacement of the tricuspid valve into the apex of the right ventricle. This valve is usually dysplastic and regurgitation is present.

RIGHT VENTRICULAR OUTFLOW DISTURBANCE

The normal pulmonic valve comprises three semilunar cusps that open in systole and close completely in diastole just like the aortic cusps. These cusps are best imaged in the high short-axis plane or right long-axis plane of the right ventricular outflow tract.

HYPOPLASTIC RIGHT HEART

There are several forms of **hypoplastic right heart syndrome**: pulmonary atresia with an intact interventricular septum, pulmonary valve fusion with an intact interventricular septum and atrial septal defect, or pulmonary atresia with a normal aortic root diameter.

The right heart is underdeveloped because of obstruction of the right ventricular outflow tract secondary to pulmonary stenosis. The tricuspid valve is small and the pulmonary infundibulum is atretic (see Figure 30-17).

Sonographic Findings. The sonographer must be careful not to call a hypoplastic right heart a hypoplastic left heart (which may be a lethal situation) (Figure 30-20). Careful assessment of the situs of the fetus, great vessel relationships,

and trabeculation pattern helps the sonographer determine right from left heart (the right heart is more trabeculated than the left). Care must also be taken to avoid mistaking the papillary muscle for the septum when a large membranous defect is present. In a fetus with a single ventricle (and essentially a hypoplastic right heart), it may be easy to confuse a large papillary muscle with the septum. In this case, it would be difficult to figure out the great vessel origin. A single ventricle usually has an associated transposition of the great arteries with a small pulmonary artery and large aorta.

TETRALOGY OF FALLOT

Tetralogy of Fallot is the most common form of cyanotic heart disease. The severity of the disease varies according to the degree of pulmonary stenosis present; the more stenosis, the greater the cyanosis. It is possible to have a mild form of pulmonary stenosis and not have any cyanosis after birth.

Tetralogy of Fallot has the following four characteristics (Figure 30-21):

1. High, membranous ventricular septal defect
2. Large, anteriorly displaced aorta, which overrides the septal defect

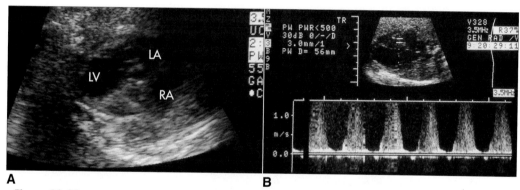

Figure 30-20   Hypoplastic right heart. Asymmetry of the ventricles **A,** with severe tricuspid regurgitation into the right atrium *(RA)*. **B,** *LA,* Left atrium; *LV,* left ventricle.

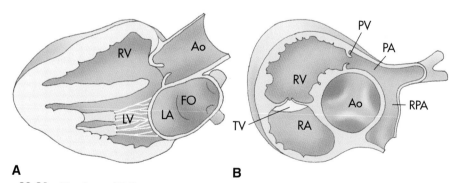

Figure 30-21   Tetralogy of Fallot. **A,** Long-axis view of the enlarged aorta *(Ao)* as it overrides the interventricular septum. The amount of aortic enlargement depends on the degree of pulmonary stenosis or atresia present. *FO,* Foramen ovale; *LA,* left atrium; *LV,* left ventricle; *RV,* right ventricle. **B,** Short-axis view of the small pulmonary artery *(PA)* displaced anteriorly by the enlarged aorta *(Ao)*. *PV,* Pulmonary valve; *RA,* right atrium; *RPA,* right pulmonary artery; *TV,* tricuspid valve.

3. Pulmonary stenosis
4. Right ventricular hypertrophy (not seen in fetal life; occurs after birth when pulmonary stenosis causes increased pressure in the right ventricle)

A large septal defect with mild to moderate pulmonary stenosis is classified as acyanotic disease, and a large septal defect with severe pulmonary stenosis is considered cyanotic disease ("blue baby" at birth).

Other congenital cardiac malformations may occur in patients with pulmonic stenosis and ventricular septal defect, including the following:

• Right aortic arch
• Persistent left superior vena cava
• Anomalies of the pulmonary artery and its branches
• Absence of the pulmonary valve
• Incompetence of the aortic valve
• Variations in coronary arterial anatomy

The prognosis for a fetus with tetralogy of Fallot is quite good with surgical intervention. One of the first surgical approaches was developed to obviate the underperfusion of the lungs. The Blalock-Taussig shunt was performed to anastomose the subclavian artery to the pulmonary artery.

The prognosis of tetralogy of Fallot with pulmonary atresia or an absent pulmonary valve does not show such a dramatic improvement (Figure 30-22, A). The absent pulmonary valve may cause congestive heart failure in the fetus. Aneurysmal dilation of the pulmonary artery and its branches may be a cause of pulmonary distress.

Sonographic Findings. Echocardiographically the demonstration of tetralogy of Fallot is distinguished on the parasternal long-axis view (see Figure 30-22). The large aorta overrides the ventricular septum. If the override is greater than 50%, the condition is called a *double-outlet right ventricle*, meaning that both great vessels arise from the right side of the heart. A septal defect is present; the size may vary from small to large. The parasternal short-axis view shows the small, hypertrophied right ventricle (if significant pulmonary stenosis is present). The pulmonary artery is usually small, and the cusps may be thickened and domed or difficult to image well.

A sample volume should be made in the high parasternal short-axis view to determine the turbulence of the right ventricular outflow tract and pulmonary valve stenosis (see Figure 30-22, C). Color flow is very helpful in this condition to actually delineate the abnormal high-velocity pattern and to direct the sample volume into the proper jet flow. If the ventricular septal defect is large, increased flow is seen in the right side of

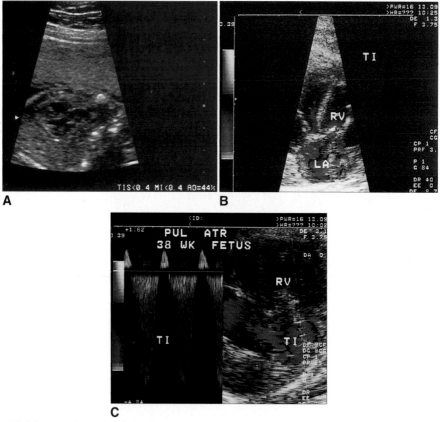

Figure 30-22 Tetralogy of Fallot. **A,** Long axis of the heart shows the aorta as it overrides the septum. **B,** Pulmonary stenosis may cause severe tricuspid regurgitation into the right atrium as the blood flow is obstructed in the right ventricular outflow tract. *LA,* Left atrium. **C,** Pulmonary atresia with tricuspid insufficiency *(TI)* is the most severe form of stenosis. *RV,* Right ventricle.

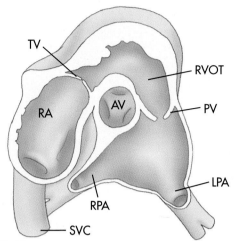

Figure 30-23 Pulmonary stenosis. The parasternal short-axis view of the domed pulmonary leaflets and some right ventricular hypertrophy are shown. *TV,* tricuspid valve; *AV,* aortic valve; *RVOT,* right ventricular outflow tract; *PV,* pulmonary valve; *LPA,* left pulmonary artery; *RPA,* right pulmonary artery; *SVC,* superior vena cava; *RA,* right atrium.

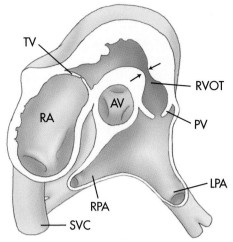

Figure 30-24 Subvalvular pulmonary stenosis. The parasternal short-axis view shows the right ventricular hypertrophy *(arrows)* with thickening of the bands of the crista supraventricularis. *TV,* tricuspid valve; *AV,* aortic valve; *RVOT,* right ventricular outflow tract; *PV,* pulmonary valve; *LPA,* left pulmonary artery; *RPA,* right pulmonary artery; *SVC,* superior vena cava; *RA,* right atrium.

the heart (increased tricuspid velocity, right ventricular outflow tract velocity, and increased pulmonic velocity). The best view for imaging the subvalvular portion of the right ventricular outflow tract is obtained with the subcostal short-axis plane. This view allows extensive visualization of the subpulmonary area so often affected in tetralogy of Fallot. In the fetus the pulmonic obstructive flow patterns are not as pronounced as in the neonatal period.

PULMONIC STENOSIS

The most common form of the right ventricular outflow tract obstruction is pulmonary valve stenosis. In pulmonic stenosis the abnormal pulmonic cusps become thickened and domed during diastole (Figure 30-23). The main pulmonary artery may be hypoplastic or there may be poststenotic dilation of the pulmonary artery. Other forms of pulmonary stenosis may show subvalvular thickening just inferior to the cusp opening.

Sonographic Findings. The domed effect is not quite as noticeable on the fetal echocardiogram, but with careful evaluation the thickness of the cusp may be compared with that of the aortic cusp. An M-mode image may be made through the area to further define cusp mobility and thickness. As with the aortic cusps, multiple degrees of stenosis and atresia may develop in the right ventricular outflow tract. The more atretic the cusp, the more hypoplastic the pulmonary artery becomes. Critical pulmonary atresia may be very difficult to image in the early second-trimester fetus because the pulmonary outflow becomes so hypoplastic that it is difficult to recognize.

When pulmonary stenosis is associated with another cardiac anomaly, such as transposition, double-outlet right ventricle, or tetralogy of Fallot, it becomes even more difficult to diagnose. Secondary findings of dilation of the right ventricular cavity and right atrial cavity (secondary to tricuspid

insufficiency) usually lead the investigator to the principal cause of the overload of the right side of the heart (pulmonic stenosis).

Color flow Doppler evaluation of the velocity is useful not only to assess the degree of obstruction but also to monitor the fetus in terms of following the course of disease (see Figure 30-22, *B*).

SUBPULMONIC STENOSIS

Subpulmonic stenosis occurs when a membrane or muscle bundle obstructs the outflow tract into the pulmonary artery (Figure 30-24).

Sonographic Findings. If the right ventricular outflow tract can be imaged adequately, the actual obstruction may be imaged. The Doppler and color flow pattern shows a turbulent obstructive pattern just before the pulmonary cusps. The velocity would not be as high as in the neonatal period but would measure at least 1.8 to 2 m/sec.

SUPRAVALVULAR PULMONIC STENOSIS

Supravalvular pulmonic stenosis is an abnormal narrowing in the main pulmonary artery. It usually is associated with Williams' syndrome and is hereditary (Figure 30-25).

Sonographic Findings. The parasternal short-axis view is best to image this condition. Prominent, dilated right and left pulmonary branch arteries may be present. Again, color flow will show a turbulent high-velocity flow pattern across the narrowed vessel.

LEFT VENTRICULAR INFLOW DISTURBANCE

Abnormalities that affect primarily the left side of the heart are listed as inflow or outflow tract disturbances. Each of these

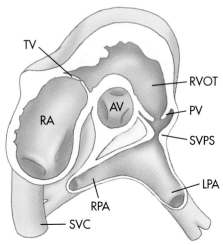

Figure 30-25   Supravalvular pulmonary stenosis. Domed pulmonary leaflets and a small pulmonary valve annulus as compared with the normal-sized aortic root. There is poststenotic dilation in the main pulmonary artery. *TV,* tricuspid valve; *AV,* aortic valve; *RVOT,* right ventricular outflow tract; *PV,* pulmonary valve; *LPA,* left pulmonary artery; *RPA,* right pulmonary artery; *SVC,* superior vena cava; *RA,* right atrium.

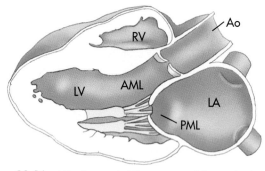

Figure 30-26   Mitral stenosis. The parasternal long-axis view shows the thickened chordae and the doming of the mitral valve apparatus. *Ao,* aorta; *LA,* left atrium; *PML,* posterior mitral leaflet; *AML,* anterior mitral leaflet; *LV,* left ventricle; *RV,* right ventricle.

lesions is presented along with technical advice on how to obtain the ideal fetal cardiac image.

CONGENITAL MITRAL STENOSIS

In normal cardiac development, the endocardial cushion forms the anterior and posterior mitral apparatus with chordae tendineae attached to two papillary muscles on the left side of the heart. When this development is interrupted in the first trimester, the mitral valve apparatus may not fully develop, causing mitral atresia or stenosis (Figure 30-26).

There are several anatomic varieties of congenital mitral stenosis. In one variety, the leaflets are thickened, nodular, and fibrotic; the commissures are rudimentary or absent; the chordae tendineae are shortened, thickened, and fused; and the papillary muscles are fibrosed. The mitral valve is a funnel-shaped, flat, or diaphragm-like structure.

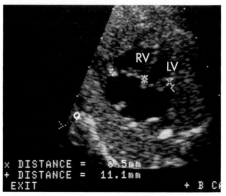

Figure 30-27   Mitral atresia. Four-chamber view shows a thickened, immobile mitral leaflet with a small left ventricular cavity. Mitral regurgitation was present. *LV,* left ventricle; *RV,* right ventricle.

The second variety consists of a "parachute" deformity of the valve. This occurs when the normal leaflets are drawn into close apposition by shortened chordae tendineae, which converge and insert into a single large papillary muscle.

The third variety of mitral stenosis consists of an anomalous arcade with obstructing papillary muscles that extend between the papillary muscles. The papillary muscles are so large that they encroach on the subvalvular area.

The last form of mitral stenosis occurs when the valve and its supporting structure are anatomically normal, but the mitral inlet is encroached upon by a circumferential supravalvular ridge of connective tissue, which arises at the base of the atrial aspect of the mitral leaflets.

Sonographic Findings. The mitral valve should be evaluated from at least two cardiac windows: the long-axis and the four-chamber views. The long-axis view allows the examiner to evaluate the mobility of the anterior and posterior mitral valve leaflets as they open into the left ventricular cavity. The four-chamber view allows comparison of the placement of the mitral valve with the normal, slightly apical displacement of the tricuspid valve. It also allows observation of the pliability of the thin leaflets as they open in diastole and close in systole. The ideal Doppler waveform should be recorded from this apical position.

Mitral Atresia. In a fetus with **mitral atresia** or congenital mitral stenosis, the examiner sees a thickened mitral orifice with restriction of leaflet amplitude. The left ventricular cavity is reduced in volume because of decreased inflow (Figure 30-27). The myocardial thickness is increased (secondary to increased left ventricular pressure overload) if associated aortic atresia is present.

Sonographic Findings. Color Doppler can be very helpful to determine how much, if any, mitral inflow is present. The apical four-chamber view is again best to obtain this assessment.

MITRAL REGURGITATION

In fetal life the presence of **mitral regurgitation** is probably from a cleft mitral valve (endocardial cushion defect) or a congenital mitral stenosis. In the presence of mitral regurgitation, the left atrial cavity would become enlarged because of the leakage of blood from the defective mitral valve.

Sonographic Findings. The color Doppler flow pattern of disturbed flow in the left atrial cavity would be seen on the apical four-chamber and probably on the parasternal long-axis view.

LEFT VENTRICULAR OUTFLOW TRACT DISTURBANCE

The normal aortic valve comprises three semilunar cusps that open in systole and close completely in diastole. The cusps are best imaged in the long-axis and short-axis planes. The aortic root is measured in the short-axis plane as the transducer bisects the right ventricular outflow tract, the pulmonary artery, and the aortic root.

Normal Doppler flow is recorded in the aortic outflow tract (either from a five-chamber view or a modified long- or short-axis view).

BICUSPID AORTIC VALVE

If the development is interrupted during the first trimester, the three aortic cusps may not fully separate. In this instance the valve may be a unicuspid valve with a central opening and aortic stenosis or a bicuspid (two-leaflet) valve with asymmetric cusps (Figure 30-28).

Sonographic Findings. In this case the raphe between the cusp tissue has not separated; thus the leaflet opens asymmetrically and may show "doming" on the parasternal long-axis view. In the fetus a bicuspid valve may be difficult to image at 18 weeks, but should be well visualized in the late second trimester at 27 weeks.

AORTIC STENOSIS

Critical Aortic Stenosis. Critical **aortic stenosis** signifies end-stage left ventricular dysfunction. At some point in the second or third trimester an infection or other viral process has

caused the aortic leaflet to thicken and close prematurely. The fetus shows a normal ascending and descending aorta with abnormal opening of the aortic cusps. The enlarged, dysfunctional left ventricle then "billows" from the increased pressure in the ventricle because the left ventricular outflow tract is blocked (Figures 30-29 and 30-30, *A*). The ventricular walls would be thin and bulge into the right ventricular cavity. The

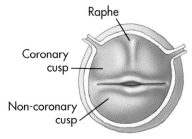

Figure 30-28   Bicuspid aortic valve showing the noncoronary cusp, and fused right and left coronary cusps with a raphe.

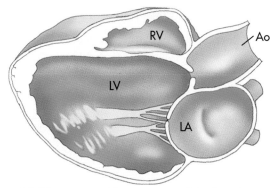

Figure 30-29   Parasternal long-axis view of the domed aortic valve, dilated left ventricle, and poststenotic dilation of the ascending aorta. *Ao,* aorta; *RV,* right ventricle; *LV,* left ventricle; *LA,* left atrium.

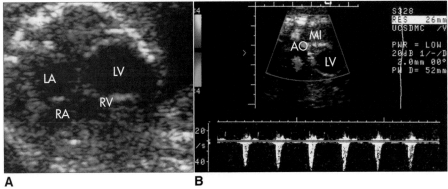

Figure 30-30   Critical aortic stenosis. **A,** Critical aortic stenosis appears in the second or third trimester. The four-chamber view shows a dilated left ventricular cavity (assumes the shape of a balloon). The ventricle is tense and quickly becomes noncompliant. *LA,* Left atrium; *LV,* left ventricle; *RA,* right atrium; *RV,* right ventricle. **B,** Color Doppler imaging shows aortic insufficiency *(blue)* and mitral insufficiency *(MI, red)*. *AO,* Aorta; *LV,* left ventricle.

parasternal long-axis and apical four-chamber views are the most helpful to image this disease.

Sonographic Findings. Color flow helps to assess the severity of the aortic stenosis to determine how much, if any, blood is flowing through the stenotic aortic leaflets (Figure 30-30, *B*).

Subvalvular or Supravalvular Aortic Stenosis. Subvalvular aortic stenosis occurs when a membrane covers the left ventricular outflow tract (Figure 30-31, *A* and *B*). Supravalvular aortic stenosis is a narrowing of the ascending aortic root.

Supravalvular aortic stenosis may be related to the Williams' syndrome (Figure 30-32). Subaortic stenosis has been described in patients with Turner's syndrome, Noonan's syndrome, and congenital rubella.

Sonographic Findings. The left ventricular outflow tract should be carefully evaluated in the parasternal long-axis, apical five-chamber, and aortic arch views to image this thin membrane. The Doppler view shows increased velocity across the obstructive membrane, whereas color flow imaging shows increased turbulence at the area of narrowing.

HYPOPLASTIC LEFT HEART SYNDROME

Hypoplastic left heart syndrome is characterized by a small, hypertrophied left ventricle with aortic and/or mitral dysplasia or atresia (Figure 30-33). This syndrome has been found to be an autosomal-recessive condition. If a couple has had one child with hypoplastic left heart syndrome, the recurrence is 4%; if two births have been affected, recurrence increases to 25%.

Although the cause of the hypoplastic left heart is unknown, it is thought to be decreased filling and perfusion of the left ventricle during embryologic development. It also may be associated with premature closure of the foramen ovale. When this closure occurs, the blood cannot cross the foramen to help the left ventricle grow. The real-time image shows a reduction in the size of the foramen ovale (the foramen should measure at least 0.6 multiplied by the diameter of the aortic root). Premature closure of the foramen would also show increased velocities across the interatrial septum (around 40 to 50 cm/sec).

The right ventricle supplies both the pulmonic and systemic circulations. The pulmonary venous return is diverted from the left atrium to the right atrium through the interatrial communication. Through the pulmonary artery and ductus arteriosus, the right ventricle supplies the descending aorta, along with retrograde flow to the aortic arch and the ascending aorta. Overload on the right ventricle may lead to congestive heart failure in utero with the development of pericardial effusion and hydrops.

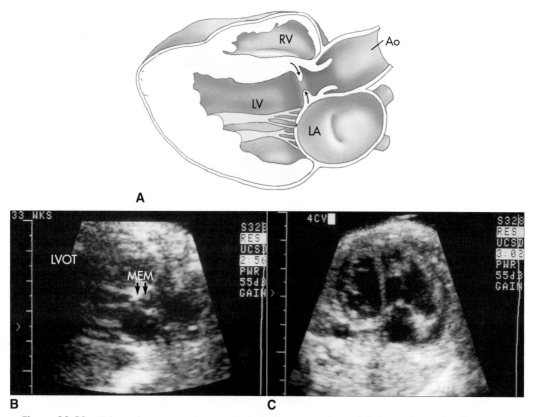

Figure 30-31 Submembranous aortic stenosis. **A,** A discrete membrane inferior to the aortic valve is shown in the parasternal long-axis view *(arrows). Ao,* aorta; *RV,* right ventricle; *LV,* left ventricle; *LA,* left atrium. **B,** Submembranous aortic obstruction. Long-axis view of the ascending aorta and left ventricle shows the thick membrane *(MEM, arrows)* that is located above the aortic cusps to cause obstruction to the left ventricular outflow tract *(LVOT).* **C,** This outflow obstruction causes the left ventricle to enlarge, as seen on this four-chamber view, and go into failure. A small pericardial effusion is seen around the heart.

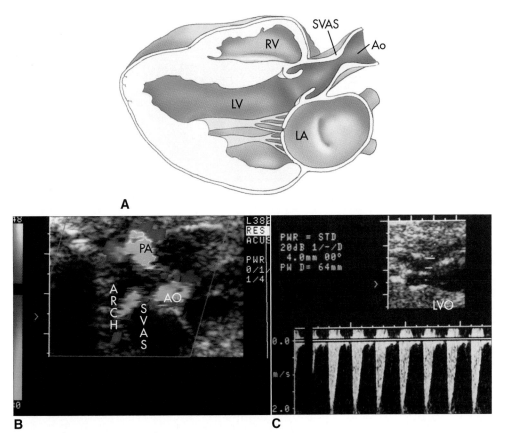

Figure 30-32 Supravalvular aortic stenosis. **A,** The parasternal long-axis view shows the hourglass narrowing of the ascending aorta superior to the aortic valve. **B,** Long-axis view of the ascending aorta *(AO)* and arch with the supravalvular narrowing *(SVAS)*. *PA,* Pulmonary artery. **C,** Doppler velocities measure 200 cm/sec, well above the normal range.

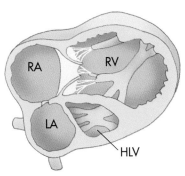

Figure 30-33 Hypoplastic left heart syndrome is characterized by a small, hypertrophied left ventricle *(HLV)* with aortic and/or mitral atresia. *LA,* Left atrium; *RA,* right atrium; *RV,* right ventricle.

Sonographic Findings. A fetus with major disturbance to the development of the mitral valve or aortic valve shows dramatic changes in the development of the left ventricle. The amount of hypoplasia depends on when the left-sided atresia developed in the valvular area (Figure 30-34). If the mitral atresia is the cause, the blood cannot fill the left ventricle to provide volume, and thus the aortic valve becomes atretic as well, with concentric hypertrophy of the small left ventricular cavity. If the cause is aortic stenosis, the myocardium shows

extreme hypertrophy from the increased pressure overload (Figure 30-35).

M-mode imaging may be used to further define the ventricular disproportion. The sonographer must be aware that even in normal fetuses, the M-mode and real-time measurements of the ventricles depend totally on the position of the fetus, position of the transducer, and angle of the cursor. Therefore, it is important to make sure the transducer is directly perpendicular to the right and left ventricles before making an M-mode measurement. This measurement is always slightly smaller than the real-time direct measurement because the detail of the endocardium is seen better on the M-mode than on the real-time image.

The prognosis for a fetus with a hypoplastic left heart is not good. This syndrome is responsible for 25% of cardiac deaths in the neonatal period. The surgeon Norwood has developed a series of surgical repairs for the hypoplastic left heart patient. His repairs are based on the development of the aorta and aortic arch. Initial palliative procedures are done, including atrial balloon septostomy, banding of the pulmonary artery (to protect the potential volume overload to the lungs), and creation of an aortopulmonary shunt. The modified Fontan surgical procedure is done to connect the left atrium to the tricuspid valve and the right atrium to the pulmonary artery. Norwood's challenge is to rebuild the hypoplastic aorta to

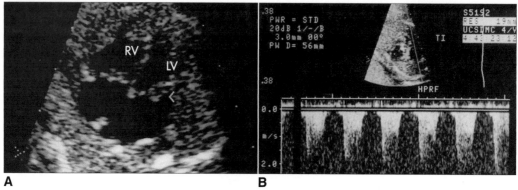

Figure 30-34 Hypoplastic left heart. **A,** Four-chamber view shows asymmetry between the right *(RV)* and left *(LV)* ventricles. The aorta and ascending aorta were also hypertrophied. **B,** Backflow of pressures from the left ventricular outflow obstruction results in severe tricuspid regurgitation.

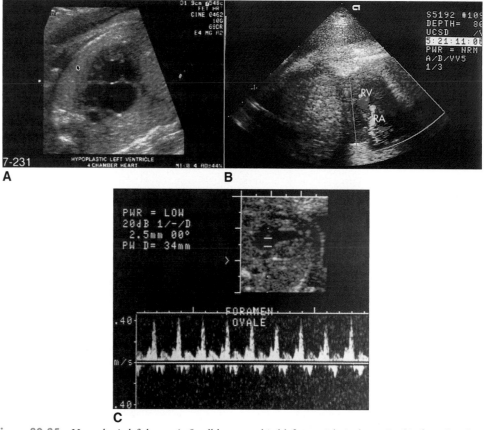

Figure 30-35 Hypoplastic left heart. **A,** Small hypertrophied left ventricle is shown in this four-chamber view. **B,** Color Doppler imaging helps to define if any inflow is going into the left ventricle or how much tricuspid regurgitation is present. *RA,* Right atrium; *RV,* right ventricle. **C,** Flow across the foramen ovale may be increased with restriction of the flap of the foramen.

improve blood flow into the left ventricle. Cardiac transplantation is another alternative for these patients.

GREAT VESSEL ABNORMALITIES

Great vessel abnormalities include interruption in the spiraling that occurs during early embryonic development. These anomalies also include complete transposition of the great arteries, corrected transposition of the great arteries, and truncus arteriosus.

TRANSPOSITION OF THE GREAT ARTERIES
Transposition of the great arteries is an abnormal condition that exists when the aorta is connected to the right ventricle and the pulmonary artery is connected to the left ventricle (Figure 30-36). The atrioventricular valves are normally

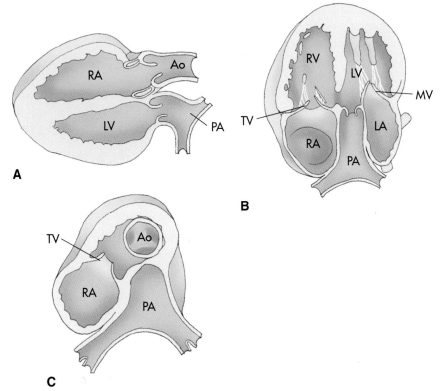

Figure 30-36   Transposition of the great arteries. **A,** Four-chamber view shows the aorta *(Ao)* anteriorly, arising from the right ventricle, and the pulmonary artery *(PA)* posteriorly, arising from the left ventricle *(LV)*. *RA,* Right atrium. **B,** Five-chamber view shows the pulmonary artery *(PA)* arising from the left ventricle *(LV)*; as the transducer follows the great artery, the bifurcation of the branch arteries is seen. *LA,* Left atrium; *MV,* mitral valve; *TV,* tricuspid valve. **C,** Short-axis view shows the aorta *(Ao)* anterior to the pulmonary artery *(PA)*.

attached and related. This occurs because of an abnormal completion of the "loop" in embryology. The great vessels originate as a common truncus and undergo rotation and spiraling; if this development is interrupted, the great arteries do not complete their spiral and thus transposition occurs. Usually the aorta is anterior and to the right of the pulmonary artery. Less frequently the two arteries are side by side or the aorta is posterior.

In the fetal heart, no hemodynamic compromise is seen in the fetus when the great arteries are transposed. The problems occur in the neonatal period when there is inadequate mixing of oxygenated and unoxygenated blood.

The prognosis for a neonate with transposition of the great arteries is quite good with surgical intervention. The survival rate is 92% at 1 year with surgical correction. Survival depends on other cardiac anomalies that may also be present.

Other associated cardiac anomalies include atrial septal defects, anomalies of the atrioventricular valves, and underdevelopment of the right or left ventricles.

Sonographic Findings. The parasternal short-axis view is the key view to image the great arteries and their normal relationship (Figure 30-37). The right ventricular outflow tract, pulmonary artery, and bifurcation should be seen anterior to the aorta in the parasternal short-axis view. In transposition this relationship is not present; it is impossible to demonstrate

the bifurcation of the pulmonary artery because the aorta would be the anterior vessel. Sometimes the double circles of the great arteries can be seen in this view.

On the modified long-axis view, the normal crisscross pattern (Figure 30-38) obtained from a normal fetal echocardiogram occurs when the transducer is swept from the left ventricular outflow tract anterior and medial into the right ventricular outflow tract. In a fetus with transposition, this crisscross sweep of the great arteries is not possible. The parallel great arteries are sometimes seen in this view as they both arise from the ventricles.

Corrected Transposition of the Great Arteries. Corrected transposition of the great arteries is a cardiac condition in which the right atrium and left atrium are connected to the morphologic left and right ventricle, respectively, and the great arteries are transposed. Therefore, these two defects essentially cancel each other out without hemodynamic consequences.

Sonographic Findings. Corrected transposition is associated with malpositions of the heart and sometimes with situs inversus. A ventricular perimembranous septal defect may be present in half of the fetuses. The pulmonary artery may be seen to override the septal defect, with pulmonary stenosis in 50%. Abnormalities of the atrioventricular valves, such as an

Ebstein type of malformation and straddling of the tricuspid valve, may be present. Atrioventricular heart block may also be recorded.

TRUNCUS ARTERIOSUS

Truncus arteriosus is a complex congenital heart lesion in which only one great artery arises from the base of the heart (Figure 30-39). From this single great artery arise the pulmonary trunk, the systemic arteries, and the coronary arteries. This defect occurs in the early embryologic period when the conotruncus fails to separate into two great arteries. The conus corresponds to the middle third of the bulbus cordis. It gives rise to the outflow tract of both ventricles and to the muscular portion of the ventricles located between the atrioventricular and semilunar valves. The truncus is the distal part of the bulbus cordis. This structure rotates and divides into the two great semilunar valvular structures that represent the aortic and pulmonic leaflets. Failure of the bulbus to divide causes a single great artery with multiple cusps within.

Associated anomalies include mitral atresia, atrial septal defect, univentricular heart, and aortic arch abnormalities. In the neonatal stage the prognosis is poor for truncus arteriosus.

Sonographic Findings. The fetal echo shows an abnormal, large, single great vessel arising from the ventricles (Figure 30-40). Usually an infundibular ventricular septal defect is present. Significant septal override is present. The truncal valve is usually dysplastic, thick, and domed. Multiple cusps are seen within the great artery. If truncal regurgitation is present, the prognosis is grim; the fetus usually develops congestive heart failure, pericardial effusion, and hydrops. Truncus arteriosus may be difficult to separate from a severe tetralogy of Fallot with pulmonary atresia (small pulmonary artery and large aorta overriding septal defect).

COARCTATION OF THE AORTA

Coarctation of the aorta is a discrete shelflike lesion present in the isthmus of the arch or, more commonly, at the site of the ductal insertion near the left subclavian artery (Figure 30-41, *A*). The coarctation may be discrete, long-segment, or tubular.

Intracardiac associated malformations are present in 90% of cases. These include aortic stenosis, aortic insufficiency,

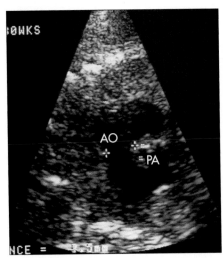

Figure 30-37   Short-axis view shows the dilated aorta *(Ao)* anterior to the hypertrophied pulmonary artery *(PA)* in this patient with transposition.

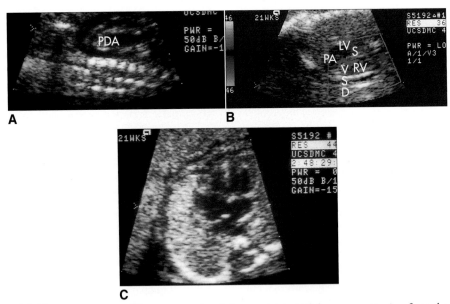

Figure 30-38   Transposition of the great arteries. **A,** Long-axis view of the aorta as it arises from the anterior right ventricle. *PDA,* Patent ductus arteriosus. **B,** A ventricular septal defect *(VSD)* is usually present in the fetus with transposition of the great vessels. *LV,* Left ventricle; *PA,* pulmonary artery; *RV,* right ventricle; *S,* septum. **C,** Four-chamber view shows the membranous septal defect.

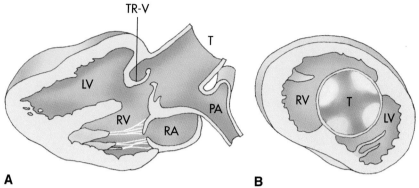

Figure 30-39   Truncus arteriosus results when the aorta and pulmonary arteries *(PA)* fail to complete their rotations and divisions early in development. A single large great artery is shown as it arises from the center of the heart on the long-axis view **(A)**. *LV,* Left ventricle; *RA,* right atrium; *RV,* right ventricle; *T,* truncus; *TR-V,* truncal valve. The short-axis view **(B)** shows the single great artery with multiple cusps within.

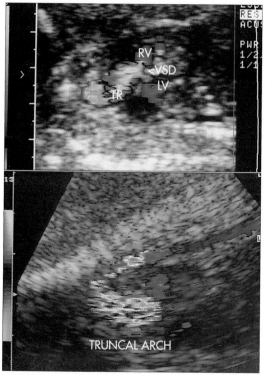

Figure 30-40   Color Doppler imaging demonstrates the single large vessel arising from both ventricles. The multiple cusps within the large vessel may be deformed and dysplastic, resulting in moderate to significant aortic insufficiency. *LV,* Left ventricle; *RV,* right ventricle; *TR,* tricuspid regurgitation; *VSD,* ventricular septal defect.

septal defects, transposition of the great arteries, truncus arteriosus, and double-outlet right ventricle. In Turner's syndrome, coarctation of the aorta and ventricular septal defects are the most common cardiac defects found.

Sonographic Findings. If a bicuspid aortic valve is suspected, the aortic arch should be carefully searched for a narrowing or coarctation of the aorta. There is a 25% association of bicuspid aortic valves in fetuses with coarctation of the

aorta. It is important to keep in mind that coarctation may be difficult to evaluate in the fetus because the ductus arteriosus is patent, so some of the blood may flow into the arch during fetal life (see Figure 30-41, *B*). Once the fetus is delivered and the ductus closes, however, the narrowed portion of the arch becomes evident.

INTERRUPTED AORTIC ARCH
Interruption of the aortic arch is characterized by complete anatomic interruption of the arch or, rarely, by an atretic fibrous remnant connecting the proximal arch with the descending aorta. The interruption occurs at one of three sites:

1. Distal to the left common carotid artery, so the left subclavian artery originates from the descending aorta
2. Just beyond the left subclavian, so that all the brachiocephalic arteries arise from the arch and none from the descending aorta
3. Distal to the innominate artery, so that the left common carotid and left subclavian arteries originate from the descending aorta

The descending aorta is really a continuation of the main pulmonary artery via the patent ductus. A ventricular septal defect is almost always present. After birth, these three items make a distinct congenital triad: interruption of the aortic arch, patent ductus arteriosus, and ventricular septal defect.

The interruption of the aortic arch also tends to occur with a bicuspid or deformed aortic valve, subaortic stenosis, biventricular origin of the pulmonary trunk, or anomalous origin of the major branches of the ascending aorta.

DUCTAL CONSTRICTION
Ductal constriction occurs when flow is diverted from the ductus secondary to tricuspid or pulmonary atresia or secondary to maternal medications given to stop early contractions. In the normal fetus the ductus arteriosus transmits about 55% to 60% of combined ventricular output from the pulmonary

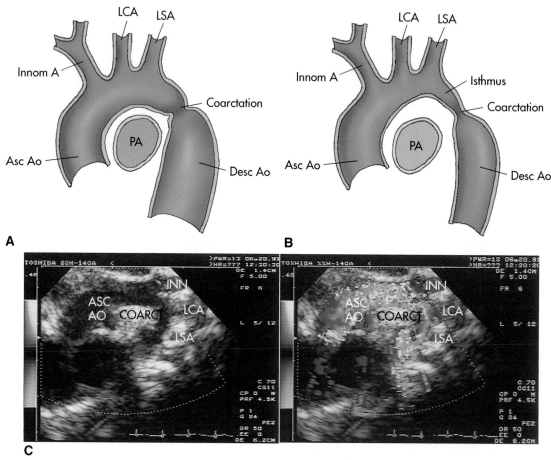

Figure 30-41   Coarctation of the aorta occurs just inferior to the insertion of the left subclavian artery *(LSA).* The coarctation may be discrete **(A)** with mild poststenotic dilation in the fetus. This narrowing usually is near the point of ductal insertion. *Asc Ao,* Ascending aorta; *INN,* innominate artery; *LCA,* left carotid artery. **B,** A long-segment narrowing of the isthmus is more likely to be found by echocardiography. **C,** A discrete narrowing was found in this 32-week fetus. Long-axis view of the aortic arch shows the narrowing at the level of the left subclavian artery. Pulsed Doppler imaging recorded velocities of 190 cm/sec. *COARCT,* Coarctation; *INN,* innominate artery.

artery to the aorta. It joins the aorta at an obtuse inferior angle, presumably because flow is directed down to the descending aorta. If aortic atresia or aortic isthmus interruption were present, a much larger proportion of the output would have to flow through the ductus to maintain ventricular output; in fact, in aortic atresia, the total output—excluding pulmonary flow—would cross the ductus. Thus, about 90% of combined ventricular output would be carried by the ductus, which could be considerably wider than normal (no change in Doppler velocities at the ductus).

In tricuspid or pulmonary atresia, no blood would be ejected from the right ventricle into the pulmonary artery. The flow through the ductus would occur from the aorta to the pulmonary arteries. Because this normally represents only about 10% of the combined ventricular output, the ductus may be quite narrow and underdeveloped (with high-velocity Doppler recordings at the level of the ductus). Furthermore, since flow is from the aorta to the pulmonary artery, the connection of the ductus with the aorta has an acute inferior angle.

CARDIAC TUMORS

Cardiac tumors of the heart are very unusual. Most of these tumors are benign and isolated. The most common tumors are rhabdomyoma (58%) and teratoma (20%), followed by fibroma, myxoma, hemangioma, and mesothelioma. Less than 10% of cardiac tumors are malignant.

RHABDOMYOMAS

Rhabdomyomas tend to be multiple and involve the septum. This tumor is associated with tuberous sclerosis (50% to 86%) (Figure 30-42). The fetus becomes symptomatic when the tumor is large and causes obstruction to the outflow tract, leading to congestive heart failure, pericardial effusion, hydrops, and death. The prognosis depends on the size of the tumor, its location, and its histologic type.

Sonographic Findings. If this mass is suspected, the sonographer should also look for associated tumor mass abnormalities in the kidneys and fetal head. The teratoma may be

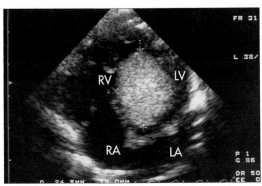

Figure 30-42   Four-chamber view of a fetus with a huge rhabdomyoma completely filling the left ventricular cavity. *LA,* Left artery; *LV,* left ventricle; *RA,* right artery; *RV,* right ventricle.

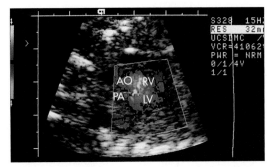

Figure 30-44   Color flow image demonstrates complete filling of the essentially "single ventricle" in a patient with transposition of the great arteries and a huge ventricular septal defect. *AO,* Aorta; *LV,* left ventricle; *PA,* pulmonary artery; *RV,* right ventricle.

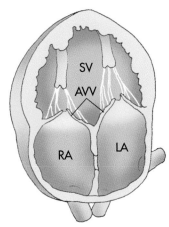

Figure 30-43   Three-chamber view shows a single inflow cavity (single ventricle *[SV]*). Two atrial cavities and atrioventricular valves *(AVV)* are present. *LA,* Left atrium; *RA,* right atrium.

intrapericardial and extracardiac. The fibroma tumors account for 12% of all cardiac tumors in the neonate. This tumor is pedunculated and may calcify.

The fetal echo shows the tumor best in the four-chamber view. Close analysis should be made to search for regurgitation and obstruction. The right and left ventricular outflow tracts should be carefully studied with Doppler to record velocities in the subvalvular and supravalvular area. Serial evaluation may be made with fetal echocardiography to follow the ventricular function and Doppler flow patterns.

COMPLEX CARDIAC ABNORMALITIES

SINGLE VENTRICLE

Single ventricle is a congenital anomaly in which there are two atria but only one ventricular chamber, which receives both the mitral and tricuspid valves (Figure 30-43). Both valves are patent, so mitral and tricuspid atresia are excluded. (Occasionally the mitral and tricuspid valves join to form a common atrioventricular valve.)

Sonographic Findings. The most common form of a single ventricle heart is a morphologic left ventricle with a small outlet chamber that represents the infundibular portion of the right ventricle. The right or left atrioventricular connection may be absent and the great arteries may be transposed, with the aorta arising above the small outlet chamber. If transposition is present, the pulmonary artery lies posterior to the aorta. The infundibulum lies at the base of the ventricle, communicating with the aorta above and the single ventricle below. If the great vessels are normal, the infundibulum communicates with the pulmonary trunk. The outlet chambers may be left-side and anterior or right-side and anterior, but they commonly lie high on the cardiac silhouette.

Pulmonary stenosis may or may not coexist. If present, the pulmonary stenosis is usually valvular or subvalvular. The pulmonary trunk is usually slightly smaller than the aortic trunk.

The four-chamber view is the most useful window in delineating the cardiac anatomy (Figure 30-44). The prominent papillary muscles should not be confused with the interventricular septum. In a single ventricle, the papillary muscles may be quite prominent. With careful transducer angulation, the chordal structures may be traced to these structures for correct delineation. The right ventricle may be just a slitlike cavity as seen on the apical four-chamber view. The position of the great arteries should be assessed, and the aorta and pulmonary arteries should be delineated clearly. Regurgitant jets may be associated with abnormal chordal connections of the atrioventricular valves. Doppler evaluation of these valves is useful in depicting any regurgitation present. Color flow imaging is especially useful in outlining the direction of jet flow for proper Doppler evaluation.

COR TRIATRIATUM

Cor triatriatum occurs when the left atrial cavity is partitioned into two compartments. This anomaly is characterized by drainage of the pulmonary veins into an accessory left atrial chamber that lies proximal to the true left atrium (Figure 30-45). The accessory chamber is believed to represent the dilated common pulmonary vein of the embryo. (This lesion has also been called stenosis of the common pulmonary vein.) The distal compartment communicates with the mitral valve and

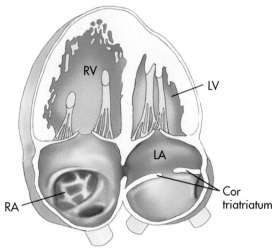

Figure 30-45   Cor triatriatum. Four-chamber view of the heart shows the pulmonary veins draining into a segment of the left atrial cavity, separated from the mitral inflow by the subdividing membrane. The amount of obstruction into the left ventricle will depend on how tight the orifice of the cor triatriatum is.

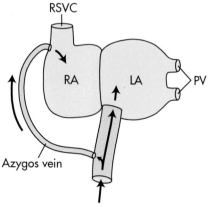

Figure 30-46   The inferior vena cava *(IVC)* communicates directly with the left atrium *(LA)*. An enlarged azygous vein arises from the anomalous IVC and communicates with the right atrium *(RA)* via a normal right superior vena cava *(RSVC)*. Inferior caval blood flows directly into the left atrium (large arrow); a portion of the IVC blood is diverted through the azygous vein into the right superior cava and right heart *(small arrow)*. *PV*, pulmonary veins.

contains the left atrial appendage and usually the fossa ovalis. The fibrous or fibromuscular diaphragm that partitions the left atrium possesses one or more openings, and the size of these openings determines the degree of left atrial obstruction.

CONGENITAL VENA CAVA TO LEFT ATRIAL COMMUNICATION

Isolated connection of the superior or inferior vena cava to the left atrium is a rare congenital malformation. The left atrium occasionally receives other systemic veins, such as the coronary sinus, the azygous vein, or the hepatic vein.

Inferior Vena Cava. When the inferior vena cava communicates with the left atrium, the vessel usually has a normal abdominal course and penetrates the diaphragm at the expected site. An enlarged azygous vein may arise from the anomalous inferior cava and ultimately communicate with the right atrium (Figure 30-46). Normally the azygous vein begins as a branch of the inferior vena cava, then proceeds upward through the aortic hiatus of the diaphragm, passes along the right side of the vertebral column, and finally arches forward to enter the superior vena cava. An enlarged azygous system can serve an important function as a conveyor of inferior vena caval blood to the right atrium even though the inferior cava itself communicates with the left atrium. Occasionally the inferior vena cava is absent and infradiaphragmatic blood reaches the right atrium entirely via the azygous system.

Superior Vena Cava. Congenital abnormalities of the superior vena cava generally fall into two categories: anomalies of position and anomalies of drainage (Figure 30-47). Anomalies of position, especially persistent left superior vena cava, are relatively more frequent than those of drainage. A left superior vena cava itself causes no physiological disturbance since it harmlessly drains into the right atrium via the coronary

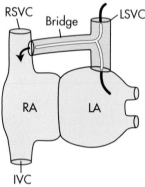

Figure 30-47   Persistent left superior vena cava *(LSVC)* communicating with the left atrium *(LA)*. The size of the bridge may vary; when very small the LSVC blood flows entirely into the left atrium. *RSVC*, right superior vena cava; *IVC*, inferior vena cava; *RA*, right atrium; *LA*, left atrium.

sinus. However, a persistent left superior vena cava assumes particular significance when it communicates with the left atrium. It also follows that when a superior vena cava drains into the left atrium, the anomalously draining vessel is likely to be a persistent left cava. A right superior vena cava usually coexists and enters the right atrium in normal fashion.

When two superior cavas are present, the right and left may be completely separate from each other or may be joined by means of an innominate vein. This "innominate bridge" can be widely patent, small, or atretic.

The intracardiac defects that may accompany caval drainage into the left atrium include atrial or ventricular septal defects, single atrium or ventricle, tetralogy of Fallot, transposition of great vessels, and complex positional anomalies of the heart. The extracardiac anomalies that have been associated with this condition include coarctation of the aorta, pulmonary arteriovenous fistula, and inferior vena cava malformations.

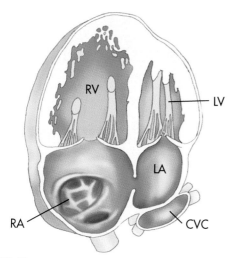

Figure 30-48 Four-chamber view of the heart showing total anomalous pulmonary venous return. In this view the veins are shown to enter the anomalous common venous chamber *(CVC)* superior to the left atrial cavity *(LA)*. RA, right atrium; RV, right ventricle; LV, left ventricle.

TOTAL ANOMALOUS PULMONARY VENOUS RETURN

The four pulmonary veins normally return blood into the left atrium from the lungs. When this fails to occur, the condition is termed **total anomalous pulmonary venous return (TAPVR).** The venous return may be totally into the right atrium or into a "common chamber" posterior to the left atrium, into the superior or inferior vena cava, or into the left subclavian vein, azygos vein, or portal vein. The venous drainage may be total or partial (Figure 30-48).

Sonographic Findings. In the fetus, TAPVR may not be evident unless the pulmonary veins are carefully recorded. The sonographer may image an enlarged right atrial cavity with the atrial septum bulging into the small left atrium. The normal pulmonary veins are seen on the four-chamber view. The right upper vein is seen near the base of the heart at the level of the septum secundum, the left upper vein is seen at the lateral atrial wall near the base of the heart, and the left lower vein is seen just above the atrioventricular junction, along the lateral atrial wall. The right lower vein is not routinely imaged in a four-chamber view. Color Doppler imaging may help identify these venous structures.

TAPVR should be suspected in all cases of atrioventricular septal defects and in asplenia and polysplenia syndromes. The prognosis is poor, with 75% dying within the first year after birth if no surgery is performed. Reconstruction of the pulmonary venous drainage into the left atrium has shown very promising survival results.

CARDIOSPLENIC SYNDROMES

Cardiosplenic syndromes are sporadic disorders characterized by a symmetric development of normally asymmetric organs or organ systems. The cardiosplenic syndromes are subdivided into asplenia and polysplenia syndromes. These two conditions are characterized by lack of the normal asymmetry of the vis-

ceral organs. The trunk tends to have two halves that are mirror images of one another. Generally speaking, asplenia is a condition of bilateral right-sidedness and polysplenia is bilateral left-sidedness.

In a fetus with asplenia, the following anomalies have been seen: the spleen is absent; the lungs are bilaterally trilobed with morphologic right bronchi on both sides; the liver is central; the stomach may be right, left, or central; the gut is malrotated; the superior vena cava is bilateral; the inferior vena cava lies to the right or left of the spine; and the aorta and cava are seen on the same side of the spine (instead of the aorta on the left and the cava on the right).

There is a high association between asplenia and congenital heart disease. Total anomalous pulmonary venous return was seen in nearly all patients, atrioventricular septal defect in 85%, single ventricle in 51%, transposition of the great arteries in 58%, and pulmonary stenosis or atresia in 70%. In less than half the patients, dextrocardia was present. Asplenia syndrome is twice as common in males.

Polysplenia syndrome is characterized by two or more spleens on both sides of the mesogastrium. Bilateral morphologic left lungs and bronchi are found in 68% of patients. The liver and stomach are on the right or left, malrotation of the bowel is found in 80%, bilateral superior vena cava is seen in half the fetuses, and the inferior vena cava is absent in 70% (blood is drained by the azygos vein, which may be on the right or left).

Cardiac malformations are frequent, but not as common as with asplenia. The most common lesions found are TAPVR (70%), dextrocardia, atrial septal defect, AVSD, transposition of the great arteries, and double-outlet right ventricle.

The prognosis of this disease depends on the severity of the cardiac lesion. Surgical intervention has increased the survival rate.

Sonographic Findings. The recognition of the cardiosplenic syndrome relies on the demonstration of both the abnormal relationship between the abdominal organs and the associated cardiac deformities. The abdominal situs must be determined clearly—with the stomach on the left, heart apex on the left, aorta on the left, and inferior vena on the right—to rule out a cardiosplenic syndrome.

ECTOPIC CORDIS

Ectopia cordis is a heart lesion that results from an abnormal development of the primitive heart outside the embryonic disk in the early stage of development (Figure 30-49).

Associated anomalies include facial and skeletal deformities, ventral wall defects, and central nervous system malformations (meningocele and cephalocele). Cardiac anomalies include tetralogy of Fallot and transposition of the great arteries. The prognosis is very poor for this fetus.

DYSRHYTHMIAS

The fetal heart undergoes multiple changes during the embryologic stages. One of these stages is the progression of the cardiac electrical system, which matures to cause a normal sinus

TABLE 30-4   SONOGRAPHIC PITFALLS FOR ARRHYTHMIAS

Heart Rate	Rhythm	Features: Atrial to Ventricular Association
40-60	Complete heart block	A-V dissociation
60-90	Atrial bigeminy	Every other atrial impulse blocked
80-110	Sinus bradycardia	Normal A-V conduction
105-185	Normal sinus rhythm	Normal A-V conduction
180-210	Sinus tachycardia	Normal A-V conduction
150-220	Ventricular tachycardia	A-V dissociation or 1:1 V-A conduction
180+	SVT (ectopic)	1:1 A-V conduction, incessant
220-260	SVT (reentrant)	A-V conduction with sudden onset and cessation
150-600	Atrial flutter	1:1 A-V conduction or 2:1, 3:1, 4:1 A-V block
Any rate	Ectopy or blocked atrial PVCs	Frequent or occasional PACs conducted

A-V, Atrioventricular; *PACs,* premature atrial contractions; *PVCs,* premature ventricular contractions; *SVT,* supraventricular tachycardia.

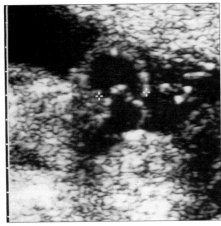

Figure 30-49   A fetus with pentalogy of Cantrell (multiple midline defects), including ectopia cordis. The heart was completely outside the thoracic cavity.

rhythm in the cardiac cycle. It is not uncommon during the course of a fetal echocardiogram to see the normal fetal heart rate decelerate from 150 beats per minute to a bradycardia stage (under 55 beats per minute), or even to pause for a few seconds. This may happen if the baby is lying on the umbilical cord or if the transducer pressure is too great. The fetus should be given a recovery time to bring the heart rate to a normal sinus rhythm. This is usually done by changing the position of the mother or releasing the pressure from the transducer.

Other changes in rhythm patterns seen during fetal development may result from premature atrial and ventricular contractions, supraventricular tachycardia, tachycardia, or atrioventricular block (Table 30-4).

ECTOPY

Premature Atrial and Ventricular Contractions. Electrical impulses generated outside the cardiac pacemaker (sinus node) can cause **premature atrial** and **ventricular** contractions, commonly called **PACs** and **PVCs**. The sinus node is located along the lateral right atrial wall. It is not clearly understood why some patients develop these ectopic premature contractions. Some investigators have tried to link them to increased amounts of caffeine, alcohol, or smoking, but none of our patients with PACs has these associations. An increased redundancy of the flap of the foramen ovale has been noted in these patients. The flap is larger than seen in the normal fetus and appears to swing with a great excursion from the left atrium into the right atrial cavity, touching the right atrial node.

The patient is usually referred for a fetal cardiac arrhythmia as heard on the routine obstetric examination by Doptone or auscultation. These techniques provide information about the ventricular rate only. To adequately assess the fetal rhythm, the ventricular and atrial rates must be analyzed simultaneously.

The atrium and ventricle may both experience extrasystoles and ectopic beats to give rise to complex echo patterns. The PACs may either be conducted to the ventricles or blocked, depending on the moment in which they occur in the cardiac cycle (Figure 30-50). Repeated PACs may lead to an increased or decreased ventricular rate. A blocked PAC must be differentiated from an atrioventricular block. This distinction relies on the demonstration of an atrial contraction that appears prematurely. PVCs are characterized by a PVC that is not preceded by an atrial contraction.

Sonographic Findings. The sonographer can help sort out the rhythm with M-mode and real-time ultrasound. To record the atrial and ventricular rates simultaneously, the four-chamber heart must be perpendicular to the transducer. The M-mode beam must dissect the ventricle and atria of the heart. It does not matter if the right or left side of the heart is more anterior. The best area to record atrial motion is usually just superior to the atrioventricular junction along the lateral wall of the atria. The atrial pattern appears to move with a box type of motion. The ventricular rate is best recorded at the level of the atrioventricular valve and is seen to move as a smooth, uniform, well-defined pattern.

If the sonographer cannot obtain adequate images from the four-chamber view, the parasternal short-axis view may be used. The M-mode beam should be directed through the right atrial wall, aortic cusps, or the left atrial wall and aortic cusps. As the aorta moves in an anterior direction, the aortic cusps open in systole and close in diastole. Thus the aortic leaflets may signify the ventricular systolic event, whereas the atrial wall signifies the atrial event.

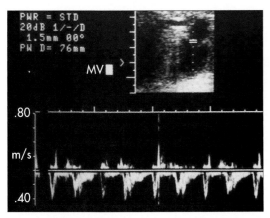

Figure 30-50 Fetus with premature atrial contractions. The fetus had normal cardiac anatomy.

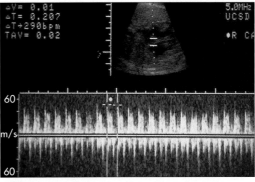

Figure 30-51 Fetus with supraventricular tachycardia showed normal conduction with a heart rate of more than 220 beats per minute.

The M-mode should be expanded to its full extent to clearly see the movement of the atrial and ventricular walls. Changes in the atrioventricular valve patterns are also noted in patients with arrhythmias. Doppler imaging of the atrioventricular valves demonstrates whether regurgitation is present during the disturbance in rhythm.

Patients with PACs and PVCs are assured that this development is a normal benign condition resulting from the immaturity of the electrical conduction system of the heart. This pattern is not associated with other cardiac anomalies.

SUPRAVENTRICULAR TACHYARRHYTHMIA

Supraventricular tachyarrhythmias include abnormal rhythms above 200 beats per minute with a conduction rate of 1:1 (Figure 30-51). These rhythm disturbances may be paroxysmal supraventricular tachycardia, paroxysmal atrial tachycardia, atrial flutter, or atrial fibrillation. In atrial flutter the atrial rate is recorded at 300 to 460 beats per minute with a normal ventricular rate. Atrial fibrillation shows the atria to beat at more than 400 beats per minute, with a ventricular rate of 120 to 200 beats per minute.

Supraventricular tachycardia occurs by automaticity or reentry mechanisms. In cases of automatic induced tachyarrhythmias, an irritable ectopic focus discharges at a high frequency. The reentry mechanism consists of an electrical impulse reentering the atria, giving rise to repeated electrical activity. Reentry may occur at the level of the sinoatrial node, inside the atrium, at the atrioventricular node, and in the His-Purkinje system. Reentry may also occur along an anomalous atrioventricular connection, such as the Kent bundle in Wolff-Parkinson-White (WPW) syndrome.

Supraventricular tachycardia is the most frequent arrhythmia caused by atrioventricular nodal reentry, occurring in 1 in 25,000 births. Viral infections or hypoplasia of the sinoatrial tract may trigger supraventricular tachycardia.

Sonographic Findings. The finding of supraventricular tachycardia in a fetus is an emergency situation. The fetus should be scanned immediately to assess signs of heart rate, ventricular and atrial size, amount of regurgitation present, ventricular function, and presence of pericardial effusion and hydrops (Figure 30-52). With supraventricular tachycardia, the fetus develops suboptimal filling of the ventricles, decreased cardiac output, and right ventricular volume overload leading to subsequent congestive heart failure.

Other cardiac anomalies associated with supraventricular tachycardia are atrial septal defects, mitral valve disease, cardiac tumors, and WPW syndrome.

Atrial flutter and fibrillation often alternate and are thought to result from a mechanism similar to that found in supraventricular tachycardia. Atrial flutter and fibrillation have been described in patients with WPW syndrome, cardiomyopathies, and thyrotoxicosis.

The fetus with this arrhythmia is usually admitted to the hospital and medically treated with antiarrhythmic drugs to control the ventricular rate, with the goal of converting the rate into normal sinus rhythm. Fetal echocardiography may be clinically useful in monitoring these patients' recovery.

ATRIOVENTRICULAR BLOCK

When the transmission of the electrical impulse from the atria to the ventricles is blocked, the condition is called an **atrioventricular block.** Normally the atria fill in ventricular diastole and empty in ventricular systole. Just before ventricular systole occurs, the pressure in the atria is at its peak (this corresponds to the p wave on the ECG). The QRS complex signifies the onset of ventricular systole, causing the pressure from the atria to open the atrioventricular valves so the left ventricle may fill. If this electrical process is blocked, the blood remains in the atria and does not cause the atrioventricular valves to open so blood can fill the ventricular cavities. This condition may be attributed to immaturity of the conduction system, absence of connection to the atrioventricular node, or an abnormal anatomic position of the atrioventricular node. The fetus may have a first-, second-, or third-degree heart block.

The fetus with a third-degree atrioventricular block has been found to have associated structural anomalies, including corrected transposition, univentricular heart, cardiac tumors, and cardiomyopathies. Patients with a connective tissue disorder, such as lupus erythematosus, have also been found to develop heart block.

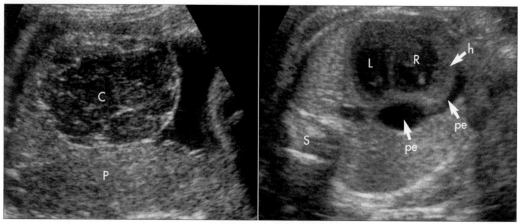

Figure 30-52　Pericardial effusion *(pe)* may be present if the arrhythmia is significant (i.e., supraventricular tachycardia). The fetus cannot withstand rapid changes in cardiac activity without developing signs of heart failure. *C,* Fetal head; *h,* heart; *L,* liver; *P,* placenta; *R,* right ventricle; *S,* spine.

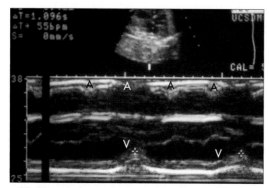

Figure 30-53　Mother with systemic lupus erythematosus presented at 20 weeks of gestation because of a "slow heart rate." The fetus was in 2:1 heart block with the atria beating twice as fast as the ventricle; every other beat was conducted. *A,* atrium; *V,* ventricle.

First- and second-degree atrioventricular blocks are not associated with any significant hemodynamic disturbance. A complete heart block may result in bradycardia, leading to decreased cardiac output and congestive heart failure during fetal life.

Sonographic Findings. The fetal M-mode echocardiogram should be performed after the normal anatomic cardiac anatomy has been demonstrated (Figure 30-53). As described in the supraventricular tachycardia section, the four-chamber and parasternal short-axis views are best used to record atrial and ventricular events simultaneously.

First-degree heart block is not seen in the fetus since the heart rate and rhythm are normal. The blockage of a normal atrial impulse can be diagnosed by demonstrating a normally timed atrial contraction that is not followed by a ventricular contraction.

Second- and third-degree heart blocks are defined by observing the relationship between the atrial and ventricular rates. In second-degree Mobitz type I block, only a few atrial impulses are not conducted; in Mobitz type II block, a sub-

multiple of atrial impulses is transmitted. In complete heart block, atrial and ventricular rates are independent of each other, with the atrial rate slower. The fetus becomes symptomatic when the cardiac output is decreased and congestive heart failure develops.

REFERENCES

1. Callen PC: *Ultrasonography in obstetrics and gynecology,* ed 3, Philadelphia, 1994, WB Saunders.
2. Roberts DJ, Genest D: Cardiac histologic pathology characteristic of trisomies 13 and 21, *Hum Pathol* 23:1130, 1992.
3. Silverman NH, Schmidt KG: Ventricular volume overload in the human fetus: observations from fetal echocardiography, *J Am Soc Echocardiography* 3:20, 1990.

SELECTED BIBLIOGRAPHY

Abuhamad A: *A practical guide to fetal echocardiography,* Philadelphia, 1997, Lippincott-Raven.

Allan LD, Sharland G, Tynan MJ: The natural history of the hypoplastic left heart syndrome, *Int J Cardiol* 25:341, 1989.

Allen L: *Manual of fetal echocardiography,* London, 1986, MTP Press Limited.

Beeby AR and others: Reproducibility of ultrasonic measurement of fetal cardiac haemodynamics, *Br J Obstet Gynaecol* 98:807, 1991.

Brand JM, Friedberg DZ: Spontaneous regression of a primary cardiac tumor presenting as fetal tachyarrhythmias, *J Perinatol* 12:48, 1992.

Brown DL: Borderline findings in fetal cardiac sonography, *Semin Ultrasound CT MRI* 19(4):329, 1998.

Brown DL and others: The peripheral hypoechoic rim of the fetal heart, *J Ultrasound Med* 8:603, 1989.

Callan NA and others: Fetal echocardiography: indications for referral, prenatal diagnoses, and outcomes, *Am J Perinatol* 8:390, 1991.

Copel J, Pilu G, Kleinman CS: Congenital heart disease and extracardiac anomalies: associations and indications for fetal echocardiography, *Am J Obstet Gynecol* 154:1121, 1986.

Copel JA, Hobbins JC, Kleinman CS: Doppler echocardiography and color flow mapping, *Obstet Gynecol Clin North Am* 18:845, 1991.

Dolkart LA, Reimers FT: Transvaginal fetal echocardiography in early pregnancy: normative data, *Am J Obstet Gynecol* 165:688, 1991.

Gembruch U, Knopfle G, Bald R and others. Early diagnosis of fetal congenital heart disease by transvaginal echocardiography, *Ultrasound Obstet Gynecol* 3:310-317, 1993.

Hornberger LK and others: Tricuspid valve disease with significant tricuspid insufficiency in the fetus: diagnosis and outcome, *J Am Coll Cardiol* 17:167, 1991.

Hornberger LK, Sanders SP, Rein AJ and others: Left heart obstructive lesions and left ventricular growth in the midtrimester fetus. A longitudinal study, *Circulation* 92:1531-1538, 1995.

Kaltman J, Di H, Tian Z and others: Impact of congenital heart disease on cerebrovascular blood flow dynamics in the fetus, *Ultrasound Obstet Gynceol* 25(1):32-36, 2005.

Moore KL: *The developing human*, Philadelphia, 1991, WB Saunders.

Perloff J: *The clinical recognition of congenital heart disease*, Philadelphia, 1970, WB Saunders Co.

Reed KL: Cyanotic disease in the fetus, *J Am Soc Echocardiography* 3:9, 1990.

Reed KL and others: Cardiac Doppler flow velocities in human fetuses, *Circulation* 73:41, 1986.

Reed KL and others: Human fetal tricuspid and mitral deceleration time: changes with normal pregnancy and intrauterine growth retardation, *Am J Obstet Gynecol* 161:1532, 1989.

Rizzo G, Arduini D, Romanini C: Accelerated cardiac growth and abnormal cardiac flow in fetuses of type I diabetic mothers, *Obstet Gynecol* 80:369, 1992.

Romero R and others: *Prenatal diagnosis of congenital anomalies,* East Norwalk, Conn, 1988, Appleton & Lange.

Rudolph AM: *Congenital diseases of the heart,* Chicago, 1974, Year Book Medical Publishers.

Rychik J: Frontiers in fetal cardiovascular disease, *Pediatric Clinics of North America* 51:6, 2004.

Rychik J, Tian T, Cohen MD and others: Acute cardiovascular effects of fetal surgery in the human, *Circulation* 110:1549-1556, 2004.

Sahn DJ, Anderson F: *Two-dimensional anatomy of the heart*, Philadelphia, 1982, John Wiley & Sons.

Sahn DJ and others: Quantitative real-time cross sectional echocardiography in the developing normal human fetus and newborn, *Circulation* 62:3, 1980.

Shime J and others: Two-dimensional and M-mode echocardiography in the human fetus, *Am J Obstet Gynecol* 143:178, 1983.

PART VI

Vascular

CHAPTER 31

Extracranial Cerebrovascular Evaluation

Mira L. Katz

KEY TERMS

amaurosis fugax – transient partial or complete loss of vision in one eye

aphasia – inability to communicate by speech or writing

ataxia – gait disturbances

bruit – noise caused by tissue vibration produced by turbulence that causes flow disturbance

collateral pathway – occurs when one vessel becomes obstructed; smaller side branches of the vessel provide alternative flow pathways

common carotid artery (CCA) – arises from the aortic arch on the left side and from the innominate artery on the right side

CVA – cerebrovascular accident

diplopia – double vision

dysarthria – difficulty with speech because of impairment of the tongue or muscles essential to speech

dysphagia – inability or difficulty in swallowing

external carotid artery (ECA) – smaller of the two terminal branches of the common carotid artery

hemiparesis – unilateral partial or complete paralysis

internal carotid artery (ICA) – larger of the two terminal branches of the common carotid artery

RIND – reversible ischemic neurologic deficit

TIA – transient ischemic attack

vertebral artery – large branch of the subclavian arteries

vertigo – sensation of objects moving about; sensation of revolving

---

The life of an individual is often dramatically affected by having a stroke. Not only is stroke a leading cause of adult disability in the United States, but approximately 275,000 of the 700,000 strokes that occur each year result in death.[26] Stroke is the third leading cause of death in the United States. Additionally the direct (hospital, physician, rehabilitation, etc.) and indirect (lost productivity, etc.) costs associated with stroke tally more than $56.8 billion for 2005 in the United States.[26]

A stroke or "brain attack" is caused by an interruption of blood flow to the brain (ischemic stroke) or by a ruptured intracranial blood vessel (intracranial hemorrhage). Approximately 80% of all known strokes are ischemic, and the remaining 20% are hemorrhagic. Because extracranial carotid artery disease is responsible for more than 50% of all strokes, carotid ultrasound becomes an important imaging modality to identify disease that may be the potential cause of a stroke. This is important because prevention remains the best treatment for a stroke.

STROKE RISK FACTORS, WARNING SIGNS, AND SYMPTOMS

Risk factors for stroke may be categorized into those that are not modifiable and those that are changeable or can be controlled. The nonmodifiable risk factors are age (the risk of stroke dramatically increases with increasing age), sex (the incidence of stroke is higher in males, although females generally have a more severe deficit), and race (African-Americans have a higher stroke risk than other races). The modifiable or controllable risk factors are hypertension, atrial fibrillation and other cardiac diseases, diabetes mellitus, elevated cholesterol, smoking, and a history of a sedentary lifestyle.

The five warning signs of stroke are listed in Box 31-1. It is important to remember that symptoms of weakness or numbness of a leg or arm on one side of the body indicate disease in the contralateral carotid system. In other words, left body symptoms implicate the right carotid system and vice versa. Ocular symptoms, however, suggest disease in the carotid system on the ipsilateral (same) side. For example, transient blindness of the right eye suggests disease of the carotid system on the right side.

Patients are classified as asymptomatic (without symptoms) or symptomatic. The asymptomatic patients are usually referred for carotid duplex imaging because they are at high risk for stroke or because of the presence of a cervical **bruit**. The classification of cerebrovascular symptoms includes the following: stroke or cerebrovascular accident (**CVA**) is a

permanent ischemic neurological deficit; reversible ischemic neurologic deficit (**RIND**) is a neurologic deficit that resolves in greater than 24 hours; transient ischemic attack (**TIA**) is an ischemic neurologic deficit that lasts less than 24 hours.

Other cerebrovascular (carotid and vertebral territory) symptoms include the following:

1. **amaurosis fugax**—transient partial or complete loss of vision in one eye, often described as a shade or curtain being lowered over the eye
2. **hemiparesis**—unilateral partial or complete paralysis
3. **dysarthria**—difficulty with speech because of impairment of the tongue or muscles essential to speech
4. **aphasia**—inability to communicate by speech or writing
5. **dysphagia**—inability or difficulty in swallowing
6. **ataxia**—gait disturbances
7. **diplopia**—double vision
8. **vertigo**—sensation of having objects move about the person or sensation of moving around in space

ANATOMY FOR EXTRACRANIAL CEREBROVASCULAR IMAGING

AORTIC ARCH

The ascending aorta originates from the left ventricle of the heart. The transverse aortic arch lies in the superior mediastinum and is formed as the aorta ascends and curves posteroinferiorly from right to left, above the left mainstem bronchus. It descends to the left of the trachea and esophagus. Three main arteries arise from the superior convexity of the arch in its normal configuration. The brachiocephalic trunk (innominate artery) is the first branch, the left common carotid artery the second, and the left subclavian artery the third branch in approximately 70% of cases.

The innominate artery divides into the right common carotid artery and the right subclavian artery, which gives rise to the right vertebral artery. The left common carotid artery originates slightly to the left of the innominate artery, followed by the left subclavian artery, which likewise gives rise to the left vertebral artery.

Anatomic variants of the major arch vessels occur frequently. The most commonly occurring variant (approximately 10%) is the left common carotid artery forming a common origin with or originating directly from the innominate artery. Less frequently, the left vertebral artery arises directly from the arch, the right subclavian artery originates from the arch distal to the left subclavian artery, the right common carotid artery originates directly from the arch, and a left innominate artery may exist, from which the left common carotid and left subclavian originate.

COMMON CAROTID ARTERY

Each **common carotid artery (CCA)** ascends through the superior mediastinum anterolaterally in the neck and lies medial to the jugular vein (Figure 31-1). The common carotid artery usually measures between 6 and 8 mm in diameter. The left common carotid is usually longer than the right because it

---

BOX 31-1   CLASSIC WARNING SIGNS OF STROKE

- Sudden numbness or weakness of face, arm, or leg, especially on one side of the body
- Sudden confusion; trouble speaking or understanding
- Sudden trouble seeing in one or both eyes
- Sudden trouble walking or experiencing dizziness, loss of balance, or coordination
- Sudden headache with no known cause

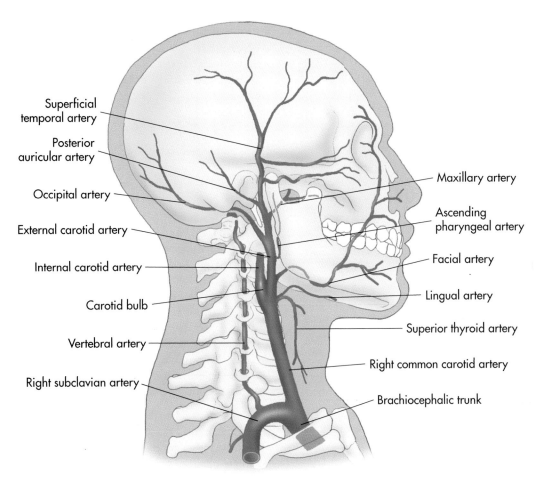

Figure 31-1   Anatomy of the extracranial carotid system. During carotid duplex imaging, the area of focus is the common carotid bifurcation because of its propensity for atherosclerotic plaque formation.

originates from the aortic arch. In the neck, the carotid artery, jugular vein, and vagus nerve are enclosed in connective tissue called the carotid sheath. The vagus nerve lies between and dorsal to the artery and vein. The CCA usually does not have branches, but occasionally it is the origin to the superior thyroid artery. The termination of the CCA is the carotid bifurcation, which is the origin of the internal carotid artery (ICA) and the external carotid artery (ECA). The CCA bifurcates in the vicinity of the superior border of the thyroid cartilage (approximately C4) in 70% of the cases, and the level of the CCA bifurcations may be asymmetric. The CCA bifurcation, however, has been described as low as T2 and as high as C1.

EXTERNAL CAROTID ARTERY

The **external carotid artery (ECA)** originates at the midcervical level and is usually the smaller of the two terminal branches of the CCA. Initially, it lies anteromedial to the ICA, but as the ECA ascends, it courses posterolaterally. In approximately 15% of the population, the ECA originates lateral to the ICA. This anatomic variation occurs more frequently on the right (3:1). The ECA usually measures 3 to 4 mm in diameter.

There are eight named branches of the ECA: the superior thyroid, ascending pharyngeal, lingual, facial, occipital, posterior auricular, and the terminal branches, the superficial temporal and the internal maxillary. The superior thyroid artery is the most commonly visualized branch of the ECA during carotid duplex imaging.

The abundant number of anastomoses between the branches of the ECA and the intracranial circulation underscore the clinical significance of the ECA as a **collateral pathway** for cerebral perfusion when significant disease is present in the ICA.

INTERNAL CAROTID ARTERY

The **internal carotid artery (ICA)** is usually the larger of the CCA terminal branches. The ICA is divided into four main segments: the cervical, petrous, cavernous, and cerebral.

The cervical portion of the ICA is evaluated during carotid duplex imaging examinations. The cervical portion of the ICA begins at the CCA bifurcation and extends to the base of the skull. The ICA lies in the carotid sheath and runs deep to the sternocleidomastoid muscle. In the majority of individuals, the ICA lies posterolateral to the ECA and courses medially as it ascends in the neck. At its origin, the cervical ICA normally

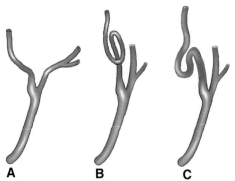

Figure 31-2 Morphologic variations of the internal carotid artery. **A,** Tortuosity: curving of the artery. **B,** Coiling: a redundant curve. **C,** Kinking: a sharp and abrupt angulation.

has a slight dilation, termed the carotid bulb. The carotid bulb may include the distal CCA, the proximal ICA, and the proximal ECA. The cervical ICA usually does not have branches and usually measures between 5 and 6 mm in diameter. With age and progressive disease, the cervical ICA may become tortuous, coiled, or kinked (Figure 31-2).

VERTEBRAL ARTERY

The vertebral arteries are large branches of the subclavian arteries. Atherosclerotic changes usually occur at the origin of the vertebral arteries. Occasionally the vertebral artery arises directly from the aortic arch (4% of cases on the left side and rarely on the right side). The two vertebral arteries are equal in size in approximately 25% of the cases; therefore, size asymmetry is common. In the majority of cases, the left vertebral artery is the dominant artery. The vertebral artery can be divided into four segments: extravertebral, intervertebral, horizontal, and intracranial.

The extravertebral segment is evaluated during the duplex imaging examination. This segment courses superiorly and medially from its subclavicular origin to enter the transverse foramen of the sixth cervical vertebra. The proximal segment of the vertebral artery is approximately 4 to 5 cm in length, and usually there are no branches. The vertebral artery ascends within the transverse foramina of the upper cervical vertebrae (intervertebral segment), emerges from the transverse foramen of the atlas (horizontal segment), and becomes the intracranial portion of the vertebral artery as it pierces the spinal dura and arachnoid below the base of the skull at the foramen magnum.

TECHNICAL ASPECTS OF CAROTID DUPLEX IMAGING

The examination is explained and a medical history (risk factors, symptoms) is obtained from the patient. Arm pressures are recorded, and a difference of ≥20 mm Hg pressure between arms suggests a proximal stenosis/occlusion of the subclavian or innominate artery on the side of the lower pressure. The presence of cervical bruits is documented by auscultation of the carotid arterial system. A bruit (noise) is caused by tissue

vibration that is produced by blood flow turbulence. Not all stenosis in the carotid arteries will cause bruits, and a bruit may be identified from a normal artery or the bruit may be transmitted (cardiac).

Suggested instrument setups for carotid duplex imaging are as follows:

1. Use a high-frequency (5-, 7- to 10-MHz) linear array transducer.
2. The image orientation is usually with the head to the left of the monitor.
3. Although color is based on the direction of blood flow (toward or away) in relation to the transducer, red is usually assigned to arteries and blue to venous blood flow.
4. Keep the Doppler sample volume size small.
5. Use a 60-degree angle (or less) to the vessel wall.
6. The color and velocity scale (pulse repetition frequency [PRF]) should be adjusted throughout the examination to evaluate the changing velocity patterns.
7. The color and Doppler wall filter is set low.
8. The color "box" width affects frame rates (number of image frames per second), so the color display should be kept as small as possible.
9. The color, image, and Doppler gain should be adjusted throughout the examination as the signal strength changes.

It is imperative that each institution develop a carotid imaging protocol that defines the standard examination (arteries to be evaluated, the number and location of the Doppler samples obtained from each artery, angle of insonation, etc.). This protocol must include information about the technique, clinical applications, indications for a complete and/or limited examination, interpretation criteria, quality assurance, and equipment maintenance. A standard complete examination usually includes evaluation of both the right and left sides, acquiring both imaging and Doppler information from the carotid and vertebral arterial systems.

PROCEDURE

Carotid imaging is performed with the patient lying in the supine position on an examination table. The patient's head is placed on a pillow and turned slightly away from the side being scanned. After applying ultrasound gel along the sternocleidomastoid muscle border on the neck, the transducer is placed above the clavicle. It is recommended that the carotid system be evaluated first by gray scale imaging to determine the location of the arteries, the CCA bifurcation, vessel tortuosity, and atherosclerotic plaque. The initial scan of the carotid arteries may be performed in a transverse or longitudinal view, depending upon the preference of the operator. Longitudinal images are displayed with the distal segment (toward the head) of the artery on the left side of the monitor and the proximal artery on the right side of the monitor. Transverse images are usually displayed on the monitor as if the observer were looking towards the patient from their feet.

In a longitudinal view, the CCA is located and followed proximally as far as the clavicle will permit. The CCA can be distinguished from the internal jugular vein because the vein changes with respiration and compresses with pressure from the transducer. Although the origin of the right CCA is often located as it arises from the innominate artery, the left CCA originates from the arch and is usually not accessible to ultrasound imaging. The origin of the left CCA may be located in some cases, however, by using a lower-frequency transducer with a smaller footprint angled inferiorly.

The ultrasound transducer is moved cephalad, following the CCA to the level of the carotid bifurcation (thyroid cartilage). Careful imaging of the CCA is important because plaque may be located in this vessel. The CCA bifurcation is a common site for the development of atherosclerotic disease. At the bifurcation, the ultrasound transducer is moved slightly anteriorly and posteriorly to image the origin of the ECA and ICA. The ICA and ECA are individually followed distally to the angle of the mandible. Multiple longitudinal views (anterior, lateral, and posterior to the sternocleidomastoid muscle) and a transverse view are required to completely assess the cervical carotid arteries because of the eccentric shape of atherosclerotic plaque. Although the lateral approach provides the best visualization of the carotid system, the distal ICA is usually best visualized from a posterior approach. The transverse view provides the best cross-sectional view of the artery; therefore, any measurement of vessel diameter or plaque should be performed from this imaging plane.

The color Doppler and Doppler interrogation of the carotid system is performed in the longitudinal plane using a 60-degree angle between the ultrasound beam and the vessel walls (placement of the Doppler sample volume parallel to the color jet has not undergone extensive validation testing). Using a constant Doppler angle permits comparison of repeated studies in the same individual. If variable angles are used (usually between 45 and 60 degrees), validation with the gold standard (arteriography or magnetic resonance angiography) must be performed for the different angles that are used when imaging the proximal ICA. Doppler angles greater than 60 degrees and less than 30 degrees are not recommended because of an increase in measurement error. The sample volume size should be small and placed in the center of the artery (or center stream). The Doppler sample volume is moved slowly throughout the length of the artery searching for the highest velocity. "Spot" Doppler checks at specified locations will result in errors because areas of increased velocity may be missed. The color Doppler display will help to guide the proper placement of the Doppler sample volume and is useful in locating sites of increased velocity (aliasing) suggesting disease. However, although color is helpful in locating an area of increased velocity, care must be taken to evaluate that area for the maximum velocity by slowly moving the sample volume in proximity to the color "jet" (change).

Doppler signals are recorded from the proximal, mid, and distal CCA; the origin of the ECA; the proximal, mid, and distal ICA; the origin of the vertebral artery; and the subclavian artery bilaterally. In addition, Doppler signals are obtained from any area of stenosis. It is important to evaluate all Doppler signals bilaterally to correctly perform and interpret a carotid duplex imaging examination in an individual patient.

At the end of the carotid duplex imaging examination, the ultrasound gel should be removed from the patient. Excess gel should be removed from the ultrasound transducer and it should be cleaned using a disinfectant.

Common sources of technical error when performing carotid duplex imaging include the following: the transmitting frequency is too high for the vessel depth, the focal zone is not appropriately set to the depth of the vessel, the angle of the color box is too steep, the color gain setting is too low, and the color velocity scale is set too high. Color and power Doppler imaging provide "roadmaps" that guide the proper placement of the Doppler sample so that the artery is properly evaluated.

NORMAL RESULTS

In the normal setting, the CCA spectral waveform will demonstrate a low resistance pattern (end-diastole above the zero baseline) because blood travels from the CCA to the brain via the ICA. The CCA Doppler signal will display a positive Doppler shift throughout the cardiac cycle. The normal color flow pattern of the CCA will have continuous color throughout the cardiac cycle. At peak systole, the color will fill the artery to the vessel walls and display an increased velocity (a lighter shade) in center stream. The Doppler spectral waveforms should be evaluated from the proximal CCA, the midportion of the CCA, and the distal CCA (just proximal to the bifurcation). The CCA spectral Doppler waveform is important because it may indicate proximal disease or suggest distal disease. When calculating the ICA to CCA peak systolic ratio, the Doppler spectral waveform that is obtained from the straight portion (mid to distal) of the CCA is used. Investigators have shown that the velocity recorded from the CCA changes along its length.[23] Errors will occur if the spectral waveform obtained from the proximal tortuous CCA (increased velocity) or the distal CCA that may include the bulb (decreased velocity) is used in the calculation of the ratio.

Proper identification of the ICA and ECA is not a problem in most patients, but it is essential to performing accurate carotid duplex imaging. The most reliable method to distinguish the ICA from the ECA is by the Doppler signal (Figure 31-3). The ICA demonstrates blood flow velocity that is continuous and above the zero baseline throughout the cardiac cycle. The shape of the waveform is smooth. The normal color pattern of the ICA will have continuous color throughout the cardiac cycle because the ICA has diastolic blood flow caused by the low peripheral resistance of the brain. Because the carotid bulb usually includes the origin of the ICA, the dilation of the proximal vessel produces a change in the blood flow characteristics. Boundary layer separation, which is a normal flow disturbance, is detected as a transient reversal of blood flow along the posterior wall of the bulb. Boundary layer separation may be visualized in the color Doppler display and in the Doppler spectral waveform.

The ECA demonstrates a more pulsatile Doppler signal (minimal diastolic flow) because it supplies blood to the skin and muscular bed of the scalp and face. The ECA usually has a faster slope to peak systole and blood flow velocity to or very close to zero in late diastole. The normal color flow pattern of

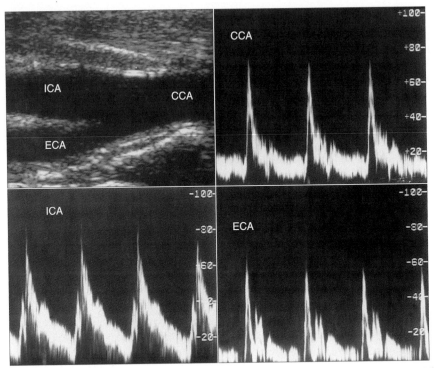

Figure 31-3 The Doppler spectral waveforms from a normal extracranial carotid arterial system. The spectral waveforms from the common carotid artery *(CCA)* and internal carotid artery *(ICA)* demonstrate low resistance. The external carotid artery *(ECA)* spectral waveform reflects a higher resistance.

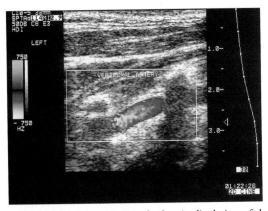

Figure 31-4 This is a color Doppler longitudinal view of the vertebral artery as it travels between the bony transverse processes. Note that the blood flow is in the correct direction (head is to the left of the image). It is important to follow the vertebral artery proximally to obtain the Doppler signal near the origin of the artery.

the ECA will reflect the higher resistance of the scalp and face. The color pattern will decrease during diastole and may disappear at end diastole. Additionally the ECA is smaller in diameter, usually originates anterior and medial at the carotid bifurcation, and has cervical branches. The superior thyroid artery is the ECA branch most visualized during a carotid duplex imaging examination.

The vertebral arteries are located by angling the transducer slightly laterally from a longitudinal view of the mid or proximal CCA. The vertebral artery lies deeper than the CCA. To reliably identify the vertebral artery, it should be followed distally and periodic shadowing should be visualized from the transverse processes of the vertebrae (Figure 31-4). The vertebral artery is accompanied by the vertebral vein, and proper identification of the artery is made by the Doppler signal. Once the vertebral artery has been correctly identified, it should be followed as far proximally as possible. The use of color Doppler will greatly assist in locating the vertebral artery and its origin and evaluating the direction of blood flow. Decreasing the color velocity scale may be helpful in locating the vertebral artery. The color flow pattern in the vertebral artery will demonstrate continuous color throughout the cardiac cycle, and the blood flow velocity is continuous and above the zero baseline throughout the cardiac cycle. The vertebral artery Doppler signal should be obtained near the origin of the vessel to identify any significant plaque formation.

Tortuous Arteries. During a carotid duplex imaging examination, encountering tortuous arteries is very common (Figures 31-5 and 31-6). Normal blood flow disturbances occur because of the curves in the arteries. There is usually an increase in the blood flow velocity associated with a tortuous vessel. Correct placement of the Doppler sample volume and adjustment of the Doppler angle may be very difficult in some arteries. Often the increased velocity obtained when scanning through a curve is because of the acute Doppler angles relative to the changing blood flow direction and not necessarily because of increased velocity of the blood flow. It is recom-

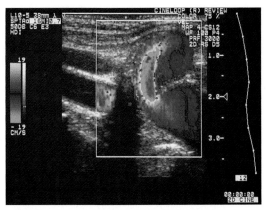

Figure 31-5   A complete loop in the proximal common carotid artery. Note the increased blood flow velocity (color Doppler aliasing) in the artery as it travels directly toward the transducer. This increased velocity may reflect the transducer-to-artery angle rather than a true increase in blood flow velocity.

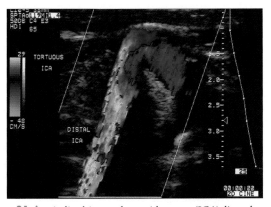

Figure 31-6   A distal internal carotid artery (ICA) dives deep away from the transducer. Doppler information from this artery cannot be taken 60 degrees to the vessel wall. It is important to note which angle was used during the examination, and to sweep the Doppler sample volume along the length of the vessel noting any increases in velocity and poststenotic turbulence.

mended that other evidence, such as poststenotic turbulence, be used to identify a stenosis in this setting. Additionally, whatever angle is used to evaluate the tortuous vessel should be documented and the same angle used for follow-up examinations in an individual patient.

PATHOLOGY

Atherosclerotic Disease. The location of any plaque visualized during the examination should be described, along with its length, surface characteristics (smooth versus irregular), and echogenicity (homogeneous, heterogeneous, calcification). The extent of plaque may be measured in a longitudinal or transverse plane by subjectively tracing the border of the plaque using the software measurement packages included on most imaging systems. Measuring plaque, however, is not a reliable method for determining the percent of narrowing. Although a plaque's surface may be described as smooth or irregular

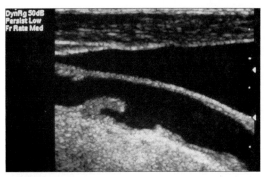

Figure 31-7   A longitudinal view of the common carotid artery. The plaque's surface is irregular.

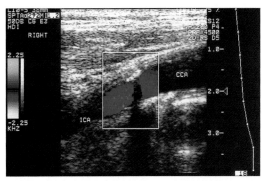

Figure 31-8   A calcified plaque near the origin of the internal carotid artery (ICA). Calcified plaques cause a drop out deep to its location. This shadow affects the gray scale and the color Doppler display. CCA, Common carotid artery.

(Figure 31-7), imaging is not a valid and reliable testing modality to identify plaque ulceration.[1,10,37] The echogenicity of plaque is usually described as homogeneous if it demonstrates a uniform level of echogenicity and texture throughout the plaque and heterogeneous if the plaque has mixed areas of echogenicity and textures. Calcification is very dense and is visualized as brightly echogenic areas in the plaque. A calcified plaque is usually visualized with an accompanying acoustic shadow that obscures imaging information deep to it (Figure 31-8). Multiple views of an artery from different scanning planes in most cases will minimize the shadowing associated with calcified plaque and allow visualization and Doppler interrogation of the artery.

It is very important for patient management to differentiate between a high-grade stenosis versus an occlusion of the ICA (Figure 31-9). An ICA occlusion is not amenable to surgical intervention. To characterize an ICA as occluded, the artery should be evaluated with Doppler, color Doppler, and power Doppler to rule out the presence of trickle flow. When determining if the ICA is occluded, the color PRF should be decreased to document the presence of any slow-moving blood flow and the color gain should be increased to enhance any blood flow that may be present. The ICA should be sampled at multiple sites with Doppler. Increasing the sample volume size may be helpful when trying to locate the presence of any

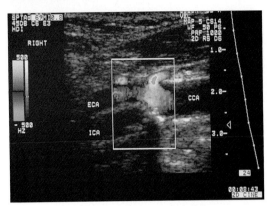

Figure 31-9 Occlusion of the internal carotid artery *(ICA)*. There is no color Doppler information, and a spectral Doppler waveform could not be located from the *ICA*. Blood flow is present in the external carotid artery *(ECA)*. The superior thyroid branch is visualized at the distal common carotid artery *(CCA)*.

blood flow. Secondary ultrasound characteristics of an ICA occlusion are echogenic material filling the lumen, lack of arterial pulsations, reversed blood flow (color display) near the proximal origin of the occlusion, the loss of diastolic blood flow in the ipsilateral CCA, an increase in blood flow velocity in the ipsilateral ECA, and increased velocity in the contralateral ICA. Occlusion of the ECA or CCA may also occur and should be documented during a carotid duplex imaging examination. At times the CCA may be occluded and the ICA and ECA may remain patent. Usually there is retrograde blood flow in the ECA that supplies the ICA; however, retrograde flow in the ICA supplying the ECA may also occur. In this imaging presentation, it is important to document the blood flow direction and the velocity in the ECA and the ICA.

Aneurysms. Aneurysms of the cervical carotid system are relatively uncommon. Most patients present with a pulsatile mass of the neck and a bruit is often noted.

Sonographic Findings. In most cases, carotid duplex imaging demonstrates a tortuous CCA. In cases of aneurysms, however, the vessel diameter will be significantly increased. The abnormal blood flow pattern demonstrated within the aneurysm by color Doppler and by the Doppler signal depends on the size of the aneurysm.

Dissection. Some of the common causes of a carotid artery dissection are blunt and penetrating trauma, acceleration-deceleration cervical injuries, and neck flexion. A carotid artery dissection occurs between the intima and medial layers of the arterial wall, creating a false lumen.

Sonographic Findings. The different blood flow patterns in the two lumens may be documented with color Doppler and spectral Doppler waveforms, depending on the elevation of the intima. In some cases, the ICA has a gradual taper ending at the base of the skull, causing a decrease in peak-systolic velocity with a high-resistance pattern. Luminal narrowing of the vessel without visualization of plaque is characteristic of a dissection.

Fibromuscular Dysplasia. Fibromuscular dysplasia (FMD) is a nonatherosclerotic disease that usually affects the media of the arterial wall. It predominantly occurs in the midsegment of the ICA, is bilateral in approximately 65% of the cases, and is usually found in females. FMD has been described as having a "string of pearls" appearance by arteriography. This pattern is caused by multiple arterial dilations separated by concentric stenosis.

Sonographic Findings. Color Doppler imaging may reveal turbulent blood flow patterns adjacent to the arterial wall, with the absence of atherosclerotic plaque in the proximal and distal segments of the ICA.

Carotid Body Tumors. Carotid body tumors are slow-growing neoplasms of the carotid body. The carotid body is a small (3- to 5-mm) chemoreceptor that lies within the adventitial layer on the posterior aspect of the carotid bifurcation. The carotid body assists in regulating heart rate, blood pressure, and respiration. The carotid body tumor is a rare, hypervascular structure that usually lies between the ICA and ECA. The blood supply to most carotid body tumors is via branches of the ECA.

Sonographic Findings. Evaluating the patient with a large mass of the neck may be challenging, and a liberal amount of acoustic gel is often necessary to maintain good skin to transducer contact. The carotid body tumor usually lies in between the ICA and ECA, may displace an artery from its normal location, and is supplied by branches of the ECA; its hypervascularity is easily identified by color Doppler imaging.

Currently the best carotid duplex imaging examinations will be achieved by proper attention to detail. The major areas to focus on when performing carotid duplex imaging examinations are summarized in Box 31-2. Attention to these technical areas and interpretation details will ensure the best carotid duplex imaging results.

INTERPRETATION OF CAROTID DUPLEX IMAGING

The accurate interpretation of a carotid duplex imaging examination depends on the quality and the completeness of the evaluation. Often the patient's body habitus will affect the quality of the image and the sonographer's ability to search the entire carotid system with Doppler. The sonographer must be prepared to switch transducers if necessary to complete the carotid examination and have a complete understanding of the equipment controls to optimize the image and Doppler information. The peak-systolic velocity, end-diastolic velocity, direction of blood flow, and shape of the Doppler spectral waveforms should be evaluated bilaterally. There should be symmetry of the Doppler spectral waveforms. Abnormal waveform shape (increased or decreased pulsatility) may be an indicator of more proximal (innominate, subclavian) or distal (intracranial) disease. Blood flow reversal is uncommon; however, it may occur in patients with aortic valve regurgitation, arrhythmias, dissections, or intraaortic balloon pumps.

To determine the degree of stenosis present, a complete Doppler evaluation of the carotid arterial system is necessary.[17] The Doppler spectral waveform should demonstrate an elevated velocity through the narrowed segment and color changes (aliasing) should be present. Poststenotic disturbances distal to the stenosis will be demonstrated by bidirectional turbulent blood flow patterns (spectral broadening). Additionally, there will be a mottled color pattern consisting of aliasing and multiple directions of blood flow. The highest velocity obtained from an ICA stenosis is used to classify the degree of narrowing. Doppler signals obtained distal to the area of poststenotic flow disturbance may be normal or diminished, and the upstroke of the distal Doppler spectral waveform may be slowed. There have been multiple diagnostic criteria (peak-systolic velocity, end-diastolic velocity, ICA/CCA ratios) for varying degrees of narrowing of the ICA suggested by various investigators.* The most important recommendation is that each institution establish its own diagnostic criteria by comparing the carotid duplex imaging results with conventional arteriography or magnetic resonance arteriography.[16,21]

The information in Table 31-1 is from the Carotid Research Laboratory at the University of Washington.[31] These diagnostic criteria have been used successfully by many investigators to categorize disease from the origin of the ICA. These well-documented diagnostic criteria are a good starting point for any institution before establishing their own diagnostic criteria (Figures 31-10 and 31-11). Internal carotid artery peak systolic velocities are normally approximately 60 to 80 cm/sec in older individuals and about 80 to 100 cm/sec in younger individuals.

Because the carotid endarterectomy trials (the North American Symptomatic Carotid Endarterectomy Trial [NASCET],[28] the Asymptomatic Carotid Atherosclerosis Study [ACAS],[15]

TABLE 31-1	DIAGNOSTIC CRITERIA FOR THE PROXIMAL INTERNAL CAROTID ARTERY*	
Diameter Reduction	Peak Systolic Velocity	End-Diastolic Velocity
<50%	<125 cm/sec	N/A
50%-79%	≥125 cm/sec	N/A
80%-99%	N/A	≥140 cm/sec
Occlusion	No signal	No signal

Courtesy Carotid Research Laboratory, University of Washington.
*60-degree angle.
N/A, Not applicable.

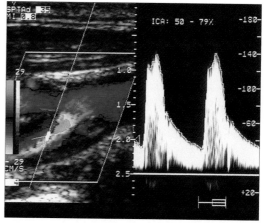

Figure 31-10 An example of a 50% to 79% diameter reduction of the internal carotid artery. The peak-systolic velocity is approximately 140 cm/sec, and the end-diastolic velocity is 35 cm/sec. The color Doppler information was used as a guide to sweep the Doppler sample volume through the area of increased velocity. Note that the Doppler signal was obtained with the sample volume parallel to the vessel walls and not the color jet.

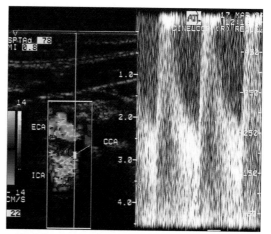

Figure 31-11 An example of a greater than 80% diameter reduction stenosis of the internal carotid artery. The peak-systolic velocity is greater than 450 cm/sec and the end-diastolic velocity is greater than 200 cm/sec. Note the aliasing of the color Doppler near the origin of the internal carotid artery *(ICA)* and the external carotid artery *(ECA)*. *CCA*, Common carotid artery.

---

*References 8, 9, 14, 16, 18, 20, 21, 24, 25, 27, 31.

TABLE 31-2 ICA/CCA PEAK-SYSTOLIC VELOCITY RATIOS FOR THE PROXIMAL INTERNAL CAROTID ARTERY

Diameter Reduction	Internal Carotid Artery/Common Diameter Carotid Artery Peak Systolic Reduction Velocity Ratio
70%-99%*	>4
60%-99%*	>3.2
>50%	>2.0

*Data from Moneta GH and others: *J Vasc Surg* 17:152, 1995; Moneta GH and others: *J Vasc Surg* 21:695, 1995.

BOX 31-3 ESSENTIAL QUESTIONS TO BE ANSWERED BY CAROTID DUPLEX IMAGING

- Is the ultrasound examination of high quality and complete?
- What level is the carotid bifurcation?
- Is disease present in the cervical carotid system?
- Where is the disease located?
- What is the percent diameter reduction of the stenosis?
- What is the length of the plaque?
- What are the characteristics of the plaque?
- Is the distal internal carotid artery (ICA) patent?
- Are the arteries tortuous or kinked?
- Are the Doppler signals from all arteries symmetric?
- Does the distal ICA Doppler signal suggest distal (intracranial) disease?
- Is the proximal CCA Doppler signal normal or does it suggest proximal disease?
- What is the direction of blood flow in the vertebral arteries?

and the European Carotid Surgery Trial [ECST)][32]) used specific thresholds for surgical treatment, ultrasound criteria for ICA stenosis greater than 70% and greater than 60% were necessary to classify patients. Investigators have found that an ICA-CCA peak-systolic velocity (PSV) ratio is useful in grading ICA stenosis greater than 70% and greater than 60%. The ratios (Table 31-2) are calculated using the highest PSV from the origin of the ICA divided by the highest PSV from the CCA (straight mid to distal segment). Again, many investigators have used different ICA-CCA ratios to document varying degrees of ICA narrowing.

In the presence of an ICA occlusion, the velocity in the contralateral ICA may be elevated. This may lead to overreading the extent of disease in the patent ICA.[7,15,38] To avoid overestimation of the ICA stenosis contralateral to an ICA occlusion, new velocity criteria have been suggested.[15] The new velocity criteria use a peak-systolic velocity of greater than 140 cm/sec (instead of greater than 125 cm/sec) for a stenosis greater than 50% diameter reduction. For a stenosis greater than 80% diameter reduction of the lumen, the new criteria use an end-diastolic velocity of greater than 155 cm/sec (instead of greater than 140 cm/sec).

The evaluation of normal vertebral arteries produces a wide variation in velocities. Absolute velocities are not useful to diagnose a stenosis. Poststenotic disturbances in the vertebral artery and changes in the waveform shape may suggest a proximal obstruction. It is important to note the direction of blood flow in the vertebral artery. A subclavian steal is present if there is reversal of vertebral artery blood flow direction secondary to a significant obstruction proximal to the origin of the vertebral artery in the ipsilateral subclavian or innominate artery. A vertebral artery Doppler signal can also display an alternating (toward and away) pattern. If an alternating pattern occurs in the vertebral artery, it may change to complete reversal of blood flow direction with arm exercise or after reactive hyperemia of the ipsilateral arm. This may be documented by monitoring the vertebral artery Doppler signal after release of a blood pressure cuff that has been inflated above systolic pressure on the ipsilateral arm for approximately 3 minutes.

The evaluation of normal subclavian arteries produces multiphasic high-resistance Doppler signals. The color flow pattern from the subclavian artery will reflect the high peripheral resistance. Blood flow will be toward (red) the transducer in peak systole, away from (blue) the transducer in early diastole, and toward (red) the transducer in late diastole. If there is a significant stenosis or occlusion of the proximal segment of this vessel, the Doppler signal distal to the stenosis will be monophasic. A difference of blood pressure in the arms greater than 20 mm Hg is usually associated with disease of the subclavian or innominate artery on the side with the lower blood pressure.

Other important information to include in the interpretation of a carotid duplex imaging examination is (1) the location of the stenosis, (2) the extent of the plaque and patency of the distal ICA, (3) the presence of tortuosity or kinking of the vessels, and (4) plaque characteristics (smooth versus irregular surface, calcification). Additionally, the report should include any variation from the protocol, if the quality of the examination was not optimal (e.g., body habitus), and any atypical Doppler waveforms.

At many institutions, carotid duplex imaging may be the only diagnostic imaging modality that is performed before a patient undergoes carotid endarterectomy. Careful imaging technique and the appropriate interpretation of the results are essential to address several important questions. The questions that should be answered by a carotid duplex imaging examination are listed in Box 31-3.

Consistency of the findings on gray scale, color Doppler, and the Doppler spectral waveforms will limit errors when interpreting carotid duplex imaging examinations. There are, however, many pitfalls in the interpretation of these examinations. The more common errors encountered when interpreting carotid duplex imaging examinations are listed in Box 31-4. Proper technique is essential to providing accurate carotid duplex imaging examinations and minimizing errors in the interpretation.

CAROTID DUPLEX IMAGING: COMMON INTERPRETATION ERRORS

INCREASED VELOCITY WITHOUT A STENOSIS
- Improper technique
- Diagnostic criteria for proximal internal carotid artery (ICA) applied to the distal ICA, common carotid artery (CCA), external carotid artery (ECA), or vertebral arteries
- Tortuous arteries
- Contralateral ICA high-grade stenosis or occlusion
- Distal arteriovenous malformation (AVM)
- Cardiac function (affects signals bilaterally)
- Decreased hematocrit (affects signals bilaterally)

NORMAL VELOCITY WITH A STENOSIS
- Improper technique
- Velocity "jet" not identified
- Very high-grade stenosis (velocity decreases)

ABSENCE OF BLOOD FLOW VELOCITY WITH ARTERIAL PATENCY
- Improper technique
- Improper setting of equipment controls
- "Pseudoocclusion" because of low volume flow
- Increased velocity missed

BLOOD FLOW VELOCITY RECORDED IN PRESENCE OF ARTERIAL OCCLUSION
- Improper technique
- ECA and branches misidentified for the ICA
- Time interval between ultrasound evaluation and arteriography

OTHER CLINICAL APPLICATIONS AND EMERGING TECHNIQUES

INTRAOPERATIVE USE OF CAROTID DUPLEX IMAGING

The assessment of the carotid endarterectomy site by duplex imaging for technical adequacy is an effective method to improve the results of the operation. Ultrasound transducers (10 MHz) designed for intraoperative use identify disturbed blood flow and anatomic abnormalities, such as residual plaque at the endarterectomy end point, thrombus, intimal flap, suture stenosis, platelet aggregation, and clamp or shunt trauma. Intraoperative carotid imaging is performed after the procedure, but before skin closure. The transducer is placed in a sterile sleeve and imaging is performed on the exposed artery. It has been established that the detection of intraoperative peak systolic velocities greater than 150 cm/sec with the presence of an anatomic defect warrants correction because of its potential to progress.[5] Several investigators have reported that the use of routine intraoperative carotid duplex imaging has had a favorable impact on the stroke rate and incidence of restenosis of the carotid artery.[2,5,12]

CAROTID DUPLEX IMAGING AFTER STENT PLACEMENT OR ENDARTERECTOMY

Carotid artery stenting is a technique that has been introduced as an alternative to carotid endarterectomy in selected

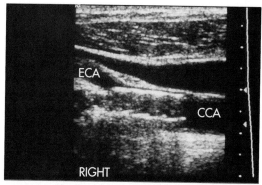

Figure 31-12   A longitudinal view of the carotid system. The bright echoes within the lumen are from the stent. The stent is placed in the distal common carotid artery *(CCA)* and extends into the bifurcation area near the origin of the external carotid artery *(ECA)*.

patients.[6] The gray scale image of a stent produces bright echoes (Figure 31-12).[33] The velocity criteria established to identify disease in the native carotid arteries may not be sensitive in identifying a stenosis after carotid artery stent placement.[32] The stent is a smaller diameter compared with the native vascular lumen, and the size difference or the lack of elasticity may cause an increase in the velocity within the stent. Other anatomic configurations, such as the carotid bulb, may cause a significant diameter change between the native vessel and the stent, which may cause an increased velocity within the stent. Duplex imaging, however, has been useful in detecting carotid artery stent occlusion. The performance of carotid duplex imaging following stent placement is in its infancy. As more experience is gained, diagnostic criteria will be developed and error in interpretation will be avoided in the future.

Carotid duplex imaging performed after carotid endarterectomy may reveal residual or recurrent stenosis in the ipsilateral ICA and disease progression in the contralateral ICA.[34] A follow-up duplex imaging examination should be performed approximately 1 to 3 months after a carotid endarterectomy. The time interval for follow-up after the initial postoperative study depends on the status of the artery after endarterectomy and the amount of disease present in the contralateral ICA. If a carotid patch is used, then imaging immediately after endarterectomy is difficult because the synthetic material often retains air, and information can only be obtained proximal and distal to the patch. The gas present in the synthetic material is usually reabsorbed within a few days and then can be evaluated.

If the operated carotid artery and the contralateral carotid artery demonstrate narrowing that is less than 50% diameter reduction, the patient is followed by carotid imaging annually. If the operated carotid artery or contralateral nonoperated carotid artery demonstrates more than a 50% diameter reduction, the next postoperative scans are performed at 6-month intervals.

CAROTID INTIMA-MEDIA THICKNESS

High resolution gray scale (B-mode) imaging is being used to measure the intima-media thickness (IMT) of the carotid

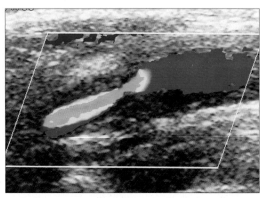

Figure 31-13   A color Doppler image of the origin of the internal carotid artery. Note the color Doppler aliasing suggesting an increased velocity associated with the plaque.

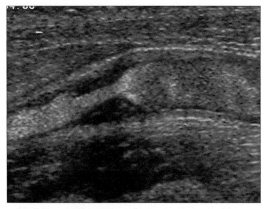

Figure 31-14   A B-flow image of the internal carotid artery shown in Figure 31-13. Note the improved visualization of the plaque versus lumen near the origin of the vessel and the improved visualization of the distal vessel.

artery to detect early atherosclerotic changes. Carotid IMT is the distance between the lumen-intima interface to the media-adventitia interface and if monitored in a consistent method can be used as a marker of the progression or regression of atherosclerotic disease.[3] Individuals with increased carotid IMT are more likely to suffer strokes and myocardial infarction than those with thinner walls.[4,29,30,40] Additionally, individuals with hypercholesterolemia have increased IMT compared with individuals with normal cholesterol levels.[19] To accurately measure carotid IMT, investigators must be experienced, use an imaging protocol, use modern equipment and a high-frequency transducer (>7 MHz), and acquire multiple samples from a longitudinal view.

NEW DEVELOPMENTS

Extended field of view,[35,41] tissue harmonic imaging,[36] echo-enhanced imaging,[8] and B-flow imaging[39] (Figures 31-13 and 31-14) are current developments in equipment capabilities that have improved the accuracy of carotid imaging. It is important to maintain state-of-the-art duplex imaging systems to provide accurate carotid evaluations for good-quality patient care.

REFERENCES

1. Arnold JAC and others: Carotid plaque characterization by duplex scanning: observer error may undermine current clinical trials, *Stroke* 30:61, 1999.
2. Baker WH and others: Intraoperative duplex scanning and late carotid artery stenosis, *J Vasc Surg* 19:829, 1994.
3. Baldassarre D and others: Carotid artery intima-media thickness measured by ultrasonography in normal clinical practice correlates well with atherosclerotic risk factors. *Stroke* 31:2426-2430, 2000.
4. Baldassarre D and others: Reproducibility validation study comparing analog and digital imaging technologies for the measurement of intima-media thickness, *Stroke* 31:1104-1110, 2000.
5. Bandyk DF and others: Intraoperative duplex scanning of arterial reconstructions: fate of repaired and unrepaired defects, *J Vasc Surg* 20:426, 1994.
6. Bowser AN and others: Outcome of carotid stent-assisted angioplasty versus open surgical repair of recurrent carotid stenosis. *J Vasc Surg* 38:432-438, 2003.
7. Busuttil SJ and others: Carotid duplex overestimation of stenosis due to severe contralateral disease, *Am J Surg* 172:144, 1996.
8. Carpenter JP, Lexa FJ, Davis JT: Determination of duplex Doppler ultrasound criteria appropriate to the North American Symptomatic Carotid Endarterectomy Trial, *Stroke* 27:695, 1996.
9. Carpenter JP, Lexa FJ, Davis JT: Determination of sixty percent or greater carotid artery stenosis by duplex Doppler ultrasonography, *J Vasc Surg* 22:697, 1995.
10. Comerota AJ and others: The preoperative diagnosis of the ulcerated carotid atheroma, *J Vasc Surg* 11:505, 1990.
11. Droste DW and others: Echocontrast-enhanced ultrasound of extracranial internal carotid artery high-grade stenosis and occlusion, *Stroke* 30:2302, 1999.
12. Dykes JR and others: Intraoperative duplex scanning reduces both residual stenosis and postoperative morbidity of carotid endarterectomy, *Am Surg* 63:50, 1997.
13. Executive Committee Asymptomatic Carotid Atherosclerosis Study: Endarterectomy for asymptomatic carotid artery stenosis, *JAMA* 273:1421, 1995.
14. Fillinger MF and others: Carotid duplex criteria for a 60% or greater angiographic stenosis: variation according to equipment, *J Vasc Surg* 24:856, 1996.
15. Fujitani RM and others: The effect of unilateral internal carotid artery occlusion upon contralateral duplex study: criteria for accurate interpretation, *J Vasc Surg* 16:459, 1992.
16. Grant EG and others: Ability to use duplex US to quantify internal carotid arterial stenoses: fact or fiction? *Radiology* 214:247, 2000.
17. Grant EG and others: Carotid artery stenosis: gray scale and Doppler US diagnosis-Society of Radiologists in Ultasound Consensus Conference. *Radiology* 229:340-346, 2003.
18. Grant EG and others: Doppler sonographic parameters for detection of carotid stenosis: is there an optimum method for their selection? *Am J Radiol* 172:1123, 1999.
19. Hodis HN and others: The role of carotid arterial intima-media thickness in predicting clinical coronary events. *Ann Intern Med* 128:262-269, 1998.
20. Hood DB and others: Prospective evaluation of new duplex criteria to identify a 70% internal carotid stenosis, *J Vasc Surg* 23:254, 1996.
21. Kuntz KM and others: Duplex ultrasound criteria for the identification of carotid stenosis should be laboratory specific, *Stroke* 28:597, 1997.

22. Lal BK and others: Carotid artery stenting: is there a need to revise ultrasound velocity criteria? *J Vasc Surg* 39:58-66, 2004.

23. Lee VS and others: Assessment of stenosis: implications of variability of Doppler measurements in normal-appearing carotid arteries, *Radiology* 212:493, 1999.

24. Moneta GH and others: Correlation of North America Symptomatic Carotid Endarterectomy Trial (NASCET) angiographic definition of 70-99% internal carotid artery stenosis with duplex scanning, *J Vasc Surg* 17:152, 1995.

25. Moneta GH and others: Screening for asymptomatic carotid internal carotid artery stenosis: duplex criteria for discriminating 60-99% stenosis, *J Vasc Surg* 21:989, 1995.

26. American Heart Association: *Heart disease and stroke statistics, 2005 update,* 2005, Dallas, American Heart Association.

27. Nehler MR and others: Improving selection of patients with less than 60% asymptomatic internal carotid artery stenosis for follow-up of carotid artery duplex scanning, *J Vasc Surg* 23:580, 1996.

28. North American Symptomatic Carotid Endarterectomy Trial Collaborators: Beneficial effect of carotid endarterectomy in symptomatic patients with high grade carotid stenosis, *N Engl J Med* 325:445, 1991.

29. O'Leary DH and others: Thickening of the carotid wall. A marker for atherosclerosis in the elderly? Cardiovascular Health Study Collaborative Research Group. *Stroke* 27:224-231, 1996.

30. O'Leary DH, Polak JF: Intima-media thickness: a tool for atherosclerotic imaging and event prediction. *Am J Cardiol* 90:18L-21L, 2002.

31. Primozich JF: Color flow in the carotid evaluation, *J Vasc Technol* 15:112, 1991.

32. Randomized trial of endarterectomy for recently symptomatic carotid stenosis: final results of the MRC European Carotid Surgery Trial (ECST), *Lancet* 351:1379, 1998.

33. Robbin ML and others: Carotid artery stents: early and intermediate follow-up with Doppler US, *Radiology* 205:749, 1997.

34. Roth SM and others: A rational algorithm for duplex scan surveillance after carotid endarterectomy, *J Vasc Surg* 30:453, 1999.

35. Sauerbrei EE: Extended field-of-view sonography: utility in clinical practice, *J Ultrasound Med* 18:335, 1999.

36. Shapiro RS and others: Tissue harmonic imaging sonography: evaluation of image quality compared with conventional sonography, *Am J Radiol* 171:1203, 1998.

37. Sitzer M and others: Color-flow Doppler-assisted duplex imaging fails to detect ulceration in high-grade internal carotid artery stenosis, *J Vasc Surg* 23:461, 1996.

38. Spadone DP and others: Contralateral internal carotid artery stenosis or occlusion: pitfall of correct ipsilateral classification—a study performed with color-flow imaging, *J Vasc Surg* 11:642, 1990.

39. Umemura A, Yamada K: B-mode flow imaging of the carotid artery. *Stroke* 32:2055-2057, 2001.

40. Vemmos KN and others: Common carotid artery intima-media thickness in patients with brain infarction and intracerebral haemorrhage. *Cerebrovasc Dis* 17:280-286, 2004.

41. Weng L and others: US extended-field-of-view imaging technology, *Radiology* 203:877, 1997.

SELECTED BIBLIOGRAPHY

Elkind MS, Sacco RL: Stroke risk factors and stroke prevention, *Sem Neurol* 18:429, 1998.

Lippert H, Pabst R: *Arterial variations in man: classification and frequency,* New York, 1985, Springer-Verlag.

Osborn AG: *Introduction to cerebral angiography,* Philadelphia, 1980, Harper & Row.

CHAPTER 32

Intracranial Cerebrovascular Evaluation

Mira L. Katz

OBJECTIVES

- Describe the intracranial arterial anatomy encountered during transcranial color Doppler imaging
- Articulate the proper instrument control settings used during transcranial color Doppler imaging
- Describe the characteristics of the Doppler waveforms from the arteries evaluated during a transcranial color Doppler examination
- List the clinical applications in which transcranial color Doppler imaging may be beneficial
- Describe the diagnostic criteria associated with the different clinical applications
- Identify common errors associated with performing and interpreting a transcranial color Doppler imaging examination

INTRACRANIAL ARTERIAL ANATOMY

INTERNAL CAROTID ARTERY
OPHTHALMIC ARTERY
POSTERIOR COMMUNICATING ARTERY
MIDDLE CEREBRAL ARTERY
ANTERIOR CEREBRAL ARTERY
ANTERIOR COMMUNICATING ARTERY
VERTEBRAL ARTERY
BASILAR ARTERY
POSTERIOR CEREBRAL ARTERY
CIRCLE OF WILLIS

TECHNICAL ASPECTS OF TRANSCRANIAL COLOR DOPPLER IMAGING

INSTRUMENTATION
TECHNIQUE

INTERPRETATION OF TRANSCRANIAL COLOR DOPPLER IMAGING

NORMAL INTRACRANIAL ARTERIAL VELOCITIES
PHYSIOLOGIC FACTORS

CLINICAL APPLICATIONS

VASOSPASM
DIAGNOSIS OF INTRACRANIAL DISEASE

ADVANTAGES AND LIMITATIONS OF TRANSCRANIAL COLOR DOPPLER IMAGING

DIAGNOSTIC PITFALLS

KEY TERMS

anterior cerebral artery (ACA) – smaller of the two terminal branches of the internal carotid artery

anterior communicating artery (ACoA) – a short vessel that connects the anterior cerebral arteries at the interhemispheric fissure

basilar artery (BA) – formed by the union of the two vertebral arteries

cerebral vasospasm – vasoconstriction of the arteries

circle of Willis – a polygon vascular ring at the base of the brain

internal carotid artery (ICA) – arises from the common carotid artery to supply the anterior brain and meninges

mean velocity – based on the time average of the outline velocity (maximum velocity envelope)

middle cerebral artery (MCA) – large terminal branch of the internal carotid artery

ophthalmic artery – first branch of the internal carotid artery

posterior cerebral artery (PCA) – originates from the terminal basilar artery and courses anteriorly and laterally

posterior communicating artery (PCoA) – courses posteriorly and medially from the internal carotid artery to join the posterior cerebral artery

subclavian steal syndrome – characterized by symptoms of brain stem ischemia associated with a stenosis or occlusion of the left subclavian, innominate, or right subclavian artery proximal to the origin of the vertebral artery

submandibular window – transducer is placed at the angle of the mandible and angled slightly medially and cephalad toward the carotid canal

suboccipital window – transducer is placed on the posterior aspect of the neck inferior to the nuchal crest

transorbital window – transducer is placed on the closed eyelid

transtemporal window – transducer is placed on the temporal bone cephalad to the zygomatic arch anterior to the ear

vertebral artery – branch of the subclavian artery

Significant progress has been made in the noninvasive evaluation of cerebrovascular disease during the past 25 years, especially in the area of extracranial vasculature. Development of a noninvasive method to interrogate the intracranial arterial system lagged because of the attention focused on surgically correctable lesions of the carotid bifurcation and the difficulty in penetrating the skull with ultrasound. Technical sophistication has progressed and experience has been gained in the past decade to allow ultrasonic evaluation of the intracranial arterial system by using transcranial color Doppler (TCD) imaging.

The TCD technique was introduced in 1982 as a method to detect cerebral arterial vasospasm after subarachnoid hemorrhage. During the past 22 years, however, TCD has been used for many different clinical applications (Box 32-1). A better understanding of intracranial arterial hemodynamics may be gained by using TCD in many different clinical settings.

The accurate interpretation of a patient's TCD examination is not possible without knowledge of the amount and the location of atherosclerotic disease in the extracranial vasculature. Carotid and vertebral duplex imaging should be performed before the TCD examination because extensive extracranial disease may cause changes in the velocity profile or direction of blood flow in a patient's intracranial arterial system.

INTRACRANIAL ARTERIAL ANATOMY

Blood supply to the brain is provided by the carotid (anterior) and vertebral (posterior) arteries. Familiarity with the anatomy of the large intracranial arteries is requisite to performing accurate TCD imaging examinations.

<table>
<tr><td>

BOX 32-1 TRANSCRANIAL COLOR DOPPLER IMAGING: CLINICAL APPLICATIONS

- Diagnosis and follow-up of intracranial vascular disease
- Assessment of intracranial collateral pathways
- Evaluation of the hemodynamic effects of extracranial occlusive disease on intracranial blood flow
- Intraoperative monitoring
- Detection of cerebral emboli
- Monitoring vasospasm in subarachnoid hemorrhage
- Screening of children with sickle cell disease
- Documentation of the subclavian steal syndrome
- Evaluation of vertebrobasilar system
- Monitoring after head trauma
- Monitoring during anticoagulative or fibrinolytic therapy
- Detection of feeders of AV malformations
- Evaluation of migraine headaches
- Monitoring evolution of cerebral circulatory arrest

</td></tr>
</table>

This chapter concentrates on the intracranial arteries that make up the circle of Willis (Figure 32-1). The extracranial portion of the carotid and vertebral arteries is described in Chapter 31.

INTERNAL CAROTID ARTERY

The **internal carotid artery (ICA)** is divided into four main segments: (1) the cervical ICA originates at the common carotid bifurcation and ends as the artery enters the carotid canal of the temporal bone at the base of the skull; (2) the petrous section of the ICA begins as the ICA enters the carotid canal within the petrous portion of the bone and continues until it crosses over the cranial portion of the foramen lacerum and passes into the cavernous sinus; (3) the cavernous segment of the ICA runs from the foramen lacerum and cavernous sinus entrance to just medial of the anterior clinoid process; and (4) the supraclinoid portion of the ICA enters the intracranial space at the anterior clinoid and continues to its termination into the middle cerebral and anterior cerebral arteries. The portion of the ICA that forms two curves (S shape) is termed the carotid siphon. The segments of the ICA that are evaluated during a TCD examination are the terminal portion of the ICA just proximal to the origin of the middle cerebral artery and anterior cerebral artery and the carotid siphon. The internal carotid siphon may be the site of atherosclerotic disease in adults.

OPHTHALMIC ARTERY

The ophthalmic artery is the first branch of the ICA and is evaluated during TCD imaging. It courses anterior laterally

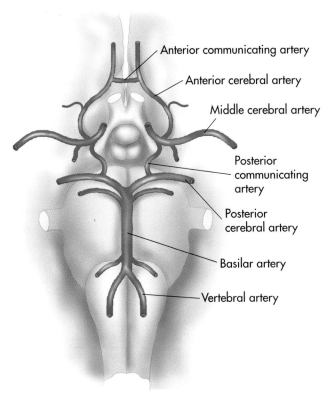

Figure 32-1 The arteries of the circle of Willis.

Labels: Anterior communicating artery; Anterior cerebral artery; Middle cerebral artery; Posterior communicating artery; Posterior cerebral artery; Basilar artery; Vertebral artery

and slightly downward through the optic foramen to supply the globe, orbit, and adjacent structures. The ophthalmic artery has three major groups of branches: the ocular branches, the orbital branches, and the extraorbital branches. The branches of the ophthalmic artery often play an important role in collateral pathways that form as a result of disease of either the internal or external carotid arteries.

POSTERIOR COMMUNICATING ARTERY

The **posterior communicating artery (PCoA)** courses posteriorly and medially from the ICA to join the posterior cerebral artery. The PCoA is variable in size and may angle upward or downward. Hypoplasia is the common PCoA anomaly. However, the PCoA can be large when the posterior cerebral artery is hypoplastic, which occurs in 15% to 25% of cases. This is termed a "fetal" origin of the posterior cerebral artery. The PCoA is usually a potential rather than an actual arterial conduit. The PCoA generally does not function as an important collateral pathway unless the patient has extensive extracranial occlusive disease bilaterally or in a patient lacking a patent anterior communicating artery. The PCoA may be evaluated during TCD imaging examinations.

MIDDLE CEREBRAL ARTERY

The **middle cerebral artery (MCA)** is the larger terminal branch of the ICA. From its origin, the MCA extends laterally and horizontally in the lateral cerebral fissure. The horizontal segment may course downward or upward. The MCA either bifurcates or trifurcates before the limen insulae (a small gyrus), where the branches turn upward into the Sylvian fissure, forming its genu ("knee"). The vessels course around the island of Reil, which is a triangular-shaped mound of cortex, and runs posterosuperiorly within the Sylvian fissure. The terminal branches of the MCA anastomose with terminal branches of the anterior cerebral and posterior cerebral arteries.

The middle cerebral artery is usually divided into four segments (M1 to M4). The M1 and the origin of the M2 branches are evaluated during TCD imaging. The main horizontal section from its origin to the limen insulae is the M1 segment. The M1 segment gives rise to numerous small lenticulostriate branches. The M2 segment is composed of the branches overlying the insular surface in the deep Sylvian fissure. The initial MCA bifurcation is the third most common site for congenital aneurysms, giving rise to approximately one fourth of all intracranial aneurysms. The anterior communicating and the posterior communicating arteries are the first and second most common sites for aneurysm formation, respectively. The MCA may also be the site for arterial stenosis and occlusion.

ANTERIOR CEREBRAL ARTERY

The **anterior cerebral artery (ACA)** is the smaller of the two terminal branches of the ICA. The ACA is a midline marker. From its origin, the ACA courses anteromedially over the optic chiasm and the optic nerve to the interhemispheric fissure (longitudinal cerebral fissure). The proximal horizontal segment of the ACA is known as the A1 segment and is connected to the contralateral A1 segment via the anterior communicating artery (ACoA). The A1 segment is evaluated during a TCD imaging examination. The contour of the A1 segment may take a horizontal course, ascend, or slightly descend. Complete absence of the A1 segment is unusual. An anomalous origin of the ACA is rare, but asymmetry between the two A1 segments is common. A direct correlation exists between size of the A1 segment and the size of the ACoA. A small or hypoplastic A1 is usually found in conjunction with a large ACoA because the contralateral A1 segment supplies most of the blood flow to both distal ACA territories. Individuals with anomalies of the A1 segment have a slightly higher incidence of ACoA aneurysms. The ACA is a rare site for stenosis or occlusion.

Distal to the ACoA, the ACAs turn superiorly and run side-by-side in the interhemispheric fissure. The ACA curves anterosuperiorly around the genu of the corpus callosum. The segment of the ACA from the ACoA to the distal ACA bifurcation (callosomarginal artery and pericallosal artery) is termed the A2 segment. The proximal portion of the A2 segments may be visualized during TCD imaging in some patients. The distal A2 segments anastomose with branches of the posterior cerebral arteries. A large medial striate artery, the recurrent artery of Heubner, is a major branch of the proximal A2 segment in approximately 80% of the cases, but this artery can also originate from the distal A1 segment.

ANTERIOR COMMUNICATING ARTERY

The **anterior communicating artery (ACoA)** is a short vessel that connects the anterior cerebral arteries (A1) at the interhemispheric fissure. The ACoA may be absent or may be a single, duplicated, or multichanneled system. The longer ACoAs are found to be curved, tortuous, or kinked. The ACoA often is the location for congenital anomalies. The ACoA frequently is a site for aneurysm formation and is the most common site for aneurysms associated with subarachnoid hemorrhage. The ACoA is short in length, and although it may be captured in the Doppler sample volume at midline, it cannot be visualized during TCD imaging.

VERTEBRAL ARTERY

The **vertebral arteries** are large branches of the subclavian arteries. Atherosclerotic changes usually occur at the origin of the vertebral arteries. The two vertebral arteries are equal in size in approximately 25% of cases; therefore, size asymmetry is common. The left vertebral artery is usually the dominant artery. The vertebral artery is divided into four segments; the extravertebral, intervertebral, horizontal, and the intracranial. During TCD examinations the intracranial segment of the vertebral artery is evaluated. The intracranial portion begins as it pierces the dura and arachnoid immediately below the base of the skull at the foramen magnum. It continues anterior and medial to the anterior surface of the medulla and unites with the contralateral vertebral artery to form the basilar artery. Several major branches arise from this segment of the vertebral artery. The anterior spinal artery and the posterior inferior cerebellar artery (PICA) are sometimes visualized during TCD imaging. The PICA is the largest branch of the vertebral artery and commonly arises approximately 1 to 2 cm proximal to the confluence of the two vertebral arteries.

BASILAR ARTERY

The **basilar artery (BA)** is formed by the union of the two vertebral arteries and is evaluated during TCD imaging. It is variable in its pathway, size, and length. It usually originates at the lower border of the pons, extends anteriorly and superiorly, and terminates by dividing into the paired posterior cerebral arteries. During its course, the basilar artery gives off several branches, including the anterior inferior cerebellar arteries, the internal auditory (labyrinthine) arteries, the pontine branches, and the superior cerebellar arteries just proximal to the posterior cerebral arteries. The basilar artery is often tortuous and may be duplicated or fenestrated.

POSTERIOR CEREBRAL ARTERY

The **posterior cerebral arteries (PCAs)** originate from the terminal basilar artery and course anteriorly and laterally. The segment of the PCA from its origin to its junction with the PCoA is termed P1, the precommunicating portion. The P1 segment is evaluated during TCD imaging. Many perforating branches that supply the brain stem and thalamus originate from this segment. The portion of the vessel extending posteriorly from the PCoA to the posterior aspect of the midbrain is the P2 segment and may be visualized during transcranial imaging. The P3 and P4 segments of the PCA are not visualized during transcranial imaging. The proximal portion of the PCA is usually asymmetric. In cases of a "fetal" origin, the P1 segment is hypoplastic or smaller than the PCoA. It is uncommon for occlusive disease to be limited to the PCA, but if it does occur, the P2 segment is most commonly affected.

CIRCLE OF WILLIS

The **circle of Willis** was first described in 1664 by Thomas Willis. The circle is composed of the A1 segments of the two ACAs, the ACoA, the two PCoAs, the two ICAs, and the P1 segment of the two PCAs. It is a polygon vascular ring at the base of the brain that permits communication between the right and left cerebral hemispheres (via the ACoA) and between the anterior and posterior systems (via the PCoAs). These communications are important when there is significant disease or occlusion of one of the major cervical arteries. Variations of the circle of Willis are common: A "classic" circle of Willis is found in only approximately 20% to 25% of cases. Significant hypoplasia or absence of the PCoA, ACoA, ACA (A1), and PCA (P1) are the most common variations.

TECHNICAL ASPECTS OF TRANSCRANIAL COLOR DOPPLER IMAGING

Color Doppler imaging is currently being used to investigate the intracranial arterial circulation. To obtain consistently reliable studies with TCD imaging the operator must appreciate the importance of proper patient positioning, use the available anatomic landmarks that are important for the accurate identification of the intracranial arteries, and be knowledgeable about the proper use of the instrument's controls. The accuracy of the examination will increase by using the gray scale image and the color display to guide the TCD evaluation.

INSTRUMENTATION

Instrument controls and control settings vary depending on the manufacturer of the color Doppler imaging system. Therefore, it is important for the operator to be familiar with the particular imaging system being used. Hard copy records of the spectral waveforms may be made using any of the standard formats, but a videocassette recording has the advantage of the audio signal in addition to the spectral waveforms.

TCD imaging is performed with a phased array imaging transducer. A 2-MHz transducer (imaging and Doppler) is ideal for this application. However, transmitting frequencies as high as 2.5 MHz have been used with success. High-quality TCD imaging depends on the proper adjustment of several instrument controls. It is important to optimize the gray scale image, know how each color control will independently affect the image, and understand how the different controls affect each other. The patient's arterial hemodynamics and the information that is relevant to the patient being evaluated may result in the adjustment of different controls.

The gray scale image is produced by echoes, which are transmitted sound waves that are reflected from tissue interfaces and returned to the ultrasound transducer. Instrument controls to consider when adjusting the gray scale image during TCD imaging are sector width, image depth, gain, focal zone, frame rate, and dynamic range.

The color Doppler display is very important during TCD imaging. It is used as a guide to correctly place the sample volume to obtain the detailed hemodynamic information from the Doppler spectral waveforms. The color Doppler information is displayed in a small area designated the color "box" in most imaging systems. The color box is moved to the area of interest on the gray scale image. During TCD imaging, the entire circle of Willis often can be captured within a small color box. If not, to maintain a good frame rate, the color box should remain small and the anterior and posterior circulations evaluated separately by moving the position of the color box. Instrument controls to consider when adjusting the color Doppler display during TCD are color gain, scale (pulse repetition frequency [PRF]), wall filter, sensitivity (ensemble length), and persistence.

The real-time display of all Doppler shift frequencies over time is the Doppler spectral waveform. Time is recorded along the horizontal axis, and velocity (frequency) is recorded on the vertical axis. Velocity is recorded in centimeters per second (cm/sec). A positive Doppler shift (toward the transducer) is displayed above the baseline and a negative Doppler shift (away from the transducer) below the baseline. Accurate recording of the intracranial Doppler spectral waveform is critical, because this is the basis for interpretation of the TCD imaging examination. Instrument controls to consider when obtaining Doppler signals are sample volume size, gain, velocity scale (PRF), baseline, wall filter, and output. During TCD imaging the Doppler power should be increased for adequate penetration. However, it should be at the lowest level necessary and applied for the shortest duration possible to obtain good clinical information. The ALARA (*as low as reasonably achievable*) principle should be applied during TCD imaging examinations.

TECHNIQUE

The standard transtemporal, transorbital, suboccipital, and submandibular windows are used for TCD imaging (Figure 32-2). Interpretation criteria previously developed with the nonimaging TCD technique are used with TCD imaging. TCD imaging, however, permits identification of structural landmarks that assist in accurately locating the intracranial arteries. Anatomic landmarks that are helpful in locating the circle of Willis when using the transtemporal approach are the petrous ridge of the temporal bone, sphenoid bone, cerebral falx, suprasellar cistern, and cerebral peduncles. When performing the suboccipital approach, the foramen magnum and the occipital bone are used as anatomic landmarks to locate the vertebrobasilar system. The globe and optic nerve are helpful anatomic landmarks for locating the ophthalmic artery and the carotid siphon when using the transorbital window.

Conventional color orientation for TCD examinations is set for shades of red indicating blood flow toward the transducer and shades of blue indicating flow away from the transducer. By keeping this color assignment constant, intracranial blood flow direction in the arteries can be readily recognized.

The TCD evaluation of the intracranial arteries is performed with a large sample volume (5 to 10 mm) to obtain a good signal to noise ratio. Intracranial arterial velocities acquired with TCD imaging are also acquired assuming a zero-degree angle. Several investigators have evaluated the potential use of angle-adjusted (corrected) velocities during TCD imaging.[12,29,39] Because the walls of the arteries cannot be visualized during TCD imaging, the operator must angle-correct

for the color display. Angle-adjusted velocities are elevated compared with velocities taken assuming a zero-degree angle. Considering that an intracranial artery is tortuous and lies in different ultrasound planes, angle adjustment is only possible for a short segment of the artery.[13] Although the data for angle adjustment appear interesting, they have not been thoroughly evaluated, and it is recommended that routine TCD imaging be performed assuming a zero-degree angle.

Additionally, with the use of TCD imaging, many investigators are reporting TCD results using peak-systolic and end-diastolic velocities instead of the traditionally accepted mean velocities (time-averaged peak velocities). Each institution will have to decide which velocity value to report and adjust diagnostic criteria accordingly.

Transtemporal Window. The **transtemporal window** approach is performed with the patient in the supine position with the head aligned straight with the body. The transducer is placed on the temporal bone cephalad to the zygomatic arch and anterior to the ear. A generous amount of acoustic gel is necessary to ensure good transducer to skin contact, especially in patients for whom angling the transducer to optimize the Doppler signal requires the footprint to be elevated from the skin's surface.

Finding this window can be difficult and at times frustrating because ultrasound penetration of the temporal bone is necessary. Other windows used during the TCD examination are usually less difficult to find because natural ostia allow easy intracranial penetration of the ultrasound beam. The transtemporal window varies in size and location with each patient and may vary in an individual from one side to the other. Attenuation of the Doppler signal occurs at the temporal bone interface, and its magnitude depends on the thickness of the bone. One study found that the power measured behind the skull was never greater than 35% of the transmitted power, and the mean value of power loss was 80%.[15] The ability to penetrate the temporal bone is influenced by the patient's age, sex, and race. Hyperostosis of the skull is commonly found in older individuals, females, and African-Americans. A transtemporal window is not located in approximately 10% to 30% of the population.

The transducer's orientation marker or light should be pointing in the anterior direction, with the transducer angled slightly superiorly. This orientation of the transducer produces an imaging plane that is a transverse oblique view. This view has the advantage of simultaneous visualization of the anterior and posterior intracranial circulation in many patients. The ipsilateral hemisphere is at the top and the contralateral hemisphere at the bottom of the monitor, with anterior being to the left side and posterior to the right side of the monitor. Although the contralateral hemisphere is visualized in many patients, each hemisphere should be separately studied through the ipsilateral ultrasound window to obtain the best artery to transducer angle. In patients with only a unilateral transtemporal window, however, evaluating the contralateral hemisphere is possible and may provide valuable information.

After locating the transtemporal window, identifying bony landmarks ensures position at the correct level within the skull

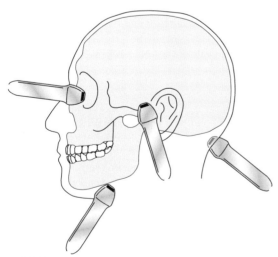

Figure 32-2 Placement of the ultrasound transducer for the four transcranial Doppler windows; transtemporal, transorbital, suboccipital, and the submandibular approaches.

to locate the circle of Willis. The reflective echo extending anteriorly is the lesser wing of the sphenoid bone, and the petrous ridge of the temporal bone extends posteriorly (Figures 32-3 and 32-4). The ipsilateral temporal lobe is at the top of the image.

Once the bony landmarks are identified, the color Doppler display is turned on (Figures 32-5 and 32-6). The terminal ICA (t-ICA) is visualized, and the direction of blood flow depends on the artery's anatomic configuration. Blood flow is usually toward the transducer, and the mean velocity is normally 39 ± 9 cm/sec. At this anatomic location, there may be mirror imaging artifact caused by the adjacent bone. The transducer is then angled anteriorly and superiorly so the MCA and anterior cerebral artery ACA can be evaluated. The MCA

courses adjacent to the sphenoid wing. The main trunk of the MCA is displayed in red because blood flow is normally toward the transducer. The mean velocity is normally 62 ± 12 cm/sec (Figure 32-7). The M2 branches are usually displayed in red but may appear blue as they curve and blood flows away from the transducer.

The ACA is displayed in shades of blue as it courses away from the transducer toward the midline. It may be necessary to angle the transducer slightly anteriorly and superiorly to visualize the ACA. The mean velocity is normally 50 ± 11 cm/sec. It may be necessary to decrease the color PRF to visualize this artery because of its lower velocity. The initial portion of the A2 segment often can be visualized and is displayed in blue extending in an anterior direction at midline.

The posterior circulation is visualized by angling the transducer slightly posteriorly and inferiorly, using the cerebral peduncles as an anatomic landmark. Normally the two cerebral peduncles are identical in size and shape and are of intermediate echogenicity. The PCA wraps around the cerebral peduncle. The color PRF may need to be decreased to visualize the PCAs because of the lower blood flow velocity. The P1 segment is displayed in red because blood flow is normally toward the

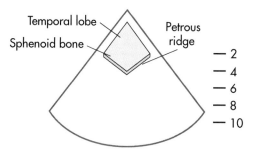

Figure 32-3 Schematic of the bony landmarks from the transtemporal approach.

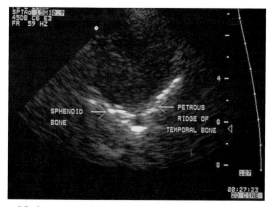

Figure 32-4 Image of the bony landmarks from the transtemporal approach.

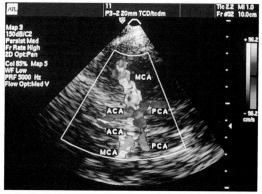

Figure 32-6 Color Doppler image of the intracranial arteries from the transtemporal approach. The ipsilateral hemisphere is at the top of the image and the contralateral hemisphere at the bottom of the image. *ACA,* Anterior cerebral artery; *MCA,* middle cerebral artery; *PCA,* posterior cerebral artery.

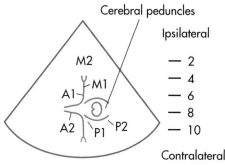

Figure 32-5 Schematic of the arteries in the circle of Willis from the transtemporal approach.

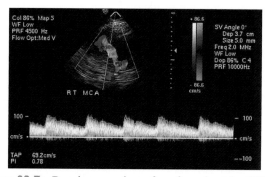

Figure 32-7 Doppler spectral waveform from the right *(RT)* middle cerebral artery *(MCA).* A zero-degree angle is used and blood flow is toward the transducer.

transducer. The normal mean velocity is 39 ± 10 cm/sec. Often the ipsilateral and contralateral P1 segments can be visualized at their origin as the basilar artery terminates. The ipsilateral P1 segment is in shades of red, and the contralateral P1 segment is displayed in shades of blue. The P2 segment may be displayed in red just distal to the origin of the PCoA, but will be displayed in blue distally as it wraps around the cerebral peduncle. The color display of the P2 segment is variable because of the vessel's anatomic course and orientation to the transducer.

The ACoA is not visualized because it is short in length. However, the PCoA is longer in length and often is visualized connecting the anterior and posterior circulations in patients (Figure 32-8). The mean peak velocity in the PCoA is 36 ± 15 cm/sec, and the direction of blood flow may be toward or away from the transducer. The color PRF may need to be decreased to visualize the PCoA. Additionally, using power Doppler imaging may be helpful in locating the PCoA because this artery often courses parallel to the skin line.

Although the anterior and posterior circulations can be simultaneously visualized in many patients, often the patient's anatomy requires separate evaluation. Minor changes in the transducer's position on the surface of the skin or its angle permit individual evaluation of either intracranial circulatory circulation.

The quality of the intracranial image depends on proper adjustment of many instrument controls. To obtain quality color Doppler images, increase the color gain to the appropriate level, maintain a small sector width and color box width to keep the highest possible frame rates, change the color PRF depending on the patient's hemodynamics or the particular intracranial artery being evaluated, and be aware of the color sensitivity and persistence settings. The color display is important because it assists in the proper placement of the Doppler sample volume. The interpretation of the TCD examination is made from the Doppler spectral waveform information. Doppler signals are obtained along the path of the artery using the color display as a road map. At each depth setting, it is important to adjust the sample volume and angle the transducer to optimize the Doppler signal. Additionally, it is important to remember that the color Doppler display is in two dimensions and tortuous intracranial arteries frequently cannot be displayed along their length as a continuous color pathway.

Suboccipital Window. When evaluating the vertebrobasilar system, the best results are obtained with the patient lying on his or her side with the head bowed slightly toward the chest. This position increases the gap between the cranium and the atlas. The orientation marker or light on the transducer should be pointing to the patient's right side. The transducer is placed on the posterior aspect of the neck inferior to the nuchal crest. The best images from this approach are acquired with the transducer slightly off midline, with the ultrasound beam directed toward the bridge of the patient's nose.

The large, circular, anechoic area seen from the **suboccipital window** is the foramen magnum, and the bright, echogenic reflection is from the occipital bone. Blood flow is normally away from the transducer in the vertebrobasilar system, and the color display appears as a blue Y. The right vertebral artery is displayed on the left side of the image and the left vertebral artery is on the right side (Figure 32-9). The basilar artery is deep to the vertebral arteries (Figure 32-10). The mean velocity is 38 ± 10 cm/sec in the vertebral arteries and 41 ± 10 cm/sec in the basilar artery. Because the posterior circulation has lower velocities than the anterior circulation, the operator may need to decrease the color PRF to visualize the vertebrobasilar system.

TCD imaging allows visualization of the confluence of the vertebral arteries into the basilar artery. Attention to the color gain setting is critical when trying to measure the exact depth of the vertebral artery confluence. Additionally, branches

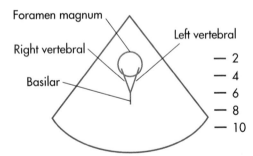

Figure 32-9   Schematic of the suboccipital approach during a transcranial Doppler imaging examination.

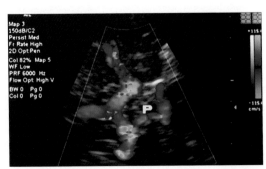

Figure 32-8   The posterior communicating artery *(P)* is visualized connecting the anterior and the posterior intracranial arterial circulations.

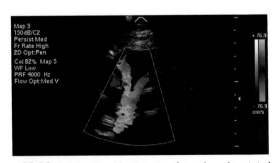

Figure 32-10   Color Doppler imaging from the suboccipital approach. Blood flow is away from transducer and displayed in blue. The right vertebral artery is on the left side of the image, and the left vertebral artery is displayed on the right side of the image. The basilar artery is deep to the vertebral arteries.

of the vertebral arteries, especially the PICA, can often be visualized and are usually displayed in red as they curve and carry blood toward the transducer. Moving the transducer slightly inferiorly on the neck and angling superiorly often allows better visualization of the distal basilar artery. The terminal portion of the basilar artery as it bifurcates into the PCAs cannot be visualized from this TCD approach.

Transorbital Window. The **transorbital window** evaluation provides information about the ophthalmic artery and the carotid siphon. Recently the U.S. Food and Drug Administration (FDA) approved certain imaging transducers on various manufacturers' equipment for the evaluation of the orbit. It is important for each operator to contact the appropriate ultrasound company and determine which transducer is approved for orbital imaging for their imaging system.

When imaging the orbit, it is important to decrease the power setting significantly before evaluating the orbit. Additionally, the examination time should be minimized. Although there are not any known observed bioeffects from the ultrasound evaluation of the eye, the power settings raise concern for ocular damage. The current FDA maximum acoustic output allowable levels (derated) for ophthalmic imaging are a spatial peak temporal average intensity of 17 mW/cm^2 and a mechanical index of 0.28.

The examination is performed with the patient in the supine position, and the transducer gently placed on the closed eyelid. A liberal amount of acoustic gel is important, and firm pressure on the eyelid is not necessary. The orientation marker on the imaging transducer should be pointed medially, toward the nose, when performing the right or left examination. Evaluation of either eye produces an image with medial (nasal) on the left side and temporal on the right side of the monitor. A variation of this technique is to have the transducer's orientation marker directed to the patient's right side when evaluating either eye. This transducer orientation will produce an image with medial (nasal) on the monitor's left when examining the left eye and medial on the monitor's right side when evaluating the right eye. The globe is visualized at the top of the monitor.

The direction of blood flow in the carotid siphon depends on which segment (parasellar, genu, or supraclinoid) is insonated (Figure 32-11). Blood flow is bidirectional at the genu, toward the transducer in the parasellar portion and away from the transducer in the supraclinoid segment. The mean velocity in the carotid siphon is 47 ± 14 cm/sec (Figure 32-12).

The **ophthalmic artery** is generally identified adjacent to the optic nerve. The color PRF should be decreased to visualize the ophthalmic artery. The ultrasound beam should be directed slightly medially along the anteroposterior plane. Blood flow is normally toward the transducer, with a mean velocity of 21 ± 5 cm/sec. The ophthalmic artery Doppler signal has a high pulsatility because this artery supplies blood to the globe and its structures.

Submandibular Window. The **submandibular window** approach is a continuation of the duplex imaging evaluation

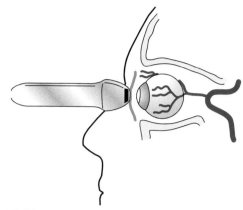

Figure 32-11   Schematic of the transorbital approach. The ophthalmic artery is a branch of the internal carotid artery.

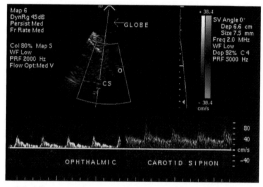

Figure 32-12   Color Doppler image of the transorbital approach. The ophthalmic Doppler spectral waveform demonstrates a high-resistance signal, and the carotid siphon *(CS)* a low-resistance signal. A mechanical index of 0.28 or less should be used when using the transorbital approach. *O,* Ophthalmic artery.

of the extracranial distal ICA. The transducer is placed at the angle of the mandible and angled slightly medially and cephalad toward the carotid canal. The transducer's orientation marker or light is pointed in a superior direction. Distal ICA blood flow is away from the transducer and is displayed in shades of blue. Careful Doppler evaluation will distinguish the ICA's low-resistance signal from the higher-resistance signal from the ECA. The mean velocity in the retromandibular portion of the ICA is normally 37 ± 9 cm/sec.

At the end of the TCD imaging examination, the ultrasound gel should be removed from the patient. Excess gel should be removed from the ultrasound transducer, and it should be cleaned using a disinfectant.

INTERPRETATION OF TRANSCRANIAL COLOR DOPPLER IMAGING

Standard interpretation criteria for TCD examinations have been reported in the literature. During the evolution of the TCD examination, however, it became apparent that important underlying physiologic variables may affect the intracranial velocities. Therefore, it is important to be aware of the factors that may affect intracranial hemodynamics and interpret each case individually.

The proper identification of the intracranial vasculature is, of course, the first step in evaluating the TCD examination. Each TCD window provides access to specific arteries. The identification of the arteries is based on the following:

1. *Depth of the sample volume.* The sample volume depth is measured in millimeters (mm) and is the distance from the face of the ultrasound transducer to the middle of the Doppler sample volume. The sample volume length should be kept large (5 to 10 mm) to achieve the best signal to noise ratio. The depth ranges at which the intracranial arteries can be located from each TCD window are listed in Table 32-1. The depths of the arteries may vary with each individual, but in most adults the artery in question will usually fall within these ranges. Midline is in the range of 70 to 80 mm in most adults.

2. *Angle of the transducer.* The angle of the transducer is also important because different arteries can be insonated at the same depth from a TCD ultrasound window. The operator's position at the head of the patient will enable the best perception of the transducer-artery angle because it permits orientation of the ultrasound transducer to the body's axes and planes.

3. *Blood flow direction.* The normal direction of blood flow in the intracranial arteries relative to the ultrasound transducer

is listed in Table 32-1. From the different approaches, Doppler spectral waveforms may demonstrate blood flow direction away from, toward, or in both directions (bidirectional). If the direction of blood flow is reversed from the established norm, it can be assumed that the artery is functioning as a collateral channel or that there may be an anatomic variant.

4. *Spatial relationship.* Understanding the spatial relationship of one artery to another is also helpful in properly identifying the intracranial arteries. Using the t-ICA bifurcation as a guide, the location of the intracranial arteries is determined with more technical ease.

5. *Traceability of an artery.* The operator should be able to "trace" the anatomic route of the artery in stepwise fashion by increasing or decreasing the depth setting of the sample volume. The Doppler sample volume can be swept slowly along the path of the color Doppler display to correctly assess the entire length of the artery.

6. *Adjacent anatomic structures.* Using the anatomic structures visualized on gray scale as a guide to correctly identify the intracranial arteries is especially important. It is the major advantage of using imaging versus the nonimaging TCD technique.

NORMAL INTRACRANIAL ARTERIAL VELOCITIES

The depths, mean velocities, and the normal direction of blood flow relative to the ultrasound transducer for the intracranial arteries from each TCD window are listed in Table 32-1.

It is customary to assume a zero-degree angle (no angle correction) when performing TCD examinations. Different investigators have reported similar velocities for the same vessels, demonstrating good interobserver agreement. Mean velocities (time-averaged peak) are usually reported for TCD examinations because this parameter is less affected by changes of central cardiovascular factors (heart rate, peripheral resistance, etc.) than systolic or diastolic values, thereby diminishing interindividual variations.

The **mean velocity** calculated during TCD imaging examinations is based on the time average of the outline velocity (maximum velocity envelope). The velocity envelope is a trace of the peak velocities as a function of time. The mean velocity can be estimated by positioning the horizontal cursor at the velocity where the area below the peak velocity and above the cursor are equal to the area below the cursor and above the peak velocity envelope in diastole (Figure 32-13). Another method to estimate the mean velocity of a TCD Doppler signal is to use the following formula:

Differences between intracranial arterial velocities are more important than the absolute values recorded from an individual. General observations of the mean velocities in the intracranial arteries are as follows:

- The velocities are highest in the MCA.
- If an ACA velocity is more than 25% greater than the MCA velocity, the ACA may be hypoplastic or stenotic or serving as a collateral vessel or there may be an MCA distribution infarction.

TABLE 32-1	INTRACRANIAL ARTERIAL IDENTIFICATION CRITERIA		
Window/Artery	Depth (mm)	Mean Velocity (cm/sec)	Direction*
Transtemporal			
MCA	30-67	62 ± 12	Toward
ACA	60-80	50 ± 11	Away
t-ICA	55-67	39 ± 9	Toward
PCA	60-75	39 ± 10	Toward
PCoA	60-75	36 ± 15	Toward, away
Transorbital			
Ophthalmic	40-60	21 ± 5	Toward
ICA siphon	60-80	47 ± 14	Bi, away, toward
Suboccipital			
Vertebral	60-85	38 ± 10	Away
Basilar	>85	41 ± 10	Away
Submandibular			
ICA	35-80	37 ± 9	Away

*Relative to the ultrasound transducer.
ACA, Anterior cerebral artery; *Bi,* bidirectional; *ICA,* internal carotid artery; *t-ICA,* terminal internal carotid artery; *MCA,* middle cerebral artery; *PCA,* posterior cerebral artery; *PCoA,* posterior communicating artery.

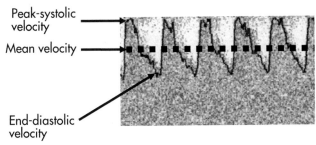

Peak-systolic velocity

Mean velocity

End-diastolic velocity

Figure 32-13 A Doppler spectral waveform from the middle cerebral artery. The arrows point to the peak-systolic velocity, the mean velocity *(dotted line)*, and the end-diastolic velocity.

• The velocities in the anterior circulation are higher than the posterior circulation.

In the asymptomatic adult patient, side-to-side asymmetry should be minimal. The difference between sides has been reported to be less than 30%.[18,35] Small differences generally do not indicate an underlying pathologic condition. If a significant side-to-side difference is noted during the examination, try repeating the side with the lower velocities. Often by repeating the evaluation and modifying the transducer-to-artery angle, the side-to-side differences found on the initial examination can be reduced. If side-to-side differences occur, they should not be considered abnormal unless they exceed 30%. Additionally, asymmetries in the intracranial vertebral arteries make it difficult to interpret asymmetric velocities from these arteries unless the differences are in a focal segment of the vessels.

The pulsatility index (PI) was first described in an attempt to quantify Doppler waveforms during the evaluation of lower extremity arterial disease.[14] Although most imaging systems will automatically calculate the PI with each Doppler display sweep, it can be calculated from the following formula:

$$PI = \frac{\text{Systolic velocity} - \text{Diastolic velocity}}{\text{Mean velocity}}$$

When using the PI, the resistance that is encountered with each cardiac cycle is considered. For example, damped blood flow distal to an obstruction will have a decreased PI (diastolic velocity greater than 50% to 60% of peak systolic). Doppler signals obtained proximal to a high resistance (i.e., increased intracranial pressure), however, will have an increased PI (pulsatile spectral waveform). The PI in the MCA is normally in the range of 0.5 to 1.1.

Spectral broadening is observed in the Doppler waveforms obtained during TCD examinations. The Doppler sample volume size used during TCD imaging is usually larger than the intracranial arteries. In fact, the sample volume often includes the entire cross-sectional lumen of an intracranial artery and its small branches. Therefore, even though spectral broadening may be used as a diagnostic criterion for moderate degrees of stenosis in the extracranial carotid arteries, it is not helpful in refining the TCD interpretation.

Various technical factors, including the operator, can contribute to TCD measurement variability. Several studies have concentrated on the interobserver and intraobserver variabil-

ity.[25,35,38] The data provided by these studies indicate that day-to-day differences found by the same examiner usually do not exceed 20%. The size of the ultrasound window and the possibility of different angles of insonation may be the major source of the variability.

PHYSIOLOGIC FACTORS

Age. TCD velocities are affected by the age of the patient. Several investigators have found lower intracranial arterial velocities with increasing age.* The downward trend in intracranial arterial velocities may be multifactorial, but primarily results from changes in cardiac output and corresponds to an age-related decrease in cerebral blood flow.

Sex. Penetration of the temporal bone with the ultrasound beam is more difficult in females than in males. However, once intracranial Doppler signals are obtained, there do not appear to be major differences in the velocity readings because of the sex of the patient. Two studies, however, have demonstrated a slight increase (3% to 5%) of MCA velocities in females.[16,17] Possible explanations for these findings are that females have lower hematocrits, the intracranial arteries may be smaller in diameter, and women have higher hemispheric cerebral blood flow than men. The small differences documented in the intracranial arterial velocities because of the sex of the patient need further investigation.

Hematocrit. Hematocrit (Hct) is the percentage of red blood cells by volume in whole blood and is a major determinant of blood viscosity. Blood viscosity is an important factor influencing intracranial arterial blood flow velocity. Intracranial arterial velocities increase in the presence of anemia (Hct <30%). If anemia is the cause for the elevated velocities, then these changes should be detected from all of the intracranial arteries. Focal or localized velocity increases suggest a different cause.

Carbon Dioxide Reactivity. Changes in arterial carbon dioxide (CO_2) partial pressure (PCO_2) have an effect on cerebral blood flow and the intracranial arterial velocities. An early study demonstrated angiographically that the diameters of the large basal arteries remain constant during changes in PCO_2.[19] Alteration of cerebral vascular resistance and changes in the TCD signals are a result of changes at the level of the arteriolar channels. Hyperventilation (a deficiency of CO_2 in the blood known as hypocapnia) causes a decrease in the MCA mean velocity and an increase in the PI. Hypoventilation (an excess of CO_2 in the blood is referred to as hypercapnia) causes an increase in MCA mean velocity and a decrease in the PI. This information suggests that general changes in the intracranial arterial velocities caused by CO_2 reactivity must be taken into account when interpreting the TCD data.

Heart Rate and Cardiac Output. Intracranial arterial velocities are also a reflection of an individual's heart rate. Most experienced TCD examiners caution against taking a reading if the patient is yawning, agitated, or experiencing pain or if

---

*References 3, 17, 19, 20, 30.

there is any other reason causing a change in the heart rate. Any cardiac arrhythmia will be reflected in the TCD recording. If there is any question concerning a change in the patient's heart rate, several display sweeps should be obtained before relying on the calculations. To compensate for extreme cases of bradycardia or tachycardia, the operator may need to adjust the instrument's Doppler display sweep time. Changes resulting from cardiac output not associated with hemodilution have little effect on the cerebral blood flow if autoregulation is intact. This suggests that TCD velocities should be relatively independent of small changes in cardiac output. Data on the relationship between cardiac output and intracranial arterial velocities are limited, and further investigation in this area is necessary.

Many parameters are involved in the accurate interpretation of TCD data. Each patient must be considered individually because of the variety of physiologic factors that affect the intracranial arterial hemodynamics (Box 32-2). The parameters that affect the intracranial velocities can be categorized into those factors that are: (1) proximal to the circle of Willis, (2) at the level of the circle of Willis, and (3) distal to the circle of Willis.

The most useful TCD results are from comparing velocities from different sample volume depths from the same artery and from comparing the velocities from the different arteries within an individual. Bilateral symmetric disease may be difficult to diagnose by TCD imaging. Correct identification of the intracranial arteries, knowledge of the normal velocity ranges, familiarity with the technique's limitations, and understanding of how cerebral hemodynamics may be affected by different physiologic parameters are essential for the accurate interpretation of TCD examinations. It is imperative that each institution develop a TCD imaging protocol that defines the standard examination (arteries to be evaluated from each window, the number of Doppler samples from each artery, etc.). This protocol must include the technique, clinical applications, indications for a complete and/or limited examination, and interpretation criteria. A standard complete examination usually includes evaluation of both the right and left sides, acquiring Doppler information from the anterior and posterior intracranial arterial systems.

CLINICAL APPLICATIONS

The clinical applications for TCD have expanded since its inception in 1982. A brief description of a variety of the clinical applications follows, with special attention to the technical nuances and the interpretation criteria used for the various clinical applications.

VASOSPASM

Cerebral vasospasm (vasoconstriction of the arteries) is a serious complication after subarachnoid hemorrhage (SAH), and is a significant cause of morbidity and mortality. The most common cause of SAH is leakage of blood from intracranial cerebral aneurysms into the subarachnoid space. Common sites for intracranial aneurysm formation are the ACoA, the MCA, and the PCoA. Early diagnosis and treatment reduce the devastating consequences of this disorder.

The hemodynamic effect of vasospasm produces an increase in blood flow velocity coupled with a pressure drop distal to the narrowed segment. Patients compensate for these changes and maintain cerebral blood flow through their collateral circulations and cerebral autoregulation. When there is increased intracranial pressure or the vasomotor reserve has been exhausted, cerebral blood flow can be reduced to critical levels resulting in ischemia or infarction.

Examinations are usually performed bedside in the intensive care unit. The important technical features when studying the patient with vasospasm associated with SAH are as follows:

- The operator must be properly positioned at the patient's bedside to make appropriate adjustments in transducer angle and be able to adjust the control settings on the equipment.
- Headphones are helpful because the high-velocity signals associated with vasospasm can be difficult to appreciate if there is extraneous background noise.
- The locations of the transtemporal window should be marked on the patient's skin, if possible, so that subsequent examinations can be performed from the same location, thereby ensuring the most reliable comparisons.
- If possible, repeat examinations should be performed by the same operator to eliminate interobserver variability.

In some patients the surgical head dressing may need to be removed to access the transtemporal window. Sterile ultrasound gel is used if the transducer is placed near a wound. TCD recording is possible through a burr hole. However, the equipment's intensity levels should be decreased because the bone no longer causes attenuation of the Doppler signal. TCD imaging in this group of patients can be challenging because of variable patient cooperation, changing cardiovascular and cerebral hemodynamics, and less than optimal testing conditions. Clip artifacts may mask localized segments of increased velocity.

BOX 32-2   INTERPRETATION OF TRANSCRANIAL COLOR DOPPLER IMAGING

PROXIMAL TO THE CIRCLE OF WILLIS
- Patient's age
- Amount and location of extracranial arterial obstruction
- Hematocrit
- Cardiac output

AT THE LEVEL OF THE CIRCLE OF WILLIS
- Vessel diameter
- Blood viscosity
- Turbulence

DISTAL TO THE CIRCLE OF WILLIS
- Infarction
- Intracranial arteriovenous malformations (AVMs)
- Increased intracranial pressure
- Change in PCO_2

Vasospasm is unusual the first 2 to 3 days after an SAH. Therefore, a TCD examination during this prespastic period serves as a valuable baseline. It allows monitoring of the rate at which vasospasm develops and provides a guide to future examinations because vessels in spasm are small and can be difficult to locate. The TCD examination should be performed daily or every other day for 2 weeks, and the highest velocity obtained from each artery should be recorded. Although a complete TCD examination is preferred, it is not always possible in these patients. Additionally, a cervical ICA signal is obtained at a depth of 45 to 60 mm (without angle adjustment) to calculate a hemispheric ratio. The frequency of follow-up studies will vary depending on the clinical symptoms and the degree of vasospasm. The PCO_2, Hct, and blood pressure should be recorded because these parameters may affect the intracranial arterial blood flow velocities. The time and the date of the examination are documented, and a graph plotting velocity versus time illustrates the time course of a patient's vasospasm. Following SAH, velocity increases begin to occur about day 3, reach a maximum between days 7 and 12, and generally resolve at 2 to 3 weeks.

MCA mean velocities of 100 to 120 cm/sec correlate with mild vasospasm as demonstrated by arteriography. Moderate vasospasm is defined by velocities in the 120- to 200-cm/sec range (Figures 32-14 and 32-15), and severe vasospasm is characterized by velocities exceeding 200 cm/sec. Mean velocities greater than 200 cm/sec indicate that the patient is at risk of reduced cerebral blood flow (CBF). A rapid increase (greater than 25 cm/day) in velocity in the first few days after the hemorrhage is associated with a poor prognosis.

The MCA/ICA (distal extracranial ICA) mean velocity ratio may be used to determine vasospasm. This hemispheric ratio accounts for a possible increase in the flow volume. The ratio increases with severe spasm resulting from increased MCA velocity as well as from reduced blood flow volume in the ipsilateral extracranial ICA caused by the increase in cerebral vascular resistance. The normal range for the MCA/ICA ratio is 1.7 ± 0.4. An MCA/ICA ratio greater than 3 corresponds to MCA vasospasm, and a ratio greater than 6 demonstrates severe vasospasm.

The sensitivity for diagnosing vasospasm by TCD depends on the skill of the operator, the presence of a good transtemporal window, anatomic consistency, a good transducer-to-artery angle, the location and the severity of the vasospasm, the presence of proximal hemodynamically significant lesions, physiologic parameters (increased intracranial pressure, blood pressure fluctuations, PCO_2 variations, Hct, etc.), the diagnostic criteria used, and the cooperation of the patient. The sensitivity of detecting vasospasm of the MCA has been reported to be from 39% to 94% and the specificity from 85% to 100%.[7,8,9,10,31] Data for detecting vasospasm in other intracranial arteries are limited but show a lower sensitivity.[24,34] *A negative TCD study does not exclude vasospasm.* Sources of error are (1) a tortuous or aberrant artery, (2) distal branch vasospasm, (3) increased intracranial pressure, and (4) reduction in volume flow (with or without infarction).

DIAGNOSIS OF INTRACRANIAL DISEASE

The ability to detect intracranial arterial stenosis, occlusion, and aneurysms is a new and potentially important addition to the noninvasive cerebrovascular examination. However, to accurately assess the intracranial vasculature, one must be cognizant of the hemodynamic changes associated with intracranial (and extracranial) disease.

Stenosis. Intracranial arterial stenoses cause characteristic alterations in the Doppler signal (audio and spectral waveform), including focal increases in velocity, local turbulence, and a poststenotic drop in velocity. These changes associated with a stenosis occur assuming that volume flow is maintained. Stenoses may also produce low-frequency enhancements around the baseline (bruit) or band-shaped enhancements symmetric with and parallel to the baseline (musical murmur).

A stenosis greater than 60% diameter reduction usually will be detected by TCD imaging. Absolute velocity criteria for the diagnosis of intracranial arterial stenoses are not reliable because of the many velocity alterations caused by nonvascular variables (age, Hct, etc.). Because absolute velocities are inaccurate, most investigators agree that a focal velocity increase of greater than or equal to 25% should raise suspicion of an arterial narrowing. Intracranial stenoses are most commonly found in the MCA and the internal carotid siphon. The status of the cerebral tissue perfused can also have considerable impact on intracranial velocity profiles. Patients with central MCA stenosis without infarction demonstrate an increased MCA velocity. However, the same patient with a cerebral infarction has diminished MCA velocity because of the decreased perfusion through the infarcted outflow bed.

Occlusion. TCD is limited in its ability to reliably identify intracranial arterial occlusion. The restriction to occlusion of the MCA is the result of inadequate transtemporal windows, anatomic variability, congenital aplasia, or severe hypoplasia of the other intracranial arteries.

MCA occlusion is suspected when an MCA Doppler signal is absent and high-quality Doppler signals are obtained from the uninvolved ipsilateral intracranial arteries (t-ICA, ACA, PCA). Locating the other ipsilateral arteries demonstrates that an adequate transtemporal window exists. An increase in the ipsilateral ACA velocity resulting from perfusion through leptomeningeal collaterals is considered corroborating evidence for an MCA occlusion.[21]

Information regarding the sensitivity and specificity of TCD in the diagnosis of intracranial stenoses and occlusion is limited.[5,10,18,22,36] The lack of reliable data is due to the overall low incidence of intracranial disease and the small number of patients who have quality intracranial arteriograms.

Aneurysm. Data are limited regarding TCD sensitivity in the diagnosis of intracranial aneurysms. Most investigators have found that detecting a patent intracranial aneurysm depends on the aneurysm's location and size and the sensitivity has been reported to be from 0% to 85%.[6,7,27,40] In one study 26 of 37 intracranial aneurysms were identified using color power

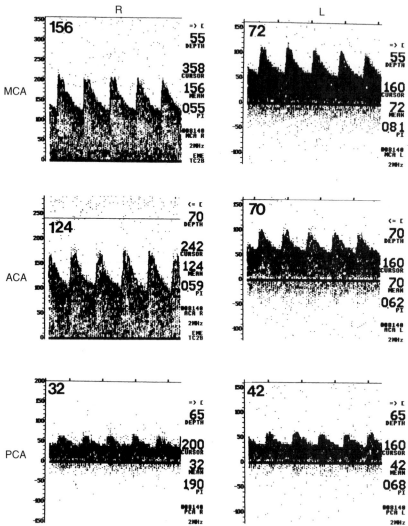

Figure 32-14 Doppler spectral waveforms from the middle cerebral artery *(MCA)*, anterior cerebral artery *(ACA)*, and the posterior cerebral artery *(PCA)* bilaterally. The Doppler spectral waveforms from the right *(R)* MCA and ACA demonstrate an increase in velocity, suggesting vasospasm in this 42-year-old patient. *L,* Left.

Doppler imaging.[41] In this exploratory study, the investigators found the following features useful in the identification of intracranial aneurysms: (1) rounded color areas projecting from an artery that appear noncontinuous at both ends with an artery; (2) color flow appearing in an unexpected area; (3) a color area that is wider than the adjacent arteries; and (4) an area with greater expansion and contraction during the cardiac cycle compared with the adjacent artery. These ultrasound characteristics may be important in the identification of intracranial aneurysms; however, the importance of proper instrument control settings cannot be overemphasized. In a recent study, investigators reported the identification of ruptured intracranial aneurysms in patients with acute subarachnoid hemorrhage using three-dimensional power Doppler imaging.[28] As technology advances, the role of TCD imaging may prove to be more useful for this clinical application in the future.

Collateral Pathways. The TCD examination reveals intracranial arterial collateral patterns in patients with extracranial arterial stenosis. An artery providing collateral circulation usually demonstrates an increased blood flow velocity. Unlike focal increases in velocity found in arterial stenosis, collateral pathways contain diffuse velocity increases throughout the length of the artery. Babikian and others have shown good correlation of TCD and arteriography in the identification of collateral patterns.[4]

The three main collateral pathways identified by TCD are (1) the ACoA providing a channel from hemisphere to hemisphere; (2) the ophthalmic artery providing a channel from the extracranial ECA to the intracranial ICA via the orbit; and (3) the PCoA allowing blood flow between the posterior and anterior circulation.

The most commonly found collateral pathway in response to significant extracranial disease is via the ACoA. The ultrasound characteristics of this collateral pathway include (1) an increase in the contralateral ACA velocity; (2) a turbulent Doppler signal with increased velocity at midline (resulting from high-velocity blood flow through the small ACoA); and (3) reversal of blood flow direction in the ipsilateral ACA.

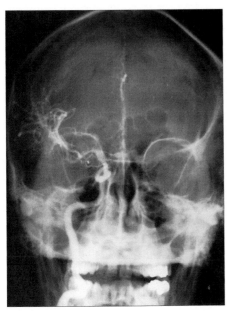

Figure 32-15 Corresponding arteriogram demonstrating vasospasm of the right middle cerebral and anterior cerebral arteries.

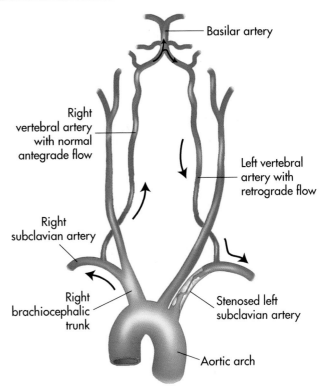

Figure 32-16 Subclavian steal. A narrowing of the left subclavian artery proximal to the vertebral artery causes a pressure drop that may cause reversal of blood flow direction in the left vertebral artery. This change in direction can be visualized in the extracranial or the intracranial vertebral arteries.

The ECA collateral pathway through the orbit is documented by reversed blood flow direction and a change to a low-resistance Doppler signal in the ophthalmic artery carrying blood flow from the ECA to the ICA. Collateral perfusion from the posterior circulation to the anterior circulation via the PCoA is the third pattern and is found most often in patients with significant bilateral extracranial carotid artery disease.

Subclavian Steal. The **subclavian steal syndrome** is characterized by symptoms of brain stem ischemia associated with a stenosis or occlusion of the left subclavian, innominate, or right subclavian artery proximal to the origin of the vertebral artery. A stenosis in this location may cause the pressure in the upper extremity to be lower than normal. The production of a pressure gradient can cause reversal of flow in the vertebral artery, especially during exercise of the involved arm (Figure 32-16). If this occurs, the vertebral artery becomes a major collateral to the upper extremity. The "stealing" of blood from the basilar artery, via retrograde vertebral artery flow, causes the patient to experience neurologic symptoms of brain stem ischemia.

If a systolic pressure differential greater than 20 mm Hg between arms is detected, a subclavian or innominate artery obstruction on the side of the lower pressure should be suspected. This physical finding is absent in rare instances and in cases of bilateral lesions.

If subclavian steal is suspected, a standard TCD examination should be performed, with special attention to the blood flow direction and the velocities in the vertebral and arteries and basilar artery. Blood flow is normally away from the transducer (suboccipital approach) in the vertebrobasilar system. If flow is toward the transducer in a vertebral artery and the basilar artery, there is evidence of a steal. Often the reversed

flow direction is found only in the vertebral artery, suggesting a possible vertebral to vertebral artery steal.

In the absence of blood flow reversal at rest or if alternating blood flow is observed, the involved upper extremity should be stressed to reduce outflow resistance, thereby revealing the hemodynamics of a potentially latent steal. The baseline examination and the subsequent changes in the spectral waveforms that occur after arm exercise or after occlusive hyperemia are recorded. To perform postocclusive reactive hyperemia, a blood pressure cuff is applied ipsilateral to the suspected stenosis/occlusion. The ipsilateral vertebral artery Doppler signal is located and monitored during inflation of the arm cuff. The blood pressure cuff is inflated above systolic pressure (greater than 20 mm Hg above systolic) for approximately 3 minutes, and any changes in the Doppler signal are noted. Then the cuff is rapidly deflated, and changes in the vertebral artery blood flow direction and velocity are recorded. This procedure is repeated while monitoring the contralateral vertebral artery and the basilar artery. A 5- to 10-minute rest period is usually sufficient for the return of baseline arterial hemodynamics between evaluations. Resting basilar artery blood flow is rarely affected, but may become abnormal if the contralateral feeding vertebral artery is also diseased.

Emboli Detection. Emboli detection has been reported during routine TCD testing in patients with carotid or cardiac disease. When monitoring the MCA for emboli, it is best to

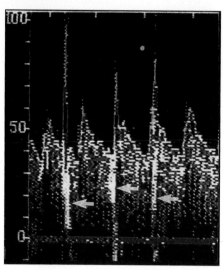

Figure 32-17   Emboli *(arrows)* recorded in the spectral Doppler waveform from a middle cerebral artery.

use the main trunk of the MCA (45 to 55 mm). A minimum of 15 to 20 minutes of monitoring is usually required, and a videotape recording is essential. The emboli rate is reported as the number of emboli per hour. Emboli cause an identifiable difference in the intensity of the returning Doppler signal (Figure 32-17); therefore, proper Doppler gain setting is critical and should be reduced so that the emboli can be detected.

The Consensus Committee of the Ninth International Cerebral Hemodynamic Symposium proposed minimal identification criteria for establishing microembolic signals.[3] An individual Doppler microembolic signal must have the following four features:

- The signal is transient, usually lasting less than 300 microseconds (μs).
- The amplitude of the signal is at least 3 decibels higher than the background blood flow signal.
- The signal is unidirectional within the Doppler spectral waveform.
- A microembolic signal is accompanied by a "snap," "chirp," or "moan" on the audio output.

In one study, bilateral MCAs were monitored for 20 minutes on each side.[26] No emboli were detected in 20 normal volunteers. However, emboli were detected in 24% (6/25) of the symptomatic patients with a carotid stenosis (mean = 2.17 signals per 20 minutes), and in 38% (9/24) of the patients with prosthetic cardiac valves (mechanical valves; mean = 17.6 signals per 20 minutes).

In another study, the MCA was monitored for 1 hour in 20 controls, 33 symptomatic patients, and 56 asymptomatic patients.[32] All patients had an extracranial ICA stenosis. There were no emboli detected in the controls. However, emboli were observed in 16% (9/56) of the asymptomatic patients and in 80% (27/33) of the symptomatic patients.

Sixty-four asymptomatic patients were followed for a mean follow-up of 72 weeks.[33] The patients had a documented unilateral 70% to 99% stenosis of the extracranial ICA by carotid

duplex imaging and did not have a history of atrial fibrillation or an artificial heart valve. The MCA was monitored for 1 hour. Thirteen percent (8/64) had two or more emboli per hour. This study demonstrated a significant association between two or more emboli per hour detected during a TCD examination and a subsequent neurologic event ($p = 0.005$). TCD imaging is currently being used to identify right-to-left shunts by detecting microbubbles.[2,11,37] To increase the sensitivity of detecting a patent foramen ovale, different patient positions have been recommended when using TCD for this clinical application.

The detection of cerebral microemboli by TCD offers new information in the diagnosis and management of patients with cerebrovascular disease. Good interobserver agreement suggests that the detection of microemboli by TCD is sufficiently reproducible to be used in the clinical setting. Adding the potential advantage of microemboli detection to TCD monitoring must be balanced with known limitations.

Predicting Stroke in Sickle Cell Disease.   TCD imaging is being used in the pediatric population, especially to screen children with sickle cell disease. Cerebral infarction in these patients is associated with an occlusion vasculopathy involving the terminal ICA, the MCA, and the ACA. Prevention of stroke may be feasible with chronic blood transfusion therapy if patients at risk can be identified.

The Stroke Prevention Trial in Sickle Cell Anemia (STOP) enrolled 130 children (ages 2 to 16) who were found to be at high risk for stroke on the basis of elevated (greater than 200 cm/sec) intracranial arterial mean velocities of the t-ICA or the MCA on two separate occasions.[1] The children were randomized to receive either standard supportive care or periodic blood transfusions. After 1 year, 10 children in the standard care group had a cerebral infarction compared with 1 child in the transfusion group. It is now recommended that children with sickle cell disease undergo screening with TCD. If the TCD examination is positive (greater than 200 cm/sec in the MCA or t-ICA), the child is at high risk for developing a stroke. In addition, positive or negative TCD results have been shown to be highly correlated between family members.[23] In children who had a sibling with a positive TCD examination, there were significant associations with elevated velocities in the other siblings with sickle cell disease.[23] The decision to start a child on chronic blood transfusion therapy is a clinical decision that should be made after careful consideration of the risks and benefits.

Technical adjustments for the evaluation of children by TCD imaging include using a smaller sample volume size (5 to 6 mm), applying different depth ranges for the intracranial arteries (these change with the age of the patient), and changing the PRF settings for the increase in intracranial arterial velocities (Figure 32-18).

Intracranial Venous Evaluation.   TCD imaging has allowed investigators to begin to explore the intracranial venous system. Several instrument adjustments are important when evaluating intracranial venous blood flow. The ultrasound evaluation of normal intracranial veins produces low-amplitude, pulsatile Doppler signals. Therefore, the color,

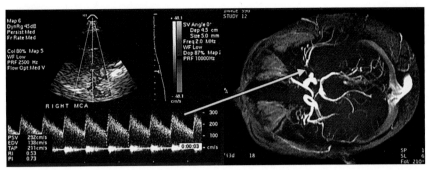

Figure 32-18 Transcranial color Doppler imaging examination and the corresponding magnetic resonance angiography in an 8-year-old patient with sickle cell disease. The mean velocity of the middle cerebral artery is greater than 200 cm/sec and corresponds to the intracranial arterial narrowing *(arrow)*.

Doppler PRF, and wall filter settings should be significantly reduced to ensure acquisition of good quality intracranial venous Doppler signals.

ADVANTAGES AND LIMITATIONS OF TRANSCRANIAL COLOR DOPPLER IMAGING

TCD imaging has several limitations (Box 32-3) and advantages when compared with the nonimaging TCD technique. Reducing the limitations and maximizing the advantages will ensure the most complete evaluation.

A limitation of the TCD imaging technique includes the operator having a sound understanding of color Doppler imaging principles. To obtain a quality study, this technique involves the proper use of more instrument controls than the nonimaging technique. Additionally, imaging systems are larger and less portable and therefore cumbersome to move for bedside examinations. The distal basilar artery is difficult to visualize with the color Doppler display because of the larger beam width. However, the basilar artery can usually be followed distally by increasing the sample volume depth and continuing as with a nonimaging examination by using the Doppler signal. The larger beam width also hampers penetration of the temporal bone when the transtemporal ultrasound window is small.

The advantages of using transcranial color Doppler imaging are that anatomic landmarks guide the proper identification of the intracranial arteries. This instills confidence in the operator and leads to improved reliability. Those who are inexperienced with the TCD technique also find the learning curve is shorter with the color Doppler imaging technique. Additionally, TCD imaging allows the identification of the large M2 branches, accurate identification of contralateral arteries if a transtemporal window can be located only on one side, easy visualization of collateral pathways, ease in following tortuous vessels, and identification of the vertebral confluence in many patients. Imaging also provides a method to document the location from which the Doppler spectral waveform is derived, which becomes important with repeat examinations, in departments where there are multiple operators and/or interpreters, and for quality improvement.

BOX 32-3   LIMITATIONS OF THE TRANSCRANIAL DOPPLER EXAMINATION

- Operator experience
- Improper instrument control settings
- An uncooperative patient or patient movement
- Absent or poor transtemporal window
- Anatomic variations
- Arterial misidentification
- Distal branch disease
- Distal basilar artery
- Misinterpretation of collateral channels or vasospasm as a stenosis
- Displacement of arteries by an intracranial mass

DIAGNOSTIC PITFALLS

Sources of error in the TCD diagnosis of intracranial arterial disease are as follows:

- Misinterpreting collateral channels or vasospasm for stenosis (vasospasm usually involves several arteries and the velocities change with time)
- The technical limitations of evaluating distal branch disease (stenosis or occlusion)
- The misinterpretation of a tortuous or displaced MCA (by hematoma or tumor) diagnosed as occlusion
- Anatomic variability (location, asymmetry, tortuosity), especially in the vertebrobasilar system
- Technical difficulty in the evaluation of the distal basilar artery
- The location and size of cerebral aneurysms
- Poor-quality arteriography leading to inaccurate correlations of the TCD results

TCD imaging offers new and important advantages to the TCD technique. Using the anatomic landmarks and proper instrument controls, a more accurate and reproducible evaluation of the intracranial arterial hemodynamics can be performed (Box 32-4). Hints to address common technical challenges associated with performing TCD examinations are located in Table 32-2. Color power imaging offers technical advantages in imaging small-caliber intracranial arteries,

Table 32-2 Transcranial Color Doppler Imaging: Technical Hints

Challenge	Action
No Doppler signal or color display Absent window, window not located, poor patient positioning, or an occluded intracranial artery	1. Undergo a systematic search for a better window. A TCD window may be located by repositioning the transducer on the skin, changing the angle of the transducer, changing the depth of the sample volume, or by changing the color control settings. 2. Check the equipment control settings to ensure that the maximum power is being used, especially when using the transtemporal window. Adjusting the color gain/PRF settings may also prove to be valuable when searching for a window. 3. Add more ultrasound gel to maintain good transducer-to-skin contact. 4. Use a lower MHz transducer (if available). 5. Reposition the patient to help in locating a Doppler signal, especially from the suboccipital window. 6. Use headphones (if available) to eliminate extraneous noise so that subtle Doppler signals may be detected.
Poor quality Doppler signal Small or poor window, improper equipment control settings, poor technique, poor patient positioning, or intercranial pathology	1. Undergo a systematic search for a better window. A TCD window may be located by repositioning the transducer on the skin, changing the angle of the transducer, changing the depth of the sample volume, or changing the color control settings. 2. Check the equipment control settings to ensure that the maximum power is being used, especially when using the transtemporal window. Adjusting the color gain/PRF settings may also prove to be valuable when searching for a window. 3. Add more ultrasound gel to maintain good transducer-to-skin contact. 4. Use a lower MHz transducer (if available). 5. Reposition the patient to help in locating a Doppler signal, especially from the suboccipital window. 6. Use headphones (if available) to eliminate extraneous noise so that subtle Doppler signals may be detected. 7. Document any changes in blood flow velocity or spectral Doppler waveform shape that may indicate intracranial pathology (may be visualized).
Multiple Doppler signals Large sample volume size, anatomic variation, or overlapping vessel	1. Use a smaller sample volume size. 2. Search for a better window by repositioning the transducer on the skin or by changing the angle of the transducer.
Background noise in Doppler signal Improper gain settings or placement of sample volume	1. Adjust the gain setting so that the Doppler spectral waveform is optimized and the background noise is minimized. 2. Carefully adjust the angle of insonation to improve the signal-to-noise ratio. 3. Change the sample volume depth setting by a small increment to improve the quality of the signal.
Artifact in Doppler signal Patient movement, transducer movement, inadequate amount of ultrasound gel	1. Take the time to put the patient at ease or answer any questions to minimize patient movement. 2. Minimize transducer movement by properly adjusting the operator's position (arm resting on examination table). 3. Adjust the gain setting so that the Doppler spectral waveform is optimized and the background noise is minimized. 4. Carefully adjust the angle of insonation to improve the signal-to-noise ratio. 5. Change the sample volume depth setting by a small increment to improve the quality of the signal.
Aliasing of Doppler or color Doppler signal Detected frequency exceeding the Nyquist limit	1. Increase the PRF settings. 2. Decrease the zero baseline to increase the scale in one direction.
"I am lost" Not following examination protocol, patient movement, unusual window, anatomic variations, or intracranial pathology	1. Undergo a systematic search for a better window. A TCD window may be located by repositioning the transducer on the skin, changing the angle of the transducer, changing the depth of the sample volume, or changing the color control settings. If an unusual window is used, check the angle of the transducer. 2. Locate the anatomic landmarks from the specific window. 3. Locate the landmark t-ICA bifurcation signal and use it to locate the other arteries when using the transtemporal window. 4. Follow the examination protocol. 5. Remember that the patient's physiologic factors and any disease of the extracranial vessels may have an effect on the intracranial Doppler waveforms (velocity and configuration). 6. Take the time to put the patient at ease or answer any questions to minimize patient movement. 7. Remember the limitations of the technique.

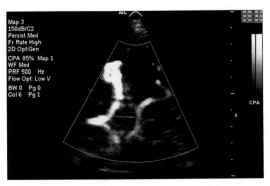

Figure 32-19   Color power Doppler imaging of the intracranial arteries. Power Doppler is helpful when trying to locate the small intracranial arteries.

BOX 32-4   TRANSCRANIAL COLOR DOPPLER IMAGING GUIDELINES

- Obtain a patient history (focus on medical history, risk factors, symptoms, and current medications)
- Obtain available laboratory values (hematocrit, intracranial pressure, blood pressure, heart rate, cardiac output)
- Be aware of the status of the extracranial vessels
- Be familiar with intracranial arterial anatomy, physiology, and pathology
- Understand how each color control affects the image and how the controls affect each other
- Use the color/power Doppler display as a guide to obtain the Doppler spectral waveform information
- Use a large Doppler sample volume (5 to 10 mm) and assume a zero-degree angle
- Be aware of the Doppler spectral waveform configuration
- Compare the Doppler spectral waveforms from the anterior and posterior circulations, and from left and right sides
- Establish institutional diagnostic criteria for the various clinical applications

---

slower-moving blood flow, and intracranial arteries that course at unfavorable angles to the ultrasound beam (Figure 32-19). Future technology may offer improved visualization of the intracranial circulation by using power Doppler imaging, three-dimensional ultrasound imaging, and color Doppler imaging with contrast enhancement.

Currently, TCD imaging is being used to evaluate cerebral hematomas, differentiate between ischemic and hemorrhagic stroke, evaluate arteriovenous malformations, and evaluate the patient with an acute stroke.

REFERENCES

1. Adams R and others: Prevention of a first stroke by transfusions in children with sickle cell anemia and abnormal results on transcranial Doppler ultrasonography, *N Engl J Med* 339:5, 1998.
2. Anzola GP and others: Transcranial Doppler and risk of recurrence in patients with stroke and patent foramen ovale, *Eur J Neurol* 10:129-135, 2003.
3. Babikian VL: Basic identification criteria of Doppler microembolic signals, *Stroke* 26:1123, 1995.
4. Babikian VL and others: Transcranial Doppler validation pilot study, *J Neuroimaging* 3:242, 1993.
5. Baumgartner RW, Mattle HP, Schroth G: Assessment of ≥50% and <50% intracranial stenoses by transcranial color-coded duplex sonography, *Stroke* 30:87, 1999.
6. Baumgartner RW and others: Transcranial color-coded duplex sonography in cerebral aneurysms, *Stroke* 25:2429, 1994.
7. Becker GM and others: Diagnosis and monitoring of subarachnoid hemorrhage by transcranial color-coded real-time sonography, *Neurosurgery* 28:814, 1991.
8. Burch CM and others: Detection of intracranial internal carotid artery and middle cerebral artery vasospasm following subarachnoid hemorrhage, *J Neuroimag* 6:8, 1996.
9. Comptom JS, Redmond S, Symon L: Cerebral blood velocity in subarachnoid haemorrhage: a transcranial Doppler study, *J Neurol Neurosurg Psychiatr* 50:1499, 1987.
10. deBray J-M and others: Transcranial Doppler evaluation of middle cerebral artery stenosis, *J Ultrasound Med* 7:611, 1988.
11. Devuyst G and others: Controlled contrast transcranial Doppler and arterial blood gas analysis to quantify shunt through patent foramen ovale, *Stroke* 35:859-863, 2004.
12. Eicke BM and others: Angle correction in transcranial Doppler sonography, *J Neuroimag* 4:29, 1994.
13. Giller GA: Is angle correction correct? *J Neuroimag* 4:51, 1994.
14. Gosling RG and others: The quantitative analysis of occlusive peripheral arterial disease by a non-intrusive ultrasound technique, *Angiology* 22:52, 1971.
15. Grolimund P: Transmission of ultrasound through the temporal bone. In Aaslid R, editor: *Transcranial Doppler sonography*, New York, 1986, Springer-Verlag.
16. Halsey JH: Effect of emitted power on waveform intensity in transcranial Doppler, *Stroke* 21:1573, 1990.
17. Halsey JH: Response: Letter to the editor, *Stroke* 22:533, 1991.
18. Hennerici M and others: Transcranial Doppler ultrasound for the assessment of intracranial arterial flow velocity, I. Examination technique and normal value, *Surg Neurol* 27:439, 1987.
19. Huber P, Handa J: Effect of contrast material, hypercapnia, hyperventilation, hypertonic glucose and papaverine on the diameter of the cerebral arteries: angiographic determination in man, *Invest Radiol* 2:17, 1967.
20. Kaps M, Seidel G, Bauer T, Behrmann B: Imaging of the intracranial vertebrobasilar system using color-coded ultrasound, *Stroke* 23:1577, 1992.
21. Kaps M and others: Transcranial Doppler ultrasound findings in middle cerebral artery occlusion, *Stroke* 21:532, 1990.
22. Kirkham FJ, Neville BGR, Levin SD: Bedside diagnosis of stenosis of middle cerebral artery, *Lancet* 1:797, 1986 (letter).
23. Kwaitkowski JL and others: Transcranial Doppler ultrasonography in siblings with sickle cell disease, *Br J Haematol* 121:932-937, 2003.
24. Lennihan L and others: Transcranial Doppler detection of anterior cerebral artery vasospasm, *J Neurol Neurosurg Psychiatr* 56:906, 1993.
25. Lippert H, Pabst R: *Arterial variations in man: classification and frequency*, New York, 1985, Springer-Verlag.
26. Markus HS, Droste DW, Brown MM: Detection of asymptomatic cerebral embolic signals with Doppler ultrasound, *Lancet* 343:1011, 1994.

27. Martin PJ and others: Intracranial aneurysms and arteriovenous malformations: transcranial colour-coded sonography as a diagnostic aid, *Ultrasound Med Biol* 20:689, 1994.

28. Perren F and others: A rapid noninvasive method to visualize ruptured aneurysms in the emergency room: three-dimensional power Doppler imaging, *J Neurosurg* 100:619-622, 2004.

29. Schoning M, Buchholz R, Walter J: Comparative study of transcranial color duplex sonography and transcranial Doppler sonography in adults, *J Neurosurg* 78:776, 1993.

30. Seibert JJ and others: Transcranial Doppler, MRA, and MRI as a screening examination for cerebrovascular disease in patients with sickle cell anemia: an 8-year study, *Pediatr Radiol* 18:138, 1998.

31. Seidel G, Kaps M, Dorndor W: Transcranial color-coded duplex sonography of intracerebral hematomas in adults, *Stroke* 24:1519, 1993.

32. Siebler M and others: Cerebral microembolism in symptomatic and asymptomatic high-grade internal carotid artery stenosis, *Neurology* 44:615, 1994.

33. Siebler M and others: Cerebral microembolism and the risk of ischemia in asymptomatic high-grade internal carotid artery stenosis, *Stroke* 26:2184, 1995.

34. Sloan MA and others: Transcranial Doppler detection of vertebrobasilar vasospasm following subarachnoid hemorrhage, *Stroke* 25:2187, 1994.

35. Spencer MP, Whisler D: Transorbital Doppler diagnosis of intracranial arterial stenosis, *Stroke* 17(5):916, 1986.

36. Stolz E, Kaps M, Dorndorf W: Assessment of intracranial venous hemodynamics in normal individuals and patients with cerebral venous thrombosis, *Stroke* 30:70, 1999.

37. Telman G and others: The positions of the patients in the diagnosis of patient foramen ovale by transcranial Doppler, *J Neuroimaging* 13:356-358, 2003.

38. Totaro R and others: Reproducibility of transcranial Doppler sonography: a validation study, *Ultrasound Med Biol* 18:173, 1992.

39. Tsuchiya T and others: Imaging of the basal cerebral arteries and measurement of blood velocity in adults by using transcranial real-time color flow Doppler sonography, *Am J Neuro Radiol* 12:497, 1991.

40. Valdueza JM and others: Venous microembolic signals detected in patients with cerebral sinus thrombosis, *Stroke* 28:1607, 1997.

41. Wardlaw JM, Cannon JC: Color transcranial "power" Doppler ultrasound of intracranial aneurysms, *J Neurosurg* 84:459, 1996.

SELECTED BIBLIOGRAPHY

Aaslid R: Transcranial Doppler examination techniques. In Aaslid R, editor: *Transcranial Doppler sonography,* New York, 1986, Springer-Verlag.

Aaslid R, Huber P, Nornes H: A transcranial Doppler method in the evaluation of cerebrovascular vasospasm, *Neuroradiology* 28:11, 1986.

Aaslid R, Markwalder T-M, Nornes H: Noninvasive transcranial Doppler ultrasound recording of flow velocity in basal cerebral arteries, *J Neurosurg* 57:769, 1982.

Ameriso SF and others: Correlates of middle cerebral artery blood velocity in the elderly, *Stroke* 21:1579, 1990.

Arnolds BJ, von Reutern G-M: Transcranial Doppler sonography: examination technique and normal reference values, *Ultrasound Med Biol* 12(2):115, 1986.

Baumgartner RW, Schmid C, Baumgartner I: Comparative study of power-based versus mean frequency-based transcranial color-coded duplex sonography in normal adults, *Stroke* 27:101, 1996.

Baumgartner RW. Transcranial color duplex sonography in cerebrovascular disease: a systematic review, *Cerebrovasc Dis* 16:4-13. 2003.

Baumgartner RW and others: Transoccipital power-based color-coded duplex sonography of cerebral sinuses and veins, *Stroke* 28:1319, 1997.

Becker GM and others: Imaging of cerebral arterio-venous malformations by transcranial color-coded real-time sonography, *Neuroradiology* 32:280, 1990.

Becker GM and others: Differentiation between ischemic and hemorrhagic stroke by transcranial color-coded real-time sonography, *J Neuroimag* 3:41, 1993.

Becker GM and others: Transcranial color-coded real-time sonography of intracranial veins: normal values of blood flow velocities and findings in superior sagittal sinus thrombosis, *J Neuroimag* 5:87, 1995.

Bogdahn U and others: Contrast-enhanced transcranial color-coded real-time sonography, *Stroke* 24:676, 1993.

Bornstein NM, Krajewski A, Norris JW: Basilar artery blood flow in subclavian steal, *Can J Neurol Sci* 15:417, 1988.

Bouma GJ, Muizelaar JP: Relationship between cardiac output and cerebral blood flow in patients with intact and with impaired autoregulation, *J Neurosurg* 73:368, 1990.

Brass LM and others: Transcranial Doppler measurements of the middle cerebral artery: effect of hematocrit, *Stroke* 19:1466, 1988.

Burns PN: Overview of echo-enhanced vascular ultrasound imaging for clinical diagnosis in neurosonology, *J Neuroimag* 7(suppl 1):S2, 1997.

Caplan LR and others: Transcranial Doppler ultrasound: present status, *Neurology* 40:696, 1990.

Creissard P, Proust F: Vasospasm diagnosis: theoretical sensitivity of transcranial Doppler evaluated using 135 angiograms demonstrating vasospasm, *Acta Neurochir* 131:12, 1994.

Fujioka KA, Gates DT, Spenser MP: A comparison of transcranial color Doppler imaging and standard static pulsed wave Doppler in the assessment of intracranial hemodynamics, *J Vasc Technol* 18:29, 1994.

Giovagnorio F, Quaranta L, Bucci MG: Color Doppler assessment of normal ocular blood flow, *J Ultrasound Med* 12:473, 1993.

Goertler M and others: Diagnostic impact and prognostic relevance of early contrast-enhanced transcranial color-coded duplex sonography in acute stroke, *Stroke* 29:955, 1998.

Grolimund P, Seiler RW: Age dependence of the flow velocity in the basal cerebral arteries—a transcranial Doppler ultrasound study, *Ultrasound Med Biol* 14(3):191, 1988.

Hennerici M, Rautenberg W, Schwartz A: Transcranial Doppler ultrasound for the assessment of intracranial arterial flow velocity, II. Evaluation of intracranial arterial disease, *Surg Neurol* 27:523, 1987.

Hu H-H and others: Color Doppler imaging of orbital arteries for detection of carotid occlusive disease, *Stroke* 24:1196, 1993.

Kaps M and others: Characteristics of transcranial Doppler signal enhancement using a phospholipid-containing echo-contrast agent, *Stroke* 28:1006, 1997.

Kaps M and others: Transcranial Doppler echo contrast studies using different colour processing modes, *Acta Neurol Scand* 95:358, 1997.

Katz ML, Alexandrov A. *A practical guide to transcranial Doppler examinations,* Littleton, CO, 2003, Summer Publishing.

Kenton AR, Martin PJ, Evans DH: Power Doppler: an advance over colour Doppler for transcranial imaging? *Ultrasound Med Biol* 22:313, 1996.

Kenton AR and others: Comparison of transcranial color-coded sonography and magnetic resonance angiography in acute stroke, *Stroke* 28:1601, 1997.

Klotzsch C and others: Transcranial color-coded duplex sonography in cerebral arteriovenous malformations, *Stroke* 26:2298, 1995.

Klotzch C, Popescu O, Berlit P: Assessment of the posterior communicating artery by transcranial color-coded duplex sonography, *Stroke* 27:486, 1996.

Lieb WE and others: Color Doppler imaging of the eye and orbit: technique and normal vascular anatomy, *Arch Ophthalmol* 109:527, 1991.

Lieb WE and others: Color Doppler imaging provides accurate assessment of orbital blood flow in occlusive carotid artery disease, *Ophthalmology* 98:548, 1991.

Lindegaard KF and others: Assessment of intracranial hemodynamics in carotid artery disease by transcranial Doppler ultrasound, *J Neurosurg* 63:890, 1985.

Lindegaard KF and others: Cerebral vasospasm diagnosis by means of angiography and blood velocity measurements, *Acta Neurochir* 100:12, 1989.

Lyden PD, Nelson TR: Visualization of the cerebral circulation using three-dimensional transcranial power Doppler ultrasound imaging, *J Neuroimag* 7:35, 1997.

Maea H and others: A validation study on the reproducibility of transcranial Doppler velocimetry, *Ultrasound Med Biol* 16:9, 1990.

Mauer M and others: Differentiation between intracerebral hemorrhage and ischemic stroke by transcranial color-coded duplex-sonography, *Stroke* 29:2563, 1998.

Nabavi DG and others: Potential and limitations of echocontrast-enhanced ultrasonography in acute stroke patients: a pilot study, *Stroke* 29:949, 1998.

Otis S, Rush M, Boyajian R: Contrast-enhanced transcranial imaging: results of an American phase-two study, *Stroke* 26:203, 1995.

Ries F: Clinical experience with echo-enhanced transcranial Doppler and duplex imaging, *J Neuroimag* 7(suppl 1):S15, 1997.

Ries F and others: A transpulmonary contrast medium enhances the transcranial Doppler signal in humans, *Stroke* 24:1903, 1993.

Ries F and others: Air microbubbles as a contrast medium in transcranial Doppler sonography, *J Neuroimag* 1:173, 1991.

Ries S and others: Echocontrast-enhanced transcranial color-coded sonography for the diagnosis of transverse sinus venous thrombosis, *Stroke* 28:696, 1997.

Ringlestein EB and others: Transcranial Doppler sonography: anatomical landmarks and normal velocity values, *Ultrasound Med Biol* 16:745, 1990.

Schoning M, Walter J: Evaluation of the vertebrobasilar posterior system by transcranial color duplex sonography in adults, *Stroke* 23:1280, 1992.

Sloan MA and others: Sensitivity and specificity of transcranial Doppler ultrasonography in the diagnosis of vasospasm following subarachnoid hemorrhage, *Neurology* 39:1514, 1989.

Sorteberg W and others: Side-to-side differences and day-to-day variations of transcranial Doppler parameters in normal subjects, *J Ultrasound Med* 9:403, 1990.

Valdueza JM and others: Venous transcranial Doppler ultrasound monitoring in acute dural sinus thrombosis: report of two cases, *Stroke* 26:1196, 1995.

Valdueza JM and others: Assessment of normal flow velocity in basal cerebral veins: a transcranial Doppler ultrasound study, *Stroke* 27:1221, 1996.

Vriens EM and others: Transcranial pulsed Doppler measurements of blood velocity in the middle cerebral artery: reference values at rest and during hyperventilation in healthy volunteers in relation to age and sex, *Ultrasound Med Biol* 15(1):1, 1989.

CHAPTER 33

Peripheral Arterial Evaluation

Mira L. Katz

KEY TERMS

anterior tibial artery – begins at the popliteal artery and travels down the lateral calf in the anterior compartment to the level of the ankle

axillary artery – continuation of the subclavian artery

brachial artery – continuation of the axillary artery

claudication – walking induced muscular discomfort of the calf, thigh, hip, or buttock

dorsalis pedis artery – continuation of the anterior tibial artery on the top of the foot

innominate artery – first branch artery from the aortic arch

ischemic rest pain – implies critical ischemia (lack of blood) of the distal limb when the patient is at rest

necrosis – the death of areas of tissue

popliteal artery – begins at the opening of the adductor magnus muscle and travels behind the knee in the popliteal fossa

profunda femoris artery – posterior and lateral to the superficial femoral artery

pseudoaneurysm – perivascular collection (hematoma) that communicates with an artery or a graft and has the presence of pulsating blood entering the collection

radial artery – branch of the brachial artery that runs parallel to the ulnar artery in the forearm

reactive hyperemia – alternative method to stress the peripheral arterial circulation

subclavian artery – originates at the inner border of the scalenus anterior and travels beneath the clavicle to the outer border of the first rib to become the axillary artery

superficial femoral artery (SFA) – courses the length of the thigh through Hunter's canal and terminates at the opening of the adductor magnus muscle

thoracic outlet syndrome – changes in arterial blood flow to the arms may be related to intermittent compression of the proximal arteries (or neural and venous structures)

tibial-peroneal trunk – takes off after the anterior tibial artery and bifurcates into the posterior tibial artery and the peroneal artery

ulnar artery – branch of the brachial artery that runs parallel to the radial artery in the forearm

---

The noninvasive evaluation of patients with peripheral arterial disease has evolved during the past 25 years. With today's sophisticated technology, an anatomic and physiologic evaluation can be obtained both at rest and after exercise. Capa-

REASONS FOR NONINVASIVE ARTERIAL TESTING

- Provides objective documentation of the severity of the arterial disease
- Aids in diagnosis of exercise-induced pain caused by occlusive arterial disease
- Supplements clinical judgment regarding healing of foot ulcers and amputation sites
- Evaluates pulsatile masses (aneurysms, pseudoaneurysms)
- Evaluates suspected arterial trauma
- Evaluates angioplasty/stent placement (planning and follow-up)
- Serves as a baseline study before operative reconstruction
- Provides postoperative follow-up, including bypass graft surveillance

bilities have advanced from simple oscillometric measurements to segmental pressures, pulse volume recordings, stress testing, and direction evaluation of arteries and bypass grafts by duplex imaging. Originally the purpose of these tests was to offer objectivity in the diagnosis of arterial disease. Indications have been expanded, and currently the noninvasive evaluation is tailored to patients' specific needs, depending on the clinical presentation and the pathologic findings being evaluated.

The noninvasive arterial evaluation complements, but does not replace, a careful history and physical examination. Noninvasive testing is important because the clinical evaluation may not always detect underlying arterial occlusive disease, especially when concomitant neuropathy or osteoarthritis is present. A prospective study of 458 diabetic patients using noninvasive techniques detected lower extremity arterial disease in 31% (128/408) of the patients who gave no history of claudication and in 21% (54/259) of the patients with a normal physical examination.[29]

The noninvasive arterial examination is an important component in the evaluation of a patient with signs and symptoms of arterial occlusive arterial disease. Although not required for diagnosis, noninvasive arterial testing is valuable to many patients and their doctors (Box 33-1).

Although indirect tests and peripheral arterial duplex imaging are discussed separately, a combination of tests may be indicated, depending on the patient and clinical presentation.

RISK FACTORS AND SYMPTOMS OF PERIPHERAL ARTERIAL DISEASE

Several risk factors have been identified to be associated with peripheral occlusive arterial disease. The risk factors are increasing age, hypertension, diabetes mellitus, elevated cholesterol, tobacco smoking, documented atherosclerosis in the coronary or carotid system, and a family history of atherosclerosis.

Symptoms of lower extremity occlusive arterial disease are claudication and rest pain. **Claudication** is defined as walking-induced muscular discomfort of the calf, thigh, hip, or buttock. Most patients describe claudication as a cramping or aching in the muscles of their legs. Claudication is relieved by stopping the walking or exercise and standing or sitting for 2 to 5 minutes. Unless the disease is progressing, the distance most patients walk to the onset of symptoms is usually constant. Approximately 25% of patients with intermittent claudication will progress to rest pain within 5 years of the onset of their claudication.

Ischemic rest pain implies critical ischemia of the distal limb when the patient is at rest. The patient usually complains of pain in the toes when lying down. The pain often awakens a patient who is sleeping. If the ischemia is severe, the patient may find relief by sitting with the affected limb in the dependent position during the day and night. This position permits gravity to assist in delivering blood flow to the foot.

The physical signs of peripheral occlusive arterial disease are elevation pallor and dependent rubor, ischemic ulcers, gangrene, bruits, and decreased peripheral pulses (femoral, popliteal, dorsalis pedis, posterior tibial, axillary, brachial, radial, ulnar). Pulses are usually compared from side to side and are graded on a scale from 0 to 3+, with 0 = no pulse, 1+ = questionable pulse, 2+ = weak pulse, and 3+ = normal pulse.

ANATOMY ASSOCIATED WITH PERIPHERAL ARTERIAL TESTING

LOWER EXTREMITY

The descending aorta is the continuation of the aorta beyond the aortic arch. The descending aorta is divided into a thoracic section and an abdominal section. The thoracic section of the aorta terminates at the aortic opening in the diaphragm. The abdominal aorta begins at the level of the twelfth thoracic vertebra as it passes through the aortic hiatus of the diaphragm. The abdominal aorta terminates in the bifurcation of the right and left common iliac arteries (approximately at the level of the fourth lumbar vertebra) (Figure 33-1). Each of the common iliac arteries bifurcates into an internal iliac artery (hypogastric artery), which supplies the pelvis, and an external iliac artery, which continues distally to supply the lower extremity. The external iliac artery terminates at the inguinal ligament, where it becomes the common femoral artery. The common femoral artery originates beneath the inguinal ligament and terminates by dividing into the superficial femoral and profunda femoris arteries. The **profunda femoris artery** is posterior and lateral to the superficial femoral artery. The profunda femoris (deep femoral) artery begins at the common femoral bifurcation and terminates in the lower third of the thigh. The profunda femoris artery supplies the muscles of the thigh and the hip joint. The **superficial femoral artery (SFA)** travels the length of the thigh, travels through Hunter's canal, and terminates at the opening of the adductor magnus muscle. The proximal SFA is superficial and dives deep in the distal portion of the thigh. The **popliteal artery** begins at the opening of the adductor magnus muscle and travels behind the knee in the popliteal fossa. Major branches off the popliteal artery are the sural and genicular arteries. The popliteal artery terminates distally into the anterior tibial artery and the tibial-peroneal trunk.

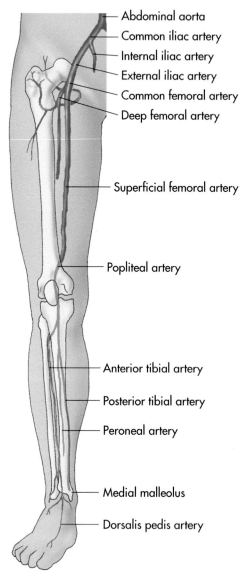

Abdominal aorta
Common iliac artery
Internal iliac artery
External iliac artery
Common femoral artery
Deep femoral artery

Superficial femoral artery

Popliteal artery

Anterior tibial artery

Posterior tibial artery

Peroneal artery

Medial malleolus

Dorsalis pedis artery

Figure 33-1   The arteries of the lower extremity.

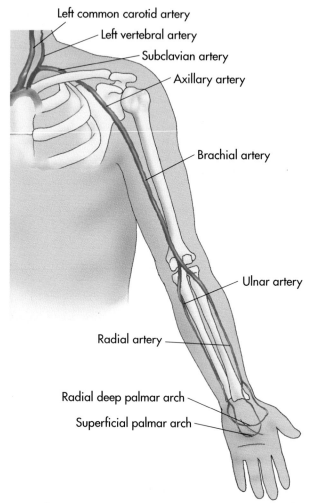

Left common carotid artery
Left vertebral artery
Subclavian artery
Axillary artery

Brachial artery

Ulnar artery

Radial artery

Radial deep palmar arch
Superficial palmar arch

Figure 33-2   The arteries of the upper extremity.

The **anterior tibial arteries** take off at the popliteal and travel down the lateral calf in the anterior compartment to the level of the ankle. The **dorsalis pedis artery** is a continuation of the anterior tibial artery on the top of the foot. The arterial branches of the anterior tibial artery join branches of the posterior tibial artery to form the plantar arch. Arising off the plantar arch are the metatarsal arteries that divide into the digital branch arteries.

The **tibial-peroneal trunk** takes off after the anterior tibial artery and bifurcates into the posterior tibial artery and the peroneal artery. The posterior tibial artery travels down the medial calf in the posterior compartment and terminates between the ankle and the heel into the medial and lateral plantar arteries. The peroneal artery is located deep within the calf and travels near the medial aspect of the fibula. The peroneal artery terminates in the distal third of the calf and its branches communicate with branches of the posterior and anterior tibial arteries.

UPPER EXTREMITY

The ascending aorta originates from the left ventricle of the heart. The transverse aortic arch lies in the superior mediastinum and is formed as the aorta ascends and curves posteroinferiorly from right to left, above the left mainstem bronchus. It descends to the left of the trachea and esophagus. Three main branches arise from the superior convexity of the arch in its normal configuration. The **innominate artery** (brachiocephalic trunk) is the first branch (divides into the right subclavian and the right common carotid artery), the left common carotid artery is the second, and the left subclavian artery the third branch in approximately 70% of cases.

The **subclavian artery** originates at the inner border of the scalenus anterior and travels beneath the clavicle to the outer border of the first rib, where it becomes the axillary artery (Figure 33-2). Major branches of the subclavian artery are the vertebral artery, thyrocervical trunk, costocervical trunk, internal mammary, and dorsal scapular.

The **axillary artery** is a continuation of the subclavian artery. It begins at the outer border of the first rib and terminates at the lower border of the tendon of the teres major muscle. The **brachial artery** is a continuation of the axillary artery. It originates at the lower margin of the tendon of the teres major muscle and usually terminates just below the antecubital fossa into the radial and ulnar arteries.

The **radial artery** begins at the brachial artery bifurcation. The radial artery travels down the forearm (thumb side) and terminates in the palm. The radial artery forms the deep palmar arch. The **ulnar artery** originates at the brachial artery bifurcation, is usually slightly larger than the radial artery, and travels down the forearm (small finger side) to the palm. The ulnar artery terminates and forms the superficial palmar arch. Both palmar arches supply blood to the digital arteries.

INDIRECT ARTERIAL TESTING

SEGMENTAL DOPPLER PRESSURES

Before beginning the examination, there should be a 15-minute rest period to allow the patient's blood pressure to stabilize and legs to recover from walking to the examination room. During this rest period, the patient's history can be obtained. The patient's history should document risk factors, current severity and location of symptoms, and previous history of arterial interventions, including arterial operations.

Segmental pressures are obtained with the patient in the supine position. The legs should be at the same level as the heart because this position prevents hydrostatic pressure artifact. Blood pressure cuffs are placed bilaterally on the upper arm (brachial pressure), proximal thigh, low thigh (above the knee), calf (below the knee), and ankle just above the medial malleoli. Using a flow detector (continuous wave Doppler transducer) on the distal limb, each cuff is independently inflated about 20 to 30 mm Hg above systolic pressure, then slowly deflated. As the cuff pressure is lowered, the systolic pressure recorded at that cuff location is the pressure at which the audible arterial Doppler signal returns. The calf and ankle pressures are recorded using the Doppler signals from both the dorsalis pedis and posterior tibial arteries. The proximal and low thigh pressures are recorded using the strongest distal Doppler signal. If no distal Doppler signals are noted (no measurable blood flow or occlusion of the distal vessels), the thigh pressures are obtained by using the Doppler signal from the popliteal artery.

A continuous wave Doppler instrument is used when performing segmental limb pressures. An 8-MHz continuous wave transducer can be used for most patients. However, if the Doppler signal is attenuated because of depth, a 5-MHz transducer may be necessary to improve penetration. A generous amount of ultrasound gel is used to ensure good transducer-to-skin contact. A transducer angle of 45 to 60 degrees is used. The pressure applied to the skin must maintain good contact, but cannot be excessive or it may obliterate the Doppler signal.

To obtain pressures comparable with direct intraarterial measurements, the blood pressure cuff must have a width 20% greater than the diameter of the limb. When the width of the cuff is small compared with the girth of the limb, the pressure in the cuff may not be completely transmitted to the arteries, and measured pressures are often falsely elevated. In a normal person, pressure measurements increase from the ankle to the proximal thigh because of the relation between constant cuff width and the increase in limb girth. Blood pressure cuffs used for segmental pressure studies should have bladders that measure 12 × 40 cm, and cuffs with longer bladders (12 × 55 cm) may be used for the proximal and distal thigh measurements.

Pressures may be falsely elevated in obese patients, and a proximal thigh pressure may be lower in extremely thin patients. The cuff-to-limb ratio should be kept in mind when the patient's legs are either abnormally large or abnormally small.

The brachial pressures should be obtained in both arms. If a difference of ≥20 mm Hg occurs between arms, an arterial obstruction (usually the subclavian artery) is suspected on the side with the lower systolic pressure. The proximal thigh pressure reading should be 30 mm Hg more than the brachial pressure because of the cuff size artifact rather than an actual increase in intraarterial pressure. A proximal thigh pressure equal to or less than the brachial pressure suggests disease at or proximal to the level of the superficial femoral artery. A pressure gradient of 20 mm Hg between adjacent segments of the limb is abnormal and indicates intercurrent disease. Pressures measured at the same level of each leg should not differ by more than 20 mm Hg. A significant pressure gradient (20 mm Hg) between the proximal and distal thigh cuffs suggests disease of the superficial femoral artery. Disease of the distal superficial femoral artery, the popliteal artery, or both, is suspected if a significant pressure gradient is present from the low thigh to the calf. Disease of the tibial arteries is suspected if a 20 mm Hg pressure gradient is present from the calf to the ankle.

When interpreting segmental pressures, it may be difficult to localize the disease when patients have multilevel disease. Proximal arterial obstruction or stenosis causing a significant pressure gradient may mask distal disease. Additionally, segmental pressure gradients cannot distinguish between a stenosis and an occlusion.

Because systemic pressures vary from person to person, and in the same patient from time to time, absolute pressures are not used to categorize or follow patients. All pressures are divided by the highest brachial pressure and expressed as a ratio, and this pressure index (PI) is used to follow patients. The ad hoc committee on reporting standards for the Society for Vascular Surgery/International Society for Cardiovascular Surgery (North American chapter) concluded that an ankle-brachial index (ABI) change of more than 0.10 should be considered significant.[42] Another study demonstrated that an ABI must change by at least 0.15 before it can be considered significant.[1] Under constant conditions and with careful measurements, these values may be appropriate.

Modest variability in measuring ankle pressures is likely to be associated with normal patient or observer variability. The importance of body temperature on recording ABIs in claudicators has been demonstrated.[9] The variability in the ankle pressure index was documented as being higher after body cooling (0.79 ± 0.04) than during routine testing (0.69 ± 0.03) or after warming (0.65 ± 0.04).

TABLE 33-1	INTERPRETATION OF ANKLE-BRACHIAL PRESSURE INDEX (ABI)	
Clinical Presentation		Ankle-Brachial Index
Normal		>0.95
Claudication		0.50-0.95
Rest pain		0.21-0.49
Tissue loss		<0.21

Resting ABIs correlate with the degree of functional disability. The ABI has been found to be 1.11 ± 0.10 in the absence of arterial occlusion, 0.59 ± 0.15 in limbs with intermittent claudication, 0.26 ± 0.13 in limbs with ischemic rest pain, and 0.05 ± 0.08 in limbs with impending gangrene.[48]

ABIs are usually divided into four main categories (Table 33-1). Most patients' clinical symptoms and their ABIs fit into these four categories, but there tends to be some overlap between groups.

Lower-extremity pressures may be artifactually elevated because of medial calcinosis, medial sclerosis, or both, with pressure indices exceeding 1.25. When this occurs, toe pressures or pulse volume recordings are particularly valuable in evaluating the patient's ischemia because these tests are not affected by a noncompliant arterial wall.

Segmental pressure measurements of the lower extremity tend to underestimate the extent of the disease. Reasons for underestimation of the disease are (1) the narrowing of the arterial lumen must be significant enough to cause a pressure change, (2) proximal disease may mask distal disease, and (3) calcified vessels may falsely elevate the pressures recorded. Indirect testing, however, provides information about the overall limb hemodynamics. This information in combination with direct testing using duplex imaging will provide the best information in most patients.

Additionally, measuring penile blood pressure in persons who have proximal arterial disease may be necessary. A penile blood pressure cuff is placed at the base of the penis, and Doppler signals from the cavernosal arteries are used to obtain a pressure.

If the arterial disease is severe, many of these patients will have sexual dysfunction. A normal potent male over the age of 40 years will have a penile-brachial pressure index of 0.75 or greater. A penile-brachial PI of less than 0.60 will usually indicate some degree of impotence.

Arterial disease in the upper extremity does not occur as often as arterial disease in the lower extremity. Disease of the upper extremity may result from the large inflow arteries (innominate, subclavian), arterial embolization (cardiac origin), **thoracic outlet syndrome** (compression of neural and vascular structures), or Raynaud's syndrome (intermittent digital ischemia in response to cold or emotional stress). Segmental Doppler pressures and pulse volume recordings may be taken at the upper arm level, the forearm, the wrist, and the digits. If a difference of 20 mm Hg or greater occurs between

arms, an arterial obstruction (usually the subclavian artery) is suspected on the side with the lower systolic pressure. There should be no more than a 10- to 15-mm Hg difference between adjacent sites on the arm. Normal digital pressures will be within 20 mm Hg of the brachial pressure. It is technically less challenging to use photoplethysmography (PPG) as the end-point detector when taking digital pressures than trying to locate the digital arteries with a Doppler transducer.

TOE PRESSURES

Toe pressures are a more accurate method of evaluating distal limb and foot perfusion in patients with falsely elevated segmental limb pressures. Toe pressures may also be used to determine if there is obstructive disease involving the pedal arch and digital arteries.

A digital cuff (2.5×9 cm bladder) is placed at the base of the big toe, and the pressure is obtained using an audible Doppler signal from a digital artery or by placing a PPG on the distal toe as an end-point detector. A toe pressure is considered normal if it is 50 mm Hg or more than 64% of the brachial pressure, whichever is higher. The mean toe PI in patients with claudication is 0.35 ± 0.15 and 0.11 ± 0.10 in patients with rest pain.

PULSE VOLUME RECORDINGS

Pulse volume recordings measure changes in segmental limb volume with each cardiac cycle. The patient is examined in the supine position, and blood pressure cuffs are placed on the patient's arms, thighs, calves, ankles, and feet. Each cuff is inflated to a preset pressure (usually 65 mm Hg) to maintain adequate contact between the cuff bladder and the limb. Accurate pulse volume tracings are only possible if the size of the blood pressure cuff (and bladder) are appropriate and if the cuff is correctly placed on the limb. The pulse volume waveforms are recorded on an analogue chart recorder.

Pulse volume recordings are interpreted qualitatively and complement the systolic segmental pressure measurements. A normal pulse volume waveform is characterized by a rapid rise to a sharp peak during systole and slower fall during diastole (Figure 33-3). The downslope of a normal pulse volume waveform contains a dicrotic notch that reflects the brief period of retrograde flow in the arteries during diastole.

Occlusive arterial disease causes changes in the amplitude and contour of the pulse volume waveform. Sequential changes in the waveform that occur with progressive occlusive arterial disease are that the dicrotic notch disappears, the upslope is slower, the peak is more rounded, and upslope and downslope times equalize (Figure 33-4). Recording of no pulse amplitude (a straight line) is possible in patients with severe occlusive arterial disease of the lower extremity.

The calf pulse volume waveform normally has greater amplitude than the thigh waveform because of cuff artifact. If the amplitude of the calf pulse volume waveform is equal to or smaller than thigh waveform, superficial femoral artery disease should be suspected.

The pulse volume recordings provide important information and are usually performed in addition to the segmental

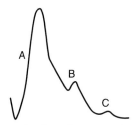

Figure 33-3 A normal pulse volume recording from the lower extremity. Note the rapid rise to a sharp peak during systole (A) and a slower fall during diastole (C). The downslope of a normal pulse volume recording contains a dicrotic notch (B) that reflects the brief period of retrograde blood flow in the arteries during diastole.

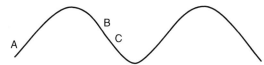

Figure 33-4 Arterial occlusive disease causes changes in the amplitude and contour of the pulse volume recording. The dicrotic notch disappears (B), the upslope is slower (A), the peak is more rounded, and the downslope time (C) equalizes to the upslope time.

pressure measurements. A discrepancy often occurs between the pulse volume waveforms and the segmental pressures when arteries cannot be compressed (systolic PI greater than 1.25). This frequently occurs when patients have diabetes mellitus. In this clinical presentation, the pulse volume waveforms provide the only accurate information about the overall hemodynamics of the limb.

ARTERIAL STRESS TESTING

In a normal individual without occlusive arterial disease, blood flow will increase with exercise because of a decrease in peripheral vascular resistance. This increase in blood flow demand will occur without a decrease in the ankle systolic pressure. Some patients will have arterial lesions that are quiescent at rest (normal resting ABIs), but limit perfusion during exercise. They maintain their normal resting pressure by forming collaterals and by decreasing peripheral vascular resistance. These patients should be stressed with either exercise or **reactive hyperemia** to further reduce peripheral resistance, thereby increasing the pressure gradient across the arterial segment and unmasking a hemodynamically significant lesion.

Contraindications to lower-extremity arterial stress testing are symptomatic cardiac disease, severe pulmonary disease, severe hypertension, inability to walk on the treadmill, and cases of calcified vessels (unreliable pressure measurements; the use of pulse volume recordings may be helpful in some patients).

After the patient's brachial and ankle pressures are recorded at rest, the cuffs are left in place and exercise testing is performed on a treadmill at 1.5 to 2 mph on a 10% to 12% grade. Continuous ECG monitoring during the exercise testing is rec-

ommended. The patient walks for 5 minutes or until symptoms develop and pain forces the patient to stop. The patient is quickly returned to the supine position, and ankle pressures are recorded immediately and repeated every few minutes until the pressure returns to baseline. The time to onset of symptoms, location and severity of the symptoms, and the total walking time are recorded and used to monitor changes in an individual patient over time.

The magnitude of the decrease in ankle pressure after exercise and the time required for the ankle pressure to return to baseline reflect the severity of the underlying arterial disease. In general, ankle pressures that fall after exercise and return to baseline within 5 minutes suggest single-segment occlusive disease. Multisegment arterial disease is usually associated with reduced ankle pressures that persist for more than 10 minutes after exercise. When a patient stops walking because of symptoms associated with arterial disease, the ankle pressure is less than 60 mm Hg. If ankle pressures are unchanged or improved after exercise, underlying arterial disease (even if present) can be excluded as a cause of the patient's symptoms.

An alternative method to stress the peripheral arterial circulation is reactive hyperemia. This testing is useful when patients cannot walk on the treadmill because of cardiac or other physical disabilities. Resting ankle and arm pressures are recorded. A thigh cuff is inflated to a suprasystolic pressure for 3 to 5 minutes, which produces ischemia and vasodilation in the periphery. On release of the thigh cuff, ankle pressures are immediately recorded and measurements are repeated until they return to baseline. Normal individuals will experience up to a 30% decrease in ankle systolic pressure immediately after release of the thigh cuff. Patients with occlusive arterial disease will have a more pronounced effect after thigh cuff release and will take longer to return to baseline pressures.

HEALING OF FOOT ULCERS AND AMPUTATIONS

Indirect arterial testing is helpful in predicting the likelihood of the healing of skin lesions. This is especially helpful in diabetic patients, who often have foot ulcers and an abnormal physical examination. Ischemic skin lesions are not likely to heal if the ankle systolic pressure is below 55 mm Hg (below 80 mm Hg in diabetic patients), the toe pressure is below 30 mm Hg, or the foot pulse volume recording fails to demonstrate pulsatile perfusion.

If a lower-extremity amputation is required, segmental pressures and pulse volume recordings assist in selecting the appropriate amputation level. Pressure measurements have been reported as both helpful and misleading in predicting amputation site healing.[5,14,28,36,45] A below-knee amputation is likely to heal in patients with low thigh region or calf systolic pressures above 50 mm Hg. In diabetics, however, the systolic pressures may be falsely elevated and amputation sites may fail to heal even though there appears to be adequate pressure.[29] The associated pulse volume recordings, however, add valuable information in diabetics and patients with calcified vessels.

Prediction of healing of forefoot and toe amputations is less precise. In general, a forefoot or toe amputation will not heal if the ankle pressure is less than 60 mm Hg or the toe pressure is less than 45 mm Hg.

In summary, the indirect methods of evaluation of the peripheral arterial systems have provided much useful information over the past several decades. These techniques are limited, however, by not establishing the exact disease location, missing disease that causes minor changes, having difficulty in differentiating the level and extent (stenosis vs. occlusion) of the disease, and not being able to accurately follow disease progression.

ARTERIAL DUPLEX IMAGING

Arterial duplex imaging provides direct anatomic and physiologic information, but it does not provide information regarding overall limb hemodynamics. Duplex imaging distinguishes between a stenosis and an occlusion, determines the length of the disease segment and patency of the distal vessels, evaluates the results of intervention (angioplasty, stent placement), aids in diagnoses of aneurysms and pseudoaneurysms, and monitors patients' postoperative course with continuing bypass graft surveillance.

Color Doppler imaging provides a guide for the accurate placement of the Doppler sample volume to obtain the arterial Doppler spectral waveforms. Additionally, color Doppler imaging reduces the time required to perform an examination by visually identifying the blood flow disturbances on initial survey. When using color Doppler to guide the examination, however, properly adjusting the controls (e.g., pulse repetition frequency, color gain, frame rate, etc.) during the study is essential for an accurate examination.

The gray scale image and color Doppler display are helpful in recognizing anatomic variations and locating plaque and calcification, but are not accurate in determining the amount of arterial narrowing. The percent narrowing of an artery is determined from the Doppler spectral waveform information. A small Doppler sample volume is used for arterial imaging, and the Doppler waveforms are obtained by maintaining a 60-degree angle to the vessel walls. If a 60-degree angle cannot be maintained, documentation of the angle used during the examination is important, especially in following the patient over time. It is best not to use an angle greater than 60 degrees because of the inherent error associated with using larger angles. The Doppler is swept through the color display looking for focal increases in velocity or blood flow disturbances. Representative Doppler signals are recorded from standard sites along the peripheral arteries. Additionally, if an area of narrowing is noted, Doppler signals proximal to the area, at the narrowing, and distal to the narrowing will provide the complete documentation necessary for an accurate interpretation.

It is imperative that each institution develop an arterial imaging protocol that defines the standard examination (arteries to be evaluated, the location of Doppler samples, etc.). This protocol must include information about the technique, clinical applications, indications for a complete and/or limited examination, and interpretation criteria. A standard complete examination for arterial occlusive disease usually includes acquiring both imaging and Doppler information from the entire extremity.

LOWER EXTREMITY

Peripheral arterial imaging begins at the level of the aortic bifurcation. Visualization of the proximal arteries is improved if patients do not take anything by mouth the morning of the examination. It is best to use a low-frequency transducer (2.0 to 3.5 MHz) for the proximal segment of the examination. The aortic bifurcation is best seen with the patient turned to the left side and with the transducer placed just in front of the right iliac crest in a longitudinal plane. The distal aorta and the origin of both common iliac arteries can usually be visualized. Doppler signals should be obtained from all three vessels at this location.

The patient should be placed in a lateral decubitus position (side being evaluated up) to evaluate the internal and external iliac arteries with the transducer placed between the iliac crest and the umbilicus. Doppler waveforms should be obtained from the internal and external iliac arteries, noting direction of blood flow and velocity. If difficulty is encountered in locating the iliac arteries from this approach, the arteries may be located by identifying the femoral arteries at the groin level and following the arteries proximally.

The patient should return to the supine position, and a higher-frequency, linear array transducer (5 to 10 MHz) should be used for evaluation of the arteries of the lower extremity. The common femoral artery is located at the level of the groin. The artery lies lateral to the common femoral vein. Imaging should be performed in the longitudinal plane, and a Doppler signal should be obtained from this artery. The vessel should be followed distally on the leg to the origin of the superficial femoral and profunda femoris (deep femoral) arteries. Doppler signals should be obtained from the origin of both the superficial femoral artery and the deep femoral artery. The superficial femoral artery is followed distally as it courses down the medial aspect of the thigh. Doppler signals should be obtained along its superficial femoral artery pathway and at areas of questionable narrowing. The distal portion of the superficial femoral artery may be easier to evaluate from the distal posterior thigh. This artery is followed distally in the limb and becomes the popliteal artery. The popliteal artery should be followed through the popliteal fossa. The popliteal artery lies deep to the vein, and a Doppler spectral waveform should be obtained from this vessel.

Following the distal popliteal artery in a longitudinal plane, the origin of the anterior tibial artery can usually be visualized diving deep on the monitor. The anterior tibial artery can only be followed for a short distance from this approach. The remainder of the vessel can be located distally by placing the transducer on the lateral calf and followed to the level of the ankle. The tibial-peroneal trunk extends into the calf from the popliteal artery. The posterior tibial and peroneal arteries are usually visualized by placing the transducer on the medial calf. The peroneal artery lies deep and runs parallel to the posterior tibial artery. These vessels are located above the malleolus and followed proximally.

UPPER EXTREMITY

Arteries of the upper extremity may also be evaluated with arterial duplex imaging. A low-frequency transducer should be used to evaluate the proximal vessels. The **subclavian artery** is evaluated from a supraclavicular and infraclavicular approach. Segments of the subclavian artery may not be visualized because of the shadowing from the clavicle. A Doppler signal should be obtained from the subclavian artery. The axillary artery may be evaluated from an infraclavicular approach or from the axilla.

The arteries in the arm should be evaluated with a higher-frequency linear array transducer. The brachial artery should be followed along the length of the upper arm. The brachial artery divides into the radial and ulnar arteries near the antecubital fossa. The radial and ulnar arteries are visualized in a longitudinal plane along the length of the forearm. These vessels are superficial and may become very small at the wrist level.

Changes in arterial blood flow to the arms may be related to intermittent compression of the proximal arteries (thoracic outlet syndrome). The patient should be sitting with the arms relaxed and alongside the body. The arterial Doppler signals should be recorded in the proximal brachial artery at rest and can then be monitored during positional maneuvers.

At the end of the peripheral arterial duplex imaging examination, the ultrasound gel should be removed from the patient. Excess gel should be removed from the ultrasound transducer, and the transducer should be cleaned using a disinfectant.

INTERPRETATION

The arterial duplex imaging examination of the lower extremities focuses on answering several important questions (Box 33-2). The duplex imaging criteria for the normal arterial evaluation of the lower extremity has been established.[19] In normal vessels, the arterial Doppler signal is triphasic from the abdominal aorta to the tibial arteries at the ankle (Figure 33-5). This characteristic waveform has a high-velocity forward flow component during systole (ventricular contraction), followed by a brief reversal of flow in early diastole (because of peripheral resistance), and a final low-velocity forward flow phase in late diastole (elastic recoil of the vessel wall). Peak-systolic velocity gradually decreases from the proximal to the distal arteries. The peak velocity in the abdominal aorta is 100 cm/sec, and the velocity gradually decreases to 70 cm/sec in the popliteal artery.

Criteria have been developed for duplex imaging used to detect abnormal arterial segments.[23] A triphasic waveform with an increase in peak velocity of 30% to 100% relative to the adjacent proximal segment indicates disease, defined as a stenosis with a narrowing of less than 50% of the diameter of the artery. A 50% to 99% diameter reduction stenosis produces a monophasic waveform with extensive spectral broadening (caused by turbulence) and a peak-systolic velocity of more than 100% relative to the adjacent proximal segment, and reduced systolic velocity is present distal to the stenosis (Figures 33-6 through 33-9). The three major changes in the

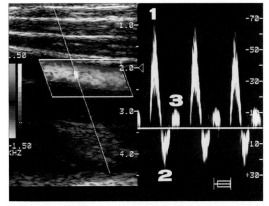

Figure 33-5 A normal color Doppler image and spectral Doppler waveform from a superficial femoral artery. The triphasic Doppler signal demonstrates a fast upstroke to peak systole *(1)*, reversal of blood flow during early diastole *(2)*, and a forward flow component during late diastole *(3)*.

BOX 33-2 ESSENTIAL QUESTIONS TO BE ANSWERED BY ARTERIAL DUPLEX IMAGING

- Is disease present in the lower extremity?
- Is the disease a stenosis, an occlusion, an arteriovenous fistula, an aneurysm, or a pseudoaneurysm?
- What is the location of the narrowing? What is the length and severity?
- What is the location of the occlusion? What is the length of the occlusion and are collaterals identified near the occlusion?
- Is there adequate inflow into the leg?
- Is an outflow vessel identified?
- Is an adequate superficial vein identified that may be used as an arterial conduit?
- Is an arteriovenous fistula identified? What is the location of the fistula?
- Is a patent arterial aneurysm identified? What is the location of the aneurysm and its dimensions?
- Is a pseudoaneurysm identified? What is the location and its dimensions? Is the neck of the pseudoaneurysm identified? What is the vessel of origin?

spectral Doppler arterial waveform that occur because of a significant stenosis are an increase in peak-systolic velocities (greater than 100%), marked spectral broadening because of turbulence, and the loss of the reversal of blood flow during diastole. The color Doppler display also provides information that identifies the presence of a significant arterial narrowing. Color aliasing, color persistence (continuous signal), and color bruit (tissue vibration caused by severe blood flow disturbance) indicate the presence of a blood flow abnormality.

No color Doppler or Doppler spectral waveform will be obtained in areas of occlusion. Damped proximal arterial Doppler spectral waveforms are obtained, which demonstrate a low velocity with little or no diastolic blood flow. The color

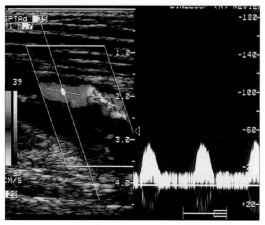

Figure 33-6 Color Doppler imaging in a patient who presented with claudication. There was a 40-mm Hg drop in pressure from the upper to the lower thigh. The Doppler signal is proximal to the narrowed segment. Peak-systolic velocity is approximately 55 cm/sec, and the waveform shape is abnormal.

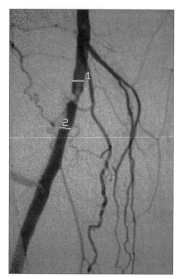

Figure 33-9 Corresponding arteriogram demonstrating the narrowing of the superficial femoral artery.

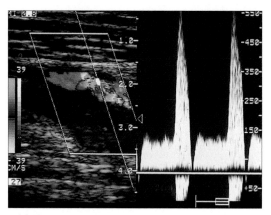

Figure 33-7 An area of increased velocity (color aliasing) was noted in the distal superficial femoral artery. At the site of the narrowing, the peak-systolic velocity increases to greater than 450 cm/sec.

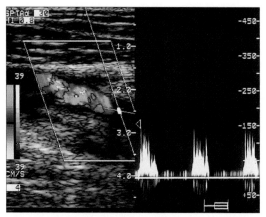

Figure 33-8 Distal to the segment of arterial narrowing, the Doppler spectral waveform is turbulent and the peak-systolic velocity is approximately 150 cm/sec.

BOX 33-3 **LIMITATIONS OF THE LOWER EXTREMITY ARTERIAL DUPLEX IMAGING EXAMINATION**

- Nonvisualization of the iliac system because of bowel gas or obesity
- Shadowing because of calcification
- Imaging of the popliteal trifurcation
- Difficulty evaluating lesions distal to tight stenoses because of low velocities in these segments

Doppler display may reveal collaterals near the occluded segment. Power Doppler imaging improves visualization of areas of tight stenosis, especially in vessels running parallel to the skin line.

Duplex imaging has been compared with lower extremity arteriography to define its accuracy.[22,24,33,46] These studies demonstrate a sensitivity of 77% to 92% and a specificity of 92% to 98% for correctly categorizing a stenosis as greater or less than 50% diameter reduction. These reports evaluated the capabilities of duplex imaging in the proximal vessels, but there is limited information about its sensitivity in the calf arteries.[17]

All studies reported high negative predictive values (87% to 98%), indicating that significant occlusive arterial disease can be excluded in patients with normal duplex imaging examinations. Limitations of the lower extremity arterial duplex imaging examination are listed in Box 33-3.

Aneurysms and Pseudoaneurysms. Arterial duplex imaging has also become valuable for evaluating patients with aneurysms and pseudoaneurysms of the extremity. Duplex imaging distinguishes between aneurysms (Figure 33-10), pseudoaneurysms (Figure 33-11), perigraft fluid collections (Figure 33-12), and hematomas. Information about the size,

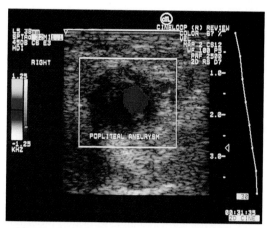

Figure 33-10 A popliteal artery aneurysm. The red represents the blood flow within the aneurysm. Blood flow within the popliteal vein is displayed in blue.

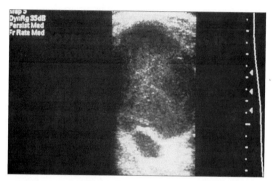

Figure 33-11 A large pseudoaneurysm from an axillofemoral bypass graft. The swirling of blood is visualized in gray scale.

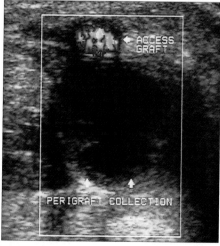

Figure 33-12 Color Doppler image of a patent access graft with adjacent perigraft collection.

location, site of communication, and presence of luminal thrombus is easily obtained in most cases.

The evaluation of arterial aneurysms by duplex imaging is considered an accurate method in determining the size, position, patency, and associated arterial blood flow dynamics.

Aneurysms may be located in the distal abdominal aorta, iliac, common femoral, and popliteal arteries. To accurately measure the size (length and width) of an aneurysm, the artery should be evaluated in both longitudinal and transverse imaging planes.

Pseudoaneurysms occur as a result of trauma, at vascular anastomoses, in angioaccess grafts, or at puncture sites (usually following cardiac catheterization).

A **pseudoaneurysm** is a perivascular collection (hematoma) that communicates with an artery or a graft and has the presence of pulsating blood entering the collection. A track (neck) of variable length connects the native vessel to the collection.

A pseudoaneurysm may be unilocular or multilocular and may partially contain thrombus. Pseudoaneurysms occur in variable sizes and the size of the pseudoaneurysm changes during each cardiac cycle. Although spontaneous thrombosis of pseudoaneurysms has been reported in the literature,[20,25,38] fatal spontaneous hemorrhage of pseudoaneurysms has also occurred.[31]

Sonographic Findings. Swirling blood within the collection is often visualized in gray scale imaging. The use of color Doppler imaging helps to identify the neck of the pseudoaneurysm. Identification of the neck of the pseudoaneurysm is important when ultrasound-guided compression therapy is attempted and color Doppler imaging permits identification of the vessel of origin, which is important when planning surgical interventions.

A spectral Doppler waveform obtained from the neck of a pseudoaneurysm displays a to-and-fro (bidirectional) pattern. During systole, blood flows from the native artery into the pseudoaneurysm and during diastole blood flow returns to the native artery. Additionally, the size (length, width, and depth) of the pseudoaneurysm should be measured. Some pseudoaneurysms are very large and it is difficult to capture the entire area in one image for measurement. The sensitivity and specificity in the identification of pseudoaneurysms range from 94% to 100%.

Compression therapy. Compression therapy of the pseudoaneurysm may be attempted if the neck of the pseudoaneurysm has been clearly identified during arterial duplex imaging. The neck of the pseudoaneurysm is the area that is compressed with pressure placed on the skin by the ultrasound transducer. The goal is to stop the blood flow into the pseudoaneurysm by occluding the neck. It is extremely important not to occlude blood flow in the native artery, so distal blood flow should be monitored during compression therapy.

A considerable amount of time and upper body strength are necessary to perform ultrasound compression therapy of pseudoaneurysms for an extended period. Compression cycles of 15 to 20 minutes are usually performed, with progress being evaluated between cycles. In most cases it will take at least 30 to 60 minutes to achieve a successful thrombosis of the pseudoaneurysm. Most investigators suggest bed rest (6 to 24 hours) after a successful compression procedure and reexamination of the area the next day. Recurrence rates have been reported for ultrasound compression, and a second attempt to compress the pseudoaneurysm may be warranted.[16]

Success rates of ultrasound compression of pseudoaneurysms have varied from 70% to 86%.[10, 13] Success varies depending on the size and age of the pseudoaneurysm and when the patient is on anticoagulation therapy. Failure to thrombose a pseudoaneurysm occurs more often in large pseudoaneurysms, if the pseudoaneurysm has been present for a prolonged period, and if the patient is or has been given anticoagulants. Additionally, some patients cannot tolerate the pain associated with the compression technique. The complications of ultrasound compression therapy of pseudoaneurysms have included occlusion of the native artery, development of deep vein thrombosis, and rupture of the pseudoaneurysm.

As an alternative to ultrasound compression therapy, some investigators have performed ultrasound-guided thrombin injection of pseudoaneurysms.* As the thrombin is injected, results are continuously monitored with color Doppler imaging. Thrombin injection is stopped when blood flow is no longer documented (visualized color Doppler). In addition, distal pulses and other signs of arterial disease are also closely monitored. Follow-up imaging can be repeated immediately and within 24 hours. Successful treatment occurs in approximately 97% of the reported patients. Complications of this technique include the thrombosis of the femoral or brachial artery. Investigators use this technique in uncomplicated pseudoaneurysms and suggest that complicated pseudoaneurysms (AVF, rapid expansion, infection, hemorrhage, etc.) should be managed surgically. Important issues associated with the successful repair of pseudoaneurysms using this technique are the size, the location and size of the neck, the thrombin dose, and the number of injections.

Transluminal Angioplasty. Lower extremity arterial duplex imaging is important in the evaluation and follow-up of patients who may be candidates for percutaneous intervention. Because duplex imaging can identify the extent and location of the arterial disease, it may eliminate the need for an arteriogram in patients who are considered candidates for balloon angioplasty but not operative reconstruction.

One study compared color Doppler imaging and arteriography in 84 lower extremities in 61 patients being evaluated for angioplasty.[12] Differentiation between a normal and diseased artery was possible, with a sensitivity of 83% and a specificity of 96%. For identifying stenosis greater than 50% diameter reduction, the sensitivity was 87% and specificity was 99%. In the detection of occluded arterial segments, the sensitivity and specificity were 81% and 99%, respectively. In this group of patients, color Doppler imaging accurately provided information in 48/51 (94%) of the arterial occlusions, including four extremities for which the original arteriogram overestimated the length of the occlusion.

A study used color Doppler imaging to evaluate 62 patients with limiting claudication.[11] Twenty-six patients were believed to be suitable candidates for percutaneous balloon angioplasty and underwent arteriography. Duplex imaging and arteriography agreed in 97% (62/64) of the femoral and popliteal segments and in 97% (93/96) of the tibial and peroneal arteries.

One hundred ten patients who had lower extremity arterial duplex imaging before arteriography were evaluated.[15] Fifty patients were selected for transluminal balloon angioplasty on the basis of the duplex imaging examination. Three of the 50 patients did not have angioplasty performed because of the lesion's location or extent. The authors concluded that duplex imaging allowed accurate prediction of which arterial lesions can be treated by transluminal balloon angioplasty and the authors therefore recommended duplex imaging as a screening test.

Duplex imaging allows accurate identification of the location, length, and severity of arterial lesions, which is important in planning the best type of intervention. Duplex imaging is also ideal in the follow-up examination of patients after intervention for lower extremity arterial disease. Although pressure measurements can be valuable when observing these patients, they cannot distinguish between restenosis of the angioplasty site and progression of proximal or distal disease, or both. Duplex imaging can identify recurrent stenosis before occlusion and, if indicated, allows for a repeat angioplasty.

Bypass Graft Surveillance. The patency of bypass grafts can be significantly prolonged if developing graft lesions are corrected before graft thrombosis. Therefore, all lower extremity bypass grafts should be monitored for technical adequacy, hemodynamic function, and development of postimplantation lesions (Figures 33-13 and 33-14). Graft abnormalities, such as myointimal stenosis, retained valve cusps, arteriovenous fistulas, degenerative aneurysmal formation, and low flow states, can be detected with arterial duplex imaging even if they are not obvious in changes in ankle pressures.[6,32] A graft surveillance program should identify bypass grafts at risk for thrombosis, provide information on the mechanism of failure, and with appropriate intervention reduce the incidence of unexpected graft failure.

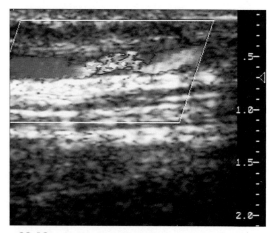

Figure 33-13 A color Doppler image of an in situ bypass graft. There is an area of increased blood flow velocity (color change) within the graft.

---

*References 8, 21, 27, 37, 39, 41, 44, 47.

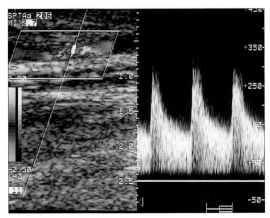

Figure 33-14 Doppler spectral waveform from the area of narrowing in the in situ bypass graft demonstrates an increase in peak-systolic velocity to approximately 300 cm/sec.

Surveillance programs by arterial duplex imaging have resulted in assisted primary patency rates of 82% to 92% at 5 years compared with 60% to 70% patency for bypasses followed clinically and 30% to 50% patency rates after secondary procedures to salvage thrombosed vein grafts.[3,4,42]

To accurately evaluate bypass grafts with arterial duplex imaging, it is important to know the location and type of graft before beginning the study. The technique is similar to the color Doppler imaging of native arteries. The entire length of the bypass graft should be evaluated with color Doppler and Doppler signals. Additionally, the inflow and outflow vessels should be evaluated and close attention paid to the proximal and distal anastomoses.

The timing of bypass graft surveillance will vary with each surgeon. Some authors suggest performing an examination after the operation before the patient is discharged from the hospital. This baseline duplex examination permits identification of bypass grafts with residual graft defects. If the baseline postoperative duplex evaluation is considered normal, follow-up examinations are performed at 4- to 6-week, 3-month, and 3- to 6-month intervals for the first postoperative year. The second postoperative year, evaluations are performed at 18 and 24 months and then on an annual basis. If graft surveillance detects a stenosis, more frequent evaluations may be performed to follow the patient or the decision to intervene may be indicated.

A change from the triphasic Doppler signal to a monophasic waveform with a decrease in peak-systolic velocity to below 45 cm/sec is diagnostic of a lesion placing the graft at risk. Additionally, repair of graft stenosis is recommended with peak systolic velocities of greater than 300 cm/sec or a peak systolic ratio of greater than 3.5.[42]

A wide range of peak velocities may be identified in normal grafts.[7] The peak-systolic velocity in a bypass graft is due to the size of the graft and the outflow resistance. A low velocity in a bypass graft may relate to a large graft diameter, poor arterial inflow, and small vessel runoff. A significant decrease in peak-systolic velocity within a graft on serial duplex imaging may be a better indicator of pending graft failure.

Other investigators suggest using a velocity ratio to determine graft stenosis. A doubling of the velocity ratio has been noted to indicate a significant graft stenosis.[40] The velocity ratio is calculated by dividing the peak-systolic velocity at the site of the flow disturbance by the peak-systolic velocity in the adjacent proximal segment. A velocity ratio greater than 2.0 was associated with a sensitivity of 95% and a specificity of 100% for detection of stenosis greater than 50% diameter reduction.

Arterial duplex imaging plays an important role in the follow-up of patients with lower extremity arterial bypass grafts. Identification of arterial lesions during the preocclusive phase is critical for prolonging the patency of the graft.

Dialysis Access Grafts. The evaluation of dialysis access grafts is an area of increasing interest. Dialysis grafts (autogenous or synthetic) are typically placed in the forearm. The Brescia-Cimino arteriovenous fistula is a direct connection of the artery and vein. The other type of dialysis access has a synthetic graft interposed between the artery and the vein (straight or loop). The most common problems associated with these grafts are caused by venous outflow obstruction, venous anastomotic stenosis, pseudoaneurysms, hematoma, perigraft fluid collection, or an arterial anastomotic stenosis. Patients are referred for evaluation and mapping of the veins before access placement or because of inadequate dialysis, suspicion of a steal, a stenosis, thrombosis, or a pseudoaneurysm. The ultrasound examination should include recording of Doppler velocity signals from throughout the native arterial system, the graft, and the venous outflow system. This evaluation should include checking for stenosis and thrombosis within the graft and the native circulation. Some investigators include volume flow calculations in the overall evaluation; however, continued research is necessary to determine the value of calculating the volume flow in this clinical setting. Typically, the access grafts will demonstrate an increased velocity that has continuous forward diastolic flow and notable spectral broadening. The velocities will be slightly lower moving toward the venous limb of the graft. Peak systolic velocities are usually in the range of 200 cm/sec or higher. Decreases in peak velocities between 100 cm/sec and 200 cm/sec are suspicious for the development of a problem (usually an outflow stenosis). No Doppler signals and intraluminal echoes are evidence for occlusion of the graft. Using an ultrasound surveillance program for the early detection and treatment of problems associated with hemodialysis access grafts has demonstrated that the patency of the access grafts can be significantly prolonged if developing graft lesions are corrected before graft thrombosis.[35,43]

GUIDELINES FOR EVALUATION

Peripheral arterial testing provides valuable information by addressing specific questions at the patient's original visit and during follow-up studies (Table 33-2).

Producing high-quality and complete examinations is key to the diagnostic value of these tests. The best peripheral arterial evaluation will be achieved by proper attention to detail.

TABLE 33-2 EVALUATION GUIDELINES BASED ON CLINICAL PRESENTATION		
Clinical Presentation	Questions	Noninvasive Test
Initial visit	Is disease present? How severe is the process? What segments are involved?	Resting segmental pressures, pulse volume tracings, exercise testing (select patients)
Focal problems	Is pulsatile mass an aneurysm or a pseudoaneurysm? What is the size/location of the aneurysm?	Duplex imaging
Before angioplasty	What is the location of the lesion? Is it a stenosis or occlusion? What is the length of the disease segment? What is the status of the runoff vessels?	Duplex imaging
After angioplasty	Was the angioplasty successful? What is the degree of improvement?	Pressure measurements and duplex imaging
Bypass graft	Is the bypass graft patent? What is the degree of improvement? Is the graft at risk for failure?	Pressure measurements and duplex imaging

BOX 33-4   ARTERIAL EVALUATION GUIDELINES

- Take a patient history.
- Be familiar with arterial anatomy, physiology, and pathology.
- When measuring ankle pressures, always use the highest brachial pressure when calculating an ankle-brachial index.
- When performing arterial duplex imaging, optimize the gray scale image.
- Understand how each color control affects the image and how the controls affect each other.
- Use a longitudinal imaging plane to obtain color Doppler information and use it as a guide to obtain the spectral Doppler waveforms.
- Use a small Doppler sample volume size and a 60-degree angle.
- Be aware of the Doppler spectral waveform velocity and its configuration.
- Establish institutional diagnostic criteria.

The major areas to focus on when performing a peripheral arterial evaluation are summarized in Box 33-4. Attention to these technical areas and interpretation details will ensure the best peripheral arterial evaluation.

REFERENCES

1. Baker JD, Dix D: Variability of Doppler ankle pressures with arterial occlusive disease: an evaluation of ankle index and brachial-ankle pressure gradient, *Surgery* 89:134, 1981.
2. Bandyk DF and others: Monitoring functional patency of in situ saphenous vein bypasses: the impact of a surveillance protocol and elective revision, *J Vasc Surg* 9:284, 1989.
3. Bandyk DF and others: Intraoperative duplex scanning of arterial reconstructions: fate of repaired and unrepaired defects, *J Vasc Surg* 20:426, 1994.
4. Bandyk DF, Cato RF, Towne JB: A low flow velocity predicts failure of femoropopliteal and femorotibial bypass grafts, *Surgery* 98:799, 1985.
5. Barnes RW, Shanik GD, Slaymaker EE: An index of healing in below-knee amputation: leg blood pressure by Doppler ultrasound, *Surgery* 79:13, 1976.
6. Barnes RW and other: Serial noninvasive studies do not herald postoperative failure of femoropopliteal or femorotibial bypass grafts, *Ann Surg* 210:486, 1989.
7. Belkin M and others: A prospective study of the determination of vein graft flow velocity: implications for graft surveillance, *J Vasc Surg* 17:259, 1994.
8. Brophy DP and others: Iatrogenic femoral pseudoaneurysms: thrombin injection after failed US-guided compression, *Radiology* 214:278-282, 2000.
9. Carter SA, Tate RB: The effect of body heating and cooling on the ankle and toe systolic pressures in arterial disease, *J Vasc Surg* 16:148, 1992.
10. Coley BD and others: Postangiographic femoral artery pseudoaneurysm: further experience with US-guided compression repair, *Radiology* 194:307, 1995.
11. Collier P and others: Improved patient selection for angioplasty utilizing color Doppler imaging, *Am J Surg* 160:171, 1990.
12. Cossman DV and others: Comparison of contrast arteriography to arterial mapping with color flow duplex imaging in the lower extremities, *J Vasc Surg* 10:552, 1989.
13. Cox GS and others: Ultrasound-guided compression repair of postcatheterization pseudoaneurysms: results of treatment in one hundred cases, *J Vasc Surg* 19:683, 1994.
14. Dean DO and others: Ultrasound-guided compression closure of postcatheterization pseudoaneurysms during concurrent anticoagulation: a review of seventy-seven patients, *J Vasc Surg* 23:28, 1996.
15. Edwards JM and others: The role of duplex scanning in the selection of patients for transluminal angioplasty, *J Vasc Surg* 13:69, 1991.
16. Feld R and others: Treatment of iatrogenic femoral artery injuries with ultrasound-guided compression, *J Vasc Surg* 16:832, 1992.
17. Hatsukami TS and others: Color Doppler imaging of infrainguinal arterial occlusive disease, *J Vasc Surg* 16:527, 1992.

18. Idu MM and others: Impact of a color-flow duplex surveillance program on infrainguinal graft patency: a five-year experience, *J Vasc Surg* 17:42, 1992.

19. Jager KA, Ricketts HJ, Strandness DE: Duplex scanning for the evaluation of lower limb arterial disease. In Bernstein EF, editor: *Noninvasive diagnostic techniques in vascular disease,* ed 3, St Louis, 1985, Mosby.

20. Johns JP, Pupa LE, Bailey SR: Spontaneous thrombosis of iatrogenic femoral artery pseudoaneurysms: documentation with color Doppler and two-dimensional ultrasonography, *J Vasc Surg* 14:24, 1991.

21. Kang SS and others: Percutaneous ultrasound guided thrombin injection: a new method for treating postcatheterization femoral pseudoaneurysms, *J Vasc Surg* 27:1032, 1998.

22. Keagy BA and others: Comparison of reactive hyperemia and treadmill tests in the evaluation of peripheral arterial disease, *Am J Surg* 142:158, 1981.

23. Kohler TR and others: Duplex scanning for diagnosis of aortoiliac and femoropopliteal disease: a prospective study, *Circulation* 76:1074, 1987.

24. Kohler TR and others: Can duplex scanning replace arteriography for lower extremity arterial disease? *Ann Vasc Surg* 4:280, 1990.

25. Kotval PS and others: Doppler sonographic demonstration of the progressive spontaneous thrombosis of pseudoaneurysms, *J Ultrasound Med* 9:185, 1990.

26. Kundell A and others: Femoropopliteal graft patency is improved by an intensive surveillance program: a prospective-randomized study, *J Vasc Surg* 21:26, 1995.

27. Liau CS and others: Treatment of iatrogenic femoral artery pseudoaneurysm with percutaneous thrombin injection, *J Vasc Surg* 26:18, 1997.

28. Malone JM and others: Prospective comparison of noninvasive techniques for amputation level selection, *Am J Surg* 154:179, 1987.

29. Marinelli MR and others: Noninvasive testing vs. clinical evaluation of arterial disease: a prospective study, *JAMA* 241:2031, 1979.

30. Mattos MA and others: Does correction of stenoses identified with color duplex scanning improve infrainguinal graft patency? *J Vasc Surg* 17:54, 1993.

31. McCann RL, Schwartz LB, Pieper KS: Vascular complications of cardiac catheterization, *J Vasc Surg* 14:375, 1991.

32. Mills JL and others: The importance of routine surveillance of distal bypass grafts with duplex scanning: a study of 379 reversed vein grafts, *J Vasc Surg* 12:379, 1990.

33. Moneta GL, Strandness DE: Peripheral arterial duplex scanning, *J Clin Ultasound* 15:645, 1987.

34. Moody AP, Gould DA, Harris PL: Vein graft surveillance improves patency in femoropopliteal bypass, *Eur J Vasc Surg* 4:117, 1990.

35. Neyra NR and others. Change in access blood flow over time predicts vascular access thrombosis, *Kidney Int* 54:1714-1719, 1998.

36. Nichols GG, Myers JL, DeMuth WE: The role of vascular laboratory criteria in the selection of patients for lower extremity amputation, *Ann Surg* 195:469, 1982.

37. Partap VA, Cassoff J: Ultrasound-guided percutaneous thrombin injection for treatment of femoral pseudoaneurysms: technical note, *Can Assoc Radiol J* 50:182-184, 1999.

38. Paulson EK and others: Femoral artery pseudoaneurysms: value of color Doppler sonography in predicting which ones will thrombose without treatment, *Am J Radiol* 159:1077, 1992.

39. Pezzullo JA and others: Percutaneous injection of thrombin for the treatment of pseudoaneurysms after catheterization: an alternative to sonographically guided compression, *AJR* 175:1035-1040, 2000.

40. Polak JF and others: Early detection of saphenous vein arterial bypass graft stenosis by color-assisted duplex sonography: a prospective study, *Am J Radiol* 154:857-861, 1990.

41. Reeder SB and others: Low-dose thrombin injection to treat iatrogenic femoral artery pseudoaneurysms, *AJR* 177:595-598, 2001.

42. Roth SM, Bandyk DF: Duplex imaging of lower extremity bypasses, angioplasties, and stents, *Semin Vasc Surg* 12:275, 1999.

43. Safa AA and others: Detection and treatment of dysfunctional hemodialysis access grafts: effect of a surveillance program on graft patency and the incidence of thrombosis, *Radiology* 199:653-657, 1996.

44. Taylor BS and others: Thrombin injection versus compression of femoral artery pseudoaneurysms, *J Vasc Surg* 30:1052-1059, 1999.

45. Wagner WH and others: Noninvasive determination of healing of major lower extremity amputation: the continued role of clinical judgment, *J Vasc Surg* 8:703, 1988.

46. Whelan JF, Barry MH, Moir JD: Color-flow Doppler ultrasonography: comparison with peripheral arteriography for the investigation of peripheral vascular disease, *J Clin Ultrasound* 20:369, 1992.

47. Wixon CL and others: Duplex-directed thrombin injection as a method to treat femoral artery pseudoaneurysms, *J Am Coll Surg* 187:464-466, 1998.

48. Yao JST: Haemodynamic studies in peripheral arterial disease, *Br J Surg* 57:761, 1970.

SELECTED BIBLIOGRAPHY

Allon M and others: Effect of preoperative sonographic mapping on vascular access outcomes in hemodialysis patients, *Kidney Int* 60:2013-2020, 2001.

Baker WH, Barnes RW: Minor forefoot amputation in patients with low ankle pressure, *Am J Surg* 133:331, 1977.

Barnes RW and others: Prediction of amputation wound healing: roles of Doppler ultrasound and digit photoplethysmography, *Arch Surg* 116:80, 1981.

Bone GE, Pomajzl MJ: Toe blood pressure by photoplethysmography: an index of healing in forefoot amputation, *Surgery* 89:569, 1981.

Carroll RM and others: Cardiac arrhythmias associated with treadmill claudication testing, *Surgery* 83:294, 1978.

Carter SA: Response of ankle systolic pressure to leg exercise in mild or questionable arterial disease, *N Engl J Med* 287:578, 1972.

Carter SA: The relationship of distal systolic pressures to healing of skin lesions in limbs with arterial occlusive disease, with special reference to diabetes mellitus, *Scand J Clin Lab Invest* 31(suppl 128):239, 1973.

Darling RC and others: Quantitative segmental pulse volume recorder: a clinical tool, *Surgery* 72:873, 1972.

Dean RH and others: Predictive value of ultrasonically derived arterial pressure in determination of amputation level, *Am Surg* 41:731, 1975.

DiPrete DA, Cronan JJ: Compression ultrasonography: treatment for acute femoral artery pseudoaneurysms in selected cases, *J Ultrasound Med* 11:489, 1992.

Dol JA, Reekers JA, Kromhout JG: Rupture of pseudo-aneurysm during attempted US-guided compression repair, *Radiology* 185:284, 1992 (letter).

Dorfman GS, Cronan JJ: Postcatheterization femoral artery injuries: is there a role for nonsurgical treatment? *Radiology* 178:629, 1991.

Fellmeth BD and others: Post-angiographic femoral artery injuries: nonsurgical repair with US-guided compression, *Radiology* 178:671, 1991.

Gibbons GW and others: Noninvasive prediction of amputation level in diabetic patients, *Arch Surg* 114:1253, 1979.

Hertz SM, Brener BJ: Ultrasound-guided pseudoaneurysm compression: efficacy after coronary stenting and angioplasty, *J Vasc Surg* 26:913, 1997.

Hopkins PN, Williams RR: A survey of 246 suggested coronary risk factors, *Atherosclerosis* 40:1, 1981.

Hummel BW and others: Reactive hyperemia vs. treadmill exercise testing in arterial disease, *Arch Surg* 113:95, 1978.

Katz ML and others: B-Mode imaging to determine the suitability of arm veins for primary arteriovenous fistulae, *J Vasc Technology* 11:172-174, 1987.

Kempczinski RF: Role of the vascular diagnostic laboratory in the evaluation of male impotence, *Am J Surg* 138:278, 1979.

Kempczinski RF: Segmental volume plethysmography in the diagnosis of lower extremity arterial occlusive disease, *J Cardiovasc Surg* 23:125, 1982.

Kinney EV and others: Monitoring functional patency of percutaneous transluminal angioplasty, *Arch Surg* 126:743, 1991.

McCabe CJ and others: The value of electrocardiogram monitoring during treadmill testing for peripheral vascular disease, *Surgery* 89:183, 1981.

Mewissen MW and others: The role of duplex scanning versus angiography in predicting outcome after balloon angioplasty in the femoropopliteal artery, *J Vasc Surg* 15:860, 1992.

Mitchell DG and others: Femoral artery pseudoaneurysm: diagnosis with conventional duplex and color Doppler US, *Radiology* 165:687, 1987.

Older RA and others: Hemodialysis access stenosis: early detection with color Doppler US, *Radiology* 207:161-164, 1998.

Polak JF and others: Determination of the extent of lower extremity peripheral arterial disease with color-assisted duplex sonography: comparison with angiography, *Am J Radiol* 155:1085, 1990.

Raines JK and others: Vascular laboratory criteria for the management of peripheral vascular disease of the lower extremities, *Surgery* 79:21, 1976.

Ramsey DE, Manke DA, Sumner DS: Toe blood pressure: a valuable adjunct to ankle pressure measurement for assessing peripheral arterial disease, *J Cardiovasc Surg* 24:43, 1983.

Rosenbloom MS and others: Risk factors affecting the natural history of intermittent claudication, *Arch Surgery* 123:867, 1988.

Rutherford RB and the Ad Hoc Committee on Reporting Standards, Society for Vascular Surgery/North American Chapter, International Society for Cardiovascular Surgery: Suggested standards for reports dealing with lower extremity ischemia, *J Vasc Surg* 4:80, 1986.

Solberg CA, Strong JP: Risk factors and atherosclerotic lesions: a review of autopsy studies, *Arteriosclerosis* 3:187, 1983.

Sumner DS, Strandness DE: The relationship between calf blood flow and ankle blood pressure in patients with intermittent claudication, *Surgery* 65:763, 1969.

CHAPTER 34

Peripheral Venous Evaluation

Mira L. Katz

KEY TERMS

anterior tibial veins – drain blood from the dorsum of the foot and anterior compartment of the calf

augmentation – blood flow velocity increases with distal limb compression or with the release of proximal limb compression

axillary vein – begins where the basilic vein joins the brachial vein in the upper arm and terminates beneath the clavicle at the outer border of the first rib

basilic vein – originates on the small finger side of the dorsum of the hand and enters the brachial veins in the upper arm

cephalic vein – begins on the thumb side of the dorsum of the hand and joins the axillary vein just below the clavicle

common femoral vein (CFV) – formed by the confluence of the profunda femoris and the superficial femoral vein; also receives the greater saphenous vein

common iliac vein – formed by the confluence of the internal and external iliac veins

deep femoral vein (DFV) – travels with the profunda femoris artery to unite with the superficial femoral vein to form the common femoral vein

gastrocnemius veins – paired veins that lie in the medial and lateral gastrocnemius muscles; terminate into the popliteal vein

greater saphenous vein (GSV) – originates on the dorsum of the foot and ascends anterior to the medial malleolus and along the anteromedial side of the calf and thigh; joins the common femoral vein in the proximal thigh

innominate veins – right vein: courses vertically downwards to join the left innominate vein below the first rib to form the superior vena cava; left vein: longer than right, courses from left chest to the right beneath the sternum to join the right innominate vein

lesser saphenous vein – originates on the dorsum of the foot and ascends posterior to the lateral malleolus and runs along the midline of the posterior calf. Vein terminates as it joins the popliteal vein.

perforating veins – connect the superficial and deep venous systems

peroneal veins – drain blood from lateral compartment of the lower leg

popliteal vein – originates from the confluence of the anterior tibial veins with the posterior and peroneal veins

posterior arch vein – main tributary of the greater saphenous vein

posterior tibial veins – originate from the plantar veins of the foot and drain blood from the posterior compartment of the lower leg

pulmonary embolism (PE) – blockage of the pulmonary circulation by foreign matter

respiratory phasicity – blood flow velocity changes with respiration

soleal sinuses – large venous reservoirs that lie in the soleus muscle and empty into the posterior tibial or peroneal veins

spontaneous – flow is present without augmentation

subclavian vein – continuation of the axillary vein joins the internal jugular vein to form the innominate vein

superficial femoral vein (SFV) – originates at the hiatus of the adductor magnus muscle in the distal thigh and ascends through the adductor (Hunter's) canal

valves – folds of the intima that temporarily close to permit blood flow in one direction only

varicose veins – dilated, elongated, tortuous superficial veins

---

Venous disease can be categorized into the acute and chronic process. Deep vein thrombosis (DVT), the acute process, may be located in the lower and/or upper extremities. Although the exact incidence or prevalence of DVT in the United States is unknown because many episodes are not clinically detected, it has been estimated that DVT affects more than 500,000 individuals annually.[8] In a recent summary, incidence rates of venous thromboembolism (first time) were estimated to be 70 to 113 cases/100,000/year. Historically, upper extremity DVT was considered an uncommon clinical event that was usually caused by compression at the thoracic inlet ("effort thrombosis"). The incidence of upper extremity DVT is on the rise, however, because of the increasing use of central venous lines.

A potentially lethal complication of acute DVT is pulmonary embolism (PE). The number of fatal PEs in the United States has been estimated to range from 50,000 to 200,000/yr.[6] Nonfatal pulmonary embolisms have been estimated to occur three times more often than fatal PE. The chronic process, postthrombotic syndrome, is a complication following DVT. It is responsible for patient morbidity caused by leg swelling, pain, hyperpigmentation, and venous ulceration.

The symptoms and signs of DVT are common and may have several possible causes (e.g., musculoskeletal disorders, ruptured Baker cyst, cellulitis). Because the clinical diagnosis of DVT is unreliable, noninvasive methods to diagnose DVT were developed. Venous duplex imaging has emerged as the valuable diagnostic test because compared with the other non-invasive techniques (nonimaging Doppler, impedance plethysmography), it is more accurate, and compared with venography, there are no risks or discomfort associated with the technique. The ability to correctly diagnose DVT is critical to patient management. Treatment of DVT with anticoagulants has reduced the occurrence of PE, relieved symptoms, and prevented extension of the DVT. Additionally, it is critical to correctly identify patients without DVT so that the patients are not exposed to the risks associated with anticoagulant therapy.

RISK FACTORS AND SYMPTOMS OF VENOUS DISEASE

In response to a wide variety of stimulus, elements within the blood alter themselves to form a thrombus or blood clot. In 1856, Rudolph Virchow presented the classic concepts on the causes of clot formation within the intact venous system.[17] The three factors associated with thrombus formation, Virchow's triad, are (1) a hypercoagulable state, (2) venous stasis (blood pools in the veins), and (3) vein wall injury (endothelium of the vein is damaged, exposing the subendothelium to blood and triggering platelet adhesion and aggregation, which promotes blood coagulation). The interplay of these three factors creates the most likely setting for the development of deep venous thrombosis.

The risk factors for DVT are listed in Box 34-1. An individual with an increasing number of risk factors is at greater risk for developing DVT.

Deep vein thrombosis and **pulmonary embolism (PE)** may be symptomatic or asymptomatic (no symptoms or signs). Severe forms of lower extremity DVT are phlegmasia alba dolens (swollen, painful white leg) and phlegmasia cerulea

---

> **BOX 34-1   RISK FACTORS FOR DEEP VEIN THROMBOSIS**
>
> - Age (greater than 40 years old)
> - Malignancy (cancer)
> - Previous deep venous thrombosis or pulmonary embolism
> - Immobilization (bed rest, paralysis of legs, extended travel)
> - Fracture of the pelvis, hip, or long bones
> - Myocardial infarction, stroke
> - Congestive heart or respiratory failure
> - Pregnancy and postpartum
> - Oral contraceptives and hormone replacement therapy
> - Extensive dissection at major surgery (especially orthopedic surgery)
> - Trauma (multiple)
> - Hereditary factors (antithrombin deficiency, Protein C and Protein S deficiencies, etc.)
> - Obesity
> - Central venous lines, pacemakers, etc.
> - Intravenous drug abuse

SYMPTOMS AND SIGNS ASSOCIATED WITH DVT AND PULMONARY EMBOLISM

DEEP VEIN THROMBOSIS
- Persistent calf, leg, or arm swelling
- Pain or tenderness of the leg (usually the posterior calf) or arm-shoulder region
- Venous distention
- Increased temperature
- Superficial venous dilation
- Homan's sign (calf discomfort on passive dorsiflexion)

SUPERFICIAL VENOUS THROMBOSIS
- Local erythema
- Tenderness or pain
- Palpable subcutaneous "cord"

PULMONARY EMBOLUS
- Dyspnea (shortness of breath)
- Chest pain
- Hemoptysis
- Sweats
- Cough

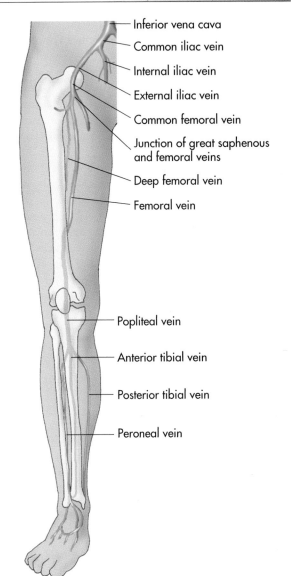

Figure 34-1   The deep veins of the lower extremity.

dolens (swollen, painful cyanotic leg). The common symptoms associated with DVT and PE are listed in Box 34-2.

The chronic venous process, postthrombotic syndrome, is caused by increased ambulatory venous pressure. Increased ambulatory venous pressure may result from venous obstruction and/or incompetent venous valves. Transmission of venous hypertension to the capillaries over time may result in damage to the capillaries and produce edema, stasis dermatitis (redness, itching, flaking skin), hyperpigmentation, and ulceration.

Additionally, varicose veins may occur in an individual. **Varicose veins** are dilated, elongated, tortuous superficial veins. Primary varicose veins are congenital, are an inherent weakness of the venous walls, and occur without coexisting deep venous disease. Secondary varicose veins occur secondary to pathology (DVT, absence of valves) of the deep venous system.

ANATOMY FOR VENOUS DUPLEX IMAGING

The peripheral veins return deoxygenated blood back to the heart. The venous systems of the lower and upper extremities consist of superficial, deep, and perforating (communicating) veins. Perforating veins provide a channel between the superficial and deep veins. Venous blood flow is normally from the superficial veins to the deep veins.

A unique feature of the venous system is the venous valve. **Valves** are folds of the intima, the innermost layer of the vein wall. Venous valves are important in maintaining unidirectional blood flow from the peripheral veins to the central veins. Venous valves are bicuspid, more numerous in the distal leg, and often located near a vein confluence. There are no venous

valves in the inferior vena cava, superior vena cava, innominate veins, or soleal sinuses.

LOWER EXTREMITY

Deep Veins. In the lower extremity, the primary route of drainage is via the deep veins of the leg (Figure 34-1). The lower extremity deep veins have corresponding arteries. The **anterior tibial veins** drain blood from the dorsum of the foot (dorsalis pedis veins) and the anterior compartment of the calf. The anterior tibial veins originate near the tibia at the ankle, lie anterior to the interosseous membrane as they ascend the lower leg, and move toward the fibula. They join at a variable level and pattern with the posterior tibial veins to become the **popliteal vein.**

The posterior tibial veins originate from the plantar (superficial and deep) veins of the foot. They run from the medial malleolus along the medial calf with the posterior tibial artery. The posterior tibial veins drain blood from the posterior compartment of the lower leg. They often unite as a single vein and receive the combined peroneal veins (tibial-peroneal trunk) before uniting with the anterior tibial veins to become the popliteal vein.

The peroneal veins course along the peroneal artery near the fibula. They lie deep to the soleus and gastrocnemius muscles and parallel the path of the posterior tibial veins. The peroneal veins drain blood from the lateral compartment of the lower leg. They unite as a single vein before joining the posterior tibial veins.

Lying within the deep muscular compartment of the calf are the soleal sinuses and the gastrocnemius (sural) veins. The **soleal sinuses** are large venous reservoirs that lie in the soleus muscle and empty into the posterior tibial or peroneal veins. The gastrocnemius veins are paired, accompany an artery, and lie in the medial and lateral gastrocnemius muscles. The gastrocnemius veins terminate in the popliteal vein.

The popliteal vein accompanies the popliteal artery. The popliteal vein originates from the confluence of the anterior tibial veins with the posterior and peroneal veins (tibial-peroneal trunk). A duplicated popliteal vein occurs in approximately 30% to 35% of the population. The popliteal vein lies superficial to the artery. In the lower popliteal fossa, the popliteal vein lies medial to the artery. The vein passes to the lateral side of the artery as it ascends through the popliteal space.

The **superficial femoral vein (SFV)** is the companion of the superficial femoral artery. The superficial femoral vein is a deep vein and is often referred to as the femoral vein. The vein originates at the hiatus of the adductor magnus muscle in the distal thigh and ascends through the adductor (Hunter's) canal. The vein courses deep to the artery and terminates in Scarpa's (femoral) triangle. The superficial femoral vein is duplicated in 20% to 30% of limbs.

The deep femoral (profunda femoris) vein travels with the profunda femoris artery, which unites with the superficial femoral vein to form the common femoral vein. The confluence of the profunda femoris vein and the superficial femoral vein is distal in the leg to the bifurcation of the common femoral artery. The deep femoral vein drains the deep muscles of the proximal thigh.

The common femoral vein lies in Scarpa's triangle medial to the common femoral artery. The common femoral vein is formed by the confluence of the profunda femoris and the superficial femoral vein and it also receives the greater saphenous vein. The common femoral vein terminates at the level of the inguinal ligament and becomes the external iliac vein.

The external iliac vein is a single vein that travels with the artery beginning at the level of the inguinal ligament. It is joined with the internal iliac vein to become the common iliac vein. The internal iliac vein is a single vein that travels with the internal iliac artery. The internal iliac vein drains the pelvis.

The **common iliac vein** is formed by the confluence of internal and external iliac veins. The right common iliac vein is shorter than the left, is oriented vertically, and ascends posterior and then lateral to its companion artery. The left common iliac vein is longer than the right, and is oriented obliquely. It lies to the medial side of the left common iliac artery and while it ascends the vein crosses beneath the right iliac artery where it joins the right common iliac vein. This anatomic feature of the left common iliac vein crossing beneath the right iliac artery causes a mild compression of the vein and has been cited as the reason for a slightly greater number of left-side deep vein thromboses. The union of the right and left common iliac veins forms the inferior vena cava. The inferior vena cava lies to the right of the aorta.

Superficial Veins. The superficial veins of the leg lie beneath the skin and between the two layers of superficial fascia. The greater (long) saphenous vein originates on the dorsum of the foot and ascends anterior to the medial malleolus and along the anteromedial side of the calf and thigh (Figure 34-2). The **greater saphenous vein (GSV)** ends as it joins the common femoral vein (saphenofemoral junction) in the proximal thigh. The greater saphenous vein is the longest vein in the body, has approximately 10 to 20 valves, and receives many tributaries.

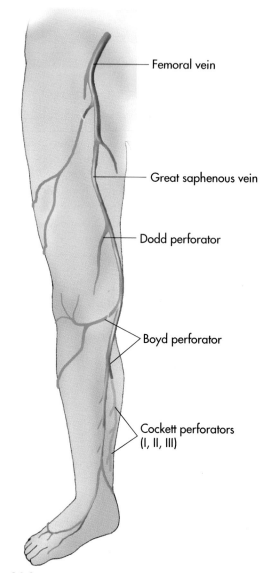

Femoral vein

Great saphenous vein

Dodd perforator

Boyd perforator

Cockett perforators (I, II, III)

Figure 34-2   The greater saphenous vein is a superficial vein. It courses along the medial thigh and calf. Many perforators join the greater saphenous vein.

The lesser (short) saphenous vein originates on the dorsum of the foot and ascends posterior to the lateral malleolus and runs along the midline of the posterior calf (Figure 34-3). The **lesser saphenous vein** terminates when it joins the popliteal vein. The level of entry of the lesser saphenous vein into the popliteal vein is variable and has even been visualized to enter the superficial femoral vein in the mid thigh. The lesser saphenous vein has approximately 6 to 12 valves and receives many tributaries.

The **posterior arch vein** is a main tributary of the greater saphenous vein in the lower leg. This vein arises posterior to the medial malleolus and terminates in the greater saphenous vein below the knee. It communicates with the deep vein by multiple perforators in the gaiter (region above the medial malleolus) area of the leg.

The **perforating veins** connect the superficial and deep venous systems. The perforating veins penetrate the deep fascia and contain valves that permit unidirectional blood flow from the superficial to the deep veins. There are many named perforators (Cockett's, Boyd's, Dodd's, Hunterian) in the lower extremity.

UPPER EXTREMITY

Deep Veins. The deep veins (superficial and deep palmar venous arches) draining the hand form the paired radial and ulnar veins (Figure 34-4). The radial veins accompany the radial artery, and the ulnar veins accompany the ulnar artery in the forearm. Near the antecubital fossa, the radial and ulnar veins join to form the brachial veins. The brachial veins are paired veins that travel with the brachial artery in the upper arm.

The **axillary vein** is a single vein. It begins where the basilic vein joins the brachial veins in the upper arm and terminates beneath the clavicle at the outer border of the first rib. The axillary vein receives the cephalic vein near its termination.

The **subclavian vein** is a continuation of the axillary vein. It extends from the outer border of the first rib to the inner end of the clavicle, where it joins the internal jugular vein to form the innominate vein. The subclavian vein lies beneath the clavicle and is inferior and anterior to the subclavian artery.

There are right and left innominate (brachiocephalic) veins. On the right side, the innominate vein courses almost vertically downward joining the left innominate vein just below the first rib to form the superior vena cava. It lies superficial and to the right of the innominate artery. The right innominate vein receives the right vertebral, internal mammary, and inferior thyroid veins. The left innominate vein is longer than the right vein. It courses from the left to the right side of the chest beneath the sternum and at a slight downward angle to join the right innominate vein to form the superior vena cava. It receives the left vertebral, internal mammary, inferior thyroid, and left superior intercostal veins.

Superficial Veins. In the upper extremity, the superficial venous system is the primary route of drainage (Figure 34-5). The superficial veins lie beneath the skin and between the two layers of superficial fascia and outside the deep investing fascia.

The cephalic vein begins on the thumb side of the dorsum of the hand. It courses along the outer border of the biceps muscle, courses along the deltopectoral groove, penetrates the deep fascia at variable levels, and joins the axillary vein just below the clavicle.

The **basilic vein** originates on the small finger side of the dorsum of the hand. The basilic vein is large, courses medially along the inner side of the biceps muscle, pierces the deep fascia, and enters the brachial veins in the upper arm, which then become the axillary vein.

TECHNICAL ASPECTS OF VENOUS DUPLEX IMAGING

LOWER EXTREMITY

Imaging Examination. The venous duplex imaging examination is explained to the patient. A history is taken from the patient focusing on risk factors, signs, and symptoms (if present) of venous disease. If the patient is symptomatic it

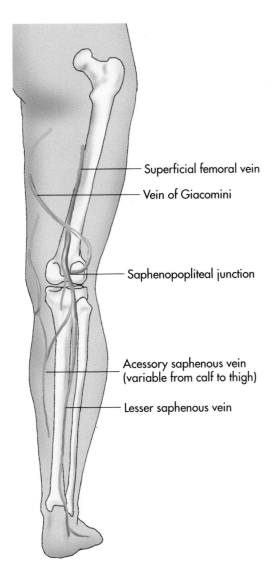

Figure 34-3 The lesser saphenous vein is a superficial vein that courses along the posterior calf. The lesser saphenous vein usually enters the popliteal vein.

Labels on figure:
- Superficial femoral vein
- Vein of Giacomini
- Saphenopopliteal junction
- Acessory saphenous vein (variable from calf to thigh)
- Lesser saphenous vein

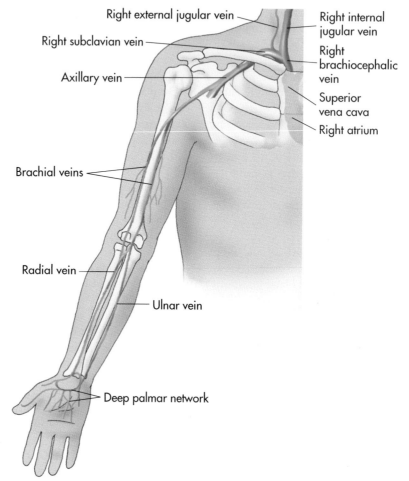

Right external jugular vein
Right subclavian vein
Axillary vein
Brachial veins
Radial vein
Ulnar vein
Deep palmar network

Right internal jugular vein
Right brachiocephalic vein
Superior vena cava
Right atrium

Figure 34-4   The deep veins of the upper extremity.

helps to locate the area of pain and to measure any limb swelling at the calf level.

Patients are evaluated in the supine position on a hospital bed or on an examination table. The bed or table should be placed in reverse Trendelenburg's (head elevated) position, which promotes venous distention and optimizes visualization of the veins. The leg being evaluated is externally rotated and the knee slightly flexed.

Ultrasound gel is placed on the leg along the anatomic route of the veins to ensure good transducer-to-skin contact. The transverse view is used to locate the veins and to perform the examination. The transverse view is mandatory for an accurate examination and interpretation when evaluating the veins in the lower extremity. The transverse view allows visualization of multiple venous segments and of the entire lumen(s) of the vein(s) during compression maneuvers.

The venous duplex examination begins by locating the **common femoral vein (CFV)** at the level of the inguinal crease. The vein is usually large at this location and easy to locate compared with the smaller veins located distally in the leg. Veins can be distinguished from arteries by the characteristics listed in Box 34-3. In general, compared with the common femoral artery, the common femoral vein will collapse with light to moderate transducer pressure on the skin

---

BOX 34-3   **IMAGING CHARACTERISTICS OF NORMAL VEINS AND ARTERIES IN THE LOWER EXTREMITY**

VEINS
- Vessel walls collapse with light or moderate pressure by the transducer on the skin
- Phasic low-velocity Doppler signals augment with distal limb compression
- Common femoral vein changes in size with respiration

ARTERIES
- Vessel does not collapse with light pressure by the transducer on the skin
- Triphasic high-velocity Doppler signal
- Pulsation of vessel walls present

---

and usually will change in size with respiration. If the artery is deformed by the compression maneuver, then the operator knows that adequate pressure has been applied to compress the vein.

After locating the vein, it is followed as far proximally as possible. The distal external iliac vein is usually the most

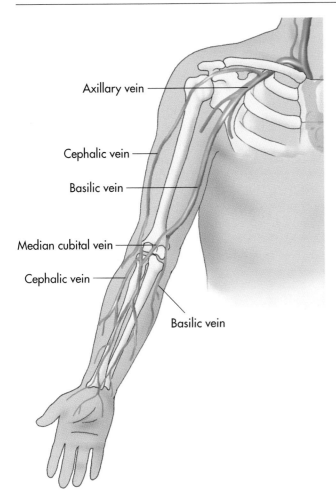

Figure 34-5   The superficial veins of the upper extremity.

proximal vein imaged. The mid and proximal external iliac and common iliac veins lie deep in the pelvis and are often obscured by the overlying bowel.

To evaluate the proximal iliac veins, a low-frequency sector transducer will usually provide the best images. During this portion of the examination it is not possible to perform accurate compression testing of the veins. The iliac veins are evaluated in a longitudinal view using color Doppler as a guide. Usually blue is the color assigned to venous blood flow. Careful attention to color control settings is critical, and evaluation of the venous Doppler signals is essential to performing an accurate examination of the veins at this level.

After the examination of the proximal veins, a higher-frequency (5 to 7.5 MHz) linear array transducer is placed at the inguinal crease in a transverse imaging plane. The transducer's orientation marker should be pointing medially or toward the patient's right side (transducer orientation may vary by institutional protocol). Using the transducer, pressure is applied to the skin to evaluate the compressibility of the vein. During each compression maneuver, the vein is observed to visualize if the vein walls "touch" each other (coapt), demonstrating the absence of intraluminal material. The lumen of the vein should reopen with release of the transducer's pressure on the skin. The amount of transducer pressure necessary to compress the

vein varies with its location and the patient's body habitus. The veins are followed distally along the length of the thigh, and transducer pressure is applied to the skin approximately every width of the transducer's footprint. It is not necessary to completely lift the transducer's footprint off the skin. The best venous imaging technique is to compress the vein by applying pressure on the skin with the transducer, then to release the pressure on the transducer and the vein's lumen will reopen, to slide the transducer distally on the limb (approximately the width of the transducer's footprint), and to reapply transducer pressure on the skin to compress the vein. Following this technique along the pathway of the venous system will provide the best results when performing venous duplex imaging.

At the level of the inguinal ligament, the common femoral vein is located and evaluated for compressibility. The transducer is moved distally on the limb, and the proximal greater saphenous vein (GSV) is compressed at the saphenofemoral junction. If superficial thrombophlebitis is suspected, the GSV should be followed along its entire length. The GSV lies beneath the skin and may be compressed by the weight of the transducer on the skin. If the saphenous vein is not visualized, reduce the pressure on the transducer to make sure that the vein is not inadvertently being compressed. This problem can be avoided by adding more gel to the leg to maintain contact and by not using any transducer pressure on the skin. The proximal greater saphenous vein is important to evaluate during venous duplex imaging because it is often the site of a clot that propagates and extends into the deep system.

While the transducer is moved distally on the leg from the common femoral vein, the origin of the superficial femoral vein (SFV) and **deep femoral vein (DFV or *profunda*)** will be visualized. The origins of the two veins are evaluated with transducer pressure applied to the skin. The compressibility of the origin of the DFV varies with patients, but can usually be evaluated with color Doppler for patency. When the vein is followed in the distal thigh, it will course deep and may be difficult to follow. The superficial femoral vein is followed along its length in the thigh. The SFV usually lies deep to the superficial femoral artery. When the vein is followed in the distal thigh, it will course deep and may be difficult to follow. The SFV can be difficult to coapt at the level of the adductor canal in the distal thigh because of the surrounding tissue. The distal SFV may be imaged and compressed from the posterior distal thigh or may be evaluated for compression by using hand pressure from the posterior distal thigh and bringing the vein toward the transducer.

The popliteal vein is evaluated from a posterior approach with the patient's knee rotated externally, with the patient in the decubitus position, or with the patient in the prone position with the foot elevated on a pillow to eliminate extrinsic compression of the vein. The popliteal vein should be followed proximally to the distal SFV and distally to the proximal calf veins. While the popliteal vein is followed along its length, it is evaluated in a transverse plane with the venous imaging compression technique. The popliteal vein usually lies superficial to the popliteal artery. Although venous aneurysms are rare vascular anomalies, popliteal venous aneurysms do occur and may be visualized during venous duplex imaging examinations.

The paired calf veins (anterior tibial, posterior tibial, and peroneal) are evaluated in the same manner (transverse view) along their length. The anterior tibial veins are small and are located in the proximal calf by placing the transducer on the lateral calf in a transverse imaging plane. The anterior tibial veins travel with the anterior tibial artery. The anterior tibial veins are located medial to the fibula in the proximal calf, travel just superior to the interosseous membrane, and gradually move in the direction of the tibia in the distal calf. The posterior tibial and peroneal veins are usually visualized by placing the transducer in a transverse imaging plane along the medial calf. The **posterior tibial veins** are located near the medial malleolus and are followed proximally in the calf. The peroneal veins are usually visualized, whereas the transducer is moved a few centimeters proximally on the calf. These veins travel along the peroneal and posterior tibial arteries. The **peroneal veins** lie deep and travel near the fibula. The posterior tibial and peroneal veins run parallel and can usually be visualized in the same imaging plane. In the upper calf, the two posterior tibial veins form a common trunk with the two peroneal veins (tibial-peroneal trunk).

In addition to the paired calf veins, there are two sets of muscular calf veins that may be visualized: the gastrocnemius and soleus calf veins. The paired gastrocnemius veins accompany an artery and can be visualized in the proximal calf as they enter the popliteal vein. The **gastrocnemius veins** lie in the muscles and are easily compressed with transducer pressure on the skin. The soleal sinuses lie deeper in the calf muscle and empty into the posterior tibial or peroneal veins. Additionally, the lesser saphenous vein runs along the posterior calf, lies just beneath the skin, is easily compressed by transducer pressure on the skin, and usually enters the popliteal vein.

Doppler. The evaluation of the lower extremity veins by Doppler is performed during the imaging examination. Doppler signals should be obtained from the longitudinal imaging plane. Angle correction of the Doppler signal is not necessary during venous duplex imaging because the actual peak velocity does not provide any clinical information. The pattern of the venous Doppler signal is what is clinically relevant. The Doppler scale should be reduced to visualize the low-velocity venous Doppler signals. Additionally, the Doppler sample volume may be increased to include the entire diameter of the lumen.

The following are the characteristics of a normal venous Doppler signal from a lower extremity:

- *Spontaneous:* Flow is present without augmentation maneuvers (usually not found in calf veins).
- *Respiratory phasicity:* Blood flow velocity changes with respiration (usually not found in calf veins). In the lower extremity, on inspiration the diaphragm descends and causes intraabdominal pressure to rise, compressing the vena cava and impeding venous outflow from the legs. With expira-

tion, the diaphragm rises, intraabdominal pressure decreases, and venous blood flow from the legs increases toward the vena cava.

- *Augmentation:* Blood flow velocity increases with distal limb compression or with the release of proximal limb compression.

Venous Doppler signals should be obtained from the common femoral vein and the popliteal vein. The signal from the common femoral vein helps to identify proximal obstruction (loss of phasicity), and the popliteal venous Doppler signal provides information about possible calf vein thrombosis (absent or decreased augmentation). During a unilateral venous imaging examination, the contralateral femoral venous Doppler signal should be documented. Venous Doppler signals may be obtained from other veins according to each institution's protocol.

UPPER EXTREMITY

Imaging Examination. The examination is explained to the patient. A history is taken from the patient, focusing on risk factors, signs, and symptoms (if present) of venous disease. Additionally, documentation of the history or presence of a line placed in the veins is critical.

The patient is evaluated in the supine position (unless contraindicated). The arm is positioned at the side of the patient. The head should be turned away from the side being examined. The internal jugular vein (IJV) is evaluated along its route in the neck in a transverse plane. The IJV can usually be compressed with transducer pressure on the skin. If the IJV cannot be compressed and if the lumen is echo free, the use of color Doppler or Doppler may be helpful. In this situation, the IJV will usually compress when the patient's head is raised. Evaluate the IJV carefully for intraluminal echoes. Often after indwelling lines or catheters are removed, there may be partial thrombus noted in the IJV. If there is an indwelling line or catheter in place, special attention should be made to image this area carefully (Figure 34-6). Compressive ultrasound technique will be limited. A clot is often visualized near the line or by its tip. The subclavian and **innominate veins** are evaluated from a supraclavicular approach. A low-frequency transducer with a small footprint will improve visualization of the central veins. Mirror imaging artifacts may occur when evaluating the central veins because of the clavicle. Normal Doppler signals from the central veins are pulsatile (right side of heart) with a phasic respiratory variation superimposed on the venous velocity pattern. The superior vena cava may be visualized from a supraclavicular or a suprasternal approach, depending on the patient.

Next, from an infraclavicular approach, the subclavian and axillary veins are evaluated in a transverse plane and the compression technique can be attempted. Shadowing from the clavicle is a problem from this approach and it may take multiple views to fully visualize the subclavian vein. The patient's arm is repositioned to allow access to the axilla. A low-frequency (5-MHz) linear array transducer is used to evaluate the veins in the arm. A higher-frequency (7.5- to 10-MHz)

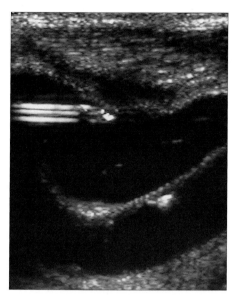

Figure 34-6 A longitudinal view of the internal jugular vein and the common carotid artery. The internal jugular vein lies superficial to the artery. The indwelling line produces bright echoes within the venous lumen. The tip of the line is against the vessel's wall. When imaging a patient who has an indwelling line, careful attention must be paid to the area surrounding the line.

linear array transducer may be used to evaluate the more superficial veins, depending on the patient. The axillary vein travels with the axillary artery and receives the cephalic vein. The axillary vein is followed distally on the arm to the confluence of the basilic vein. Distally on the arm, the axillary vein becomes the brachial vein after the entrance of the basilic vein. The brachial veins travel with the brachial artery and the veins tend to be small.

Near the antecubital fossa, the radial and ulnar veins can be visualized as they travel with their respective arteries along the length of the forearm. Although they are often small in diameter, they can usually be evaluated without too much difficulty. The forearm veins should compress with transducer pressure on the skin. The radial and ulnar veins can usually be followed to the wrist level.

The cephalic and basilic veins are the superficial veins in the upper extremity. The **cephalic vein** is a superficial vein and is not accompanied by an artery. This vein travels along the lateral aspect of the biceps muscle and may be followed from the axillary vein to the level of the wrist. The basilic vein is a superficial vein, is usually large, does not travel with an artery, and travels along the medial side of the arm and enters the brachial vein.

Doppler. The evaluation of the upper extremity veins by Doppler imaging is a critical part of the venous imaging examination. Color Doppler is very helpful in locating the central veins and in the identification of filling defects from a clot. Doppler signals should be obtained from the longitudinal plane. Angle correction of the Doppler signal is not necessary during venous duplex imaging because the actual peak veloc-

ity does not provide any clinical information. Additionally, the Doppler sample volume may be increased to include the entire lumen of the vein, and the Doppler scale should be reduced to visualize the low-velocity venous Doppler signals. The pattern of the venous Doppler spectral waveform is what is important and extremely critical in the examination of the views of the upper extremity.

The following are the characteristics of a normal venous Doppler signal from an upper extremity:

- *Spontaneous:* Flow is present without augmentation maneuvers.
- *Pulsatility:* Pulsatile signals should be present in the jugular, subclavian, innominate, and superior vena cava because of retrograde transmission of right atrial pressure.
- *Respiratory phasicity:* Blood flow velocity changes with respiration. In the upper extremity (central veins), the venous Doppler signal will increase with inspiration and decrease with expiration.
- *Augmentation:* Blood flow velocity increases with distal limb compression or with release of proximal limb compression (limited in the upper extremity examination).

Venous Doppler signals should be obtained from the superior vena cava and jugular, innominate, subclavian, and axillary veins. When evaluating the upper extremity, it is helpful to compare the Doppler signals from the right and left side. During a unilateral venous imaging examination, the contralateral internal jugular or subclavian venous Doppler signal should be documented. Lack of pulsatility in the central veins suggests venous obstruction.

At the end of the venous duplex imaging examination, the ultrasound gel should be removed from the patient. Excess gel should be removed from the ultrasound transducer, and the transducer should be cleaned using a disinfectant.

Some general tips when performing venous duplex imaging are listed in Table 34-1. The best quality and most reliable examination will be obtained by careful attention to venous anatomy and imaging technique.

INTERPRETATION OF VENOUS DUPLEX IMAGING

It is imperative that each institution develop a venous imaging protocol that defines the standard examination (veins to be evaluated during a lower and upper extremity examination, the locations for Doppler signal documentation). This protocol must include the technique, clinical applications, indications for a complete and/or limited examination, and interpretation criteria. The interpretation criteria for venous duplex imaging (Table 34-2) are based on three components: the patent vein is free of echogenic material, compresses fully with transducer pressure on the skin (Figures 34-7 and 34-8), and exhibits a normal (Figure 34-9) venous Doppler signal.

Consistency of the findings on gray scale imaging, by compression technique, and with color Doppler and/or the venous Doppler spectral waveform will limit errors when interpreting venous duplex imaging examinations.

TABLE 34-1 VENOUS DUPLEX IMAGING TIPS

Challenge	Action
Nonvisualization of veins	Veins may collapse easily with pressure from the transducer. If a vein cannot be visualized, less pressure should be applied on the transducer. Release of the transducer's pressure on the skin will enable the vein to be visualized from the correct anatomic position.
Veins do not compress	If a vein segment appears patent but does not compress, transducer pressure may be applied from a different site on the skin or by repositioning the patient. Often an adjacent bone or tendon prevents compression of the vein.
Pressure assessment	Adequate pressure has been applied to compress a vein if the adjacent artery is compressed by the compression maneuver.
Imaging in a longitudinal plane	Be aware of multiple veins or vein segments. They are common and may be missed if imaging only in a longitudinal plane.
Imaging limitations	Obesity, extensive edema, leg wounds, calcified arteries, anatomic structures (clavicle), and casts will limit the venous duplex imaging study or may affect the quality of the examination. Use transducers of different frequency and use different imaging planes to improve visualization of the veins.
Color Doppler limitations	Color Doppler may obscure a nonoccluding thrombus. If evaluating the vein in the longitudinal plane, visualization of a nonoccluding thrombus depends on the angle of the imaging plane and the accurate setting of the instrument controls.
Venous Doppler	Angle correction is not necessary during venous duplex imaging. The actual peak velocity is not critical. The pattern of the Doppler spectral waveform is what is important during venous imaging. Doppler signals are taken in the longitudinal plane, and the sample volume may be increased to the size of the diameter of the vein.
Upper extremities	During upper extremity imaging: use color Doppler to help locate the central veins; the central veins should have a pulsatile and phasic signal; compare the Doppler signals from right and left sides; and be aware of mirror imaging artifact because of the clavicle.

TABLE 34-2 INTERPRETATION CRITERIA OF VENOUS DUPLEX IMAGING

Gray Scale/ Compression	Doppler Signal	Color Doppler
Normal		
No intraluminal echoes Vein compresses	*Normal:* Phasic, augments with distal compression (pulsatile for upper extremities)	Color fills lumen
Abnormal: Nonocclusive		
Vein lumen partially filled with echoes Vein partially compresses	May be normal or abnormal	Defect in color as it is displayed around thrombus; may appear normal if thrombus is small or if instrument controls are not adjusted properly
Abnormal: Occlusive		
Vein filled with intraluminal echoes Vein does not compress	*Abnormal:* Absence of Doppler signal, a continuous signal, absent or reduced phasicity, and the lack of pulsatility in the central veins of the upper extremity	Absence of color

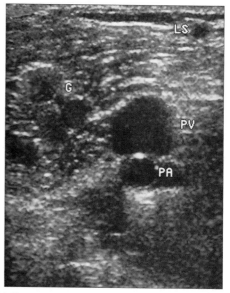

Figure 34-7 Transverse view at the popliteal fossa without transducer pressure. The popliteal vein *(PV)* lies superficial to the popliteal artery *(PA)*. The lesser saphenous *(LS)* vein lies just below the skin line. A set of paired gastrocnemius *(G)* veins are located on either side of the accompanying artery.

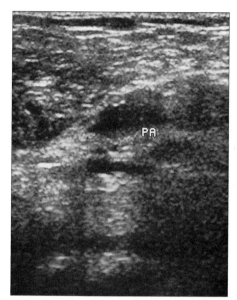

Figure 34-8 Transverse view at the popliteal fossa with transducer pressure on the skin. The vein walls collapse suggesting no evidence of venous thrombosis in the lesser saphenous, popliteal, or gastrocnemius veins. The popliteal artery *(PA)* is still visualized and does not collapse.

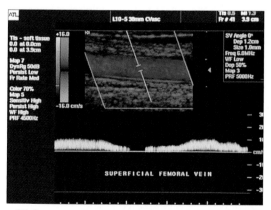

Figure 34-9 Normal venous Doppler signal of the superficial femoral vein. Note that the color fills the lumen of the vein by using a low-color pulse repetition frequency. The venous spectral Doppler waveform demonstrates a low velocity and the phasic characteristic of a normal venous Doppler signal.

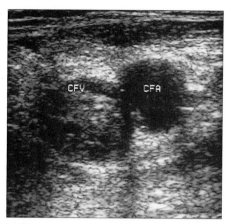

Figure 34-10 The common femoral artery *(CFA)* and vein *(CFV)* are visualized in a transverse view with transducer pressure on the skin. The vein walls do not coapt and echogenic material fills the lumen of the vein suggesting thrombosis.

TABLE 34-3	TECHNICAL ADJUSTMENTS FOR VENOUS DUPLEX IMAGING
Challenge	Action
Vein does not compress; lumen is echo free	**Technique:** Move the transducer on the skin to attempt compression from a different approach. Use the correct transverse plane, and check for adequate pressure. **Patient Position:** Repositioning the patient's extremity often results in being able to compress the vein. **Anatomy:** At times the depth of the vessel and the surrounding tissue will make vein compression impossible.
Vein compresses; lumen is filled with echoes	**Equipment:** Gain settings too high **Technique:** Use the correct transverse plane to make sure that there is complete compression of the venous lumen.

There are, however, many pitfalls in the interpretation of these examinations. Proper technique is essential to providing accurate venous duplex imaging examinations and minimizing errors in interpretation.

If inconsistent findings are obtained when performing a venous duplex imaging examination, there are several technical and equipment adjustments that should be considered before the final interpretation (Table 34-3).

It is important to remember that the most significant diagnostic criterion during venous imaging is how the vein responds to transducer pressure. To check if adequate pressure was used during the examination, look at the effects of the compression on the artery. Adequate pressure was used if the artery is deformed during the compression maneuver.

If the vein does not compress and the lumen is echo-free, try repositioning the extremity. If the vein still does not compress, remember that visualization of the thrombus is quite variable. At times the thrombus is very echogenic and may blend into the surrounding tissue (Figure 34-10), and at other times the clot is anechoic. A vein may not compress because the clot is present in the lumen but is not visualized with gray scale imaging. Additionally, trying to determine the age of the thrombus by the degree of its echogenicity is unreliable (Figure 34-11).

A free-floating clot may also be visualized moving freely within the lumen during venous duplex imaging (Figure 34-12). When this phenomenon occurs, the compression technique is not performed at that level on the limb. Usually the

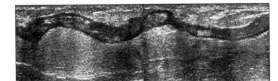

Figure 34-11   A longitudinal view of the basilic vein demonstrates venous thrombosis of mixed echogenicity.

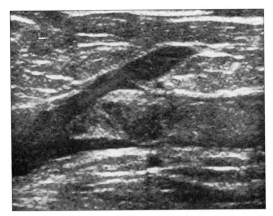

Figure 34-12   A longitudinal view of the femoral vein. A free-floating clot is visualized within the lumen of the vein. Blood flows around the tip of the thrombus. Distally in the vein (*right side of the image*), the clot attaches to the vein walls.

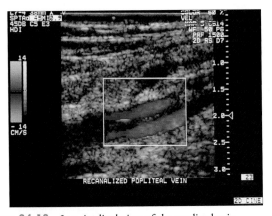

Figure 34-13   Longitudinal view of the popliteal vein demonstrating recanalization of the venous thrombosis. The color Doppler display demonstrates blood flow channels.

free-floating clot becomes attached to the walls of the vein distally and the compression technique can be resumed.

In follow-up studies, the resolution of a clot varies dramatically from patient to patient. Complete resolution of an extensive clot may occur at 3 months, 6 months, or 1 year, or it may never occur in an individual patient. Recanalization of veins occurs often, and blood flowing through small channels can be documented with color Doppler imaging (Figure 34-13).

In a review of more than 30 studies, the results of venous duplex imaging compared with venography demonstrate a good sensitivity for the detection of DVT.[4] In symptomatic

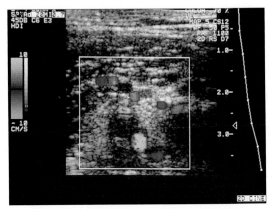

Figure 34-14   A transverse view at the level of the popliteal fossa with transducer pressure. The popliteal vein and several of the gastrocnemius veins in the proximal calf do not compress, suggesting deep vein thrombosis.

patients, the sensitivity for proximal DVT ranges from 89% to 100%. The specificity for DVT is greater than 90%. Additionally, good results have been reported for proximal disease in the asymptomatic high-risk patient. The sensitivity in these patients ranges from 63% to 100%, with a specificity of greater than 90%. It is important to note that the distribution and magnitude of DVT may vary, depending on the type of patient. Screening high-risk patients has demonstrated an increase in the number of nonoccluding thrombi compared with symptomatic patients.[5]

Evaluation of the calf veins remains more problematic. The size and number of the veins makes the examination technique more challenging. There are reports in the literature of a sensitivity of greater than 80% for detecting DVT in the calf veins. This has improved in recent years with the better resolution obtained with the use of state-of-the-art imaging systems and color Doppler imaging in select patients (Figure 34-14).

COMBINED DIAGNOSTIC APPROACH

A recent and controversial approach to the diagnostic evaluation of DVT has been to use a combined approach of ultrasound imaging, D-dimer assays, and a detailed clinical risk assessment score.[1,3,16,18,20] The assays measure D-dimer, which is a fibrin-specific degradation product that detects cross-linked fibrin resulting from endogenous fibrinolysis. The precise role of using D-dimer assays in conjunction with venous ultrasound has not been clearly established. The D-dimer assays have not been standardized, and results are variable depending on the thrombus size, location, and interpretation of the results. Algorithms for diagnosing DVT using a clinical risk assessment score, venous imaging of the entire leg, and D-dimer testing have been proposed, and they will probably become more widely used in the future in an attempt to limit costs and improve efficiency in the diagnosis of DVT.

VEIN MAPPING

The purpose of superficial vein mapping is to determine the vein's suitability for use as a bypass conduit and to identify its anatomic route. Vein mapping is usually performed before lower extremity arterial bypass or coronary bypass operations. The accurate mapping of the location of the veins is important when the surgeons plan an in situ bypass graft of the lower extremity or when harvesting the vein. Preoperative vein mapping avoids exposing inadequate veins, which in turn decreases operative time and the possibility of wound complications from unnecessary incisions.

A high-frequency linear array transducer provides the best resolution for evaluating the superficial veins of the lower (greater and lesser saphenous veins) and upper extremities (cephalic and basilic veins). Light transducer pressure on the skin is critical because the superficial veins lie below the skin line and are easily compressed with minimal pressure from the transducer. The patient should be in the supine position. The bed may be placed in the reverse Trendelenburg's position to promote venous distention if necessary.

The imaging begins at the groin level in a transverse plane. The common femoral vein should be located and followed distally on the limb. The saphenofemoral junction is usually located a few centimeters distally on the leg from the inguinal ligament. The greater saphenous vein travels along the anteromedial side of the thigh and calf, has many branches, and usually has valves. The anatomy of the greater saphenous vein is variable, and a double system for short segments of the vein is common.

If an adequate greater saphenous vein is not located in either leg, the lesser saphenous vein should be evaluated bilaterally. The lesser saphenous vein extends from posterior to the lateral malleolus and terminates at variable levels of the popliteal vein, has branches, and usually has valves. If the superficial veins on the lower extremity are not adequate, the superficial veins on the arms may be evaluated for their suitability. If the arm veins are difficult to visualize, try using a tourniquet on the upper arm to promote venous dilation.

Confirm the patency of the vein along its length by using the compression technique. The size of the vein, the presence of thickened walls, calcification, recanalization, and stenotic valves should also be documented. Mark the vein's path and its branches on the skin using an indelible marker. When marking the skin, make sure that the vein is centered in the ultrasound image. The challenge in vein mapping is to use enough ultrasound gel to provide a good image, but not more than what is necessary or the excess gel will make it difficult to mark the skin.

VENOUS REFLUX TESTING

The purpose of venous reflux testing is to identify the presence and the location of incompetent venous valves. The evaluation of venous reflux by duplex imaging is performed using a low-frequency (5 MHz) linear array imaging transducer. The examination is performed with the patient standing, holding onto a frame for support, and with full body weight placed on the opposite leg. Although venous valves may be visualized at different locations in many individuals, the gray scale image is not used for determining valvular incompetence. The absence or presence of venous reflux is measured from the venous spectral Doppler waveform.

A longitudinal view of the saphenofemoral junction is located. The Doppler sample volume size is adjusted to the vein's width. The Doppler sample volume is positioned in the femoral vein distal to the saphenofemoral junction and distal limb compression is performed. In the presence of incompetent valves, sudden release of the distal compression produces retrograde blood flow (reflux), which is recorded and measured on the spectral Doppler waveform display (Figure 34-15). The valves are considered incompetent if retrograde blood flow is present and lasts longer than 1 second. Absence of retrograde blood flow indicates competent valves. The examination is repeated with the sample volume located in the greater saphenous vein distal to the saphenofemoral junction. The popliteal and the lesser saphenous veins are selectively evaluated in a similar manner with the imaging transducer located over the popliteal fossa. Depending on the patient, any vein, including the perforators, may be evaluated for venous reflux.

Duplex imaging provides the ability to quantify reflux in the individual (deep, superficial, perforating) veins of the thigh and calf. It is technically difficult to operate the imaging system, hold the transducer on the patient's leg, and compress the patient's distal limb to test for venous reflux. Two examiners are necessary to ensure proper testing, or a distal automatic cuff compression-release device must be used. A cuff compression-release device is used on the leg distal to the imaging transducer and ensures standard compression pressure and timing of the release.

To perform a complete venous duplex imaging examination for reflux takes approximately 30 minutes per extremity. With the addition of color Doppler imaging, the identification of the veins with reflux is immediate, and individual vein Doppler sample volume placement is not necessary. Although using color Doppler to test for venous reflux may reduce the examination time and technical difficulty, appropriate color control settings are essential for an accurate diagnosis. The venous

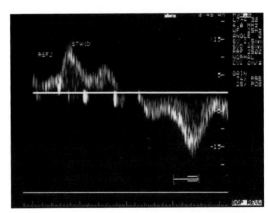

Figure 34-15 The Doppler spectral waveform obtained during a venous reflux test. Reversal of blood flow that lasts longer than 1 second is obtained with release of distal compression, suggesting venous reflux.

duplex imaging examination for venous reflux provides accurate information about the individual veins. It does not provide information about the limb's overall venous hemodynamics.

CONTROVERSIES IN VENOUS DUPLEX IMAGING

COMPLETE VERSUS LIMITED EXAMINATION

Why examine the entire leg in a symptomatic patient? The standard technique for venous duplex imaging of the lower extremity in symptomatic patients has been to evaluate the veins from the level of the inguinal ligament to and including the calf veins. A limited venous ultrasound of the lower extremity has been defined multiple ways in the literature. Investigators have described a limited examination as an evaluation limited to the common femoral and popliteal veins, imaging limited to the full length of the femoral and popliteal veins, imaging limited to the common femoral vein, and imaging limited to the popliteal vein. It has been suggested that a "two-point" venous duplex examination in symptomatic patients would detect a clot in a high percentage of the cases and significantly reduce the examination time.[11] The abbreviated study employs compression of the veins at the level of the common femoral and popliteal veins.

In a prospective study of 53 symptomatic patients (56 limbs), the results of a limited examination were compared with the routine venous imaging examination.[11] The limited examination was performed before the routine examination. During the limited examination, the CFV from the inguinal ligament to the deep femoral (profunda) takeoff and the popliteal vein above and below the knee to the level of its trifurcation were visualized. Limited venous evaluations were performed in transverse and longitudinal views.

Of the 56 cases, 7 (12%) demonstrated deep vein thrombosis by limited and routine venous examinations. Both techniques failed to visualize an isolated iliac vein clot that was depicted by CT scan. The average time for the limited examination was 8.3 minutes, and for the routine examination the average time was 18.0 minutes.

In another study the investigators performed 755 venous duplex imaging examinations in 721 symptomatic patients (1024 limbs).[7] Acute DVT was visualized in one or more veins in 131 (17.4%) of 755 examinations. DVT was limited to a single vein in 28 (21.4%) of 131 examinations in which DVT was detected. There was isolated thrombus in the CFV in 8 examinations (6.1%), in the SFV in 6 examinations (4.6%), and in the popliteal vein in 14 examinations (10.7%). These investigators concluded that DVT limited to a single vein occurs frequently and that adoption of an abbreviated venous duplex imaging examination may be potentially dangerous for patients.

At the current time, it is recommended that the routine venous duplex imaging examination be performed in most cases. The abbreviated or limited venous duplex examination may have a role in the symptomatic, critically ill patient or in symptomatic patients with limited mobility. The limited venous duplex examination should not be performed when screening patients at high risk for DVT.

UNILATERAL VERSUS BILATERAL

Why examine the asymptomatic leg in a patient with unilateral symptoms? Traditionally, only the symptomatic limb was evaluated in a patient when the accepted diagnostic test for DVT was venography. However, it was customary to study both lower extremities when vascular laboratories were using nonimaging Doppler and plethysmographic techniques that relied on the comparison of the venous hemodynamics from one limb with the other for an accurate interpretation.

In a prospective bilateral venous duplex imaging study of the proximal veins in 206 patients with unilateral symptoms, the diagnosis of DVT was made in 37 (18%) of the 206 patients.[13] No patient was found to have thrombosis in the asymptomatic limb. These investigators suggest that unilateral imaging will not subject the patients to any risks, but will improve cost effectiveness.

Another study retrospectively reviewed the bilateral venous duplex imaging examinations in 1694 symptomatic patients.[15] Two hundred forty-eight of the patients had acute DVT. There was no case of acute DVT in the asymptomatic limb if the symptomatic limb was normal. These investigators recommend that patients with unilateral symptoms undergo unilateral venous duplex imaging because treatment in these patients would not have been altered, and unilateral imaging improves cost efficiency.

In a prospective study of 488 patients referred for venous duplex imaging, DVT was present in 121 of 488 (25%) patients.[10] There were 245 patients with unilateral signs and symptoms of DVT. Deep venous thrombosis was present in 65 of the 245 patients with unilateral signs and symptoms. If only the symptomatic leg was evaluated, three patients with DVT of the contralateral asymptomatic limb would have been missed. Additionally, 18 patients with unilateral symptoms were found to have DVT bilaterally. In these 18 patients the diagnosis of DVT would have been made, but the extent of the disease would not have been appreciated. This may affect the patient in the future if follow-up venous imaging is performed for new signs and symptoms. These investigators conclude that bilateral venous duplex imaging should be performed on all patients with unilateral symptoms.

Currently, it is recommended to image the contralateral asymptomatic extremity if DVT is visualized in the symptomatic extremity. This procedure will document the patency of the femoral vein (access for percutaneous placement of vena caval filters) and the presence of any DVT that may prove to be helpful in follow-up studies. If DVT is not detected in the symptomatic limb, then DVT in the asymptomatic, contralateral limb occurs in approximately 1% of patients with unilateral symptoms. A protocol for this clinical situation should be established by each institution.

BILATERAL SYMPTOMS

Why perform venous duplex imaging in patients with bilateral leg symptoms? It has been suggested in the literature that patients with symptoms of bilateral edema of the lower extremity may have cardiac disease as the dominant cause of their leg swelling. Other causes of bilateral lower extremity symptoms may be peripheral arterial disease, venous stasis, trauma, or venous thrombosis.

In a study of 488 patients evaluated with venous duplex imaging, 149 had bilateral signs and symptoms of DVT.[10] Of the 149 patients 35 (23%) were found to have proximal DVT by venous duplex imaging. Ten patients had unilateral DVT, and 25 patients had bilateral DVT. These investigators conclude that bilateral venous duplex imaging should be performed in patients with bilateral signs and symptoms of DVT.

In a prospective study of 500 symptomatic patients who were referred for venous duplex imaging, there were 50 patients with bilateral symptoms.[14] No DVT was diagnosed in the 50 patients with bilateral symptoms, although the overall detection rate of DVT was 17.4% in this patient population. On the basis of the patient's medical history, a possible alternative cause for the patient's symptoms was found in 34 of the 50 patients. Alternative causes for symptoms included cardiac disease in 18 patients, peripheral arterial disease in 6 patients, and superficial thrombophlebitis or cellulitis in 12 patients. The remaining 16 patients had no history that could explain the development of the bilateral symptoms. These investigators suggest that DVT in the patient with bilateral symptoms is rare and venous duplex imaging should not be performed if the patient's medical history indicates a more likely alternative cause.

CALF VEIN IMAGING

Why examine the calf veins in patients at high risk for developing DVT or in patients suspected of DVT? This controversy centers on three distinct points. Calf veins can be difficult to image in many patients. Physicians often do not treat an isolated calf clot, and patients with calf clot are unlikely to have signs or symptoms of pulmonary embolism. Additionally, patients can be followed serially with venous duplex imaging for propagation of the clot, which occurs in approximately 20% of the cases.

Critical to the direct evaluation of the calf veins is the knowledge of venous anatomy and the use of proper technique. Improvement in equipment's gray scale resolution and color Doppler capability have also made the identification of calf veins possible. Evaluation of the calf veins adds approximately 10 minutes to the examination of the lower extremity. Evaluation of the calf veins for DVT provides the clinician with the option to initiate treatment. Additionally, imaging of the calf veins documents calf clot that provides an explanation for a patient's symptoms or provides important information in the high-risk patient being screened for DVT.

ASSESSMENT OF PULMONARY EMBOLUS

Why examine the lower extremities with venous duplex imaging if the patient has signs and symptoms of a pulmonary embolus? Clinicians not wishing to order pulmonary arteriography in patients have determined that if venous duplex imaging detects DVT in patients suspected of PE, then anticoagulation therapy may be initiated.[12] Because the majority of pulmonary emboli originate from the lower extremity, using venous duplex imaging to clarify an indeterminate lung scan may also help to confirm a clinical suspicion of PE. However, it has been shown that approximately half of the patients with documented pulmonary embolism by pulmonary arteriography do not have clots in their legs.[9] Therefore, a negative venous duplex imaging study of the legs does not exclude the diagnosis of PE and further work-up in these patients is necessary. Venous duplex imaging should not be used as the first or the only diagnostic test for the diagnosis of pulmonary embolus.

TERMINOLOGY

Why use the term *superficial* femoral vein when describing the deep venous system in the thigh? The term *superficial* femoral vein is often used to describe the deep venous system in the thigh in venous duplex imaging reports. A survey was conducted to evaluate if this terminology was causing confusion among referring clinicians and potentially being hazardous to patients.[2] The survey was sent to family practitioners and general internists in San Diego County, California, in 1994. Physicians were asked how they would treat a 56-year-old woman with leg pain and a venous duplex imaging report that read "Occluding thrombus of the distal superficial femoral vein. The thrombus appears acute."

Seventy-five percent (46 out of 61) of the surveys were returned. Only 24% (11 out of 46) of the clinicians who responded to the survey chose to administer anticoagulant agents to the patient. Additionally, in the same study, 110 surveys were sent to the medical directors of vascular laboratories. Of the returned surveys, 93% (79 out of 85) used the term *superficial femoral vein* in venous duplex imaging reports.

The term *superficial femoral vein* is often used in venous duplex imaging reports. Many primary care physicians, however, do not universally understand this nomenclature. It may be advisable to use the term *femoral vein* in venous duplex imaging reports when describing the deep venous system in the thigh.

IMAGING GUIDELINES

Producing high-quality and complete venous duplex examinations is key to its diagnostic value. The best examinations will be achieved by proper attention to detail. Technical areas and interpretation details that will ensure the best venous duplex imaging results are listed in Box 34-4.

BOX 34-4   VENOUS DUPLEX IMAGING GUIDELINES

- Take a patient history
- Be familiar with venous anatomy, physiology, and pathology
- Optimize the gray scale
- Use a transverse view for compression technique
- Use a longitudinal view to obtain Doppler signals. Use a large Doppler sample volume size, a zero-degree angle, and a low-velocity scale
- Use a longitudinal view to obtain color Doppler images
- Upper extremities: document pulsatility in the Doppler signal and compare the right and left sides
- Establish institutional diagnostic criteria

REFERENCES

1. Anderson DR and others: Combined use of clinical assessment and D-dimer to improve the management of patients presenting to the emergency department with suspected deep vein thrombosis (the EDITED study), *J Thromb Haemost* 1:645-651, 2003.

2. Bundens WP and others: The superficial femoral vein: a potentially lethal misnomer, *JAMA* 274:1296, 1995.

3. Caprini JA and others: Laboratory markers in the diagnosis of venous thromboembolism, *Circulation* 109:I4-I8, 2004.

4. Comerota AJ, Katz ML, Hashemi HA: Venous duplex imaging for the diagnosis of acute deep venous thrombosis, *Haemostasis* 23:61, 1993.

5. Comerota AJ and others: The comparative value of noninvasive testing for diagnosis and surveillance of deep vein thrombosis, *J Vasc Surg* 7:40, 1988.

6. Dalen JE and others: Venous thromboembolism: scope of the problem, *Chest* 89:370S, 1986.

7. Frederick MG and others: Can the US examination for lower extremity deep vein thrombosis be abbreviated? A prospective study of 755 examinations, *Radiology* 199:45, 1996.

8. Kahn SR: The clinical diagnosis of deep venous thrombosis: integrating incidence, risk factors, and symptoms and signs, *Arch Intern Med* 158:2315, 1998.

9. Killewich LA, Nunnelee JD, Auer AI: Value of lower extremity venous duplex examination in the diagnosis of pulmonary embolism, *J Vasc Surg* 17:934, 1993.

10. Naidich JB and others: Suspected deep venous thrombosis: is US of both legs necessary? *Radiology* 200:429, 1996.

11. Pezzullo JA, Parkins AB, Cronan JJ: Symptomatic deep vein thrombosis: diagnosis with limited compression US, *Radiology* 198:67, 1996.

12. Rosen MP and others: Compression sonography in patients with indeterminate or low probability lung scans: lack of usefulness in the absence of both symptoms of deep vein thrombosis and thromboembolic risk factors, *Am J Roentgenol* 166:285, 1996.

13. Sheiman RG, McArdle CR: Bilateral lower extremity US in the patient with unilateral symptoms of deep vein thrombosis: assessment of need, *Radiology* 194:171, 1995.

14. Sheiman RG, Weintraub JL, McArdle CR: Bilateral lower extremity US in the patient with bilateral symptoms of deep vein thrombosis: assessment of need, *Radiology* 196:379, 1995.

15. Strothman G and others: Contralateral duplex scanning for deep venous thrombosis is unnecessary in patients with symptoms, *J Vasc Surg* 22:543, 1995.

16. Tick LW and others: Practical diagnostic management of patients with clinically suspected deep vein thrombosis by clinical probability test, compression ultrasonography, and D-dimer test, *Am J Med* 113:630-635, 2002.

17. Virchow R: Neuer fall von todlicher emboli der lungenarterie, *Virchows Arch Pathol Anat* 10:225, 1856.

18. Wells PS and others: Evaluation of D-Dimer in the diagnosis of suspected deep-vein thrombosis, *NEJM* 349:1227-1235, 2003.

19. White RH: The epidemiology of venous thromboembolism, *Circulation* 107:I4-I8, 2003.

20. Zierler BK: Ultrasonography and diagnosis of venous thromboembolism, *Circulation* 109:I9-I14, 2004.

SELECTED BIBLIOGRAPHY

Aldridge SC and others: Popliteal venous aneurysm: report of two cases and review of the world literature, *J Vasc Surgery* 18:708, 1993.

Anderson FA, Spencer FA: Risk factors for venous thromboembolism, *Circulation* 107:I9-I16, 2003.

Atri M and others: Accuracy of sonography in the evaluation of calf vein thrombosis in both postoperative surveillance and symptomatic patients, *Am J Roentgenol* 166:1361, 1996.

Beecham RP and others: Is bilateral lower extremity compression sonography useful and cost-effective in the evaluation of suspected pulmonary embolism? *Am J Roentgenol* 161:1289, 1993.

Kearon C: Natural history of venous thromboembolism, *Circulation* 107:I22-I30, 2003.

Neglen P, Raju S: A comparison of descending phlebography and duplex Doppler investigation in the evaluation of reflux in chronic venous insufficiency: a challenge to phlebography as the "gold standard," *J Vasc Surg* 16:687, 1992.

Ruoof BA and others: Real-time duplex ultrasound mapping of greater saphenous vein before in situ infrainguinal revascularization, *J Vasc Surg* 6:107, 1987.

Shah DM and others: The anatomy of the greater saphenous venous system, *J Vasc Surg* 3:273, 1986.

Strandness DE and others: Long-term sequelae of acute venous thrombosis, *JAMA* 250:1289, 1983.

Van Bemmelen PS and others: Quantitative segmental evaluation of venous valvular reflux with duplex ultrasound scanning, *J Vasc Surg* 10:425, 1989.

Welch HJ and others: Duplex assessment of venous reflux and chronic venous insufficiency: the significance of deep venous reflux, *J Vasc Surg* 24:755, 1996.

PART VII

Gynecology

CHAPTER 35

Normal Anatomy and Physiology of the Female Pelvis

Tamara L. Salsgiver and Sandra L. Hagen-Ansert

KEY TERMS

amenorrhea – an absence of menstruation

anteflexed – refers to the position of the uterus when the uterine fundus bends forward toward the cervix

anteverted – refers to the position of the uterus when the uterus is tipped slightly forward so that the cervix forms a 90-degree angle or less with the vaginal canal; most common uterine position

broad ligament – a broad fold of peritoneum draped over the fallopian tubes, uterus, and the ovaries; extends from the sides of the uterus to the sidewalls of the pelvis, dividing the pelvis from side to side and creating the vesicouterine pouch anterior to the uterus and the rectouterine pouch posteriorly; it is divided into the mesometrium, mesosalpinx, and mesovarium

cardinal ligament – wide bands of fibromuscular tissue arising from the lateral aspects of the cervix and inserting along the lateral pelvic floor; a continuation of the broad ligament that provides rigid support for the cervix; also called the *transverse cervical ligaments*

coccygeus muscles – one of two muscles in the pelvic diaphragm; located on the posterior pelvic floor where it supports the coccyx

corpus luteum – an anatomic structure on the surface of the ovary, consisting of a spheroid of yellowish tissue that grows within the ruptured ovarian follicle after ovulation; acts as a short-lived endocrine organ that secretes progesterone to maintain the decidual layer of the endometrium should conception occur

dysmenorrhea – pain associated with menstruation

estrogen – a steroidal hormone secreted by the theca interna and granulosa cells of the ovarian follicle that stimulates the development of the female reproductive structures and secondary sexual characteristics; promotes the growth of the endometrial tissue during the proliferative phase of the menstrual cycle

false pelvis – portion of the pelvis found above the brim; that portion of the abdominal cavity cradled by the iliac fossae; also called the *greater* or *major pelvis*

follicle-stimulating hormone (FSH) – a hormone secreted by the anterior pituitary gland that stimulates the growth and maturation of graafian follicles in the ovary

gonadotropin – a hormonal substance that stimulates the function of the testes and the ovaries; in the female, FSH and LH are gonadotropins

gonadotropin-releasing hormone (GnRH) – a hormone secreted by the hypothalamus that stimulates the release of the follicle-stimulating hormone (FSH) and luteinizing hormone (LH) by the anterior pituitary gland

iliacus muscle – paired triangular, flat muscles that cover the inner curved surface of the iliac fossae; arise from the iliac fossae and join the psoas major muscles to form the lateral walls of the pelvis

iliopectineal line – a bony ridge on the inner surface of the ilium and pubic bones that divides the true and false pelves; also called the *pelvic brim* or *linea terminalis*

levator ani – one of two muscles of the pelvic diaphragm that stretch across the floor of the pelvic cavity like a hammock, supporting the pelvic organs and surrounding the urethra, vagina, and rectum; a broad thin muscle that consists of the pubococcygeus, iliococcygeus, and puborectalis

luteinizing hormone (LH) – a hormone secreted by the anterior pituitary gland that stimulates ovulation and then induces luteinization of the ruptured follicle to form the corpus luteum

menarche – refers to the onset of menstruation and the commencement of cyclic menstrual function; usually occurs between 11 and 13 years of age

menopause – refers to the cessation of menstruation

menorrhagia – abnormally heavy or long periods

menses – the periodic flow of blood and cellular debris that occurs during menstruation

mesometrium – the portion of the broad ligament below the mesovarium, composed of the layers of peritoneum that separate to enclose the uterus

mesosalpinx – the upper portion of the broad ligament that encloses the fallopian tubes

mesovarium – the posterior portion of the broad ligament that is drawn out to enclose and hold the ovary in place

obturator internus muscle – a triangular sheet of muscle that arises from the anterolateral pelvic wall and surrounds the obturator foramen; passes through the lesser sciatic foramen and inserts into the medial aspect of the greater trochanter of the femur; serves to rotate and abduct the thigh

oligomenorrhea – abnormally light menstrual periods

oocyte – an incompletely developed or immature ovum

ovarian ligament – a paired ligament that extends from the inferior/medial pole of the ovary to the uterine cornua; also called the *utero-ovarian ligament*

ovum – the female egg; a secondary oocyte released from the ovary at ovulation

perimetrium – a serous membrane enveloping the uterus; also called the *serosa*

piriformis muscle – a flat, pyramidal muscle arising from the anterior sacrum, passing through the greater sciatic notch to insert into the superior aspect of the greater trochanter of the femur; serves to rotate and abduct the thigh

polymenorrhea – an abnormally frequent recurrence of the menstrual cycle; a menstrual cycle of less than 21 days

postmenopause – time period of life after menopause

premenarche – time period in young girls before the onset of menstruation

progesterone – a steroidal hormone produced by the corpus luteum that helps prepare and maintain the endometrium for the arrival and implantation of an embryo

psoas major muscle – paired muscles that originate at the transverse process of the lumbar vertebrae and extend inferiorly through the false pelvis on the pelvic sidewall, where it unites with the iliacus muscle to form the iliopsoas muscle before inserting into the lesser trochanter of the femur; serves to flex the thigh towards the pelvis

rectouterine recess (pouch) – area in the pelvic cavity between the rectum and the uterus that is likely to accumulate free fluid; also known as the *posterior cul-de-sac* and the *pouch of Douglas*

retroflexed – refers to the position of the uterus when the uterine fundus bends posteriorly upon the cervix

retroverted – refers to the position of the uterus when the entire uterus is tipped posteriorly so that the angle formed between the cervix and vaginal canal is greater than 90 degrees

round ligaments – paired ligaments that originate at the uterine cornua, anterior to the fallopian tubes, and course anterolaterally within the broad ligament to insert into the fascia of the labia majora; hold the uterus forward in its anteverted position

space of Retzius – located between the anterior bladder wall and the pubic symphysis; contains extraperitoneal fat

striations – parallel longitudinal lines commonly seen in muscle tissue when imaged sonographically; appear as hyperechoic parallel lines running in the long axis of the hypoechoic muscle tissue

suspensory (infundibulopelvic) ligament – paired ligaments that extend from the infundibulum of the fallopian tube and the lateral aspect of the ovary to the lateral pelvic wall; also called the *infundibulopelvic ligament*

true pelvis – pelvic cavity found below the brim of the pelvis; also called the *minor* or *lesser pelvis*

uterosacral ligaments – posterior portion of the cardinal ligament that extends from the cervix to the sacrum

vesicouterine recess (pouch) – area in the pelvic cavity between the urinary bladder and the uterus; also known as the *anterior cul-de-sac*

Understanding the anatomy and physiology of the female genital organs is important for understanding the pathophysiology of the female pelvis. There are many pelvic landmarks, ligaments, and muscular structures within the pelvis that are important to know to differentiate normal reproductive organs from muscular and vascular structures.

Traditionally, two approaches are used to evaluate the female pelvis sonographically: transabdominal and endovaginal. A transabdominal approach requires a full urinary bladder for use as an "acoustic window" and typically necessitates the use of a 3.5- to 5-MHz transducer for adequate penetration. An endovaginal examination is performed with an empty bladder and allows the use of a higher-frequency transducer, typically 7.5 to 10 MHz. It is generally recommended that a complete pelvic examination consist of a transabdominal scan followed by an endovaginal examination. The transabdominal scan offers a wider field of view for a general screening of the pelvic anatomy. The endovaginal examination will usually offer a more detailed study, but is limited in its field of view and depth of penetration. The approach used, however, will depend on the patient's age and sexual status. Endovaginal examinations are typically contraindicated in patients who are not sexually active.

When using a transabdominal scanning technique, a distended urinary bladder is essential. An adequately filled bladder will tilt the uterus posteriorly and push the bowel up out of the pelvic cavity and into the lower abdominal cavity, making visualization of the uterine fundus and adnexa easier. An overly distended bladder, on the other hand, will often push the uterus too far posteriorly, making the pelvic structures difficult to see. An overdistended bladder may also cause compression and distortion of the pelvic organs. If the bladder appears overly distended, throwing the pelvic structures too deep, it may be necessary to have the patient partially void.

When endovaginal ultrasound is used to evaluate the pelvic structures, the patient should empty her bladder completely before the endovaginal transducer is inserted into the vaginal canal. With the urinary bladder empty, the uterus and iliac vessels become the primary landmarks used to evaluate and image the pelvic organs.

This chapter presents a discussion of the normal anatomy and physiology of the female genital organs. The sonographically significant muscular structures and pelvic ligaments will also be discussed because a basic understanding of these structures is essential to performing an adequate pelvic ultrasound examination.

PELVIC LANDMARKS

EXTERNAL LANDMARKS

The external genitalia in the female, also known as the *vulva* or the *pudendum*, consist of the mons pubis, labia majora, labia minora, clitoris, urethral opening, and vestibule of the vagina (Figure 35-1). (The vagina itself is the part of the female genitalia that forms a canal from the orifice through the vestibule to the uterine cervix. It is behind the bladder and in front of the rectum.) These external structures are important to recognize when using translabial and endovaginal scanning techniques. The mons pubis is a pad of fatty tissue and thick skin that overlies the symphysis pubis and is covered by pubic hair after puberty. The labia are folds of skin at the opening of the vagina, the labia majora being the thicker external folds and the minora being the thin folds of skin between the labia majora. The clitoris is located anterior to the urethra and is usually partially hidden between the labia majora. Posterior to the clitoris, the urethral opening and vestibule of the vagina can normally be identified between the labia minora. The most posterior orifice is the anus.

THE BONY PELVIS

The bony pelvis consists of four bones: two innominate (coxal) bones, the sacrum, and the coccyx. The innominate bones make up the anterior and lateral margins of the bony pelvis, whereas the sacrum and coccyx form the posterior wall. Anatomically, the pelvis is divided into two continuous compartments (the true and false pelves) by an oblique plane that passes through the pelvic brim. This plane of division passes from superior border of the sacrum to the superior margin of the pubic symphysis and corresponds to the **iliopectineal line** (Figure 35-2). The **false pelvis,** also known as the greater or major pelvis, is located above the brim. The false pelvis communicates with the abdominal cavity superiorly and with the

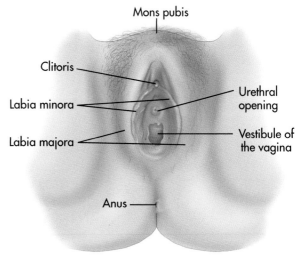

Figure 35-1 External genitalia as viewed in the lithotomy position.

pelvic cavity inferiorly. The **true pelvis,** also known as the lesser or minor pelvis, is the area below the pelvic brim.

THE PELVIC CAVITY AND PERINEUM

The true pelvis, situated inferior to the caudal portion of the parietal peritoneum, is considered the pelvic cavity (Figure 35-3 and Box 35-1). The posterior wall of the pelvic cavity is formed by the sacrum and coccyx, whereas the margins of the posterolateral wall are formed by the piriformis and **coccygeus muscles** (see Figure 35-6). The anterolateral walls of the pelvic cavity are formed by the hip bones and the obturator internus muscles, which rim the ischium and pubis (see Figure 35-10). The lower margin of the pelvic cavity, the pelvic floor, is formed by the **levator ani** and coccygeus muscles and is known as the pelvic diaphragm. The area below the pelvic floor is the perineum.

MUSCLES OF THE PELVIS

There are several primary muscle groups in the pelvis that the sonographer must be able to identify. These muscles serve as landmarks that may be used to help differentiate the reproductive organs and should be recognized sonographically to prevent misidentifying the muscles as a mass (Box 35-2). The pelvic muscles vary in shape, but typically appear hypoechoic with characteristic hyperechoic **striations** when viewed in their long axis. The pelvic muscles are easiest to locate and identify sonographically if classified by their region. The major pelvic muscles can be differentiated as muscles of the abdominal wall, those running through the false pelvis, and those found within the true pelvis.

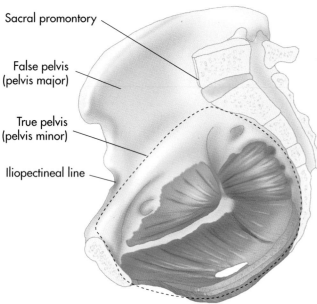

Figure 35-2   Sagittal plane through the lateral pelvis. The true pelvis is the most inferior portion of the body cavity. It is separated from the false pelvis by the pelvic brim, which corresponds with the iliopectineal line and the sacral promontory.

Labels on figure: Sacral promontory; False pelvis (pelvis major); True pelvis (pelvis minor); Iliopectineal line

> **BOX 35-1**   **PELVIC CAVITY**
>
> - *Posterior:* Occupied by rectum, colon, and ileum
> - *Anterior:* Occupied by bladder, ureters, ovaries, fallopian tubes, uterus, and vagina

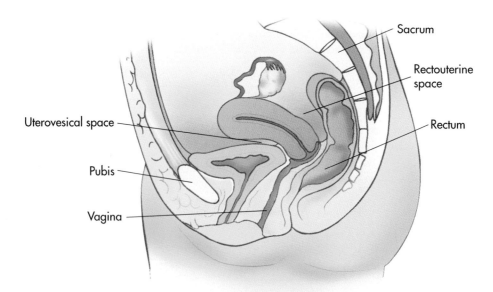

Figure 35-3   Sagittal plane through the female pelvis. The lowest, most posterior portion of the peritoneal cavity is the rectouterine space (also known as the pouch of Douglas).

Labels on figure: Sacrum; Rectouterine space; Rectum; Uterovesical space; Pubis; Vagina

THE ABDOMINAL WALL

The muscles of the anterior abdominal wall extend superiorly from the xyphoid process to the symphysis pubis inferiorly. These muscles include the paired rectus abdominis muscles anteriorly and the external obliques, internal obliques, and transversus abdominis muscles anterolaterally (Figure 35-4). These muscles are described in greater depth in Chapter 13.

MUSCLES OF THE FALSE PELVIS

The muscles of the false pelvis include the psoas major and iliacus muscles. The **psoas major muscles** originate at the transverse process of the lumbar vertebrae and descend inferiorly through the false pelvis on the pelvic sidewalls. In the false pelvis, they join with the **iliacus muscles** to form the iliopsoas muscles. The iliopsoas muscles pass anterior to the hip and insert into the lesser trochanters on the posterior aspect of the femurs (Figure 35-5). Note that the iliopsoas muscles pass outside the pelvic bones and do not enter the true pelvis.

MUSCLES OF THE TRUE PELVIS

The muscles found within the true pelvis include the piriformis muscles, obturator internus muscles, and the muscles of the pelvic diaphragm. The **piriformis muscles** are flat, triangular muscles that arise from the anterior sacrum and pass though the

greater sciatic notch on the posterior aspect of the innominate bone to insert into the superior aspect of the greater trochanter of the femur (Figures 35-6 and 35-7). The **obturator internus muscles** are triangular sheets of muscle that arise from the anterolateral pelvic wall and surround the obturator foramen. They pass out of the pelvic cavity through the lesser sciatic foramen where they insert into the superior aspect of the greater trochanter of the femur (see Figures 35-6 and 35-7). The pelvic diaphragm is formed by the levator ani and coccygeus muscles and makes up the floor of the true pelvis (Figure 35-8). The **levator ani** is a group of three muscles that extend across the pelvic floor like a hammock. This group of muscles consists of the pubococcygeus muscles, the iliococcygeus muscles, and the puborectalis muscles. The pubococcygeus muscles are the most anterior and medial of the three levator ani muscles. They extend from the pubic bones anteriorly to the coccyx posteriorly and surround the urethra, vagina, and rectum. The iliococcygeus muscles extend from the anterolateral pelvic wall to the coccyx posteriorly. The puborectalis muscles arise from the lower part of the pubic symphysis and surround the lower part of the rectum, forming a sling. The levator ani, in addition to forming the floor of the pelvis, also has an important role in rectal and urinary continence.

BLADDER AND URETERS

The urinary bladder is located in the anterior portion of the pelvic cavity, posterior to the pubic symphysis (see Figure 35-2 and Box 35-3). The function of the bladder is to collect and store urine until it empties through the urethra. When the bladder is empty or only slightly filled, it remains entirely within the true pelvis; as it becomes distended, it rises up behind the lower anterior abdominal wall and pushes the peritoneum away from the wall.

The ureters are the two tubes that carry urine from the kidneys to the urinary bladder (Box 35-4). As the ureters descend inferiorly from the kidneys, they run anteriorly and

---

BOX 35-2

PELVIC MUSCLES

- *Psoas major:* Pelvic sidewall
- *Iliacus:* Pelvic sidewall
- *Piriformis:* Posterolateral wall
- *Obturator internus:* Anterolateral pelvic sidewall
- *Levator ani:* Pelvic floor (diaphragm)
- *Coccygeus:* Posterior pelvic floor (diaphragm)

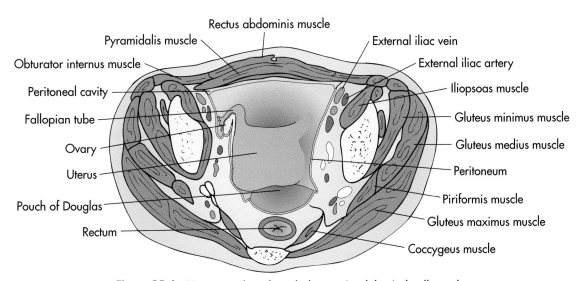

Figure 35-4   Transverse plane through the anterior abdominal wall muscles.

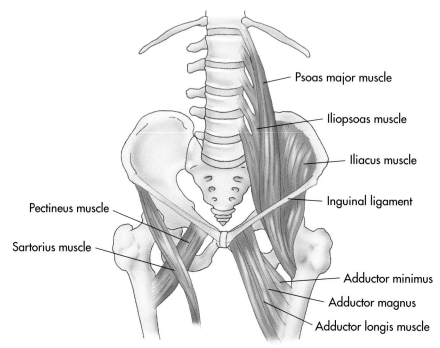

Figure 35-5 Anterior diagram of the psoas major muscle extending from the abdominal cavity into the false pelvis. The iliacus muscle joins the psoas muscle to form the iliopsoas muscle along the sidewall of the false pelvis.

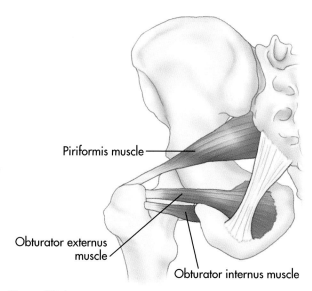

Figure 35-6 Posterior view of the piriformis and obturator internus muscles.

medially, passing anterior to the psoas major muscles, behind the peritoneum, and along the lateral aspect of the cervix and upper portion of the vagina, where they enter the bladder at the trigone. As the ureters descend from the retroperitoneal cavity, they pass anterior to the internal iliac arteries and posterior to the ovaries and uterine arteries. The ureters are not normally visualized sonographically but may be identified by the visualization of "ureteral jets" in the posteroinferior portion of the urinary bladder as it fills. The ureteral jets are identified by a swirling of urine, which is easily identified with color Doppler. The urinary bladder and ureters are discussed in detail in Chapter 10. Pregnancy, uterine fibroids, and ovarian masses can lead to compression of the ureters, resulting in hydronephrosis.

VAGINA

The vagina is a collapsed muscular tube that extends from the external genitalia to the cervix of the uterus. It lies posterior to the urinary bladder and urethra, and anterior to the rectum and anus (Figure 35-9). It is normally directed upward and backward, forming a 90-degree angle with the uterine cervix. It measures approximately 9 cm in length and is longest along its posterior wall (Box 35-5). The vaginal canal is a potential space in which the anterior and posterior walls usually touch. It is the passageway for the products of menstruation and is easily distended during sexual intercourse and childbirth. The vagina has a mucous membrane lining its muscular walls. This membrane receives secretions from the vaginal wall, the mucous glands of the cervix (around ovulation), and the vestibular glands of the vagina (during sexual excitement).

The uterine cervix protrudes into the upper portion of the vaginal canal forming four archlike recesses called fornices. The posterior vaginal wall attaches higher on the cervix, and the fornices are blind pockets formed by the inner surface of the vaginal walls and outer surface of the cervix. It is a continuous ring-shaped space with the posterior fornix running deeper than its anterior counterpart. This design aids in easing the use of the endovaginal probe and concomitant visualization of the cervix and uterus (Figure 35-10).

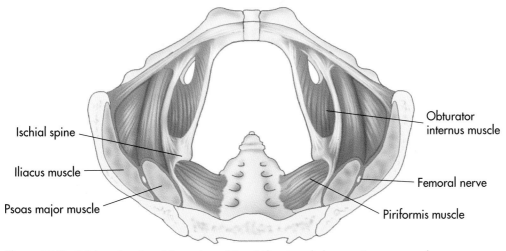

Ischial spine

Iliacus muscle

Psoas major muscle

Obturator internus muscle

Femoral nerve

Piriformis muscle

Figure 35-7   Pelvic cavity viewed from above. The piriformis and obturator internus muscles pass out from the pelvis through the sciatic foramina to attach to the greater tuberosity of the femur.

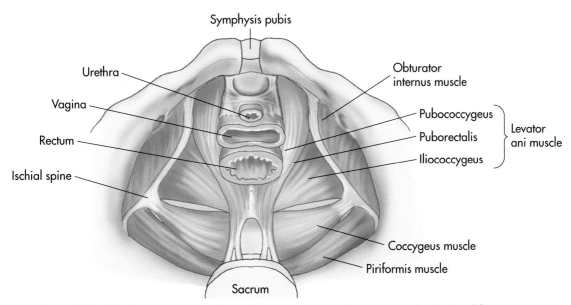

Symphysis pubis

Urethra

Vagina

Rectum

Ischial spine

Obturator internus muscle

Pubococcygeus

Puborectalis

Iliococcygeus

Levator ani muscle

Coccygeus muscle

Piriformis muscle

Sacrum

Figure 35-8   The floor of the pelvis is formed by the coccygeus and levator ani muscles (as viewed from above).

BOX 35-3   BLADDER

- *Apex:* Located posterior to pubic bones
- *Base:* Anterior to vagina, superior surface related to uterus
- *Neck:* Rests on upper surface of urogenital diaphragm; inferolateral surfaces relate to retropubic fat, obturator internus, levator ani muscles, and pubic bone

BOX 35-4   URETERS

- Cross the pelvic inlet anterior to bifurcation of common iliac arteries
- Run anterior to internal iliac arteries and posterior to the ovaries
- Run anteriorly and medially under the base of the broad ligament where they are crossed by the uterine artery
- Run anterior and lateral to the upper vagina to enter the posteroinferior bladder

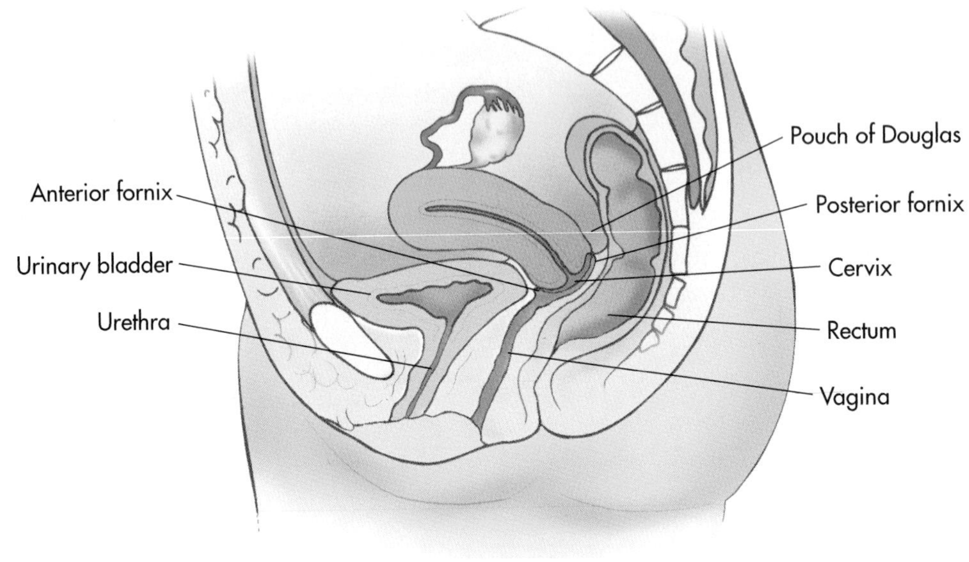

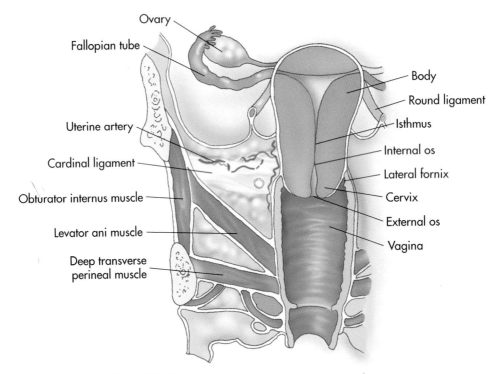

Figure 35-9 Lateral view of the pelvis demonstrating the relationship of the anterior and posterior fornices to the cervix and vagina.

Figure 35-10 Coronal view of the vagina, cervix, and uterus.

UTERUS

NORMAL ANATOMY

The uterus and vagina are derived from the embryonic müllerian (paramesonephric) ducts as they elongate, fuse, and form a lumen between the 7th and 12th weeks of embryonic development. The uterus is pear-shaped and is the largest organ in the normal female pelvis when the urinary bladder is empty (Box 35-6). The average menarcheal uterus measures approx-

imately 6 to 8 cm in length and 3 to 5 cm in anteroposterior and transverse dimensions. The size of the uterus varies with age and parity (Box 35-7 and Table 35-1).

The uterus consists of a fundus, body, and cervix (Figure 35-11). The fundus is the widest and most superior portion of the uterus. At the lateral borders of the fundus are the cornua, where the fallopian tubes enter the uterine cavity. The body or corpus (Box 35-8) lies between the fundus and the cervix and is the largest portion of the uterus. The uterine cavity is cen-

TABLE 35-1	UTERINE SIZE				
	Length (cm)	Width (cm)	AP (cm)	Volume (ml)	Cervix/Corpus Ratio
Adult (nulliparous)	6-8	3-5	3-5	30-40	1:2
Adult (parous)	8-10	5-6	5-6	60-80	1:2
Postmenopausal	3-5	2-3	2-3	14-17	1:1

From Warwick W, editor: *Gray's anatomy,* New York, 1994, Churchill-Livingstone.

BOX 35-5 VAGINA

- Extends upward and backward from the vulva
- Upper half lies above pelvic floor
- Lower half lies within perineum
- Area of vaginal lumen surrounding the cervix is divided into four fornices
- Arterial supply is from vaginal and uterine arteries; drains into the internal iliac vein

---

BOX 35-8 BODY OF THE UTERUS

- Posterior to the vesicouterine pouch and the superior surface of the bladder
- Anterior to the rectouterine pouch (of Douglas), the ilium, and colon
- Medial to the broad ligaments and uterine vessels
- Uterine cavity is funnel shaped in coronal plane; "slitlike" in a sagittal plane

---

BOX 35-6 UTERUS

- Hollow, pear-shaped organ
- Divided into fundus, body, and cervix
- Usually anteflexed and anteverted
- Covered with peritoneum except anteriorly below the os where peritoneum is reflected onto bladder
- Supported by levator ani muscles, cardinal ligaments, and uterosacral ligaments
- Round ligaments hold uterus in anteverted position

BOX 35-9 CERVIX

- Projects into vaginal canal
- *Endocervix:* Cervical canal; communicates with uterine cavity by the internal os; the vagina by the external os
- *Exocervix:* Continuous with the vagina

BOX 35-10 LAYERS OF THE UTERUS

- *Perimetrium:* Serous outer layer of the uterus; serosa
- *Myometrium:* Muscular middle layer of the uterus composed of thick, smooth muscle supported by connective tissue
- *Endometrium:* Inner mucous membrane of the uterine body

BOX 35-7 UTERINE SIZE

- *Premenarchal:* 1.0 to 3.0 cm long by 0.5 to 1.0 cm wide
- *Menarchal:* 6.0 to 8.0 cm long by 3.0 to 5.0 cm wide
- *With multiparity:* Increases size by 1.0 to 2.0 cm
- *Postmenopausal:* 3.5 to 5.5 cm long by 2.0 to 3.0 cm wide

---

trally located within the pelvis and is a potential space for fluid to accumulate, allowing for dynamic changes during the menstrual cycle and pregnancy. The cervix (Box 35-9) is the lower cylindrical portion of the uterus that projects into the vaginal canal (see Figure 35-11). The surface of the cervix is divided into an exocervix and an endocervix. The exocervix is a squamous epithelium continuous with the vagina. The surface of the endocervix is made up of columnar cells, which excrete mucus. The cervix is constricted at its upper end by the internal os and at its lower end by the external os. The isthmus is the outer transition point between the body of the uterus and the cervix. This is the point where the uterus bends either anteriorly (anteversion) or posteriorly (retroversion) with an empty bladder.

The uterine wall consists of three histologic layers: the serosa or **perimetrium**, the myometrium, and the endometrium (see Figure 35-11). The external layer, the serosa, reflects on the anterior surface of the uterus at the isthmus. The muscular middle layer, the myometrium, is the thickest layer of the uterus and is primarily smooth muscle that is longitudinal and circular (Box 35-10). The mucous membrane lining the uterine cavity is the endometrium.

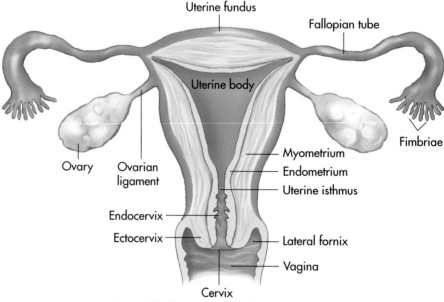

Figure 35-11   Normal female pelvic anatomy.

ENDOMETRIUM

The endometrium consists primarily of two layers: the superficial functional layer (zona functionalis) and the deep basal layer (zona basalis). The functional layer is a superficial layer of glands and stroma (supporting tissue) that shed with **menses.** The basal layer is a thin layer of the blind ends of endometrial glands that regenerates new endometrium after menses. The endometrium changes dynamically in response to the cyclic hormonal flux of ovulation and varies in sonographic appearance and histologic structure, depending on the patient's menstrual status and the period of life in which it is studied.

UTERINE LIGAMENTS

The uterus is supported in its midline position by paired broad ligaments, round ligaments, uterosacral ligaments, and cardinal ligaments (Figure 35-12 and Box 35-11). The **broad ligaments** are a double-fold of peritoneum that drape over the fallopian tubes, uterus, and ovaries (Figure 35-13). They extend from the lateral sides of the uterus to the sidewalls of the pelvis. The broad ligaments provide a small amount of support for the uterus and contain the uterine blood vessels and nerves. The upper fold of the broad ligament, known as the **mesosalpinx**, encloses the fallopian tube as it extends from the cornua of the uterus. The posterior portion of the broad ligament that is drawn out to enclose the ovary is the **mesovarium**.

The **round ligaments** are fibrous cords that occur in front of and below the fallopian tubes between the layers of broad ligament. These two cords commence on each side of the superior aspect of the uterus and course upward and lateral to the inguinal canal and insert into the labia majora and help to hold the uterine fundus and body in a forward position. The cervix is the only portion of the uterus that is firmly supported. It is fixed in position by the **cardinal** and **uterosacral ligaments.** The cardinal ligaments are a continuation of the broad ligaments that extend across the pelvic floor laterally. The uterosacral ligaments originate at the lateral uterine isthmus and extend downward along the sides of the rectum to the third and fourth bones of the sacrum.

POSITIONS OF THE UTERUS

The position of the uterus is variable. The average uterine position is considered to be anteverted and anteflexed. The uterine position is described as **anteverted** when the cervical canal forms a 90-degree angle or less with the vaginal canal and **anteflexed** when the body and fundus of the uterus are curved forward upon the cervix (Figure 35-14 and Box 35-12). In the nulliparous female, the round ligaments help to hold the uterus in an anteverted, anteflexed position. In multiparous females, the entire uterus may tip backward rather than

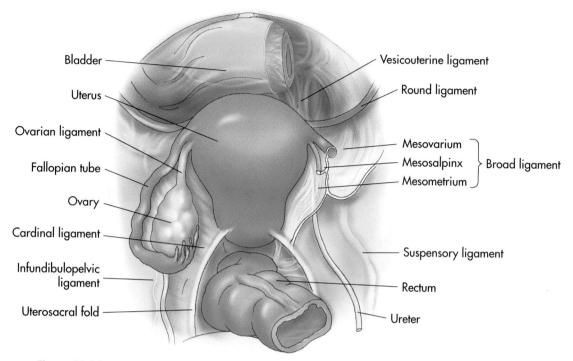

Figure 35-12 View of the pelvic cavity from above, looking inferiorly, showing the attachment of the round ligament and broad ligament to the uterus.

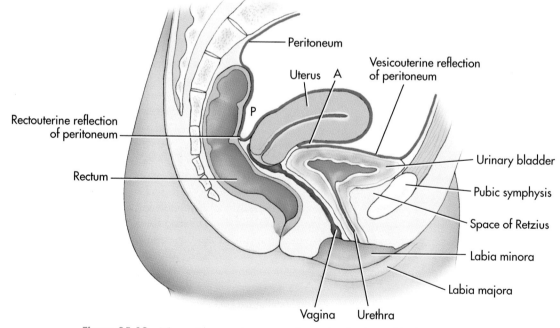

Figure 35-13 The peritoneum drapes over the uterine fundus and body to divide the pelvis into an anterior (A) and posterior (P) section. The peritoneum extends laterally from the uterus, forming the broad ligaments and creating the mesosalpinx as it folds over the fallopian tubes. The mesovarium is another fold of the peritoneum, which forms posterior to the broad ligament as it folds over the ovary.

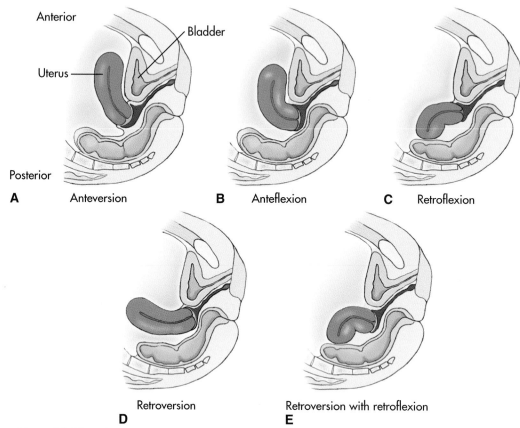

Figure 35-14   The uterus may be found in one of several positions: **A,** Anteversion (entire uterus tipped forward). **B,** Anteflexion (body and fundus folded anteriorly towards the cervix). **C,** Retroflexion (body and fundus folded posteriorly upon the cervix). **D,** Retroversion (entire uterus tilted backwards). **E,** Retroversion with retroflexion (entire uterus tilted backward with fundus and body folded posteriorly upon the cervix).

> **BOX 35-12   UTERINE POSITIONS**
>
> - *Anteversion:* Most common position; fundus and body bent forward towards the cervix (degree of anteversion is dependent on bladder distention)
> - *Dextroversion or levoversion:* Normal variant in absence of pelvic masses
> - *Retroversion:* Entire uterus tilted posteriorly
> - *Retroflexion:* Fundus and body bent backwards towards the cervix

forward and is described as a **retroverted** position. The term retroverted is used to describe the uterine position when the cervical canal forms an angle less than 90 degrees with the vaginal canal. The uterine fundus or body may also curve backward upon the cervix, and the position is described as **retroflexed.** It is not uncommon to see a uterus that has variations of version and flexion. For example, a common variation from the average uterine position is retroverted and retroflexed. Another variation to the normal uterine position is for the entire uterus to tilt either to the right (dextro) or to the left (levo) of midline. An abnormal dropping of the uterus (uterine prolapse) occurs if the uterine ligaments and pelvic floor muscles are weak, allowing the uterus to protrude into the vagina. It is also important to recognize that filling of the bladder will affect uterine position. A full urinary bladder will tip the average anteverted, anteflexed uterus backward.

FALLOPIAN TUBES

The fallopian tubes or oviducts are coiled, muscular tubes that open into the peritoneal cavity at their lateral end. They are approximately 10 to 12 cm in length and 1 to 4 mm in diameter (Box 35-13). The fallopian tubes lie superior to the utero-ovarian ligaments, round ligaments, and tubo-ovarian blood vessels. They are contained in the upper margin of the broad ligament and extend from the cornua of the uterus laterally, where they curve over the ovary.

The fallopian tubes are divided into four anatomic portions (Figure 35-15): the infundibulum (lateral segment), ampulla (middle segment), isthmus (medial segment), and interstitial portion (segment that passes through the uterine cornua). The interstitial portion is the narrowest segment of the fallopian tube. The tube widens as it extends laterally, with the infundibulum being the wide, trumpet-shaped, lateral portion. The infundibulum is often referred to as the fimbriated end of the fallopian tube because it contains fringelike extensions, called fimbriae, which move over the ovary directing the ovum

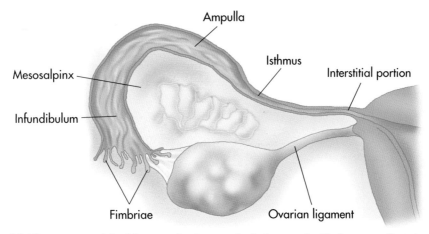

Figure 35-15 Diagram of the fallopian tube showing the fimbriae, infundibulum, ampulla, isthmus, and interstitial portions.

TABLE 35-2	NORMAL OVARIAN VOLUME BY MENSTRUAL STATUS			
Group	Mean Volume (cm^3)	Standard Deviation	No. of Ovaries Evaluated	95% Confidence Interval (cm^3)*
Premenarcheal	3.0	2.3	32	0.2 to 9.1
Menstruating	9.8	5.8	866	2.5 to 21.9
Postmenopausal	5.8	3.6	100	1.2 to 14.1

From Cohen HL, Tice HM, Mandel FS: *Radiology* 177:189, 1990.
*Calculated on the basis of cube root values, then transformed back to cubic centimeters.

BOX 35-13   FALLOPIAN TUBES

- *Infundibulum:* Funnel-shaped lateral tube that projects beyond the broad ligament to overlie the ovaries; "free edge" of the funnel has fimbriae (fingerlike projectors draped over the ovary)
- *Ampulla:* Widest part of the tube where fertilization occurs
- *Isthmus:* Hardest part; lies just lateral to the uterus
- *Interstitial portion:* Pierces the uterine wall at the cornua
- *Length:* 12 cm; blood is supplied by ovarian arteries and veins

into the fallopian tube after ovulation. The ampulla is the longest and most coiled portion of the fallopian tube and is the area in which fertilization of the ovum most often occurs because it is the most distensible region of the tube. The innermost region of the fallopian tube, with its mucosal layer, runs directly into the mucosal layer of the uterus (the endometrium). The continuous nature of the endometrium and the endocervical canal is important to realize as a pathway for organisms, infection, and hemorrhage to occur because it is the most distensible.

The normal fallopian tubes are difficult to distinguish sonographically from the surrounding ligaments and vessels.

Doppler interrogation may help differentiate prominent blood vessels from the fallopian tubes.

OVARIES

POSITION AND SIZE OF THE OVARIES
The ovaries are almond-shaped structures, measuring approximately 3 cm long in a menarcheal female (Table 35-2 and Box 35-14). They usually lie posterior to the uterus at the level of the cornua. They are suspended from the posterior aspect of the broad ligament in a fold of peritoneum called the **mesovarium**. The ovaries are usually located medial to the external iliac vessels and anterior to the internal iliac vessels and ureter (Box 35-15). The ovarian arteries have a double supply of blood. The primary blood supply to the ovaries is from the ovarian arteries, which arise from the lateral aspect of the abdominal aorta, below the renal arteries. The ovarian artery anastomoses with the uterine artery, providing additional blood to the ovary (Box 35-16).

NORMAL ANATOMY
The ovaries consist of an outer layer or cortex, which surrounds the central medulla. The cortex consists primarily of follicles in varying stages of development and is covered by a layer of dense connective tissue, the tunica albuginea. The tunica albuginea is surrounded by a single, thin layer of cells known as the germinal epithelium. The central medulla is composed

---

BOX 35-14   OVARIES

- Almond shaped
- Attached at posterior aspect of the broad ligament by mesovarium
- Lie in ovarian fossa
- Fossa is bounded by external iliac vessels, ureter, and obturator nerve
- Dual blood supply; receives blood from ovarian artery and uterine artery
- Blood drained by ovarian vein into inferior vena cava on the right and into renal vein on the left

---

BOX 35-15   VARIABLE POSITIONS OF THE OVARIES

- Anterior to the internal iliac artery and vein
- Medial to the external iliac artery and vein
- Ellipsoid shape with long axis oriented vertically
- Location highly variable as ligaments loosen, especially after pregnancy

---

BOX 35-16   PELVIC VASCULATURE

- *External iliac arteries:* Medial psoas border
- *External iliac veins:* Medial and posterior to the arteries
- *Internal iliac arteries:* Posterior to ureters and ovaries
- *Internal iliac veins:* Posterior to arteries
- *Uterine arteries and veins:* Between the layers of the broad ligaments, lateral to the uterus
- *Arcuate arteries:* Arclike arteries that encircle the uterus in the outer third of the myometrium
- *Radial arteries:* Branches of the arcuate arteries that extend from the myometrium to the base of the endometrium
- *Straight and spiral arteries:* Branches of the radial arteries that supply the zona basalis of the endometrium
- *Ovarian arteries:* Branch laterally off the aorta, run within the suspensory ligaments and anastomose with the uterine arteries
- *Ovarian veins:* Right vein drains into the IVC directly, whereas the left drains into the left renal vein

---

of connective tissue containing blood, nerves, lymphatic vessels, and some smooth muscle at the region of the hilum.

The ovaries produce the reproductive cell, the **ovum,** and two known hormones: **estrogen,** secreted by the follicles, and **progesterone,** secreted by the **corpus luteum.** These steroidal hormones are responsible for producing and maintaining secondary gender characteristics, preparing the uterus for implantation of a fertilized ovum, and development of the mammary glands in the female.

OVARIAN LIGAMENTS

The ovaries are supported medially by the **ovarian ligaments,** originating bilaterally at the cornua of the uterus, and laterally by the **suspensory (infundibulopelvic) ligament,** extending from the infundibulum of the fallopian tube and ovary to the sidewall of the pelvis. The ovary is also attached to the posterior aspect of the broad ligament via the mesovarium (see Figure 35-15).

PELVIC VASCULATURE

The common iliac arteries course anterior and medial to the psoas muscles, providing blood to the pelvic cavity and lower extremities. The common iliac arteries normally bifurcate into the external and internal iliac (hypogastric) arteries at the level of the superior margin of the sacrum (Figure 35-16 and Box 35-16). The external iliac arteries course along the pelvic brim and continue inferiorly as the common femoral arteries, supplying blood to the lower extremities. The internal iliac arteries extend into the pelvic cavity, along the posterior wall and provide multiple branches that perfuse the pelvic structures to include the urinary bladder, uterus, vagina, and rectum. The ovarian veins follow a slightly different course as the left ovarian vein drains into the left renal vein, whereas the right ovarian vein drains directly into the IVC.

Blood is supplied to the uterus by the uterine artery, which arises from the anterior branch of the internal iliac artery (Figure 35-17). From the internal iliac artery, the uterine artery crosses above and anterior to the ureter, extending medially in the base of the broad ligament to the uterus at the level of the cervix. The uterine artery is tortuous and spirals up the sides of the uterus within the broad ligament to the cornua, where it courses laterally to anastomose with the ovarian artery. The uterine artery gives off many branches that perforate the serosa and carry blood to the myometrium (Figure 35-18). These branches anastomose extensively anteriorly and posteriorly within the myometrium, forming arcuate (arclike) vessels that encircle the uterus. The arcuate vessels can often be identified sonographically as anechoic tubular structures in the outer third of the myometrium.

Blood is supplied to the endometrium by the radial arteries that "radiate" from the arcuate arteries within the myometrium. The radial arteries extend through the myometrium to the base of the endometrium, where straight and spiral arteries branch off the radial arteries to supply the zona basalis of the endometrium. The spiral arteries will lengthen during the regeneration of the endometrium after menses to traverse the endometrium and supply the zona functionalis. Blood from the spiral arteries is shed during menses. The pelvic vessels supply blood to the functional layer of the endometrium.

PHYSIOLOGY

THE MENSTRUAL CYCLE

A female's reproductive years begin around 11 to 13 years of age at the onset of menses (menstruation) and end around age

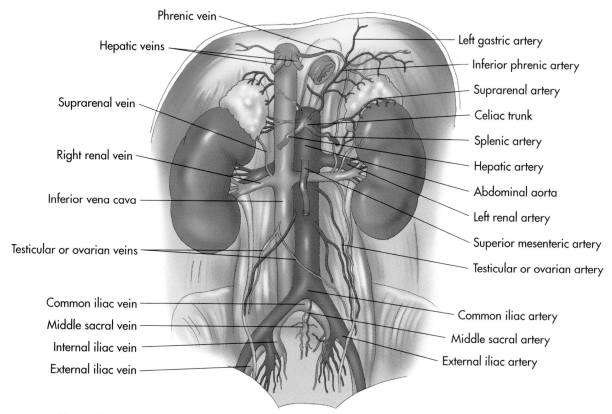

Figure 35-16 Blood is supplied to the pelvic cavity by the external and internal iliac arteries; the iliac veins drain the pelvis. The ureter enters the pelvis and courses anterior to the internal iliac artery to empty into the posterior base of the bladder.

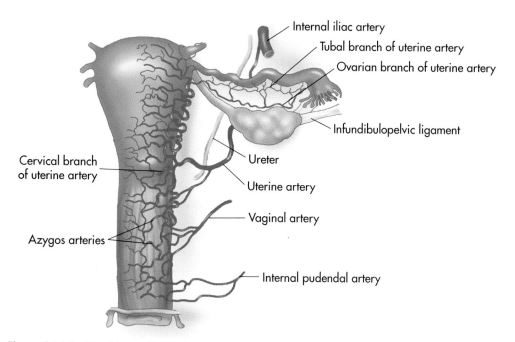

Figure 35-17 Blood is supplied to the uterus and vagina by the uterine artery (arising from the internal iliac artery) and the vaginal artery (arising from the uterine artery). The ovaries receive blood from branches of the uterine artery and from the ovarian arteries arising from the abdominal aorta.

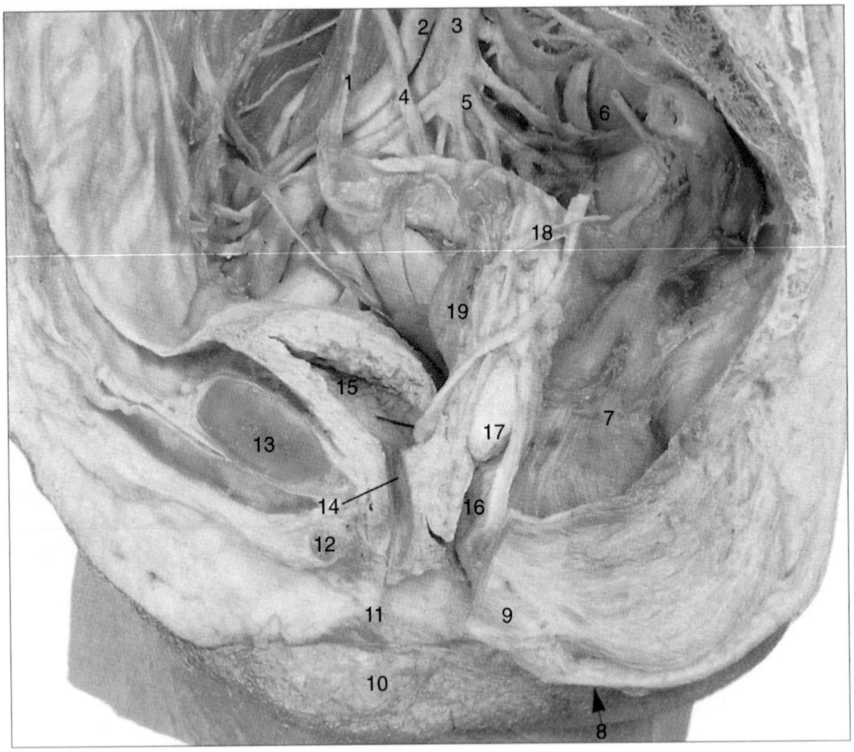

1. Ovarian vessels
2. External iliac artery
3. External iliac vein
4. Ureter
5. Internal iliac vessels and branches
6. Piriformis
7. Rectum
8. Anus
9. Perineal body
10. Labium majora
11. Labium minora
12. Clitoris
13. Pubic symphysis
14. Urethra
15. Bladder
16. Vagina
17. Cervix of uterus
18. Left uterine artery
19. Body of uterus

Figure 35-18   Female pelvic vessels and viscera, seen on the right side in a sagittal section, after removal of most of the peritoneum.

> **BOX 35-17   MENSTRUAL STATUS**
>
> - *Premenarche:* Prepuberty
> - *Menarche:* Menstruating approximately every 28 days
> - *Menopause:* Cessation of menses

50, when menses ceases. The average menstrual cycle is approximately 28 days in length, beginning with the first day of menstrual bleeding. The length of the menstrual cycle can, however, vary considerably from one woman to another. When the menstrual cycle occurs at intervals of less than 21 days, it is called polymenorrheic, and when the cycle is prolonged more than 35 days, it is called oligomenorrheic.

Menstrual status is described using the terms premenarche, menarche, and menopause (Box 35-17). **Premenarche** is the physiologic status of prepuberty, the time before the onset of menses. **Menarche** is the state after reaching puberty in which menses occurs normally every 28 days. **Menopause** refers to the cessation of menses. The menstrual cycle is regulated by the hypothalamus and is dependent upon the cyclic release of estrogen and progesterone from the ovaries.

FOLLICULAR DEVELOPMENT AND OVULATION

During the menarchal years, an ovum is released once a month by one of the two ovaries. This process is known as ovulation. Ovulation normally occurs midcycle on about day 14 of a 28-

day cycle. It is speculated that ovum release alternates between the two ovaries; one month from the right, the next month from the left. All ova begin development during embryonic life and remain in suspended animation within a preantral follicle as an immature **oocyte** until the onset of menarche. Each female ovary contains approximately 200,000 oocytes at the time of birth. Some of these oocytes will mature and be released from the ovaries during ovulation, whereas others will degenerate (Figure 35-19).

The process of ovulation is regulated by the hypothalamus within the brain. When a young girl reaches puberty, the hypothalamus begins the pulsatile release of the **gonadotropin-releasing hormones (GnRHs),** which stimulate the anterior pituitary gland to secrete varying levels of **gonadotropins** (primarily **follicle-stimulating hormone [FSH]** and **luteinizing hormone [LH]).**

The secretion of the follicle-stimulating hormone (FSH) by the anterior pituitary gland causes the ovarian follicles to develop during the first half of the menstrual cycle. This phase of the ovulatory cycle, known as the follicular phase, begins with the first day of menstrual bleeding and continues until ovulation on day 14 (Figure 35-20). As the ovarian follicles grow, they fill with fluid and secrete increasing amounts of estrogen. Although typically 5 to 8 preantral follicles will begin to develop, only one usually reaches maturity each month. This mature follicle is known as a graafian follicle and is typically 2 cm in size right before ovulation. As the estrogen level in the blood rises with follicle development, the pituitary gland is inhibited from further production of FSH and begins secret-

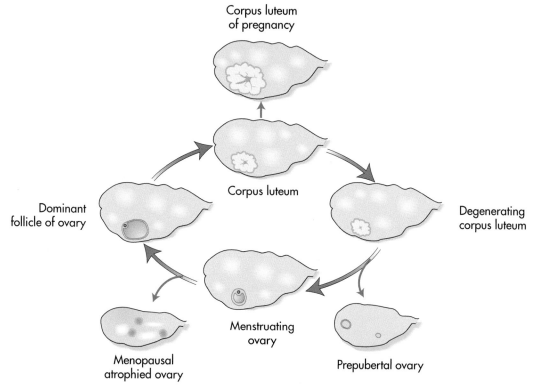

Figure 35-19   Cyclic changes of the ovary. The prepubertal ovary contains small preantral follicles in an arrested state of development. At the onset of puberty, the hypothalamus stimulates the pituitary gland that secretes follicle-stimulating hormone (FSH). The FSH causes several follicles to develop. One of these follicles persists to become the dominant (graafian) follicle, while the others degenerate. The dominant follicle fills with fluid and begins to secrete estrogen. As the estrogen level increases, the pituitary gland begins secreting luteinizing hormone (LH). Midcycle, the luteinizing hormone will surge, causing ovulation. The collapsed follicle lining begins to multiply and creates the corpus luteum. The corpus luteum secretes progesterone and, if pregnancy occurs, will continue for up to 3 months. If pregnancy does not occur, the corpus luteum degenerates. The progesterone levels decline, menstruation occurs, and the cycle repeats itself until the onset of menopause when the ovary atrophies.

ing luteinizing hormone (LH). The luteinizing hormone level will typically increase rapidly 24 to 36 hours before ovulation in a process known as the LH surge. This surge is often used as a predictor for timing ovulation for conception. The LH level usually reaches its peak 10 to 12 hours before ovulation. It is the LH surge, accompanied by a smaller FSH surge, that triggers ovulation on about day 14.

Ovulation is the explosive release of an ovum from the ruptured graafian follicle. The rupture of the follicle is associated with small amounts of fluid in the posterior cul-de-sac midcycle. Some women can tell when they're ovulating because at midcycle they have pain, typically a dull ache on either side of the lower abdomen lasting a few hours. The term "mittelschmerz," from the German word meaning *middle pain*, is often used to describe this sensation. After ovulation, the ovary enters the luteal phase. This phase begins with ovulation and is about 14 days in length. It is interesting to note that the luteal phase does not usually vary in length. When a menstrual cycle is less than or greater than 28 days, it is the follicular phase that is altered. Menstruation almost always occurs 14 days after ovulation. During the luteal phase, the cells in the

lining of the ruptured ovarian follicle begin to multiply and create the corpus luteum, or yellow body. This process is known as luteinization and is stimulated by the LH surge. The corpus luteum immediately begins secreting progesterone. Nine to eleven days after ovulation, the corpus luteum degenerates, causing the progesterone levels to decline. As the progesterone levels decline, menstruation occurs and the cycle begins again. Should conception and implantation occur, the human chorionic gonadotropin (hCG) produced by the zygote causes the corpus luteum to persist, and it will continue to secrete progesterone for 3 more months until the placenta takes over. Box 35-18 summarizes the phases of the menstrual cycle.

ENDOMETRIAL CHANGES

The varying levels of estrogen and progesterone throughout the course of the menstrual cycle induce characteristic changes in the endometrium. These changes correlate with ovulatory cycles of the ovary. The typical endometrial cycle is identified and described in three phases, beginning with the menstrual phase (see Figure 35-20). The menstrual phase lasts approximately 1 to 5 days and begins with the declining progesterone

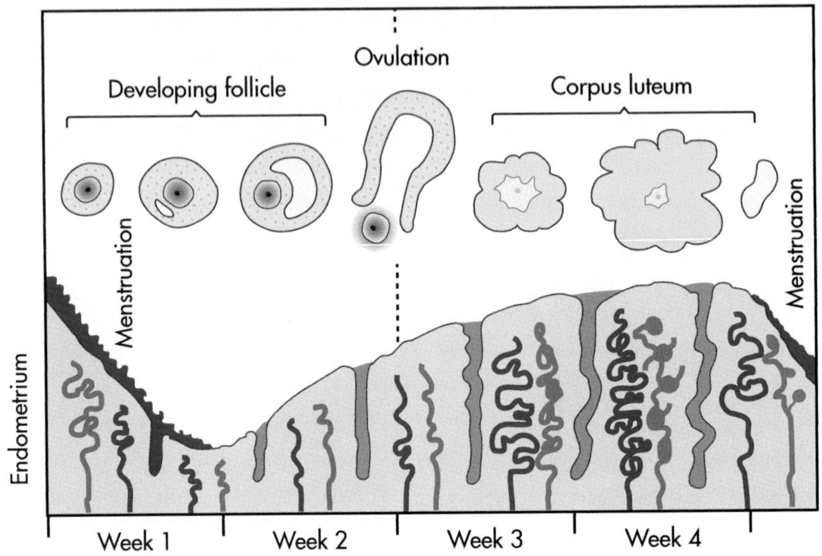

Figure 35-20   The average menstrual cycle is approximately 28 days, beginning with the first day of bleeding. As the menstrual lining is shed, the pituitary gland begins secreting follicle-stimulating hormone (FSH), which causes 5 to 8 preantral ovarian follicles to develop. As the ovarian follicles grow, they fill with fluid and secrete increasing amounts of estrogen. This estrogen stimulates the superficial layer of the endometrium to regenerate and grow. As the estrogen level in the blood rises, the pituitary gland is inhibited from further production of FSH and begins secreting luteinizing hormone (LH). The LH surges 24 to 36 hours before ovulation and is accompanied by a smaller FSH surge that triggers ovulation on about day 14. Ovulation occurs as the follicle ruptures, releasing the mature ovum. After ovulation, the cells lining the ruptured ovarian follicle begin to multiply and create the corpus luteum. The corpus luteum immediately begins secreting progesterone. Progesterone causes the spiral arteries and endometrial glands to enlarge as the endometrium prepares for implantation should conception occur. Without conception, the corpus luteum degenerates 9 to 11 days after ovulation, causing the progesterone levels to decline. Declining progesterone levels cause the spiral arterioles to constrict, resulting in decreasing blood flow to the endometrium with ischemia and shedding of the functionalis. As menstruation occurs, the menstrual cycle begins again.

BOX 35-18   THE MENSTRUAL CYCLE

PROLIFERATIVE PHASE
- Days 1 to 14
- Corresponds to the follicular phase of ovarian cycle
- Menstruation occurs on days 1 to 4
- Thin endometrium
- Estrogen level increases as ovarian follicles develop
- Increasing estrogen levels cause uterine lining to regenerate and thicken
- Ovulation occurs on day 14

SECRETORY PHASE
- Days 15 to 28
- Corresponds to the luteal phase of ovarian cycle
- Ruptured follicle becomes corpus luteum
- Corpus luteum secretes progesterone
- Endometrium thickens
- If no pregnancy, estrogen and progesterone decrease
- Menses on day 28

levels, causing the spiral arterioles to constrict. This causes a decreased blood flow to the endometrium, resulting in ischemia and shedding of the zona functionalis. These first 5 days coincide with the follicular phase of the ovarian cycle. As the follicles produce estrogen, the estrogen stimulates the superficial layer of the endometrium to regenerate and grow. This phase of endometrial regeneration is called the proliferative phase and will last until luteinization of the graafian follicle around ovulation. With ovulation and luteinization of the graafian follicle, the progesterone secreted by the ovary causes the spiral arteries and endometrial glands to enlarge. This will prepare the endometrium for implantation, should conception occur. The endometrial phase after ovulation is referred to as the secretory phase and extends from approximately day 15 to the onset of menses (day 28). The secretory phase of the endometrial cycle corresponds to the luteal phase of the ovarian cycle.

The sonographic appearance of the endometrium changes dramatically among the three phases of the endometrial cycle and should be correlated to the patient's menstrual status (Figure 35-21). During menses, it is not uncommon to see varying levels of fluid and debris within the uterine cavity; likewise, the thickness of the endometrium will decrease with menstruation, becoming a thin echogenic line during the early

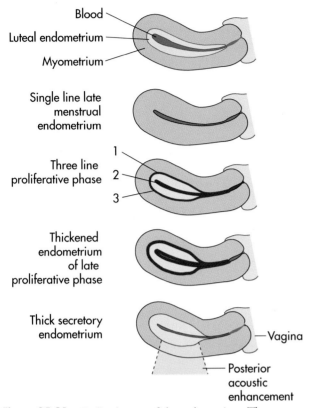

Blood
Luteal endometrium
Myometrium

Single line late menstrual endometrium

Three line proliferative phase
1
2
3

Thickened endometrium of late proliferative phase

Thick secretory endometrium
Vagina
Posterior acoustic enhancement

Figure 35-21 Cyclic changes of the endometrium. The menstrual cycle begins with approximately 5 days of bleeding. During menses, varying levels of fluid and debris may be seen within the uterine cavity. The thickness of the endometrium decreases with menstruation, becoming a thin echogenic line during the early proliferative phase. As regeneration ensues, the endometrium thickens and appears hypoechoic with a "three-line" sign. The outer echogenic line surrounding the hypoechoic functionalis represents the zona basalis, whereas the central echogenic line represents the uterine cavity. As ovulation nears, the endometrium becomes isoechoic with the myometrium. The secretory phase occurs after ovulation when the endometrium reaches its thickest dimension and becomes hyperechoic.

proliferative phase. As regeneration of the endometrium occurs during the proliferative phase, the endometrium will thicken to an average of 4 to 8 mm in the proliferative phase, when measured as a double layer from anterior to posterior. The endometrium characteristically appears hypoechoic with the appearance of the "three-line" sign. The three echogenic lines seen in the proliferative endometrium represent the zona basalis anteriorly and posteriorly, with the central line representing the uterine cavity. Right before ovulation, the endometrium averages 6 to 10 mm and becomes isoechoic with the myometrium. After ovulation, during the secretory phase, the endometrium reaches its thickest dimension, averaging 7 to 14 mm, and becomes echogenic, blurring the "three-line" appearance. The endometrium in anovulatory patients (e.g., those on the birth control pill, postmenopausal patients, etc.) will usually appear as a thin, echogenic line. Postmenopausal patients who are not on hormone replacement therapy (HRT) should have an endometrial thickness of less

than 5 mm. Postmenopausal patients on HRT or taking tamoxifen (a drug used as an adjuvant palliative therapy to help in the prevention of breast cancer) may demonstrate normal endometrial thicknesses of up to 8 mm.

ABNORMAL MENSTRUAL CYCLES

Several terms are used to describe abnormal menstrual cycles and should be familiar to the sonographer (Box 35-19). The term **menorrhagia** is used to describe abnormally heavy or long periods and is often associated with uterine fibroids, intrauterine contraceptive devices (IUDs), or hormonal imbalances. Persistent menorrhagia can lead to anemia. The term **oligomenorrhea** describes abnormally short or light periods and is often associated with polycystic ovary syndrome (PCOS). Oligomenorrhea can also be caused by emotional and physical stress, chronic illnesses, tumors that secrete estrogen, poor nutrition and eating disorders, such as anorexia nervosa, and heavy exercise. Many patients complain of **dysmenorrhea** or painful periods. Dysmenorrhea is often associated with endometriosis. The term **amenorrhea** refers to the absence of menstruation. Amenorrhea is considered primary when menarche is delayed beyond 18 years of age and secondary when there is a cessation of uterine bleeding in women who have previously menstruated. Amenorrhea may be due to a congenital vaginal or cervical stenosis or may a result from an infection, trauma, ovarian dysfunction, or other endocrine disturbances that affect ovarian function, such as pituitary disease.

PELVIC RECESSES AND BOWEL

The peritoneal cavity contains two potential spaces formed by the caudal portion of the parietal peritoneum (Box 35-20). These potential spaces are sonographically significant in that fluid may accumulate or pathology may be present in these locations. The **vesicouterine recess (pouch),** or anterior cul-de-sac, is located anterior to the fundus of the uterus between the urinary bladder and the uterus, whereas the **rectouterine recess (pouch),** or posterior cul-de-sac, is located posterior to the uterus between the uterus and the rectum. The rectouterine pouch is often referred to as the pouch of Douglas and is normally the most inferior and most posterior region of the peritoneal cavity. One additional area that is sonographically significant is the retropubic space (also called the **space of Retzius**). It can be identified between the anterior bladder wall

---

BOX 35-20

PELVIC RECESSES

- *Vesicouterine pouch:* Anterior cul-de-sac; anterior to the fundus between the uterus and bladder
- *Rectouterine pouch:* Posterior cul-de-sac; posterior to the uterine body and cervix, between the uterus and rectum
- *Retropubic space:* Space of Retzius; between bladder and symphysis pubis

---

and the pubic symphysis. This space normally contains sub-cutaneous fat, but a hematoma or abscess in this location may displace the urinary bladder posteriorly.

It is normal to observe a small accumulation of free fluid throughout the menstrual cycle in the posterior cul-de-sac (see Figure 35-3). The greatest quantity of free fluid in the cul-de-sac normally occurs immediately following ovulation when the mature follicle ruptures. A small amount of fluid in the posterior cul-de-sac is considered normal; however, there is no sonographic means of confirming that the fluid is related to ovulation. Hemorrhage or infection within the fluid may be related to a ruptured cyst, ascites, a ruptured corpus luteum cyst, ectopic pregnancy, or pelvic inflammatory disease.

SELECTED BIBLIOGRAPHY

Anderson DM: *Mosby's medical, nursing, & allied health dictionary,* ed, 6, St Louis, 2002, Mosby.

Berman MC, Cohen HL: *Obstetrics and gynecology,* ed 2, Philadelphia, 1997, Lippincott-Raven Publishers.

Callen PW: *Ultrasonography in obstetrics and gynecology,* ed 4, Philadelphia, 2000, WB Saunders.

Curry RA, Tempkin BB: *Sonography: introduction to normal structure and function,* ed 2, Philadelphia, 2004, WB Saunders Co.

Doubilet PM, Benson CB: *Atlas of ultrasound in obstetrics and gynecology,* Philadelphia, 2003, Lippincott, Williams & Wilkins.

Lyons EA, Gratton D, Harrington C: Transvaginal sonography of normal pelvic anatomy, *Radiol Clin North Am* 30:663, 1992.

Nyberg D and others: *Transvaginal ultrasound,* St Louis, 1992, Mosby.

Rosen DJD and others: Transvaginal ultrasonographic quantitative assessment of accumulated cul-de-sac fluid, *Am J Obstet Gynecol* 166:542, 1992.

Rumack CM, Wilson SR, Charboneau JW: *Diagnostic ultrasound,* ed 3, St Louis, 2005, Mosby.

CHAPTER 36

The Sonographic and Doppler Evaluation of the Female Pelvis

Barbara J. Vander Werff and Sandra L. Hagen-Ansert

OBJECTIVES

- Demonstrate how to take a patient history specific to a pelvic ultrasound examination
- Define the terms *premenarche, menarche,* and *menopause*
- Describe the sonographic technique used to evaluate the uterus and adnexal area
- Distinguish between the appropriate cases for transabdominal and endovaginal scans
- Name the contraindications for endovaginal sonography
- Describe the disinfectant technique for transducers
- Discuss the differences among longitudinal, sagittal, transverse, and coronal planes
- Describe the scan orientation for transabdominal and endovaginal ultrasonography
- Name the important muscles in the pelvic cavity
- Discuss quantitative Doppler measurements
- Define the sonographic appearance of the uterus and adnexal area

PATIENT PREPARATION AND HISTORY

PERFORMANCE STANDARDS FOR THE ULTRASOUND EXAM

SONOGRAPHIC TECHNIQUE
TRANSABDOMINAL (TA) ULTRASONOGRAPHY
ENDOVAGINAL (EV) ULTRASONOGRAPHY

SONOGRAPHIC EVALUATION OF THE PELVIS
BONY PELVIS
MUSCLES OF THE PELVIS
PELVIC VASCULARITY
UTERUS
ENDOMETRIUM
FALLOPIAN TUBES
OVARIES
RECTOUTERINE RECESS AND BOWEL
SONOHYSTEROGRAPHY
THREE-DIMENSIONAL ULTRASOUND

KEY TERMS

adnexa – structure or tissue next to or near another related structure; the ovaries and the fallopian tubes are adnexa of the uterus

anteverted – tipped forward

arcuate vessels – small vessels found along the periphery of the uterus

cornu, cornua – any projection like a horn; refers to the fundus of the uterus where the fallopian tube arises

coronal – refers to a horizontal plane through the longitudinal axis of the body to image structures from anterior to posterior

endometrium – inner lining of the uterine cavity, which appears echogenic to hypoechoic on ultrasound, depending on the menstrual cycle

internal os – inner surface of the cervical os

introitus – an opening or entrance into a canal or cavity, as the vagina

menarche – state after reaching puberty in which menses occur normally every 21 to 28 days

menopause – when menses have ceased permanently

menstruation – days 1 to 4 of the menstrual cycle; endometrial canal appears as a hypoechoic central line representing blood and tissue

myometrium – middle layer of the uterine cavity that appears very homogeneous with sonography

parity – pregnancy

Pourcelot resistive index – Doppler measurement that takes the highest systolic peak minus the highest diastolic peak divided by the highest systolic peak

premenarche – time before the onset of menses

proliferative phase (early) – days 5 to 9 of the menstrual cycle; endometrium appears as a single thin stripe with a hypoechoic halo encompassing it; creates the "three-line sign"

proliferative phase (late) – days 10 to 14 of the menstrual cycle; ovulation occurs; the endometrium increases in thickness and echogenicity

pulsatility index (PI) – Doppler measurement that uses peak systole minus peak diastole divided by the mean

retroverted – bending backwards

sagittal – refers to a vertical plane through the longitudinal axis of the body that divides it into two portions

S/D ratio – difference between peak systole and end diastole

secretory (luteal) phase – days 15 to 28 of the menstrual cycle; the endometrium is at its greatest thickness and echogenicity with posterior enhancement

sonohysterography – (saline infused sonography or SIS) technique that uses a catheter inserted into the endometrial cavity, with the insertion of saline solution or contrast medium, to fill the endometrial cavity for the purpose of demonstrating abnormalities within the cavity or uterine tubes

translabial – across or through the labia

transperineal – across or through the perineum

Ultrasonography has proven to be an important diagnostic tool for the evaluation of pelvic anatomy and pathology in adult and pediatric populations. The noninvasive nature of sonography with its high-resolution imaging capabilities and ability to separate fluid from soft tissue structures in multiple imaging planes has proved clinically useful.

In the pediatric population, transabdominal ultrasound is used in a variety of clinical circumstances. These include evaluation of ambiguous genitalia, pelvic masses, and disorders of puberty, and to further evaluate pelvic or lower abdominal pain that may result from appendicitis.

The size, location, contour, vascularity, and physiologic state of pelvic organs are easily obtained using both transabdominal and endovaginal ultrasound. The information obtained complements the clinical evaluation and aids the process of forming differential considerations.

Color and spectral Doppler have evolved to play a role in assessing normal and pathologic blood flow. Sonohysterography can provide more detailed evaluation of the endometrium. Sonography also plays an important role in guiding interventional procedures.

The role of the sonographer is to gather the clinical history, identify the referring physician's indications for the study *(working diagnosis),* review the previous imaging results, and tailor the ultrasound exam to each patient. Critical thinking by the sonographer produces valid, reliable, and reproducible results that are the basis of an effective diagnostic medical sonographic practice.

PATIENT PREPARATION AND HISTORY

A complete history is critical to adequately tailor the ultrasound exam and correlate ultrasound findings with the proper differential consideration. It is useful for the sonographer to use a routine patient questionnaire requesting the following information: date of last menstrual period, gravidity, parity, physiologic menstrual status, hormone regimen, symptoms, history of cancer, family history of cancer, past pelvic surgeries, laboratory tests, previous Pap or biopsy results, and pelvic examination findings. Review of previous examinations (ultrasound, CT, MRI, PET) should be done before the start of the ultrasound exam to determine if a mass was previously present and to assess if there has been any change in size or internal characteristics.

The patient's menstrual status is described by using the terms premenarche, menarche, and menopause. **Premenarche** is the physiologic status of prepuberty, the time before the onset of menses. **Menarche** is the state after reaching puberty in which menses occur normally every 21 to 28 days. **Menopause** is when menses have ceased permanently. Perimenopause or premenopause is a transitional stage of 2 to 10 years before complete cessation of the menstrual cycle. This is the stage where there is a gradual decrease of estrogen and the menstrual cycles become shorter, longer, or irregular.

The sonographer should carefully explain the examination to the patient after the clinical history has been taken. If both the transabdominal (TA) and endovaginal (EV) examinations are going to be performed, the patient should be told that the pelvic ultrasound examination will be performed in two parts. The first is the transabdominal approach, in which the transducer is carefully scanned across her lower abdomen after warm gel has been applied, and the second is the endovaginal approach, which is an internal ultrasound and similar to a pelvic examination. The sonographer should tell the patient that she will be allowed to empty her bladder completely after the first part of the examination is completed. After receiving a brief explanation of the entire ultrasound examination, the patient is placed in the supine position. Ideally the scanning should be performed on a gynecologic ultrasound examination table, which can be modified for the EV examination.

By understanding all of the patient's clinical history and by talking and listening to the patient, the sonographer can gain a perspective as to what questions the ultrasound examination needs to answer and can tailor a plan of how to accomplish this. Once the scanning begins, the sonographer adds the information gained to develop a clinical and diagnostic image for each patient.

PERFORMANCE STANDARDS FOR THE ULTRASOUND EXAM

Four major organizations have determined standards for the pelvic ultrasound examination: the Society of Diagnostic Sonography, the American Institute of Ultrasound in Medicine, the American College of Obstetrics & Gynecology, and

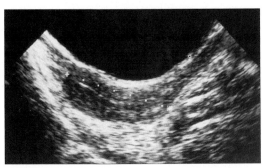

Figure 36-3 Sagittal image of an overdistended bladder compressing the uterine cavity.

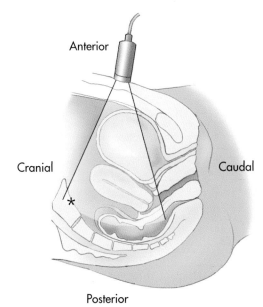

Anterior

Cranial

Caudal

Posterior

Figure 36-4 Longitudinal plane is oriented with the patient's head toward the left of the image and the feet to the right.

The uterus should then be identified in its long axis. This may not be in a true anatomic sagittal plane because the uterus can normally deviate toward either the right or the left. A somewhat oblique angulation through the distended bladder may be necessary to visualize the entire uterus and cervix. Anatomic orientation is correct for longitudinal scans (Figure 36-4) when the left side of the screen represents cephalic anatomy (toward the patient's head) and the right side of the screen represents caudal anatomy (toward the patient's feet). Once the long axis has been established, parallel sagittal scans are then obtained to the right and left to evaluate the uterine margins and the adnexa. The adnexal area may be imaged by scanning obliquely from the contralateral side and scanning through the fluid-filled bladder. In many instances, the adnexal area can be visualized by scanning directly over the adnexal area. Gentle pressure with the transducer on the pelvic area may be necessary to bring the area of interest within the focal zone. The iliac vessels can be used as a landmark to identify the lateral adnexal borders.

BOX 36-2
TRANSABDOMINAL PELVIC ULTRASOUND PROTOCOL

Survey the pelvic area before images are made.

LONGITUDINAL
Midline: Distended urinary bladder, uterus, endometrium, cervix, vagina (Figure 36-6)
Measure length of uterus from the fundus to the cervix
Angle right of midline: Bladder, uterus, area of right ovary (Figure 36-7)
Angle left of midline: Bladder, uterus, area of left ovary (Figure 36-8)
Look at both right and left adnexal areas in true pelvis (iliacus muscle is lateral border)

TRANSVERSE
Low: Distended urinary bladder, vagina, cervix
Mid: Bladder, body of uterus, endometrium; look for ovaries (Figure 36-9)
High: Fundus of uterus, endometrium; look for ovaries lateral to cornu of uterus

---

By again identifying the true sagittal plane of the uterus and cervix, and then rotating the transducer 90 degrees, the axial or axial-coronal (transverse) images can be obtained. Again, angulation from the contralateral side or direct visualization may help to image the adnexa. Anatomic correlation is correct for axial scans when the left side of the screen correlates with the right side of the patient (Figure 36-5). Applying gentle pressure on the transducer or placing the free hand on the abdomen helps move overlying bowel gas to bring the area of interest within the focal zone. The ovaries tend to travel cephalad with increasing bladder distention and may come to lie superior to the uterine fundus. When this occurs it may be necessary to have the patient empty her bladder before the exam can be completed.

Documentation and scanning techniques should be methodical and become routine for viewing by both the sonographer and the physician. A routine protocol consists of longitudinal and transverse scans of the uterus (to include the **myometrium** and **endometrium**), cervix, rectouterine recess (cul-de-sac), right adnexa, and left adnexa (Box 36-2; Figures 36-6 to 36-9). Measurements of normal structures and pathology are made in the length, width, and depth dimensions. Additional information may be obtained by the Doppler evaluation of all pelvic anatomy and pathology.

If pathology is present, documentation of the right upper quadrant (Morison's pouch and subphrenic area) and bilateral renal areas must be obtained. The evaluation of these areas demonstrates the presence or absence of free fluid, hydronephrosis, or anatomic variants related to pelvic findings.

It is important to have adequate bladder filling for all TA exams. The examination is routinely begun with a TA exam to

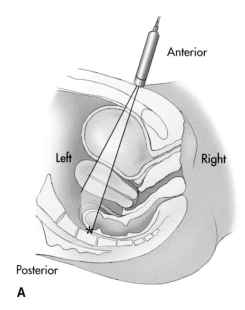

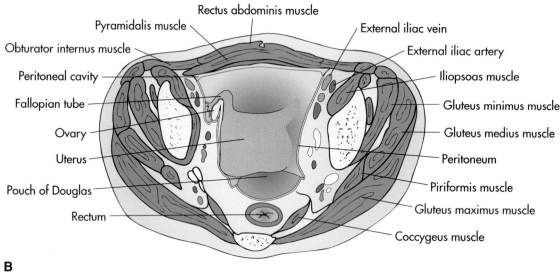

Figure 36-5 A, Transverse plane is 90 degrees to the longitudinal plane. The right of the patient is located on the left side of the image. **B,** Cross section of the female pelvis just below the junction of the sacrum and coccyx. The anterior inferior spine of the ilium and the greater sciatic notch are shown. The uterine artery and vein and the ureter are shown dissected beyond the uterine wall. The bladder is anterior to the uterus. The ovaries are cut through their midsections at this level.

look for large masses, fluid collections, or any obvious abnormalities. The survey of the pelvis is made to identify the uterus and ovaries. Then scan both the right and left flanks, and document the sagittal and transverse the liver–right kidney interface and the spleen–left kidney interface. The patient is then instructed to void and the EV scan is performed.

ENDOVAGINAL (EV) ULTRASONOGRAPHY

The inclusion of the endovaginal transducer in standard gynecological sonography protocols has improved the effectiveness of the pelvic exam. This exam has allowed the sonographer and physician a better visual survey by shortening the distance from the transducer to the ovaries, uterus, and adnexal regions. The resolution of pelvic structures has improved and the ability to

zoom in on smaller objects has been enhanced. This advance in technology brings with it more frequent detection of small tissue differences.

Patient Instructions. After the transabdominal study is completed, the patient is asked to empty her bladder completely. If the bladder is very full from all the fluids ingested before the examination, the patient may void and think the bladder is "empty" because it had been difficult to hold so much urine during the transabdominal examination. Ask the patient to wait a few seconds after her bladder has been emptied and try to void again; this technique is usually successful in completely emptying the bladder. If the bladder is not completely empty, reverberation artifacts may obscure

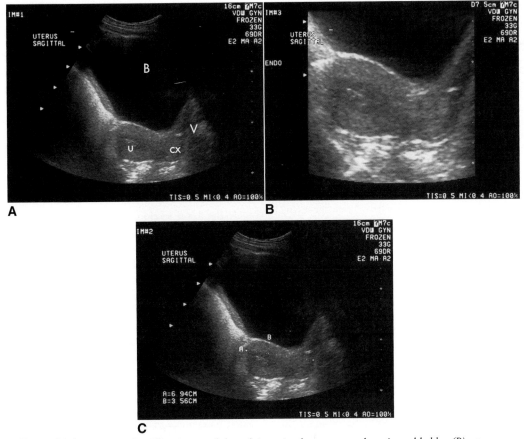

Figure 36-6 **A,** Sagittal midline image of the pelvic cavity demonstrates the urinary bladder *(B)*, uterus *(u)*, cervix *(cx)*, and vagina *(V)*. **B,** The image is magnified to better view the myometrium and endometrial canal within the uterus. **C,** Measurements of the length *(A)* and anteroposterior *(B)* dimension of the uterus are shown.

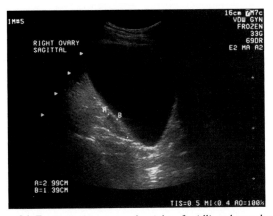

Figure 36-7 Sagittal image to the right of midline shows the bladder with the right ovary posterior. The ovarian length *(A)* and depth *(B)* are measured.

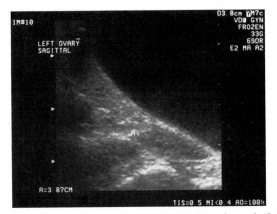

Figure 36-8 Sagittal image to the left of midline shows the left ovary posterior to the urinary bladder. The length *(A)* is measured.

crucial structures, and problem areas may be pushed too far away from the transducer. This is also an opportune time to reiterate the endovaginal procedure, obtain a verbal consent, and answer any questions the patient may have.

An adequate explanation of the procedure is essential. Many patients are apprehensive at any mention of an "inter-nal" examination, and the referring physician may not have explained the possibility of having one. It is important to explain why it is necessary to perform the endovaginal exam and to stress that the examination is a simple, usually pain-less procedure and that only part of the probe is inserted. Many labs will require a verbal or written consent from the

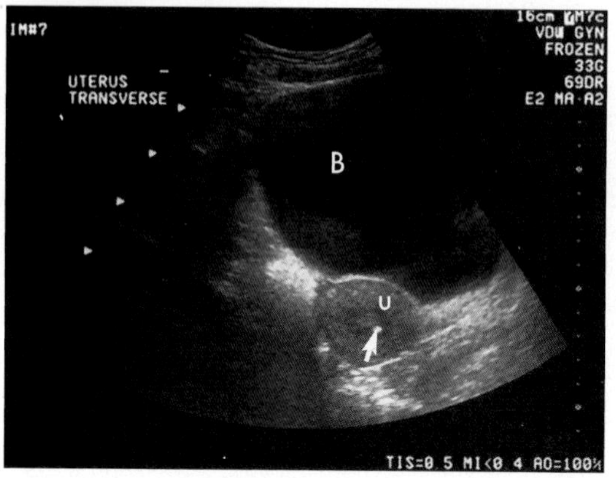

Figure 36-9   Transverse image of the bladder *(B)* with the uterus *(u)* posterior. The endometrial cavity *(arrow)* is well seen in the center of the uterine cavity.

patient and examiner for the endovaginal examination. If the examiner is a male, it is essential to have a female staff member in the room during the entire examination to act as a chaperone.

Endovaginal ultrasonography is performed using transducer frequencies of 7.5 MHz or more. These higher frequencies have better near-field resolution, which often permits greater detail of the uterus and adnexal anatomy. The primary disadvantage of high-frequency endovaginal ultrasound is the limited field of view and penetration (8 to 10 cm) because of the high frequency of the transducer and limited movement of the probe within the vagina. EV is often the preferred method of evaluation because it provides optimal visualization of the pelvic organs and should always be performed in women with suspected endometrial disorders, a strong family history of ovarian cancer, or a suspected pelvic mass. Contraindications include patient refusal, lack of patient tolerance (usually secondary to intense pelvic pain), and age, both premenarchal and menopausal. It is not recommended that an endovaginal examination be performed in patients who have never been sexually active, have an intact hymen, or have a narrow vaginal canal. If a patient experiences discomfort with an attempted insertion of the transducer, the examination should be discontinued.

Probe Preparation. The EV transducer is prepared with coupling gel on the transducer face and then covered with a protective sheath, usually a plastic sheath. It is a good idea to use latex-free plastic sheaths to prevent any allergic reactions for latex-sensitive patients. Instruct the patient that only a short portion of the end of the transducer is introduced into the vaginal canal, because the length of the probe can be intimidating. After the protective sheath has been put on, any air bubbles should be eliminated to prevent artifacts. A sterile external lubricant is then applied to the outside of the protective covering. This provides lubrication for insertion of the probe and is important especially in older women. If the examination is performed on an infertility patient, the use of water to lubricate the transducer is pre-

ferred because water does not have a negative effect on sperm mobility.

Examination Technique. After the patient has completely voided, she is asked to undress from the waist down, given a gown, and covered with a sheet. The patient position should be supine, knees gently flexed, and hips elevated slightly on a pillow or folded sheets and feet flat on the table, approximately shoulder length apart. The head and shoulders are slightly elevated with a pillow. A slightly reversed Trendelenburg's position may be helpful in lowering the pelvic organs to enhance visualization and detect free intraperitoneal fluid that gravitates to the posterior cul-de-sac. Current ultrasound scanning tables allow the lower section to be dropped with stirrups added to provide for ease of patient positioning. It is important that the patient's buttocks be at the end of the table with the patient's heels in the stirrups. This elevation is necessary to provide adequate mobility of the transducer handle. Being able to easily position the patient, cart, ultrasound equipment, and sonographer chair enhances the ergonomic position and reduces musculoskeletal stress on the sonographer. The height adjustment of the scanning table may permit the sonographer to sit or stand during the EV exam. The use of a chair with arms to rests on takes the strain off the examiner's shoulder and elbow.

Scan Orientation. The most accepted method of orientation used during endovaginal scanning is such that the left side of the screen corresponds to the cephalic and right side of the patient, while the right side of the screen corresponds to the caudal and left side of the patient (Figures 36-10 and 36-11). This method of orientation is the same one for radiography and conventional ultrasound. Residual fluid in the bladder is a helpful orientation landmark and should always appear in the right upper corner of the screen in the sagittal plane. For an **anteverted** uterus, the cervix would be seen on the right side of the screen, whereas the fundus of the uterus is found on the left side of the screen. In the case of a retroverted uterus, the cervix would be seen on the left with the fundus on the right.

Scanning Planes. When inserting the transducer in the sagittal plane, the flat part of the transducer is along the top surface of the handle so that the beam is projected in the midline anteroposterior aspect of the body. From the sagittal plane, the transducer is limited in motion because of the vagina. True parasagittal planes are never obtained, but angulation from this central point is considered sagittal imaging (Figure 36-12, *A*). As in the TA examination, oblique angulation is often necessary to visualize the entire uterus and cervix. It is often necessary to advance the transducer slightly, angling anterior to visualize the fundus, and then withdraw slightly, away from the external os, while angling posterior to see the cervix and rectouterine recess (Figure 36-12, *B*). The uterus is surveyed by scanning from the midline to the right and left. Angulation and tilting of the transducer directs the sound beam to visualize the adnexa in an oblique sagittal plane. Applying manual external pressure (either by the sonographer

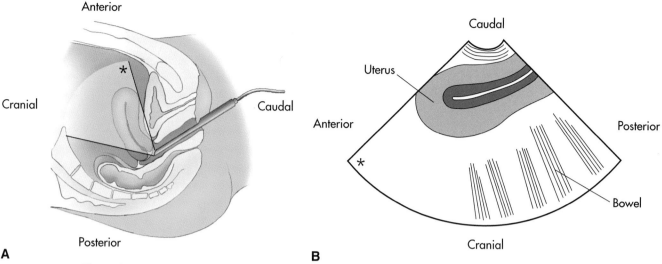

Figure 36-10   A, Endovaginal sagittal plane. The notch of the transducer is along the top surface of the handle so the beam is projected in the midline anteroposterior aspect of the body. **B,** The bladder is emptied, so only the uterine cavity and endometrial canal are seen.

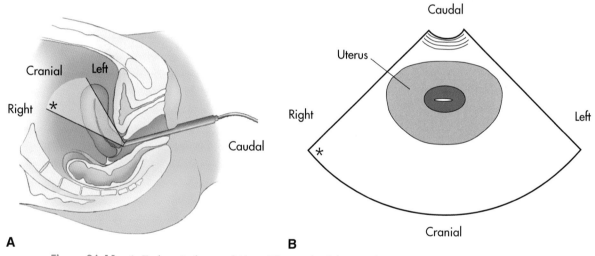

Figure 36-11   A, Endovaginal coronal plane. The notch of the transducer is rotated toward the sonographer so the beam may image the uterus in a coronal view. **B,** Coronal view of the uterus with the endometrial canal centrally located.

or the patient) to the outer abdominal wall may help displace the bowel and bring the ovaries into the focal zone, helping to visualize and delineate the borders of the ovaries.

When the transducer is rotated 90 degrees from the sagittal plane, image orientation represents the coronal plane (Figure 36-12, *C*). Rotating the transducer 360 degrees is possible. If the uterus is retroverted, better resolution may be obtained by inverting the transducer 180 degrees. The image should be inverted to properly document the retroverted uterus. It may also help to rotate the transducer 180 degrees in the coronal plane to better image the left ovary. The sonographer should check the orientation to guarantee that the left side of the screen represents the right side of the patient and again invert the image as necessary.

A helpful technique for locating the ovary is to first obtain a coronal image of the uterine fundus and then to angle the probe out to the **cornua** and ovarian ligament. Once this region is identified, the ovary can usually be identified by slowly sweeping the beam anteriorly and posteriorly.

By sweeping from the cervix through the lower, mid, and fundal portions of the uterus, the entire organ can be evaluated and measurements can be taken. For an anteverted uterus, the sweep will be posterior to anterior. A retroverted uterus will be anterior to posterior.

Scan Technique. The orientation of the endovaginal probe is controlled by probe rotation and angulation. The probe can be rotated up to 90 degrees, angled or pointed in any direc-

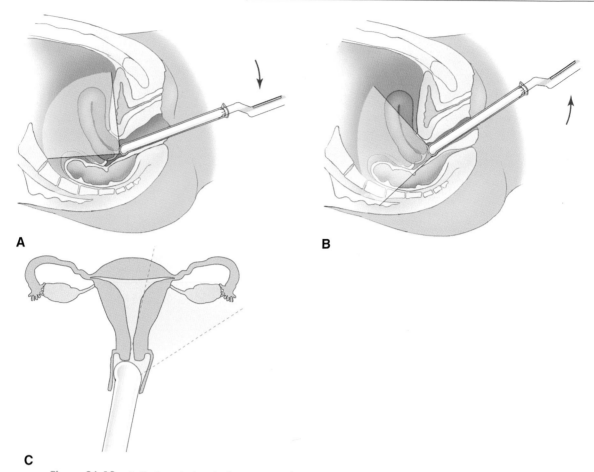

Figure 36-12 **A,** Endovaginal sagittal scanning with anterior angulation to better visualize the fundus of a normal anteflexed uterus. **B,** Endovaginal sagittal scanning with posterior angulation to better visualize the cervix and rectouterine recess. **C,** The probe is rotated 90 degrees to record the axial (transverse) images.

tion, and inserted or withdrawn to allow structures to be placed in the focal zone of the transducer rotation (Box 36-3; Figures 36-13 to 36-16). Varying the depth of the transducer may optimize the imaging of a structure in that field of view. Movement of the transducer is centered around the **introitus.** Any tilting movement of the transducer handle produces reciprocal motion at the probe tip. Rotation of the probe along its long axis provides 360-degree longitudinal visualization of the pelvis. Pushing or pulling the probe can bring the tip close to a region of interest and provide a method of indirect palpation, allowing evaluation of focal tenderness or fixation.

The insertion of the transducer into the vagina should be done in real time so the sonographer can watch the anatomy, because real time appears to ensure proper orientation. The probe may be inserted or guided by the patient, sonographer, or physician. It should not be inserted beyond the external cervical os. To maintain patient dignity and privacy, the patient should be properly draped at all times, and all practitioners who will be observing the examination should be present from the beginning of the examination.

Scan Protocol. Before recording any images, a complete pelvic survey should be performed. This survey is performed by slowly sweeping the beam in a sagittal plane from the midline through both adnexa to the lateral pelvic sidewalls. The probe is then rotated to the coronal plane, and the beam swept from the cervix to the fundus of the uterus. The survey will orient the sonographer to the relative positions of the uterus and ovaries and identify any obvious masses. After the survey, standard views are obtained. These include the following:

- Sagittal plane: Cervix, endocervical canal, posterior cul-de-sac, uterus (midline, right, and left), endometrium, right ovary and adnexa, and left ovary and adnexa.
- Coronal plane: Vagina, cervix and posterior cul-de-sac, uterine corpus and endometrium, uterine fundus and endometrium, right ovary and adnexa, and left ovary and adnexa.

Length, width, and axial measurements of the uterus and ovaries should be documented. The thickness of the endometrium should be measured in the sagittal plane (Figure 36-17). By sweeping side to side through the endometrium, the thickest portion can be identified and any areas of focal irregularity can be evaluated. It may be helpful to either zoom or decrease the field of view to obtain an accurate measurement.

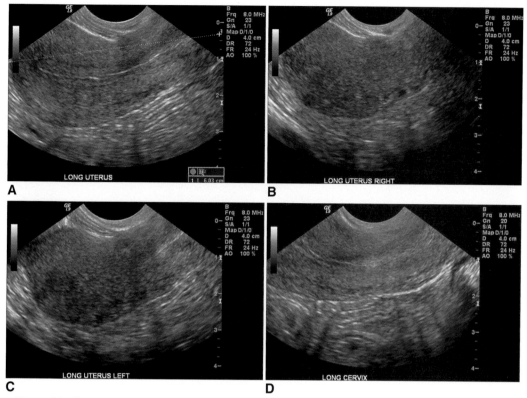

Figure 36-13 **A,** The uterus is imaged from the cervix to the fundus, showing the endometrial stripe; measure the long axis of the uterus. **B,** The probe should be angled slowly to the right of the uterus. **C,** The probe is then angled slightly to the left of the uterus. **D,** Withdraw the probe slightly to image the cervix.

BOX 36-3 ENDOVAGINAL SCANNING PELVIC PROTOCOL

Survey the pelvic area before images are made.

SAGITTAL: UTERUS
Image the uterus from cervix to fundus, endometrial cavity: measure the long axis (Figure 36-13, *A*).
Angle slowly to right of uterus (Figure 36-13, *B*).
Angle slowly to left of uterus (Figure 36-13, *C*).
Pull probe out slightly to image cervix (Figure 36-13, *D*).

CORONAL: UTERUS
Rotate transducer 90 degrees; image uterine fundus, body, and cervix with endometrial canal (Figure 36-14, A-E).
Look for free fluid surrounding uterine cavity.

SAGITTAL: OVARIES
Follow the fundus of the uterus to the area of the cornu to image the ovaries; the internal iliac vessels serve as their posterior border (Figures 36-15, A and 36-16, A). Color imaging may be used to separate vascular structures from the ovary (Figures 36-15, C and 36-16, C). Look for follicles surrounding the periphery of the ovary.
Measure long axis.

CORONAL: OVARIES
Rotate transducer 90 degrees once sagittal plane of ovary is obtained (Figures 36-15, B and 36-16, B).
Measure width and depth (Figure 36-15, B).

Any internal fluid should not be included in the endometrium measurement. Additional views of pathology or areas indicated should be obtained and measured in three dimensions.

Obtaining the standard images indicates that the entire organ and regions imaged have been carefully assessed in real time in two orthogonal planes. Any pathology or variant of normal must be assessed and appropriate images recorded. Color flow Doppler, power Doppler, and pulsed Doppler are added to the examination, depending on the clinical situation and pathology demonstrated on gray scale.

Translabial (transperineal) sonography prevents any potential complications of the endovaginal approach and is well tolerated by the patient. A 3.5 to 5.0 curvilinear transducer is covered with a plastic sheath and placed at the vaginal introitus and oriented in the direction of the vagina. Partial bladder filling may assist visualization of the cervix. Transperineal sonography is technically more challenging. Rectal gas and the pubic symphysis may obscure visualization and the identification of anatomic landmarks. These limitations can be overcome by elevation of the hips (as in endovaginal scanning), better application of the transducer on the perineum, or changes in the orientation of the probe. The endovaginal probe may also be placed at the vaginal introitus or slightly inserted within. This can assist in imaging the lower cervical area and distal vagina. Transrectal examinations may also be helpful if the endovaginal approach is not feasible or if the region of interest lies in the cul-de-sac.

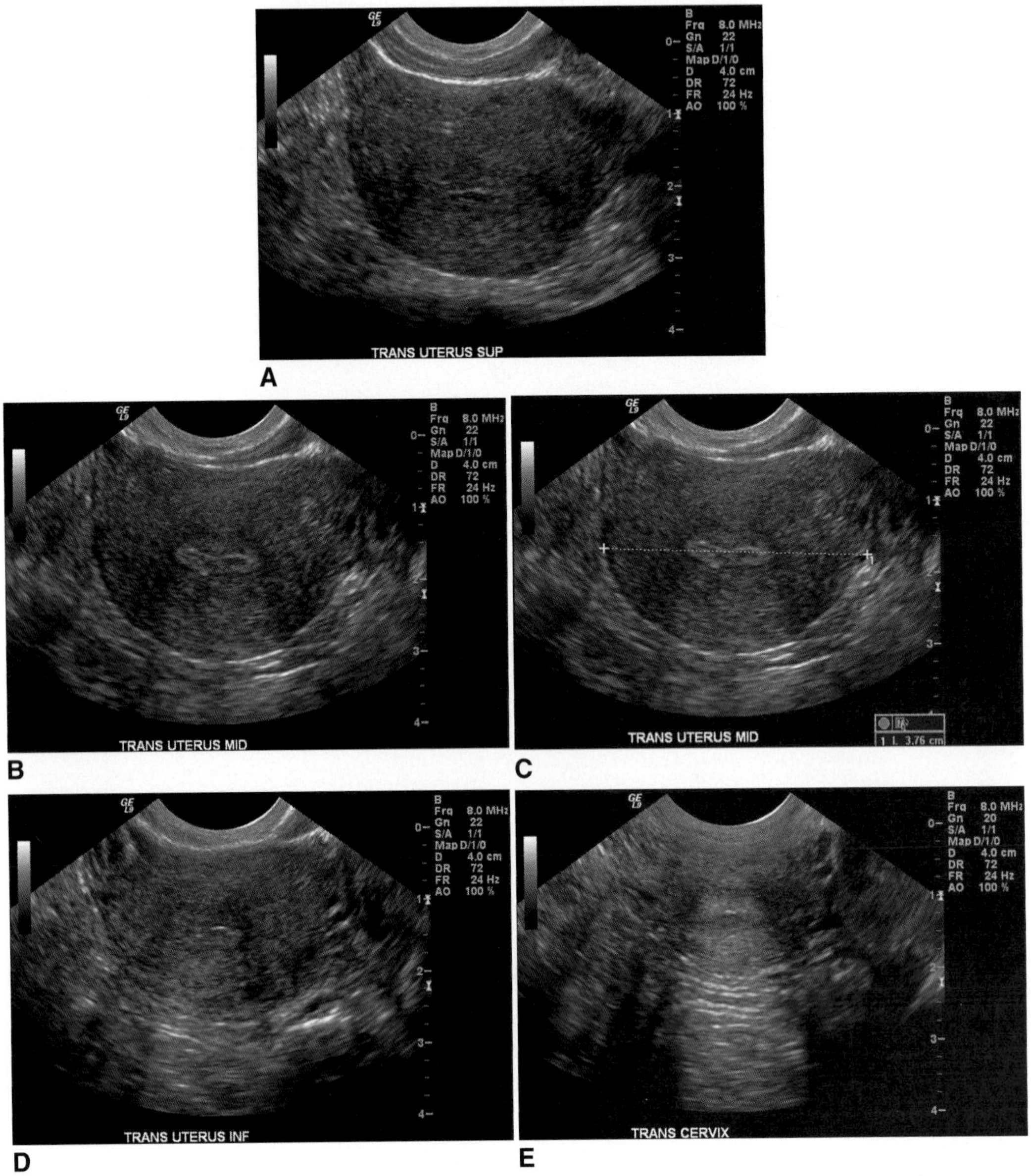

Figure 36-14 **A,** Rotate the probe 90 degrees; image the uterine fundus, body, and cervix with the endometrial stripe. This is the fundus of the uterus. **B,** The probe is angled caudally to image the miduterine cavity. **C,** The width of the uterus is measured. **D,** The probe is angled slightly more caudal to image the lower uterine segment. **E,** The probe is withdrawn slightly to image the cervix.

Disinfectant Technique. The use of an intracavitary device requires the prevention of cross contamination between patients. After completing the EV exam, the plastic sheath should be removed. This can be done easily with the gloved scanning hand by sliding the sheath off into the glove, removing the glove, and disposing of both into the waste container. The transducer should then be wiped clean with the facility disinfectant (be sure to read the vendor's recommendation for cleaning transducers) and dried with a towel. The transducer should then be soaked in a disinfectant between uses for at least the minimum recommended amount of time from the equipment manufacturer (10 to 20 minutes). Disinfection for extended times can cause damage or degradation to the trans-

ducer face. Most disinfectants are glutaraldehyde based (e.g., Cidex), and care should be taken when handling these caustic and toxic chemicals. Staff members must wear gloves, and some manufacturers recommend the use of safety goggles. There are various safety "stations" that are commercially available, which contain the required venting for this toxic chemical. Emergency eyewash stations should be available on-site. After the transducer has been soaked in a Cidex-type of solution, it is important to rinse the transducer with water and dry it before applying the coupling gel and protective plastic sheath. It is advisable to contact the probe manufacturer if information regarding the type of disinfectant and immersion time limit is not provided in the manual.

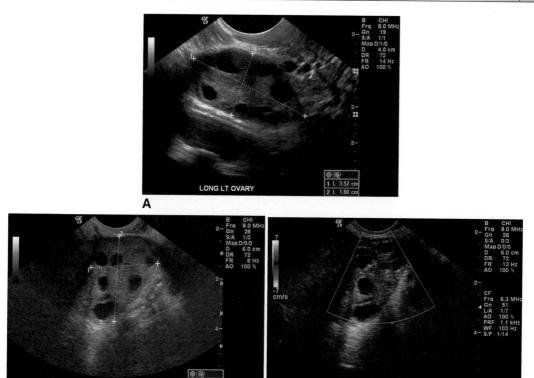

Figure 36-15   A, Long axis of the left ovary well demarcated by small follicles. The length and depth is measured. **B,** Transverse measurement of the left ovary. **C,** Color Doppler shows normal flow within the ovarian tissue.

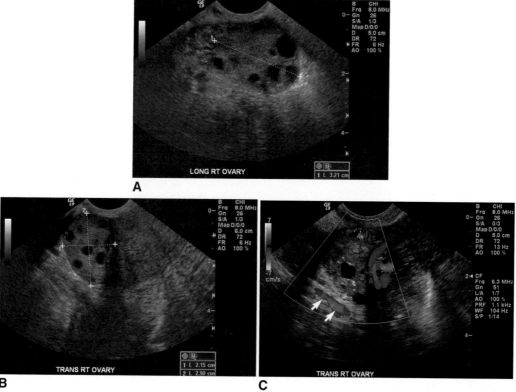

Figure 36-16   A, Long axis of the right ovary again well demarcated by follicles. The length is measured. **B,** Transverse of the right ovary with measurements. **C,** Transverse of the right ovary with color Doppler showing normal flow patterns. The iliac vessels are seen *(arrows)*.

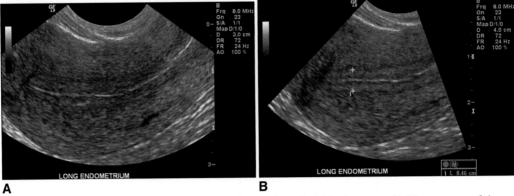

Figure 36-17   A, Longitudinal image of the endometrial canal within the uterus. **B,** Measurement of the endometrial canal is made from leading edge to leading edge.

SONOGRAPHIC EVALUATION OF THE PELVIS

BONY PELVIS

Ultrasound is essentially absorbed by bone. The shadow is produced because no sound is returned to the transducer since it is virtually all absorbed. The bony pelvis resembles a ring or funnel in shape. Anteriorly the pubic symphysis is formed by the articulation of the pubic bones with each other. The transabdominal study is begun just superior or cephalad to this midline landmark. Posteriorly the connection between the os ilium and the sacrum is formed by the sacroiliac joint on either side. Sonographically the sacrum may appear as a bright line with an overlying bowel shadow. This is more apparent in infants, children, and thin patients.

MUSCLES OF THE PELVIS

The filled urinary bladder displaces the bowel and acts as an acoustic window for evaluating three major groups of muscles. Pelvic muscles may be mistaken for ovaries, fluid collections, or masses. A symmetric bilateral arrangement indicates that they are muscles (Figure 36-18). The rectus abdominis muscles insert on the pubic rami and are paired parasagittal straps in the abdominal wall; they appear as hypoechoic structures with echogenic striations. The rectus sheath separates the sonographic appearance of the rectus abdominis muscle from surrounding fat and bowel as a bright linear echogenic reflector (Figure 36-19).

Obturator Internus Muscles. In the lesser or true pelvis, the urinary bladder, reproductive organs, levator ani, and obturator internus muscles can be identified. Sonographically, sections of the obturator internus muscle are seen at the posterior lateral corners of the bladder at the level of the vagina and cervix. This muscle is hypoechoic, ovoid, and surrounded by the obturator fascia, which serves as a tendinous attachment for the levator ani muscle (Figure 36-20).

Pelvic Floor Muscles. The levator ani muscle is best visualized sonographically in a transverse plane with caudal angu-

lation at the most inferior aspect of the bladder. It is a hypoechoic, hammock-shaped area that is medial, caudal, and posterior to the obturator internus (Figure 36-21). The two other muscles of the lesser pelvis, the coccygeus and piriformis, are located deep, cranially, and posteriorly. They are not routinely visualized on ultrasound examination and are not distinguished from other surrounding muscles. The piriformis muscles are located on either side of the midline posterior to the upper half of the uterine body and fundus. This is the most common muscle to be mistaken for the ovary.

Iliopsoas Muscles. The iliopsoas muscles can be seen in the greater pelvis. The iliopsoas muscle is a combination of the iliacus muscle and the psoas major. The psoas major originates bilaterally at the paravertebral lumbar region and courses caudally. The iliacus muscle is contiguous with and arises posterior to the psoas major at the level of the superior two thirds of the iliac fossa. Together, they form the iliopsoas muscle, which continues in the caudal direction, coursing anterolaterally to its insertion on the lesser trochanter of the femur.

The sonographic appearance of this muscle varies greatly depending on its development. On ultrasound examination, the iliopsoas muscle is discretely marginated and hypoechoic (Figure 36-22). The separation of the iliacus and psoas muscles can often be determined by the bright echogenic line representing the interposed fascial sheath. Both longitudinal and transverse images may be obtained through the urinary bladder midline with lateral angulation. Endovaginally, the positions of these muscles are deep and beyond the field of view.

PELVIC VASCULARITY

Pelvic vascularity can easily be evaluated using real-time and Doppler imaging. The use of color Doppler techniques (color flow, power, and pulsed) permits the vessel to be localized, allows the sample gate to be placed exactly in the area of interest, and reduces examination time. The quantitative waveform is displayed and analyzed in one of the following indices:

A/B ratio (A equals peak systolic and B equals end diastolic)
Pourcelot resistive index (A − B/A)
Pulsatility index (PI) (A − B/mean)

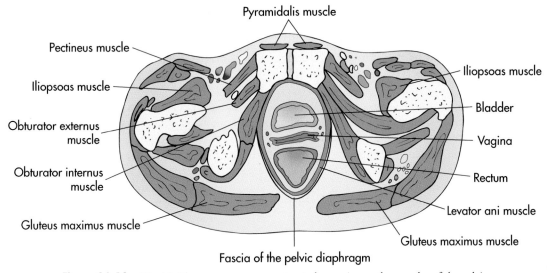

Figure 36-18   The bladder serves as an acoustic window to image the muscles of the pelvis.

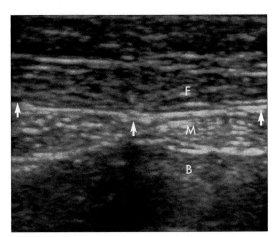

Figure 36-19   The rectus abdominis muscle is visualized with a 5-MHz linear transducer. *Arrows* represent the rectus sheath, which separates the muscle *(M)* from surrounding fat *(F)* and bowel *(B)*.

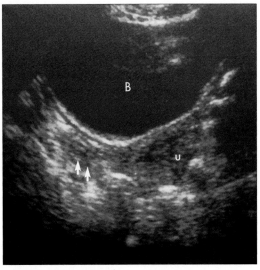

Figure 36-20   The obturator internus muscle *(arrows)* is visualized with the transabdominal sector transducer as hypoechoic-ovoid muscles lateral to the bladder *(B)*. Angle the transducer through a distended bladder from the contralateral side to demonstrate these muscles. *u,* Uterus.

Because the Doppler velocities are assessed as ratios, the waveform values are angle independent. (Remember that to obtain accurate Doppler velocities, it is critical to have the Doppler as parallel to the flow as possible; however, when ratios are determined, the difference in flow between systole and diastole is assessed and therefore the angle is not as critical.)

Imaging with transabdominal and endovaginal ultrasound, the internal iliac vessels can almost always be visualized and used as a landmark for the lateral pelvic wall and ovary. This vessel is commonly seen lateral and deep to the ovary (Figure 36-23). The internal iliac vessel has classic characteristic blood flow, demonstrating parabolic flow with an even distribution of velocities throughout the waveform. The pulsatility and slow movement of blood flow can often be appreciated on gray scale imaging. It is important to differentiate the vessels from an ovarian cyst because of its proximity to the ovary. If uncertain, the sonographer can use Doppler technique or rotate on the structure to elongate a vessel into a tube.

The arteries may be noted anterior to the veins in the pelvis. To assess the uterine vessels, the sonographer interrogates just lateral to the cervix and lower uterine segment at the level of the **internal os.** Uterine flow in the nonpregnant female usually shows a resistive pattern with a resistive index (RI) of 0.88 in the **proliferative phase,** decreasing slightly beginning the day before ovulation.

The vagina has two sources of blood. The anterior surface of the vagina and cervix is supplied with blood from a branch off the uterine artery before it reaches the uterus. The posterior surface of the vagina is supplied with blood from a branch off the internal iliac vessel (see Figure 36-23).

The ovary receives its blood supply from the aorta. The ovarian arteries also have a tortuous course from the lateral posterior border of the ovary to anastomose, with the uterine artery in the broad ligament adjacent to the cornual area (see Figure 36-23). This is considered the ovarian branch of the uterine artery, which is the most consistent and successful area for assessing ovarian Doppler flow. The blood flow of the functional ovary varies with the menstrual cycle. The changes in resistive index (RI) are thought to be a result of hormone-mediated changes in vessel wall compliance, allowing increased blood flow to the ovary in the late follicular and early luteal phases. A low-velocity, highly resistive flow pattern is shown during the follicular phase of the menstrual cycle. At ovulation, the maximal velocity increases and the RI decreases. The RI reaches 0.44 ± 0.004, and 4 to 5 days later it rises slightly before menstruation. The nonresistive flow pattern during ovulation probably results from the neovascularization of the follicle and subsequent corpus luteum. A normal pregnancy causes persistent low-resistive corpus luteal flow throughout the first trimester.

UTERUS

The uterine muscle consists of three layers, and the outer serosa of the uterus is not visualized sonographically. The middle layer is the myometrium of the uterus. This layer should have a homogeneous echotexture with smooth-walled borders. Any areas of increased or decreased echotexture should be noted and measured. The inner layer is the endometrium. This layer is thin, compact, and relatively hypovascular. The endometrium is hypoechoic and surrounds the relatively echogenic endometrial stripe, creating a subendometrial halo. The thin outer layer is separated from the intermediate layer by the arcuate vessels.

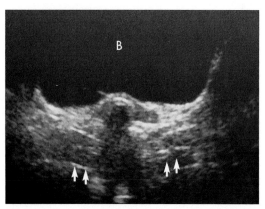

Figure 36-21 The levator ani muscle *(arrows)* is visualized with the transabdominal sector transducer as hypoechoic, hammock-shaped muscles medial, caudal, and posterior to the obturator internus. Angle from the most superior aspect of the urinary bladder *(B)* caudally to demonstrate these muscles.

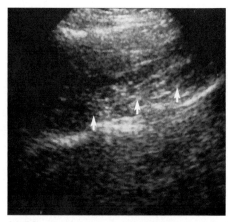

Figure 36-22 Sagittal image of the iliopsoas muscle *(arrows)*.

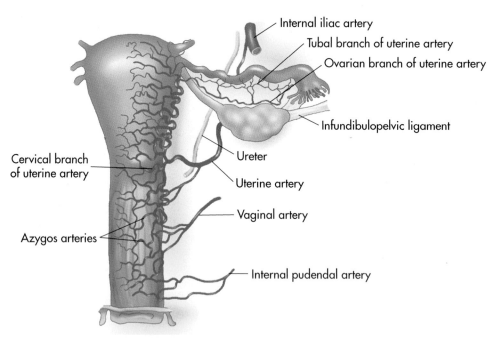

Figure 36-23 Diagram demonstrating the blood supply to the female pelvis.

The normal **arcuate vessels** are often seen in the periphery of the uterus and should not be mistaken for pathology (Figure 36-24). The radial arteries arise as multiple branches from the arcuate arteries and travel centrally to supply the rich capillary network in the deeper layers of the myometrium and the endometrium. Before entering the endometrium, the radial arteries give rise to the straight and spiral arteries of the endometrium (Figure 36-25). These vessels are most often demonstrated between 1 and 3 weeks after the onset of the last menses. Just before the onset of menses and during menses, these vessels are less apparent. The vasodilating actions of estrogens on the uterus during midcycle, and the vasoconstricting hormonal influences during the late luteal phase before menses explain the normal dynamic changes of these vessels. Calcifications may be seen in the arcuate arteries in postmenopausal women and appear as peripheral linear echoes with shadowing. This is a normal aging process that may be accelerated in diabetic patients. Echogenic foci in the inner layer of the myometrium, which are usually nonshadowing, are thought to represent dystrophic calcification related to previous instru-

mentation. Although they are of no clinical significance, they should be distinguished from calcified leiomyomas. Uterine perfusion (the vascular blood flow within the myometrium) can be assessed by Doppler sonography of the uterine arteries. The Doppler waveform usually shows a high-velocity, high-resistance pattern.

The body of the uterus is separated from the cervix by the isthmus at the level of the internal os and is identified by the narrowing of the canal. Tissue echogenicity surrounding the cervical canal should appear homogeneous. One can frequently visualize cervical inclusion cysts, known as nabothian cysts, near the endocervical canal. These are generally less than 1 to 2 cm wide and are anechoic smooth-walled structures with acoustic enhancement posteriorly; they are of no clinical significance (Figure 36-26).

The cervix is fixed in the midline, but the uterine body is mobile and may lie obliquely on either side of the midline. Flexion refers to the axis of the uterine body relative to the cervix, whereas version refers to the axis of the cervix relative to the vagina. The uterus is usually anteverted and anteflexed.

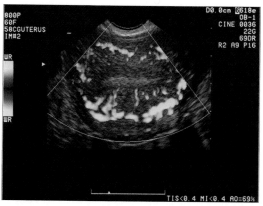

Figure 36-24 Endovaginal coronal view of the uterus with color Doppler that outlines the vascularity of the uterine cavity. The arcuate arteries are in the periphery of the uterine myometrium.

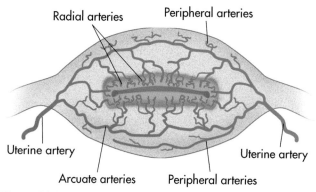

Figure 36-25 The blood is supplied to the uterus from the uterine artery, which bifurcates into the arcuate artery, radial arteries, and peripheral arteries. These vessels are very tortuous and have many anastomotic sites.

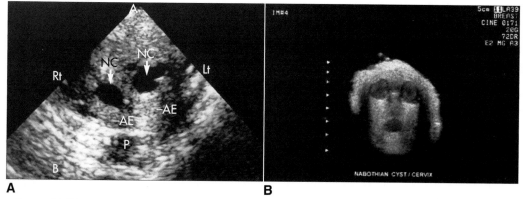

Figure 36-26 **A,** Endovaginal midline coronal view of the cervix with nabothian cysts. Naboth's cysts are often multiple and demonstrated in the coronal plane. *A,* Anterior; *AE,* acoustic enhancement; *B,* bowel; *Lt,* left side of patient; *NC,* Naboth's cyst; *P,* posterior; *Rt,* right side of patient. **B,** Endovaginal coronal view of the cervical area demonstrating multiple nabothian cysts.

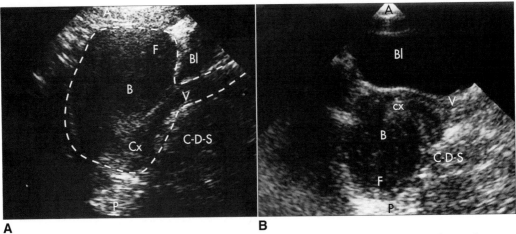

A   **B**

Figure 36-27   A, Transabdominal longitudinal scan of an anteflexed uterus. Anteflexion is abnormal bending forward of part of an organ. *A,* Anterior; *B,* body of uterus; *Bl,* bladder; *C-D-S,* cul-de-sac; *Cx,* cervix of uterus *F,* fundus of uterus; *P,* posterior; *V,* vagina. **B,** Transabdominal longitudinal scan of a retroflexed uterus. Retroflexion is abnormal backward-bending of part of an organ. *A,* Anterior; *B,* body of uterus; *Bl,* bladder; *C-D-S,* cul-de-sac; *cx,* cervix of uterus; *F,* fundus of uterus; *P,* posterior; *V,* vagina.

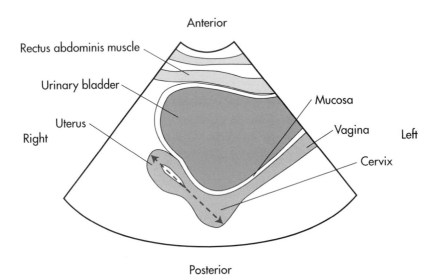

Figure 36-28   The length of the uterus is measured on the longitudinal image from the fundus to the cervix.

The uterus may also be retroflexed when the body is tilted posteriorly or retroverted when the entire uterus is tilted backward (Figure 36-27).

The fundus of a retroverted or retroflexed uterus is difficult to assess by transabdominal sonography. It may appear hypoechoic because it is situated a distance from the transducer and may mimic a mass in the rectouterine space. This can be confused for a fibroid. Endovaginal sonography is close to the posteriorly located fundus and is much better for assessing the retroverted or retroflexed uterus. As discussed earlier, it is necessary to use all three motions of the endovaginal transducer to optimize the image.

The transabdominal technique is the best way to measure the cervical-fundal dimension of the uterus in the longitudinal plane. Oblique angulation may be necessary to elongate

and measure the entire length of the longitudinal plane of the uterus. Its length is always measured from the distal end of the fundus to the distal end of the cervix (Figure 36-28). Either transabdominal or endovaginal scanning technique may be used to measure the width and anteroposterior dimensions of the uterus (Figure 36-29). Because of the proximity of the uterus to the broad ligament and surrounding vessels, it may be difficult to delineate the lateral borders of the uterus. Color Doppler technique or changing postprocessing controls may help delineate these borders.

The size and shape of the normal uterus varies throughout life and is related to age, hormonal status, and **parity.** Neonatally the uterus is pear-shaped secondary to maternal hormonal stimulation (Figure 36-30). Prepubertally the cervix occupies two thirds of the uterine length and the uterus is about 1 to

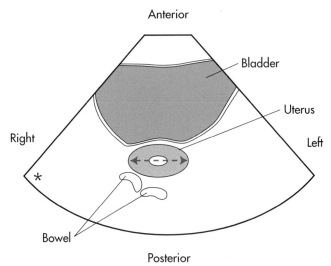

Figure 36-29   The width of the uterus is measured on the transverse image at the widest diameter of the body.

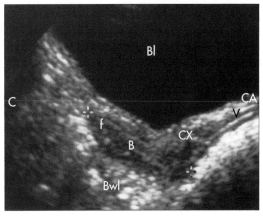

Figure 36-31   Transabdominal sagittal scan of a 6-year-old prepubertal uterus. The cervix occupies two thirds of the entire uterine length, but loses the pear shape of a neonatal uterus. *B*, body of uterus; *Bl*, bladder; *Bwl*, bowel; *C*, cephalic; *CA*, caudal; *CX*, cervix of uterus; *f*, fundus of uterus; *V*, vagina.

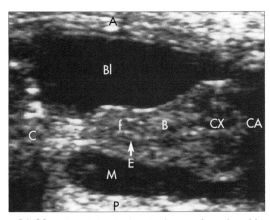

Figure 36-30   Transabdominal sagittal scan of a 1-day-old neonatal uterus. The cervix occupies two thirds of the entire uterine length secondary to maternal hormonal stimulation. *A*, Anterior; *B*, body of uterus; *Bl*, bladder; *C*, cephalic; *CA*, caudal; *CX*, cervix of uterus; *E*, endometrial canal; *f*, fundus of uterus; *M*, meconium; *P*, posterior.

3 cm in length and 0.5 to 1 cm in width and diameter (Figure 36-31). The nulliparous cervix occupies one third of the uterine length and is about 6 to 8 cm in length and 3 to 5 cm in width and diameter; add 2 cm for multiparous dimensions. The postmenopausal cervix occupies two thirds of the uterine length. The uterus is about 3 to 5 cm in length and 2 to 3 cm in width and diameter.

ENDOMETRIUM

Sonographic images of the endometrium disclose a characteristic appearance at each phase of the menstrual cycle. To optimally visualize and delineate the endometrium, endovaginal scanning is performed.

The sonographic appearance of the endometrial canal is seen as a thin echogenic line as a result of specular reflections from the interface between the opposing surfaces of the endometrium. The endometrium consists of a superficial functional layer and a deep basal layer.

During **menstruation** (days 1 to 4), the endometrial canal appears as a hypoechoic central line representing blood and tissue and reaching 4 to 8 mm, including the basal layer. This is surrounded by a hyperechoic basal endometrial echo. If menstrual flow is heavy, the entire endometrial cavity can appear anechoic (Figure 36-32). During this phase of early menses, acoustic enhancement posterior to the endometrium may appear. As menses progress (days 3 to 7), the hypoechoic echo that represented blood disappears and the endometrial stripe is a discrete thin hyperechoic line, which is usually only 2 to 3 mm.

In the early **proliferative phase** (days 5 to 9), the endometrial canal appears as a single thin stripe. The functionalis layer is seen as a hyperechoic halo encompassing it. The basalis layer of the endometrium represents the thin surrounding hyperechoic outermost echo. This complex creates the three-line sign (Figure 36-33). Early in the proliferative phase (days 5 to 9), the endometrial complex is thin, measuring 6 mm and becomes thicker, 10 mm, from days 10 to 14 before ovulation. The thin surrounding hyperechoic layer of endometrium represents the innermost layer of the myometrium and is not included in the measurement. In the later proliferative phase (days 10 to 14), ovulation occurs.

During the **secretory (luteal) phase** (days 15 to 28), the endometrium is at its greatest thickness and echogenicity with posterior enhancement (Figure 36-34). The posterior enhancement is thought to be attributable to the increased vascularity of the endometrium. The functionalis layer becomes isoechoic with the basalis layer. The endometrial complex measures 7 to 14 mm during the secretory phase (Figure 36-35).

The endometrial thickness is measured from the highly reflective interface of the basalis layer of the endometrium and myometrium in the sagittal view. This sonographic measurement includes both the anterior and posterior layers of the endometrium (Figure 36-36). The surrounding

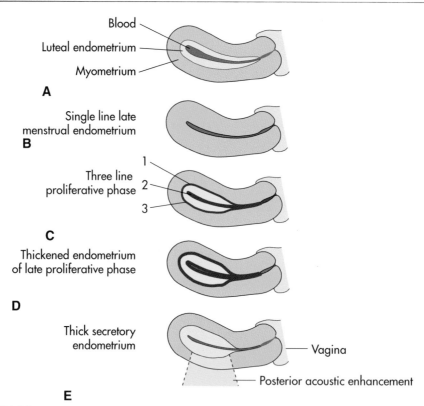

Blood

Luteal endometrium

Myometrium

A

Single line late
menstrual endometrium

B

1
Three line
proliferative phase 2
3

C

Thickened endometrium
of late proliferative phase

D

Thick secretory
endometrium

Vagina

Posterior acoustic enhancement

E

Figure 36-32 Endometrial changes through a normal menstrual cycle. **A,** Endometrium (days 1 to 4) of early menses. The hypoechoic central cavity represents blood and tissue. This is surrounded by a hyperechoic endometrial echo. **B,** Endometrium (days 3 to 7) as menses progress. The hypoechoic area that represented blood is sloughed. **C,** Proliferative phase (days 5 to 9) endometrium presents as the three-line sign. The thin endometrial center cavity is surrounded by a hypoechoic halo (the functionalis). The thin surrounding echogenic layer represents the basalis. **D,** The endometrium of the late proliferative phase (days 10 to 14) increases in thickness and echogenicity, representing the basalis. **E,** The secretory endometrium is at its greatest thickness and echogenicity with posterior acoustic enhancement.

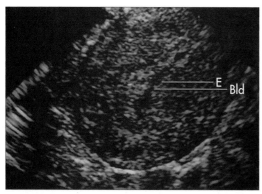

Figure 36-33 Endovaginal scan of the endometrium during menses (see Figure 36-32 correlation). *Bld,* Blood and tissue; *E,* endometrial echo.

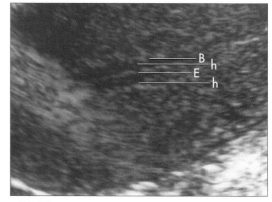

Figure 36-34 Endovaginal scan of the endometrium during late proliferative (early secretory) phase (see Figure 36-32 correlation). *B,* Basalis.

hypoechoic area represents the innermost layer of myometrium and is not included in the measurement. Similarly, fluid presenting within the endometrial cavity should not be included in the measurement of the endometrial complex (Figure 36-37). With the use of electronic calipers and endovaginal scanning, measurements of endometrial

thickness have been found to be within 1 mm of measurements from pathology examinations.

In all stages of a female's life, the normal measurement of the endometrium varies depending on hormonal status. In an infant, the endometrium may appear thick and echogenic because of maternal hormonal stimulation. In the child-

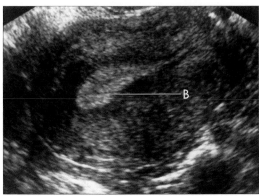

Figure 36-35   Endovaginal scans of the endometrium during proliferative phase (see Figure 36-32 correlation). *B*, Echogenic basalis; *E*, endometrial echo; *h*, halo (functionalis).

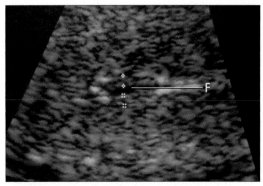

Figure 36-38   Endovaginal sagittal uterus. Fluid that is within the endometrial cavity is excluded from the measurement. Measure the anterior and posterior layers separately and add together. *F*, Fluid.

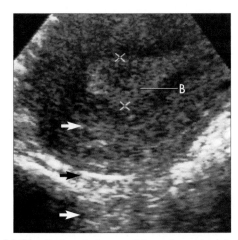

Figure 36-36   Endovaginal scan of the endometrium during the secretory phase (see Figure 36-32 correlation). The basalis *(B)* is at its greatest thickness and echogenicity with posterior acoustic enhancement *(arrows)*.

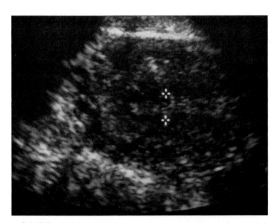

Figure 36-37   Endovaginal sagittal uterus. The endometrial measurement includes both the anterior and posterior layers of the endometrium. The hypoechoic area surrounding the endometrium is not included.

bearing ages, the endometrium varies between 4 and 14 mm. During menopause the endometrium becomes atrophic because it is no longer under hormonal control. Sonographically, the postmenopausal endometrial complex is seen as a thin echogenic line measuring less than 8 mm unless a hormone regimen is followed. The literature conflicts somewhat as to what the normal cut-off measurement is for the nonhormonally stimulated endometrium. The range clinically accepted as being normal is between 4 and 10 mm (Figure 36-38). Patients with postmenopausal bleeding and an endometrial double-layer thickness greater than 5 mm should have further evaluation.

FALLOPIAN TUBES

The normal fallopian tube can be difficult to identify by transabdominal or endovaginal sonography unless it is surrounded by fluid or dilated. Developmental abnormalities are rare. The normal fallopian tube is a tubular structure of approximately 8 to 10 mm in width and running posterolateral from the uterus to near the ovaries. It is divided into intramural, isthmic, infundibular, and ampullary portions. In the transverse view transabdominally, or the coronal view endovaginally, the fallopian tube region can be followed laterally from either side of the cornua at the fundal level of the uterus to the ovaries. The high resolution of endovaginal scanning allows improved visualization of the fallopian tube. It is not unusual to visualize the region of the proximal tube and surrounding ligaments. If the tubes are distended with or surrounded by a sufficient amount of fluid, they can be easily outlined by the contrasting fluid. The patient is placed in reverse Trendelenburg's position to use any fluid in the peritoneum as a contrast agent (Figure 36-39).

OVARIES

The sonographic approach to evaluate the ovary is often initially performed transabdominally. The transabdominal approach is especially important when the ovary is in an obscure location (i.e., high in the pelvis) so as to determine a general location to interrogate endovaginally. Transabdominal

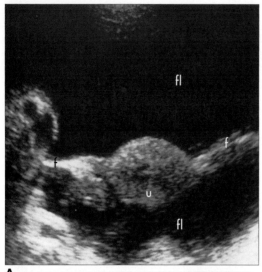

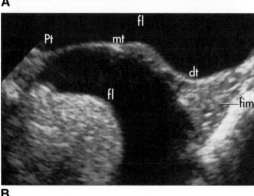

Figure 36-39 **A,** Transabdominal transverse scan of uterus and fallopian tubes. *f,* Fallopian tube; *fl,* free-fluid. *u,* uterus. **B,** Endovaginal coronal scan of fallopian tube surrounded by free fluid within peritoneum. *dt,* Distal tube; *fim,* fimbriae; *fl,* free fluid; *mt,* mid (ampulla) tube; *Pt,* proximal (isthmus) tube.

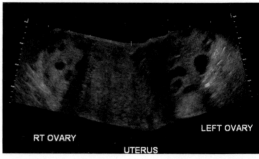

Figure 36-40 EV image of the prominent ovaries with multiple follicles present allows the visualization of the ovaries to be easily seen with sonography. The bladder is somewhat full in this endovaginal image. The uterus separates the two ovaries.

evaluation is also necessary to evaluate a large adnexal mass and determine its origin. The ovary is very mobile and can move considerably in the pelvis, depending on bladder volume and whether women have had a previous pregnancy. Uterine location influences the position of the ovaries. The ovaries are elliptical in shape, with the long axis usually oriented vertically. Endovaginal scanning is superior for characterizing the ovary and its contents and for visualizing ovaries that are not risible transabdominally.

Typically the ovary is located just lateral to the uterus and anteromedial to the internal iliac vessels, which can be used as a landmark to localize the ovary. Endovaginally, the ovaries are easiest to locate in the coronal plane lateral to the cornua. However, it is not uncommon to find the ovaries located above the uterus or posterior in the rectouterine cul-de-sac area.

Sonographically, the normal ovary appears as an ovoid medium-level echogenic structure; follicular cysts may be seen peripherally in the cortex. The appearance of the ovary changes with age and the menstrual cycle. During the proliferative phase, many follicles develop and increase in size until about day 8 or 9 of the menstrual cycle. This is caused by stimula-

tion of follicle-stimulating hormone (FSH) and luteinizing hormone (LH). At that time one follicle becomes dominant and increases in size to about 2 to 2.5 cm at the time of ovulation. The other follicles become atretic. If the fluid is not reabsorbed in the nondominant follicles, a follicular cyst develops.

Following ovulation, the corpus luteum develops and, if fertilization has not occurred, involutes before menstruation. Sonographically, these cysts are unilocular, anechoic structures with well-defined thin walls and posterior acoustic enhancement. Corpus luteum cysts may have a thicker wall and a peripheral rim of color around the wall on color Doppler.

The best sonographic marker for the ovary is identification of a follicular cyst, which has the classic appearance of being thin walled and anechoic with through-transmission posteriorly. The normal range in diameter of a mature graafian follicle is 1.8 to 2.4 cm. These cysts may be present in normal premenarchal, menstruating, and menopausal ovaries (Figure 36-40).

The ovary is measured in the sagittal or longitudinal plane at its longest length and anteroposterior dimension (see Figures 36-14, *D* and 36-15, *B*). In transverse or coronal scans, the width is measured at the widest point. With the use of color Doppler technique, a vessel and a cyst can easily be distinguished. Because of the variability in shape, ovarian volume is considered the best method for determining ovarian size. The volume of the ovary is calculated using the formula for a prolate ellipse: $0.523 = \text{length} \times \text{thickness} \times \text{width}$. The mean volume for a premenarchal ovary is 3 cm³, with an upper limit of 8 cm³; for a normal menstruating ovary, 9.8 cm³, with an upper limit of 21.9 cm³; and for a postmenopausal ovary, 5.8 cm³, with an upper limit of 8 cm³.

Due to its smaller size and lack of follicles, the postmenopausal ovary may be difficult to see on ultrasound. Scanning must be done slowly to look for peristalsis, so that stationary loops of the bowel are not mistaken for the ovary. Changes in imaging parameters (e.g., decreased frame averaging) may also help. The absence of a uterus following hysterectomy may also make it more difficult to visualize the ovaries. A difference in size of one ovary greater than twice the volume of the contralateral ovary should also be considered abnormal. Small anechoic cysts (less than 3 cm in diameter) may be seen in some postmenopausal ovaries. These may disappear or change in size over time. Surgery is generally recommended for postmenopausal women who have cysts greater than 5 cm and for those who have cysts containing septations or solid nodules.

Occasionally, echogenic ovarian foci are seen in the normal ovary. These are usually tiny (1 to 3 mm) and are nonshadowing foci, which can be peripheral or diffuse. They are thought to represent inclusion cysts and associated calcifications. These are insignificant findings and do not need further follow-up. Focal calcifications may occasionally be seen and are thought to be a stromal reaction to previous hemorrhage or infection. The calcifications are suggested for follow-up to rule out an early neoplasm.

The ovarian arteries arise from the aorta laterally, slightly inferior to the renal arteries. After giving off branches to the ovary, they continue to anastomose with the branches of the uterine artery. The ovarian veins leave the ovarian hilum and communicate with the uterine plexus of veins. The right ovarian vein drains into the inferior vena cava, and the left ovarian vein drains directly into the left renal vein.

RECTOUTERINE RECESS AND BOWEL

The rectouterine recess (posterior cul-de-sac) is the most posterior and inferior reflection of the peritoneal cavity. It is located between the rectum and vagina and is also known as the pouch of Douglas. The posterior cul-de-sac is frequently the initial site for intraperitoneal fluid collection. In asymptomatic women, fluid can normally be seen in the cul-de-sac during all phases of the menstrual cycle. Possible causes include follicular rupture and retrograde menstruation. Pathologic fluid collections may be seen in association with ascites, blood from ruptured ectopic pregnancy or hemorrhagic cyst, or pus resulting from an infection. Endovaginal scanning is better at demonstrating echoes within the fluid and helping to identify the type of fluid along with the clinical indications.

Gas and fluid-filled bowel loops are poorly defined, echo-free mobile structures that usually demonstrate peristalsis under observation. Solid material in the bowel is hyperechoic and may produce shadowing, as does gas (Figure 36-41). An empty bowel can look like an irregular bull's-eye with a thin, sharp, hypoechoic outline on a cross section. When rectal gas obscures the cul-de-sac and it is necessary to differentiate a mass from bowel, a saline or water enema may delineate the rectosigmoid, posterior uterus, and cul-de-sac in a transabdominal view.

Fluid-filled small bowel loops can appear cystic, but are easily identified by their swirling activity demonstrated on real-time imaging. Fluid may accumulate in the small bowel with rapid oral hydration. An endovaginal search for ovaries is often aided by the movements of bowel outlining the ovary. Immobile, dilated, or distorted bowel should be further investigated.

SONOHYSTEROGRAPHY

Sonohysterography, also known as *saline infused sonography (SIS),* involves the instillation of sterile saline solution into

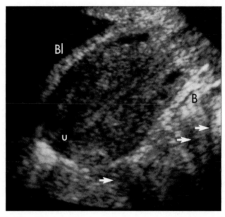

Figure 36-41 Endovaginal sagittal uterus *(u). B,* Bowel. Peristalsis is often observed in the cul-de-sac. Solid material in bowel is hyperechoic and produces shadows posteriorly *(arrows).* The bladder *(Bl)* is always oriented in the upper left corner.

the endometrial cavity. This is used when the endometrium exceeds the normal thickness or shows focal areas of thickness for the patient's clinical picture. The patient is prepared in the same manner as for a pelvic examination. A sterile speculum is inserted by the physician and the cervix is cleansed with an antiseptic solution. A very small catheter (5 to 7 French) filled with saline solution or contrast medium (Albunex) is inserted into the uterine cavity to the level of the uterine fundus. The catheter should be prefilled with saline before insertion to minimize air artifact. The speculum is removed with the catheter in place, and the endovaginal transducer is inserted into the vagina. A hysterosalpingography catheter may have a balloon to prevent retrograde leakage of saline into the vagina. Use fluid to inflate the balloon to minimize air artifact in the lower uterine segment. The balloon should be placed as close to the internal os as possible. The tip of the catheter may be localized on ultrasound, and then 10 to 15 ml of sterile normal saline is injected to distend the endometrial cavity while under continuous sonographic evaluation.

The uterus is surveyed with ultrasound in sagittal and coronal planes to delineate the entire endometrial cavity (Figure 36-42). Appropriate images are recorded or cine clips may be recorded in the sagittal and coronal planes. This technique is clinically useful to outline the endometrial cavity to determine the presence of polyps, tumors, or hyperplasia. In addition, the cornu of the uterus may be demonstrated with the interstitial area of the fallopian tube. The examination is contraindicated in patients with pelvic inflammatory disease.

The procedure is usually performed on premenopausal women between days 6 and 10, or soon after the cessation of bleeding in women with irregular cycles. Postmenopausal women who are not on sequential hormone replacement can have the procedure performed at any time. In most cases, there is no special patient preparation. Prophylactic antibiotic can be given for women with chronic pelvic inflammatory disease and women with a history of mitral valve prolapse or other cardiac disorders.

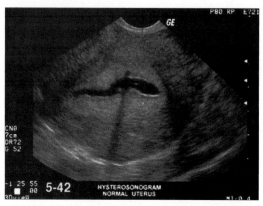

Figure 36-42 Endovaginal hysterosonogram of the uterus with a small amount of saline solution injected into the endometrial cavity.

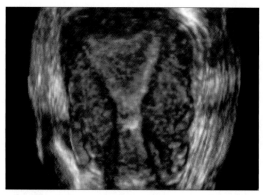

Figure 36-43 3-D reconstruction of the uterus showing a coronal image of the endometrium.

THREE-DIMENSIONAL ULTRASOUND

Three-dimensional ultrasound (3-D ultrasound) is a newer technology that allows imaging from volume sonographic data rather than conventional planar data. Volume data are generally obtained by acquiring many slices of conventional ultrasound data, identifying the location of the slices in space, and reconstructing them into a volume. That data can then be viewed as a 3-D object and displayed using a variety of formats to rotate and view the images from different angles for optimal visualization of anatomy and pathology (Figure 36-43). An additional approach to acquiring volume data is to use multidimensional arrays. Display of 3-D data is challenging. Currently the most common methods include multiplanar display of perpendicular slices through the volume and volume rendering. The display can be optimized to emphasize soft tissue or be changed to optimize vessels. Volume editing can be performed to eliminate or mask structures that obscure the areas of interest. Archived volume data may be further reviewed after the patient exam has been completed, permitting the reviewer to "rescan" the patient in the computer workstation. Volumes often require significant storage media and currently may be stored on magnetic optical disks, CD-ROMs or hard drives or transferred to computer networks with Internet capabilities.

The current AIUM guidelines regarding 3-D sonography state that because it is still a developing technology, its role is restricted to that of an adjunct of, not a replacement for, 2-D ultrasound. Continued work will likely show that the most promise for 3-D ultrasound in the pelvis is its ability to provide unique planes for improved evaluation of organs, tubal morphology, tumor invasion, accurate volume estimation, and guidance for invasive procedures. Sonohysterography also benefits from volume scanning. The exact location of a polyp, fibroid, or adhesion is readily identified.

As the 3-D technology becomes available in many more clinical sites, additional benefits will be identified. Four-dimensional ultrasound data are another new technology that allows 3-D imaging in a real-time mode versus computerized imaging postcapture. These technologies are exciting areas in development along with efforts of improved resolution and application.

SELECTED BIBLIOGRAPHY

ACR standard for the performance of ultrasound examination of the female pelvis, *ACR Res* 23, 2004.

Andolf E, Jorgensen C: A prospective comparison of transabdominal and endovaginal ultrasound with surgical findings in gynecologic disease, *J Ultrasound Med* 9:71-75, 1990.

Arger PH: Endovaginal ultrasound in postmenopausal patients, *Radiol Clin North Am* 30:759, 1992.

Callen PW: *Ultrasonography in obstetrics and gynecology,* ed 4, Philadelphia, 2000, Saunders.

Cohen HL, Tice HM, Mandel FS: Ovarian volumes measured by US: bigger than we think, *Radiology* 177:189, 1990.

Coleman BG and others: Endovaginal and transabdominal sonography: prospective comparison, *Radiology* 168:639, 1988.

Cullinan JA, Fleischer AC, Kepple DM and others: Sonohysterography: a technique for endometrial evaluation, *Radiographics* 1995;15:501-514.

Debose TJ, Hill LW, Hennigan HW: Sonography of arcuate uterine blood vessels, *J Ultrasound Med* 4:229, 1985.

Dodson MG: *Endovaginal ultrasound,* New York, 1991, Churchill Livingstone.

Evers JLH, Heineman MJ: *Gynecology: a clinical atlas,* St Louis, 1990, Mosby.

Fleischer AC and others: Endovaginal scanning of the endometrium, *J Clin Ultrasound* 18:337, 1990.

Goldstein SR: Incorporating endovaginal ultrasonography into the overall gynecologic examination, *Am J Obstet Gynecol* 162:625, 1990.

Granberg S and others: Endometrial thickness as measured by endovaginal ultrasound for identifying endometrial abnormality, *Am J Obstet Gynecol* 164:47, 1991.

Greimanis MG, Jones AF: Endovaginal ultrasonography, *Radiol Clin North Am* 30:955, 1992.

Grunfeld L and others: High resolution endovaginal ultrasonography of the endometrium: a noninvasive test for endometrial adequacy, *Obstet Gynecol* 78:200, 1991.

Kurjak A, Zalud I: Doppler and color flow imaging. In Nyberg and others, editors: *Endovaginal ultrasound,* St Louis, 1992, Mosby.

Lyons EA, Gratton D, Harrington C: Endovaginal sonography of normal pelvic anatomy, *Radiol Clin North Am* 30:663, 1992.

Mendelson EB, Bohm-Velez M, Joseph N and others: Gynecologic imaging: comparison of abdominal and endovaginal sonography, *Radiology* 166:321-324, 1988.

Nasri MN and others: The role of vaginal scan in measurement of endometrial thickness in postmenopausal women, *Br J Obstet Gynaecol* 8:470, 1991.

Nyberg D and others: *Endovaginal ultrasound,* St Louis, 1992, Mosby.

Occhipinti K, Jutcher R, Rosenblatt R: Sonographic appearance and significance of arcuate artery calcification, *J Ultrasound Med* 10(2):97-100, 1991.

Rumack CM, Wilson SR, Charboneau JW: *Diagnostic ultrasound,* vol. 1, ed 3, St Louis, 2005, Mosby.

Timor-Tritsch IE, Rottem S: Endovaginal ultrasonographic study of the fallopian tube, *Obstet Gynecol* 70:424, 1987.

Timor-Tritsch IE and others: The technique of endovaginal sonography with the use of a 6.5 MHz probe, *Am J Obstet Gynecol* 158:1019, 1988.

Varner E and others: Endovaginal sonography of the endometrium in postmenopausal women, *Obstet Gynecol* 78:195, 1991.

Winer-Muram HT and others: The sonographic features of the peripubertal ovaries, *Adolesc Pediatr Gynecol* 2:160, 1989.

CHAPTER 37

Pathology of the Uterus

Barbara J. Vander Werff and Sandra L. Hagen-Ansert

KEY TERMS

adenomyosis – benign invasive growth of the endometrium that may cause heavy, painful menstrual bleeding

cervical polyp – hyperplastic protrusion of the epithelium of the cervix; may be broad based or pedunculated

cervical stenosis – acquired condition with obstruction of the cervical canal

curettage – scraping with a curet to remove the contents of the uterus, as is done following inevitable or incomplete abortion; to produce abortion; to obtain specimens for use in diagnosis; and to remove growths, such as polyps

dysmenorrhea – pain in association with menstruation

ectocervix – a portion of the canal of the uterine cervix that is lined with squamous epithelium

ectopic pregnancy – pregnancy occurring outside the uterine cavity

endometrial carcinoma – malignancy characterized by abnormal thickening of the endometrial cavity; usually includes irregular bleeding in perimenopausal and in postmenopausal women

endometrial hyperplasia – condition that results from estrogen stimulation to the endometrium without the influence of progestin; frequent cause of bleeding (especially in postmenopausal women)

endometrial polyp – pedunculated or sessile well-defined mass attached to the endometrial cavity

endometritis – infection within the endometrium of the uterus

Gartner's duct cyst – small cyst within the vagina

hematometra – obstruction of the uterus and/or the vagina characterized by an accumulation of blood

hydrometra – obstruction of the uterus and/or the vagina characterized by an accumulation of fluid

intramural leiomyoma – most common type of leiomyoma; deforms the myometrium intrauterine contraceptive device (IUCD), a device inserted into the endometrial cavity to prevent pregnancy

leiomyoma – most common benign gynecologic tumor in women during their reproductive years

metrorrhea – irregular, acyclic bleeding

nabothian cyst – benign tiny cyst within the cervix

pyometra – obstruction of the uterus and/or the vagina characterized by an accumulation of pus

sonohysterography – injection of sterile saline into the endometrial cavity under ultrasound guidance; also known as saline infused sonography (SIS)

squamous cell carcinoma – most common type of cervical cancer

submucosal leiomyoma – type of leiomyoma found to deform the endometrial cavity and cause heavy or irregular menses

subserosal leiomyoma – type of leiomyoma that may become pedunculated and appear as an extrauterine mass

tamoxifen – an antiestrogen drug used in treating carcinoma of the breast

---

Sonography is traditionally applied in the female pelvis to delineate the size, texture, vascularity, and structure of pelvic anatomy. The examination may also supply information on the morphology of malfunctioning organs that seem normal on pelvic examination. Small, nonpalpable submucosal myomas or polyps may cause abnormal bleeding. The localization of intrauterine contraceptive devices (IUCDs) may be assessed by pelvic ultrasound examination. The homogeneity of the myometrium is assessed, and the thickness of the endometrial cavity is measured, in addition to the length and width of the uterus and cervix. Both transabdominal and endovaginal sonography are important in these evaluations. Transabdominal imaging furnishes a survey of anatomy, whereas endovaginal imaging provides better characterization of internal architecture of the vagina, cervix, and uterus. Color and spectral Doppler sonography can also play a role in assessing normal and pathologic blood flow, as well as identify vessels separate from fluid-filled structures. Newer techniques include sonohysterography, a process in which a small catheter, under ultrasound guidance, introduces sterile saline into the endometrium to provide a detailed evaluation of an intracavitary, endometrial, or submucosal lesion. Other imaging modalities used to evaluate pelvic anatomy and pathology include magnetic resonance imaging (MRI) and computed tomogra-

phy (CT). These two modalities are particularly useful in the staging of malignant disease.

PATHOLOGY OF THE CERVIX AND THE VAGINA

BENIGN CONDITIONS

Unless endovaginal ultrasound is used, the cervix can present a challenge to obtaining good sonographic images. The cervix lies posterior to the bladder between the lower uterine segment and the vaginal canal. The cervical canal extends from the internal os, where it joins the uterine cavity, to the external os, which projects into the vaginal vault. It is a cylindrical portion of the uterus that enters the vagina and measures 2 to 4 cm in length. With endovaginal scanning, after the patient empties her bladder, the transducer is inserted into the vagina with the patient supine, knees gently flexed, and hips elevated on a pillow. After the uterine cavity has been examined, the probe should be slowly pulled back to image the internal and external cervical os. In the sagittal view, the handle of the transducer is slowly moved upward to better image the cervix (see Chapter 36). With gentle rotation and angulation of the transducer, coronal images are also obtained.

The most common finding is the presence of **nabothian cysts** (Figure 37-1) (Box 37-1), which result from chronic cervicitis and are seen frequently in middle-aged women. This cyst results from an obstructed dilated transcervical gland and is also called epithelial inclusion cyst.

On sonographic evaluation, these lesions appear along the cervical canal as discrete, round, fluid-filled anechoic struc-

BOX 37-1	**NABOTHIAN CYSTS**

- Benign cysts in cervix
- Chronic inflammatory retention cysts
- Asymptomatic

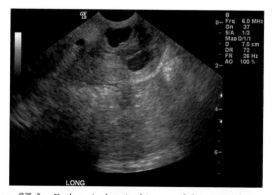

Figure 37-1 Endovaginal sagittal image of the cervix shows multiple very small nabothian cysts just inferior to the endometrial cavity in the center of the cervix with increased through-transmission beyond. The areas of shadowing represent poor contact or air bubbles between the transducer and the vaginal wall.

tures, usually measuring less than 2 cm; they may be multiple. Occasionally, nabothian cysts may have internal echoes that may be caused by hemorrhage or infection.

Clinical findings of irregular bleeding may be the result of **cervical polyps.** This benign condition arises from the hyperplastic protrusion of the epithelium of the endocervix or **ectocervix.** Chronic inflammation is the most likely factor. The polyps may be pedunculated, projecting out of the cervix, or broad based. Women in their late middle age are more likely to develop polyps.

A small percentage of **leiomyomas** (myoma tumors) occur in the cervix (Figure 37-2). When the myomas are small, the patient is asymptomatic, but as the mass enlarges, bladder or bowel obstruction may result. The myoma may be pedunculated (Figure 37-3) and prolapse into the vaginal canal. Sonography may assist in determining the location of the stalk and the thickness of the stalk. Fluid infusion with sonohysterography enhances this visualization.

Cervical stenosis is an acquired condition with obstruction of the cervical canal at the internal or external os resulting from radiation therapy, previous cone biopsy, postmenopausal cervical atrophy, chronic infection, laser or cryosurgery, or cervical carcinoma. The menopausal patient may be asymptomatic even though the stenosis can produce a distended, fluid-filled uterus (Figure 37-4), the result of an accumulation of uterine

secretions, fluid (hydrometra), pus (pyometra), or blood (hematometra). Intracavitary fluid collection can be readily seen on ultrasound and may be an indirect indicator of cervical stenosis. Premenopausal patients may experience abnormal bleeding, oligomenorrhea or amenorrhea, cramping, **dysmenorrhea,** or infertility.

CERVICAL CARCINOMA

Squamous cell carcinoma is the most common type of cervical cancer. Precursors to this disease are the cervical dysplasia classified as mild, moderate, or severe. When the full thickness of the epithelium is composed of undifferentiated neoplastic cells, the lesion is referred to as carcinoma in situ. The detection of these abnormalities is attributed to screening with Papanicolaou (PAP) smears because most of the early lesions are asymptomatic. Advanced cervical cancer is usually evident clinically (Box 37-2 and Figure 37-5). Sonography may demonstrate a solid retrovesical mass, which may be indistinguishable from a cervical myoma. Endovaginal, translabial, and transrectal ultrasonography demonstrate bladder, ureteral,

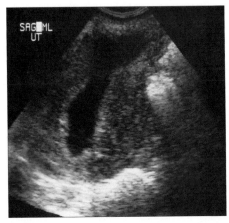

Figure 37-4 A 63-year-old asymptomatic woman on cyclic hormone replacement therapy demonstrates a large endometrial fluid collection. She underwent dilation for cervical stenosis, and bloody fluid was drained.

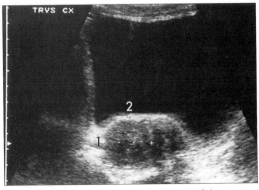

Figure 37-2 Transabdominal transverse view of the cervix reveals a 3-cm cervical myoma.

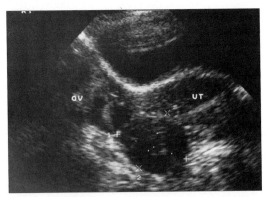

Figure 37-3 Transabdominal view of the uterus *(UT)* and ovary *(OV)* with a 4-cm hypoechoic pedunculated myoma *(mass outlined by calipers).* The pedicle is not visible on this image.

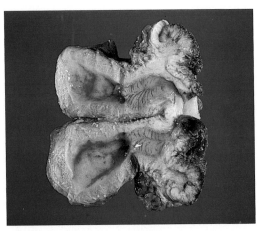

Figure 37-5 Gross pathologic findings of cervical squamous cell carcinoma.

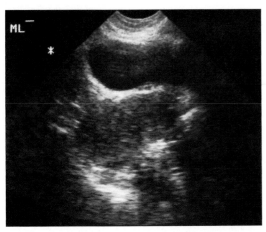

Figure 37-6 Transabdominal image of the distended urinary bladder and lower uterine segment. The cervical area is enlarged and hypoechoic with decreased through-transmission. The patient was found to have cervical carcinoma at surgery.

BOX 37-2   CERVICAL CARCINOMA

- Affects women of menstrual age
- *Clinical:* Vaginal discharge or bleeding
- *Sonographic findings:* Retrovesical mass, obstruction of ureters, invasion of bladder

---

vaginal, and rectal involvement and may be used in staging cervical cancer; however, CT and MRI are preferable. CT and MRI are superior for evaluating lymphatic spread for staging. Areas of increased echogenicity or hypoechoic areas with an irregular outline signify changes compatible with cervical carcinoma (Figure 37-6). Multiple cystic areas within a solid cervical mass are a rare cervical neoplasm arising from the endocervical glands termed *adenoma malignum* or *minimal deviation adenocarcinoma*. Ultrasound is also helpful in guiding biopsies of the cervix and vagina.

Translabial or transperineal sonography may be used instead of or with the endovaginal approach to help define the cervical area. A 5.0- to 7.5-MHz sector or curvilinear transducer is covered with a plastic sheath and applied to the vestibule of the vagina in the sagittal plane. Partial bladder filling may assist visualization of the cervical area. Rotation of the transducer obliquely in a counterclockwise direction shows the coronal images and defines the second plane for visualization. Positioning the patient with the hips elevated, as in the endovaginal approach, helps to displace rectal gas and identify anatomy. Limitations can be overcome by elevation of the hips, better application of the transducer to the perineum, or changes in the orientation of the probe.

THE VAGINAL CUFF

A vaginal cuff is seen in hysterectomy patients after surgery. The upper size limit of a normal vaginal cuff is 2.1 cm. If the cuff is larger than this or contains a well-defined mass or areas of high echogenicity, it should be regarded with suspicion for malignancy, especially in the patient who has a previous history of cancer. Nodular areas in the vaginal cuff may be due to post-irradiation fibrosis.

THE VAGINA

The vagina runs anterior and caudal from the cervix, between the bladder and rectum. Occasionally, sonography is used to characterize a vaginal mass, such as a **Gartner's duct cyst.** These are the most common cystic lesions of the vagina and usually are found incidentally during sonographic examination. The most common congenital abnormality of the female genital tract is an imperforate hymen resulting in obstruction. Obstruction of the uterus and/or the vagina may result in an accumulation of fluid (hydrometra), blood (hematometra), or pus (pyometra).

Solid masses of the vagina are rare. As in carcinoma of the cervix, sonography is not used for diagnosis of carcinoma of the vagina, but it may play a role in staging. When found, the lesion is usually vaginal adenocarcinoma and rhabdomyosarcoma. The lesions appear as a solid mass, occasionally with areas of necrosis. Translabial scanning may be used to best evaluate the vaginal area.

RECTOUTERINE RECESS

The rectouterine recess (posterior cul-de-sac) is the most posterior and inferior reflection of the peritoneal cavity. It is located between the rectum and vagina. It is also called the pouch of Douglas. Because of its location, it is frequently the site for intraperitoneal fluid collections. As little as 5 ml of fluid has been detected by endovaginal sonography. Fluid in the cul-de-sac is a normal finding in asymptomatic women and can be seen during all phases of the menstrual cycle. Pathological fluid collections may be associated with ascites, blood resulting from a ruptured **ectopic pregnancy,** hemorrhagic cyst, or pus resulting from an infection. Pelvic abscesses and hematomas can also occur in the cul-de-sac. Sonographic characteristics help to differentiate these findings.

PATHOLOGY OF THE UTERUS

The uterus lies in the true pelvis between the urinary bladder anteriorly and the rectosigmoid colon posteriorly. Uterine position is variable and changes with the degrees of bladder and rectal distention. The body of the uterus may lie obliquely on either side of the midline. This may mimic a mass on physical exam. Flexion refers to the axis of the uterine body relative to the cervix. Version refers to the axis of the cervix relative to the vagina. The uterus is usually anteverted and anteflexed. It may also be retroflexed (when the body tilts posteriorly) or retroverted (when the uterine fundus tilts backward). Endovaginal sonography has proven to be excellent for assessing the retroverted or retroflexed uterus because the transducer is close to the posteriorly located fundus. The size and shape of the normal uterus are related to age, hormonal status, and parity.

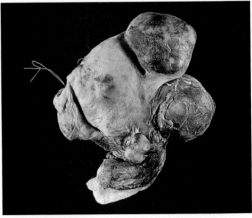

Figure 37-7   Gross pathologic findings of the uterine cavity with multiple subserosal myoma tumors arising from its walls.

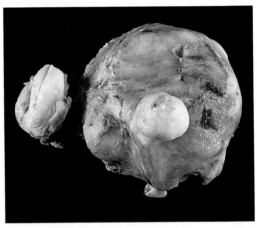

Figure 37-8   Gross pathologic findings of the uterus with the encapsulated leiomyoma in the submucosal area.

Common differential considerations for the uterus are seen in Box 37-3.

LEIOMYOMAS

Leiomyomas, commonly called myomas, are the most common gynecologic tumors, occurring in approximately 20% to 30% of women over the age of 30 years. They are more common in African-American women.

Myoma tumors are composed of spindle-shaped, smooth muscle cells arranged in a whorl-like pattern with variable amounts of fibrous connective tissue, which can degenerate into a number of different histologic subtypes (Figure 37-7). The tumors consist of nodules of myometrial tissue and are usually multiple. The myoma is encapsulated (Figure 37-8) with a pseudocapsule and separates easily from the surrounding myometrium. With atrophy and vascular compromise as a result of outgrowing their blood supply, fibrotic changes and degeneration of the myomas occur. Liquefaction, necrosis, hemorrhage, and ultimate calcification may take place. Hyalinization (development of an albuminoid mass in a cell or tissue) occurs most often, making the myomas appear more lucent or hypoechoic than myometrium. Ten percent of myomas contain calcification, and a similar number have areas of hemorrhage. Other myomas contain tissue that has undergone necrosis and liquefaction and become myxoid in texture.

Myomas are estrogen-dependent and may increase in size during pregnancy, although about one half of all myomas show little change during pregnancy. Myomas identified in the first trimester are associated with an elevated risk of pregnancy loss, and this risk is higher in patients with multiple myomas. They rarely develop in postmenopausal women, and most stabilize or decrease in size following menopause because of a lack of estrogen stimulation. They may increase in size in postmenopausal patients who are undergoing hormone replacement therapy. Tamoxifen has also been reported to cause growth in leiomyomas. A rapid increase in myoma size, especially in a postmenopausal patient, should raise the possibility of sarcomatous change.

Clinically, myomas cause uterine irregularity and enlargement with the sensation of pelvic pressure and sometimes pain. Patterns of irregular bleeding, menometrorrhagia, or heavy menstrual bleeding (menorrhagia) are the primary clinical problems with myomas. The tumor may contribute to infertility by distorting the fallopian tube or endometrial cavity; if located in the lower uterine segment or cervix, the tumor may interfere with normal vaginal delivery. Because of the increased estrogen during pregnancy, the tumor grows and may bleed within, causing pain. Box 37-4 summarizes the characteristics of leiomyomas.

Leiomyomas can affect any portion of the uterine wall; however, the tumor may also be uncommonly found in the lower uterine segment, the cervix, and in the broad ligament. Leiomyomas are either **submucosal** (displacing or distorting the endometrial cavity with subsequent irregular or heavy

menstrual bleeding), **intramural** (confined to the myometrium, the most common type), or **subserosal** (projecting from the peritoneal surface of the uterus). Sometimes subserosal leiomyomas become pedunculated and appear as extrauterine masses (Box 37-5 and Figure 37-9).

The signs and symptoms of leiomyomas depend on their size and location. Submucosal myomas may erode into the endometrial cavity and cause irregular or heavy bleeding, which may lead to anemia (Figure 37-10). Fertility may be affected by submucosal or intramural myomas, which may impede sperm flow, prevent adequate implantation, or cause recurrent miscarriages.

Uncommonly, a pedunculated subserosal lesion develops a long stalk and is migratory; it can implant into the blood supply of the broad ligament, omentum, or the bowel mesentery. Endovaginal sonography is often helpful in showing the uterine origin of the mass and identifying the stalk. Occasionally a pedunculated myoma becomes adherent to surrounding structures and develops an auxiliary blood supply. It is particularly important to diagnose submucosal leiomyomas because they are a well-established cause of dysfunctional

> ## BOX 37-4   CHARACTERISTICS OF LEIOMYOMAS
>
> - Most common pelvic tumor
> - Smooth muscle cell composition
> - Fibrosis occurs after atrophic or degenerative changes
> - Degeneration occurs when myomas outgrow their blood supply; calcification
> - May be pedunculated
> - *Clinical:* Enlarged uterus, profuse and prolonged bleeding, pain

> ## BOX 37-5   UTERINE LOCATIONS OF LEIOMYOMAS
>
> SUBMUCOSAL
> Erode into endometrial cavity—heavy bleeding; infertility
>
> INTRAMURAL
> May enlarge to cause pressure on adjacent organs; infertility
>
> SUBSEROSAL
> May enlarge to cause pressure on adjacent organs

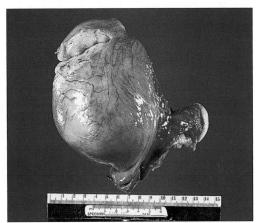

Figure 37-9 Gross pathologic findings of a pedunculated subserosal myoma of the uterus.

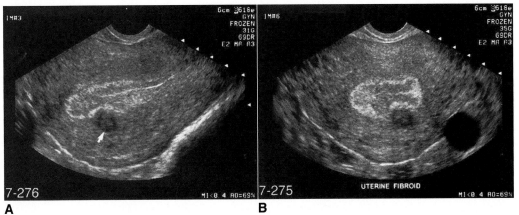

A **B**

Figure 37-10 Sagittal **(A)** and coronal **(B)** endovaginal images of the uterus with a small submucosal myoma indenting the endometrial cavity *(arrow)*. A follicular cyst is seen along the posterior border slightly compressing the uterine wall.

uterine bleeding, infertility, and spontaneous abortion. Submucosal leiomyomas can be removed hysteroscopically.

Sonographic Findings. Leiomyomas have variable sonographic appearances. The earliest sonographic finding of myomas is the demonstration of uterine enlargement or irregular uterine wall contour with a heterogeneous myometrial texture pattern. The sonographer should also look for contour distortion along the interface between the uterus and the bladder (Figure 37-11). The myoma alters the normal homogeneous myometrial texture pattern. Discrete myomas usually are hypoechoic but can be hyperechoic if they contain dense fibrous tissue. Bright clusters of echoes occur with calcific deposits and produce typical distal acoustic shadowing

(Figure 37-12). Some myomas demonstrate an area of acoustic attenuation without a discrete mass, making it impossible to estimate size. The attenuation is thought to be caused by dense fibrosis within the substance of the tumor. The ultrasound technique and gain controls often must be manipulated to provide increased penetration, or a lower frequency may be necessary to fully evaluate the uterus. If extensive calcification is present, the uterus and adnexa may be difficult to image because of shadowing. In such cases, endovaginal imaging is helpful in visualizing the ovaries. Myomas as small as 0.5 cm can be detected by endovaginal sonography and their relationship to the endometrial cavity defined precisely. Larger myomas cause heterogeneous uterine

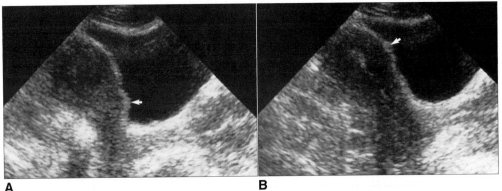

Figure 37-11   **A** and **B,** Transabdominal longitudinal views of the uterus reveal subtle myomas *(arrows).* These slightly echogenic masses distort the contour between the bladder and the uterus.

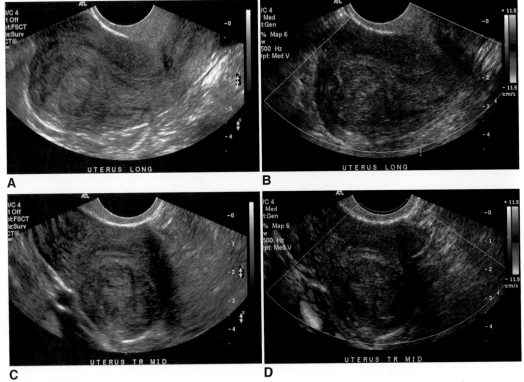

Figure 37-12   **A-D,** Endovaginal images of the uterine cavity with a large myoma posterior to the endometrium.

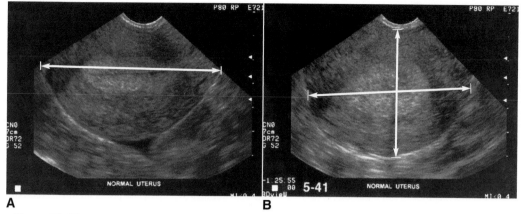

Figure 37-13   Endovaginal images of the uterus for measurement. **A,** Sagittal image should measure the uterus at the longest point from the fundus to the cervix. **B,** Coronal image at the level of the fundus measures the anteroposterior dimension and the width of the uterus.

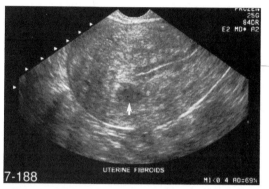

Figure 37-14   Endovaginal sagittal image of the uterus with a small myoma tumor *(arrow)* just posterior to the endometrial stripe. The tumor is not large enough to displace the endometrium.

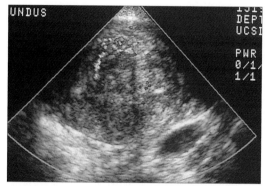

Figure 37-15   Endovaginal sagittal image of the uterus in a pregnant women with a 13-cm myoma. No flow within the myoma was seen on color Doppler imaging.

enlargement and are better outlined by transabdominal sonography.

The sonographic study should include measurement of the uterus in three dimensions: (1) cervix to fundus, (2) widest transverse diameter at fundus, and (3) widest anteroposterior diameter (Figure 37-13). The texture of the myoma (calcific, complex, or anechoic), size, and location are described. Individual myomas are measured if they are discrete. The shape of the endometrial complex and its thickness are also described; alterations in the endometrial border will be evident if a myoma is present (Figure 37-14). This is especially important in women with a history of abnormal bleeding. Myomas can be associated with endometrial infection or cancer. Blood debris and polyps can artifactually widen the endometrium; therefore, definitive diagnosis of the cause of abnormal bleeding requires an endometrial biopsy or sonohysterography.

Cystic degeneration of myomas causes lucencies that are well visualized with endovaginal sonography. Cystic degeneration often occurs during pregnancy and causes pain. Doppler should be used to assess the vascularity of myomas as a possible predictor of growth. Sonography

shows thin vessels with low-velocity flow within myomas. In cases of cystic degeneration, these vessels with low-velocity flow are not seen (Figure 37-15). Giant leiomyomas with multiple cystic spaces due to edema have also been described.

Although ultrasound is used to identify myomas in women with abnormal bleeding, uterine enlargement, or infertility, MRI, with its tissue differentiation characteristics, is more sensitive for evaluating the location, size, and number of myomas.

UTERINE CALCIFICATIONS

Myomas are the most common cause of uterine calcifications. A less common cause is arcuate artery calcification in the periphery of the uterus (Figure 37-16). These calcifications are thought to occur as a consequence of cystic medial necrosis within these vessels and indicate underlying disease, such as diabetes mellitus, hypertension, and chronic renal failure.

Sonographic Findings. Calcifications may occur as focal areas of increased echogenicity with shadowing or as a curvilinear echogenic rim.

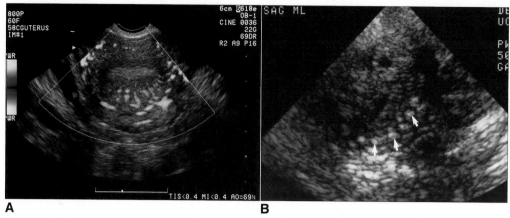

Figure 37-16   A, Color Doppler image of normal arcuate artery flow within the periphery of the uterus. **B,** Endovaginal sagittal view of the uterus demonstrates multiple echogenic foci in the region of the arcuate vessels. These are consistent with arcuate artery calcifications *(arrows).*

ADENOMYOSIS

Adenomyosis is a benign disease, commonly diffuse, with global infiltration of the endometrium. Adenomyosis is the ectopic occurrence of nests of endometrial tissue within the myometrium and is more extensive in the posterior wall. On occasion, adenomyosis may be focal with discrete masses or be identified with adenomyomas in the wall of the uterus. The exact cause is unknown, but the most commonly accepted theory suggests that a compromise of the natural barrier between the endometrium and myometrium occurs, allowing the growth of ectopic endometrial bands and stroma within the uterine myometrium. The tissue penetration usually reaches a depth of at least 2.5 mm from the basal layer of the endometrium. Because this ectopic tissue arises from the stratum basalis component of the endometrium, it does not bleed in response to cyclical hormone stimulation. Adenomyosis may arise from multiple pregnancies and deliveries with subsequent uterine shrinking. Elevated estrogen levels may also promote the growth of myometrial islands of endometrial tissue.

Adenomyosis is often classified into diffuse and focal forms. The more common form is diffuse adenomyosis. It represents a reactive hypertrophy of the myometrial muscle, which produces uterine enlargement, but never to the extent seen with leiomyomas. Focal adenomyosis is sometimes called *adenomyoma,* referring to isolated implants that typically cause reactive hypertrophy of the surrounding myometrium and produce diffuse uterine enlargement. Less common than the diffuse form, focal adenomyosis (adenomyoma) lacks a hypoechoic border that is seen with fibroids, not endometriosis. Adenomyosis can be appropriately managed with hormone therapy.

Clinically, both adenomyosis and endometriosis are identical with respect to structure and function, but are usually regarded as separate and distinct processes. Patients with adenomyosis are often multiparous and older than patients with endometriosis. The patient presents with heavy, painful abnormal menses, and, on physical examination, the uterus is found to range from normal to three times normal size and is globular in contour, boggy, and somewhat tender.

An estimated 60% of women with adenomyosis experience abnormal uterine bleeding (hypermenorrhea), prolonged/profuse uterine bleeding (menorrhagia), or irregular, acyclic bleeding **(metrorrhea).** Approximately 25% of patients with adenomyosis also suffer from pelvic pain during menstruation (dysmenorrhea). Currently, only 10% to 20% of adenomyosis cases are correctly diagnosed before surgery. This low rate is thought to exist because many adenomyosis patients are asymptomatic in the absence of other uterine pathology, and its presence may be overshadowed by associated pathology, such as leiomyomas, endometriosis, endometrial polyps, and so on.

Sonographic Findings. Sonographically, the diagnosis of adenomyosis may be difficult. The most common finding of extensive adenomyosis is diffuse uterine enlargement. There may be thickening of the posterior myometrium, with the involved area being slightly more anechoic than normal myometrium (Figure 37-17). Typically, adenomyosis involves the inner two thirds of the myometrium, where a slight decrease in echo content of the involved areas may be observed.

Hemorrhage in the islands of endometrial tissue appears as small hypoechoic myometrial cysts. This has previously been described as a Swiss cheese or honeycomb pattern. Lesions of this size are at the limit of ultrasound resolution. The fluid nature of these lesions produces increased posterior acoustic enhancement rather than the degree of attenuation that is normally seen posterior to the uterus. Further evaluation using signal processing (preprocessing and postprocessing) is helpful to better distinguish the contour and border differentiation of any coexisting pathology, such as leiomyomas. Doppler studies have also proven helpful in differentiating uterine pathology, as color flow studies of uterine masses show that myomas and sarcomas typically demonstrate a feeding artery, but adenomyosis rarely demonstrates feeding arteries.

Calcifications resulting from prior instrumentation are seen along the inner myometrium and cervix (Figure 37-18). Localized adenomyomas may be seen by endovaginal sonography as inhomogeneous, circumscribed areas in the myometrium,

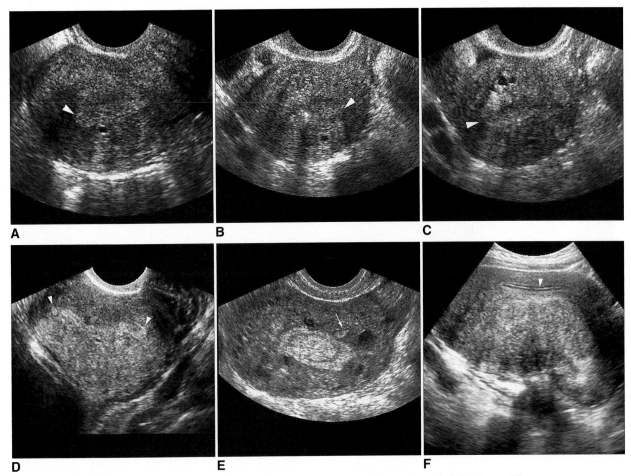

Figure 37-17 Adenomyosis on endovaginal scans—spectrum of appearances. **A,** Subendometrial cyst *(arrow)*. **B,** Cysts with heterogeneity in both anterior and posterior myometrium. **C,** Cysts with heterogeneity in anterior myometrium. **D,** Myometrial heterogeneity with ill-defined endometrial borders *(arrowheads)*. **E,** Multiple subendometrial cysts and echogenic nodule *(arrow)*. **F,** Large area of myometrial heterogeneity producing a focal mass effect and displacing endometrium *(arrowhead)*. This may mimic a fibroid. (From Rumack C, Wilson S, Charboneau W: *Diagnostic ultrasound,* ed 3, St Louis, 2005, Mosby.)

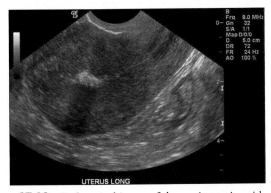

Figure 37-18 Endovaginal image of the uterine cavity with a bright echogenic echo in the endometrium. Shadowing is present beyond the calcification.

having indistinct margins and containing anechoic lacunae. They may be difficult to distinguish from leiomyomas, and these two conditions frequently occur together.

Adenomyosis is not reliably diagnosed by ultrasonography, and caution is advised because these findings are also similar in appearance to uterine myomas, muscular hypertrophy, myometrial contractions, endometritis, endometrial carcinoma, and the presence of increased endometrial secretions.

Localized adenomyomas may be seen by endovaginal sonography as inhomogeneous, circumscribed areas in the myometrium, having indistinct margins and containing anechoic cavities. They are usually difficult to distinguish from leiomyomas, and these two conditions frequently occur together. The presence of myomas has been shown to limit the ability to diagnose the severity of adenomyosis. Adenomyosis is not reliably diagnosed by ultrasonography, but is well characterized by MRI, which currently is thought by many to be the best technique for the presurgical diagnosis of adenomyosis. The MRI hallmark is the appearance of diffuse or focal widening of the junctional zone or the appearance of an indistinctly bordered myometrial mass (Figure 37-19).

ARTERIOVENOUS MALFORMATIONS

Uterine arteriovenous malformations (AVMs) consist of a vascular plexus of arteries and veins without an intervening

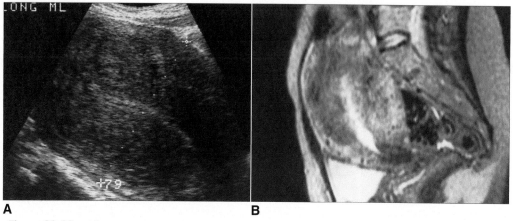

Figure 38-19   Adenomyosis. **A,** Endovaginal view of the uterus demonstrates an enlarged heterogeneous uterus. **B,** MRI shows an enlarged uterus with heterogeneous decreased signal intensity throughout the myometrium.

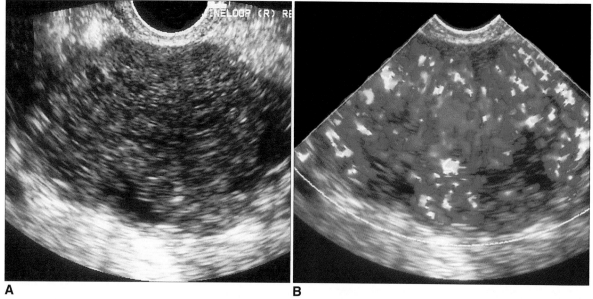

Figure 38-20   Uterine arteriovenous malformation. **A,** Transverse endovaginal images shows a textural inhomogeneity in the uterine fundus. **B,** Color Doppler image shows a floridly colored mosaic pattern with apparent flow reversals and areas of color aliasing. (From Huang M, Muradali D, Thurston WA: Uterine arteriovenous malformations (AVMs): ultrasound and Doppler features with MRI correlation, *Radiology* 206:115-123, 1998.)

capillary network. They are rare, usually involving the myometrium and rarely the endometrium. They can be congenital but most are teratogenic (acquired) due to pelvic trauma, surgery, and gestational trophoblastic neoplasia. Clinically, women of childbearing years have metrorrhagia with blood loss and anemia. Diagnosis is critical because dilation and **curettage** may lead to catastrophic hemorrhaging.

Sonographic Findings. Sonographically, serpiginous, anechoic structures are seen within the pelvis. Uterine AVMs may appear as subtle myometrial inhomogeneity, tubular spaces within the myometrium, intramural uterine mass, endometrial or cervical mass, or sometimes as prominent parametrial vessels. Color Doppler is diagnostic to show

blood flow within the anechoic structures (Figure 37-20). There may be a florid colored mosaic pattern with apparent flow reversals and areas of color aliasing. Spectral Doppler shows high-velocity, low-resistance arterial flow coupled with high-velocity venous flow, with an arterial component. Treatment and confirmation include angiography with embolic therapy.

UTERINE LEIOMYOSARCOMA

Leiomyosarcoma is rare, accounting for 1.3% of uterine malignancies (Figure 37-21). The tumor is derived from smooth muscle in the wall of the uterus (the same as leiomyomas) and is thought to arise from preexisting leiomyoma (Box 37-6).

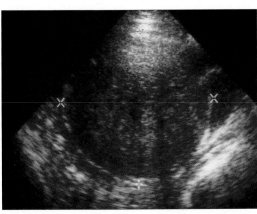

Figure 38-21 A 61-year-old woman with lower abdominal "fullness" and frequency of urination. Endovaginal ultrasound showed a large heterogeneous mass in the uterus. A large leiomyosarcoma was found at surgery.

TABLE 37-1	ENDOMETRIAL THICKNESS RELATED TO PHASES OF MENSTRUAL CYCLE
Phase of Menstrual Cycle	**Endometrial Thickness* (mm)**
Menstrual	2-3
Early proliferative	4-6
Periovulatory	6-8
Secretory	8-15

Data from Goldberg BB, Kurtz AB: *Ultrasound measurements,* St Louis, 1990, Mosby.
*Measured as full thickness, anteroposterior (AP), from outer border to outer border of hypoechoic interface.

BOX 37-6   LEIOMYOSARCOMA

- Rare, solid tumor arising from the myometrium or endometrium
- Commonly in fundus of uterus
- Can affect any age
- Rapid growth
- *Sarcoma botryoides:* Very rare condition in children characterized by grapelike clusters of tumor mass

---

Frequently, patients are asymptomatic, although uterine bleeding may occur.

Sonographic Findings. Leiomyosarcoma may resemble myomas or endometrial carcinoma with features of solid or mixed-solid and cystic texture. Clinically the enlargement of a myoma in the perimenopausal or postmenopausal patient raises concern about the development of a malignancy.

PATHOLOGY OF THE ENDOMETRIUM

The endometrial canal is the landmark for the identification of the long axis of the uterus. The echogenicity of the endometrial tissue is compared with the homogeneous, medium-level echogenicity of the middle layer of the myometrium. A hypoechoic layer of inner myometrium surrounds the endometrium. Progressive thickening and increased reflectivity of the endometrium occurs in the majority of patients until it is shed during menstruation. In the immediate preovulatory and postovulatory periods (approximately 2 days), an additional inner hypoechoic layer appears secondary to edema.

The endometrium should be measured perpendicular to the long axis of the uterus. The hypoechoic halo surrounding the endometrium should not be included in the measurement because this represents the inner compact layer of myometrium. Fluid, if present, should not be included in endometrial measurements (Table 37-1).

Improved resolution with endovaginal sonography is better able to image and see subtle abnormalities within the endometrium. Knowledge of the normal sonographic appearance of the endometrium allows for earlier recognition of the pathologic conditions where the endometrium is thickened, irregular, or poorly defined. An abnormally thick endometrium results from a variety of conditions, including early intrauterine pregnancy, gestational trophoblastic disease, endometrial hyperplasia, secretary endometrium, estrogen replacement therapy, polyps, or endometrial carcinoma. Many endometrial pathologies, such as hyperplasia, polyps, and carcinoma, can cause abnormal bleeding, especially in the postmenopausal patient.

Many menopausal patients with breast cancer receive tamoxifen therapy. This is a partial estrogen receptor antagonist. The effects on the uterus include epithelial metaplasia, hyperplasia, and even carcinoma. In these patients, TV scanning may show thickened, irregular cystic endometrium. These patients frequently have biannual serial ultrasound exams of their uterus and endometrium. A biopsy is performed in suspicious cases.

SONOHYSTEROGRAPHY

Sonohysterography (saline infused sonography) has been shown to be of great value in further evaluating the abnormally thickened endometrium because it can distinguish between focal and diffuse endometrial abnormalities. After performing routine endovaginal scanning to orient the sonographer to the patient's anatomy and pathology, the doctor should explain the procedure to the patient and obtain consent. A sterile speculum is inserted into the vagina and the cervix is cleansed with an antiseptic solution. A hysterosalpingography catheter is inserted into the uterine cavity to the level of the uterine fundus. The catheter is prefilled with sterile saline before insertion to minimize air artifact. The speculum is removed and the endovaginal transducer is inserted into the vagina. The catheter is identified in the endometrial cavity by locating the saline filled balloon, and the saline is slowly injected through the catheter under sonographic visualization. The uterus is scanned systematically in sagittal and coronal planes to delineate the entire endometrial cavity. Appropriate images are obtained under the direction of the physician performing the procedure. A sweep of the fluid-filled endometrium in both planes can be captured on cine clips to further document the presence of any pathology.

In premenopausal women the procedure is performed midmenstrual cycle, usually between days 6 to 10. This will prevent the possibility of disrupting an early pregnancy and prevent blood clots artifactually filling some of the endometrial cavity. For women with irregular cycles, the procedure is performed soon after the cessation of bleeding, if possible. In postmenopausal women the procedure can be performed at any time or shortly after the monthly bleeding period if they are on sequential hormone replacement therapy. The procedure is *not* performed in women with acute pelvic inflammatory disease. In most cases there is no special patient preparation. Prophylactic antibiotics are given to women with chronic pelvic inflammatory disease and to women with a history of mitral valve prolapse or other cardiac disorders.

Sonographic Findings. Sonographically, after the saline is injected, the endometrial canal fills with saline and the borders are clearly identified (Figure 37-22). Any projections or filling defects can be delineated and confirmed in the sagittal and coronal planes. By using color Doppler, a vascular pedicle can be identified in polyps. The catheter is slowly removed while injecting a small amount of the saline to help distinguish the cervical area.

ENDOMETRIAL HYPERPLASIA

Endometrial hyperplasia (Box 37-7) is the most common cause of abnormal uterine bleeding in both premenopausal and postmenopausal women. Hyperplasia develops from unopposed estrogen stimulation. It appears as thickening of the endometrium. In premenopausal women, if the endometrium measures more than 14 mm (double thickness), hyperplasia is suggested (Figure 37-23). In asymptomatic postmenopausal women, 8 mm (double thickness) is the upper limit of normal. However, women on sequential estrogen and progesterone replacement regimens may have endometrial thickness up to 15 mm during the estrogen phase; the thickness decreases after progesterone is added. Ideally a woman using sequential hormones should be studied at the beginning or end of her hormone cycle, when the endometrium is theoretically at its thinnest (Figure 37-24). Common hormonal regimens in menopausal women can be seen in Box 37-8. Hyperplasia is less common during the reproductive years, but may occur with persistent anovulatory cycles, with polycystic ovarian disease, and in obese women with increased production of endogenous estrogens. Hyperplasia may also be seen in women with estrogen-producing tumors, such as granulose cell tumors and thecomas of the ovary. Because hyperplasia has a nonspecific sonographic appearance, an endometrial biopsy is necessary for diagnosis. A sonohysterography can also be performed to evaluate the internal structure of the endometrial canal.

The majority of women with postmenopausal uterine bleeding have endometrial atrophy. On endovaginal sonogra-

---

BOX 37-7 **ENDOMETRIAL HYPERPLASIA**

- Follows prolonged endogenous or exogenous estrogenic stimulation
- May be precursor of endometrial cancer
- *Sonographic findings:* Abnormal thickening of endometrium

BOX 37-8 **COMMON HORMONAL REGIMENS IN MENOPAUSAL WOMEN**

1. No hormones.
2. Unopposed estrogen (usually Premarin): These women generally have had hysterectomies; if uterus is intact, unopposed estrogen is associated with increased risk for endometrial hyperplasia or carcinoma.
3. Continuous/combined estrogen and progesterone (Premarin and Provera): This combination produces endometrial atrophy after 3 to 6 months. Usually there is no risk of endometrial cancer; however, women may have "breakthrough" bleeding during the month and/or annoying progesterone side effects (i.e., irritability, depression, bloating, and breast tenderness).
4. Sequential estrogen and progesterone (Premarin first half then Provera second half of month): Women have predictable withdrawal bleeding at end of each month.

In the United States, regimens 2 and 4 are most commonly used.

BENEFICIAL EFFECTS

Estrogen
Alleviates menopausal symptoms (hot flashes, night sweats, painful intercourse)
Reduces risk of osteoporosis, vertebral and hip fractures
Reduces risk of heart attacks, strokes

Progesterone
Produces endometrial atrophy; reduces risk of endometrial hyperplasia/cancer

NEGATIVE EFFECTS

Estrogen
Increases risk of endometrial hyperplasia/cancer

Progesterone
Increases risk of breast cancer
Irritability, depression, breast tenderness in some women

---

phy, an atrophic endometrium is thin, measuring less than 5 mm. If the postmenopausal patient has irregular bleeding, 5-mm thickness may warrant a sonohysterography procedure.

Sonographic Findings. The endometrium is usually diffusely thick and echogenic with well-defined margins. Focal or asymmetrical thickening can occur. Small cysts representing dilated cystic glands may be seen within the endometrium. Although cystic changes within a thickened endometrium are more frequently seen in benign conditions, they can also be seen in endometrial carcinoma.

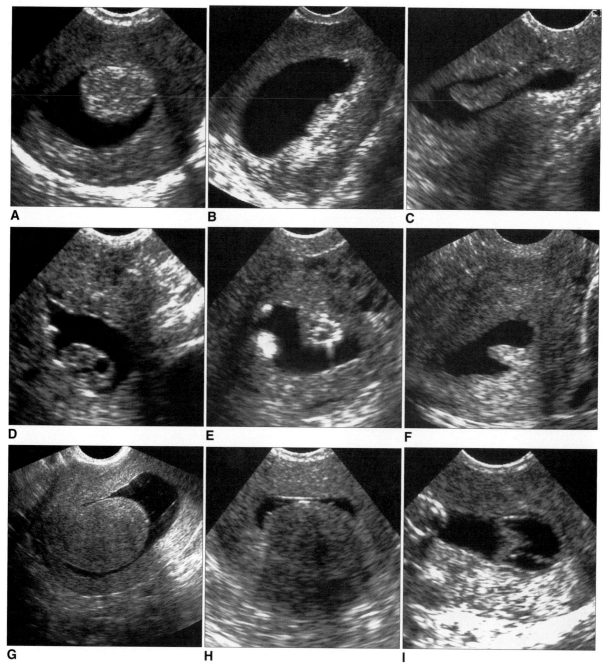

Figure 37-22 Sonohysterograms. **A,** Well-defined, round echogenic polyp. **B,** Carpet of small polyps. **C,** Polyp on a stalk. **D,** Polyp with cystic areas. **E,** Small polyp. **F,** Small polyp. **G,** Hypoechoic submucosal fibroid. **H,** Hypoechoic attenuating submucosal fibroid. **I,** Endometrial adhesions. Note bridging bands of tissue within the fluid-filled endometrial canal. (From Rumack C, Wilson S, Charboneau W: *Diagnostic ultrasound,* ed 3, St Louis, 2005, Mosby.)

ENDOMETRIAL POLYPS

Patients with **endometrial polyps** usually are asymptomatic, but some polyps may be the cause of uterine bleeding. Histologically, polyps are overgrowths of endometrial tissue covered by epithelium. They contain a variable number of glands, stroma, and blood vessels. Approximately 20% of endometrial polyps are multiple. They may be pedunculated, broad based, or have a thin stalk. They typically cause diffuse or focal endometrial thicken-

ing. They are more frequently seen in perimenopausal and postmenopausal women. In menstruating women, they may be associated with menometrorrhagia or infertility. In postmenopausal women, especially those being investigated for bleeding, the major differential considerations are hyperplasia, submucosal myomas, or, less commonly, endometrial carcinoma.

Sonographic Findings. Sonographically, polyps appear toward the end of the luteal phase and are represented by a hypoechoic region within the hyperechoic endometrium. They initially may appear as nonspecific echogenic endometrial thickening. The polyp may be diffuse or focal and may also appear as a round echogenic mass within the endometrial cavity (Figure 37-25). Cystic areas representing histologically dilated glands may be seen within a polyp. A feeding artery in the pedicle may be seen with color Doppler. Individual polyps are better visualized when outlined by intracavitary fluid. Sonohysterography is a valuable technique when endovaginal sonography is unable to differentiate an endometrial polyp from a submucosal leiomyoma.

ENDOMETRITIS

Endometrial thickening or fluid may indicate endometritis. **Endometritis** is an infection within the endometrium of the uterus. It occurs most often in association with PID, in the postpartum state, or following instrumentation invasion. In patients with pelvic infection, the uterus is the route for infection to the tubes and adnexa. Postpartum patients may develop endometritis after prolonged labor, vaginitis, premature

rupture of the membranes, or retained products of conception. Clinically, the patient has intense pelvic pain (Box 37-9).

Sonographic Findings. Sonographically the endometrium appears prominent, irregular, or both, with a small amount of endometrial fluid (Figure 37-26). Pus may be demonstrated in the cul-de-sac as echogenic particles or debris (Figure 37-27). Enlarged ovaries with multiple cysts and indistinct margins may be seen secondary to periovarian inflammation. Dilation of the fallopian tube shows fluid-filled tubular shapes in a folded configuration and well-defined echogenic walls. A thickened tubal wall (5 mm or more) is indicative of acute disease. These should be distinguished from a fluid-filled bowel by gentle compression on the pelvic wall to look for peristalsis or movement in the bowel lumen.

As the infection worsens, periovarian adhesions may form and fuse the inflamed tube and ovary, called the tubo-ovarian complex. Further progression results in a tubo-ovarian abscess that appears as a complex multiloculated mass with septations, irregular shaggy margins, and scattered internal echoes. There can be posterior enhancement and a fluid-debris level. Gas bubbles are present in rare cases; however, these also are seen in normal postpartum patients. In the immediate postpartum period, the presence of retained tissue is difficult to distinguish from inflammatory debris or blood clots. The sonographic

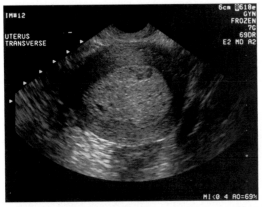

Figure 37-23 Endovaginal coronal image of the uterus with a very prominent endometrium measuring more than 23 mm. On biopsy the patient had endometrial hyperplasia.

> **BOX 37-9   ENDOMETRITIS**
>
> - Inflammation of the endometrium
> - *Clinical:* Low back pain and fever; lower abdominal pain; dysmenorrhea; menorrhagia; sterility; constipation
> - *Sonographic findings:* Endometrium appears prominent or irregular; pus may be seen in the cul-de-sac; enlarged ovaries with multiple cysts secondary to periovarian inflammation; dilated fallopian tubes

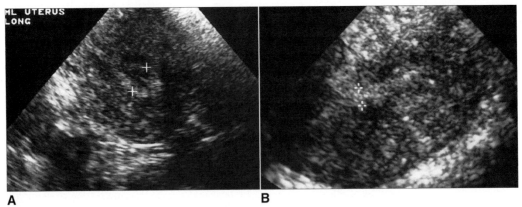

Figure 37-24 Normal variation in endometrial thickness from cyclic hormone replacement in a 62-year-old woman. **A,** Day 9, three-layer endometrium, 10-mm thick. **B,** Day 3, 4-mm thick endometrium. Women taking sequential hormones should be examined after the progesterone phase of the cycle, when the endometrium is theoretically at its thinnest. (From Levine D, Gosink BB. In Nyberg DA and others, editors: *Endovaginal ultrasound,* St Louis, 1992, Mosby.)

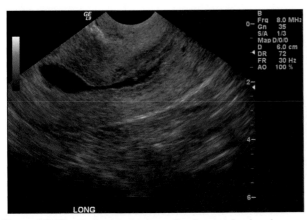

Figure 37-25   Endovaginal image of endometrial polyp shows a focal thickening within the endometrial cavity.

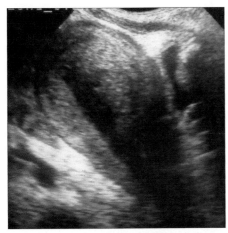

Figure 37-26   The enlarged uterus with an edematous complex endometrium in a patient who presented 10 days postoperatively with intense pelvic pain. She was diagnosed with endometritis.

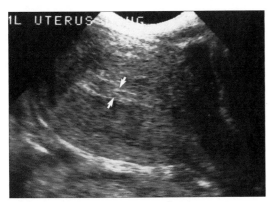

Figure 37-27   Endometritis in a 31-year-old woman. A endovaginal sagittal view of the uterus 3 days postpartum demonstrates a slightly irregular endometrium *(arrows)*.

appearance can be similar to that of other adnexal masses, so clinical correlation is very important. Sonography can also be useful in following the response to antibiotic therapy or in guided endovaginal aspirations and drainage. If the aspirate is purulent, catheter drainage is used. In chronic PID, fibrosis

and adhesions may make identification of pelvic organs difficult. Torsion of the tube is uncommon, but it occurs in association with chronic hydrosalpinx.

SYNECHIAE

Intrauterine synechiae (endometrial adhesions, Asherman's syndrome) are found in women with posttraumatic or postsurgical histories. This includes uterine curettage and may be a cause of infertility or recurrent pregnancy loss.

Sonographic Findings. Ultrasonography may demonstrate bright echoes within the endometrial cavity in this condition. The diagnosis is difficult unless fluid is distending the endometrial cavity. This is best seen during the secretory phase when the endometrium is more hyperechoic. Synechiae are more easily seen in the gravid uterus.

Sonohysterography is an excellent technique for demonstrating adhesions and should be performed in all cases of suspected adhesions. Adhesions appear as bridging bands of tissue that distort the cavity or as thin, undulating membranes. Thick, broad-based adhesions may prevent distention of the uterine cavity. Adhesions can be divided under hysteroscopy.

ENDOMETRIAL CARCINOMA

Endometrial carcinoma is the most common gynecologic malignancy in North America, and its incidence has been rising. Most endometrial malignancies are adenocarcinomas occurring in postmenopausal patients. The most common clinical presentation is uterine bleeding, although only 10% of women with postmenopausal bleeding will have endometrial carcinoma. There is a strong association with replacement estrogen therapy. In the premenopausal woman, anovulatory cycles and obesity are also considered risk factors. The earliest change of endometrial carcinoma is a thickened endometrium (Figure 37-28). An abnormally thick endometrium also is associated with endometrial hypertrophy and polyps.

Recent studies of patients with postmenopausal bleeding show that an endometrial thickness (double layer) of less than 5 mm reliably excludes significant endometrial abnormality.[1-4] At present, most investigators believe biopsies should be performed for all symptomatic patients. In the future, however, endovaginal ultrasonography may be used to follow symptomatic patients with normal endometrial thickness for whom biopsy is contraindicated or who do not wish to undergo an invasive procedure.

Although increased endometrial thickness is an early finding in endometrial carcinoma, enlargement with lobular contour of the uterus and mixed echogenicity are correlated with more advanced stages of the disease. The risk of malignancy increases with the presence of a large endometrial fluid collection or clinical symptoms, such as abdominal pain or bleeding.

Sonographic Findings. Endovaginal examination is helpful in screening for early changes of endometrial hyperplasia or carcinoma by accurately measuring endometrial thickness. Sonographically, a thickened endometrium (greater than 4 to 5 mm) must be considered cancer until proven otherwise. Demonstration of myometrial invasion is clear evidence for endometrial carcinoma. Endovaginal ultrasonography

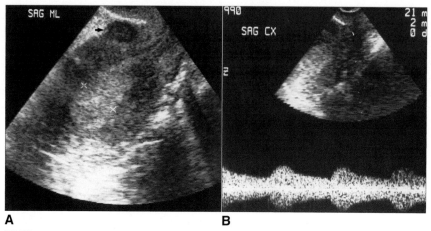

Figure 37-28 Endometrial carcinoma in a 52-year-old woman. **A,** Sagittal view of the uterus demonstrates a 2-cm thick endometrium. A small myoma *(arrow)* is also present. **B,** Doppler examination of the uterine artery shows abnormal increased diastolic flow (resistive index, 0.5).

> ### BOX 37-10 ENDOMETRIAL CARCINOMA
>
> - Associated with estrogen stimulation
> - *Clinical:* Postmenopausal bleeding
> - *Sonographic findings:* Prominent endometrial complex; enlarged uterus with irregular areas of low-level echoes

demonstrates myometrial invasion as thickening and irregularity of the central endometrial interface with echogenic or hypoechoic patterns combined with infiltration of hyperdense structures in the myometrium (Box 37-10). Cystic changes within the endometrium are more commonly seen in endometrial atrophy, hyperplasia, and polyps, but can also be seen with carcinoma.

Endometrial carcinoma may obstruct the endometrial canal, resulting in **hydrometra** or **hematometra.** The level of myometrial invasion (superficial versus deep) also can be detected by endovaginal ultrasonography, although contrast-enhanced MRI is more sensitive. Intactness of the subendometrial halo (the inner layer of myometrium) usually indicates superficial invasion, whereas obliteration of the halo is indicative of deep invasion. Magnetic resonance imaging is also valuable in evaluating extrauterine extension and involvement of lymph nodes.

Tamoxifen, a nonsteroidal antiestrogen compound, is widely used for adjuvant therapy in premenopausal and postmenopausal women with breast cancer. An increased risk of endometrial carcinoma, hyperplasia, and polyps has been reported in patients on tamoxifen therapy. On sonography, tamoxifen-related endometrial changes are nonspecific and similar to those described in hyperplasia, polyps, and carcinoma. Because it may be difficult to distinguish the endometrial-myometrial border in many of these patients, sonohysterography is valuable.

Sonography may be helpful in staging carcinoma and in distinguishing between tumors limited to the uterus (stages I and II) and those with extrauterine extension (stages III and IV). Both MRI and CT are useful in staging by demonstrating lymphadenopathy and distant disease (stages III or IV). Endometrial biopsy is usually required for a definite diagnosis.

Doppler Evaluation. The role of color and spectral Doppler in the diagnosis of endometrial carcinoma is controversial. Doppler ultrasonography of the uterine artery may help distinguish benign from malignant endometrial thickening. Pulsed Doppler is used to evaluate the resistive index (RI = peak systolic − end diastolic/peak systolic) or pulsatility index (PI = peak systolic − end diastolic/mean). The technique of this examination is discussed in Chapter 36. Low-resistance flow (RI < 0.4) has been found in patients with endometrial carcinoma and high-resistance flow (RI > 0.5) in normal or benign endometria. If a pulsatility index is used, the cutoff is 1. Intratumoral neovascularity is a more sensitive marker of endometrial carcinoma than resistive index alone.

SMALL ENDOMETRIAL FLUID COLLECTIONS

Small endometrial fluid collections also occur with ectopic pregnancy, endometritis, degenerating myomas, and recent abortion (Figure 37-29).

Sonographic Findings. Endovaginal sonography, with its improved resolution, sometimes shows tiny endometrial fluid collections not seen on transabdominal scans. These small endometrial fluid collections (less than 2 ml) are common in women during the menstrual phase of the cycle. They are seen in postmenopausal women, especially during the menstrual phase in women taking sequential hormones. In a uterus with a fluid collection, the anteroposterior diameter of the fluid should be subtracted from the endometrial measurement for a true assessment of endometrial thickness.

LARGE ENDOMETRIAL FLUID COLLECTIONS

Large endometrial fluid collections should be regarded with suspicion. Obstruction of the genital tract results in the accu-

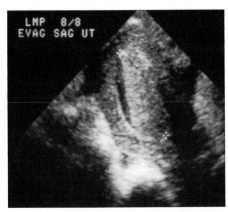

Figure 37-29 Endovaginal image in a 23-year-old woman after a dilation and curettage demonstrates a central fluid collection with a fluid debris level representing a hematometra.

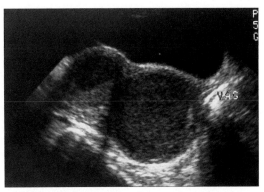

Figure 37-30 Large endometrial fluid collection. Endovaginal ultrasound image of obstructed right horn of a bicornuate uterus. This 63-year-old asymptomatic woman, placed on cyclic hormone replacement therapy, demonstrates a large endometrial fluid collection. She subsequently underwent dilation for cervical stenosis, and bloody fluid was drained. Biopsy was unremarkable. (From Levine D, Gosink BB. In Nyberg DA, and others, editors: *Endovaginal ultrasound,* St Louis, 1992, Mosby.)

mulation of secretions, blood, or both in the uterus. Before menstruation, the accumulation of secretions is referred to as hydrometrocolpos. Following menstruation, hematometrocolpos results from the presence of retained menstrual blood. The obstruction may be congenital, imperforate hymen (most common), vaginal septum, vaginal atresia, or a rudimentary uterine horn. Hydrometra and hematometra may also be acquired as a result of cervical stenosis from endometrial or cervical tumors or from postirradiation fibrosis. They may also be caused by uterine, cervical, tubal, or ovarian carcinoma. Hyperplasia and polyps also cause endometrial fluid collections, so these collections also indicate increased risk of endometrial carcinoma. However, large amounts of endometrial fluid also are associated with benign conditions, such as congenital anomalies (Figure 37-30) or cervical stenosis from prior instrumentation or childbirth.

The patient typically complains of abdominal pain and has a globular abdominal mass. She usually has little or no vaginal bleeding. The presence of fever suggests infection of the blood collection. Lab results show an elevated white blood count. In simple hematometra the uterine cavity returns to normal promptly after dilation and curettage. **Pyometra** is more likely to occur with uterine cancer. Abnormal development of the vagina or uterus may result in a cystic uterine or vaginal collection of mucus in children. When menstruation begins, the collection consists of blood.

Sonographic Findings. The sonographic picture of large endometrial cavity fluid collections is that of a centrally cystic, round, moderately enlarged uterus. This may contain echogenic material if pus or blood is present.

INTRAUTERINE CONTRACEPTIVE DEVICES

LOST INTRAUTERINE DEVICE

Intrauterine contraceptive devices (IUCDs) are devices placed in the uterine cavity during menses for the purpose of birth control. Proper placement is verified by weekly digital palpation of the string in the cervix, performed by the patient. If the string is not felt in the cervix, the IUCD may have been expelled or more likely the string has fallen off or retracted into the uterus. A pregnancy test is performed. If it is negative, the gynecologist explores the uterine cavity with a sterile hooked probe. If no string is found or if the pregnancy test is positive, an ultrasound examination is performed. Sonography can demonstrate malposition, perforation, and incomplete removal of the IUCD. Eccentric position of an IUCD suggests myometrial penetration. If the IUCD is not seen by sonography, a radiograph should be done. The IUCD may be difficult to see with coexisting intrauterine abnormalities, such as blood clots or an incomplete abortion. In the first trimester, the IUCD can usually be removed safely under ultrasound guidance. After the first trimester, an IUCD is very difficult to visualize. Patients with IUCDs are at increased risk for ectopic pregnancy and pelvic inflammatory disease. In these women, tubo-ovarian abscess (TOA) may be unilateral; more commonly, though, it is bilateral.

Sonographic Findings. Transabdominal and endovaginal scanning demonstrate the IUCD. The device appears as highly echogenic linear structures in the endometrial cavity within the uterine body. Do not confuse them with the normal, central endometrial echoes. An analysis of in vivo and in vitro transabdominal images of the many types of IUCDs previously used in the United States found that the shafts of all of them appeared as a double line. This is because of entrance-exit reflections of sound waves when scanned perpendicular to the uterine cavity with high-resolution equipment. Posterior shadowing occurs when the ultrasound beam is entirely interrupted. This requires that the scanning plane be placed perpendicular to the IUCD.

The Copper 7 is shaped like a 7, with a copper wire spiraled around the vertical shaft. The Tatum T and Progestasert are T-shaped (Figures 37-31 and 37-32), and the Lippes loop is serpentine. Occasionally a thick midcycle endometrium

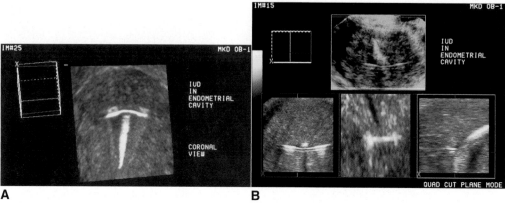

Figure 37-31   **A,** Three-dimensional reconstruction of a safety coil intrauterine contraceptive device located within the uterine cavity. **B,** X, Y, and Z axes of the IUCD.

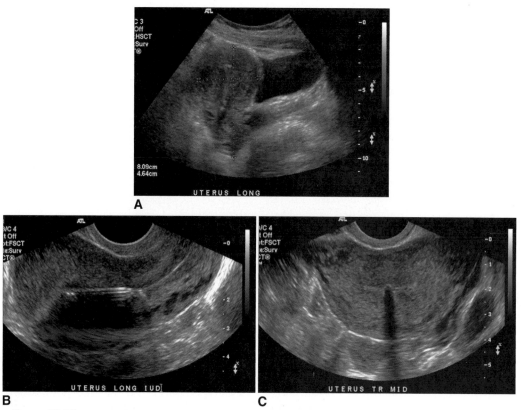

Figure 37-32   IUCD device in uterine cavity. **A,** Transabdominal longitudinal midline image shows the IUCD implanted within the central uterine cavity. **B,** Endovaginal long shows the IUCD with shadowing posterior. **C,** EV transverse image of the IUCD shadowing within the uterine cavity.

obscures the bright IUCD echo when transabdominal ultrasonography is used. If no intrauterine IUCD is identified on ultrasound examination and the pregnancy test is negative, a thin metal probe is inserted into the uterine cavity to mark it, and abdominal x-ray films are obtained to search for the IUCD in an extrauterine location (Figure 37-33). Perforation of the uterus by an IUCD almost always occurs at the time of insertion. The displaced IUCD may not be suspected until an abscess or painful bowel involvement occurs.

When a pregnancy is present, either transabdominal or endovaginal ultrasound examination demonstrates both gestational age and the location of the IUCD. Occasionally a string is visible in the external os of a pregnant uterus. Approximately 50% of pregnancies abort on extraction of the IUCD. With endovaginal scanning, the location of the IUCD can be detected relative to the sac, and it may be possible to predict which pregnancy will be disrupted. Intrauterine contraceptive devices are always external to fetal membranes.

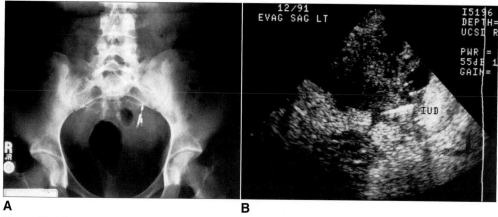

A   **B**

Figure 37-33   Extrauterine location of IUCD in a 25-year-old woman with abdominal pain. Patient was unable to feel the string of the IUCD. **A,** Plain film of the abdomen shows the extrauterine location of the IUCD. **B,** Left parasagittal view demonstrates a linear echogenic focus consistent with the IUCD located outside the uterus.

REFERENCES

1. Carlson JA Jr and others: Clinical and pathologic correlation of endometrial cavity fluid detected by ultrasound in the postmenopausal patient, *Obstet Gynecol* 77:119, 1991.
2. Goldstein SR and others: Endometrial assessment by vaginal ultrasonography before endometrial sampling in patients with postmenopausal bleeding, *Am J Obstet Gynecol* 163:119, 1990.
3. Karlsson B, Granberg S, Wikland M and others: Endovaginal ultrasonography of the endometrium in women with postmenopausal bleeding: a Nordic multicenter study, *Am J Obstet Gynceol* 172:1488-1494, 1995.
4. Varner RE and others: Endovaginal sonography of the endometrium in postmenopausal women, *Obstet Gynecol* 78:195, 1991.

SELECTED BIBLIOGRAPHY

Aartsen EJ: Fluid detection in the uterus during and after irradiation for carcinoma of the cervix: clinical implications, *Eur J Surg Oncol* 16:42, 1990.

Atri M, Nazarnia S, Aldis AE and others: Endovaginal US appearance of endometrial abnormalities, *RadioGraphics* 14:483-492, 1994.

Becker E Jr, Lev-Toaff AS, Jaufman EP and others: The added value of transvaginal sonohysterography over transvaginal sonography alone in women with known or suspected leiomyoma, *J Ultrasound Med* 21:237-247, 2002.

Bernaschek G and others: *Endosonography in obstetrics and gynecology,* Berlin, 1990, Springer-Verlag.

Blask ARN and others: Obstructed uterovaginal anomalies: demonstration with sonography. I, Neonates and infants, *Radiology* 179:79, 1991.

Bromley B, Shipp TD, Benacerraf B: Adenomyosis: sonographic findings and diagnostic accuracy, *J Ultrasound Med* 10:529-534, 2000.

Burks DD and others: Uterine inner myometrial echogenic foci: relationship to prior dilatation and curettage and trans-cervical biopsy, *J Ultrasound Med* 10:487, 1991.

Caoili EM, Hertzberg BS, Liewer MA and others: Refractory shadowing from pelvic masses on sonography: a useful diagnostic sign for uterine leiomyomas, *AJR* 174:97-101, 2000.

Cotran RS and others: *Robbins pathologic basis of disease,* Philadelphia, 1989, WB Saunders.

Davis PC, O'Neill MJ, Yoder IC and others: Sonohysterographic findings of endometrial and subendometrial conditions, *Radiographics* 22:803-816, 2002.

Doubilet PM: Society of Radiologists in Ultrasound consensus conference statement on postmenopausal bleeding. Commentary, *J Ultrasound Med* 20:1037-1042, 2001.

Fedele L, Bianchi S, Dorta M and others: Endovaginal ultrasonography in the differential diagnosis of adenomyoma versus leiomyoma, *Am J Obstet Gynecol* 167:603-606, 1992.

Goldberg BB and others: *Ultrasound measurements,* St Louis, 1990, Mosby.

Granberg S and others: Endometrial thickness as measured by endovaginal ultrasonography for identifying endometrial abnormality, *Am J Obstet Gynecol* 164:47, 1991.

Grunfeld L and others: High-resolution endovaginal ultrasonography of the endometrium: a noninvasive test for endometrial adequacy, *Obstet Gynecol* 78:200, 1991.

Hata K and others: Sonographic findings of uterine leiomyosarcoma, *Gynecol Obstet Invest* 30:242, 1990.

Hertzberg BS, Kliewer MA, George P and others: Lipomatous uterine masses: potential to mimic ovarian dermoids on endovaginal sonography, *J Ultrasound Med* 14:689-692, 1995.

Karasick S and others: Imaging of uterine leiomyomas, *Am J Roentgenol* 158:799, 1992.

Kliewer MA, Hertzberg BS, George PY: Acoustic shadowing from uterine leiomyomas: sonographic-pathologic correlation, *Radiology* 196:99-102, 1995.

Kupfer MC and others: Endovaginal sonographic appearance of endometriomata: spectrum of findings, *J Ultrasound Med* 11:129, 1992.

Kurjak A and others: The characterization of uterine tumors by endovaginal color Doppler, *Ultrasound Obstet Gynecol* 1:50, 1991.

Kurman RJ. *Blaustein's pathology of the female genital tract,* ed 4, New York, 1994, Springer-Verlag.

Lin MC and others: Endometrial thickness after menopause of hormone replacement, *Radiology* 180:427, 1991.

Lyons EA and others: Characterization of subendometrial myometrial contractions throughout the menstrual cycle in normal fertile women, *Fertil Steril* 55:85, 1991.

Occhipinti K and others: Sonographic appearance and significance of arcuate artery calcification, *J Ultrasound Med* 10:97, 1991.

Platt JF, Bree RL, Davidson D: Ultrasound of the normal non-gravid uterus; correlation with gross and histopathology, *J Clin Ultrasound* 18:15-19, 1990.

Rosati P and others: Longitudinal evaluation of uterine myoma growth during pregnancy: a sonographic study, *J Ultrasound Med* 11:511, 1992.

Rumack CM, Wilson SR, Charboneau JW: *Diagnostic ultrasound*, ed 3, St Louis, 2005, Mosby.

Wachsberg RH and others: Gas within the endometrial cavity at postpartum US: a normal finding after spontaneous vaginal delivery, *Radiology* 183:431, 1992.

CHAPTER 38

Pathology of the Ovaries

Barbara J. Vander Werff and Sandra L. Hagen-Ansert

OBJECTIVES

- Describe the effect of hormones on the ovarian cycle
- Define the characteristics of the simple ovarian cyst
- Discuss the sonographic findings of the common cystic and the complex ovarian masses
- Discuss the sonographic findings of the common solid ovarian masses
- Describe a functional ovarian cyst
- List the characteristics found in polycystic ovarian disease
- Discuss the benign pelvic masses found in neonates and adolescent girls
- Describe the sonographic findings in ovarian neoplasms
- Differentiate between mucinous and serous types of tumors
- Discuss the sonographic findings in a dermoid tumor
- Define the Doppler parameters used in ovarian torsion
- Discuss the role of ultrasonography with infertility patients

ANATOMY OF THE OVARIES

NORMAL SONOGRAPHIC APPEARANCE

SONOGRAPHIC EVALUATION OF THE OVARIES

SIMPLE CYSTIC MASSES
COMPLEX MASSES
SOLID TUMORS
DOPPLER OF THE OVARY

BENIGN ADNEXAL CYSTS

FUNCTIONAL OVARIAN CYSTS
OVARIAN SYNDROMES
OTHER BENIGN OVARIAN CYSTS

ENDOMETRIOSIS

OVARIAN TORSION

SONOGRAPHIC EVALUATION OF OVARIAN NEOPLASMS

OVARIAN CARCINOMA

DOPPLER FINDINGS IN OVARIAN CANCER

EPITHELIAL TUMORS

MUCINOUS CYSTADENOMA
MUCINOUS CYSTADENOCARCINOMA
SEROUS CYSTADENOMA
SEROUS CYSTADENOCARCINOMA
OTHER EPITHELIAL TUMORS

GERM CELL TUMORS

TERATOMA
IMMATURE AND MATURE TERATOMAS
DYSGERMINOMA
ENDODERMAL SINUS TUMOR

STROMAL TUMORS

FIBROMA AND THECOMA
GRANULOSA
SERTOLI-LEYDIG CELL TUMOR
ARRHENOBLASTOMA
METASTATIC DISEASE

CARCINOMA OF THE FALLOPIAN TUBE

OTHER PELVIC MASSES

KEY TERMS

androgen – substance that stimulates the development of male characteristics, such as the hormones testosterone and androsterone

corpus luteum cyst – a small endocrine structure that develops within a ruptured ovarian follicle and secretes progesterone and estrogen

cystadenocarcinoma – a malignant tumor that forms cysts

cystadenoma – a benign adenoma containing cysts

dermoid tumor – benign tumor comprised of hair, muscle, teeth, and fat

endometriosis – a condition that occurs when functioning endometrial tissue invades other sites outside the uterus

estrogen – the female hormone produced by the ovary

follicular cyst – benign cyst within the ovary that may occur and disappear on a cyclic basis

functional cyst – results from the normal function of the ovary

Meigs' syndrome – benign tumor of the ovary associated with ascites and pleural effusion

mucinous cystadenocarcinoma – malignant tumor of the ovary with multilocular cysts

mucinous cystadenoma – benign tumor of the ovary that contains thin-walled multilocular cysts

ovarian carcinoma – malignant tumor of the ovary that may spread beyond the ovary and metastasize to other organs via the peritoneal channels

ovarian torsion – partial or complete rotation of the ovarian pedicle on its axis

paraovarian cyst – cystic structure that lies adjacent to the ovary

polycystic ovarian syndrome (PCOS) – endocrine disorder associated with chronic anovulation

pulsatility index (PI) – peak-systolic velocity minus end-diastolic velocity divided by the mean velocity

resistive index (RI) – peak-systolic velocity minus the end-diastolic velocity divided by the peak-systolic velocity

serous cystadenocarcinoma – most common type of ovarian carcinoma; may be bilateral with multilocular cysts

serous cystadenoma – second most common benign tumor of the ovary; unilocular or multilocular

simple ovarian cyst – smooth, well-defined cystic structure that is filled completely with fluid

surface epithelial-stromal tumors – gynecologic tumors that arise from the surface epithelium and cover the ovary and the underlying stroma

theca-lutein cysts – multilocular cysts that occur in patients with hyperstimulation (hydatidiform mole and infertility patients)

Ultrasonography is clinically useful to characterize adnexal masses, evaluate abnormal bleeding, assess infertility, monitor follicular growth, perform endovaginal needle aspiration and biopsy, and screen for ovarian carcinoma. Both transabdominal and endovaginal sonography are important in these evaluations. Transabdominal imaging furnishes a global survey of anatomy, whereas endovaginal imaging provides better characterization of internal architecture of the ovary, vascular anatomy, and adnexal area. It is important to note that information from the clinical pelvic examination is required for optimal interpretation of the ultrasound studies, thus necessitating good communication between the referring physician and the sonologist.

A woman will ovulate nearly 400 times in her reproductive life, and a quarter of a million follicles will be stimulated to varying degrees over this time. It is not surprising that an organ as dynamic as the ovary can form more than 100 different types of tumors, both benign and malignant. These masses are described on ultrasound examination as primarily cystic, complex, or predominantly solid; however, the final diagnosis is left to the pathologist. Precise diagnosis on the basis of ultrasonography alone is usually impossible. The primary role of sonography is to indicate the need for surgical or medical intervention.

ANATOMY OF THE OVARIES

The ovaries are paired, almond-shaped structures situated one on each side of the uterus close to the lateral pelvic wall (Figure 38-1). The ovaries can be quite variable in position and are influenced by the uterine location and the ligament attachments. In the anteflexed midline uterus, the ovaries are usually identified laterally or posterolaterally. When the uterus lies to one side of the midline, the ipsilateral ovary often lies superior to uterine fundus. In a retroverted uterus, the ovaries tend to be lateral and superior, near the uterine fundus. When the uterus is enlarged, the ovaries tend to be displaced more superiorly and laterally. Following hysterectomy, the ovaries tend to be located more medially and directly superior to the vaginal cuff. They can be located high in the pelvis or in the cul-de-sac. Superiorly or extremely laterally placed ovaries may not be visualized by the endovaginal approach because they are out of the field of view. Ovaries are ellipsoid in shape, with their craniocaudad axes paralleling the internal iliac vessels, which lie posterior and serve as a reference point.

NORMAL SONOGRAPHIC APPEARANCE

The normal ovary has a homogeneous echotexture, which may exhibit a central, more echogenic medulla. Small anechoic or cystic follicles may be seen peripherally in the cortex (Figure 38-2). The appearance of the ovary varies with age and the menstrual cycle (Figure 38-3). During the reproductive years, three phases are recognized ultrasonically during each menstrual cycle. During the early proliferative phase, many follicles develop and increase in size until about day 8 or 9 of the menstrual cycle. This is due to stimulation by both follicle-stimulating hormone (FSH) and luteinizing hormone (LH). At that time one follicle becomes dominant, reaching up to 2.0 to 2.5 cm at the time of ovulation. The cumulus oophorus may occasionally be detected as an eccentrically located, cystlike, 1-mm internal mural protrusion. Although visualization of the cumulus indicates a mature follicle and imminent ovulation, no reproducible sonographic sign is reliable. The other follicles become atretic. A **follicular cyst** develops if the fluid in the nondominant follicles is not reabsorbed. Usually the dominant follicle disappears immediately after rupture at ovulation. Occasionally the follicle decreases in size and develops a wall that appears crenulated (scalloped). The occurrence of fluid in

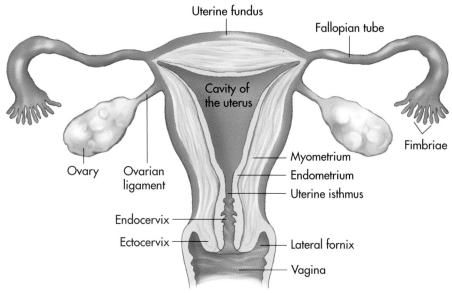

Uterine fundus

Fallopian tube

Cavity of
the uterus

Myometrium

Endometrium

Uterine isthmus

Fimbriae

Ovary

Ovarian
ligament

Endocervix

Ectocervix

Lateral fornix

Vagina

Figure 38-1   Normal anatomy of the female pelvis. Note the relationship of the ovaries to the lateral walls of the uterus and the position of the fallopian tubes to the ovaries.

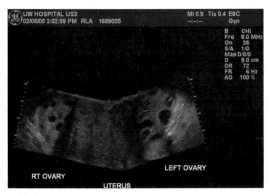

Figure 38-2   Normal endovaginal image of the ovaries with multiple follicles.

the cul-de-sac is commonly seen after ovulation and peaks in the early luteal phase. Following ovulation in the luteal phase, a mature corpus luteum develops and may be identified sonographically as a small hypoechoic or isoechoic structure peripherally within the ovary. It may appear irregular with echogenic crenulated walls and contain low-level echoes. Less frequent appearances include a typical "ring" color flow Doppler pattern around the wall of an isoechoic corpus luteum. In the absence of fertilization, the corpus luteum begins to undergo involutional changes on postovulatory days 8 or 9 and disappears shortly before or with the onset of menstruation.

Multiple small, punctate, echogenic foci are commonly seen in the normal ovary. These foci are reported to be a common finding with endovaginal ultrasound examination. They are generally very small (1 to 2 mm) and located in the periphery. The foci are nonshadowing and can be multiple. A possible source of these foci of specular reflection is from the walls of tiny unresolved cysts below the spatial resolution of ultrasound. More central punctate echogenic foci are thought to represent stromal reaction to previous hemorrhage or infec-

tion. Since they do not indicate significant underlying disease, no follow-up is necessary.

Following menopause the ovary atrophies and the follicles disappear with increasing age. For this reason, the postmenopausal ovary may be very difficult to visualize sonographically because of the smaller size and lack of discrete follicles. A stationary loop of the bowel may mimic a small shrunken ovary, so scanning must be done slowly to look for peristalsis. After a hysterectomy, the ovaries can be difficult to visualize with ultrasound. The use of both transabdominal and endovaginal approaches increases the chance of visualization.

Because of the variability in ovarian shape and size, the volume measurement is the best method for determining overall ovarian size. The volume measurement is based on the prolate ellipse formula ($0.523 \times$ length $\times$ width $\times$ height). In the adult menstruating female, a normal ovary may have a volume as large as 22 cc^3, with a mean ovarian volume of 9.8 $\pm$ 5.8 cc. An ovarian volume of more than 8.0 cc is definitely considered abnormal for the postmenopausal patient. An ovarian volume more than twice that of the opposite side should also be considered abnormal, regardless of the actual size. Three-dimensional (3-D) ultrasound techniques may provide the most accurate method of ovarian volume measurement by allowing accurate determination of the ovarian long axis and objective calculation of stromal and cystic volume components. Further development in this technology will define more future applications.

SONOGRAPHIC EVALUATION OF THE OVARIES

SIMPLE CYSTIC MASSES

The ovary's function is to mature oocytes until ovulation under the influence of luteinizing hormone and follicle-stimulating hormone from the pituitary. At the same time, the ovary

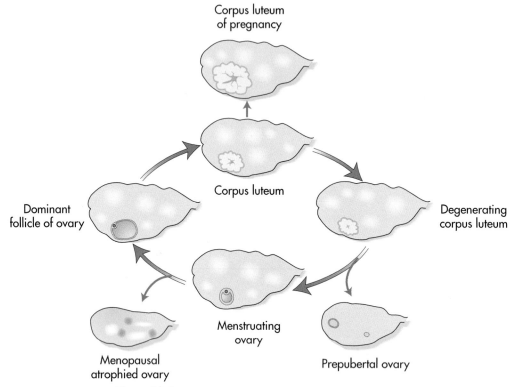

Figure 38-3   Diagram of cyclic changes of the normal ovary.

synthesizes **androgens** (male hormones) and converts them to **estrogens** (female hormones). Finally, it produces progesterone after ovulation to sustain early pregnancy until the placenta can do so at 10 to 12 weeks of gestation.

Usually only one follicle enlarges from 3 mm to approximately 24 mm over about 10 days in the mid- and late-follicular phases of the cycle. This is followed by ovulation. The resulting corpus luteum or an abnormal unruptured follicle can persist as a webbed cystic structure from 1 to 10 cm in size. These so-called functional cysts may produce discomfort and/or delayed menses but can be observed to regress within 8 weeks with serial ultrasound studies. If a cyst greater than 6 cm persists more than 8 weeks, surgical intervention is usually considered necessary.

Ultrasonically guided needle aspiration has become popular for deflating recurrent **simple ovarian cysts** in carefully selected cases. The majority of ovarian masses are simple cysts, most of which are benign. Sonographic criteria for a simple cyst include a thin smooth wall, anechoic contents, and acoustic enhancement (Figure 38-4, *A*). In premenopausal women these cysts usually are functional. The differential considerations of simple adnexal cysts include functional cyst, paraovarian cyst, cystadenoma, cystic teratoma, endometrioma, and rarely tubo-ovarian abscess (TOA) (Box 38-1).

Small anechoic cysts may be seen in postmenopausal ovaries. They can disappear or change in size over time. Serial sonographic studies can monitor the size or any changes. Surgery is generally recommended for postmenopausal cysts greater than 5 cm and for those containing internal septations and/or solid nodules.

BOX 38-1   COMMON CYSTIC OR COMPLEX OVARIAN MASS

- Follicular cyst
- Corpus luteum cyst of pregnancy
- Cystic teratoma
- Paraovarian cyst
- Hydrosalpinx
- Endometrioma (low-level echoes)
- Hemorrhagic cyst

COMPLEX MASSES

Any simple cyst that hemorrhages may appear as a complex mass (Box 38-2). In patients of reproductive age, the classic differential considerations of a complex adnexal mass are ectopic pregnancy, endometriosis, and pelvic inflammatory disease (PID) (Figure 38-4, *B*). Dermoids and other benign tumors can appear in a similar fashion.

SOLID TUMORS

Mixed solid to cystic ovarian masses are typical of all the epithelial ovarian tumors; the most common are the serous types: **cystadenoma** and **cystadenocarcinoma** (Figure 38-4, *C*). During the peak fertile years, only 1 in 15 is malignant; this ratio becomes 1 in 3 after age 40.

The more sonographically complex the tumor, the more likely it is to be malignant, especially if associated with ascites. The epithelium of serous tumors is tubal in type, and there

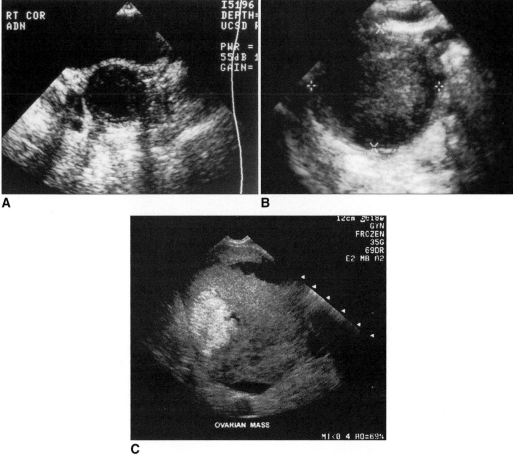

Figure 38-4 **A,** Simple ovarian cyst. Endovaginal coronal image of the corpus luteum cyst (just posterior to the bladder) in the right adnexal area. The cyst is well defined and anechoic, with increased through-transmission. **B,** Complex ovarian cyst. Endovaginal coronal image of a simple cyst that has hemorrhaged; this mass had resolved spontaneously when the patient was rescanned 2 weeks later. The borders of the mass are well defined; there are low-level internal echoes within the mass. On real-time imaging, swirling of these echoes could be seen. **C,** Solid mass. Endovaginal sagittal image of a large, solid ovarian mass in a 56-year-old woman. The mass has irregular borders with a heterogeneous texture and decreased through-transmission.

BOX
38-2
COMMON COMPLEX MASSES

- Cystadenoma
- Dermoid cyst
- Tubo-ovarian abscess
- Ectopic pregnancy
- Granulosa cell tumor

BOX
38-3
COMMON SOLID MASSES

- Solid teratoma
- Adenocarcinoma
- Arrhenoblastoma
- Fibroma
- Dysgerminoma
- Torsion

---

may be one or multiple cysts. One fourth of them are bilateral, and most occur in women over age 40. They are large and often fill the pelvic cavity.

The differential considerations of a solid-appearing adnexal mass include pedunculated fibroid, dermoid, fibroma, thecoma, granulosa cell tumor, Brenner tumor, and metastasis. Tubo-ovarian abscess, ovarian torsion, hemorrhagic cysts, and ectopic pregnancy also may appear solid. Solid adnexal masses are often difficult to diagnose because normal ovarian size varies widely. However, an ovary with a volume twice that of the opposite side is generally considered abnormal. When a solid mass is found, care should be taken to identify a connection with the uterus to differentiate an ovarian lesion from a pedunculated fibroid (Box 38-3).

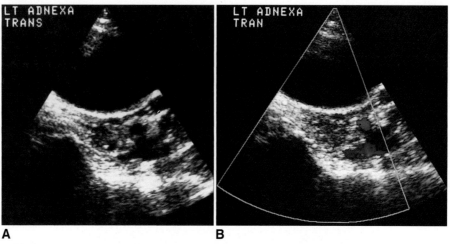

Figure 38-5 Usefulness of color Doppler to distinguish cysts from vessels. **A,** Transabdominal transverse view of the left adnexa demonstrates multiple hypoechoic regions adjacent to the adnexa. **B,** Color Doppler demonstrates flow within these areas consistent with vessels.

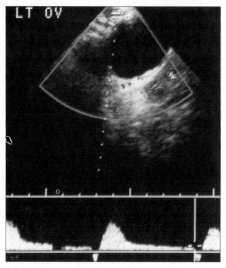

Figure 38-6 Simple cyst. Coronal view of the right ovary in an asymptomatic 52-year-old woman demonstrates a 3-cm simple cyst. Ovarian artery Doppler shows a normal resistive pattern with low diastolic flow. (From Levine D, Gosink BB. In Nyberg DA and others, editors: *Endovaginal ultrasound,* St Louis, 1992, Mosby.)

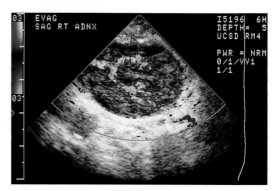

Figure 38-7 Endovaginal color Doppler view of the right adnexa in a woman during the luteal phase. Note the prominent flow to the ovary during this phase of the cycle.

DOPPLER OF THE OVARY

When any abnormality of the ovary is detected, including a cyst, Doppler examination should be performed. In the case of cysts, color Doppler is helpful in differentiating a potential cyst from adjacent vascular structures (Figure 38-5). Color also can be used to localize flow for pulsed Doppler, which should be obtained on all ovarian masses. Pulsed Doppler interrogation of the adnexal branch of the uterine artery, the ovarian artery, or intratumoral flow is performed to determine the resistive index or pulsatility index (Figure 38-6). Patients with normal menstrual cycles are best scanned in the first 10 days of the cycle; this avoids confusion with normal changes in intraovarian blood flow because high diastolic flow occurs in the luteal phase (Figure 38-7).

A debate in the literature exists regarding the value of an RI in distinguishing between benign and malignant adnexal masses. The largest study in the literature uses a cutoff of greater than 0.4 as a normal RI in a nonfunctioning ovary.[7] Other investigators employ a PI of greater than 1 as normal.[1,5] Intratumoral vessels, low-resistance flow, and absence of a normal diastolic notch in the Doppler waveform are all signs that are worrisome for malignancy. However, abnormal waveforms can be seen in inflammatory masses, metabolically active masses (including ectopic pregnancy), and corpus luteum cysts. The most significant problem in the use of an RI is that it is not a sensitive indicator of malignancy. One study found a low RI in only 25% of malignant lesions.[8]

The color Doppler central distribution of the small arteries within an ovarian mass may be an important factor in malignancy. Two pulsed Doppler indices have been analyzed, comparing the relative amount of diastolic to systolic components of their arterial waveforms. The **pulsatility index (PI)** is calculated as peak-systolic velocity minus end-diastolic velocity divided by the mean velocity. The **resistive index (RI)** is the peak-systolic velocity minus the end-diastolic velocity divided by the peak-systolic velocity. Although these indices have different cut-off values, increased diastolic flow suggests neovascularity and the likelihood of malignancy. The cut-off value for the PI is 1.0 and the value for the RI is 0.4, with malignancy considered more likely below and benign disease more likely above these values. Inflammatory masses, active endocrine tumors, and trophoblastic disease (ectopic pregnancies) may give low indices, thus mimicking cancer.

A mass showing a complete absence of or very little diastolic flow (very elevated RI and PI values) is usually benign. A diastolic notch in early diastole may also be a sign of benign disease. This finding is not often noted and its absence has no diagnostic value.

The PI and RI values may vary considerably in the fertile patient during the menstrual cycle, and this can complicate the pulsed Doppler analysis. In the first 7 days, the flow to the ovaries has the greatest resistance with the lowest diastolic flow and the indices are at their highest. Later in each cycle, the diastolic flow increases, particularly to the dominant ovary and may lower the indices sufficiently to falsely suggest a malignant process. A Doppler study can be performed at any time during the cycle. If the indices are in the benign range, they do not need repeating. However, if a suspicious mass is present and the indices suggest possible malignancy and are expected to affect management, a repeat study should be performed to confirm the abnormal indices in the first week of another cycle.

BENIGN ADNEXAL CYSTS

FUNCTIONAL OVARIAN CYSTS

Functional cysts result from the normal function of the ovary. They are the most common cause of ovarian enlargement in young women. Functional cysts include follicular, corpus luteum, hemorrhagic, and theca-lutein cysts. Hormonal therapy is sometimes administered to suppress a cyst. Most cysts measure less than 5 cm in diameter and regress during the subsequent menstrual cycle. A follow-up ultrasound examination in 6 weeks usually documents change in size.

Follicular Cysts. A follicular cyst forms when a mature follicle fails to ovulate or involute (Box 38-4). These cysts are usually unilateral, asymptomatic, and less than 2 cm in size, but they can be as large as 20 cm in diameter. They regress spontaneously and are frequently detected incidentally on sonographic examinations.

Corpus Luteum Cysts. Corpus luteum cysts result from failure of absorption or from excess bleeding into the corpus luteum. These cysts usually are less than 4 cm in diameter and are unilateral. They are prone to hemorrhage and rupture. The presenting feature is often pain. If the ovum is fertilized, the corpus luteum continues as the corpus luteum of pregnancy during the first trimester of pregnancy, when maximum size is reached by 10 weeks, and resolution occurs by 16 weeks (Box 38-5).

Sonographic Findings. Because of the hemorrhagic nature of these cysts, they usually appear as complex masses with central blood clot and echogenic septations (Figure 38-8). This appearance is difficult to distinguish from ectopic pregnancy and endometriosis. They may exhibit posterior acoustic enhancement, depending on the content.

BOX 38-4   FOLLICULAR CYSTS

- Occur when a dominant follicle does not succeed in ovulating and remains active though immature
- Usually unilateral
- Thin-walled, translucent, watery fluid, may project above or within surface of the ovary
- May grow 1 to 8 cm
- Usually disappear spontaneously by resorption or rupture
- *Clinical:* Asymptomatic to dull, adnexal pressure and pain, abnormal ovarian function, torsion of the ovary resulting in severe pain
- *Sonographic findings:* Simple cyst

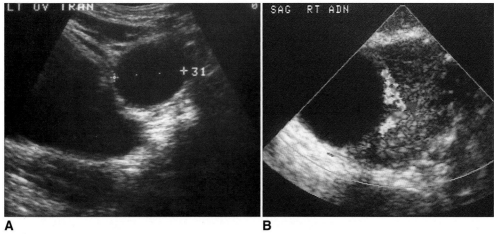

A   **B**

Figure 38-8 Hemorrhagic corpus luteum cyst. Transabdominal, **A,** and endovaginal, **B,** views of the right adnexa demonstrate a 3.5-cm cystic mass with internal echoes. The acoustic enhancement posterior to this mass confirms the cystic nature of the mass.

Duplex Doppler reveals prominent diastolic flow in corpus luteum cysts. This low-velocity waveform is present throughout the luteal phase of the cycle. They may also have a peripheral rim of color around the wall of color Doppler, sometimes termed the "ring of fire."

Hemorrhagic Cysts. Internal hemorrhage may occur in follicular cysts or more commonly in corpus luteal cysts. The patient may present with an acute onset of pelvic pain.

Sonographic Findings. The sonographic picture is variable depending on the amount of hemorrhage and the clot formation (Figure 38-9). The internal characteristics are better visualized by endovaginal scanning, but transabdominal scanning should also be performed for a global view. An acute hemorrhagic cyst is usually hyperechoic and may mimic a solid mass. It usually has a smooth posterior wall and shows posterior acoustic enhancement indicating its cystic component. Diffuse low-level echoes may be seen but are more commonly seen in endometriomas. As time goes on, the internal pattern becomes more complex. The clotted blood becomes more echogenic and may show a fluid level. Echogenic free intraperitoneal fluid in the cul-de-sac can help confirm the diagnosis of a ruptured or leaking hemorrhagic cyst. This may mimic a ruptured ectopic pregnancy, so it is very important to know if the patient had a positive pregnancy test.

Theca-Lutein Cysts. **Theca-lutein cysts** are the largest of the functional cysts and appear as very large, bilateral, multiloculated cystic masses. They are associated with high levels of human chorionic gonadotropin (hCG). They are seen most frequently in association with gestational trophoblastic disease (30%). Similar cysts occur in normal pregnancies, especially multiple gestations, and in some patients being treated with infertility drugs, particularly Pergonal (Box 38-6). These cysts may undergo hemorrhage, rupture, and torsion (Figure 38-10).

OVARIAN SYNDROMES

Ovarian Hyperstimulation Syndrome. Ovarian hyperstimulation syndrome (OHS) is a frequent iatrogenic complication of ovulation induction. This hyperstimulation can result in mild, moderate, and severe forms. In the mild form, the patient presents with pelvic discomfort, but no significant weight gain. The ovaries are enlarged, but measure less than 5 cm in diameter (Figure 38-11). With severe hyperstimulation, the patient has severe pelvic pain, abdominal distention, and notably enlarged ovaries, measuring greater than 10 cm in diameter. There can also be associated ascites, pleural effusions, and numerous large, thin-walled cysts throughout the periphery of the ovary. When treated, this condition usually resolves within 2 to 3 weeks.

Polycystic Ovarian Syndrome. Polycystic ovarian syndrome (PCOS), which includes Stein-Leventhal syndrome (infertility, oligomenorrhea, hirsutism, and obesity), is an endocrine disorder associated with chronic anovulation (Box 38-7). An imbalance of LH and FSH results in abnormal estrogen and androgen production. The serum LH level is high and the FSH level is low. An elevated LH/FSH ratio is characteristic. Pathologically the ovaries are rounded, usually two to five times normal size, with an increased number of follicles. Clinically, PCOS encompasses a spectrum of findings from hyperandrogenism in lean, normally menstruating women to obese women with severe hirsutism and oligomenorrhea or amenorrhea, as originally described by Stein and Leventhal. Manifestations of unopposed estrogenic hyperplasia and endometrial carcinoma occur in a significant proportion of patients, so long-term follow-up is recommended. PCOS is a common cause of infertility and a higher-than-usual rate of early pregnancy loss.

Sonographic Findings. On ultrasound examination, the ovaries appear normal or enlarged with echogenic stroma (Figure 38-12). The number of small follicles is often increased bilaterally (0.5 to 0.8 cm), usually to more than five in each

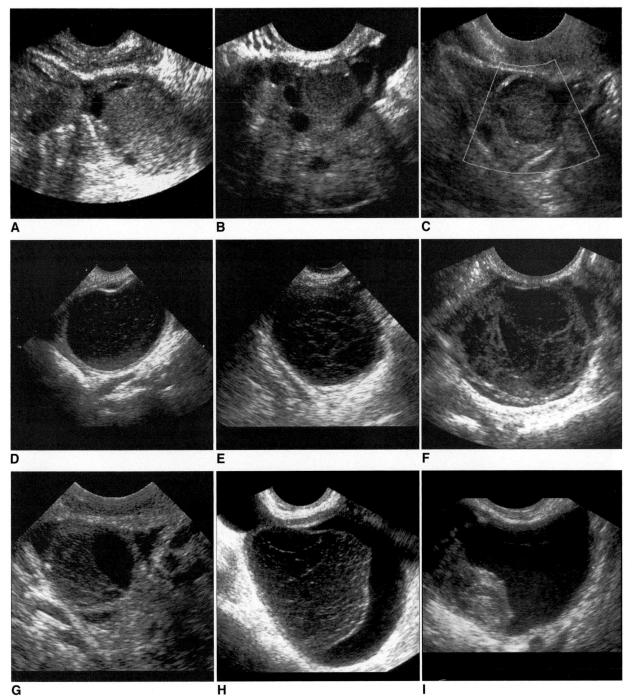

Figure 38-9 Hemorrhagic cysts on endovaginal scans—spectrum of appearances. **A,** Acute hyperechoic hemorrhagic cyst. **B,** Acute hemorrhagic cyst mimicking a solid lesion. **C,** Color Doppler shows peripheral ring of vascularity, but not vascularity within the cyst. **D,** Large cyst containing multiple internal low-level echoes. **E,** Reticular pattern of internal echoes and septations within cyst. **F,** Reticular pattern. **G, H,** and **I** show variations in clot retraction. The clot in **I** suggests a solid mass. Lack of color Doppler signal supports its benign nature. (From Rumack C, Wilson S, Charboneau W: *Diagnostic ultrasound,* ed 3, St Louis, 2005, Mosby.)

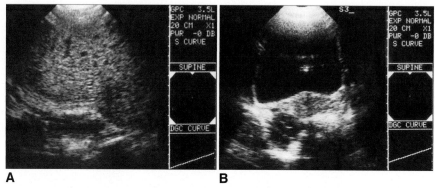

Figure 38-10 A, A patient in her 15th week of pregnancy came to the clinician with size larger than dates. The ultrasound examination showed an enlarged uterus completely filled with grapelike clusters. **B,** Evaluation of both ovaries demonstrated enlargement with multiple septations, suggesting the presence of bilateral theca-lutein cysts with the molar pregnancy.

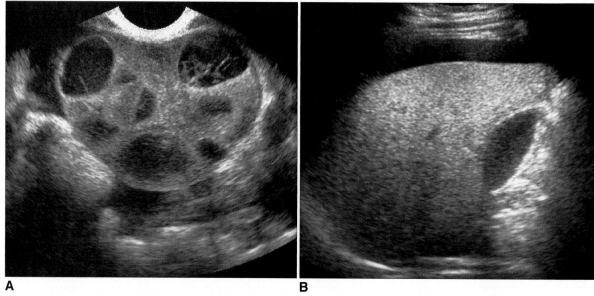

Figure 38-11   Ovarian hyperstimulation. **A,** Endovaginal image showing a notably enlarged and round ovary with multiple complicated cysts. **B,** Sagittal image in the right upper quadrant showing large volume of free intraperitoneal fluid. (From Rumack C, Wilson S, Charboneau W: *Diagnostic ultrasound,* ed 3, St Louis, 2005, Mosby.)

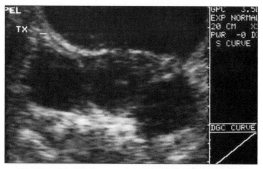

Figure 38-12   Polycystic ovaries. Transabdominal transverse image of the enlarged ovaries as they lie adjacent to the uterine cavity and posterior to the bladder.

ovary. The ovaries have a more rounded shape, with the follicles usually located peripherally. This is called the "string of pearls." Small cysts of variable size can also occupy both the subcapsular and stromal parts of the ovary. Endovaginal ultrasonography is more sensitive for detecting these small follicles than is transabdominal scanning. The diagnosis of PCOS is usually made biochemically, but sonography is useful. Serial studies show the follicles persist because ovulation does not occur.

Ovarian Remnant Syndrome. Infrequently, a cystic mass may be seen in a patient who has a history of bilateral oophorectomy. This usually results in a technically difficult surgery (due to adhesions), in which a small amount of residual ovarian tissue has been unintentionally left behind. The residual ovarian tissue can become functional and produce cysts with a thin rim of ovarian tissue in the wall.

OTHER BENIGN OVARIAN CYSTS

Peritoneal Inclusion Cysts. Peritoneal inclusion cysts are lined with mesothelial cells and are formed when adhesions trap peritoneal fluid around the ovaries, resulting in a large adnexal mass. Clinically, most patients have pelvic pain and/or a pelvic mass.

Sonographic Findings. Peritoneal inclusion cysts (benign cystic mesothelioma) are multiloculated cystic adnexal masses. The diagnosis must include the presence of an intact ovary either within or on the margin of the cyst. The fluid may contain echoes as a result of hemorrhage or proteinaceous fluid (Figure 38-13). Predominantly these occur in premenopausal women with a history of abdominal surgery. The cyst may also occur in patients with a history of trauma, pelvic inflammatory disease, or endometriosis. The risk of recurrence after surgical resection is 30% to 50%. Do not confuse with hydrosalpinx, which appears as a tubular or ovoid cystic structure with visible folds, where the ovary lies outside of the cystic structure.

Paraovarian Cysts. **Paraovarian cysts** account for approximately 10% of adnexal masses (Box 38-8). They arise from the broad ligament and usually are of mesothelial or paramesonephric origin. They may occur at any age, but are more common in the third and fourth decades of life. A specific diagnosis of a parovarian cyst is possible only by demonstrating a normal ipsilateral ovary close to, but separate from, the cyst. The cyst may undergo hemorrhage, torsion, or rupture similar to other cystic masses.

Sonographic Findings. Paraovarian cysts have thin, deformable walls that are not surrounded by ovarian stroma. They are difficult to distinguish from ovarian cysts and may contain small nodular areas and occasionally have septations. Paraovarian cysts vary in size and can become large enough to extend into the upper abdomen. Paraovarian cysts can arise anywhere in the adnexal structures, and if they fill the pelvis, their point of origin may not be clear (Figure 38-14). Their size does not change with the hormonal cycle.

Fluid Collections in Adhesions. Fluid collections in adhesions can create cystic structures of odd shapes throughout the abdomen. Omental cysts tend to be higher in the abdomen, and urachal cysts are midline in the anterior abdominal wall peritoneum above the bladder. Any tumor may have cystic elements, and the sonographer should demonstrate if the tumor is a "simple" cyst or a complex mass.

Benign Cysts in Fetuses and Adolescents. Small simple cysts (1 to 7 mm) normally occur in fetuses and newborn girls because of stimulation by maternal hormones. In premenarchal girls, small follicles (less than 9 mm) are common. Larger cysts also are seen in otherwise healthy premenarchal girls. These may be followed closely if they are regressing, as long as the

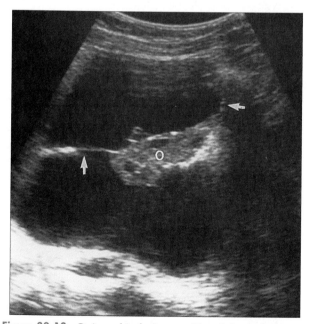

Figure 38-13 Peritoneal inclusion cyst. Transabdominal scan shows multiple fluid-filled cystic areas with linear septations *(arrows)* representing adhesions attached to normal ovary (O). (From Rumack C, Wilson S, Charboneau W: *Diagnostic ultrasound,* ed 3, St Louis, 2005, Mosby.)

BOX 38-8	**PARAOVARIAN CYSTS**

- Usually simple
- Can bleed or torse
- Wolffian duct remnants
- Ten percent of all adnexal masses
- Located in broad ligament
- *Clinical:* Asymptomatic
- *Sonographic findings:* Simple cyst adjacent to ovary

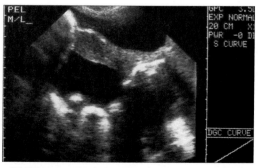

Figure 38-14 Paraovarian cyst. Transabdominal longitudinal scan of the paraovarian cyst seen posterior to the uterus and bladder. Anterior reflections from the bowel loops are shown posterior to the cyst.

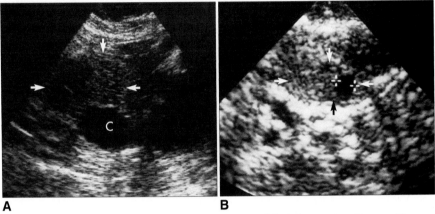

Figure 38-15   Disappearing ovarian cyst. **A,** Transverse view of the left ovary in a 63-year-old woman demonstrates a 4.7-cm simple cyst *(C)*. **B,** Follow-up examination 6 months later shows near-complete resolution of the cyst, now 0.3 cm. *Arrows* indicate the margins of the left ovary. (From Levine D, Gosink BB. In Nyberg DA and others, editors: *Endovaginal ultrasound,* St Louis, 1992, Mosby.)

child's growth and development appear normal. Occasionally, ovarian cysts produce symptoms of precocious puberty in young girls. These may arise spontaneously or in association with other hormonal derangements.

Simple Cysts in Postmenopausal Women. Palpable ovaries in postmenopausal women are of concern. However, the cause of ovarian enlargement is often a simple adnexal cyst. In postmenopausal women, small (up to 3 cm) simple cysts of the ovaries are seen in approximately 15% of patients. These cysts commonly change in size and often disappear completely (Figure 38-15).

A large majority of ovarian malignancies are epithelial in origin and most are cystic. In the past, the occurrence of any ovarian cyst in a postmenopausal woman was considered abnormal and an indication for surgery. However, several retrospective studies have evaluated simple ovarian cysts and concluded that simple cystic lesions of the ovary, especially cysts less than 5 cm in diameter, are not likely to be malignant. It has therefore been recommended that if the resistive index is normal (greater than 0.4), these simple adnexal cysts be followed sonographically rather than surgically removed.

ENDOMETRIOSIS

Endometriosis is a common condition in which functioning endometrial tissue is present outside the uterus. The ectopic tissue can be found almost anywhere in the pelvis, including the ovary, fallopian tube, broad ligament, the external surface of the uterus, and scattered over the peritoneum, cul-de-sac, and even the bladder. The endometrial tissue cyclically bleeds and proliferates. In the diffuse form, this leads to disorganization of the pelvic anatomy with an appearance similar to pelvic inflammatory disease (PID) or chronic ectopic pregnancy. Two forms of endometriosis have been described: diffuse and localized (endometrioma). The diffuse form is more common and consists of endometrial plantings within the peritoneum and is rarely diagnosed by sonography. The localized form consists of a discrete mass called an *endometrioma,* or *chocolate cyst,* and can frequently be found in multiple sites. The patient with an endometrioma is usually asymptomatic.

There are two possible explanations for endometriosis. The first is that of the chronic reflux of menstrual fluid through the tubes and into the pelvis, which may in some women produce implantation and proliferation of endometrial cells with cyclic bleeding. The second theory involves the evolution of endometrial activity in susceptible cells that retain the embryonic capacity to differentiate in response to chronic irritation (for example, by menstrual fluid) or to hormonal stimulation. The resulting tissue bleeds and proliferates in response to cyclic hormones, producing pain, scarring, and distortion of adherent pelvic organs and endometrium-lined collections of blood known as endometriomas in the ovary. These may become moderately enlarged and create a surgical emergency by rupturing or by causing the ovary to twist on the vessels that supply it (torsion).

Sonographic Findings. Endometriosis may appear as bilateral or unilateral ovarian cysts with patterns ranging from anechoic to solid, depending on the amount of blood and its organization (Figure 38-16). The ovaries are typically adherent to the posterior surface of the uterus or stuck in the cul-de-sac and may be intimately associated with the rectosigmoid colon and difficult to define. Obscured organ borders and multiple irregular cystic masses are also suggestive of either disseminating cancer or pelvic infection, and the clinical picture and serial sonographic studies determine when and if exploratory surgery is indicated.

The endometrioma is a well-defined unilocular or multilocular, predominantly cystic mass containing diffuse homogeneous, low-level internal echoes (Figure 38-17). It is better characterized on endovaginal scanning. Occasionally a fluid-fluid level can be seen. Small linear hyperechoic foci may be present in the wall and are thought to be cholesterol deposits accumulating in the cyst wall. Clinical symptoms help to differentiate endometriosis from a hemorrhagic ovarian cyst, ovarian neoplasm, or tubo-ovarian abscess.

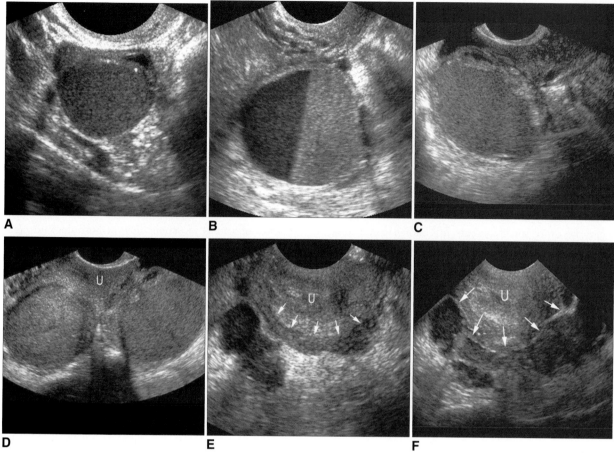

Figure 38-16 Endometriosis—spectrum of appearances. Endovaginal scans. Images **A** to **D** show uniform low-level echoes within a cystic ovarian mass. **A,** Typical peripheral echogenic foci. **B,** A fluid-filled level. **C,** Avascular marginal echogenic nodules. **D,** Bilateral disease. **E,** Endometriotic plaque on the posterior surface of the uterus *(arrows)* filling the pouch of Douglas (**F**) *(arrows)*. *U*, Uterus. (From Rumack C, Wilson S, Charboneau W: *Diagnostic ultrasound,* ed 3, St Louis, 2005, Mosby.)

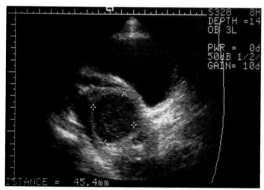

Figure 38-17 Endometrioma. A well-defined mass with homogeneous low-level echoes is seen in this 43-year-old woman.

OVARIAN TORSION

Torsion of the ovary is caused by partial or complete rotation of the ovarian pedicle on its axis. Torsion usually occurs in childhood and adolescence and is common in association with adnexal masses. **Ovarian torsion** produces an enlarged ede-

---

> ### BOX 38-9   OVARIAN TORSION
>
> - Usually associated with a mass
> - Hypoechoic, enlarged ovary, with or without peripheral follicles
> - Absent blood flow on Doppler examination
> - Free fluid in cul-de-sac
> - Surgical emergency

matous ovary, usually greater than 4 cm in diameter. The classically described appearance is of multiple tiny follicles around a hypoechoic mass, but the most common presentation is that of a completely solid adnexal mass. Free fluid often is present in the pelvis. Doppler examination usually reveals absent blood flow to the torsed ovary (Box 38-9). Occasionally, however, blood flow can be detected to torsed ovaries. This is thought to be the result of the dual blood supply of the ovary or because of venous thrombosis, leading to symptoms before arterial thrombosis occurs.

Ovarian torsion is an unusual but serious problem because it accounts for 3% of gynecologic operative emergencies. Ovarian torsion is an acute abdominal condition requiring prompt diagnosis and surgical intervention. The ovarian pedicle partially or completely rotates on its axis, compromising the lymphatic and venous drainage. This causes edema and eventual loss of arterial perfusion and infarct. Torsion typically involves not only the ovary but also frequently the fallopian tube. It is most common in women during the fertile years and even occurs during pregnancy in 20% of the cases. Torsion may present at any time in female life, from childhood to the postmenopausal period. Occasionally the lead point is an ovarian mass. Once torsion has occurred, there is a 10% increased incidence of torsion occurring in the contralateral adnexa. Torsion of a normal ovary usually occurs in children and younger females with mobile adnexa, preexisting ovarian cyst or mass, or pregnancy.

Clinically, acute severe unilateral pain is typically the presenting symptom in patients with torsion. Intermittent pain may precede the acute pain by weeks. These symptoms can be mimicked by many other pelvic or lower abdominal processes, and therefore quite frequently torsion is part of a differential diagnostic list. The patient may also have fever, nausea, and vomiting. A palpable mass is felt in more than 50% of patients. The right ovary is three times more likely to torse than the left.

Sonographic Findings. As a general rule, ovarian torsion is very unlikely when the ovary is normal in size and texture with sonography. The torsed ovary is typically enlarged and heterogeneous in appearance, owing to edema, hemorrhage, and/or necrosis (Figure 38-18). There is often a lead mass, but in some cases the lead mass is not appreciated because it is mixed in with the necrosis and hemorrhage of the torsed mass. Torsed masses are often large (greater than 4 cm in diameter), vary in their appearance from cystic to solid, and vary in echogenicity from relatively anechoic to markedly hyperechoic. A palpable mass may be present. Torsion occurs more frequently on the right side, and the pain may mimic an acute appendicitis.

The differentiation of torsion from other adnexal masses is often not possible unless there is clinical suspicion. The sono-graphic picture varies, depending on the duration and degree of vascular compromise. The ovary is enlarged and may have multiple cortical follicles. Free fluid in the cul-de-sac is a common finding. Color and spectral Doppler may show absent flow in the affected ovary. However, Doppler findings may vary on the degree and chronicity of the torsion and whether or not there is an associated adnexal mass. If torsion is intermittent, a "hyperemic" increased diastolic flow during the times when torsion is not present may be seen. This could be related to the dual ovarian arterial blood supply from the ovarian artery and ovarian branches of the uterine artery. Different appearances include target, ellipsoid, or tubular structures with internal heterogeneous echoes. Doppler may show the presence of circular, coiled twisted vessels, known as the *whirlpool sign.* The presence of arterial or venous flow or both does not exclude the diagnosis of torsion. Comparison with the appearance of morphology and flow patterns in the contralateral ovary helps in the evaluation.

SONOGRAPHIC EVALUATION OF OVARIAN NEOPLASMS

Ultrasound screening finds adnexal cysts in 1% to 15% of postmenopausal women. Only 3% of ovarian cysts less than 5 cm are malignant. Therefore, a cyst greater than 5 cm is recommended to be surgically removed. In the postmenopausal woman, the ovaries are enlarged; if a mass is seen, it may be mixed texture to solid with papillae within. Well-defined anechoic lesions are more likely to be benign, whereas lesions with irregular walls, thick irregular septations, mural nodules, and solid echogenic elements favor malignancy. Doppler examination shows a low-resistive pattern. Extension beyond the ovary into the omentum or peritoneum and liver metastases should be evaluated. Malignant ascites may also be present. Unilocular or thinly septated cysts are more likely to be benign. Multilocular, thickly septated masses and masses with solid nodules are more likely to be malignant. In advanced stages, peritoneal carcinomatosis with malignant ascites and peritoneal implants can be seen.

Any change in ovarian echogenicity or volume of more than 20 ml should be considered suspicious. In postmenopausal women, the ovaries become atrophic and often do not have follicles. Thus the ovary can be difficult to identify. Only women receiving hormone replacement therapy continue to have normal-sized ovaries. Abnormal ovaries suggestive of malignancy are defined as enlarged echogenic ovaries (more than twice the size of normal ovaries or greater than 2 SDs above the norm [for the woman's age]).

Although ultrasound is able to identify masses and subtle changes in ovaries, it is not often able to distinguish benign from malignant. Doppler imaging has been studied to determine whether it can detect the neovascularity of malignant masses. Pulsed Doppler imaging is then performed to analyze the vascular component. When evaluating the soft tissue from the margins of the abnormal ovary or mass, care must be taken so that the sample volume does not obtain flow patterns from adjacent normal structures.

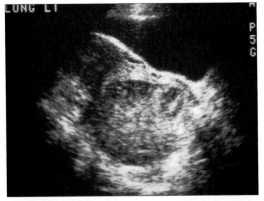

Figure 38-18   Ovarian torsion. Transabdominal view of the distended bladder lying anterior to the enlarged ovary in this 5-day-old girl. Decreased Doppler flow was apparent during the real-time examination.

OVARIAN CARCINOMA

Ovarian cancer is often detected by a combination of physical examination and laboratory and imaging findings. Every year **ovarian carcinoma** kills more women than cancer of the uterine cervix and body combined and is the fourth leading cause of cancer death. The American Cancer Society estimates that there were 25,400 new cases of ovarian cancer in the United States in 2003 and that about 15,000 women die from this disease annually. Approximately 1 in 70 women develop the disease. Ovarian carcinoma is the leading cause of death from gynecologic malignancy (25%) in the United States. Sixty percent of the ovarian malignancies occur in women between 40 and 60 years of age. About 80% of cases involve women over 60 years of age, with the risk of cancer increasing with age. New chemotherapeutic and surgical techniques have done little to decrease mortality, so continued efforts are being directed at developing methods of early diagnosis. The 5-year survival rate is between 20% and 30% overall (stages I through IV).

Ovarian malignancy is a "silent" cancer. Because of its relative absence of symptoms early in the disease, ovarian cancer commonly is not detected until advanced, either having spread beyond the capsule but still within the pelvis (stage II) or into the abdomen (stage III). At the time of initial detection, 50% of women present with stage III spread. The adnexal finding on physical examination is variable, ranging from almost "normal" to slightly enlarged firm irregular ovaries to pelvic masses. In advanced disease, ascites and omental masses may be palpated. The blood chemistry test CA 125 is helpful in some patients, but has been disappointing as a screening test because of its inability to detect many cases of ovarian cancer. It has many false-positive and false-negative results, and elevated levels are found in only 50% of patients with stage III ovarian cancer. If a baseline level is known, however, such as for patients who have undergone resection of primary ovarian cancer, then an elevated follow-up level has greater significance.

Ovarian cancer can present as either a complex, cystic, or solid mass, but is more likely predominantly cystic. As many as 20% are bilateral. Differential diagnoses include endometriosis, hemorrhagic ovarian cyst, ovarian torsion, PID, and benign ovarian neoplasms (e.g., serous cystadenoma, mucinous cystadenoma, dermoid, fibroma, and thecoma). An exophytic fibroid or a nongynecologic mass may also appear in the adnexa and resemble an ovarian neoplasm. The likelihood of malignancy is increased by the greater the amount of solid tissue in a complex ovarian mass and the presence of complex ascites.

Most ovarian cancers are detected as masses. The size of the mass, age of the patient, and ultrasound characteristics of the mass relate directly to its potential for being malignant. Masses less than 5 cm in their longest axis are much more likely to be benign, whereas masses larger than 10 cm are much more likely to be malignant. Increasing age also correlates with an increased incidence of malignancy. The incidence of ovarian cancer is greatly increased in women who have had breast and colon cancer. This appears primarily related to genetic mutations in the BRCA1 and BRCA2 genes and less commonly in the MSH2 and MLH1 genes.

The primary clinical problem with this disease is the asymptomatic and undetectable nature of the cancer in the earliest stages. Often the patient will seek medical attention after ascites has initiated abdominal distention. The 5-year survival rate for stage IV ovarian cancer is 5%; stage I tumors diagnosed early and confined to the capsule show a survival rate of 90% at 5 years.

The strongest risk factor is a family history of ovarian or breast cancer. Women with carcinoma of the breast have increased risk of developing ovarian cancer, and women with ovarian cancer are three to four times more likely to develop breast cancer. Other risk factors include increasing age, nulliparity, infertility, uninterrupted ovulation, and late menopause. About 3% to 5% of women with a family history of ovarian cancer will have a hereditary ovarian cancer syndrome. The three main hereditary syndromes associated with ovarian cancer are the breast-ovarian, nonpolyposis colorectal, and site-specific ovarian cancer syndrome. They have an earlier age of onset than do other ovarian cancers.

Clinical symptoms include vague abdominal pain, swelling, indigestion, frequent urination, constipation, and weight change (ascites). Over 70% of the women first seen by their doctors are in advanced stages of the disease. Although the median age of diagnosis is 63 years, the peak age ranges between 55 and 59 years, although it may also affect women in their forties.

Ovarian cancer[4] arises primarily from epithelial tumors (60% to 70%), including serous cystadenocarcinoma (50%), endometrioid tumor similar to endometrial adenocarcinoma (15% to 30%), mucinous cystadenocarcinoma (15%), clear cell carcinoma (5%), Brenner tumor (2.5%), and undifferentiated tumor (less than 5%). Germ cell tumors contribute 15% to 30% of the malignancies and are more common in girls and young women (age 4 to 27 years), including mature teratoma, dysgerminoma, immature teratoma, transdermal sinus tumor, malignant mixed germ cell tumor, choriocarcinoma, and embryonal carcinoma. Metastases (5% to 10%) and stromal tumors (5%) are the remaining tumors that contribute to ovarian cancer.

On laparotomy, the cancer is classified into one of the following stages:

STAGE I: Limited to ovary
  a. Limited to one ovary
  b. Limited to two ovaries
  c. Positive peritoneal lavage (ascites)
STAGE II: Limited to pelvis
  a. Involvement of uterus/fallopian tubes
  b. Extension to other pelvic tissues
  c. Positive peritoneal lavage (ascites)
STAGE III: Limited to abdomen-intraabdominal extension outside pelvis/retroperitoneal nodes/extension to small bowel/omentum
STAGE IV: Hematogenous disease (liver parenchyma)/spread beyond abdomen

The treatment for ovarian carcinoma includes surgery and chemotherapy initially, followed by a second laparotomy in 6 months and follow-up CA 125 blood tests and computerized tomography (CT) scans.

The CA 125 test is a serum marker for ovarian cancer; it is elevated in more than 80% of epithelial ovarian cancers. It has not been found effective as a screening tool because only 50% of stage I malignant ovarian tumors have CA 125 levels higher than 35 U/ml, and the method has a high false-positive rate that is attributed to nonmalignant gynecologic disease. It is also insensitive to mucinous and germ-cell tumors. Levels of CA 125 may be elevated in benign conditions, such as endometriosis, pelvic inflammatory disease, uterine fibroids, pregnancy, and in other types of cancer not arising from the ovaries.

Sonographic Findings. Sonographically, ovarian cancer usually presents with an adnexal mass (Figure 38-19). Ultrasonography can detect morphologic characteristics of the tumor, but cannot (with the exception of dermoid cysts) dis-

tinguish benign from malignant tumors. In general, well-defined, smooth bordered anechoic lesions are more likely to be benign. Lesions with irregular walls, thick, irregular septations, mural nodules, and solid echogenic elements are frequently malignant. Mixed cystic and solid masses are the most frequent presentation of the common epithelial tumors of the ovary. Ascites, extension to adjacent organs, peritoneal implants, lymphadenopathy, and hepatic metastases support the diagnosis of malignant disease (Figure 38-20).

DOPPLER FINDINGS IN OVARIAN CANCER

Abnormal tumor vascularity and abnormal RI or PI are also worrisome for malignancy. The results of the many studies using Doppler are quite variable. It is difficult to compare

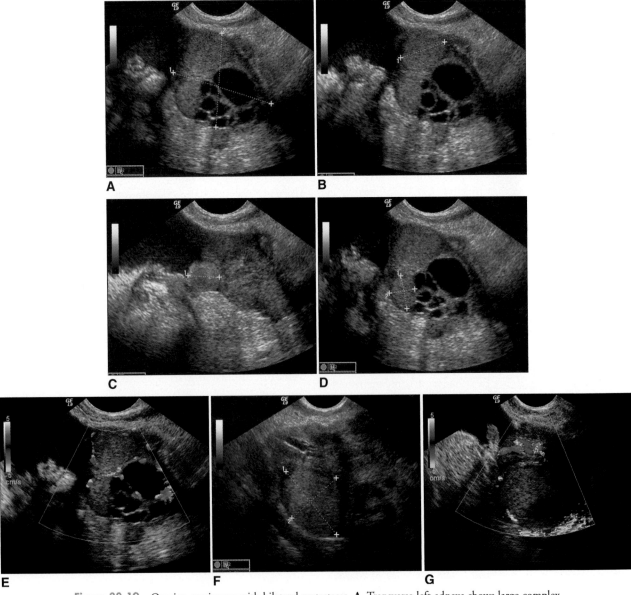

Figure 38-19   Ovarian carcinoma with bilateral metastases. **A,** Transverse left adnexa shows large complex mass. **B,** Transverse left adnexa. **C,** Transverse left adnexa shows nodule superior to uterine fundus. **D,** Transverse left adnexa shows uterus, mass, ovaries, and vascular structures. **E,** Color Doppler of increased vascular flow. **F,** Right transverse of large mass. **G,** Increased vascularity demonstrated with color Doppler.

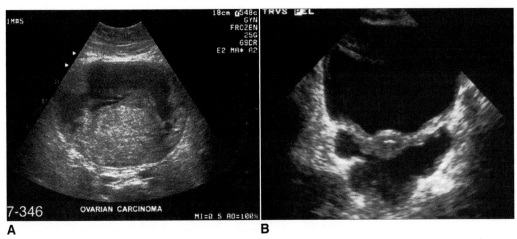

Figure 38-20   Ovarian carcinoma. **A,** A large, solid mass was found in the left adnexa in this 49-year-old woman whose presenting symptom was a palpable mass. **B,** Complications of advanced stages of ovarian carcinoma led to malignant ascites. This transabdominal transverse image shows the distended urinary bladder anterior to the uterus as it is surrounded by massive ascites.

studies because of many factors, such as the lack of standardization of equipment, technical settings and techniques, and differences in various patient populations. Absence of flow within a lesion usually indicates a benign lesion. This is based on the premise that malignant masses, because of internal neovascularization, will have high diastolic flow, which can be seen on spectral Doppler waveforms. Malignant tumor growth is dependent on angiogenesis with the development of abnormal tumor vessels. This leads to decreased vascular resistance and higher diastolic flow velocity.

Contrast imaging in ultrasound will enable us to image the anatomical area better and give the physician more confidence in determining whether an exam is abnormal or normal. It might allow us to distinguish between benign and malignant lesions. Vascular contrast agents consist of surfactant coated or encapsulated gas microbubbles less than 10 U/m in diameter. These agents are injected into the bloodstream via a peripheral vein and then circulate through the body. The vascular contrast agent Echovist, used to diagnose ovarian malignancies, shows increased brightness of power Doppler signal and the amount of recognizable vascular areas after contrast administration. The contrast agent enhancement was significantly higher in malignant than benign adnexal masses. There was also an increase in the number of recognizable vessels after contrast agent administration. Contrast agent uptake times were significantly shorter in malignant than benign tumors. For differentiation of benign from malignant tumors, the kinetic properties of the contrast agent, such as uptake and washout times, have significant potential in diagnosis.

EPITHELIAL TUMORS

Gynecologic tumors that arise from the surface epithelium and cover the ovary and the underlying stroma are termed **surface epithelial-stromal tumors**. This group accounts for 65% to 75% of all ovarian neoplasms and 80% to 90% of all ovarian malignancies. The two most common types are serous and mucinous tumors. Serous tumors are the most common and comprise 30% of all ovarian neoplasm. Mucinous tumors account for 20% to 25% of ovarian neoplasms. The benign or low-malignancy potential form is termed *adenoma* and the malignant form is termed *adenocarcinoma*. The prefix *cyst* is added if the lesion is cystic, and *fibroma* is added if the tumor is more than 50% fibrous. Mucinous tumors are less frequently bilateral than are the serous type.

Some investigators believe that benign-appearing tumors (which are anechoic, thin walled, have no septation, and are acoustically enhanced) can be aspirated safely.[2,6]

Metastatic spread is primarily intraperitoneal, although direct extension to surrounding structures and lymphatics is not uncommon. Hematogenous spread usually occurs late in the course of the disease.

Sonographic Findings. Serous and mucinous tumors vary greatly in size, but can be very large. They often fill the pelvis and extend into the abdomen. In general the serous tumors are smaller than mucinous tumors (Figure 38-21).

MUCINOUS CYSTADENOMA

Mucinous cystadenoma is a type of epithelial tumor that is lined by the mucinous elements of the endocervix and bowel. It constitutes 20% to 25% of all benign ovarian neoplasms. When benign, it is a mucinous cystadenoma; when malignant, it is a cystadenocarcinoma. This type of tumor is usually found in a woman between the ages of 13 and 45 years old. A reported 80% to 85% of mucinous tumors are benign. These tumors can be very large, measuring 15 to 30 cm in diameter, and weigh more than 100 pounds. They can fill the entire pelvis and abdomen. The tumor is usually benign and unilateral (5% bilateral) (Box 38-10).

Sonographic Findings. In 75% of patients with mucinous tumors, ultrasound examination shows simple or septate thin-walled multilocular cysts (Figure 38-22). They often contain internal echoes with compartments differing in echogenicity caused by the mucoid material in the dependent portions.

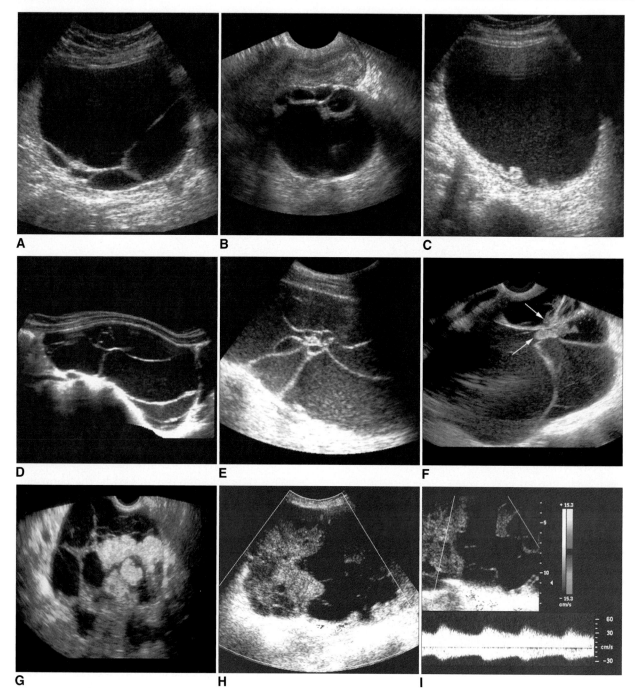

Figure 38-21   Epithelial ovarian neoplasms—spectrum of appearances. **A, B,** and **C** show serous cystadenomas. In **A,** septations within a cystic mass are fairly thin. In **B,** septations are thicker, and in **C,** there are low-level echogenic particles and small mural nodules. **D** and **E** are mucinous cystadenomas, and **F** is a mucinous cystadenocarcinoma. Large size and septations are characteristic; septal nodularity is marked in **F** *(arrows)*. **G, H,** and **I** are images in a single patient with a serous cystadenocarcinoma. Extensive nodularity shows vascularity confirming the morphologic suspicion of a malignant mass. There is high diastolic flow resulting in a low resistive index. (From Rumack C, Wilson S, Charboneau W: *Diagnostic ultrasound,* ed 3, St Louis, 2005, Mosby.)

BOX 38-10

MUCINOUS CYSTADENOMA

- Unusually large (15 to 30 cm)
- Most common cystic tumor
- Usually unilateral
- Cyst filled with sticky, gelatin-like material
- Multilocular cystic spaces
- Benign type more common than malignant
- *Clinical:* Pressure, pain, increased abdominal girth
- *Sonographic findings:* Simple or septate thin-walled multilocular cysts

MUCINOUS CYSTADENOCARCINOMA

Mucinous cystadenocarcinoma most frequently occurs in women 40 to 70 years old and accounts for 5% to 10% of all primary malignant ovarian neoplasms; 15% to 20% are bilateral when malignant (Box 38-11); 10% occur in menopausal women. These tumors can also become very large and are more likely than the benign form to rupture. If the tumor ruptures, it is associated with pseudomyxoma peritoneum. This causes loculated ascites with mass effect.

Sonographic Findings. On ultrasound examination, malignant cysts tend to have thick, irregular walls and septations with papillary projections and echogenic material (Figures 38-23 and 38-24). They generally have a similar sonographic appearance to that of serous cystadenocarcinomas.

Penetration of the tumor capsule or rupture may lead to the mucoid ascites that appears as hypoechoic fluid with bright

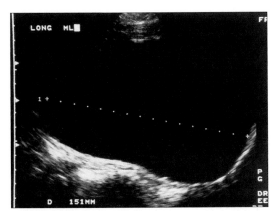

Figure 38-22 Mucinous cystadenoma. A 37-year-old woman presented with pelvic pressure and fullness. A large pelvic mass was found on pelvic examination. The ultrasound image shows a huge "cystic"-appearing mass with smooth borders extending beyond the patient's umbilicus.

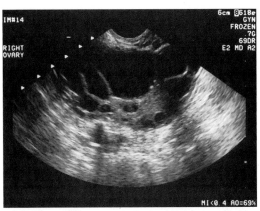

Figure 38-23 Mucinous cystadenocarcinoma. A large septated mass with thick, irregular walls was found in this 33-year-old woman.

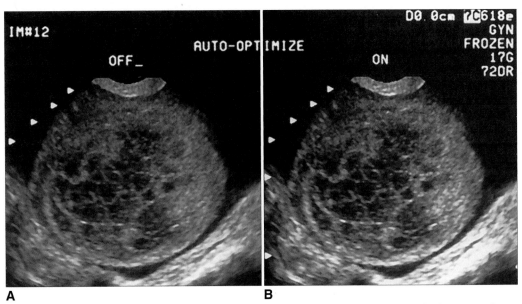

A   **B**

Figure 38-24 Mucinous cystadenocarcinoma. Adjustments in equipment focus may help the sonographer determine the thickness of the septations within the large ovarian mass.

punctate echoes. This condition, known as pseudomyxoma peritonei, can be seen in mucinous cystadenomas and cystadenocarcinomas or mucinous tumors of the appendix and colon. It may contain multiple septations and low-level echogenic material that fills much of the pelvis and abdomen.

SEROUS CYSTADENOMA

Serous cystadenoma is the second most common benign tumor of the ovary (after the dermoid cyst) and represents 20% to 25% of all benign ovarian neoplasms. This tumor is usually unilateral (20% are bilateral) (Box 38-12).

Sonographic Findings. Serous tumors are usually unilocular or multilocular with thin septations (Figure 38-25). The size is smaller than the mucinous cysts (up to 20 cm); borders are irregular with a loss of capsular definition. Multilocular cysts contain a small amount of solid tissue in chambers of varying size with occasional internal septum or mural nodules.

BOX 38-11

MUCINOUS CYSTADENOCARCINOMA

- Bilateral
- May occur in menopausal women (10%)
- Large, likely to rupture—ascites
- *Clinical:* Pelvic pressure, pain when ruptured
- *Sonographic findings:* Ascites appears as hypoechoic fluid with bright punctate echoes; thick, irregular walls and septations

---

BOX 38-12

SEROUS CYSTADENOMA

- Usually unilateral
- Smaller than mucinous cysts
- Multilocular cysts with septations
- *Clinical:* Pelvic pressure, bloating
- *Sonographic findings:* Multilocular cyst—may have nodule

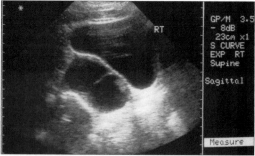

Figure 38-25 Serous cystadenoma. Multilocular mass with septations is seen in this ovarian mass posterior to the bladder.

SEROUS CYSTADENOCARCINOMA

Serous cystadenocarcinoma constitutes 60% to 80% of all ovarian carcinomas. More than half of these tumors are bilateral.

Sonographic Findings. Serous cystadenocarcinomas are smaller than mucinous cysts, but still may be quite large, with irregular borders and a loss of capsular definition (Box 38-13). The tumor may be accompanied by bilateral ovarian enlargement. Multilocular cysts contain chambers of varying size with septated, internal papillary projections. Calcifications may be present. Solid elements or bilateral tumors suggest malignancy (Figure 38-26). Ascites forms secondary to peritoneal surface implantation and is frequently seen. The tumor may spread to the lymph nodes (e.g., periaortic, mediastinal, and supraclavicular).

OTHER EPITHELIAL TUMORS

Less common varieties of epithelial tumors are endometrioid, clear cell, Brenner (transitional cell), and undifferentiated carcinoma. Endometrioid tumors are nearly all malignant and are the second most common epithelial malignancy. Approximately 25% to 30% are bilateral and occur most frequently postmenopausal; peak age ranges from 50 to 60 years. Clear cell tumors are considered to be of müllerian duct origin and a variant of the endometrioid carcinoma. Clear cell tumors are nearly always malignant and are bilateral about 20% of the time. Peak age ranges from 50 to 70 years. Transitional cell tumor, also known as *Brenner tumor,* is uncommon. The Brenner tumor is found in 1.5% to 2.5% of patients; peak age ranges from 40 to 70 years. It is nearly always benign and 6% to 7% are bilateral; 30% are associated with cystic neoplasms in the ipsilateral ovary.

Sonographic Findings. These types of epithelial tumors cannot be distinguished sonographically; however, they are more frequently found unilaterally. They are usually small and present as a nonspecific, complex, predominantly cystic mass. Occasionally the tumor may contain hemorrhage or necrosis. The Brenner tumors are hypoechoic, solid masses that may contain calcifications in the outer wall. They are composed of dense fibrous stroma and appear similar to ovarian fibromas and thecomas.

GERM CELL TUMORS

Germ cell tumors are derived from the primitive germ cells of the embryonic gonad. They account for 15% to 20% of ovarian neoplasms, with approximately 95% being benign

---

BOX 38-13

SEROUS CYSTADENOCARCINOMA

- External papillary mass adhesions and infection lead to bilateral involvement
- Loss of capsular definition and tumor fixation; calcifications
- Peritoneal implants; ascites; metastases to omentum, lymph nodes, liver, and lungs
- *Clinical:* Pelvic fullness, bloating
- *Sonographic findings:* Cystic structure with septations and/or papillary projections; internal and external papillomas usually present

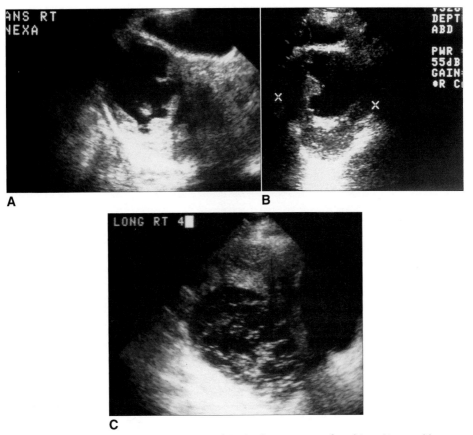

Figure 38-26 Serous cystadenocarcinoma. **A** and **B,** A 14-cm mass was found in a 62-year-old woman. This mass had papillary projections within. **C,** In another patient the ovarian mass showed multiple thick septations within. Massive ascites was seen throughout the pelvic cavity.

cystic teratomas. Besides teratomas, germ cell tumors include dysgerminoma, embryonal cell carcinoma, choriocarcinoma, and transdermal sinus tumor. These types are rare and occur mainly in adolescents and are the most common ovarian malignancy in this age group. Germ cell tumors often occur as mixed tumors with elements of two or three varieties of germ cell tumors. They are associated with elevated alpha-fetoprotein (AFP) and hCG levels.

Clinical symptoms include pelvic and/or abdominal pain and a palpable mass (average diameter is 15 cm).

Sonographic Findings. The germ cell tumor is usually unilateral; 40% of tumors will calcify. The tumor ranges in texture from homogeneously solid (3%), predominantly solid (85%), to predominantly cystic (12%).

TERATOMA

Dermoid Tumors. Dermoid tumors are the most common ovarian neoplasm, constituting 20% of ovarian tumors. Up to 15% are bilateral. About 80% occur in women of childbearing age, but may occur at any age.

They are composed of well-differentiated derivatives of the three germ layers: ectoderm, mesoderm, and endoderm. In 10% of cases, the tumor is diagnosed during pregnancy. A rare dermoid that is composed of thyroid tissue is termed a stroma ovarii (thyroid tissue) and may produce insuppressible thyro-

> **BOX 38-14   DERMOID TUMORS**
>
> - Size ranges from small to 40 cm
> - Unilateral, round to oval mass
> - Contains fatty, sebaceous material, hair, cartilage, bone, teeth
> - *Clinical:* Asymptomatic to abdominal pain, enlargement and pressure; pedunculated, subject to torsion
> - *Sonographic findings:* Cystic/complex/solid mass, echogenic components; acoustic shadowing

toxicosis. Malignant degeneration into squamous cell carcinoma is uncommon (2%) in teratomas, usually in older women.

Sonographic Findings. Dermoids have a spectrum of sonographic appearances, depending on which elements (ectoderm, mesoderm, or transderm) are present. Teeth, bones, and fat can be seen on plain films (Box 38-14). Clinical findings include abdominal mass and/or pain secondary to torsion or hemorrhage.

Ultrasonography demonstrates a completely cystic mass, a cystic mass with an echogenic mural nodule representing a "dermoid plug" (Figure 38-27, *A*), a fat-fluid level (Figure 38-27, *B*), high-amplitude echoes with shadowing (e.g., teeth or bone), or a complex mass with internal septations (Figure

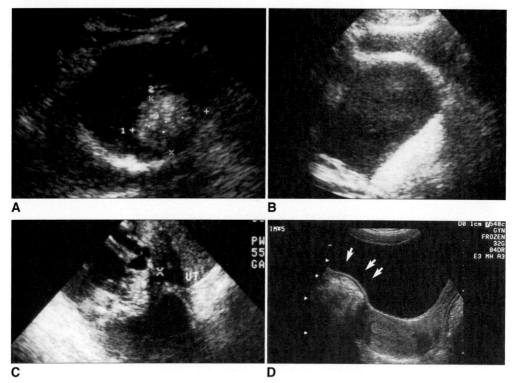

Figure 38-27 Dermoid tumor. Spectrum of appearances on ultrasound examination. **A,** Cystic dermoid with an echogenic mural nodule. **B,** Cystic dermoid with a fat-fluid level. **C,** Complex pattern of a dermoid tumor. *UT,* Uterus. **D,** Calcification and shadowing are shown in this dermoid tumor as it indents the bladder wall *(arrows).*

38-27, *C* and *D*). Echogenic dermoids may often be confused with bowel, as the mass may have characteristics similar to those of bowel tissue. If a palpable pelvic mass is present that is not identified on ultrasonography, an echogenic dermoid must be considered. Indentation on the bladder wall will be a clue that a pelvic mass is present. The calcification within the pelvic cavity is also shown on the radiograph (Figure 38-28).

The term "tip-of-the-iceberg" refers to a mixture of matted hair and sebum producing ill-defined acoustic shadowing that obscures the posterior wall of the lesion (Figure 38-29). The "dermoid mesh" refers to multiple linear hyperechoic interfaces floating within the cyst and represent hair.

Acute hemorrhage into an ovarian cyst or an endometrioma may be so echogenic that it resembles a dermoid or a dermoid plug (Figure 38-30). Posterior sound enhancement is usually seen where a dermoid plug usually causes attenuation. Other pitfalls include a pedunculated fibroid or an appendicolith in a perforated appendix.

IMMATURE AND MATURE TERATOMAS

Immature teratomas are uncommon and occur in girls and young women 10 to 20 years of age. These are rapidly growing, solid malignant tumors with many tiny cysts (Figure 38-31). alpha fetoprotein is elevated in 50% of patients. The tumor is unilateral and small in size, although it may grow to a larger dimension.

Sonographic Findings. On ultrasound examination, the texture of immature teratomas ranges from cystic to complex;

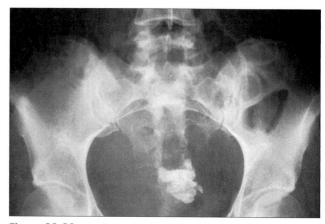

Figure 38-28 Radiograph of a 17-year-old girl with a calcified dermoid tumor shown within the pelvic cavity.

the teratoma usually is solid with internal echoes. Calcifications are commonly seen.

DYSGERMINOMA

Dysgerminoma is a rare malignant germ cell tumor that is bilateral in 15% of cases. The mass constitutes 1% to 2% of primary ovarian neoplasms and 3% to 5% of ovarian malignancies. An entirely solid ovarian mass in a woman less than 30 years of age is usually a dysgerminoma. The dysgerminoma and the serous cystadenoma are the two most common ovarian neoplasms seen in pregnancy.

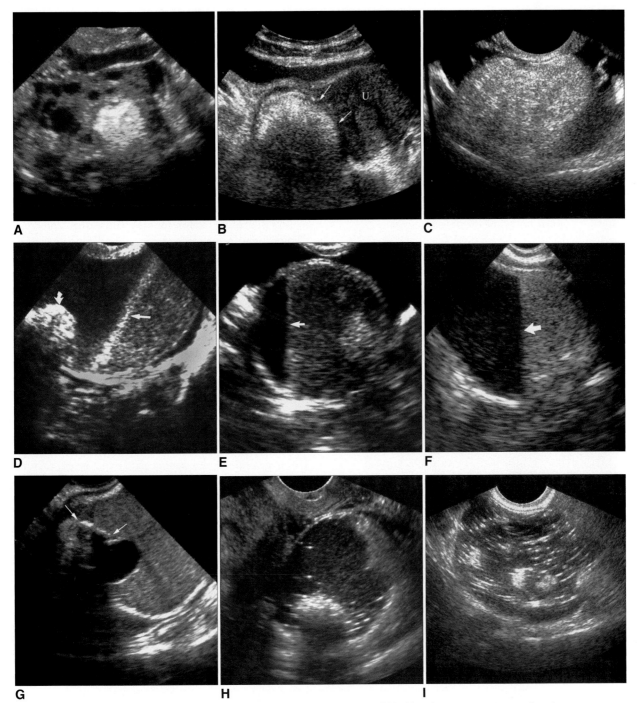

Figure 38-29 Dermoid cysts—spectrum of appearances. **A,** Small, highly echogenic mass in an otherwise normal ovary. **B,** Transverse transabdominal scan showing the uterus (U). In the right adnexal region there is a highly echogenic and attenuating mass *(arrows)*. This is a tip-of-the-iceberg sign. **C,** A highly echogenic intraovarian mass with no normal ovarian tissue. **D,** Mass of varying echogenicity with hair-fluid level *(straight arrow)* and highly echogenic fat-containing dermoid plug *(curved arrow)* with shadowing. **E,** Predominantly echogenic mass with fat-fluid level *(arrow)*. **F,** Mass with fat-fluid level *(arrow)*. **G,** Mass containing uniform echoes, small cystic area, and calcification *(arrows)* with shadowing. **H,** Combination of dermoid mesh and dermoid plug appearances. **I.** Dermoid mesh, multiple linear hyperechogenic interfaces floating within cystic mass. (From Rumack C, Wilson S, Charboneau W: *Diagnostic ultrasound,* ed 3, St Louis, 2005, Mosby.)

Sonographic Findings. Dysgerminoma is a hyperechoic solid mass with areas of hemorrhage and necrosis on ultrasound examination. It may show a speckled pattern of calcifications. In a postmenopausal patient, a fibroma or thecoma is most likely.

ENDODERMAL SINUS TUMOR

Endodermal sinus tumors are rare rapidly growing tumors also called *yolk sac tumors.* The lesion usually occurs in women under 20 years of age and is almost always unilateral. Increased serum AFP may be seen. Endodermal sinus tumor has a poor prognosis and is the second most common malignant ovarian germ cell neoplasm after dysgerminoma. The sonographic appearance is similar to that of the dysgerminoma.

STROMAL TUMORS

Sex cord-stromal tumors typically are solid adnexal masses that arise from the sex cords of the embryonic gonadal and/or ovarian stroma. This category includes granulosa cell tumor, thecoma, fibroma, and Sertoli-Leydig cell tumors (androblastoma). This group accounts for 5% to 10% of all ovarian neoplasms and 2% of all ovarian malignancies. Thecomas and

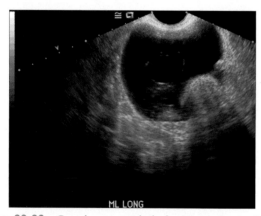

Figure 38-30 Complex mass with shadowing consistent with a dermoid plug mass.

fibromas are the most common of these. They are benign solid hypoechoic adnexal masses that occur in middle-aged women.
Sonographic Findings. Stromal tumors are often so hypoechoic as to appear cystic, but there is lack of through-transmission.

FIBROMA AND THECOMA

Both of these arise from the ovarian stroma and are pathologically similar. Tumors with an abundance of thecal cells are called thecomas, and those with an abundance of fibrous tissue are called fibromas. Thecomas are usual benign and unilateral, comprising 1% of all ovarian neoplasms, and 70% occur in postmenopausal women. They frequently show signs of estrogen production.

Fibromas compromise 4% of ovarian neoplasms. Unlike thecomas, they are rarely associated with estrogen production. Clinical signs include lack of symptoms if the tumor is small; if large, increasing pressure and pain are apparent. Ascites has been reported in up to 50% of patients with fibromas larger than 5 cm in diameter. Associated ascites along with pleural effusion, referred to as **Meigs' syndrome**, occurs in 1% to 3% of patients with fibroma, but is not specific, as it can occur with other ovarian neoplasms as well. The tumor is found in postmenopausal women. Fibromas occurring with basal cell nevus syndrome are commonly bilateral and calcified and occur in women with a mean age of 30 years.
Sonographic Findings. Fibromas are usually unilateral (90%), and their size ranges from small to melon size, with a variable sonographic appearance. A hypoechoic mass with posterior attenuation is seen from the homogeneous fibrous tissue. The larger tumors are pedunculated and prone to torsion, edema, and cystic degeneration (Figure 38-32).

GRANULOSA

A granulosa is a feminizing neoplasm composed of cells resembling the graafian follicle. It is the most common hormone-active estrogenic tumor of the ovary, but is rarely found (1% to 3%). It is more common after menopause (50%) but is also seen in the reproductive ages (45%) and in adolescence (5%). Clinical symptoms of estrogen production may include precocious puberty or vaginal bleeding and full breasts. Pain, pressure, and fullness may also be present. The tumor may twist

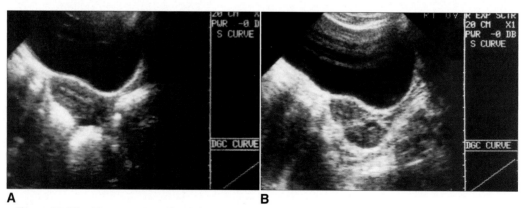

Figure 38-31 Teratoma. A small, solid mass was incidentally found posterior to the uterus in this 2-year-old girl. **A,** Transabdominal, midline (bladder and uterus). **B,** Midline, slightly to the left, to show the uterus and teratoma in the area of the left ovary.

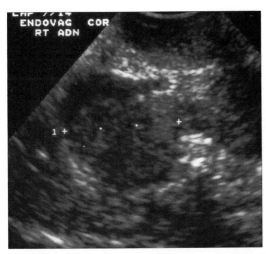

Figure 38-32   Fibroma. A 65-year-old woman presented with fullness in her abdomen. A homogeneous, well-defined mass was found in the right ovary. At surgery an endometrioid cyst adenofibroma was removed.

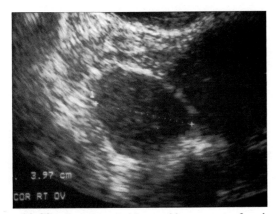

Figure 38-33   Granulosa. A 46-year-old woman was found to have a grapefruit-size mass on pelvic examination. The ultrasound image showed a well-defined, homogeneous mass in the right ovary, which was surgically removed.

on itself to cause torsion or rupture, leading to Meigs' syndrome. Malignant transformation is rare, but when it occurs, the lesion spreads via the lymphatics and bloodstream.

Sonographic Findings. On ultrasound examination, adult granulose cell tumors have a variable appearance. A mass without torsion is similar to an endometrioma or cystadenoma, with low-level homogeneous echoes (Figure 38-33); if torsion occurs, a multilocular cyst containing blood or fluid is seen. The solid masses may have an echogenicity similar to that of uterine fibroids. The size may range up to 40 cm in diameter; the mass is usually unilateral. Endometrial glandular hyperplasia may be apparent. Metastases are uncommon and appear as peritoneal-based masses.

SERTOLI-LEYDIG CELL TUMOR

Sertoli-Leydig cell tumors (also called *androblastomas*) are rare. They generally occur in women under 30 years and constitute less than 0.5% of ovarian neoplasms. Almost all are unilateral,

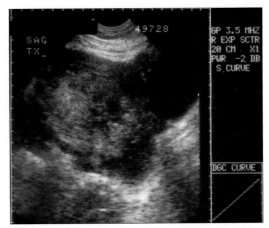

Figure 38-34   Metastatic disease. A complex, solid-appearing mass was found in this 42-year-old woman 6 months after she was diagnosed with adenocarcinoma of the colon.

and malignancy occurs in 10% to 20% of these tumors. Clinically, symptoms of virilization occur in about 30% of patients. Occasionally, these tumors may be associated with estrogen production.

Sonographic Findings. Sonographically, the tumor usually appears as solid hypoechoic masses.

ARRHENOBLASTOMA

Arrhenoblastoma is a masculinizing ovarian tumor that occurs in females 15 to 65 years of age, with a peak incidence at 25 to 45 years. Clinical features are the same as for other pelvic masses, with the addition of amenorrhea and infertility. This mass may experience malignant transformation in 22% of patients.

Sonographic Findings. The tumor is a solid mass with cystic components; it is lobulated and well encapsulated. In 95% of patients the mass is unilateral, and the size ranges from 2 to 30 cm.

METASTATIC DISEASE

The ovaries are more involved with metastatic disease than any other pelvic organ, and these metastases often mimic the appearance of advanced stage II to III primary ovarian cancer. Approximately 5% to 10% of ovarian neoplasms are metastatic in origin. Metastatic cancer can arise from the breast, upper gastrointestinal tract, and other pelvic organs by direct extension or lymphatic spread. Krukenberg tumors are "drop" metastases to the ovaries from the gastrointestinal tract, primarily from the stomach, but also from the biliary tract, gallbladder, and pancreas. These masses are typically solid. Cystic metastatic masses appear to result more commonly from rectosigmoid colon cancers. Regardless of the site of origin, when there are metastases to the ovaries these malignancies are often widespread, with metastasis to the peritoneum (including ascites) and to the mesentery. The ovary is a common site of metastasis from carcinoma of the bowel (Krukenberg's tumor), breast, and endometrium and from melanoma and lymphoma.

Sonographic Findings. Metastatic disease to the ovaries frequently is bilateral and is often associated with ascites (Figure 38-34). Metastases are usually completely solid or

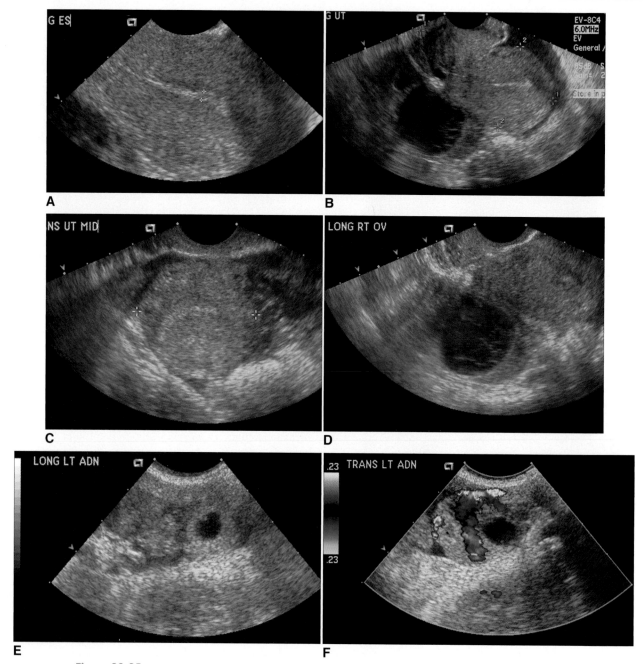

Figure 38-35   Ectopic pregnancy. **A,** Endovaginal sagittal image showing the empty uterus in a patient who presented with vaginal bleeding and elevated hCG levels. **B,** Complex mass seen posterior to uterus. **C,** Transverse image of uterus. **D,** Sagittal image of complex mass posterior to uterus. **E,** Sagittal image of gestational sac in the adnexal area. **F,** Increased color Doppler flow surrounding the ectopic pregnancy "ring of fire."

solid with a "moth-eaten" cystic pattern that occurs when they become necrotic. Lymphoma involving the ovary is usually diffuse and disseminated and is also frequently bilateral. Sonographically, the mass appears as a solid hypoechoic tumor similar to lymphoma elsewhere in the body.

CARCINOMA OF THE FALLOPIAN TUBE

Carcinoma of the fallopian tube is the least common (less than 1%) of all gynecologic malignancies. Adenocarcinoma is the most common histological finding. It occurs most frequently in postmenopausal women with pain, vaginal bleeding, and a pelvic mass. The tumor usually involves the distal end, but it may involve the entire length of the tube.

Sonographic Findings. Sonographically, carcinoma of the fallopian tube appears as a sausage-shaped, complex mass, with cystic and solid components often with papillary projections. The clinical and sonographic findings are similar to those of ovarian carcinoma.

OTHER PELVIC MASSES

Not all pelvic masses are gynecologic in origin. Pelvic kidneys, omental cysts, distended impacted feces in the rectosigmoid colon, a distended bladder, hydroureters, colonic cancer or masses, diverticular abscesses, and retroperitoneal masses can all be identified by ultrasound examination. In addition, the use of ultrasound in detecting an ectopic pregnancy has been well documented (Figure 38-35). The location, size, consistency, and source of adnexal masses can be defined by a flexible combination of endovaginal and transabdominal scanning. It is of key importance to try to distinguish solid ovarian masses from pedunculated myomas by identifying the uterine connection and searching for an ovary. Any fluid present in the pelvis can be used to outline dependent portions of the pelvic organs by tilting the patient, using an endovaginal approach, or both. Large palpable tumors rising out of the pelvis are best viewed with transabdominal technique.

Ultrasound examination is useful in defining symptomatic or palpable masses, as described previously. It allows the surgeon to observe functional-appearing cysts without resorting to immediate surgery and to plan strategy for surgical exploration and treatment when necessary. Obvious signs of malignancy, such as sonolucent liver metastases or nodular peritoneum outlined by ascites, assist in preoperative assessment. With current equipment, excellent resolution is available, and the experienced sonographer may frequently identify the tumor by its texture if the clinical context is understood. However, histologic diagnosis is the job of the pathologist.

REFERENCES

1. Bourne T and others: Endovaginal colour flow imaging: a possible new screening technique for ovarian cancer, *Br Med J* 299:1367, 1989.
2. Bret PM and others: Endovaginal US-guided aspiration of ovarian cysts and solid pelvic masses, *Radiology* 185:377, 1992.
3. Cohen HL and others: Ovarian cysts are common in premenarchal girls: a sonographic study of 101 children 2-12 years old, *Am J Roentgenol* 159:89, 1992.
4. Dahnert W: *Radiology review manual,* ed 3, Baltimore, 1996, Williams and Wilkins.
5. Fleischer AC, Kepple DM, Vasquez J: Conventional and color Doppler endovaginal sonography in gynecologic infertility, *Radiol Clin North Am* 30:693, 1992.
6. Granberg S and others: Comparison of endovaginal ultrasound and cytological evaluation of cystic ovarian tumors, *J Ultrasound Med* 10:9, 1991.
7. Kurjak A and others: Evaluation of adnexal masses with endovaginal color ultrasound, *J Ultrasound Med* 10:295, 1991.
8. Levine D and others: Sonography of adnexal masses: poor sensitivity of resistive index for identifying malignant lesions, *Am J Roentgenol* 162:1355, 1994.

SELECTED BIBLIOGRAPHY

Brammer HM III and others: From the archives of the AFIP: malignant germ cell tumors of the ovary: radiologic-pathologic correlation, *Radiographics* 10:715, 1990.

Buy J-N and others: Epithelial tumors of the ovary: CT findings and correlation with US, *Radiology* 178:811, 1991.

Fleischer AC: Ultrasound imaging-2000: assessment of utero-ovarian blood flow with endovaginal color Doppler sonography: potential clinical applications in infertility, *Fertil Steril* 55:684, 1991.

Fleischer AC and others: Assessment of ovarian tumor vascularity with endovaginal color Doppler sonography, *J Ultrasound Med* 10:563, 1991.

Fleischer AC and others: Color Doppler sonography of benign and malignant ovarian masses, *Radiographics* 12:879, 1992.

Helvie MA and others: Ovarian torsion: sonographic evaluation, *J Clin Ultrasound* 17:327, 1989.

Hilgers TW and others: Assessment of the empty follicle syndrome by endovaginal sonography, *J Ultrasound Med* 11:313, 1992.

Kurjak A and others: New scoring system for prediction of ovarian malignancy based on endovaginal color Doppler sonography, *J Ultrasound Med* 11:631, 1992.

Pache TD and others: How to discriminate between normal and polycystic ovaries: endovaginal US study, *Radiology* 183:421, 1992.

Rosado WM and others: Adnexal torsion: diagnosis by using Doppler sonography, *Am J Roentgenol* 159:1251, 1992.

Rottem S and others: Classification of ovarian lesions by high-frequency endovaginal sonography, *J Clin Ultrasound* 18:359, 1990.

Rumack CM, Wilson SR, Charboneau JW, *Diagnostic ultrasound,* ed 3, St Louis, 2005, Mosby.

Shimizu H and others: Characteristic ultrasonographic appearance of the Krukenberg tumor, *J Clin Ultrasound* 18:697, 1990.

Siegel MJ: Pediatric gynecologic sonography, *Radiology* 179:593, 1991.

Takahashi K and others: Endovaginal ultrasound is an effective method for screening in polycystic ovarian disease, *Gynecol Obstet Invest* 30:34, 1990.

Zalud I and others: The assessment of luteal blood flow in pregnant and nonpregnant women by endovaginal color Doppler, *J Perinat Med* 18:215, 1990.

CHAPTER 39

Pathology of the Adnexa

Barbara J. Vander Werff and Sandra L. Hagen-Ansert

KEY TERMS

adenomyosis – benign invasive growth of the endometrium into the muscular layer of the uterus

Chlamydia trachomatis – an organism that causes a great variety of diseases, including genital infections in men and women

endometrioma – localized tumor of endometriosis most frequently found in the ovary, cul-de-sac, rectovaginal septum, and peritoneal surface of the posterior wall of the uterus

endometriosis – a condition that occurs when functioning endometrial tissue invades sites outside the uterus

endometritis – infection within the endometrium of the uterus

hydrosalpinx – fluid within the fallopian tube

myometritis – infection within the myometrium of the uterus

oophoritis – infection within the ovary

parametritis – infection within the uterine serosa and broad ligaments

pelvic inflammatory disease (PID) – all-inclusive term that refers to all pelvic infections (endometritis, salpingitis, hydrosalpinx, pyosalpinx, and tubo-ovarian abscess)

periovarian inflammation – enlarged ovaries with multiple cysts and indistinct margins

pyosalpinx – retained pus within the inflamed fallopian tube

salpingitis – infection within the fallopian tubes

tubo-ovarian abscess (TOA) – infection that involves the fallopian tube and the ovary

tubo-ovarian complex – fusion of the inflamed dilated tube and ovary

Pelvic inflammatory disease (PID) and endometriosis are diffuse disease processes of the female pelvic cavity. They can be caused by sexually transmitted diseases and are most commonly associated with gonorrhea and chlamydia. PID and endometriosis have very different clinical presentations and pathologies. However, early in the disease the clinical presentation of both endometriosis and PID is nonspecific and may mimic functional bowel disease.

PID is an inclusive term that refers to all pelvic infections (e.g., endometritis, salpingitis, hydrosalpinx, pyosalpinx, **periovarian inflammation**, **tubo-ovarian complex,** and tubo-ovarian abscess). The infection usually occurs bilaterally and may be found in the endometrium (**endometritis**), the uterine wall (**myometritis**), the uterine serosa and broad ligaments (**parametritis**), the ovary (**oophoritis**), and the most common location, the oviducts (salpingitis) (Figure 39-1). Ultrasound has limited value during acute PID. In the setting of chronic

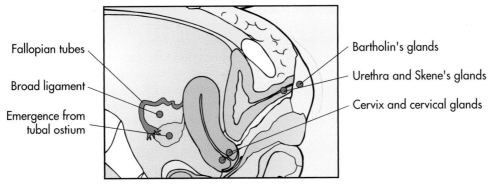

Figure 39-1 Pelvic inflammatory disease may be found in the endometrium, the uterine wall, the uterine serosa and broad ligaments, the ovary, and the fallopian tubes.

PID, ultrasound can identify dilated fallopian tubes (hydrosalpinx or pyosalpinx), abscess, and complex intraperitoneal fluid.

Endometriosis is the presence of endometrial glands or stroma in abnormal locations. It occurs most commonly in two forms: adenomyosis of the uterus and endometriosis of the adnexa. In many cases, endometriosis is diagnosed on clinical grounds and is not detectable by ultrasound. When identified sonographically, it presents as an adnexal mass or masses (endometriomas) of variable echogenicity, shape, and size.

PELVIC INFLAMMATORY DISEASE

The occurrence of **pelvic inflammatory disease (PID)** is becoming more common. PID occurs in 11% of women during reproductive age (17% in African-Americans) and affects 1 million American women each year, with the highest occurrence among teenagers. Risk factors include early sexual contact, multiple sexual partners, history of sexually transmitted disease, previous history of PID, intrauterine contraceptive device (IUCD), and douching, because douching may push bacteria into the upper genital tract. Although sexually transmitted diseases, such as gonorrhea and chlamydia, are the most common forms of infection, other routes of infection are possible, such as direct extension from appendiceal, diverticular, or postsurgical abscess collections that have ruptured into the pelvis, the string from an IUCD, and puerperal and postabortion complications. Other types of invasive instrumentation procedures in the pelvic cavity may leave the route more open to bacterial invasion. PID is usually found as a bilateral collection of fluid and pus within the pelvic cavity, except when it is caused by direct extension of an adjacent inflammatory process, in which case it is most commonly unilateral (Box 39-1).

Infrequently, particularly in patients with PID resulting from gonorrhea, a pelvic infection may ascend the right flank, causing a perihepatic inflammation. The pain may mimic liver, gallbladder, or right renal pain. Perihepatic inflammation can be detected sonographically by scanning along the liver margin and identifying a hypoechoic rim between the liver and the adjacent ribs. This perihepatic inflammation is called the Fitz-Hugh-Curtis syndrome.

> ### BOX 39-1   PELVIC INFLAMMATORY DISEASE
>
> - Inflammatory disease (acute or chronic); infection spreads to pelvis
> - Large, palpable, bilateral complex mass; ovary may be seen separate from mass
> - Free fluid in cul-de-sac
> - Doppler image shows increased vascularity and diastolic flow
> - Associated with infertility and endometritis

Sexually transmitted PID is spread via the mucosa of the pelvic organs through the cervix into the uterine endometrium (**endometritis**) and out the fallopian tubes (acute salpingitis) to the area of the ovaries and peritoneum. As the tube becomes obstructed, it fills with pus (pyosalpinx). In the setting of extensive PID, the margins of the ovaries and other pelvic structures can become difficult to distinguish from each other.

The bacterial infection may arise from ***Chlamydia trachomatis*** and *Neisseria gonorrhea*. Other bacteria that have been found in PID patients include aerobes (*Streptococcus* sp., *Escherichia coli*, *Haemophilus influenzae*), anaerobes (*Bacteroides, Peptostreptococcus,* and *Peptococcus*), *Mycobacterium tuberculosis*, *Actinomycetes* sp. in IUCD users, and herpesvirus hominis type 1.

If the pregnancy test result is positive in a woman with previously treated PID, a careful evaluation of the adnexa is indicated even if a normal intrauterine pregnancy is detected. From the previous fallopian tube damage, the incidence of an ectopic pregnancy is significantly increased. The possibility of a rare heterotopic pregnancy (a concomitant intrauterine and extrauterine pregnancy) increases.

Clinically, patients may present with intense pelvic pain and tenderness described as dull and aching, with constant vaginal discharge. Other symptoms include fever, pain in the right upper abdomen, painful intercourse, and irregular menstrual bleeding. A history of infertility may also be present. Lab tests may show an elevated white blood cell count (WBCs) in PID, particularly when caused by chlamydial infection. The patient may be asymptomatic or the disease may produce only minor symptoms, even though it can seriously damage the reproductive organs. A palpable mass may be present on clinical examination.

The sonographic findings may be normal early in the course of the disease (Box 39-2). As the disease progresses or becomes chronic, a variety of findings may occur. Differential considerations may include hematoma, dermoid cyst, ovarian neoplasm, and endometriosis.

SALPINGITIS, HYDROSALPINX, AND PYOSALPINX

Salpingitis is an inflammation of a fallopian tube (Box 39-3). This condition may be acute, subacute, or chronic. Clinical signs may range from asymptomatic to pelvic fullness or discomfort, or a low-grade fever. An obstructed tube filled with serous secretions is a **hydrosalpinx**; this can occur as a result of PID, endometriosis, or postoperative adhesions. The dilated tube may show a pointed beak at the swollen end of the tube near the isthmus where the tube enters the uterus. If the dilated

tube becomes infected, it is called **pyosalpinx.** The likelihood of recurrent infection and ectopic pregnancy increases significantly. Infected or hemorrhagic pelvic fluid may also be present. Infection can obscure normal tissue planes, making anatomy unclear. Severe pain requires gentle use of ultrasound probes in acute PID, and in some cases a full bladder for transabdominal study is intolerable.

Sonographic Findings. Sonographically, the normal fallopian tube is generally not visualized unless fluid surrounds it. If outlined by ascitic fluid, it is a thin, less than 5-mm hypoechoic tissue band originating from the uterine fundus and can be imaged in an axial-coronal view. The sonographer can try to follow the dilated fallopian tube as it enters the cornu of the uterus (at the fundus). Careful oblique angulations of the transducer are necessary to trace the pathway of the tube. If fluid, pus, or products of conception fill the tube, detection is easier (Figure 39-2). If the lumen is outlined and shows irregularity and multiple diverticula, a pathologic state is probable.

If distinct tubular structures are instead seen, hydrosalpinx (dilated tubes) is diagnosed. Hydrosalpinx has variable presentations, from subtle dilated tubular structures to massive tortuous cystic areas. Although both tubes may be damaged, they may be asymmetric in size, with only the more dilated tube appreciated sonographically. Although contrast-enhanced salpingography is the definitive test, ultrasound appears accurate in identifying this process, particularly when performed endovaginally. Hydrosalpinx may present as echogenic fluid or fluid-debris levels (Figure 39-3) indicating infection (pyosalpinx).

Severe and chronic pyosalpinx often contain thick, echogenic mucoid pus, which does not transmit sound as well as serous fluid or blood. A pyosalpinx can appear as a complex mass. An EV ultrasound is particularly useful for identifying the tubular nature and folds of the dilated tube, thus avoiding the mistaken diagnosis of a mass.

> **BOX 39-2**
> ## SONOGRAPHIC FINDINGS OF PELVIC INFLAMMATORY DISEASE
>
> - *Endometritis:* Thickening or fluid in the endometrium
> - *Periovarian inflammation:* Enlarged ovaries with multiple cysts, indistinct margins
> - *Salpingitis:* Nodular thickening, irregularity of tube with diverticula
> - *Pyosalpinx or hydrosalpinx:* Fluid-filled irregular fallopian tube with or without echoes
> - *Tubo-ovarian abscess:* Complex mass with septations, irregular margins, and internal echoes; usually in cul-de-sac

---

> **BOX 39-3**
> ## SALPINGITIS, HYDROSALPINX, AND PYOSALPINX

	DESCRIPTION	CLINICAL	SONOGRAPHIC FINDINGS
Salpingitis	Inflammation of fallopian tube Acute, subacute, or chronic	Asymptomatic to pelvic fullness or discomfort Low-grade fever	Dilated tube Tortuous
Hydrosalpinx	Obstructed tube filled with serous secretions Occurs secondary to PID, endometriosis, or postoperative adhesions	Asymptomatic to pelvic fullness or discomfort Low-grade fever	Walls become thin secondary to dilation Appearance of multicystic or fusiform mass Follow dilated tubes from fundus of uterus Look for pointed "beak" at swollen end of tube near isthmus Bilateral Ampullary portion more dilated than interstitial part of tube
Pyosalpinx	Retained pus in oviduct with inflammation	Asymptomatic to pelvic fullness or discomfort Low-grade fever	May appear as complex mass Pus within dilated tube very thick and echogenic–poor sound transmission

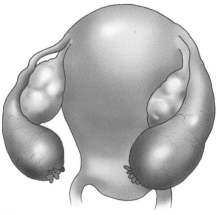

Figure 39-2 Salpingitis is an inflammation of the fallopian tubes that causes nodular dilation. This infection may be unilateral or bilateral.

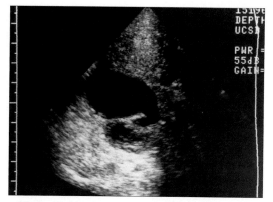

Figure 39-4 Endovaginal coronal image of a patient with acute salpingitis. The wall appears slightly thickened and very dilated.

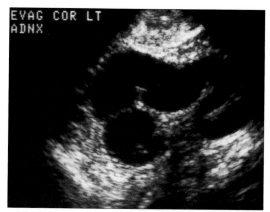

Figure 39-3 Endovaginal coronal image of the very dilated fallopian tube. When swollen with fluid, the tube bends and curls in the adnexal area.

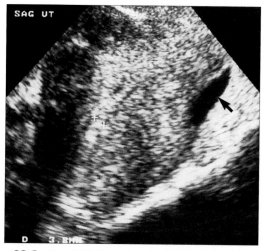

Figure 39-5 Free fluid. Sagittal view of the uterus in an asymptomatic, postmenopausal female demonstrates a small fluid collection *(arrow)* posterior to the uterus.

Acute salpingitis is evident as a thick-walled nodular hyperemic tube (Figure 39-4). The unhealthy dilated tubes usually surround the ovaries like two crescents of ring sausage encircling the posterior surface of the uterus and filling the cul-de-sac.

The sonographer should be sure not to confuse the dilated tube with a dilated ureter or prominent vessel. Occasionally, prominent blood vessels may be present in the adnexa. Although these may initially be misinterpreted as a hydrosalpinx, color or pulsed Doppler imaging will show blood flow in an adnexal blood vessel and no flow in a hydrosalpinx. Evaluation of the kidneys for possible hydronephrosis and trying to trace the dilated ureter to the bladder should help. The ovaries may be difficult to delineate because of surrounding tissue, edema, and pus. In addition to hydrosalpinx or pyosalpinx, sonographic findings of PID include fluid in the cul-de-sac (Figure 39-5), mild uterine enlargement, and endometrial fluid or thickening. Transabdominal and endovaginal ultrasound can reveal the presence of pelvic intraperitoneal fluid in the cul-de-sac. Pelvic fluid may frequently have internal echoes, septations, and fluid levels, a sign that the fluid is not simple but rather may be infected or hemorrhagic (Figure 36-6).

Any simple cyst that hemorrhages may appear as a complex mass. In patients of reproductive age, the classic differential diagnosis of a complex adnexal mass is ectopic pregnancy, endometriosis, and PID. Dermoids and other benign tumors can appear in a similar fashion.

TUBO-OVARIAN ABSCESS (TOA)

The adhesive, edematous, and inflamed serosa may further adhere to the ovary and/or other peritoneal surfaces, which distorts anatomy. As the infection worsens, periovarian adhesions may form. The ovary cannot be separated from the inflamed dilated tube and is called the tubo-ovarian complex. In trying to determine if an adnexal mass is separate from the ovary, gentle pushing with the endovaginal transducer can be used to identify separate or contiguous movement. Periovarian adhesions fuse the inflamed ovary and tube, and the ovary cannot be separated from the tube. This causes a further loculation of pus known as a **tubo-ovarian abscess (TOA).** This may be unilateral abscess or bilateral and appears as a complex mass in the posterior cul-de-sac.

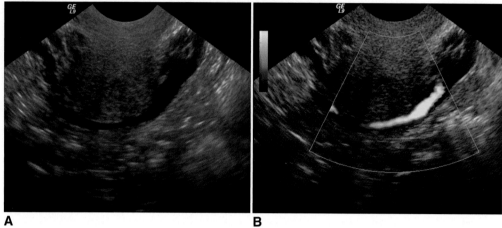

Figure 39-6   A, Endovaginal transverse image of the uterus with sonolucent structure posterior. **B,** Power Doppler shows the structure to be vascular in origin, not free fluid.

The tubo-ovarian complex or abscess usually responds well to antibiotic treatment without the need for surgical drainage. Serial ultrasound images during treatment allow observation of resolution and can indicate which patients need prolonged intravenous antibiotics and which patients may benefit more from removal of the involved tissue. Sonographic guidance can be used to assist in percutaneous or endovaginal drainage, for culture and sensitivity or complete drainage, and thus hasten recovery.

Sonographic Findings. A pelvic abscess is usually a complex mass in the cul-de-sac that distorts pelvic anatomy (Figure 39-7). It can involve the ovary alone or the fallopian tube and ovary as a tubo-ovarian abscess. The TOA appears as a complex multiloculated mass with variable septations, irregular margins, and scattered internal echoes. The ovaries are often difficult to recognize as separate from the mass because of surrounding tissue, edema, and pus (Figure 39-8). As noted, TOAs usually are bilateral, but may be unilateral if an IUCD is present or if there is direct extension from an abdominal abscess. There is usually posterior acoustic enhancement. Occasionally a fluid-debris level or gas may be seen within the mass. Gas within the abscess may appear as hyperechoic, punctate echoes that exhibit a comet tail shadowing effect. Drainage of the collection of pus may be done with interventional sonography (Figure 39-9). Recognizable ovarian tissue may be seen within the inflammatory mass by endovaginal sonography (Figures 39-10 through 39-13).

The sonographic appearance may be indistinguishable from other adnexal masses, and clinical correlation is necessary for the correct diagnosis. The endovaginal approach is helpful in assessing the extent of the disease. Dilated tubes, periovarian inflammatory change, and the internal characteristics of tubo-ovarian abscesses are better defined with endovaginal scanning.

PERITONITIS

Peritonitis is the inflammation of the peritoneum, the serous membrane lining the abdominal cavity and covering the viscera. This inflammation is caused by infectious organisms that gain access by way of rupture or perforation of the viscera or associated structures; via the female genital tract; by piercing the abdominal wall; via the bloodstream or lymphatic vessels; via surgical incisions; or by failure to practice antiseptic techniques during surgery. If the infectious process spreads to involve the bladder, ureter, bowel, and adnexal area, it becomes pelvic peritonitis.

Sonographic Findings. If the abscess collection has gas-forming bubbles within, it may be difficult to delineate well with sonography because the beam is reflected from the area of interest. The sonographer should look for loculated areas of fluid within the pelvis, the paracolic gutters, and mesenteric reflections. Evaluation of the space between the right kidney and liver and the left kidney and spleen should also include a check for fluid.

ENDOMETRIOSIS AND ENDOMETRIOMA

Endometriosis is one of the most common gynecological diseases. It is defined as the presence of functioning endometrial tissue in abnormal locations (Box 39-4). The ectopic tissue can be found almost anywhere in the body including the ovaries, fallopian tubes, broad ligaments, the external surface of the uterus, and scattered over the peritoneum, bowel, or bladder, especially in the dependent parts of the pelvis or cul-de-sac (Figure 39-14). The incidence of endometriosis is found in up to 15% of premenopausal women. It affects women in their third to fourth decade of life and is dependent on normal hormonal stimulation. Clinical findings include severe dysmenorrhea, chronic pelvic pain from peritoneal adhesions and bleeding, or dyspareunia.

The cause may arise from peritoneal seeding from retrograde travel of endometrial cells through fallopian tubes, metaplastic transformation of peritoneal epithelium into endometrial tissue, or through traumatic spread from uterine surgery or amniocentesis.

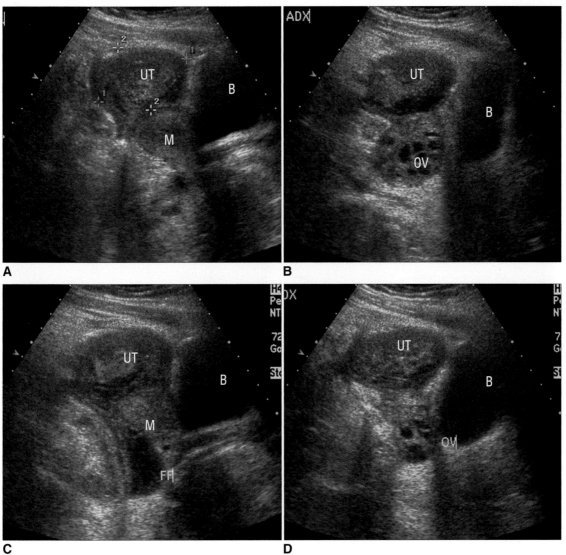

Figure 39-7 **A,** Transabdominal midline sagittal image of the bladder (B), uterus (UT), and complex mass (M) that is displacing the uterus anteriorly. **B,** The scan over the right adnexal area shows the uterus (UT) with the right ovary posterior (OV). The bladder (B) is seen inferiorly. **C,** The scan over the midline of the pelvis demonstrates the mass (M) posterior to the uterus (UT). Free fluid (FF) is seen adjacent to the complex mass. **D,** The scan over the left adnexal area shows the left ovary (OV) and uterus (UT).

BOX 39-4   ENDOMETRIOSIS

	DESCRIPTION	CLINICAL	SONOGRAPHIC FINDINGS
Endometriosis	Presence of functional ectopic endometrial glands and stroma outside the uterine cavity.	Not distinctive Complaints of dysmenorrhea with pelvic pain Premenstrual dyspareunia Sacral backache during menses Infertility	Bilateral or unilateral ovarian cysts Cysts are anechoic to solid, depending on amount of blood Ovaries adherent to posterior uterus or in cul-de-sac; difficult to define Obscured organ borders Focal mass is endometrioma ("chocolate cyst") with low-intensity echoes and acoustic enhancement

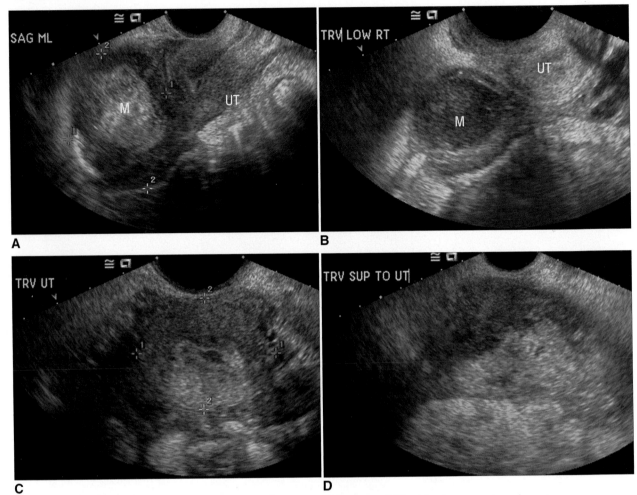

Figure 39-8 **A,** Endovaginal sagittal midline image of the uterus (UT) with a large complex echogenic mass (M) adjacent to the uterine cavity. **B,** The complex mass (M) is clearly separate from the uterus (UT). **C,** Endovaginal image of the uterus. **D,** Endovaginal image superior to the uterine fundus shows the complex mass.

Endometriosis has two forms: internal and external. Internal endometriosis occurs within the uterus **(adenomyosis).** External endometriosis is outside the uterus and may be found in the pouch of Douglas; surface of the ovary, fallopian tube, and uterus broad ligaments; or rectovaginal septum.

The more common form of endometriosis is the external, or indirect, form. The disease process for the external form varies in extent from small foci to widespread sheets of tissue to focal discrete masses. The endometrial tissue in endometriosis cyclically bleeds and proliferates as stimulated by changes in hormonal influence.

The second less common form of endometriosis, known as the internal or direct form, is called adenomyosis. It remains confined within the uterus, invading the junctional zone and the myometrium. The true prevalence of endometriosis is unknown because most cases are asymptomatic.

Endometriosis can be either diffuse or localized. The diffuse form is most common and is rarely diagnosed by sonography because the implants are so small. The diffuse form leads to disorganization of the pelvic anatomy with an appearance similar to PID (Figure 39-15) or chronic ectopic pregnancy.

The localized form consists of a discrete mass called an **endometrioma,** or "chocolate cyst." Endometriomas are usually asymptomatic and can frequently be multiple and have a unique sonographic appearance. These may become moderately enlarged and may create a surgical emergency by rupturing or by causing the ovary to twist on the vessels that supply it and cause torsion.

Two possible explanations for the cause of endometriosis are presented. The first is that the chronic reflux of menstrual fluid through the tubes and into the pelvis may in some women produce implantation and proliferation of endometrial cells with cyclic bleeding. The second theory involves the evaluation of endometrial activity in susceptible cells that retain the embryonic capacity to differentiate in response to hormonal stimulation. The resulting tissue bleeds and proliferates with resultant production of pain, scarring, and endometrium-lined collections of blood known as endometriomas.

Endometriosis may occur in any menstruating female. Clinical symptoms include painful periods (dysmenorrhea) or painful intercourse (dyspareunia); lower abdominal, pelvic, and back pain; irregular bleeding; and infertility secondary to

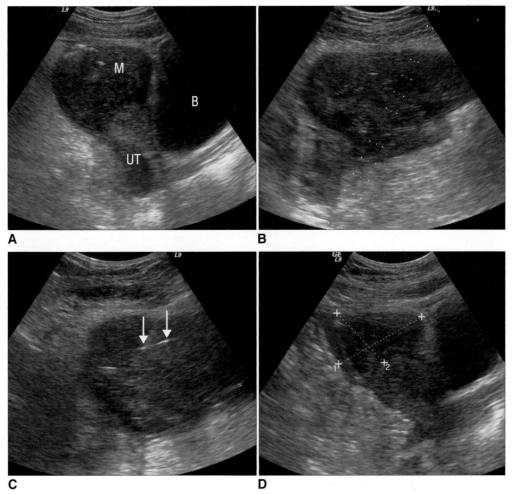

Figure 39-9 **A,** TA sagittal midline image of the pelvis shows the distended urinary bladder (B), the complex mass (M) anterior to the uterus (UT). **B,** TA transverse image over the complex mass. **C,** A drainage catheter is inserted into the mass *(arrows).* **D,** The mass is slightly decreased in size; the catheter may be left in place for several days to drain the pus accumulation.

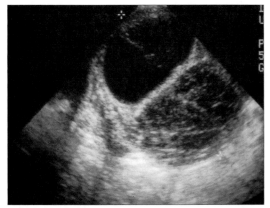

Figure 39-10 Endovaginal sagittal image in a 24-year-old female who had pelvic pain. A complex mass was seen in the right adnexa secondary to a hemorrhagic corpus lutein cyst.

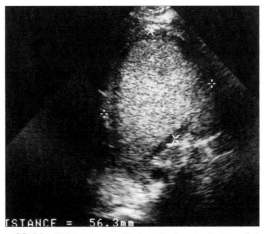

Figure 39-11 Pelvic abscess. Endovaginal sagittal view of the cul-de-sac demonstrates a 6-cm complex fluid collection in a 37-year-old intravenous drug abuser with multiple complex fluid collections in the pelvis. This abscess was drained endovaginally.

adhesions and fibrosis. Differential diagnosis would include hemorrhagic ovarian cyst, TOA, cystic ovarian neoplasm, solid ovarian tumor, or ectopic pregnancy. Clinically, most women with an acute hemorrhagic cyst or abscess present with acute pelvic pain, whereas women with an endometrioma are asymptomatic or have more chronic discomfort associated with their menses.

Symptoms depend on the location and extent of the disease, but there is no direct relationship between the extent of disease and severity of symptoms. Patients can be asymptomatic if the condition is confined to the ovaries, or they can suffer severe pain if it is widespread. Although typically associated with infertility, endometriosis may even be identified in a pregnant patient.

Sonographic Findings. Endometriomas may appear as bilateral or unilateral ovarian cysts with patterns ranging from

anechoic to solid, depending on the amount of blood and its organization. The ovaries typically adhere to the posterior surface of the uterus or are stuck in the cul-de-sac and may be difficult to define. Obscured organ borders and multiple irregular cystic masses are also suggestive of either disseminating cancer or pelvic infection. Endometriosis is rarely detected sonographically unless a focal mass called an endometrioma is present.

An endometrioma often appears as a well-defined, predominantly cystic mass with transabdominal ultrasound, but, with endovaginal ultrasound, uniform internal echoes are usually seen. The most common presentation is of a "choco-

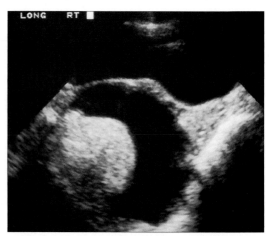

Figure 39-13   A 23-year-old female came to the emergency department with fever, vaginal discharge, and acute pelvic pain that persisted for 3 days. The transabdominal sagittal image shows the full bladder with the tubular vagina just posterior. The large complex tubo-ovarian abscess has both cystic and solid components and has pushed the uterus *(not seen)* away from the midline.

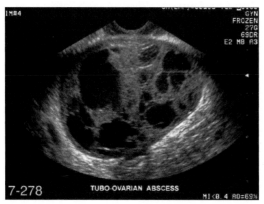

Figure 39-12   Endovaginal image in a 27-year-old female who presented with fever and intense pelvic pain shows a huge complex collection within the adnexal area consistent with a tubo-ovarian abscess.

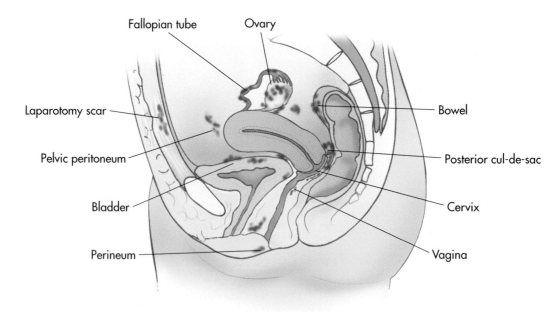

Figure 39-14   Possible pelvic sites of endometriosis.

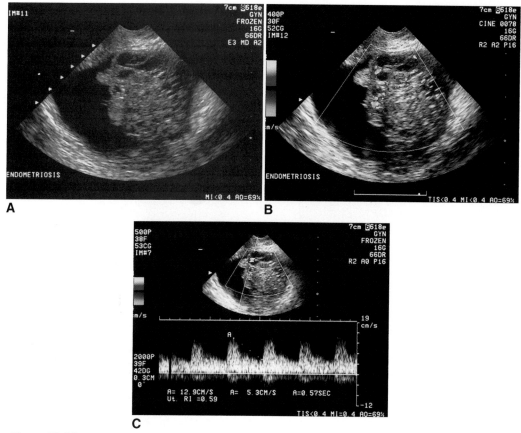

Figure 39-15 A 34-year-old female with pelvic fullness. **A,** The endovaginal coronal image shows a complex mass in the right adnexal area. **B,** Color Doppler imaging shows increased flow from the bleeding within the tissue. **C,** The spectral Doppler tracing shows a low-resistance flow pattern.

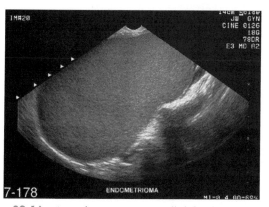

Figure 39-16 An endometrioma is a well-defined homogeneous mass with low-intensity echoes and acoustic enhancement.

late cyst" with low-intensity echoes and acoustic enhancement (Figure 39-16). The echogenicity of endometriomas can vary from cystic to solid, and their size varies widely from less than 1 cm to more than 10 cm in diameter. The masses are the result of multiple episodes of bleeding. Fluid-fluid levels and internal septations are frequently seen. Some endometriomas are multiloculated, often with varied internal echo patterns and interconnecting loculations. Endometriomas may be multiple and present in both adnexa. Endometriomas can have a similar appearance to inflammation (abscess), trophoblastic tissue (ectopic pregnancy), and dermoids.

Other appearances include an enlarged multicystic ovary with a thick wall and internal septations or a cyst with fluid-debris levels (because of different degrees of organization of the hemorrhage). Small linear hyperechoic foci may be present in the wall of the cyst and are thought to be caused by cholesterol deposits accumulating in the cyst wall. Endometriomas may also demonstrate microcalcification (Figure 39-17). Ovarian abscesses or hemorrhagic ovarian cysts may demonstrate sonographic appearances similar to endometriomas; however, the clinical picture is usually different.

INTERVENTIONAL ULTRASOUND

Ultrasound guided percutaneous biopsy and abscess drainage have become valuable diagnostic and therapeutic procedures (see Chapter 15). Interventional biopsy has also decreased patient costs by obviating the need for an operation and lengthy hospital stay. Contraindications to needle biopsy include uncorrectable coagulopathy, lack of a safe biopsy route, and an uncooperative patient. A patient's bleeding history can be evaluated with a platelet count, INR, prothrombin time, and partial thromboplastin time. Evaluation of the patient's use of aspirin, Coumadin, or heparin should also be used to screen for

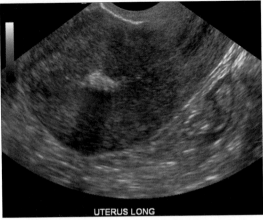

Figure 39-17 Endovaginal sagittal view of the uterus in a different patient demonstrates endometrial calcification *(arrow)* with shadowing. This woman had a history of previous dilation and curettage.

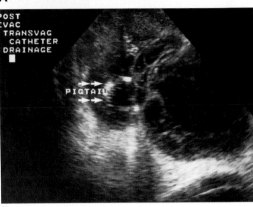

Figure 39-18 Hematometra in a 23-year-old woman 4 weeks after a dilation and curettage. **A,** Transabdominal longitudinal view of the uterus demonstrates a central fluid collection with a fluid debris level *(arrows)*. **B,** Endovaginal image in the same patient again demonstrates the pigtail catheter *(arrows)*. The fluid is monitored by ultrasound guidance.

an increased risk of bleeding. If these values are abnormal, the procedure should be delayed if deemed necessary after consulting with the patient's doctor. Transabdominal or endovaginal guidance is used for aspiration of benign-appearing cysts. Endovaginal drainage is helpful in TOAs; other pelvic abscesses, such as appendicitis and diverticulitis; and drainage of postoperative fluid collections (Figure 39-18). Transrectal drainage is used for deep pelvic abscesses. Endovaginal ultrasonography also is used in obtaining biopsies for benign and malignant solid pelvic masses and to drain recurrent malignant collections. Biopsy kits can be used with the endovaginal transducers to allow direct visualization of the region of interest.

Ultrasonically guided needle drainage of abscesses and stable hematomas, either through the abdominal wall or the vagina, is diagnostic and therapeutic. Recurrent tumor masses may be biopsied in a similar fashion. The endovaginal ultrasound and needle guide make entering the anterior or posterior cul-de-sacs safer and easier for pelvic fluid aspiration, biopsies, or radiation needle placement.

POSTOPERATIVE USES OF ULTRASOUND

Pain and the development of a pelvic mass after pelvic surgery can indicate complications, such as postoperative bleeding, hematomas, or abscess formation. Although postoperative masses are not always dangerous, more than one surgeon has made the diagnosis of severely distended bladder by ordering an ultrasound for a postoperative pelvic mass. Ultrasound can be used to distinguish a distended, fluid-filled bladder from a fluid collection in the operative site. The ability to palpate specific structures with the endovaginal probe and avoid the abdominal wound is valuable in determining the site of pain in a postoperative pelvis. Resolving hematomas often appear to be of a solid consistency and can be followed as they shrink.

An expert combination of endovaginal and transabdominal techniques is essential as new gynecologic applications of ultrasound continue to be found for screening, diagnosis, and therapy of pelvic pathology in a female patient. The inclusion of translabial and the perineal approaches to gynecological imaging allows another field of view for the sonographer to evaluate the pelvic structures. Three-dimensional imaging will surely add additional understanding of ovarian pathologies.

SELECTED BIBLIOGRAPHY

Abbitt PL, Goldwag S, Urbanski S: Endovaginal sonography for guidance in draining pelvic fluid collections, *Am J Roentgenol* 154:849, 1990.

Bennett JD and others: Deep pelvic abscesses: transrectal drainage with radiologic guidance, *Radiology* 185:825, 1992.

Bisset RA, Rhan AN: *Differential diagnosis in abdominal ultrasound,* ed 2, Philadelphia, 2002, WB Saunders.

Callen P: *Ultrasonography in obstetrics and gynecology,* ed 4, Philadelphia, 2000, WB Saunders.

Carlson JA Jr and others: Clinical and pathologic correlation of endometrial cavity fluid detected by ultrasound in the postmenopausal patient, *Obstet Gynecol* 77:119, 1991.

Fedele L and others: Endovaginal ultrasonography in the differential diagnosis of adenomyoma versus leiomyoma, *Am J Obstet Gynecol* 167:603, 1992.

Hall R: Pelvic inflammatory disease and endometriosis. In Berman MC, Cohen HL, editors: *Obstetrics & gynecology*, ed 2, Philadelphia, 1997, JB Lippincott.

Johnson PT, Jurtz AB: *Case review obstetric and gynecologic ultrasound*, ed 1, St Louis, 2001, Mosby.

Kupfer MC, Schwimer SR, Lebovic J: Endovaginal sonographic appearance of endometriomata: spectrum of findings, *J Ultrasound Med* 11:129, 1992.

Kurjak A, Zalud I, Alfirevic Z: Evaluation of adnexal masses with endovaginal color ultrasound, *J Ultrasound Med* 10:295, 1991.

Nosher JL, Winchman HK, Needell GS: Endovaginal pelvic abscess drainage with US guidance, *Radiology* 165:872, 1987.

Patten RM and others: Pelvic inflammatory disease: endovaginal sonography with laparoscopic correlation, *J Ultrasound Med* 9:681, 1990.

Sanders RC: *Clinical sonography*, ed 3, Philadelphia, 1998, Lippincott.

Schneider S, Craig M, Branning P: Improved sonographic accuracy in the presurgical diagnosis of diffuse adenomyosis, *JDMS* 18:71-77, 2002.

Van Sonnenberg E and others: US-guided endovaginal drainage of pelvic abscesses and fluid collections, *Radiology* 181:53, 1991.

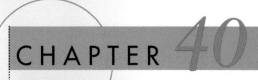

CHAPTER *40*

The Role of Ultrasound in Evaluating Female Infertility

Carol Mitchell and Valjean MacMillan

OBJECTIVES

- Define *infertility*
- List the female pelvic organs to be imaged in an infertility work-up
- State anatomic variations or pathologies that need to be defined when imaging an infertility patient
- State treatment options for infertile couples
- List complications that may occur because of infertility treatments

KEY TERMS

assisted reproductive technology (ART) – technologies employed to assist the infertility patient to become pregnant. These methods include in vitro fertilization, gamete intrafallopian transfer, zygote intrafallopian transfer, and artificial insemination.

basal body temperature – the morning body temperature taken orally before the patient does any activity

embryo transfer – a technique that follows IVF in which the fertilized ova are injected into the uterus through the cervix

gamete intrafallopian tube transfer (GIFT) – a human fertilization technique in which male and female gametes are injected through a laparoscope into the fimbriated ends of the fallopian tubes. Recently, this has been performed under ultrasound guidance.

gonadotropin – a hormonal substance that stimulates the function of the testes and ovaries

human chorionic gonadotropin (hCG) – a glycoprotein secreted from placental trophoblastic cells. This chemical component is found in maternal urine when pregnant.

intrauterine insemination – the introduction of semen into the vagina or uterus by mechanical or instrumental means rather than by sexual intercourse

in vitro fertilization (IVF) – a method of fertilizing the human ova outside the body by collecting the mature ova and placing them in a dish with a sample of spermatozoa

ovarian hyperstimulation syndrome (OHS) – a syndrome that presents sonographically as enlarged ovaries with multiple cysts, abdominal ascites, and pleural effusions. Often seen in patients who have undergone ovulation induction postadministration of follicle-stimulating hormone or a GnRH analogue followed by hCG.

ovarian induction therapy – controlled ovarian stimulation with clomiphene citrate or parenterally administered gonadotropins

postcoital test (PCT) – a clinical test done within 24 hours after intercourse to assess sperm motility in cervical mucus

zygote intrafallopian tube transfer (ZIFT) – a human fertilization technique in which the zygotes are injected through a laparoscope into the fimbriated ends of the fallopian tubes. Recently, this has been performed under ultrasound guidance.

Ultrasound has come to play an important role in the management and guidance of treatment for the infertile patient. By definition, infertility is the inability to conceive within 12 months with regular coitus. It is estimated that infertility affects one in seven couples in America. Approximately 40% of the cases of infertility are attributable to the female, 40% to the male, and the remaining 20% are combined male/female or unexplained factors. Traditionally, infertility has been divided into cervical, endometrial/uterine, tubal, ovulatory, peritoneal, and male factor causes. Male factor causes of infertility are an inadequate number of sperm and decreased motility of sperm, obstruction of the spermatic ducts or vas deferens, and scrotal varicoceles. This chapter will focus on female factors, including discussion of cervical, uterine/endometrial, tubal, ovulatory, and peritoneal causes of infertility.

As reproductive technologies continue to advance, it is important for the sonographer to be aware of the different treatment plans and the role that ultrasound plays in evaluating the infertile patient because many of these patients will come to the ultrasound lab very knowledgeable about their procedures. The sonographer should be compassionate toward each patient's situation.

EVALUATING THE CERVIX

The role of the cervix in fertility is to provide a nonhostile environment to harbor sperm. The cervix does this with glands that secrete mucus and crypts that hold the sperm. In certain instances, the mucus produced is hostile to sperm. The cervical mucus is evaluated by the **postcoital test** (PCT) performed within 24 hours of intercourse. The cervical mucus is aspirated from the cervix and evaluated under the microscope to look for the number and motility of the sperm collected in the mucus. The most common cause of "hostile" mucus is inaccurate timing, either too late or too early in relation to ovulation.

Ultrasound can be used to evaluate the cervical length during pregnancy to assess for cervical incompetence. However, in the nongravid uterus, the length of and any opening in the cervix are difficult to assess. Hysterosalpingography (HSG) can be used to evaluate the internal os diameter. A diameter less than 1 mm by HSG may indicate cervical stenosis.

EVALUATING THE UTERUS

When evaluating the uterus of the infertility patient, the sonographer has two main objectives: (1) to assess the structural anatomy and (2) to assess the endometrium. Assessing for structural anatomy refers to evaluating the uterine shape (i.e., unicolis, bicornuate, congenital malformations) (Figure 40-1) and evaluating echogenicity. Is the uterus uniform in echogenicity? Are there any masses suggestive of fibroids that may impede implantation of the fertilized egg (Figure 40-2)? When assessing the endometrium, the sonographer wants to evaluate the thickness and echogenicity characteristics and to include evaluation for any intracavitary lesions.

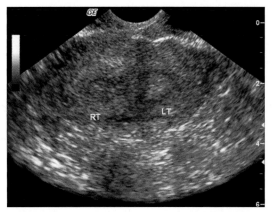

Figure 40-1   A bicornuate uterus. *RT,* right. *LT,* left.

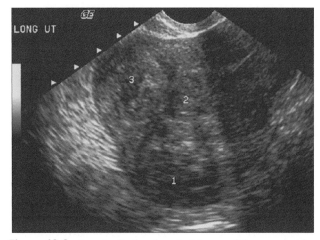

Figure 40-2   Longitudinal endovaginal image of the uterus with multiple fibroids.

CONGENITAL UTERINE ANOMALIES

It is estimated that congenital uterine anomalies occur in 1% of women. Congenital uterine anomalies are the result of defects in müllerian duct development, fusion, or resorption and are associated with renal anomalies. Although there are seven classes used to describe uterine anomalies, this chapter will discuss only the ones that ultrasound is best suited to evaluate. The congenital anomalies most easily assessed with ultrasound are evaluation for the bicornuate uterus and uterus didelphys. While these two entities are difficult to accurately confirm with ultrasound, ultrasound is good at depicting the two endometrial interfaces in the transverse plane. This finding should alert the sonographer to further evaluate the pelvic anatomy for two versus one cervix and vagina. Didelphys uterus is not usually associated with fertility problems, but bicornuate uterus is associated with a low incidence of fertility complications.

A uterine anomaly that is associated with a high incidence of infertility is the septate uterus. This congenital anomaly presents with two uterine cavities and a single fundus. In this case, the septum causes a problem for implantation. If the pregnancy implants along the septum, the pregnancy may be at an increased risk of failure because of inadequate blood supply from the septum. For these patients, the septum can be removed hysteroscopically to improve implantation and fertility success, so this is an important diagnosis to make.

On ultrasound, the septate uterus will appear as two endometrial cavities without a fundal notch compared with the bicornuate and didelphys uterus, which have two endometrial cavities, a wide uterine body, and a fundal notch (see Figure 40-1). The septate uterus should not be confused with a uterine cavity filled with myomatous tumors, as seen in Figure 40-2. The T-shaped uterus is another uterine anomaly to evaluate. This congenital anomaly is caused by exposure to diethylstilbestrol (DES) in utero. DES was a medication given to women to treat for threatened abortion from 1950 to 1970. The T-shaped uterus also is at risk for cervical incompetence, and there is no treatment known for this type of congenital anomaly. Because many uteruses imaged will not fit completely into one of these categories, the anatomy needs to be described as thoroughly as possible and may not be given a label immediately. MRI and HSG are other imaging methods that are better suited to evaluating the wide range of uterine anomalies.

EVALUTING THE ENDOMETRIUM

The endometrium can be measured throughout the menstrual cycle to look for appropriate changes. In the first half of the menstrual cycle, the mucosa begins to proliferate because of increasing estrogen levels. On ultrasound exam, the proliferative endometrial phase is seen as a triple line sign consisting of the hypoechoic mucosa and the echogenic interface where they meet in the center of the uterus (Figure 40-3). After ovulation, progesterone is secreted by the corpus luteum. This secretion of progesterone begins the secretory phase of the endometrial cycle. During the secretory phase, the endometrium becomes thickened and very echogenic as a result of stromal edema, and there is loss of the triple line sign (Figure 40-4). If there is not enough progesterone produced in the luteal phase, the endometrial lining may be thinner than expected on ultrasound evaluation. This lack of progesterone production is known as "luteal phase deficiency" and has been associated with infertility and early pregnancy loss. The endometrial

appearance has particular importance for planning for infertility treatment with embryo transfer.

Other things that can make the endometrium appear irregular or more echogenic than normal are submucosal fibroids and polyps. Saline infusion sonography (SIS) can be used in these situations to further delineate the anatomical structure of the endometrium. SIS can demonstrate fibroids and polyps by outlining the endometrial cavity. Fibroids tend to have a broad base and are more isoechoic to the uterine myometrium. They also tend to have circumferential flow around them (Figures 40-5 and 40-6). Polyps tend to have a narrow base attachment to the endometrium (a stalk) with a vascular pedicle feeding them (Figure 40-7). Fibroids and polyps are things that can potentially impede implantation, and therefore if found they can be removed to enhance fertility. SIS can also be used to evaluate the uterine cavity for synechiae, which are scars from uterine trauma (Figure 40-8). Synechiae are typically seen on ultrasound as linear strands of tissue extending from one wall of the uterine cavity to the other.

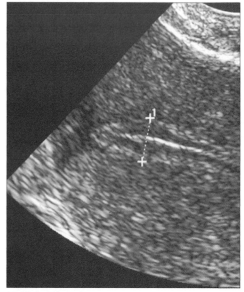

Figure 40-3 Longitudinal image of the proliferative endometrium.

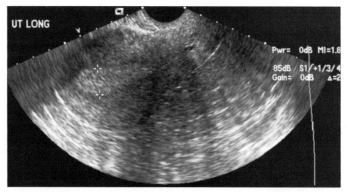

Figure 40-4 Longitudinal image of the secretory endometrium.

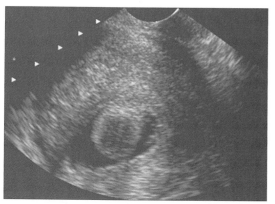

Figure 40-5 Submucosal fibroid with saline infusion sonography (SIS).

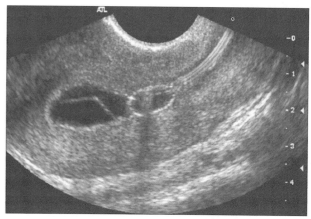

Figure 40-8 Uterine synechia with SIS.

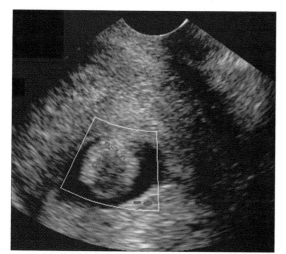

Figure 40-6 Submucosal fibroid with saline infusion sonography (SIS) and color Doppler showing circumferential flow.

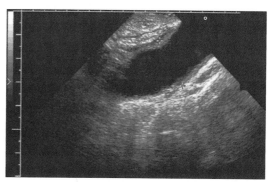

Figure 40-9 A hydrosalpinx.

EVALUATING THE FALLOPIAN TUBES

The fallopian tubes can be examined by ultrasound for hydrosalpinx and to assess patency. A hydrosalpinx is a fallopian tube containing fluid (Figure 40-9). On ultrasound, this appears as multiple cystic tubular structures in the adnexa. Tubal patency is assessed by injecting saline into the tube and looking for spillage of fluid into the cul-de-sac or by using contrast to evaluate for spillage. Before performing a saline or contrast study of the fallopian tubes, it is recommended that an endovaginal ultrasound to assess pelvic anatomy and an SIS exam of the uterine cavity be performed. The endovaginal exam allows the sonographer to see where the ovaries are in relation to the uterus and to assess for mobility of the tube and ovary. This is done by using probe pressure and hand palpation of the lower abdomen. After performing the endovaginal ultrasound, it is recommended that an SIS be performed to evaluate the structure of the endometrial cavity. Because of the expense of contrast imaging, most centers prefer to start with a saline injection for evaluation of a tube patency, and then if it is indeterminate, to move on to contrast imaging. To perform a saline infusion assessment of the fallopian tube, a catheter is placed through the cervix and advanced to the area where the endometrium is seen to invaginate into the cornu. At this point the balloon tip of the catheter is inflated, and 3 to 5 cc of sterile saline is injected to assess for patency. The approximate

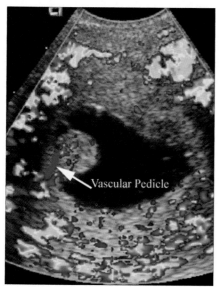

Figure 40-7 A polyp with SIS. Note the color Doppler demonstrating the vascular pedicle.

position of the fallopian tube is going to be between the ovary and the cornu. The sonographers are looking for spillage of saline into the posterior cul-de-sac. If this is seen, patency is inferred. If no spillage is noted and the patient complains of pain during injection, it may be because the tube is blocked. Obstruction of the fallopian tube can be caused by adhesions.

Before the use of ultrasound to assess for patency, there were two nonsurgical methods: the Rubin's test and hysterosalpingography (HSG). The Rubin's test involves insufflation of the fallopian tube with carbon dioxide gas, and HSG involves inserting a catheter through the cervix and then injecting contrast medium to assess the uterine cavity and fallopian tube anatomy under x-ray imaging. A surgical method used to evaluate the fallopian tubes is laparoscopy.

EVALUATING THE OVARIES

During the ovarian follicular phase, there are several follicles on the ovary less than 5 mm in diameter (Figure 40-10). A follicle is selected to develop into a dominant follicle in response to follicle-stimulating hormone (FSH) and an increase in estradiol. The dominant follicle will grow at a rate of approximately 2 to 3 mm/day until it reaches an average diameter of 22 mm (Figure 40-11). Once reaching a mean diameter of 22 mm, the dominant follicle will rupture. Rupture may be associated with an increase or decrease in size. Sonographic findings associated with ovulation are echoes within the fluid left behind (corpus luteum cyst) or free fluid in the peritoneal cavity. However, the best predictor of ovulation is the **basal body temperature** because the basal body temperature will rise after ovulation. At this time, luteinizing hormone (LH) rises just before ovulation and can also be found in the patient's urine.

One condition that can inhibit the release of FSH and LH is polycystic ovarian syndrome (PCOS). PCOS often occurs with the clinical triad of (1) oligomenorrhea, (2) hirsutism, and (3) obesity. With PCOS, follicles begin to grow but do not develop normally. In this syndrome, the immature follicles continue to produce estrogen and androgen. This production of estrogen and androgen inhibits the pituitary gland's function and prevents normal ovulation. This is due to the pituitary gland producing more LH than FSH, which causes the follicles to remain in an arrested state of development, leading to no mature ova being released with ovulation. Suggested causes of PCOS are obesity, diabetes, and thyroid, adrenal, or pituitary gland dysfunction. When obesity is a factor, more estrogen is produced, leading to decreased production of FSH and LH, which results in the abnormal cycle. With glandular dysfunction and diabetes as the cause of PCOS, the hormonal cycle is unbalanced and leads to the start of this syndrome. Women with PCOS may present with irregular bleeding, thickened endometrium, or endometrial carcinoma as a result of the chronic elevation of estrogen. Because of the chronic elevations of androgens, some women may have hirsutism.

Sonographic Findings. The sonographic findings of this syndrome may present in two ways. The first is a round ovary with multiple small immature follicles on the periphery. Usually these follicles are less than 1 cm in size. This has been described as the "string of pearls" sign (Figure 40-12), with the periphery of the ovary representing the neck and the multiple small cysts around the outside representing a string of pearls. The second is a normally appearing ovary. When evaluating for PCOS, endovaginal sonography is the preferred method and is more sensitive for detecting this syndrome.

PERITONEAL FACTORS

Peritoneal factors may be the cause for as many as 25% of infertility cases. Peritoneal factors are adhesions and endometriosis. Adhesions are bands of scar tissue that can

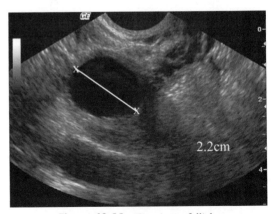

Figure 40-11 Dominant follicle.

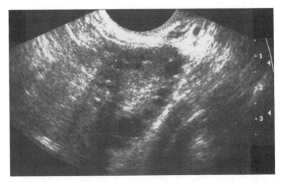

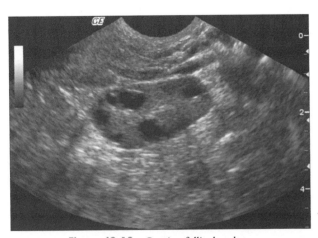

Figure 40-10 Ovarian follicular phase.

Figure 40-12 A polycystic ovary and the "string of pearls" sign.

obstruct the fimbriated end of the fallopian tube. Sometimes fluid will collect in between these adhesions, resulting in a peritoneal inclusion cyst. Endometriosis is caused by the ectopic placement of endometrial tissue outside the uterus. This tissue, just as the endometrium, undergoes cyclical changes and results in cyclical bleeding. The most common site of endometriosis is the ovaries, and often it is bilateral. The gold standard for evaluating pelvic adhesions and endometriosis is laparoscopy.

TREATMENT OPTIONS

OVARIAN INDUCTION THERAPY

Ovarian induction therapy refers to a treatment in which ovarian stimulation is achieved in a controlled setting. The first step in this process is to obtain a baseline endovaginal ultrasound of the ovaries to rule out an ovarian cyst and assess for the presence of a dominant follicle. This is important because if a cyst measuring greater than 2 cm is detected, it could represent persistent follicular activity that could interfere with response to ovarian stimulation medication. The presence of follicular activity is further evaluated by correlating the sonographic findings with serum estradiol levels. If serum estradiol is elevated and a large ovarian cyst is present, then oral contraceptives may be indicated to suppress follicular activity before starting ovarian stimulation therapy.

Ovarian induction therapy is usually accomplished by administering clomiphene citrate (Clomid) or human menopausal **gonadotropin** (Pergonal) on days 3 to 5 in a normal menstrual cycle. The administration of these medications is expected to result in the enlargement of multiple follicles compared with a single dominant follicle in a naturally occurring menstrual cycle. Once therapy has started, ultrasound is used to monitor the number and size of follicles in days 8 to 14 (follicular phase) of the menstrual cycle. When evaluating the number and size of follicles, the sonographer needs to count and measure all follicles greater than 1 cm in longitudinal and transverse planes (Figure 40-13). When follicles are asymmetrical (i.e., oblong in shape), they need to be measured in three

planes to determine a mean size. The optimal mean measurement of a follicle is between 15 and 20 mm. During this time ultrasound is correlated with the serum estradiol levels to determine the approximate time of ovulation. Correct measurement of the follicles is important because **human chorionic gonadotropin (hCG)**, a substitute for LH, may need to be given intramuscularly to trigger ovulation.

MONITORING THE ENDOMETRIUM

The endometrium is also evaluated during ovarian stimulation by assessing the thickness and echogenicity pattern of the endometrial cavity. A normal endometrial response associated with ovarian stimulation is an increasing thickness from 2 to 3 mm to 12 to 14 mm. To measure the endometrial thickness, the sonographer should image the uterus endovaginally and in the longitudinal plane. Calipers should measure from the anterior endometrial interface to the posterior endometrial interface (Figure 40-14). This is referred to as the "double-layer" thickness. Also important to evaluate is the echogenicity pattern. A normal pattern is trilaminar. This would be similar to the echographic pattern of the periovulatory endometrium. A thin endometrium (less than 8 mm in diameter) and an abnormal echographic pattern have been associated with decreased fertility. Another ultrasound method for assessing uterine receptivity is color and spectral Doppler of the uterine arteries. Steer and others found that in assessing uterine receptivity one should look for a mean pulsatility index (PI) of 2.00 to 2.99 in the uterine arteries.[3] This was done by imaging the ascending branch of the right and left uterine arteries lateral to the cervix with an endovaginal transducer. Color Doppler was used to assist in identifying these vessels.

IN VITRO FERTILIZATION AND EMBRYO TRANSFER

In vitro fertilization (IVF) is a method of fertilizing the human ova outside the body. Mature ova are collected and mixed in a dish with a sample of spermatozoa. The resulting embryos are then placed back into the uterus. The treatment plan for IVF consists of ovarian monitoring, needle aspiration of oocytes, incubation of oocytes, fertilization, and transferring

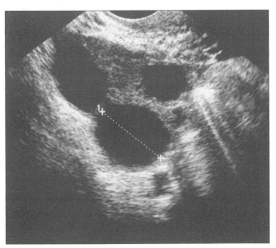

Figure 40-13   Enlargement of multiple ovarian follicles.

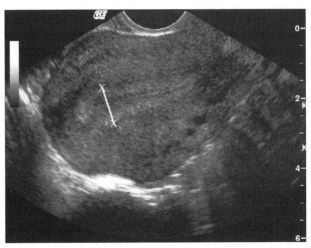

Figure 40-14   Endometrial measurement.

the embryos into the uterus. The ovarian monitoring is performed as described in the ovarian induction therapy section, with one difference: instead of evaluating for two optimal follicles, four follicles are identified before triggering evaluation. Oocyte retrieval can be accomplished laparoscopically or by transabdominal or endovaginal ultrasound guidance. The scope of this chapter will be confined to discussion of the transabdominal and endovaginal methods. Thus what follows next will be a discussion of how ultrasound is used to guide for oocyte retrieval.

The decision to use transabdominal or endovaginal sonography to guide for oocyte retrieval is dependent upon the patient's anatomy. Endovaginal sonography is used as a guide to locate the ovaries when the ovaries are more posterior in location, such as in the cul-de-sac. The endovaginal transducer is covered with a protective sheath (e.g., condom or transducer cover) and the needle guide is attached. Sterile gel should be placed in the tip of the protective sheath. If using an ultrasound machine with needle guide software, turn on the needle guide function. This function will show where the needle will go in relationship to the image. Once the transducer is prepared, it is inserted into the vagina and the ovary imaged. A 30-cm, 18-gauge needle is placed in the guide and introduced endovaginally following the outlined needle path, and under ultrasound imaging one will see the needle tip go into the desired follicle. Some centers prefer using a scored needle tip, which is more easily seen on ultrasound. Once the needle tip is in the follicle, the fluid in the follicle and ovum are aspirated. Occasionally the ovum may be stuck to a wall; therefore, a buffer solution is injected into the follicle to flush out the cavity and then is reaspirated to maximize the potential for ovum retrieval.

Once the oocytes are retrieved, they are fertilized in a dish and incubated for 48 to 74 hours before **embryo transfer** into the uterus. Embryo transfer can be done laparoscopically or by ultrasound guidance. This chapter will focus on how ultrasound is used to guide the embryo transfer. Ultrasound is first used to map the endometrial cavity. This is done by using the trace function on the ultrasound machine and tracing the endometrial interface from cervix to the apex of the fundus to determine the length of the uterine cavity. Optimal placement of the embryos is considered to be within 1 to 1.5 cm of the apex of the fundus; therefore, it is important for the clinician to know the length of the uterine cavity to ensure proper placement of the embryos. After the endometrium is mapped, using transabdominal ultrasound guidance, a catheter is inserted through the cervix and placed within 1 to 1.5 cm of the fundus of the uterine cavity. The embryos are then slowly released, and a transfer air bubble will be seen on ultrasound after the embryos are released from the catheter. Coroleu and others reported that after embryo transfer, the catheter is checked under a stereomicroscope to ensure that all embryos are transferred.[2]

Recently, ultrasound has been used to guide **gamete intrafallopian tube transfer (GIFT)** and **zygote intrafallopian tube transfer (ZIFT).** GIFT and ZIFT techniques are used for patients who have at least one functional fallopian tube and for whom the cause of infertility is unexplained or due to cervical factors. The GIFT procedure requires ovarian stimulation and oocyte retrieval. The oocytes are then mixed with sperm in a dish and then transferred through a catheter into the fallopian tube. Therefore, fertilization takes place within the woman's body (in vivo) versus in a dish (in vitro). The ZIFT procedure requires ovarian stimulation and oocyte retrieval. The oocytes are mixed with the sperm in a dish. With ZIFT, the oocytes are fertilized in the dish and then zygotes are placed into the woman's fallopian tube. In this case, fertilization takes place outside of the woman's body (in vitro). Traditionally these techniques were done laparascopically and the gametes or zygote were placed in the fimbriated end of the fallopian tube. With ultrasound guidance, a catheter is placed through the cervix and into the cornua of the uterus. The gametes or zygote are then released into the isthmic portion of the fallopian tube. The ultrasound guidance method is more cost effective, but the success rates have not been as high as the traditional laparoscopic method. The success rates per cycle for both GIFT and ZIFT have been reported as 22% to 28%.[1]

INTRAUTERINE INSEMINATION

Intrauterine insemination is a technique used to treat male factor infertility. With intrauterine insemination, a catheter containing sperm preparation is placed into the uterine fundus. The sperm preparation may be from a donor, and this is referred to as artificial insemination using donor sperm (AID). Sometimes ultrasound is used to guide for this procedure.

COMPLICATIONS ASSOCIATED WITH ASSISTED REPRODUCTIVE TECHNOLOGY

Complications associated with **assisted reproductive technology (ART)** include **ovarian hyperstimulation syndrome (OHS),** multiple gestations, and ectopic pregnancy. OHS is a syndrome that presents sonographically as enlarged ovaries with multiple cysts, abdominal ascites, and pleural effusions. This syndrome is often seen in patients who have undergone ovulation induction after administration of follicle-stimulating hormone or a GnRH analogue followed by hCG. This syndrome is more common in patients with a history of polycystic ovarian syndrome and can be graded based on patient symptoms. In mild cases of OHS, patients complain of lower abdominal pain and back pain. On ultrasound exam, a mild case of OHS will demonstrate enlarged ovaries (5 to 10 cm) with multiple cysts. More severe cases of OHS will present with leg edema, ascites, pleural effusions, hypotension, and polycythemia. Sonographic findings in severe OHS cases will demonstrate enlarged ovaries with multiple cysts, ascites, and pleural effusions (Figure 40-15).

Patients who undergo in vitro fertilization are at an increased risk for having multiple gestations. It is estimated that about 25% of in vitro fertilization pregnancies result in a multiple gestation. The concern with multiple gestations is that if there are three or more fetuses, there is an increased risk

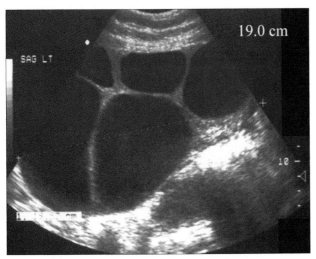

Figure 40-15   An enlarged ovary with multiple cyst in a patient with OHS.

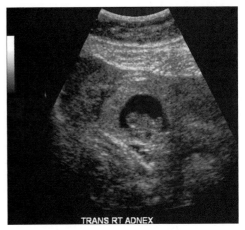

Figure 40-17   A live heterotopic pregnancy in the same patient in Figure 40-16.

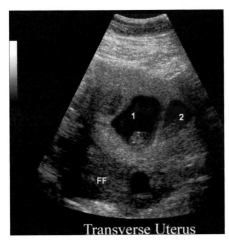

Figure 40-16   An intrauterine twin pregnancy. *FF,* free fluid.

of fetal and/or neonatal morbidity and mortality. Therefore, pregnancies that have three or more fetuses are often counseled about fetal reduction options. Fetal reduction is performed by injecting potassium chloride into the chest or fetal heart.

Patients who undergo assisted reproductive technologies are at an increased risk for ectopic pregnancy. An ectopic pregnancy is a pregnancy that is implanted outside of the uterus. These patients are also at risk for having a heterotopic pregnancy. A heterotopic pregnancy is an ectopic pregnancy coexisting with an intrauterine pregnancy (Figures 40-16 and 40-17). This used to be a rare occurrence (1:30,000). However, with the advancement in ART, the estimated occurrence is 1:6,000 in this patient population. The incidence of a heterotopic pregnancy with an intrauterine multiple gestation is 1:10,000, but in the ART patient subgroup this risk may increase to 1:100. In this patient population, when an intrauterine pregnancy is visualized, it is important to carefully image the adnexa, not just for ovarian pathology, but also to evaluate for a heterotopic pregnancy.

REFERENCES

1. Beckman CRB, Ling FW, Laube DW: *Obstetrics and gynecology,* ed 4, Philadelphia, 2002, Lipincott Williams & Wilkins.
2. Coroleu B, Carrearas O, Veiga A: Embryo transfer under ultrasound guidance improves pregnancy rates after in vitro fertilization, *Human Reproduction* 15:616-620, 2000.
3. Steer CV, Campbell S, Tan SL and others: The use of transvaginal color flow imaging after in vitro fertilization to identify optimum uterine conditions before embryo transfer, *Fertil Steril* 57:372-376, 1992.

SELECTED BIBLIOGRAPHY

Barnhart K, Coutifaris C: The use of ultrasound in the evaluation and treatment of the infertile woman. In Benson C, Arger P, Bluth E, editors: *Ultrasonography in obstetrics and gynecology: a practical approach,* ed 1, New York, 2000, Thieme.

Benson CM and others: Multifetal pregnancy reduction of both fetuses of a monochorionic pair by intrathoracic potassium chloride injection of one fetus, *J Ultrasound Med* 17:447, 1998.

Buttram VC: The American Fertility Society classification of adnexal adhesions, distal tubal occlusion, tubal occlusion secondary to tubal ligation, tubal pregnancies, müllerian anomalies and intrauterine adhesions, *Fertil Steril* 49:955, 1988.

Cohen DJ: The endometrium. In Thurmond AS, Jones MJ, Cohen DJ, editors: *Gynecologic, obstetric, and breast radiology: a text/atlas of imaging in women,* Cambridge, Mass, 1996, Blackwell Science.

Doherty CM, Silver B, Binor Z: Transvaginal ultrasonography and the assessment of luteal phase endometrium, *Am J Obstet Gynecol* 168:1702, 1993.

Fleischer AC, Vasquez JM, Parsons AM: Transvaginal sonography in gynecologic infertility. In: Fleischer AC, Maning FA, Jeanty P, editors: *Sonography in obstetrics & gynecology: principles and practice,* ed 6, New York, 2001, McGraw-Hill.

Hann LE, Crivello M, McArdle C and others: In vitro fertilization: sonographic perspective, *Radiology* 163:665, 1987.

Hill J: Assisted reproduction and the multiple pregnancy: increasing the risks for heterotopic pregnancy, *J Diag Med Sonogr* 19: 258-260, 2003.

Klein NA, Olive DL: Management of endometriosis associated in fertility. In Schlaff WD, Rock JA, editors: *Decision making in reproductive endocrinology,* Boston, 1993, Blackwell Scientific.

Levi CS, Hold SC, Lyon EA: Normal anatomy of the female pelvis. In Callen PW: *Ultrasonography in obstetric and gynecology,* ed 4, Philadelphia, 2000, Saunders.

Pache TD, Wladimiroff JW, Hop WC: How to discriminate between normal and polycystic ovaries: transvaginal US study, *Radiology* 1992; 183:421-423.

Parsons AK: *The use of ultrasound in the work-up of infertility,* American Institute of Ultrasound in Medicine, Laurel, Md, Syllabus update in Ob/gyn ultrasound, II, June 1-3, p. 87.

Sebire NJ, Sepulveda W, Jeanty P: Multiple gestations. In Nyberg D, McGahan JP, Pretorius DH, editors: *Diagnostic imaging of fetal anomalies,* Philadelphia, 2003, Lippincott Williams & Wilkins.

Takahashi K and others: Transvaginal ultrasound is an effective method for screening in polycystic ovarian disease, *Gynecol Obstet Invest* 30:34, 1990.

Thurmond AS: Imaging of female infertility, *Radiol Clin N Am* 41:757-767, 2003.

Thurmond AS: Sonographic imaging in infertility. In Callan P, editor: *Ultrasonography in obstetrics and gynecology,* ed 4, Philadelphia, 2000, WB Saunders Co.

Tufekci EC, Girit S, Bayirli E: Evaluation of tubal patency by transvaginal sonosalpingography, *Fertil Steril* 57:336-340, 1992.

PART VIII

Foundations of Obstetric Sonography

CHAPTER 41

The Role of Ultrasound in Obstetrics

Sandra L. Hagen-Ansert

OBJECTIVES

- List at least 10 indications for obstetric ultrasound examination
- List maternal risk factors that increase the chances of producing a fetus with congenital anomalies
- Recount four important questions to ask the patient before beginning the obstetric ultrasound examination
- Describe the biologic effects of diagnostic medical ultrasound energy
- Describe the four steps of the first-trimester sonography protocol
- Describe the six steps of the second- and third-trimester sonography protocol

RECOMMENDATIONS FOR OBSTETRIC AND GYNECOLOGIC SONOGRAPHY

MATERNAL RISK FACTORS

PATIENT HISTORY

THE SAFETY OF ULTRASOUND

THE SAFETY OF DOPPLER FOR THE OBSTETRIC PATIENT

GUIDELINES FOR ANTEPARTUM OBSTETRIC ULTRASOUND EXAMINATION

FIRST TRIMESTER
SECOND AND THIRD TRIMESTERS

KEY TERMS

abruptio placenta – bleeding from a normally situated placenta as a result of its complete or partial detachment after the 20th week of gestation

amniocentesis – aspiration of a sample of amniotic fluid through the mother's abdomen for diagnostic analysis of fetal genetics, maturity, and/or disease

amnion – smooth membrane enclosing the fetus and amniotic fluid; it is loosely fused with the outer chorionic membrane except at the placental insertion of the umbilical cord where the amnion is contiguous with the membranes surrounding the umbilical cord

anencephaly – a neural tube defect where absence of the brain, including the cerebrum, the cerebellum, and basal ganglia, may be present

cerclage – the ligatures around the cervix uteri to treat cervical incompetence during pregnancy

cervix – inferior segment of the uterus, which is normally more than 3.5 cm long during pregnancy, decreasing in length during labor

chorion – cellular, outermost extraembryonic membrane, composed of trophoblast lined with mesoderm; the outer chorion (villous chorion) develops villi, which are vascularized by allantoic vessels and give rise to the placenta; the inner chorion (the smooth chorion) is fused with the amnion except at the placental cord insertion

cordocentesis – insertion under sonographic guidance of a thin needle into the vessels of the umbilical cord usually at the site of placental insertion to obtain a fetal blood sample, deliver fetal drug therapy, or assess fetal well-being

corpus luteum – a functional structure within the normal ovary, which is formed from cells lining the graafian follicle after ovulation; the corpus luteum produces estrogen and progesterone and may become enlarged and appear cystic during early pregnancy

ductus venosus – vascular structure within the fetal liver that connects the umbilical vein to the inferior vena cava and allows oxygenated blood to bypass the liver and return directly to the heart

embryo – developing individual from implantation to the end of the ninth week of gestation

embryonic age (conception age) – age of embryo stated as time from day of conception

gestational age – length of pregnancy defined in the United States as number of weeks from first day of last normal menstrual period (LNMP)

gestational sac – structure lined by the chorion that normally implants within the uterine deciduas and contains the developing embryo

hydatidiform mole – abnormal conception in which there is partial or complete conversion of the chorionic villi into grapelike vesicles

incompetent cervix – a condition in which the cervix dilates silently during the second trimester; without intervention, the membranes bulge through the cervix, rupture, and the fetus drops out, resulting in a premature preterm delivery

intrauterine growth restriction (IUGR) – reduced growth rate (symmetrical IUGR) or abnormal growth pattern (asymmetrical IUGR) of the fetus; resulting in a small for gestational age (SGA) infant

lower uterine segment – thin expanded lower portion of the uterus that forms in the last trimester of pregnancy

macrosomia – exceptionally large infant with excessive fat deposition in the subcutaneous tissue; most frequently seen in fetuses of diabetic mothers

maternal serum alpha-fetoprotein (MSAFP) – one of several biochemical tests used to assess fetal risk for aneuploidy or fetal defect; a component of the "triple screen," the normal value of MSAFP varies with gestational age; assessment of gestational age is essential to accurate interpretation of results

oligohydramnios – reduced amount of amniotic fluid

placenta – organ of communication where nutrition and products of metabolism are interchanged between the fetal and maternal blood systems; forms from the chorion frondosum with a maternal decidual contribution

placenta previa – placental implantation encroaches upon the lower uterine segment; if the placenta presents first in late pregnancy, bleeding is inevitable

polyhydramnios – excessive amount of amniotic fluid

trimester – a 40-week pregnancy is divided into three 13-week periods from the first day of the last normal menstrual period (weeks 1 through 12, first trimester; weeks 13 through 26, second trimester; week 27 to term, third trimester)

umbilical cord – connecting lifeline between the fetus and placenta; it contains two umbilical arteries, which carry deoxygenated fetal blood, and one umbilical vein, which carries oxygenated fetal blood encased in Wharton's jelly

yolk sac – a circular structure within the gestational sac seen sonographically between 4 and 10 weeks of gestational age; the yolk sac supplies nutrition, facilitates waste removal, and is the origin of early hematopoietic stem cells in the embryo; it lies between the chorion and the amnion

zygote – products of conception from fertilization through implantation; the zygotic stage of pregnancy lasts for approximately 12 days after conception

----

Sonography is the primary tool used to evaluate the developing fetus during pregnancy. Obstetric sonography allows the clinician to assess the development, growth, and well-being of the fetus. When an abnormal condition is recognized prenatally, obstetric management may be altered to provide optimal care for the fetus and child. The visualization of pregnancy with ultrasound has revolutionized obstetrics. Conditions that were previously detected only at delivery are now diagnosed early in pregnancy and monitored with ultrasound. Prenatal diagnosis has led to prenatal treatments performed under ultrasound visualization. Prenatal parental education and counseling are facilitated by sharing sonographic images and diagnostic results. Though obstetric sonography is popular in many aspects of our culture, including books, television, and family gatherings, its value lies in its medical use.

The sonographer performing fetal studies must understand both sonographic and obstetric principles. This allows the sonographer to accurately and thoroughly compile pertinent information and to provide an optimal sonographic assessment of the fetus. The sonographer has a responsibility to obstetrical patients and clinicians to provide competent, safe, and appropriate examinations. In accordance with the recommended guidelines, the sonographer should establish a systematic scanning protocol encompassing all criteria of the guidelines. An organized approach to scanning ensures completeness and reduces the risk of missing a detectable birth defect.

This chapter describes the medical indications for obstetric sonography examinations; reviews practice guidelines as outlined by the American College of Radiology (ACR), the American Institute of Ultrasound in Medicine (AIUM), and the American College of Obstetricians and Gynecologists (ACOG); and describes the risk factors associated with congenital fetal anomalies.

RECOMMENDATIONS FOR OBSTETRIC AND GYNECOLOGIC SONOGRAPHY

The sonographer needs to be aware of the indications for obstetric sonography and to understand the medical complications associated with each indication. The national practice guidelines produced by ACR, AIUM, and ACOG recommend specific components of a minimum obstetrical antepartum sonography examination. Sonographers must strive to meet the minimum requirements recommended for each antepartum examination. In addition, components may be altered or added to serve the interests of the patient or the referring clinician. It is often the responsibility of the sonographer, under the general direction of a physician, to apply knowledge, competence, and critical thinking to determine and perform appropriate examination components based on the specific indication for the study and the clinical history of the mother. For example, in addition to the standard recommended components, additional attention to specific anatomy may be indicated with specific maternal disease states during pregnancy.

There are recommended indications for obstetric sonography examinations that are often incorporated into diagnosis codes and billing codes. These indications were first defined in 1983 and do not include a recommendation for "routine" obstetric sonography examinations in asymptomatic pregnancies with known dates. The indications for obstetric and gynecologic studies as detailed by the National Institute of Child Health and Human Development and National Institutes of

Health Consensus Report on Safety of Ultrasound are as follows:

1. Estimation of **gestational age** for patients with uncertain clinical dates or verification of dates for patients who are to undergo scheduled elective repeat cesarean delivery, indicated induction of labor, or other elective termination of pregnancy. Sonographic confirmation of dating permits proper timing of cesarean delivery or labor induction to avoid premature delivery.

2. Evaluation of fetal growth, for example, when the patient has an identified cause for uteroplacental insufficiency, such as severe preeclampsia, chronic hypertension, chronic renal disease, or severe diabetes mellitus, or for other medical complications of pregnancy in which fetal mal-nutrition (e.g., **intrauterine growth restriction [IUGR]** or **macrosomia**) is suspected. Following fetal growth permits assessment of the impact of a complicating condition of the fetus and guides pregnancy management.

3. Vaginal bleeding of undetermined cause in pregnancy. Sonography often allows determination of the source of bleeding and status of the fetus.

4. Determination of fetal presentation when the presenting part cannot be adequately determined in labor or the fetal presentation is variable in late pregnancy. Accurate knowledge of presentation guides management of delivery.

5. Suspected multiple gestation based on detection of more than one fetal heart beat pattern, fundal height larger than expected for dates, or prior use of fertility drugs. Pregnancy management may be altered in multiple gestation.

6. Adjunct to **amniocentesis.** Sonography permits guidance of the needle to avoid the **placenta** and fetus, to increase the chance of obtaining amniotic fluid, and to decrease the chance of fetal loss.

7. Significant discrepancy between uterine size and clinical dates. Sonography permits accurate dating and detection of such conditions as oligohydramnios and polyhydramnios, along with multiple gestation, IUGR, and anomalies.

8. Pelvic mass detected clinically. Sonography can detect the location and nature of the mass and aid in the diagnosis.

9. **Hydatidiform mole** suspected on the basis of clinical signs of hypertension, proteinuria, or the presence of ovarian cysts felt on pelvic examination or failure to detect fetal heart tones with a Doppler ultrasound device after 12 weeks. Sonography permits accurate diagnosis and differentiation of this neoplasm from fetal death.

10. Adjunct to cervical **cerclage** placement. Sonography aids in timing and proper placement of the cerclage for patients with **incompetent cervix.**

11. Suspected ectopic pregnancy or when pregnancy occurs after tuboplasty or prior ectopic gestation. Sonography is a valuable diagnostic aid for this complication.

12. Adjunct to special procedures, such as **cordocentesis**, intrauterine transfusion, shunt placement, in vitro fertilization, embryo transfer, or chorionic villi sampling. Sonography aids instrument guidance that increases the safety of these procedures.

13. Suspected fetal death. Rapid diagnosis enhances optimal management.

14. Suspected uterine abnormality (e.g., clinically significant leiomyomata, congenital structural abnormalities, such as bicornuate uterus or uteri didelphys). Serial surveillance of fetal growth and state enhances fetal outcome.

15. Intrauterine contraceptive device (IUCD) localization. Sonography guidance facilitates removal, reducing chances of IUCD-related complications.

16. Ovarian follicle development surveillance. This facilitates treatment of infertility.

17. Biophysical evaluation for fetal well-being after 28 weeks of gestation. Assessment of amniotic fluid, fetal tone, body movements, breathing movements, and heart rate patterns assists in management of high-risk pregnancies.

18. Observation of intrapartum events (e.g., version or extraction of second twin and manual removal of placenta). These procedures may be done more safely with the visualization provided by sonography.

19. Suspected **polyhydramnios** or **oligohydramnios.** Confirmation of the diagnosis and identification of the cause of the condition in certain pregnancies is necessary.

20. Suspected **abruptio placentae.** Confirmation of diagnosis and extent of abruption assists in clinical management.

21. Adjunct to external version from breech to vertex presentation. The visualization provided by sonography facilitates performance of this procedure.

22. Estimation of fetal weight and presentation in premature rupture of the membranes or premature labor. Information provided by sonography guides management decisions on timing and method of delivery.

23. Abnormal **maternal serum alpha-fetoprotein (MSAFP)** value for clinical gestational age when drawn. Sonography provides an accurate assessment of gestational age for the MSAFP comparison standard and indicates several conditions (e.g., twins, **anencephaly**) that may cause elevated AFP values.

24. Follow-up observation of identified fetal anomaly. Sonography assessment of progression or lack of change assists in clinical decision making.

25. Follow-up evaluation of placenta location for identified **placenta previa.**

26. History of previous congenital anomaly. Detection of recurrence may be permitted, or psychologic benefit to patients may result from reassurance of no recurrence.

27. Serial evaluation of fetal growth in multiple gestation. Sonography permits recognition of discordant growth, guiding patient management and timing of delivery.

28. Evaluation of fetal condition in late registrants for prenatal care. Accurate knowledge of gestational age assists in pregnancy management decisions for this group.

MATERNAL RISK FACTORS

Maternal risk factors that increase the chances of producing a fetus with congenital anomalies include increased maternal age, abnormal triple screen biochemistry values, maternal disease (e.g., diabetes mellitus and systemic lupus erythematosus), and a pregnant uterine cavity that is either too small or too large for dates. Other risk factors include a previous child born with a chromosomal disorder or exposure to a known teratogenic drug or infectious agent known to cause birth defects. Some anomalies are caused by a reduced or increased number of fetal chromosomes. These anomalies, the most common of which is Down syndrome, trisomy 21, are called aneuploidies. Other anomalies are thought to have both genetic and environmental causes. For example, neural tube defects have a genetic component, but are influenced by the maternal environment, especially a lack of adequate folic acid before pregnancy and during the early embryonic period. Assessment of maternal risk may include discussion of both genetic and family history; environmental triggers, such as maternal disease and nutrition; and available testing. Genetic counselors are trained to assist patients in determining risks before or during pregnancy. With adequate counseling and environmental factor control, some anomalies may be prevented.

PATIENT HISTORY

There are several important questions the sonographer should ask the patient before beginning the obstetric sonography evaluation. The sonographer first tries to determine the clinical dates of the pregnancy. It is important to document the clinical date reported by the patient and the date determined by the earliest sonographic examination. An accurate clinical date facilitates correlation of the obstetric measurements with the expected gestational age. It is important to ask if the patient has any latex allergies. Many ultrasound laboratories use only latex-free materials to prevent any allergic reactions.

The first date of the last menstrual period (LMP or LNMP) is the standard way to date a pregnancy in the United States. Human pregnancy lasts 266 days plus or minus 10 days. If conception occurs on day 14 from the LNMP, the pregnancy duration from LNMP is 280 days or 40 weeks. In reality the assessment of gestational age is often not precise. Many women have irregular periods, conceive within three months of coming off birth control pills when ovulation is irregular, or do not record dates. Even with a known menstrual date, conception may occur from day 6 to day 27, which is a difference of 3 weeks in gestational age as determined by sonography. The sonographer first asks the patient the first day of her last menstrual period and inputs this date into the ultrasound machine. If the patient does not remember the date of her last normal menstrual period, the sonographer may ask for the expected date of confinement. The sonographer should also ask if there have been previous sonographic examinations performed before 26 weeks and the estimated date of confinement determined by the earliest sonographic examination. By recording this information, the sonographer can provide an estimation of the clinical dates and their accuracy. It is ultimately the responsibility of the obstetrician following the pregnancy to determine the clinical gestational age, however.

The sonographer also needs to know if the patient is currently taking any medication or has experienced clinical problems with the pregnancy, such as bleeding, decreased fetal movement, or pelvic pain. If the patient has had problems with previous pregnancies, such as incompetence cervix, fibroids, fetal macrosomia or growth restriction, or congenital or chromosomal fetal anomalies, this information must be documented.

THE SAFETY OF ULTRASOUND

United States government census bureau prenatal statistics estimate that approximately 65% of all pregnant women in the United States are examined with sonography. Ultrasound imaging has been used in pregnancy since the 1950s without apparent side effects. The first studies conducted to determine the safety of ultrasound in pregnancy were small and hampered by imprecise dosimetry and poorly matched control groups. Physicists and researchers have made tremendous strides in defining the variables of importance in bioeffects and the types of tissue interactions and damage that may occur. Using human epidemiology studies, animal experiments, and in vitro studies of tissue and cells, scientists continue to study the safety of ultrasound, but challenges remain. Existing human studies are not large enough to document small increases in normally occurring anomalies that may occur as the result of sonography. Similarly, it is difficult to determine potential long-term effects of prenatal ultrasound imaging. Animal experiments and therapeutic applications document that high-intensity ultrasound may modify biologic structures and functions. Studies in pregnancy with animals and humans have suggested possibilities of growth differences (reduction in animals), increased non-right handedness, and delayed speech. In the best interests of our patients, it is important that sonographers remember the following when performing obstetrical sonography:

1. There are theoretical effects of ultrasound energy on the fetus; there are potential biological effects that have not been documented.
2. The energy produced by ultrasound equipment today is higher than that produced by earlier equipment. Doppler imaging produces higher energy. There is not a long history of safety with energy at the level in use today.
3. The studies of ultrasound bioeffects are not definitive, and continued research is essential.
4. Sonographers have a responsibility to be knowledgeable regarding ultrasound bioeffects and to use the least amount of energy necessary to produce the clinical information needed.

The major biologic effects of ultrasound are believed to be thermal (a rise in temperature) and cavitation (production and collapse of gas-filled bubbles). Sonographers can minimize thermal effects by not staying in one spot, especially over fetal bone, for long periods of time and also by extending the focus of the beam as deep into the body as reasonable to obtain adequate images. Cavitation is dependent on the presence of gas preexisting within tissue. Sonographers who work with newborns may choose to be cautious of long examinations through newborn lungs filled with gas.

The American Institute of Ultrasound in Medicine (AIUM) has a committee of scientists, clinicians, sonographers, and engineers who regularly review and summarize information regarding bioeffects. The AIUM statement on clinical safety adopted in 1997 is as follows:

> Diagnostic ultrasound has been in use since the late 1950s. Given its known benefits and recognized efficacy for medical diagnosis, including use during human pregnancy, the American Institute of Ultrasound in Medicine herein addresses the clinical safety of such use: There are no confirmed biological effects on patients or instrument operators caused by exposures from present diagnostic ultrasound instruments. Although the possibility exists that such biological effects may be identified in the future, current data indicate that the benefits to patients of the prudent use of diagnostic ultrasound outweigh the risks, if any, that may be present.

THE SAFETY OF DOPPLER FOR THE OBSTETRIC PATIENT

Doppler ultrasound provides a noninvasive and expedient method to assess the physiology and pathophysiology of the fetal and maternal circulations when such examinations are required for diagnosis of a malady. In most cases, pulsed wave Doppler is used in the fetus rather than continuous wave Doppler. Doppler may be used to detect flow in the maternal vessels, the fetal vessels (umbilical artery and vein, aorta and inferior vena cava, renal arteries, and cerebral vessels), the fetal **ductus venosus,** the fetal heart, and the placenta. Specific applications of Doppler are presented in the respective chapters. The benefits of Doppler imaging most likely outweigh the risks when there are specific indications requiring Doppler interrogation. Fetal sonography with or without Doppler should be performed only when there is a valid medical reason, and the lowest possible ultrasonic exposure settings should be used to obtain the necessary diagnostic information.

GUIDELINES FOR ANTEPARTUM OBSTETRIC ULTRASOUND EXAMINATION

In the late 1980s in response to concerns about variability in quality and practices, obstetrical examination guidelines were introduced by three professional organizations. The American Institute of Ultrasound in Medicine published obstetrical standards in 1986, which were revised in 1991. The American College of Obstetrics and Gynecology published standards in 1988 and the American College of Radiology followed in 1990 with revisions in 1995. In 2003 these three organizations collaborated and jointly published the current version of the *Practice Guidelines for the Performance of an Antepartum Obstetric Ultrasound Examination (AIUM guidelines).* The purpose of the current guidelines is to provide practitioners with information regarding the minimum criteria for a complete examination. The guidelines are often cited as a legal standard, though this use was not intended. While it is not possible to detect all fetal anomalies with sonography, adherence to practice guidelines and referral of any suspicious studies for further evaluations will optimize the possibilities of detection.

It is important that all sonographers strive to consistently meet or exceed minimum standards during every obstetric sonographic examination. Quality standards include not only the components of the examination protocol but also qualifications of personnel performing the examination, documentation, equipment specifications, fetal safety, quality control, safety, infection control, and patient education concerns.

Although no mechanism exists to absolutely ensure technical competence, the standard of practice for personnel in sonography is national board certification. The purpose of certification or registry is to assure the public that the person performing sonography has the necessary knowledge, skills, and experience to provide this service.

Documentation standards require that there is a permanent record maintained of the measurements and anatomic findings. Images need to be labeled with the patient's name, date, and image orientation if appropriate. A written report of the examination must be maintained in the patient records. Fetal echocardiography is often stored on a real-time format for future reference and review. A written report by the physician should outline the findings of the study. Real-time sonography with transabdominal and endovaginal transducers is essential to confirm fetal life and to permit the sonographer to view fetal anatomy and movements and to obtain biometric parameters used to determine fetal age and growth.

Transducer frequency selection and equipment settings should balance optimal imaging resolution and penetration. The lowest possible exposure setting should be used according to the ALARA (as low as reasonably achievable) principle. Policies and procedures related to patient information, infection control, quality control, and safety should be developed and implemented in every laboratory. Policies typically address personnel and patient safety, and may include policies that address musculoskeletal injury concerns for the sonographer. A monitor mounted on the wall for patient viewing provides ergonomic protection for the sonographer in obstetric laboratories.

FIRST TRIMESTER

Indications for first-**trimester** sonography are shown in Box 41-1. Either a transabdominal or endovaginal transducer may be used for the examination of the first-trimester embryo and fetus. If a transabdominal examination is not definitive, an endovaginal or transperineal examination is required. A transabdominal examination may provide an overview of the entire pelvic cavity and enable the sonographer to image the uterus from the **cervix** to the fundus, evaluate the ovaries and adnexal areas for abnormal collections of fluid or a mass, and look for the presence of free fluid. The endovaginal transducer provides a more limited view of the pelvic cavity but allows excellent visualization of the **embryo, yolk sac, amnion, chorion,** and **gestational sac.**

> **BOX 41-1 INDICATIONS FOR FIRST-TRIMESTER SONOGRAPHY**
>
> - To confirm the presence of an intrauterine pregnancy
> - To evaluate a suspected ectopic pregnancy
> - To define cause of vaginal bleeding
> - To evaluate pelvic pain
> - To estimate gestational (menstrual) age
> - To diagnose or evaluate multiple pregnancy
> - To confirm cardiac activity
> - As an adjunct to chorionic villus sampling, amniocentesis, embryo transfer, IUCD removal
> - To evaluate maternal pelvic masses and/or uterine abnormalities
> - To evaluate suspected hydatidiform mole

> **BOX 41-2 INDICATIONS FOR SECOND- AND THIRD-TRIMESTER SONOGRAPHY**
>
> - Evaluation of gestational age
> - Evaluation of fetal growth
> - Vaginal bleeding
> - Abdominal/pelvic pain
> - Incompetent cervix
> - Determination of fetal presentation
> - Suspected multiple gestation
> - Adjunct to amniocentesis
> - Significant discrepancy between uterine size and clinical dates
> - Pelvic mass
> - Suspected hydatidiform mole
> - Adjunct to cervical cerclage placement
> - Suspected ectopic pregnancy
> - Suspected fetal death
> - Suspected uterine abnormality
> - Evaluation of fetal well-being
> - Suspected amniotic fluid abnormalities
> - Suspected placental abruption
> - Adjunct to external cephalic version
> - Premature rupture of membranes and/or premature labor
> - Abnormal biochemical markers
> - Follow-up evaluation of a fetal anomaly
> - Follow-up evaluation of placental location for suspected placenta previa
> - History of previous congenital anomaly
> - Evaluation of fetal condition in late registrants for prenatal care

Sample Protocol

1. The uterus and adnexa should be evaluated for the presence of a gestational sac.
   - If a gestational sac is seen, its location (intrauterine or extrauterine) should be noted.
   - The gestational sac should be recorded when the embryo is not identified during the **zygote** or implantation stage of pregnancy. Caution must be used in diagnosing a gestational sac without the presence of a yolk sac or embryo since intrauterine fluid collections may appear similar.
   - The presence or absence of a yolk sac and an embryo should be noted.
   - The crown-rump length is the most accurate measurement of gestational age during the first trimester and should be recorded when an embryo is present.
   - The earliest structure seen within the gestational sac is the yolk sac (the yolk sac will indicate the presence of an intrauterine pregnancy).
   - The embryo is seen at 4 weeks as a echogenic curved structure adjacent to the yolk sac.
   - The blood tests (hCG levels) should be positive at 7 to 10 days embryonic age (conception age).
   - The placenta is seen as a thickened density (trophoblastic reaction) along part of the margin of the gestational sac.
   - The bowel herniates out from the fetal abdomen at 8 to 11 weeks, then returns to the abdominal cavity.
2. Presence or absence of cardiac activity should be reported.
   - Cardiac motion is usually seen when the embryo is 5 mm or greater in length.
   - The fetal heart rate is much faster than the mother's heart rate. The fetal heart rate changes according to fetal development stages; early in embryologic development the heart rate is slow (90 beats per minute). The rate may go up to 180 beats per minute in the middle of the first trimester, before returning to 120 to 160 beats per minute throughout the remainder of the pregnancy.
3. Fetal number should be documented.
   - Count only the embryo and yolk sac to determine multiple pregnancies. The membrane structure and the number of amniotic and chorionic membranes should be documented in all multiple pregnancies. The chorionicity is most reliably documented during the first trimester.
4. Evaluation of the uterus, adnexal structures, and cul-de-sac should be performed.
   - It is important to document the texture of the ovaries and the presence of **corpus luteum** or other adnexal masses; look for inhomogeneous uterine texture that may represent leiomyomatous growth that may be stimulated by the hormonal changes of pregnancy.

SECOND AND THIRD TRIMESTERS

The indications for second- and third-trimester sonography are shown in Box 41-2. The guidelines for the second- and third-trimester ultrasound examination include a biometric and anatomic survey of the fetus. The guidelines suggest the following:

1. Fetal life, number, presentation, and activity should be documented.
   - In multiple gestations, the following individual studies should be performed on each fetus: amnionicity, chorionicity, comparison of fetal sizes, amount of amniotic fluid (increased, decreased, or normal) on each side of the membrane, and fetal genitalia (when visualized).

2. Estimation of the quantity of amniotic fluid. Abnormal fluid amounts should be described.
   - In early pregnancy the amniotic fluid is produced by the placenta; the fetal kidneys begin to produce urine, which contributes to the production and replacement of amniotic fluid as the fetus swallows and urinates. The fluid increases in volume until the 34th week of gestation.
   - Experienced observers may subjectively estimate amniotic fluid volume. Semiquantitative methods, including the four quadrant amniotic fluid index (AFI), the single deepest pocket, and the 2-diameter pocket may be used.
   - Too much fluid is termed *hydramnios (polyhydramnios);* too little fluid is called *oligohydramnios.*

3. Placental localization, appearance, and relationship to the internal cervical os should be recorded. The **umbilical cord** should be imaged and the number of vessels should be evaluated when possible.
   - The cervix is normally 3 to 4 cm long. The maternal bladder must be adequately filled to see the cervical os in the **lower uterine segment**. The sonographer should document that the lower end of the placenta is away from the cervical os to rule out placenta previa.
   - An overdistended maternal urinary bladder or a contraction in the lower uterine cavity can give a false impression of placenta previa.
   - Placental location in early pregnancy may not correlate well with its location at the time of delivery.
   - Endovaginal or transperineal imaging may be necessary to document cervical length when it appears shortened or if there is history of regular uterine contractions.

4. The crown-rump length measured during the first trimester is the most accurate method to assess gestational age. During the second and third trimester, there are multiple sonographic parameters that can be used to estimate gestational age. The variability of these measurements increases as the pregnancy progresses. If the clinical gestational age and sonographic parameters demonstrate significant discrepancies, the possibility of fetal growth abnormalities, such as macrosomia or IUGR, is suggested. Biometric parameters that may be used include the following:
   - Biparietal diameter (BPD) is measured in an axial plane that includes the thalamus and cavum septum pellucidum. The cerebellar hemispheres should not be visible in the image where the BPD is measured. The biparietal measurement is taken from the outer edge to the inner edge of the skull. The head shape may normally be more rounded (brachycephaly) or elongated (dolichocephaly), shapes, which will make the measurement of the head circumference more accurate than the measurement of the biparietal diameter.
   - Head circumference is measured at same level as BPD, around the outer perimeter of the calvarium. The head circumference is not affected by head shape.
   - Femur length, the femoral diaphysis length, is reliably measured after the 14th week of gestation. The most accurate measurements are taken when the femoral shaft is perpendicular to the acoustic beam.
   - Abdominal circumference is measured on a transverse view at the level of the junction of the umbilical vein and portal sinus. The circumference should be measured at the skin line on a true transverse view of the fetal abdomen where the portal sinus, fetal stomach, and umbilical vein are visible. Abdominal circumference is used to estimate fetal weight.
   - Fetal weight may be estimated by using the abdominal circumference measurement in mathematical formulations with other sonographic parameters. The best fetal weight estimates yield significant errors. Interval growth may be determined by sonographic measurements at least 3 weeks apart.

5. Uterine, adnexal, and cervical evaluation should be performed to document the presence, location, and size of uterine or adnexal masses, which may complicate obstetric management. The normal maternal ovaries may not be imaged during the second and third trimester.

6. Fetal anatomy may be adequately assessed after 18 weeks of gestation. Anatomy may be difficult to image because of fetal movement, size, or position; maternal scars; or increased wall thickness. When anatomy is not seen because of technical limitation, the sonographer should note the reason. A follow-up examination may be ordered.

The guidelines recommend that the following anatomy be documented during a standard obstetric sonography examination. More detailed studies may be performed if the anatomy appears questionable or abnormal. Documentation and images of the required anatomy should be retained. Anatomic areas recommended include the following:

1. Head and neck
   - Cerebellum
   - Choroid plexus
   - Cisterna magna
   - Lateral cerebral ventricles
   - Midline falx
   - Cavum septi pellucidi
2. Chest
   - Four-chamber view of the fetal heart
   - If technically feasible, an extended basic cardiac examination that includes both outflow tracts may be attempted
3. Abdomen
   - Stomach (presence, size, and situs)
   - Kidneys
   - Bladder
   - Umbilical cord insertion into the fetal abdomen
   - Umbilical cord; number of vessels
4. Spine
   - Cervical, thoracic, lumbar, and sacral spine
5. Extremities
   - Presence or absence of arms and legs
6. Gender
   - Medically indicated in low-risk pregnancies only for assessment of multiple pregnancies

Referral or Targeted Study. The patient who requires a more in-depth investigation of fetal anatomy or condition based on risk factors or questionable sonographic findings is referred for a targeted study. The targeted obstetrical examination often includes additional measurements and counseling. The targeted study is best performed by sonographers and sonologists with considerable expertise and experience in recognizing fetal anomalies and in understanding the complexities of birth defects.

SELECTED BIBLIOGRAPHY

AIUM practice guideline for the performance of an antepartum obstetric ultrasound examination published June 4, 2003, available at *http://www.aium.org,* accessed 11/2/2004.

American College of Obstetrics and Gynecology: *Ultrasound in pregnancy,* Tech Bull 116, Washington, DC, May 1988, The College.

American College of Radiology: *ACR standard for the performance of antepartum obstetrical ultrasound,* Richmond, VA, 1995, The College.

American Institute of Ultrasound in Medicine: Bioeffects consideration for the safety of diagnostic ultrasound, *J Ultrasound Med* 7(suppl):53, 1998.

Andrist LS, Schroedter W, editors: Standards for assurance of minimum entry-level competence for the diagnostic ultrasound professional, *J Diag Medical Ultrsnd* 17:307-311, 2001.

Callen PW, editor: *Ultrasonography in obstetrics and gynecology,* ed 4, Philadelphia, 2000, WB Saunders.

Carstensen EL: Acoustic cavitation and the safety of diagnostic ultrasound, *Ultrasound Med Biol* 13:597, 1987.

Consensus Development Conference: *Diagnostic ultrasound imaging in pregnancy,* Pub No 84-667, Washington, DC, 1984, United States Department of Health and Human Services.

Kremkau WF: Biologic effects and possible hazards, *Clin Obstet Gynecol* 10:395, 1983.

Rados C: *FDA cautions against ultrasound keepsake images,* FDA Consumer Magazine, Washington, DC, U.S. Food and Drug Administration Office of Public Affairs, January/February 2004 available at *http://www.fda.gov/fdac/features/2004/104_images.html;* Accessed 1/3/05.

Reece EA and others: The safety of obstetric ultrasonography concern for the fetus, *Obstet Gynecol* 76:139, 1990.

Reece EA, Goldstein I, Hobbins JC: *Fundamentals of obstetric & gynecologic ultrasound,* Norwalk, CT, 1994, Appleton & Lange.

CHAPTER 42

Clinical Ethics for Obstetric Sonography

Jean Lea Spitz

OBJECTIVES

- Identify multiple sources of moral beliefs in a pluralistic society
- Differentiate morality from ethics
- Describe the application of nonmaleficence, beneficence, justice, veracity, and autonomy in a sonographic setting
- Define the principle of beneficence in clinical ethics
- Define the principle of respect for autonomy in clinical ethics
- Identify beneficence-based obligations to the fetal patient
- Identify ethical issues in competence and referral in sonography examinations
- Identify ethical issues in routine obstetric sonography screening
- Identify ethical issues in disclosure of results in sonographic examinations
- Identify ethical issues in the confidentiality of findings

KEY TERMS

autonomy – self-governing or self-directing freedom and especially moral independence; the right of persons to choose and to have their choices respected

beneficence – bringing about good by maximizing benefits and minimizing possible harm

confidentiality – holding information in confidence; respect for privacy

ethics – the study of what is good and bad and of moral duty and obligation; systematic reflection on and analysis of morality

informed consent – providing complete information and assuring comprehension and voluntary consent by a patient or subject to a required or experimental medical procedure

integrity – adherence to moral and ethical principles

justice – the ethical principle that requires fair distribution of benefits and burdens; an injustice occurs when a benefit to which a person is entitled is withheld or when a burden is unfairly imposed

morality – the protection of cherished values that relate to how persons interact and live in peace

nonmaleficence – refrain from harming oneself or others

respect for persons – incorporates both respect for the autonomy of individuals and the requirement to protect those with diminished autonomy

veracity – truthfulness, honesty

MORALITY AND ETHICS DEFINED

HISTORY OF MEDICAL ETHICS

PRINCIPLES OF MEDICAL ETHICS

NONMALEFICENCE
BENEFICENCE
AUTONOMY
VERACITY AND INTEGRITY
JUSTICE

CONFIDENTIALITY OF FINDINGS

Ethical codes are important regulators in healthcare. Patient trust is built on the expectation that health care professionals will follow established ethical principles and guidelines. Medical ethics promote excellence and protect patients by encouraging practitioners to reflect on, communicate, and demonstrate optimal care.

Sonographers have ethical responsibilities to their patients and colleagues. The principles of nonmaleficence, beneficence, autonomy, respect for persons, veracity and integrity, and justice must be implemented in the sonography laboratory to ensure ethical practice. Sonographers who regularly participate in ethical discussions and discourse within their environment may best meet these requirements. A code of ethics for sonographers has been adopted by the Society of Diagnostic Medical Sonography. This code has elements consistent with principles of nonmaleficence, beneficence, autonomy, veracity, justice, and confidentiality.

MORALITY AND ETHICS DEFINED

Ethics is defined as systematic reflection on and analysis of morality. **Morality** concerns right and wrong conduct (what we ought or ought not do) and good and bad character (the kinds of persons we should become and the virtues we should cultivate in doing so). Morality reflects duties and values. Freedom and autonomy are also integral to morality because values can be expressed. All aspects of morality, duties, values, and rights are of importance for the clinical ethics in sonography.

In a pluralistic, multicultural society such as the United States, moral beliefs and behavior vary widely. Morality is learned through personal experiences and family traditions, and from normative behavior within communities, ethnic and racial groups, or geographic regions. Religions disagree about conduct and character, and religious ethics provide an inadequate foundation for secular professional ethics in a culturally diverse society. National identity and history also contribute to beliefs, as do the laws of the states and the federal government. These many sources of moral beliefs can sometimes cause conflict. Well-intentioned health care providers may disagree among themselves or with patients on moral directions. When these disagreements are discussed and analyzed, a collaborative and ethical resolution of the conflict can be achieved. It is this kind of discussion, reflection, and discourse on morality that constitutes ethics.

Whereas morality has to do with the protection of cherished values, ethics is a discipline of study that seeks to articulate clear, consistent, coherent, and practical guidelines for conduct and character. Ethics tries to answer the key question "What is good?" To be applicable to a medical context like sonography, ethics must transcend moral pluralism by offering an approach with minimal ties to any substantive prior belief about moral conduct and character. This is what philosophical ethics attempts to do because it requires only a commitment to the results of rational discourse in which all substantive commitments about what morality ought to be are open to question. Every such substantive claim requires intellectual justification in the form of a rigorous ethical analysis and argument. Philosophic ethics therefore properly serves as the foundation for medical ethics, especially in an international context.

HISTORY OF MEDICAL ETHICS

Medical ethics has evolved since the beginnings of time when health care knowledge was shared orally and healers exemplified a community's moral code. Prince Hammurabi of Babylon recorded the responsibilities of health care providers in 1727 BC, and early Hindu writers at about the same time cautioned healers to treat patients with respect, gentleness, and dignity. Fundamental principles of Western medical ethics were first recorded in ancient Greece in about the fifth century BC. Hippocrates cautioned his students, "*primum non nocere,*" which famously means, "First, do no harm." In ethics, this is known as the *ethical principle of nonmaleficence.* Hippocrates's teachings emphasized choosing treatments based on knowledge to best benefit patients, treating patients like one would treat a family member, upholding confidentiality and practicing personal piety. Ethical norms, elements, or principles were refined through the centuries. Thomas Percival (1740-1805) wrote a treatise that substantially changed medical ethics. Previously a patient was someone who paid for treatment, but Percival redefined patient as anyone needing care. He also foresaw a team approach in health care and public health. Percival emphasized patient care by all professionals and ordered competitive or professional interests secondary to the needs of the patient.

Modern medical ethics were codified after the Nuremberg trials, which judged the atrocities done in medical experimentation by Nazi doctors. The judges in the Nuremberg trial issued a verdict that included a section on permissible human experimentation. That section, which became known as the Nuremberg code, was incorporated into regulatory policy in the United States. The same protections were adopted internationally and published within the Helsinki report in 1964. The Nuremberg code emphasized individual rights and autonomy and this has become a key element of modern ethics.

Basic principles of medical ethics have been incorporated into research regulations, professional codes, and clinical practices throughout the world. The ethical codes of different professional groups may differ slightly in definition and emphasis, but the basic principles of autonomy, justice, beneficence, nonmaleficence, integrity, and respect for persons are universal.

The *Code of Ethics for the Profession of Diagnostic Medical Sonography* is adopted and maintained by the Society of Diagnostic Medical Sonography.

PRINCIPLES OF MEDICAL ETHICS

NONMALEFICENCE

The principle of **nonmaleficence** directs the sonographer to not cause harm. The application of the principle of nonmaleficence requires the sonographer to obtain appropriate education and clinical skills to ensure competence in performing each examination required. Ensuring an appropriate level of competence imposes a rigorous standard of education and continuing education. Two problems result when obstetric sonographers do not maintain a baseline level of competence in the techniques and interpretation of sonographic imaging: (1) They may cause unnecessary harm to the pregnant woman or fetal patient, for example, from mistaken impressions of fetal anomalies; (2) they may undermine the **informed consent** process regarding the management of pregnancy by reporting in an incomplete or inaccurate manner to the physician who, in turn, reports them to the pregnant women.

Sonographers also need to be accountable for and participate in regular assessment and review of protocols, equipment, procedures, and results to ensure that patients are not harmed by outdated procedures or poorly functioning equipment. Appropriate oversight and approval of protocols by research or hospital committees also contribute to patient safety. Protocols and diagnostic criteria should be established by peer review. Sonographers may also contribute to safety of patients by sharing with others and publishing peer-reviewed information about mistakes made or lessons learned.

The sonographer must practice emergency procedures and strive to ensure patient safety in all procedures and circumstances. Sonographers must refrain from substance abuse or any activity that may alter their judgment or ability to provide safe and effective patient care.

Because ultrasound energy poses a theoretical risk to the fetus, the principle of nonmaleficence requires sonographers to perform all examinations with ALARA, an energy exposure that is as low as reasonably possible to achieve the desired results. Sonographers need to read the current medical literature to stay abreast of new developments related to patient safety.

BENEFICENCE

Protections for patients and subjects based on the ethical principle of nonmaleficence only partially explain what is in the patient's interests because medicine, and therefore sonography, seeks to benefit patients, not simply avoid harming them. The use of obstetric ultrasound, like other medical interventions, must be justified by the goal of seeking the greater balance of clinical "goods" over "harms," not simply avoiding harm to the patient at all cost. This ethical principle is called **beneficence** and is a more comprehensive basis for ethics in sonography than is nonmaleficence.

Goods and harms are to be defined and balanced from a rigorous clinical perspective. The goods that obstetric sonography should seek for patients are preventing early or premature death (not preventing death at all costs); preventing and managing disease, injury, and handicapping conditions; and alleviating unnecessary pain and suffering. Pain and suffering are unnecessary and therefore represent clinical harms to be avoided when they do not contribute to seeking the good of the beneficence-based clinical judgment. *Pain* is a physiologic phenomenon involving central nervous system processing of tissue damage. *Suffering* is a psychological phenomenon involving blocked intentions, plans, and projects. Pain often causes suffering, but one can suffer without being in pain.

The principle of beneficence obligates the obstetric sonographer to seek the greatest benefit in the care of pregnant patients. Beneficence encourages sonographers to go beyond the minimum standard protocol and to seek additional images and information if achievable and in the best interests of patients. Beneficence requires sonographers to focus on small comforts for the patient, respecting their privacy and the inclusion of family. Kindness and attention to small details minimize suffering caused by frustration or anger. Beneficence, like nonmaleficence, requires competency, knowledge, and excellent sonographic skills to ensure that the patient and the fetus receive the greatest benefit from the examination.

Fetal interests in sonography are understood exclusively in terms of beneficence. This principle explains the moral (as distinct from legal) status of the fetus as a patient and generates the serious ethical obligations owed by physicians and sonographers to the fetus. In the technical language of beneficence,

the sonographer has beneficence-based obligations to the fetal patient to protect and promote fetal interests and those of the child it will become, as these are understood from a rigorous clinical perspective. The clinical good to be sought for the fetal patient includes prevention of premature death, disease, and handicapping conditions and of unnecessary pain and suffering. It is appropriate therefore to refer to fetuses as patients, with the exception of previable fetuses that are to be aborted.

In clinical practice, beneficence may have to be balanced against other ethical principles. A health professional's duty of beneficence may suggest one course of action and the patient may choose another. In these cases beneficence must be balanced by respect for a person's autonomy. The principles of veracity and integrity may on occasion conflict with beneficence when truth-telling will cause undue stress and complications. The principle of justice or fair distribution of benefits may conflict with beneficence for individual patients who need extra resources. Fortunately in most situations it is in the patients' best interests to respect their autonomy, to tell the truth, and to distribute benefits justly.

AUTONOMY

In the twentieth century, **autonomy,** or the right to self-determination, has become a key ethical principle. **Respect for persons** incorporates both respect for the autonomy of individuals and the requirement to protect those with diminished autonomy. Patients, including pregnant women, have their own perspective on their interests that should be respected as much as the clinician's perspective on the patient's interests. A patient's perspective on her interests is shaped by wide-ranging and sometimes idiosyncratic values and beliefs. *Autonomy* refers to a person's capacity to formulate, express, and carry out value-based preferences. The ethical principle of respect for autonomy obligates the sonographer to acknowledge the integrity of a patient's values and beliefs and of her value-based preferences; to avoid interfering with the expression or implementation of these preferences; and, when necessary, to assist in their expression and implementation. This principle generates the autonomy-based obligations of the sonographer.

Informed consent is an autonomy-based right. Each health professional has autonomy-based obligations regarding the informed consent process. This process must include discourse about what sonography examinations can and cannot detect, the sensitivity and frequency of false-negatives and false-positives of the sonography techniques employed, and the difficult and sometimes uncertain interpretation of sonographic images. In the face of medical uncertainty about the clinical good and harm of routine ultrasound, it is obligatory to inform pregnant patients about that uncertainty and to give them the opportunity to make their own choices about how that uncertainty should be managed. In routine examinations it is also important to inform the woman of the possibility of confronting an anomaly that will lead her to decide whether to terminate the pregnancy or take it to term.

The sonographer respects the patient's autonomy by providing a detailed explanation of the examination, including appropriate choices such as the right to view the screen or to determine the gender of the fetus. Respect for maternal autonomy dictates responding frankly to requests from the pregnant woman for information about the fetus's gender. The pregnant woman should be made aware of the uncertainties of ultrasound gender identification as part of the disclosure process. The sonographer can use his or her own experience to help the pregnant woman understand these uncertainties. A second choice that may be presented during obstetric examinations is the choice to view the images. This choice concerns the phenomenon of apparent bonding of pregnant women and their families to the fetus as a result of seeing the sonographic images. Such bonding often enriches pregnancies that will be taken to term, but can at other times complicate decisions to terminate a pregnancy.

A current ethical issue is the nonmedical use of sonography, the videotaping or photography of "baby pictures." There is nothing intrinsically wrong with the practice if it is a side product of a legitimate ultrasound examination. However, when videotaping or photography is performed to generate revenue, this practice trivializes medical sonography and may result in harm because problems that could be diagnosed could be missed. It is the responsibility of sonographers to ensure that women have the information necessary to make informed choices.

It is an autonomy-enhancing strategy for a woman to be allowed to insert a vaginal probe herself to make the experience more comfortable and less threatening. It is also a sonographer's obligation to respect a patient's right to refuse a procedure.

Maternal interests are protected and promoted by both autonomy-based and beneficence-based obligations of the sonographer to the pregnant woman. Fetuses are incapable of having their own perspective on their interests because the immaturity of their central nervous system renders them incapable of having the requisite values or beliefs. Thus there can be no autonomy-based obligations to the fetus. The pregnant woman also has beneficence-based obligations to the fetal patient when the pregnancy will be taken to term. She is expected to protect and promote the fetal patient's interests and those of the child it will become. When a pregnant woman elects to have an abortion, however, these obligations do not exist. A sonographer with moral objections to abortion should keep two things in mind: First, the moral judgment and decision of the pregnant woman to end her pregnancy should not be criticized or commented on in any way; her autonomy demands respect in the form of the sonographer and physician being neutral to her judgment and decision. Second, the sonographer is free to follow his or her conscience and to withdraw from further involvement with patients who elect abortion. Physicians should as a matter of office policy respect this important matter of individual conscience on the part of the sonographer.

VERACITY AND INTEGRITY

Telling the truth is an ethical principle that most sonographers have been taught from a young age. Yet, the vast majority of us will on occasion tell "white lies" in kindness or to escape unwanted consequences. The universal acceptance and even cultural preference in some countries for "white lies" is evidence of the difficulty adhering to the principle of veracity. **Veracity** means truthfulness. **Integrity** means adherence to moral and ethical principles. Integrity is related to the word *integrate* meaning *to bring together*. In terms of honesty, integrity means that there is no difference between what you think, what you say, and what you do: they all come together in ethical behavior.

In medical care, patients properly rely for their protection on the personal and professional integrity of their clinicians. A crucial aspect of that integrity on the part of physicians is willingness to refer to specialists when the limits of their own knowledge are being approached. Integrity should also be one of the fundamental virtues of sonographers and thus a standard for judging professional character. Like other virtues, such as self-sacrifice and compassion, integrity directs sonographers to focus primarily on the patient's interests as a way to blunt mere self-interest. Sonographers must avoid conflicts of interest and situations that exploit others, create unreasonable expectations, or misrepresent information.

Veracity with respect to abilities and limitations is absolutely essential among sonographers. If a practitioner asks a sonographer to perform an examination that they are not competent to do, it is essential for the sonographer to be truthful about his or her limitations to protect the patient. A sonographer asked by a patient or a colleague must accurately represent his or her level of competence, education, and credentials.

The disclosure of the results of an abnormal sonographic examination raises significant clinical ethical issues for sonographers. Sonographers are justified in disclosing findings of normal anatomy directly to the pregnant woman. When the images reveal abnormal findings, sonographers must not act "dumb" or tell the patient that they do not know what they are seeing. Veracity is upheld by telling the patient in a nonalarming way the procedure for diagnosis, that "multiple eyes need to look at some of the images," and that the physician will determine the results. Disclosure of, and discussion about, abnormal findings by sonographers is inappropriate because it is not in the best interest of the patient. If the disclosure and discussion are to respect and enhance maternal autonomy and avoid unnecessary psychological harm to the pregnant woman, the discussion should occur in a setting where the alternatives and choices available to manage a pregnancy are presented. Sonographers, neither by training nor experience, can claim the clinical competence to engage in such discussions. Physicians can and therefore should.

Sonographers must strive to supply patients and colleagues with complete and accurate information. The sonographer's integrity is an essential safeguard for the patient's autonomy. At times the sonographer will need to become an advocate, even a vigorous advocate, for disclosure of information to a patient. In such cases sonographers must address their concerns not to the patient but to the practitioner involved. Failure to make patient disclosures undermines professional integrity and the moral authority of health care professionals. When the sonographer disagrees with the clinical judgment of his or her supervising physician, professional communication and discussion of the matter need to occur. The best interests of the health care team and the patient are enhanced by such conversations.

JUSTICE

Justice is the ethical principle that requires fair distribution of benefits and burdens; an injustice occurs when a benefit to which a person is entitled is withheld or when a burden is unfairly imposed. Justice means simply that sonographers must strive to treat all patients equally. In practical terms, justice requires that translators be used when necessary to ensure adequate and appropriate communication with all patients. Sonographers should strive to ensure that disabled patients have access to reasonable accommodations and pathways, and that obese patients have comfortable chairs, gowns, and stretchers. Children, adults, and geriatric patients need to feel equally welcome and cared for within the sonography laboratory.

Justice is served when protocols are standardized. Men and women with similar symptoms should receive similar tests and interventions. If a group is denied services or asked to assume an undue burden to obtain care provided to others, justice is not being served.

Justice and autonomy are the ethical principles that determine the timing of routine obstetrical sonography examinations. The information obtained from a sonogram enhances women's choices. It is an injustice to provide these choices to some women and not to others. Sonography results, such as risk for an abnormality, are relevant to the woman's decision about whether she will seek an abortion. In pregnancies that will be taken to term, routine sonography during the second trimester can enhance a pregnant woman's autonomy. If anomalies are detected and she does not choose abortion, she may begin to prepare herself for the decisions that she will confront later about the management of those anomalies in the intrapartum and postpartum periods. Providing this information early in pregnancy permits a pregnant woman ample time to deal with its psychologic and other sequelae before she must confront such decisions.

The principle of justice infers that health care professionals should act in accordance with the best interest of the community. As health care costs increase, insurance costs skyrocket, and bankruptcy becomes associated with chronic illness, the societal aspects of medical justice are receiving more attention. The traditional focus of medical ethics is the individual patient. In some cases, however, the costs and benefits of treating one patient may place an undue burden on others. An individual ethical focus may be in conflict with a society focus when an individual uses a disproportionate amount of health care without paying for it. This forces others to pay for the service, a burden society accepts if the service is considered essential. As the benefit of the service decreases as in experimental protocols, or the cost of the service increases, the conflict grows. If the resources used are not replaced, others may be deprived of similar services. The solution to such conflicts is not clear politically, socially, or ethically. What is clear,

however, is that the community aspect of justice will receive more attention in the future. Sonographers can support community interests by performing only medically indicated procedures prescribed by a clinician.

CONFIDENTIALITY OF FINDINGS

Confidentiality concerns the obligation of caregivers to protect clinical information about patients from unauthorized access. The obligation of confidentiality derives from the principles of beneficence (patients will be more forthcoming) and respect for autonomy (the patient's privacy rights are protected). Others, including the pregnant woman's spouse and/or sex partner and family, should be understood as third parties to the patient-sonographer relationship. Diagnostic information about a woman's pregnancy is confidential. It can be justifiably disclosed to third parties *only* with the pregnant woman's *explicit permission*. Federal regulations, including the Health Insurance Portability and Accountability Act (HIPAA), determine acceptable conditions for releasing confidential information. To prevent awkward situations, sonographers and their supervising physicians should establish policies and procedures that reflect this analysis of the ethics of confidentiality.

The ethics of confidentiality when the pregnant woman is less than the age of 18 years should be the same as when the patient is 18 years of age and older. The law, however, may complicate matters because pregnancy does not emancipate a minor in every jurisdiction and different jurisdictions give different levels of protection to the privacy of the physician-patient relationship when the patient is under the age of 18 years.

ACKNOWLEDGEMENT

The author would like to acknowledge the work of Frank A. Chervenak and Laurence B. McCullough on the sixth edition of this book.

SELECTED BIBLIOGRAPHY

Annas G, Grodin M, editors: *The Nazi doctors and the Nuremberg code: human rights in human experimentation,* New York, 1992, Oxford University Press.

Beauchamp TL and others: *Medical ethics: the moral responsibilities of physicians,* Englewood Cliffs, NJ, 1984, Prentice-Hall.

Beauchamp TL and others: *Principles of biomedical ethics,* ed 3, New York, 1989, Oxford University Press.

Beauchamp TL, Childress JF: *Principles of biomedical ethics,* ed 4, New York, 1994, Oxford University Press.

Boodt CL: A historical review of the SDMS code of ethics, *J Diagn Med Sonography* 20(4):238, 2004.

Campbell S and others: Ultrasound scanning in pregnancy: the short-term psychological effects of early real time scans, *J Psychosomat Obstet Gynecol* 1:57, 1986.

Chervenak FA and others: Perinatal ethics: a practical analysis of obligations to mother and fetus, *Obstet Gynecol* 66:442, 1985.

Chervenak FA and others: Ethics in obstetric ultrasound, *J Ultrasound Med* 8:493, 1989.

Chervenak FA and others: Prenatal informed consent for sonogram (PICS): an indication for obstetrical ultrasound, *Am J Obstet Gynecol* 161(4):857, 1989.

Dunn CM, Chadwick GL: *Protecting study volunteers in research: a manual for investigative sites,* ed 2, Boston, 2002, Thomson Centerwatch.

Eddy DM: The individual vs society: Is there a conflict? *JAMA* 265 (11):1446, 1991.

Eddy DM: The individual vs society: Resolving the conflict, *JAMA* 265(18):2399, 1991.

Ewigman BG and others: Effect of prenatal ultrasound screening on perinatal outcome, *N Engl J Med* 329:483, 1993.

McCullough LB: Methodological concerns in bioethics, *J Med Phil* 11:17, 1986.

McCullough LB and others: *Ethics in obstetrics and gynecology,* New York, 1994, Oxford University Press.

Purtilo R: *Ethical dimensions in the health professions,* ed 2, Philadelphia, 1993, WB Saunders.

Skupski DW and others: Is routine ultrasound screening for all patients? *Clin Perinat* 21:707, 1994.

Society of Diagnostic Medical Sonography, Plano, TX, www.sdms.org (code of ethics).

Warren MA: *Gendercide: the implications of sex selection,* Totowa, NJ, 1985, Rowman and Littlefield.

CHAPTER 43

The Normal First Trimester

Sandra L. Hagen-Ansert

OBJECTIVES

- Explain the early development of the embryo
- Explain the role of serum human chorionic gonadotropin
- Delineate the differences between transabdominal and endovaginal scanning
- List the goals for sonography in the first trimester
- Define the sonographic characteristics of the yolk sac, embryo, amnion and chorion, and gestational sac
- Describe when the herniation of bowel occurs in the embryo
- Describe the sonographic measurements performed in the first trimester
- Identify the methods of gestational assessment in the first trimester

KEY TERMS

amniotic cavity – cavity in which the fetus exists; forms early in gestation; fills with amniotic fluid to protect the fetus

chorionic cavity – surrounds the amniotic cavity; the yolk sac is within the chorionic cavity

corpus luteum cyst – the small yellow endocrine structure that develops within a ruptured ovarian follicle and secretes progesterone and estrogen

crown-rump length (CRL) – most accurate measurement of the embryo in the first trimester

decidua basalis – the villi on the maternal side of the placenta or embryo; unites with the chorion to form the placenta

decidua capsularis – the villi surrounding the chorionic sac

diamniotic – multiple pregnancy with two amniotic sacs

dichorionic – multiple pregnancy with two chorionic sacs

double decidual sac sign – interface between the decidua capsularis and the echogenic, highly vascular endometrium

embryologic age (conceptual age) – age calculated from when conception occurs

embryonic period – time between 6 and 12 weeks of gestation

endovaginal (EV) transducer – high-frequency transducer that is inserted into the vaginal canal to obtain better definition of first-trimester pregnancy

hematopoiesis – production and development of blood cells

human chorionic gonadotropin (hCG) – hormone secreted by the trophoblastic cells (developing placental cells) of the blastocyst; laboratory test indicates pregnancy when values are elevated

IUP – intrauterine pregnancy

menstrual age (gestational age) – length of time calculated from the first day of the last normal menstrual period (LMP) to the point at which the pregnancy is being assessed

monoamniotic – multiple pregnancy with one amniotic sac

monochorionic – multiple pregnancy with one chorionic sac

MSD – mean sac diameter

primary yolk sac – first site of formation of red blood cells that will nourish the embryo

secondary yolk sac – formed at 23 days when the primary yolk sac is pinched off by the extra embryonic coelom

yolk stalk – the umbilical duct connecting the yolk sac with the embryo

zygote – fertilized ovum resulting from union of male and female gametes

EARLY DEVELOPMENT
A NOTE ON TERMINOLOGY
EMBRYONIC DEVELOPMENT

LABORATORY VALUES IN EARLY PREGNANCY

SONOGRAPHIC TECHNIQUE AND EVALUATION OF THE FIRST TRIMESTER
SONOGRAPHIC VISUALIZATION OF THE EARLY GESTATION

DETERMINATION OF GESTATIONAL AGE
GESTATIONAL SAC SIZE
YOLK SAC SIZE
CROWN-RUMP LENGTH

MULTIPLE GESTATIONS

Ultrasonography has become an important component in evaluating obstetric patients in the first trimester. Sonography during the first trimester offers the clinician a wealth of information that may affect clinical management or aid in diagnosis of conditions that require emergency treatment. Although the ability to image the first-trimester pregnancy with ultrasound may seem routine, the potential for false-positive and false-negative diagnoses for any given pathology is substantial. Extreme care should always be taken when sonographically evaluating the first-trimester pregnancy.

EARLY DEVELOPMENT

A NOTE ON TERMINOLOGY

It is especially important to have a clear understanding of terminology when discussing embryology. Embryologists use *conceptual age*, also known as **embryologic age,** to assess gestational age, with conception as the first day of the pregnancy. Clinicians and sonographers use *gestational age*, also known as *menstrual age*, to date the pregnancy, with the first day of the last menstrual period as the beginning of gestation. Thus the gestational age would add 2 weeks onto the conceptual age. In the first 9 menstrual weeks, the conceptus is called an *embryo*. After the first 9 weeks, the embryo is called a *fetus*.

EMBRYONIC DEVELOPMENT

All embryonic dates in this chapter reflect menstrual age rather than **embryologic age (conceptual age).** The *gestational age* (age known as postmenstrual age) is calculated by adding 2 weeks (14 days) to conceptual age. Menstrual age refers to the length of time calculated from the first day of the last normal menstrual period (LMP) to the point at which the pregnancy is being assessed. During a 28-day menstrual cycle, a mature ovum is released at day 14. The ovum is swept into the distal fallopian tube via fimbria; fertilization occurs within this

region 1 to 2 days after ovulation. Meanwhile, the follicle that released the mature ovum hemorrhages and collapses to form the corpus luteum, which begins to secrete progesterone and some estrogen (Figure 43-1).

The fertilized ovum, which should now be referred to as a **zygote,** undergoes rapid cellular division to form the 16-cell morula. Further cell proliferation brings the morula to the blastocyst stage, which contains trophoblastic cells and the "inner cell mass," which forms the embryo. The blastocyst typically enters the uterus 4 to 5 days after fertilization, with implantation occurring 7 to 9 days after ovulation. During implantation, proteolytic enzymes produced by the trophoblasts erode endometrial mucosa and maternal capillaries, resulting in a primitive blood exchange network between mother and conceptus.

When implantation is complete, the trophoblast goes on to form primary villi, which initially circumvent the early gestational sac. Within the conceptus, the inner cell mass matures into the bilaminar embryonic disc, the future embryo, and the primary yolk sac. At approximately 23 days menstrual age, the **primary yolk sac** is pinched off by the extra embryonic coelom, forming the **secondary yolk sac.** The secondary yolk sac is the yolk sac seen sonographically throughout the first trimester. The amniotic and chorionic cavities also develop and evolve during this period of gestation.

The embryonic phase is between weeks 6 through 10. It is during this phase that all major internal and external structures begin to develop (Table 43-1). Although the organ function remains minimal, the cardiovascular system is the first organ to develop rapidly, with the initial heart beat between $5\frac{1}{2}$ and 6 weeks. The embryo's appearance changes from the flat, disklike configuration to a C-shaped structure, and it develops a humanlike appearance (Figure 43-2). During this period of embryogenesis the **crown-rump length (CRL)** develops rapidly, measuring 30 mm by the end of the 10th week.

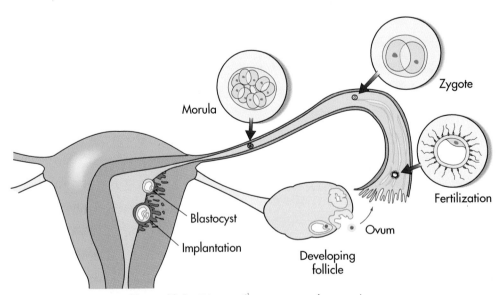

Figure 43-1 Diagram illustrates normal conception.

TABLE 43-1	NORMAL EMBRYONIC DEVELOPMENT	
Menstrual Age	**Embryonic Observations**	
Week 5	Prominent neural folds and neural groove are recognizable.	
Day 36	Heart begins to beat.	
Week 6	Anterior and posterior neuropores close and neural tube forms.	
Day 41	Upper and lower limb buds are present.	
Day 42	Crown-rump length is 4.0 mm.	
Day 46	Paddle-shaped hand plates are present. Lens pits and optic cups have formed.	
Day 48	Cerebral vesicles are distinct.	
Day 50	Oral and nasal cavities are confluent.	
Day 52	Upper lip is formed.	
Day 54	Digital rays are distinct.	
Day 56	Crown-rump length is 16.0 mm.	
Week 9	Cardiac ventricular septum is closed. Truncus arteriosus divides into aorta and pulmonary trunk. Kidney collecting tubules develop.	
Day 58	Eyelids develop.	
Day 64	Upper limbs bend at elbows. Fingers are distinct.	
Week 10	Glomeruli form in metanephros.	
Day 73	Genitalia show some female characteristics, but are still easily confused with male.	
Day 80	Face has human appearance.	
Day 82	Genitalia have male and female characteristics, but are still not fully formed.	
Day 84	Crown-rump length is 55 mm.	
Month 7	Ossification is complete throughout vertebral column.	
Month 8	Ossification centers appear in distal femoral epiphysis.	

From Neiman HL: Sonoembryology. In Nyberg DA and others, editors: *Endovaginal ultrasound*, St Louis, 1990, Mosby.

The last 2 weeks of the first trimester (weeks 11 and 12) constitute the beginning of the fetal period. At this time there is rapid continued growth of the organs. It is also noted that during this period of time, the fetal head is disproportionately larger than the rest of the fetus, constituting one half of the crown-rump length. As the fetal body grows, the body growth accelerates and this relative proportionality becomes less pronounced.

LABORATORY VALUES IN EARLY PREGNANCY

The laboratory values particular to pregnancy can be very useful in sonographic evaluation of the first trimester. An intimate relationship between the sonographic findings and quantitative serum **human chorionic gonadotropin (hCG)** levels normally exists during early pregnancy. Gestational sac size and hCG levels increase proportionately until 8 menstrual weeks, at which time the gestational sac is approximately 25 mm mean sac diameter (**MSD**) and an embryo should be easily detected by either transabdominal or endovaginal sonography. After 8 weeks, hCG levels plateau and subsequently decline while the gestational sac continues to grow.

Because the quantitative hCG levels correlate with the gestational sac size in normal pregnancies, the sonographer or clinician is able to use this objective assessment to establish if the pregnancy is normal or abnormal when the embryo is too small to be imaged with ultrasound. Discriminatory hCG level for detecting an intrauterine sac varies somewhat from lab to lab and to the standard against which the hCG is calibrated. However, when the hCG level and sonographic findings are combined, the accuracy is improved to rule in an intrauterine pregnancy or ectopic pregnancy. A normal gestational sac can be consistently demonstrated when the hCG level is 1800 mIU/ml (Second International Standard) or greater when using transabdominal sonography. This detection threshold is significantly reduced by endovaginal sonography and may be as low

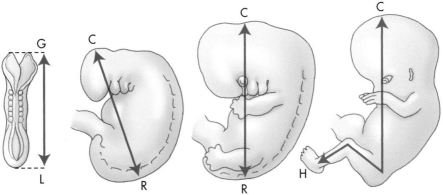

Figure 43-2   Diagram that shows the relationship of the neural tube development to the crown-rump length in the first trimester. Note the size of the embryo's head relative to the body.

as 500 mIU/ml. Many laboratories will use hCG levels of 1000 to 2000 mIU/mL as the number to indicate a normal pregnancy (Box 43-1).

Abnormal pregnancies demonstrate a low hCG level relative to gestational sac development, and it has been shown that hCG levels fall before spontaneous expulsion of nonviable gestations. The sonographer must be aware that when the hCG

level is elevated and the gestational sac is not seen within the uterus, an ectopic pregnancy should be considered.

The best method for assessment of the early gestation is to use the hCG levels along with the gestational sac measurement to determine if the pregnancy correlates with the normal values for the particular gestational age.

SONOGRAPHIC TECHNIQUE AND EVALUATION OF THE FIRST TRIMESTER

Imaging the first-trimester pregnancy with ultrasound has rapidly progressed over the past decade with the development of **endovaginal (EV) transducers**, which allow the gravid uterus and adnexa to be visualized with greater detail than that achieved with transabdominal techniques by allowing higher frequencies to be used (5 to 8 MHz) and the transducer placed closer to anatomic structures. With endovaginal transducers, the pelvic anatomy is imaged in both sagittal and coronal/semi-coronal planes. Such coronal imaging of the pelvis is unique within sonography, and the images should not be misconstrued as transverse sections (Figure 43-3).

Although endovaginal sonography has gained overall acceptance within the ultrasound community because of its improved image quality, transabdominal (TA) and transvesical

---

BOX 43-1   BETA-hCG LEVELS DURING PREGNANCY

Menstrual Weeks	hCG Levels in mIU/ml
3	35-50
4	45-426
5	518-7340
6	61,080-56,500
7-8	7,650-229,000
10-12	25,700-288,000

Note: hCG rates will likely decrease after the first trimester when the placenta takes over.

Note: Even if levels are rising, the failure for the levels to double every few days is not a good sign and the pregnancy will likely end in miscarriage. If test is low or borderline, another test will be ordered in a few days.

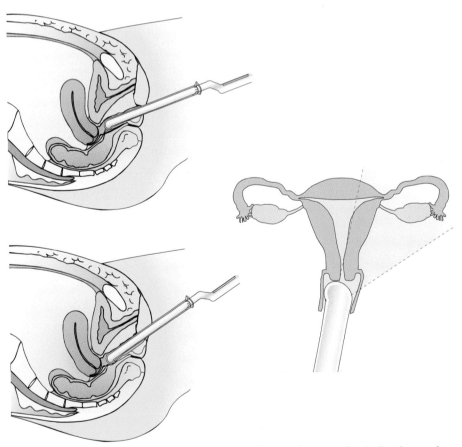

Figure 43-3   Schematic demonstrating endovaginal transducer techniques of sagittal and coronal-semicoronal anatomic planes.

sonography should not be overlooked. The transabdominal-transvesical approach allows visualization of a larger field of anatomy, which is important when specific anatomic relationships are in question. For instance, the size, extent, and anatomic relationships of a large pelvic mass with surrounding structures can only be determined with transabdominal techniques. The patient must have a full bladder to image the uterus and adnexal area.

The following goals have been outlined (i.e., ACR/AIUM/ACOG) for sonography in the first-trimester pregnancy:

- Visualization and localization of the gestational sac (intrauterine or ectopic pregnancy) (Figure 43-4)
- Identification of embryonic demise or living embryonic gestation
- Identification of embryos that are still alive but at increased risk for embryonic or fetal demise
- Determination of the number of embryos and the chorionicity and amnionicity in multifetal pregnancies
- Estimation of the duration or menstrual age of the pregnancy (Figure 43-5)

- Early diagnosis of fetal anomalies, including identification of embryos that are more likely to be abnormal based on secondary criteria (for example, abnormal yolk sac)

SONOGRAPHIC VISUALIZATION OF THE EARLY GESTATION

During the 5th week of embryonic development, the intrauterine pregnancy (**IUP**) can be visualized sonographically. It appears as a 1- to 2-mm sac with an echogenic ring having a sonolucent center. The anechoic center represents the chorionic cavity. The circumferential echogenic rim seen surrounding the gestational sac represents trophoblastic tissue and associated decidual reaction. The echogenic ring around the gestational sac can be divided embryologically into several components. The villi on the myometrial or burrowing side of the conceptus are known as the **decidua basalis**. The villi covering the rest of the developing embryo are referred to as the **decidua capsularis** (Figure 43-6). The interface between the decidua capsularis and the echogenic, highly vascularized endometrium forms the **double decidual sac sign,** which has been reported to be a reliable sign of a viable gestation. The

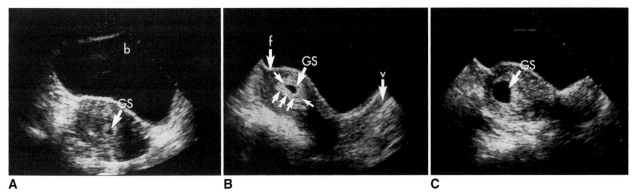

Figure 43-4 Sagittal transabdominal scans demonstrating the appearance of the gestational sac from 4 to 6 weeks gestation. **A,** A 4-week gestational sac *(GS)* noted within the fundus of the uterus. *b,* Maternal bladder. **B,** A 5-week gestational sac *(GS)* with the characteristic trophoblastic ring *(arrows)*. *f,* Fundus of uterus; *v,* vagina. **C,** A 6-week gestational sac *(GS)* within the fundus of the uterus.

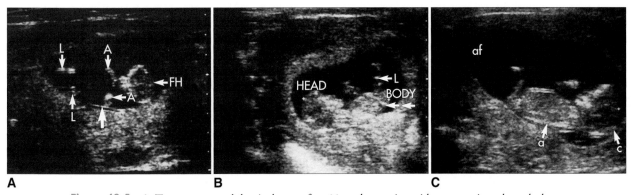

Figure 43-5 **A,** Transverse transabdominal scan of an 11-week gestation with cross sections through the upper and lower limbs *(L)*; fetal head *(FH)*; and amnion *(A)*. **B,** A fetus at 11½ weeks of gestation. *Arrows,* body; *L,* leg. **C,** A fetus at 12 weeks of gestation. Note the fetal arm and leg in this profile view. *a,* Abdomen; *af,* amniotic fluid; *c,* cranium.

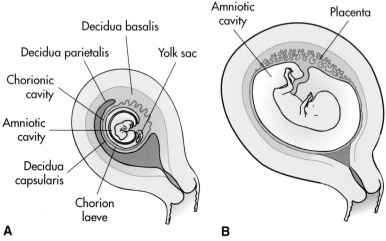

A   **B**

Figure 43-6   Schema showing the relation of the fetal membranes and the wall of the uterus. **A,** End of the second month. Note the yolk sac in the chorionic cavity between the amnion and chorion. At the abembryonic pole, the villi have disappeared (chorion laeve). **B,** End of the third month. The amnion and chorion have fused and the uterine cavity is obliterated by fusion of the chorion laeve and the decidua parietalis.

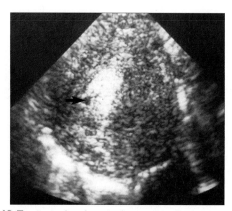

Figure 43-7   Sagittal endovaginal sonogram demonstrating a very early gestational sac, approximately 5 weeks of gestation *(arrow)*. Note the fluid center, which at this time represents chorionic cavity and the eccentric placement in relation to the very echogenic endometrial cavity.

BOX 43-2   SONOGRAPHIC FEATURES OF A NORMAL GESTATIONAL SAC

- *Shape:* Round or oval
- *Position:* Fundal or middle portion of uterus; a center position relative to endometrium (double decidua sac or intradecidua finding)
- *Contour:* Smooth
- *Wall (trophoblastic reaction):* Echogenic; 3 mm or more in thickness
- *Internal landmarks:* Yolk sac present when gestational sac is larger than 10 mm; embryo present when gestational sac is larger than 18 mm
- *Growth:* 1 mm/day (range: 0.7 mm to 1.5 mm/day)

From Nyberg DA, Hill LM: Normal early intrauterine pregnancy: sonographic development and hCG correlation. In Nyberg DA and others, editors: *Endovaginal ultrasound,* St Louis, 1992, Mosby.

---

gestational sac is eccentrically placed in relation to the endometrial cavity, secondary to its implantation. Typically, a fundal location is noted (Figure 43-7).

The normal sonographic features of a gestational sac include a round or oval shape; a fundal position in the uterus, or an eccentrically placed position in the middle portion of the uterus; smooth contours; and a decidual wall thickness greater than 3 mm. A yolk sac that can be seen with an MSD greater than 10 mm (definitely by 20 mm). An embryo that can be seen with an MSD greater than 18 mm (definitely by 25 mm) (Box 43-2). Once the gestational sac is sonographically imaged, rapid growth and development occur. The gestational sac size grows at a predictable rate of 1 mm/day in early pregnancy.

Often the first intragestational sac anatomy seen is the sonographic yolk sac (secondary yolk sac), which is routinely visualized between 5 and 5 1/2 weeks of gestation. Invariably the observer sees the yolk sac before the beating embryonic heart, which may be normal because embryonic heart motion begins at approximately 5 1/2 weeks. The yolk sac may be used as a landmark to image the embryo, given the connection between yolk sac and embryo.

At this point in gestation, rapid embryonic development increases gestational sac size, leading to better defined intragestational sac anatomy. Between 5 1/2 and 6 weeks of gestation, the amniotic cavity and membrane, chorionic cavity, yolk sac, and embryo should be seen.

Yolk Sac.   The yolk sac is routinely the earliest intragestational sac anatomy seen, normally from 5 weeks of gestation. The secondary or sonographic yolk sac has essential functions in embryonic development, including (1) provision of nutri-

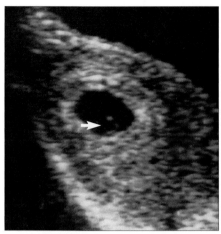

Figure 43-8 Sonogram demonstrating an approximate 6-week gestational sac with normal-appearing secondary or sonographic yolk sac *(arrow)*.

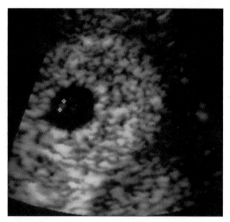

Figure 43-9 Sonogram at approximately $5^1/_2$ weeks of gestation with calipers placed on embryo with positive fetal heart motion. The crown-rump length of this trilaminar embryonic disk is approximately 2 mm. Although yolk sac was present, it is not demonstrated in this image.

ents to the developing embryo, (2) **hematopoiesis**, and (3) development of embryonic endoderm, which forms the primitive gut.

Initially the yolk sac is attached to the embryo via the yolk stalk, but with amniotic cavity expansion, the yolk sac, which lies between the amniotic and chorionic cavities, detaches from the yolk stalk at approximately 8 weeks of gestation (Figure 43-8).

Typically, the yolk sac resorbs and is no longer seen sonographically by 12 weeks. Persistent yolk sac does occur and may be visualized at the placental umbilical cord insertion where the amniotic and chorionic membranes are fused.

Embryo. At the beginning of the 5th week, the bilaminar embryonic disk undergoes gastrulation and is converted into the trilaminar (three germ layer) embryonic disk. It is at this point that organogenesis begins.

Sonographically, the early embryo is usually not identified until heart motion is detected at approximately $5^1/_2$ weeks when the crown-rump length (CRL) is approximately 2 mm. At this stage, the embryo is seen between the secondary yolk sac and the immediate gestational sac wall. Because the amniotic cavity is still relatively small, it appears that no space lies between the yolk sac and embryo (Figure 43-9).

Between the 5th and 6th weeks of gestation, identification of the amniotic membrane may not be possible using transabdominal techniques. Using endovaginal transducers, the amniotic membrane that separates the **amniotic** and **chorionic cavities** is routinely seen after $5^1/_2$ weeks. Although with normal gain settings the chorionic cavity (extraembryonic coelom) may appear sonolucent, increased overall gain settings may fill the fluid with low-level echoes, which correspond to a thicker consistency of the chorionic cavity in relation to the amniotic cavity (Figure 43-10). Later the amniotic cavity expands and the chorionic cavity decreases in size, with eventual chorioamniotic fusion occurring at approximately 16 to 17 weeks.

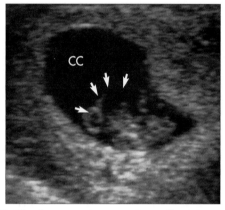

Figure 43-10 Sonogram demonstrating a $7^1/_2$-week gestation with surrounding amniotic membrane *(arrows)*. *Arrows,* Yolk sac; *CC,* chorionic cavity.

General Embryology and Sonographic Appearances: 6 to 12 Weeks. The time between 6 and 12 weeks of gestation is often considered the **embryonic period**. Although controversial, it is generally believed that the fetal period begins after 10 weeks of gestation. A distinct embryologic pattern of development occurs through the embryologic and fetal periods and is outlined in Tables 43-1 and 43-2.

At the beginning of the 6th week of gestation, the trilaminar embryonic disk folds into a C-shaped embryo (Figure 43-11). While embryonic folding continues, the embryonic head, caudal portions, and lateral folds form, resulting in a constriction or narrowing between embryo and yolk sac, creating the **yolk stalk**. While embryonic folding occurs, the dorsal aspect of the yolk sac is incorporated into the embryo, developing the foregut, midgut, and hindgut, and forming the entire gastrointestinal tract, liver, biliary tract, and pancreas. At the same time, the yolk stalk, connecting stalk, and allantois are brought together by the expanding amnion, which acts as an epithelial covering, forming the umbilical cord (Figure 43-12).

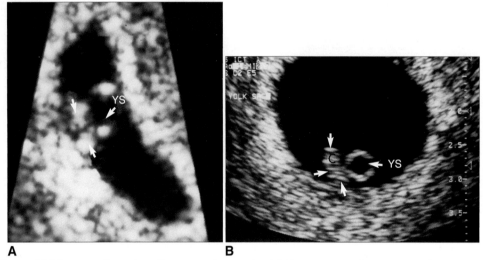

Figure 43-11   **A,** A 5¹/₂-week embryo. Note the straight, disklike appearance *(arrows); YS,* yolk sac. **B,** A 6.2-week gestation is seen at the beginning stages of embryonic "curling." **C,** Embryonic cranium; *YS,* yolk sac.

TABLE 43-2	SEQUENTIAL APPEARANCE OF EMBRYONIC STRUCTURES	
Menstrual Week of Appearance		Structures
4-5		Gestational sac
5		Yolk sac
5.5-6		Fetal heart beat
6		Fetal pole
7		Single ventricle
7.5		Spine
7.5		Lower limbs
8		Upper limbs
9		Falx
9		Body movements
9.2		Limb movements
9.5		Midgut herniation
9.5		Choroid plexus
9.5		Hindbrain
12		Fingers
12		Jaw
12.5		Toes

The limb buds are embryologically recognizable during the 6th week of gestation, as is the embryonic tail, which is not unlike that of a tadpole (Figure 43-13). The spine is also developing during the embryonic period, particularly in the 5th through 7th weeks of gestation. The spine, which develops from ectoderm, initially evolves from the primitive neural tube, which closes about the 6th week of gestation; sonographically parallel echogenic lines can be demonstrated at 7 to 8 weeks of gestation (Figure 43-14).

Throughout the first trimester, the sonographer or sonologist should be able to observe general differences in embryonic appearances. For example, the linear trilaminar disk seen at 5¹/₂ weeks rapidly changes through the 7th week of gestation, when

the cranial neural folds and closure of the neural pore are completed, forming a cranial vault that is recognizable sonographically (Figure 43-15).

The skeletal system begins to develop during the 6th week, with the upper limbs forming first, followed by the lower limbs. The hands and feet develop later in the first trimester and are completely formed by the end of the 10th week of gestation. Sonographically, limb buds can be detected, generally from the 7th week on; the fingers and toes are recognizable at 11 weeks using endovaginal sonography.

The embryonic face undergoes significant evolution starting in the 5th week of gestation, with palate fusion beginning around the 12th week of gestation. Sonographically, the embryonic face cannot presently be seen with diagnostic detail. By the 9th week, the maxilla and mandible are noted as brightly echogenic structures; further bony palate development is often visualized from the 10th week (Figure 43-16).

Physiologic Herniation of Bowel. The anterior abdominal wall is developed by 6 weeks of gestation from the fusion of four ectomesodermal body folds. Simultaneously, the primitive gut is formed as a result of the incorporation of the dorsal yolk sac into the embryo. The midgut, derived from the primitive gut, develops and forms the majority of the small bowel, cecum, ascending colon, and proximal transverse colon. Because the midgut is in direct communication with the yolk sac, amniotic cavity expansion pulls the yolk sac away from the embryo, forming the yolk stalk.

As amniotic expansion occurs, the midgut elongates faster than the embryo is growing, causing the midgut to herniate into the base of the umbilical cord. Until approximately 10 weeks of gestation, the midgut loop continues to grow and rotate before it descends into the fetal abdomen at about the 11th week.

Sonographically, this transition of the bowel within the base of the umbilical cord can readily be visualized. The small bowel

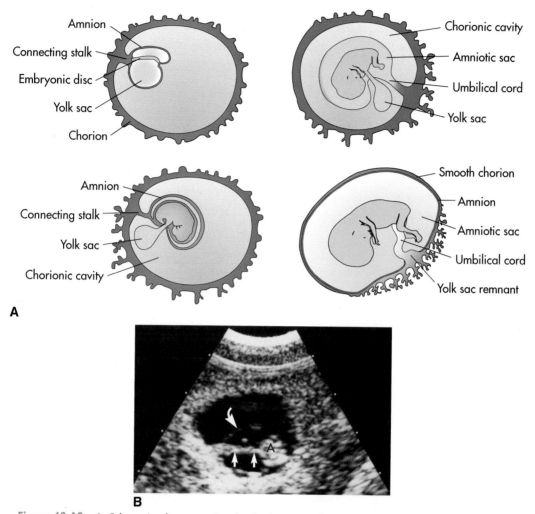

Figure 43-12   **A,** Schematics demonstrating the development of amnion, yolk sac, and embryo. **B,** Sonogram of a transverse axis through the embryonic abdomen at approximately 8 weeks, demonstrating amniotic membrane *(curved arrow)*. *Arrows,* Umbilical cord; *A,* embryonic abdomen.

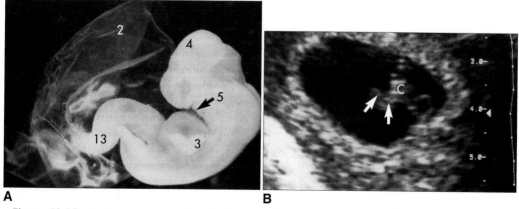

Figure 43-13   **A,** Embryo at approximately 6 weeks of gestation, demonstrating early limb buds *(3)* and embryonic tail *(13)*. *2,* Amnion; *4,* cranium; *5,* heart. (From England MA: *Color atlas of life before birth,* St Louis, 1983, Mosby.) **B,** Corresponding sonogram of a 6-week gestation, demonstrating embryonic tail *(arrows)*. *C,* Embryonic cranium.

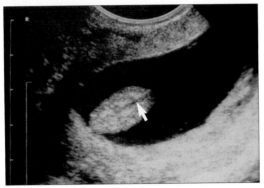

Figure 43-14   Sonogram of an 8-week embryo demonstrating parallel echogenic lines with the sonolucent center representing spine (*arrow*).

appears as an echogenic mass within the base of the umbilical cord; little echogenic bowel is seen within the embryonic or fetal abdomen. After 12 weeks of gestation, the echogenic umbilical cord mass is no longer visualized and echogenic bowel is seen within the fetal abdomen. Recent data suggest that normally the echogenic umbilical cord mass should not exceed 7 mm at any gestational age and never measure less than 4 mm. It is important that this normal embryologic event not be confused with pathologic processes, such as omphalocele or gastroschisis (Figure 43-17).

Embryonic Cranium. Although the embryonic cranium undergoes dramatic changes from the 6th to 11th week of gestation, specific anatomy can be sonographically visualized. Around the 6th week of gestation, three primary brain vesicles develop: the prosencephalon, the mesencephalon, and the rhombencephalon (Figure 43-18). Because of rapid cell prolif-

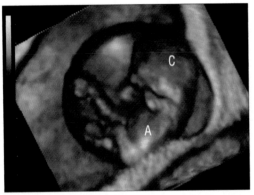

Figure 43-15   Sonogram demonstrating a 7- to 7½-week gestation. Note morphologic distinction between embryonic cranium (*C*) and embryonic abdomen (*A*).

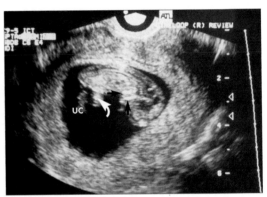

Figure 43-16   Sonogram of a 10-week embryo, demonstrating echogenic structures representing maxilla and mandible (*arrow*). Also note limb bud (*curved arrow*). *UC,* Umbilical cord.

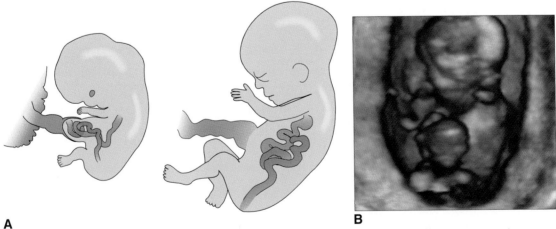

A   **B**

Figure 43-17   A, Schematic demonstrating normal gut migration. The bowel normally migrates into the base of the umbilical cord between 8 and 12 menstrual weeks (6 to 10 embryonic weeks). The bowel returns to the abdominal cavity by 12 menstrual weeks. **B,** Sonogram of a 10-week gestation demonstrating echogenic "mass" at the base of the umbilical cord. Note that there is no echogenic material within embryonic abdomen.

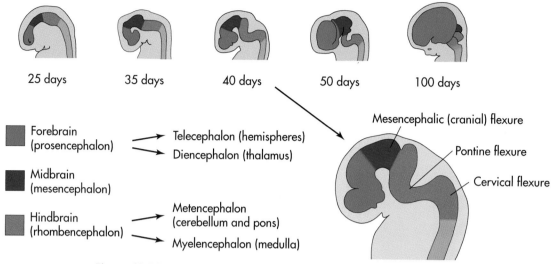

Figure 43-18   Schematic demonstrating embryonic development of the brain.

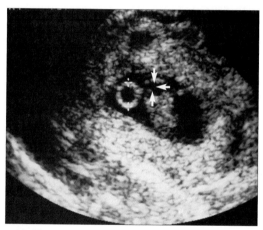

Figure 43-19   Sonogram of an 8½-week gestation demonstrating the cystic rhombencephalon within the fetal cranium *(arrows)*. Note yolk sac between calipers.

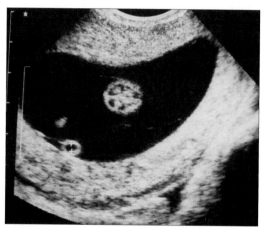

Figure 43-20   Axial plane sonogram of a 10-week embryo demonstrating cerebral falx and choroid plexus. Note the lateral ventricles and choroid plexus occupy the entire cranial vault at this gestational age.

eration in relation to cranial vault space, flexures of the developing brain occur.

The rhombencephalon divides into two segments: the cephalic portion or metencephalon and the caudal component or myelencephalon. Once the rhombencephalon divides with its corresponding flexure, the cystic rhomboid fossa forms. The cystic rhomboid fossa can sonographically be imaged routinely from the 8th to 11th week of gestation (Figure 43-19). With increasing gestational age, further evolution of the cerebellum, medulla, and medulla oblongata encloses the rhomboid fossa to form the primitive fourth ventricle and part of the cerebral aqueduct of Sylvius. This cystic structure, seen within the posterior aspect of the embryonic cranium, should not be confused with pathology, such as Dandy-Walker malformation.

The cerebral hemispheres may be seen at around 9 weeks of gestation. The echogenic choroid plexus, which fills the lateral cerebral ventricles, can be visualized. Sonolucent cere-

bral spinal fluid can be demarcated around the choroid plexus. It is important to note that the lateral ventricles completely fill the cerebral vault at this time in gestation. The cerebral hemispheres are relatively small compared with the rest of the brain, although this relationship rapidly changes at the beginning of the second trimester. The cerebral falx and midline may also be seen in axial views of the embryonic brain (Figure 43-20).

Embryonic Heart. The heart is the first organ to function within the embryo. The embryonic heart starts beating at approximately 35 days (5 to 5½ weeks) when the endocardial heart tubes fuse to form a single heart tube. Complex embryonic evolution occurs so that, by the end of the 8th week of gestation, the heart has obtained its adult configuration.

Embryonic cardiac activity should always be seen by 46 menstrual days. Embryonic cardiac rates vary with gestational

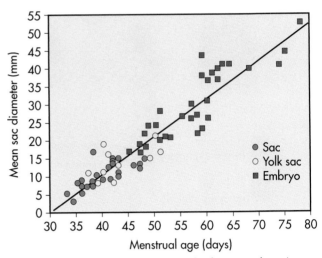

Figure 43-21 Graph correlating growth of gestational sac size, yolk sac size, and embryo length in relation to mean sac diameter and menstrual days. (Redrawn from Hadlock FP, Shah YP, Kanon DJ, Lindsey JV: Fetal crown-rump length: reevaluation of relation to menstrual age (5-18 weeks) with high resolution real time US, *Radiology* 182:501, 1992.)

age. Rates of 90 to 115 beats per minute at 6 weeks increase to rates of 140 to 160 beats per minute at 9 weeks, with rates of approximately 140 beats per minute through the remainder of the late first and second trimesters (Box 43-3).

Although with present technology, detailed morphologic anatomy of the first-trimester heart cannot be seen, further development of high-frequency transducers and ultrasound technology may allow more anatomy to be visualized in the future.

DETERMINATION OF GESTATIONAL AGE

It is widely accepted that the most accurate gestational dating during pregnancy is the use of ultrasound within the first trimester. Two parameters for sonographic gestational dating may be used: (1) crown-rump length (CRL) and (2) gestational sac size.

GESTATIONAL SAC SIZE

Mean gestational sac size correlates closely with menstrual age during early pregnancy (Figure 43-21). As a rule, the gestational sac size remains accurate through the first 8 weeks of gestation. Sonographically, the gestational sac size or mean sac diameter is determined by the average sum of the length, width, and height of the gestational sac. These measurements are obtained in both sagittal and coronal/semicoronal sonographic planes. When measuring the mean sac diameter, the sonographer should only measure gestational sac fluid space, not including the echogenic decidua (Figure 43-22).

To calculate mean sac diameter (MSD), the following formula should be used:

$$\text{Length (mm)} + \text{Width (mm)} + \text{Height (mm)}/3 = \text{MSD}$$

$$\text{MSD (mm)} + 30 = \text{Menstrual age (days)}$$

$$\text{Menstrual age (days) divided by 7} = \text{Menstrual age (weeks)}$$

It is important to note that precise standard deviations for gestational sac size have not been determined, although linear regression analysis demonstrates excellent correlation of mean sac diameter and menstrual age.

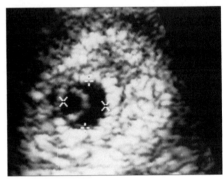

Figure 43-22 Sagittal sonogram of an approximate 6-week gestational sac demonstrating caliper placement for appropriate mean sac diameter measurement. Coronal images would also be taken for a third dimension.

YOLK SAC SIZE

Visualization of the yolk sac predicts a viable pregnancy in more than 90% of cases. Conversely, failure to visualize the yolk sac, with a minimum of 8 mm MSD, using endovaginal sonography, should provoke suspicion of abnormal pregnancy. Transabdominal studies have shown that the yolk sac should be seen within mean sac diameters of 10 to 15 mm and should always be visualized with a mean sac diameter of 20 mm.

The growth rate of the yolk sac has been reported to be approximately 0.1 mm/ml of growth of the MSD when the MSD is less than 15 mm, and 0.03 mm/ml of growth of the MSD through the first trimester. The normal diameter of the yolk sac should never exceed 5.6 mm. Enlarged yolk sacs have ominous outcomes (Figure 43-23).

CROWN-RUMP LENGTH

Determination of first-trimester gestational dates by direct measurement of the embryo using the CRL was first reported

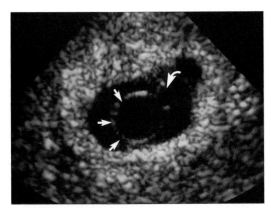

Figure 43-23 Sonogram demonstrating an enlarged yolk sac, measuring approximately 9 mm *(arrows)*. Also note enlarged or hydropic amniotic sac *(curved arrow)*. Although embryonic heart motion was initially detected, follow-up studies diagnosed embryonic demise at $8^1/_2$ weeks gestation.

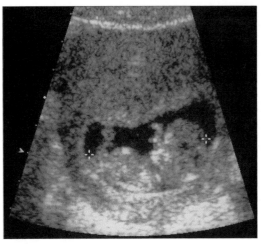

Figure 43-25 Sonogram demonstrating crown-rump length measurement on an 8-week embryo.

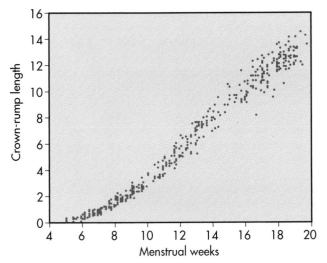

Figure 43-24 Graph demonstrating crown-rump length versus menstrual age. (From Nyberg DA and others: Distinguishing normal from abnormal gestational sac growth in early pregnancy, *J Ultrasound Med* 6:23, 1987.)

in 1975. This produced gestational dating standard deviations of plus or minus 5 to 7 days, by far the most accurate dating parameters within obstetric biometry. Hadlock and others reevaluated CRL data using modern equipment and determined gestational age standard deviation to be plus or minus 8% throughout the first trimester, essentially unchanged from the original data (Figure 43-24).

CRL measurements can be obtained as early as $5^1/_2$ weeks using endovaginal sonography. The main sonographic observation of implementing direct embryonic measurement is the visualization of embryonic heart motion, which is crucial because CRL measurement at this gestational age would be less than 1 mm.

CRLs may be used up to 12 weeks of gestation, when the fetus begins to "curl" into the fetal position, making measurement of length more difficult (Figure 43-25).

MULTIPLE GESTATIONS

The sonographic diagnosis of multiple gestations within the first trimester is valuable information for the obstetrician. A multiple-gestation pregnancy is, by definition, high risk, with significant increases in morbidity and mortality rates in relation to singleton pregnancies. Overall, twin gestations have a 7 to 10 times greater mortality rate than singletons.

Using endovaginal sonography, multiple gestations can readily be diagnosed at very early gestational ages, between $5^1/_2$ and $6^1/_2$ weeks. Sonographic identification of multiple gestational sacs with incorporated yolk sacs, amniotic membranes, and ideally, embryos with cardiac motion allows definitive diagnosis. The literature contains data concerning the identification of chorionicity and amnionicity in twin pregnancies.

Fortunately, dizygotic (two ova) twin pregnancies, which comprise 70% of all twins, are by definition **dichorionic** and **diamniotic**.

Sonographic Findings. Sonographically, dichorionic and diamniotic twins appear as two separate gestational sacs with individual trophoblastic tissue, which allows the appearance of a thick dividing membrane. As pregnancy progresses, this membrane becomes thinner secondary to the diminished space between the two sacs, so this diagnosis may be more difficult later in gestation. In a dichorionic-diamniotic pregnancy, each sac has an individual yolk sac, amniotic membrane, and embryo (Figure 43-26).

Monochorionic-diamniotic twins appear to be contained within one chorionic sac; two amnions, two yolk sacs, and two embryos are identified (Figure 43-27). The most crucial diagnosis for the sonographic observer to make is that of the monozygotic, **monoamniotic-monochorionic** twin gestation. This type of twinning has a mortality rate of approximately 50%. Sonographic visualization would include one gestational sac with one amniotic membrane, containing one or two yolk sacs and two embryos within the single amniotic membrane (Figure 43-28).

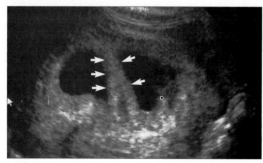

Figure 43-26 Sonogram demonstrating a diamniotic-dichorionic pregnancy. Note the thick membrane separating the two gestational sacs *(arrows)*.

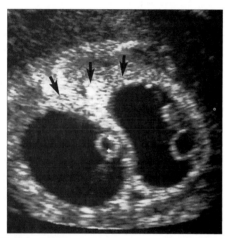

Figure 43-27 Sonogram demonstrating early monochorionic-diamniotic pregnancy. Note two yolk sacs and two embryos with single chorion-placenta *(arrows)*.

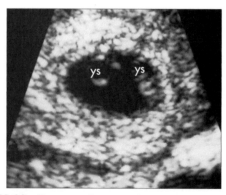

Figure 43-28 Sonogram demonstrating monoamniotic monochorionic pregnancy. Note two yolk sacs *(ys)* with no separating amniotic membrane.

SELECTED BIBLIOGRAPHY

Bateman BG, Nunley WC, Kolp LA and others: Vaginal sonography findings and hCG dynamics of early intrauterine and tubal pregnancies, *Obstet Gynecol* 75:421, 1990.

Bohm-Velez M, Mendelson EB: Endovaginal sonography: applications, equipment and technique. In Nyberg DA, Hill LM, Bohm-

Velez M and others, editors: *Endovaginal ultrasound,* St Louis, 1992, Mosby.

Bowerman RA: Sonography of fetal midgut herniation: normal size criteria and correlation with crown-rump length, *J Ultrasound Med* 5:251, 1993.

Bromley B, Harlow BL, Laboda LA: Small sac size in the first trimester: a predictor of poor fetal outcome, *Radiology* 178:375, 1991.

Callen P: *Ultrasonography in obstetrics and gynecology,* ed 4, Philadelphia, 2000, WB Saunders Co.

Cyr DR, Mack LA, Nyberg DA and others: Fetal rhombencephalon: normal ultrasound findings, *Radiology* 166:691, 1988.

Cyr DR, Mack LA, Schoenecker SA and others: Bowel migration in the normal fetus: US detection, *Radiology* 1986:161, 1986.

Dubose TJ, Cunyus JA, Johnson LF: Embryonic heart rate and age, *J Diag Med Sonogr* 6:151, 1990.

Ectopic pregnancy/United States, 1987, *MMWR* 1990:401-404, 1990.

England MA: *Color atlas of life before birth/normal fetal development,* Chicago, 1983, Mosby.

Frates MC, Benson CB, Doubilet PM: Pregnancy outcome after first trimester sonogram demonstrating fetal cardiac activity, *J Ultrasound Med* 12:383, 1993.

Hadlock FP, Shah YP, Kanon DJ, Lindsay JV: Fetal crown-rump length: reevaluation of relation to menstrual age (5-18 weeks) with high resolution real time US, *Radiology* 182:501, 1992.

Hertzberg BS, Bowie JD, Carroll BS and others: Normal sonographic appearance of the fetal neck late in the first trimester: the pseudomembrane, *Radiology* 171:427, 1989.

Hertzberg BS, Mahony BS, Bowie JD: First trimester fetal cardiac activity: sonographic documentation of a progressive early rise in heart rate, *J Ultrasound Med* 7:573, 1988.

Kurjak A, Zalud I: Doppler and color flow imaging. In Nyberg DA, Hill LM, Bohm-Velez M, and others, editors: *Endovaginal ultrasound,* St Louis, 1992, Mosby.

Laboda LA, Estroff JA, Benaceraff BR: First trimester bradycardia: a sign of impending fetal loss, *J Ultrasound Med* 8:561, 1989.

Lemire RJ, Loeser JD, Leech RW and others: *Normal and abnormal development of the human nervous system,* Hagerstown, MD, 1975, Harper & Row.

Levi CS: Sonographic evaluation of multiple gestation pregnancy. In Fleischer AC, editor: *Principles and practices of ultrasonography,* East Norwalk, CT, 1991, Appleton & Lange.

Lindsay DJ, Lovett IS, Lyons EA and others: Yolk sac diameter and shape at endovaginal ultrasound: predictors of pregnancy outcome in the first trimester, *Radiology* 183:115, 1992.

Lyons EA, Levi CS, Dashefsky SM: The first trimester. In Rumack CM and others, editors: *Diagnostic ultrasound,* ed 2, St Louis, 1998, Mosby.

Moore KL: *The developing human: clinically oriented embryology,* ed 4, Philadelphia, 1988, WB Saunders.

Neiman HL: Sonoembryology. In Nyberg DA, Hill LM, Bohm-Velez M and others, editors: *Endovaginal ultrasound,* Philadelphia, 1992, Mosby.

Nyberg DA, Filly RA, Mahony BS and others: Early gestation: correlation of hCG levels and sonographic identification, *Am J Roentgenol* 144:951, 1985.

Nyberg DA, Hill LM: Normal early intrauterine pregnancy: sonographic development and hCG correlation. In Nyberg DA, Hill LM, Bohm-Velez M and others, editors: *Endovaginal ultrasound,* St Louis, 1992, Mosby.

Nyberg DA, Mack LA, Harvey D and others: Value of the yolk sac in evaluating early pregnancies, *J Ultrasound Med* 7:129, 1988.

Nyberg DA, McGahan JP, Pretorius DH and others: *Diagnostic imaging of fetal anomalies,* Lippincott Williams & Wilkins, 2003, Philadelphia.

Peisner DB, Timor-Tritsch IE: The discriminatory zone of beta-hCG for vaginal probes, *J Clin Ultrasound* 18:280, 1990.

Rempen A: Diagnosis of viability in early pregnancy with vaginal sonography, *J Ultrasound Med* 9:711, 1990.

Rizk B, Tan SL, Morcos S and others: Heterotopic pregnancies after in vitro fertilization and embryo transfer, *Am J Obstet Gynecol* 164:161, 1991.

Robinson HP: "Gestational sac" volumes as a journal by sonar in the first trimester of pregnancy, *Br J Obstet Gynecol* 82:100, 1975.

Sadler TW: *Langman's medical embryology,* ed 5, Baltimore, 1985, Williams & Wilkins.

Schats R, Jansen CAM, Wladimiroff JW and others: Embryonic heart activity: appearance and development in early human pregnancy, *Br J Obstet Gynecol* 97:989, 1990.

Shenker L, Astle C, Reed K and others: Embryonic heart rates before the seventh week of pregnancy, *J Reprod Med* 31:333, 1986.

Timor-Tritsch IE, Farine D, Rosen MG: A close look at early embryonic development with high-frequency transvaginal transducer, *Am J Obstet Gynecol* 159:676, 1988.

Townsend R: Membrane thickness in ultrasound prediction of chorionicity of twins, *J Ultrasound Med* 7:327, 1988.

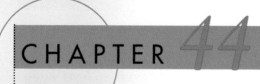

CHAPTER 44

First-Trimester Complications

Sandra L. Hagen-Ansert

KEY TERMS

acrania – partial or complete absence of the cranium

anembryonic pregnancy (blighted ovum) – ovum without an embryo

anencephaly – congenital absence of the brain and cranial vault with the cerebral hemispheres missing or reduced to small masses

bowel herniation – during the first trimester the bowel normally herniates outside the abdominal cavity between 8 and 12 weeks

cephalocele – protrusion of the brain from the cranial cavity

complete abortion – complete removal of all products of conception, including the placenta

corpus luteum cyst – a physiologic cyst that develops within the ovary after ovulation and secretes progesterone and prevents menses if fertilization occurs; may persist until the 16th to 18th week of pregnancy

cystic hygroma – fluid-filled structure (often with septations), initially surrounding the neck, may extend upward to the head or laterally to the body

ectopic pregnancy – pregnancy outside the uterus

gastroschisis – congenital fissure that remains open in the wall of the abdomen just to the right of the umbilical cord;

bowel and other organs may protrude outside the abdomen from this opening

gestational trophoblastic disease – condition in which trophoblastic tissue overtakes the pregnancy and propagates throughout the uterine cavity

heterotopic pregnancy – simultaneous intrauterine and extrauterine pregnancy

holoprosencephaly – failure of forebrain to divide into cerebral hemispheres, which results in a single large ventricle with varying amounts of cerebral cortex that has been known to occur with trisomies 13 to 15 and trisomy 18

incomplete abortion – retained products of conception

iniencephaly – a congenitally deformed fetus in which the brain substance protrudes through a fissure in the occiput, so that the brain and spinal cord occupy a single cavity

interstitial pregnancy – pregnancy occurring in the fallopian tube near the cornu of the uterus; also known as cornual pregnancy

omphalocele – congenital hernia of the umbilicus that is covered with a membrane; the cord may be seen in the middle of the mass

pseudogestational sac – decidual reaction that occurs within the uterus in a patient with an ectopic pregnancy

Turner's syndrome – a nonlethal genetic abnormality in which chromosomal makeup is 45 XO instead of the normal 46 XX or XY. Cystic hygroma often is seen in affected fetuses in the first trimester. Survivors tend to be short in stature with low-set ears, webbing of the neck, shield-shaped chest, and infertility as a result of an endocrine disorder caused by failure of the ovaries to respond to pituitary hormone.

ventriculomegaly – dilation of the ventricular system without enlargement of the cranium

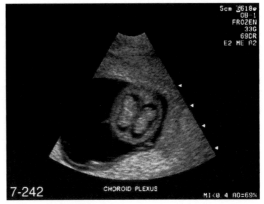

Figure 44-1   Endovaginal axial scan of the choroid plexus in a first-trimester fetus.

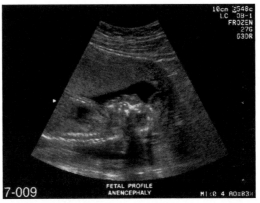

Figure 44-2   Fetal profile of an anencephalic fetus in the second trimester. The fetus is lying in a vertex position with the spine down. The face is pointing toward the anterior placenta; the skull is absent from the fetal forehead to the top of the cranium.

DIAGNOSIS OF EMBRYONIC ABNORMALITIES IN THE FIRST TRIMESTER

Normal embryologic processes that are sonographically visible in the first-trimester embryo have been described in Chapter 43. These normal processes should not be mistaken for anomalies, and the sonographer should be aware of the pathology that can be diagnosed in the first trimester. Many of the abnormalities are seen at the end of the first trimester, but are more clearly identified as the fetus matures into the second trimester. Other less common abnormalities, such as ectopia cordis, malformations of the skeleton, and complications of multifetal pregnancies, will be discussed in their respective chapters.

CRANIAL ANOMALIES

Although the embryonic head can be sonographically identified by 7 weeks, the cerebral hemisphere continues to evolve through the second trimester. The dominant structure seen within the embryonic cranium in the first trimester is that of the choroid plexus, which fills the lateral ventricles that in turn fill the cranial vault (Figure 44-1). Thus the diagnosis of hydro-

cephalus in the first trimester is impossible. However, anomalies of cranial organization, such as holoprosencephaly, have been described in the first trimester. The rhombencephalon-hindbrain is a cystic structure within the posterior aspect of the embryonic cranium that should not be confused with an abnormality. A diagnosis of hydranencephaly, which is brain necrosis from occlusion of the internal carotid arteries, has been reported during the first trimester that sonographically demonstrated loss of all intracranial anatomy. In the first trimester, anencephaly should be diagnosed with caution. Reports have shown normal amounts of brain matter seen in the first-trimester embryo with anencephaly, unlike classic sonographic appearances in the second and third trimesters (Figure 44-2). Ossification of the cranial vault is not complete in the first trimester; the resulting false cranial border definition may give rise to a false-negative diagnosis.

Extreme caution is advised if an embryonic cranial abnormality is suspected (Table 44-1). Because traditional cranial anatomy can be visualized after 12 to 14 weeks of gestation, the sonogram should be repeated at this time to either confirm or rule out abnormality.

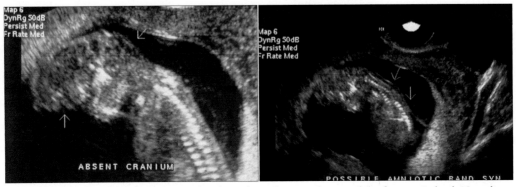

Figure 44-3 Acrania. Patient presented with an elevated maternal serum alpha-fetoprotein level. Note the amnion *(arrows)* along the back of the fetus. The amniotic band syndrome was the probable cause for acrania in this fetus.

TABLE 44-1	CRANIAL ANOMALIES IN THE FIRST TRIMESTER
Anomaly	**Sonographic Findings**
Acrania	– Abnormal mineralization of bony structures (lack of echogenicity) – Abnormally shaped "Mickey Mouse" head
Anencephaly	– Absence of cranium superior to orbits with preservation of base of skull and face – Brain may project from open cranium
Cephalocele	– Midline cranial defect – Herniation of brain and meninges
Iniencephaly	– Defect in occiput involving the foramen magnum – Extreme retroflexion of spine – Open spinal defect
Ventriculomegaly	– Dilation of ventricular system without enlargement of the cranium – Compression of choroid plexus – Increased cerebrospinal fluid – Dangling choroid in dilated lateral ventricle
Holoprosencephaly	– Failure of prosencephalon to differentiate into cerebral hemispheres and lateral ventricles between 4th and 8th weeks – Complete to partial failure of cleavage of prosencephalon – Facial dysmorphism – Remember, before 9 weeks, brain appears to be single ventricle until falx cerebri develops after 9 weeks
Dandy-Walker malformation	– 6th-7th week of gestation – Cystic dilation of 4th ventricle – Dysgenesis or agenesis of cerebellar vermis and hydrocephaly – Elevated tentorium

Acrania. **Acrania** is the partial or complete absence of the cranium. It is thought to be the predecessor of anencephaly. The ossification of the cranium begins after 9 weeks. Sonography is able to demonstrate abnormal mineralization of the bony structures: well-mineralized bone is very echogenic and easily imaged with sonography. Acrania has been reported as

early as the 12th week of gestation. When this abnormality occurs, the fetus has an abnormally shaped head, referred to as a "Mickey Mouse" head (Figure 44-3).

Anencephaly. **Anencephaly** is the congenital absence of the brain and cranial vault, with the cerebral hemispheres either missing or reduced to small masses. This abnormality may be seen near the end of the first trimester when there is an absence of the cranium superior to the orbits with preservation of the base of the skull and facial features. The brain may be seen as it projects from the open cranial vault.

Cephalocele. A **cephalocele** is a midline cranial defect in which there is herniation of the brain and meninges. The cephalocele may also involve the occipital, frontal, parietal, orbital, nasal, or nasopharyngeal region of the head. The prevalence of the lesion is geographical. In the Western Hemisphere the defect is primarily occipital, whereas in the Eastern Hemisphere the frontal defect is more common.

Iniencephaly. **Iniencephaly** is a rare, lethal anomaly of the cranial development whose primary abnormalities include (1) a defect in the occiput involving the foramen magnum, (2) retroflexion of the spine where the fetus looks upward with its occipital cranium directed toward the lumbar spine, and (3) open spinal defects.

Ventriculomegaly. **Ventriculomegaly**, or dilation of the ventricular system without enlargement of the cranium, may be seen near the end of the first trimester. The normal lateral ventricle is quite prominent in the first trimester. Look for compression and thinning of the choroid plexus as the increased cerebrospinal fluid accumulates in the ventricular system. The choroid plexus is shown to be "dangling" in the dilated dependent lateral ventricle (Figure 44-4).

Holoprosencephaly. **Holoprosencephaly** is a malformation sequence that results from failure of the prosencephalon to differentiate into cerebral hemispheres and lateral ventricles between the fourth and eighth gestational weeks. The anomaly

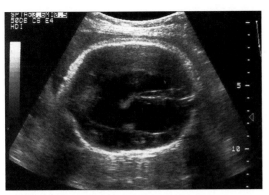

Figure 44-4 Ventriculomegaly caused by spina bifida. The near field, lateral ventricles choroid plexus "dangles" into the far field dilated ventricle.

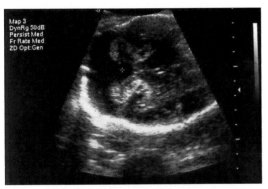

Figure 44-5 Dandy-Walker cyst. Note the splayed cerebellar hemispheres. (Courtesy Ginny Goreczky, Maternal Fetal Center, Florida Hospital, Orlando, Fla.)

ranges from complete to partial failure of cleavage of the prosencephalon with variable degrees of facial dysmorphism. Holoprosencephaly is divided into three types: alobar, semilobar, and lobar. Alobar is the most serious and consists of a single ventricle, small cerebrum, fused thalami, agenesis of the corpus callosum, and falx cerebri. It is important to remember that before 9 weeks, the normal fetal brain appears to have a "single" ventricle until the falx cerebri develops after 9 weeks.

Dandy-Walker Malformation. This malformation results from a cystic dilation of the fourth ventricle with dysgenesis or complete agenesis of the cerebellar vermis and frequently hydrocephaly. The abnormality occurs around the 6th to 7th week of gestation. Sonographically, a large posterior fossa cyst that is continuous with the fourth ventricle, an elevated tentorium, and dilated third and lateral ventricles may be seen (Figure 44-5).

Spina Bifida. Spina bifida may be detected at the end of the first trimester appearing as spinal irregularities or a bulging within the posterior contour of the fetal spine.

ABDOMINAL WALL DEFECTS
Although the diagnoses of omphalocele, gastroschisis, and limb-body wall complex have been reported in the first trimester, such diagnoses should be made with care.

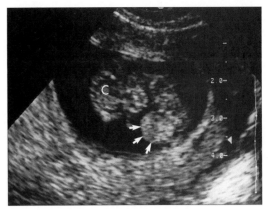

Figure 44-6 Sonogram of a 9-week gestation demonstrating herniated liver contents into the base of the umbilical cord *(arrows)*, consistent with first-trimester omphalocele. This was confirmed at 14 weeks' gestation. *C*, Embryonic cranium.

Abdominal wall defects must be distinguished from normal physiologic midgut herniation. As stated previously, normal **bowel herniation** appears sonographically as an echogenic mass at the base of the umbilical cord between 8 and 12 weeks. Because the liver is never herniated into the base of the umbilical cord, normally, any evidence of the liver outside the anterior abdominal wall should be considered abnormal (Figure 44-6). Although the diagnosis of **gastroschisis** in the first trimester may be more difficult, reports have shown the bowel to be separate and eviscerated from the umbilical cord and its attachment to the fetus. The bowel-only **omphaloceles** that have been reported to be highly associated with chromosomal abnormalities cannot be differentiated from normal physiologic bowel migration and should be diagnosed after 12 to 14 weeks.

OBSTRUCTIVE UROPATHY
The fetal urinary bladder becomes sonographically apparent at 10 to 12 weeks of gestation. Obstructive uropathy, especially when it occurs at the level of the urethra, results in a very large urinary bladder and is well imaged with sonography. The bladder may be so large as to extend out of the pelvis into the fetal abdomen and may present as a cystic mass. Bladder outlet obstruction has been diagnosed at the end of the first trimester.

CYSTIC HYGROMA
Cystic hygroma is one of the most common abnormalities seen sonographically in the first trimester (Figure 44-7). Cystic hygromas, especially those seen in the first trimester, are highly associated with chromosomal abnormalities. In fetuses detected with cystic hygroma in the second and third trimesters, **Turner's syndrome** is the most common karyotype abnormality. However, in fetuses with cystic hygroma in the first trimester, trisomies 21, 18, and 13 were most prevalent. If the hygroma resolves by 18 weeks, most fetuses are chromosomally normal, whereas all persistent hygromas are karyotypically abnormal. If cystic hygroma or nuchal thickening is

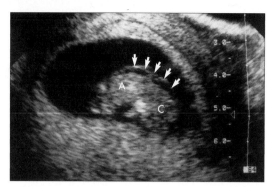

Figure 44-7 A 9-week embryo demonstrating sonolucent cystic hygroma with nuchal thickening *(arrows)*. Genetic analysis demonstrated trisomy 18. *A*, Embryonic abdomen; *C*, embryonic cranium.

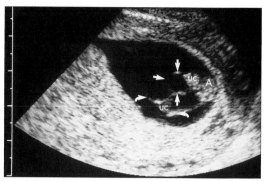

Figure 44-9 An 8.5-week gestation demonstrating umbilical cord cyst *(arrows)*. This cyst resolved by 14 weeks' gestation and went on to normal delivery. *A*, Embryonic abdomen; *UC*, umbilical cord; *curved arrows*, amniotic membrane.

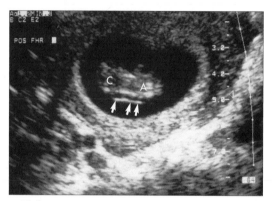

Figure 44-8 A 9-week embryo demonstrating the "hammocking" effect of the embryo lying on top of the amniotic membrane *(arrows)*. This may give a false impression of cystic hygroma/nuchal thickening. *A*, Embryonic abdomen; *C*, embryonic cranium.

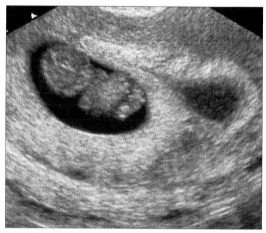

Figure 44-10 Endovaginal scan of a 10-week pregnancy; the gestational sac and embryo are clearly visible. The placenta is anterior; the prominent hypoechoic area visible between the gestational sac and the placenta represents a subchorionic hemorrhage.

seen in the first trimester, genetic counseling and further sonographic monitoring are required.

Cystic hygromas visualized in the first trimester may vary in size, but all appear on the posterior aspect of the fetal neck and upper thorax. Soft tissue thickening may also be present and should be considered as nuchal thickening. Although cystic hygroma and nuchal thickening may be concordant, differentiation may be difficult. A potential diagnostic pitfall for the sonographer is misinterpreting the hypoechoic or sonolucent embryonic skin surface in the region of the posterior neck. This has been described as the pseudomembrane sign and should not be confused with cystic hygroma, encephalocele, cervical meningomyelocele, teratoma, or hemangioma. Caution should also be observed in differentiating the pseudomembrane from the normal amniotic membrane on which the embryo is lying (Figure 44-8).

FIRST-TRIMESTER UMBILICAL CORD CYSTS

Sonographic identification of first-trimester umbilical cord cysts has been reported. One study found a 0.4% incidence of umbilical cord cysts between 8 and 12 weeks of gestation.[10] Cyst size varied with a range of 2.0 to 7.5 mm, and embryos

whose cysts resolved by the second trimester progressed to normal delivery. Differential considerations of umbilical cord cysts include (1) amniotic inclusion cysts, (2) omphalomesenteric duct cysts, (3) allantoic cysts, (4) vascular anomalies, (5) neoplasms, and (6) Wharton's jelly abnormalities. Umbilical cord cysts that persist through the second trimester or are associated with other abnormalities warrant further investigation and genetic evaluation (Figure 44-9).

PLACENTAL HEMATOMAS AND SUBCHORIONIC HEMORRHAGE

The embryonic placenta, or frondosum, may become detached, resulting in the formation of a hematoma, which typically causes vaginal bleeding (Figure 44-10). Most of these hemorrhages are contiguous with a placental edge, which is consistent with the second- or third-trimester placental marginal abruption. Although no risk factors have been associated with first-trimester placental separation, it has been reported to have a 50% or greater fetal loss rate.[7] Although the prog-

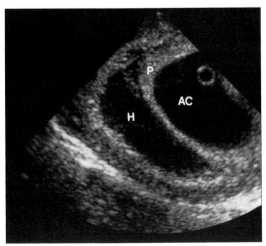

Figure 44-11   An 8-week gestation demonstrating subchorionic hematoma *(H)*. This embryo went on to normal delivery. *AC,* Amniotic cavity; *P,* edge of placenta.

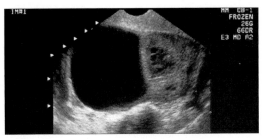

Figure 44-12   Endovaginal scan of the adnexal area in a patient in her first trimester shows a large corpus luteum cyst with internal septations and debris.

nosis seems to depend on the size of the hematoma, no specific volumes have been correlated in the first trimester with fetal outcomes. Improved outcomes do seem to be consistent with smaller hematomas (Figure 44-11).[7]

Sonographically, placental hematomas may be difficult to distinguish from subchorionic hemorrhages. The placental hematomas do not cause symptoms, bleeding, or spotting because they are within the chorionic sac without communication with the endometrium.

FIRST-TRIMESTER PELVIC MASSES

OVARIAN MASSES

The **corpus luteum cyst** is by far the most common ovarian mass seen in the first trimester of pregnancy. Corpeus luteum cysts secrete progesterone necessary to preserve the embryo. The corpus luteum cyst typically measures less than 5 cm in diameter and does not contain septations. Occasionally, corpus luteum cysts are large, reaching sizes of more than 10 cm, with internal septations and echogenic debris, which are thought to be secondary to internal hemorrhage (Figure 44-12). Because of high metabolic activity, color flow imaging may demonstrate a ring of increased vascularity surrounding the corpus luteum, displaying low-resistance (high-diastolic) waveforms on pulsed Doppler imaging. Such findings are similar to decidual flows characterized in ectopic pregnancies, but are intraovarian in location (Table 44-2).

A hemorrhagic corpus luteum cyst cannot be differentiated from other pathologic cysts, such as ovarian cancer or dermoid (Figure 44-13). As the pregnancy progresses, corpus luteum cysts regress and are typically not seen beyond 16 to 18 weeks of gestation. If ovarian cystic masses persist beyond 18 weeks of gestation or increase in size, surgical removal is often required because benign and malignant processes cannot be distinguished using sonography. A high incidence of torsion of ovarian masses during the second and third trimesters has been

TABLE 44-2	FIRST-TRIMESTER PELVIC MASS	
Condition	Sonographic Findings	Differential Considerations
Corpus luteum cyst	> 5 cm in size – Internal septations and debris (secondary to hemorrhage) – Increased vascularity surrounding corpus luteum	– Dermoid – Ovarian cancer
Uterine leiomyoma	– Increased hormones stimulate growth – May compress gestational sac – Various sonographic patterns: hypoechoic, echogenic, isoechoic when compared with myometrium – Increased size causes uterine endometrial deformity	– Uterine contractions – Dermoid

reported.[10] All persistent ovarian masses in pregnancy should be followed closely.

UTERINE MASSES

Uterine leiomyomas or fibroids are common throughout pregnancy. If fibroids coexist with a first-trimester pregnancy, the fibroid should be identified in relation to the placenta. Fibroids may increase in size throughout the first trimester and early second trimester because of estrogen stimulation. A rapid increase in fibroid size may lead to necrosis of the leiomyoma, giving rise to significant maternal symptoms that may require myomectomy. Rapidly growing fibroids may compress the gestational sac, causing spontaneous abortion (Figure 44-14).

Sonographically, fibroids may be hypoechoic, echogenic, or isoechoic in relation to myometrium. They typically cause deformity or displacement of the uterus, endometrium, or both. Fibroids are high-acoustic attenuators, which give rise to poor acoustic transmission (Figure 44-15). It may be difficult to differentiate fibroid from focal uterine contraction, although preliminary data suggest that color Doppler imaging shows a more hypovascular appearance with uterine contractions than with fibroids. Fibroids may also be differentiated from focal myometrial contractions by observing the focal lesion over

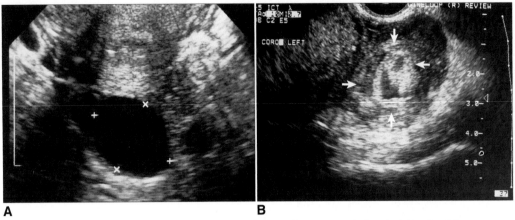

A   **B**

Figure 44-13   A, Sonogram demonstrating a typical corpus luteum cyst *(calipers)* within the right ovary in an 8-week gestation. Sonographic characteristics of this cyst are simple, which is typical. **B,** Sonographic example of hemorrhagic corpus luteum cyst *(arrows).* This may be difficult to differentiate from hematosalpinx, distal tubal ectopic pregnancy, ovarian ectopic pregnancy, or ovarian neoplasms.

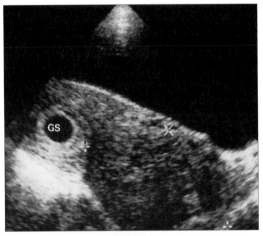

Figure 44-14   Sagittal sonogram demonstrating an 8-cm fibroid/leiomyoma *(calipers)* coexisting with a 6-week gestational sac *(GS).* This fibroid continued to grow, compressing this young gestation and causing demise.

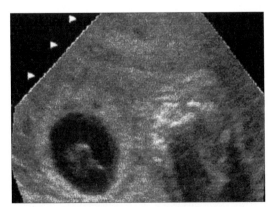

Figure 44-15   Endovaginal 3-D scan of an early pregnancy that shows the gestational sac on the left of the image with the echogenic fibroid (with shadowing) to the right.

time (typically 20 to 30 minutes); the myometrial contraction should disappear, whereas a fibroid would still be present (see Table 44-2).

ECTOPIC PREGNANCY

Ectopic pregnancy is one of the most emergent diagnoses made with ultrasound. An ectopic pregnancy is the location of the pregnancy outside the normal location of the uterus. Approximately 10% of maternal deaths are related to ectopic pregnancy. The occurrence of ectopic pregnancy also has an effect on the future fertility of a patient and increases the risk of a repeat ectopic pregnancy. The incidence of ectopic pregnancy has increased in recent years. Associated risk factors include previous pelvic infections, use of intrauterine contraceptive devices (IUCDs), fallopian tube surgeries, infertility treatments, and a history of ectopic pregnancy.

Clinical findings are nonspecific and may vary. Pelvic pain has been reported in 97% of patients, although pain may be consistent with other pathologic processes, such as appendicitis or pelvic inflammatory disease. Other clinical findings associated with ectopic pregnancy are vaginal bleeding and a palpable adnexal mass. These clinical findings are found in nearly 45% of patients.

Pathologically, ectopic pregnancy is diagnosed by the invasion of trophoblastic tissue within the fallopian tube mucosa. This causes the bleeding often associated with ectopic pregnancy, which may cause hematosalpinx, hemoperitoneum, or both.

Ectopic pregnancy occurs within the fallopian tube in approximately 95% of cases. Other sites, such as the ovary, broad ligament, peritoneum, and cervix, account for the remaining cases (Figure 44-16). When an ectopic pregnancy is found in the interstitial portion of the fallopian tube near the uterine cornu, there is increased risk for massive hemorrhage with rupture that may lead to a hysterectomy or even death.

Correlating clinical findings with sonographic findings in ectopic pregnancy is imperative for diagnosis. Specific assays for human chorionic gonadotropin (hCG) allow the sonographer/sonologist to have expectations of sonographic findings. The beta subunit of human chorionic gonadotropin (beta-hCG) is quantified from maternal blood by two preparations: the First International Reference Preparation (1st IRP) or the Second International Standard (2IS). It is crucial that the sonographer understand which hCG assay a particular institution or laboratory is using. Quantification of hCG is directly correlated with gestational age throughout the first trimester. Generally the 1st IRP has hCG quantities double those of the 2IS.

Given the complexities of hCG testing, it is vital that the sonographer have a good understanding of the discriminatory level of hCG and sonographic findings. Simply put, the discriminatory level of hCG in pregnancy should be thought of as a minimum level of hCG in normal intrauterine or ectopic pregnancy. Using endovaginal techniques, the hCG discriminatory level in detecting an intrauterine pregnancy has been shown to be 800 to 1000 IU/L based on the 2IS and 1000 to 2000 IU/L based on the 1st IRP.

If discriminatory levels of beta-hCG are met or surpassed and no intrauterine gestational sac is seen, an ectopic pregnancy should be suspected. Caution should be taken if beta-hCG levels are below discriminatory levels. Ectopic gestations do not produce hCG at normal levels (hCG levels double every other day) and 90% of ectopic gestations are not viable, and so may not reflect typical correlation between gestational age and hCG levels. Ectopic pregnancy may have a similar appearance to an early intrauterine pregnancy. Thus in nonemergent cases, serial beta-hCG levels are preferred because trending of these levels would demonstrate a continuing pregnancy if hCG levels rise normally or slowly or plateau, whereas falling hCG levels may indicate missed or incomplete abortion.

SONOGRAPHIC FINDINGS IN ECTOPIC PREGNANCY

The sonographic appearances of ectopic pregnancy have been well documented with both transabdominal and endovaginal techniques (Figure 44-17). The most important finding when scanning for ectopic pregnancy is to determine if there is a normal intrauterine gestation (reducing the probability of an ectopic pregnancy) or if the uterine cavity is empty and an adnexal mass is present (Table 44-3). Again the expectation of visualizing a normal intrauterine gestation is directly correlated to beta-hCG levels. Although the visualization of an intrauterine gestational sac that includes embryonic heart motion firmly makes the diagnosis of intrauterine pregnancy, earlier gestations (5 to 6 weeks) normally may not demonstrate these findings. As many as 20% of patients with ectopic pregnancy demonstrate an intrauterine saclike structure known as the **pseudogestational sac.**

Although difficult, differentiating between normal early gestation and pseudogestational sac often is possible (Figure

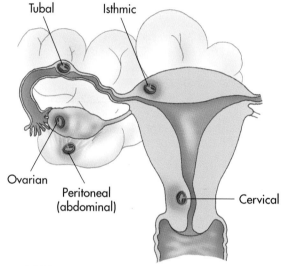

Figure 44-16 Schematic demonstrating sites of ectopic pregnancy.

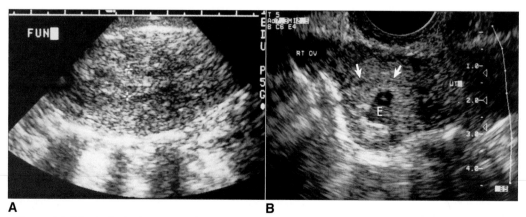

Figure 44-17 **A,** Sagittal sonogram demonstrating an empty uterus with normal endometrial canal *(calipers).* **B,** Coronal sonogram demonstrating uterus *(UT)* and right ovary *(RT OV),* with an echogenic concentric ring and embryo seen centrally with fetal heart motion. Consistent with ectopic pregnancy. *Arrows,* Decidua/trophoblastic villi; *E,* embryo.

TABLE 44-3 | NORMAL VERSUS ECTOPIC PREGNANCY

Condition/Sonographic Findings	Differential Considerations
Empty uterus	– Normal early intrauterine pregnancy (3 to 4 weeks) – Recent spontaneous abortion
Normal intrauterine pregnancy – Yolk sac present – Burrowed gestational sac eccentrically positioned in uterus (usually in the fundus) – No internal echoes seen within the gestational sac – Peritrophoblastic flow around sac – Low-resistive flow pattern	
Ectopic pregnancy with pseudogestational sac – "Intrauterine" saclike structure – Yolk sac not present – Pseudosac seen in central location in uterus – Homogeneous echoes within pseudosac – No peritrophoblastic flow – High resistive pattern	– Intrauterine debris – Incomplete spontaneous abortion – Intrauterine blood
Ectopic pregnancy – Pseudogestational sac – Extrauterine sac in adnexa with thickened echogenic ring – Gestational sac or yolk sac	– Incomplete spontaneous abortion – Intrauterine blood or fluid in cul-de-sac
Heterotopic pregnancy – Simultaneous intrauterine pregnancy and ectopic pregnancy (see findings above for IUP and ectopic pregnancy)	– Normal IUP and pelvic mass
Interstitial pregnancy – Found in segment of fallopian tube – Rupture with hemorrhage – Eccentric intrauterine gestational sac with incomplete myometrial mantel surrounding sac	– Ectopic pregnancy – Pelvic mass
Nonviable intrauterine pregnancy – Pseudogestational sac of ectopic pregnancy	– Embryo, no cardiac motion/nonliving intrauterine pregnancy – Embryo, cardiac motion/living intrauterine pregnancy

44-18). The following guidelines may be helpful: (1) pseudogestational sacs do not contain either a living embryo or yolk sac; (2) pseudogestational sacs are centrally located within the endometrial cavity, unlike the burrowed gestational sac, which is eccentrically placed; (3) homogeneous level echoes are commonly observed in pseudogestational sacs, unlike normal gestational sacs. These findings are most commonly observed using endovaginal techniques.

Color Doppler imaging and spectral analysis may also be helpful in distinguishing normal from pseudogestational sac with the demonstration of peritrophoblastic flow associated with intrauterine pregnancy. Typically, peritrophoblastic flow demonstrates a low-resistance (high-diastolic) pattern, with fairly high peak velocities (approximately 20 cm/sec). The decidual cast of the endometrium, as seen in pseudogestational sac, typically demonstrates a high-resistance pattern (low-diastolic component) with low peak velocities.

The adnexa should always be sonographically examined when evaluating for ectopic pregnancy. The identification of a live embryo within the adnexa is the most specific for ectopic gestation. Unfortunately, this occurs roughly only 25% of the time. It is important to note that only approximately 10% of

live ectopic pregnancies are identified using transabdominal sonography (Figure 44-19).

The identification of an extrauterine sac within the adnexa is one of the most frequent findings of ectopic pregnancy. It has been reported that more than 71% of patients with ectopic pregnancy demonstrate an extrauterine sac or ring, although this study did include living extrauterine ectopic fetuses.[3] The extrauterine gestational sac has sonographic appearances and characteristics similar to the intrauterine gestational sac. Extrauterine gestational sacs often demonstrate a thickened echogenic ring, separate from the ovary, which represents trophoblastic tissue or chorionic villi; there is a possibility that the embryo or yolk sac will be seen (Figure 44-20).

Color flow imaging and Doppler waveforms may also help diagnose extrauterine gestational sacs. One study reported color flow detection in and around 95 of 106 ectopic gestations with a Doppler resistive index of less than 0.40.[5] The positive predictive value of this technique was 96.8%, with sensitivity and specificity of 89.3% and 96.3%, respectively. Other studies must be performed to correlate these criteria.

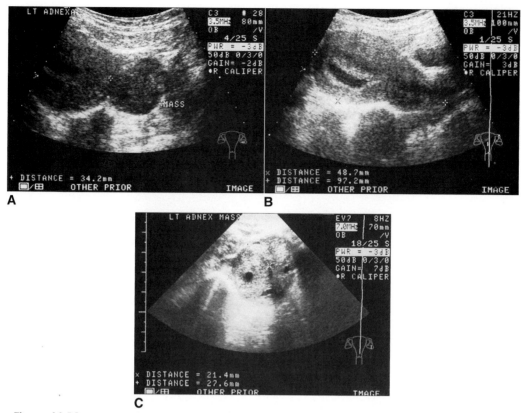

Figure 44-18   A young female in her first trimester presented in the emergency room with elevated human chorionic gonadotropin levels, bleeding, and pelvic pain. **A,** The transabdominal scan clearly shows a mass in the left adnexal area separate from the uterus. **B,** The longitudinal scan of the uterus shows the pseudogestational sac in the fundus of the uterus. **C,** An endovaginal scan shows a gestational sac within the left adnexal area.

ADNEXAL MASS WITH ECTOPIC PREGNANCY

The risk of ectopic pregnancy can be greater than 90% when intrauterine gestation is absent and there is a corresponding adnexal mass. Complex adnexal masses, aside from extrauterine gestational sacs, often represent hematoma within the peritoneal cavity, which is usually contained within the fallopian tube (hematosalpinx) or broad ligament. In early gestational ectopic pregnancy, a hematoma may be the only sonographic sign of ectopic pregnancy. It should be distinguished, however, from an ovarian cyst, such as the corpus luteum, which is typically hypoechoic, although a hemorrhagic corpus luteum cyst may mimic an extrauterine gestational sac or a distal hematosalpinx.

Often, ovarian processes, such as corpus luteum cysts and endometriomas, can be differentiated based on their location within the ovary, and one can often visualize surrounding ovarian tissue. Although this does not rule out the rare ovarian ectopic gestation, correlation with beta-hCG should help differentiate the two.

It has been reported that approximately 80% of patients with ectopic pregnancy demonstrate at least 25 ml of blood within the peritoneum, caused by blood escaping from the distal tube (fimbria). Approximately 60% of women with an ectopic pregnancy demonstrate intraperitoneal fluid, using endovaginal sonography (Figure 44-21). Studies have correlated an increased risk of ectopic pregnancy with moderate to large quantities of free intraperitoneal fluid and an associated adnexal mass.[13]

The presence of echogenic free fluid has been shown to be very specific for hemoperitoneum and to be highly correlated with ectopic pregnancy. A 92% risk of ectopic pregnancy with echogenic free fluid has been reported, with 15% of cases demonstrating echogenic free fluid to be the only sonographic finding (Figure 44-22).[6] When fluid is present, the sonographer should also look at the abdominal gutters and the right and left upper quadrants to evaluate the extent/volume of fluid present. The combination of an adnexal mass and free pelvic fluid is the best sonographic correlation in the diagnosis of ectopic pregnancy.

Although intrauterine and adnexal findings are crucial in diagnosing ectopic pregnancy, it is clear that the previously described sonographic findings are not routine. One report states that 52.5% of cases with ectopic pregnancy could not accurately demonstrate an adnexal mass or masses.[8] Of that 52.5%, less than half (25.5%) were overshadowed by coexisting findings, such as bowel segments that were echogenic or had isoechoic acoustic properties, that did not allow sonographic demarcation of tissue from surrounding ovary or adnexa. Another study demonstrated that in 74% of ectopic pregnancies a confident diagnosis was made of an intrauterine

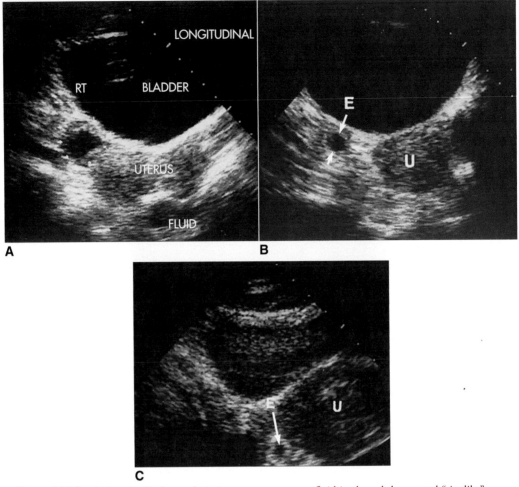

Figure 44-19 **A,** Longitudinal scan depicting an empty uterus, fluid in the cul-de-sac, and "ringlike" cystic mass anterior to the uterus representing an ectopic gestational sac. *RT,* Right. **B** and **C,** Transverse representations of ectopic gestational sacs *(E).* In **C** the ectopic sac is in close proximity to the uterine wall. *U,* Uterus.

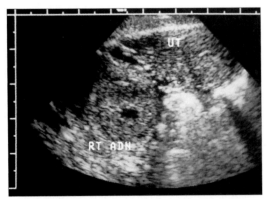

Figure 44-20 Coronal section demonstrating empty uterus *(UT),* and a right adnexal *(RT ADN)* mass with an echogenic ring and sonolucent center consistent with gestational sac. This is consistent with ectopic pregnancy with extrauterine sac.

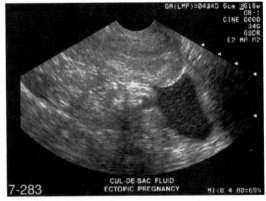

Figure 44-21 Endovaginal scan of the lower uterine segment shows the hypoechoic fluid collection in the cul-de-sac secondary to a ruptured ectopic pregnancy. Low-level echoes are suggestive of blood.

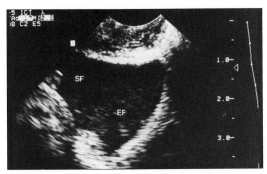

Figure 44-22 Endovaginal sonogram demonstrating echogenic free intraperitoneal fluid in an ectopic gestation. *EF,* Echogenic fluid; *SF,* simple fluid.

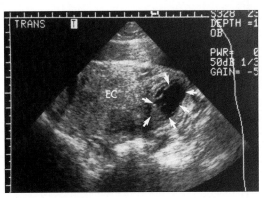

Figure 44-23 Sonogram of an 8.5-week gestation demonstrating the cystic rhombencephalon within the fetal cranium *(arrows)*. *EC,* Endometrial cavity.

pregnancy using endovaginal techniques, and that 26.3% of ectopic pregnancies had a normal endovaginal sonogram at initial presentation.[9] The definition of normal endovaginal sonogram in this study was no adnexal masses or pelvic fluid identified and no evidence of intrauterine gestation.

These findings reiterate the need for meticulous scanning when looking for evidence of ectopic pregnancy and for an understanding of the limitations of all ultrasound techniques.

HETEROTOPIC PREGNANCY

Fortunately, simultaneous intrauterine and extrauterine pregnancies are extremely uncommon, even in patients undergoing an infertility work-up. The sonographic observer should be aware that ovulation induction and in vitro fertilization with embryo transfer lead to not only higher risk of **heterotopic pregnancy** but also to an overall increase in ectopic pregnancies, including bilateral ectopic pregnancies (see Table 44-3).

INTERSTITIAL PREGNANCY

Interstitial pregnancy, or cornual pregnancy, is potentially the most life-threatening of all ectopic gestations (see Table 44-3). This is because of the location of the ectopic pregnancy, which lies in the segment of the fallopian tube that enters the uterus. This site involves the parauterine and myometrial vasculature, creating life-threatening hemorrhage when rupture occurs. Interstitial pregnancies have been reported to occur in approximately 2% of all ectopic pregnancies. Sonographic identification of an interstitial ectopic pregnancy is difficult, but it has been described as an eccentrically placed gestational sac within the uterus that has an incomplete myometrial mantle surrounding the sac (Figure 44-23).

CERVICAL PREGNANCY

Cervical pregnancy has a reported incidence of 1 in 16,000 pregnancies. Sonographic demonstration of a gestational sac within the cervix suggests a cervical pregnancy, although a spontaneous abortion may have a similar appearance. Color Doppler may show peritrophoblastic flow in a cervical ectopic pregnancy compared with lack of flow in a spontaneous abortion. Cervical ectopic pregnancies have an increased risk of

complete hysterectomy because of uncontrollable bleeding caused by increased vascularity of the cervix.

OVARIAN PREGNANCY

An ovarian pregnancy is also very rare, accounting for less than 3% of all ectopic pregnancies. The sonographic diagnosis of ovarian pregnancy may be difficult; reported cases have demonstrated complex adnexal masses that involve or contain the ovary. Thus distinguishing ovarian pregnancy from a hemorrhagic ovarian cyst or from other ovarian processes may be difficult.

ABNORMAL PREGNANCY: SONOGRAPHIC FINDINGS

Sonographic differentiation of normal and abnormal appearances of the first-trimester pregnancy may be subtle. Distinguishing living from nonliving gestations is crucial, but demonstration of a living embryo does not necessarily mean a normal outcome. Recent data prospectively looked at 556 pregnancies between 6 and 13 weeks of gestation and identified embryonic heart motion. Overall the pregnancy loss rate after identification of an intrauterine pregnancy with positive cardiac motion was 8.8%. If sonographic abnormalities were detected (subchorionic hematoma being the most frequent), the loss rate was 15.2% compared with 8.8% when sonogram findings were normal. It is of interest that the loss rate after a normal sonogram was similar in symptomatic patients (10.6%) and asymptomatic patients (9.1%).[4]

Obviously, identifying an intrauterine pregnancy with or without cardiac activity is the first conclusive sonographic sign of normality or abnormality. With endovaginal sonography, a living embryo should be detected by 46 menstrual days. Other sonographic appearances allow the ultrasound clinician to differentiate normal and abnormal findings within the gestational sac period. To conclusively demonstrate normal or abnormal findings, more than one sonogram may be necessary. These are discussed throughout this chapter and are outlined in Table 44-2.

TABLE 44-4 SONOGRAPHIC FINDINGS FOR ABNORMAL PREGNANCY IN THE FIRST TRIMESTER

Condition	Sonographic Findings
Embryonic bradycardia	> 60 beats per minute
Embryonic tachycardia	> 170 beats per minute
Complete abortion	– Empty uterus – No adnexal mass – No free fluid in pelvis – Positive hCG levels with rapid decline
Incomplete abortion	Variable findings: – Intact gestational sac with nonviable embryo to collapsed sac – Thickened endometrium > 5 mm – Retained embryonic parts
Anembryonic pregnancy	– Large >18 mm, empty gestational sac with failure to develop – No yolk sac, amnion, or embryo
Molar pregnancy – Hyperemesis – Increased hCG levels – Bleeding – Preeclampsia	– Uterus larger than dates – "Snowstorm" of multiple tiny clusters of grapelike echoes within the uterine cavity – Theca lutein cysts may be present

EMBRYONIC BRADYCARDIA AND TACHYCARDIA

The variations in embryonic cardiac rate during the first trimester range between 90 and 170 beats per minute (Table 44-4). Embryonic cardiac rates of less than 90 beats per minute at any gestational age within the first trimester have been shown to be a poor prognostic finding. In fact, no reported embryo has survived beyond the second trimester with this finding. The fetus with a heart rate greater than 170 beats per minute shows signs of tachycardia, which may lead to heart failure and fetal hydrops (pleural effusion, pericardial effusion, and ascites).

EMBRYONIC OLIGOHYDRAMNIOS AND GROWTH RESTRICTION

Growth delay and oligohydramnios within the first trimester have poor outcomes. If the gestational sac is 4 mm less than the crown-rump length, embryonic oligohydramnios may be suspected, with universal demise as the outcome.

Embryonic growth restriction can be determined only by relative sonographic dating, either by reliable menstrual history or by growth delay of the embryo or gestational sac in relation to serial sonograms. Chromosome abnormalities, such as triploidy, have been associated with embryonic growth restriction and embryonic oligohydramnios.

FIRST-TRIMESTER BLEEDING

SUBCHORIONIC HEMORRHAGE

The most common occurrence of bleeding in the first trimester is from subchorionic hemorrhage.

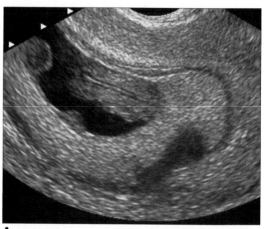

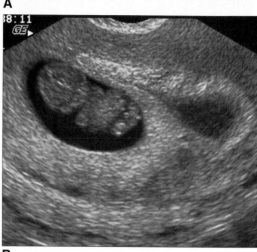

Figure 44-24 Subchorionic hemorrhages are shown in **(A)** 8-week gestation and **(B)** 10-week gestation. (From Henningsen C: *Clinical guide to ultrasonography,* St Louis, 2004, Mosby.)

These low-pressure bleeds result from the implantation of the fertilized ovum into the uterine myometrial wall. The hemorrhage is found between the uterine wall and the membranes of the fetus and is not associated with the placenta. This finding distinguishes a subchorionic hemorrhage from an abruptio placentae. Clinical findings may include bleeding or spotting and uterine contractions. If the hemorrhage becomes large enough, it may lead to a spontaneous abortion.

Sonographic Findings. An early bleed may appear echogenic as the red blood cells actively fill the area of hemorrhage. With time, the hemorrhage becomes more anechoic and may be seen between the uterine wall and the fetal membrane (Figure 44-24). Color flow Doppler will demonstrate the avascular nature of the hemorrhage.

COMPLETE ABORTION

Characteristics for the sonographic diagnosis of **complete abortion** consist of an empty uterus with no adnexal masses or free fluid and a positive beta-hCG levels. Clinical findings are characterized by bleeding and cramping in the first trimester. Correlation between the serum beta-hCG level and

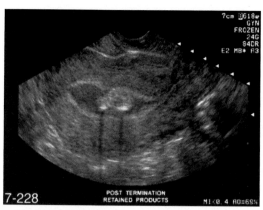

Figure 44-25 Endovaginal scan of a patient who presented with fever, pain, and bleeding secondary to an abortion 2 days previously. The endometrial cavity is distended, with retained products of conception casting small shadows into the myometrial cavity.

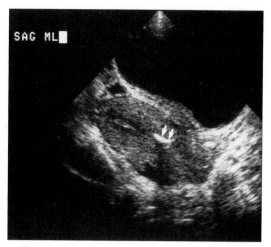

Figure 44-26 Transabdominal sagittal sonogram demonstrates an echogenic focus, causing acoustic shadowing *(arrows)*. This patient had a positive pregnancy test and was experiencing vaginal bleeding. The echogenic source most likely represents retained products, possibly skeletal structures.

the findings in the uterus can be used to confirm whether or not the sonographic indications of a first-trimester pregnancy have been met. Recall that the gestational sac is identified sonographically at 4.5 weeks' gestation. The sac grows approximately 1 mm per day. The yolk sac should be seen when the gestational sac reaches 8 mm in size, and the embryo is seen when the mean sac diameter is greater than 16 mm. The embryo likewise should grow at a rate of 1 mm per day. Cardiac activity should be noted by 5.5 to 6.5 weeks (see Table 44-4).

Serial hCG levels demonstrate rapid decline. Caution should be taken when a positive pregnancy test and an empty uterus are seen, given the possibility that an early normal intrauterine pregnancy between 3 and 5 weeks of gestation may be present. Consequently, serial hCG levels should always be obtained.

INCOMPLETE ABORTION

Incomplete abortion may show several sonographic findings, ranging from an intact gestational sac with a nonliving embryo to a collapsed gestational sac that is grossly misshapen (Figure 44-25). Often, women who are clinically undergoing abortion or who have had elective termination require follow-up sonography to determine if retained products of conception are present. Sonographic signs of retained products may be subtle; a thickened endometrium greater than 5 mm may be the only sonographic evidence of such a diagnosis. Obvious embryonic parts, which may or may not cause acoustic shadowing, are obvious evidence of retained products of conception (Figure 44-26). It can sometimes be difficult to distinguish retained parts of conception from blood clots.

ANEMBRYONIC PREGNANCY (BLIGHTED OVUM)

By definition, **anembryonic pregnancy,** or **blighted ovum,** is a gestational sac in which the embryo fails to develop (see Table 44-4). The typical sonographic appearance of anembryonic pregnancy is of a large, empty gestational sac that does not demonstrate a yolk sac, amnion, embryo, or cardiac activity

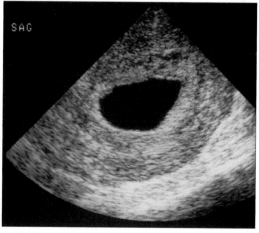

Figure 44-27 Endovaginal sonogram in a sagittal plane demonstrating a large empty gestational sac that does not contain yolk sac, amnion, or embryo. This is consistent with anembryonic pregnancy.

(Figure 44-27). The sac size typically is clearly abnormally large (greater than 18 mm mean sac diameter); no intragestational sac anatomy is seen. Box 44-1 outlines several sonographic intrauterine findings associated with abnormal pregnancies.

GESTATIONAL TROPHOBLASTIC DISEASE

Gestational trophoblastic disease is a proliferative disease of the trophoblast after a pregnancy. It represents a spectrum of disease from a relatively benign form, hydatidiform mole, to a more malignant form, invasive mole, or choriocarcinoma. The clinical hallmark of gestational trophoblastic disease is vaginal bleeding in the first or early second trimester. The serum levels of beta-hCG are dramatically elevated, often greater than 100,000 IU/ml. The patient may also experience symptoms of hyperemesis gravidarum or preeclampsia. Maternal serum

BOX 44-1 SONOGRAPHIC FINDINGS OF GESTATIONAL SACS ASSOCIATED WITH ABNORMAL INTRAUTERINE PREGNANCIES

EMBRYO
Absence of cardiac motion in embryos 5 mm or larger
Absence of cardiac motion after $6\frac{1}{2}$ menstrual weeks

YOLK SAC AND AMNION
Large yolk sac or amnion without a visible embryo
Calcified yolk sac

LARGE GESTATIONAL SAC
>18 mm lacking a living embryo
> 8 mm lacking a visible yolk sac

SHAPE
Irregular or bizarre

POSITION
Low

TROPHOBLASTIC REACTION
Irregular
Absent double decidual sac finding
Thin trophoblastic reaction < 2 mm
Intratrophoblastic venous flow

GROWTH
Gestational sac growth of < 0.6 mm/day
Absent embryonic growth

hCG CORRELATION
Discrepancy in sac size with hCG levels

From Nyberg DA, Laing FC: In Nyberg DA and others, editors: *Transvaginal ultrasound,* St Louis, 1992, Mosby.

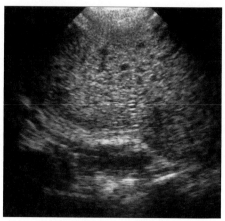

Figure 44-28 Longitudinal scan of the pregnant uterus in a patient who presented larger than appropriate for dates and with bleeding. The uterus is filled with tiny grapelike clusters of tissue, which represent a hydatidiform mole.

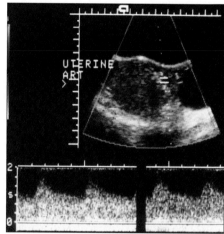

Figure 44-29 Color and spectral Doppler of the molar pregnancy shows high-velocity flow throughout the abnormal tissue.

alpha-fetoprotein levels will be notably low in pregnancies complicated by a complete hydatidiform mole. The clinical examination may reveal a uterus that is larger in size than dates with bilateral fullness that may represent ovarian enlargement of theca lutein cysts.

In the United States, gestational trophoblastic disease affects approximately 1 out of every 1500 to 2000 pregnancies. Associations with women over age 40 and with molar pregnancy have been reported. Genetic studies indicate that a complete hydatidiform mole has a normal diploid karyotype of 46XX, which is usually entirely derived from the father and has proven malignant biologic potential. A partial mole, in contrast, is karotypically abnormal, with triploidy being the most prevalent abnormality.[11]

Sonographic Findings. The sonographic appearance of molar pregnancy varies with gestational age. The characteristic "snowstorm" appearance of a hydatidiform mole, which includes a moderately echogenic soft tissue mass filling the uterine cavity and studded with small cystic spaces representing hydropic chorionic villi, may only be specific for a second-trimester mole (Figure 44-28). Sonographic identification of

the disease in the first trimester has been considered difficult. The appearance of first-trimester molar pregnancy may simulate a missed abortion, incomplete abortion, blighted ovum, or hydropic degeneration of the placenta associated with missed abortion (Figure 44-29). It may also be seen as a small echogenic mass filling the uterine cavity without the characteristic vesicles. The vesicles or cystic spaces may be too small to be seen by ultrasound in the first trimester. Increased blood flow is seen with color Doppler, whereas spectral Doppler shows low-resistive waveforms with high diastolic flow.

The primary treatment of molar pregnancy is uterine curettage followed by serial measurements of serum hCG levels. The serum hCG level falls toward normal within 10 to 12 weeks after evacuation. The reported incidence of residual disease after curettage is approximately 20%. The use of ultrasound for direct visualization of the uterine content to ensure complete evacuation during the curettage procedure has been shown to substantially reduce the incidence of residual gestational trophoblastic disease.[2]

A partial mole on sonography has an identifiable placenta, although the placental tissue is grossly enlarged and engorged with cystic spaces, which represent the hydropic villi. A fetus or fetal tissue may also be identified, but often the fetus is aborted in the first trimester. If the fetus is present, careful analysis should be made to look for structural defects as triploid fetuses usually exist with a partial mole.

Bilateral theca lutein cysts have been reported in as many as half of the molar pregnancies. These engorged ovaries may rupture or torque, causing extreme pain for the patient. The theca lutein cysts are well demonstrated on sonography as enlarged ovaries with multiple cystic areas throughout.

An invasive hydatidiform mole occurs when the hydropic villi of a partial or complete mole invades the uterine myometrium and may further penetrate the uterine wall. This may occur along with the molar pregnancy or may progress after the evacuation of the molar tissue has occurred. Clinically the patient presents with persistent heavy bleeding and very elevated hCG levels. The sonographic appearance shows an enlarged uterus with multiple focal areas of grapelike clusters throughout the uterus.

Choriocarcinoma is a malignant tumor that arises from the trophoblastic epithelium. This tumor most commonly metastasizes to the lungs, liver, and brain. The benign hydatidiform mole and mole with coexistent fetus are considered to have a malignant potential, whereas the partial mole does not have a malignant potential. Clinical symptoms include vaginal bleeding in addition to dyspnea, abdominal pain, and neurologic symptoms depending on where the metastasis has spread.

REFERENCES

1. Bateman BG and others: Vaginal sonography findings and hCG dynamics of early intrauterine and tubal pregnancies, *Obstet Gynecol* 75:421, 1990.
2. Cyr DR and others: Sonography as an aid in molar pregnancy evaluation. Presented to the 35th Annual Convention of the American Institute of Ultrasound in Medicine, Atlanta, vol 10, Baltimore, 1991, American Institute of Ultrasound in Medicine.
3. Fleisher AC and others: Ectopic pregnancy: features at transvaginal sonography, *Radiology* 174:375, 1990.
4. Frates MC, Benson CB, Doubilet PM: Pregnancy outcome after first trimester sonogram demonstrating fetal cardiac activity, *J Ultrasound Med* 12:383, 1993.
5. Kurjak A, Zalud I, Schulman H: Ectopic pregnancy: transvaginal color Doppler of trophoblastic flow in questionable adnexa, *J Ultrasound Med* 10:685, 1991.
6. Nyberg DA and others: Extrauterine findings of ectopic pregnancy at transvaginal US: importance of echogenic fluid, *Radiology* 178:823, 1991.
7. Nyberg DA, Laing FC, Filly RA: Threatened abortion: sonographic distinction of normal and abnormal gestation sacs, *Radiology* 158:397, 1986.
8. Parvey HR, Maklad W: Pitfalls in the transvaginal sonographic diagnosis of ectopic pregnancy, *J Ultrasound Med* 3:139, 1993.
9. Russell SA, Filly RA, Damato N: Sonographic diagnosis of ectopic pregnancy with endovaginal probes: what really has changed? *J Ultrasound Med* 3:145, 1993.
10. Skibo LK, Lyons EA, Levi CS: First trimester umbilical cord cyst, *Radiology* 182:719, 1992.
11. Sommerville M and others: Ovarian neoplasms and the risk of ovarian torsion, *Am J Obstet Gynecol* 164:577, 1991.
12. Szulman AE, Surti U: The syndromes of hydatidiform mole. II. Morphologic evolution of the complete and partial mole, *Am J Obstet Gynecol* 132:20, 1978.
13. Thorson MK and others: Diagnosis of ectopic pregnancy: endovaginal vs. transabdominal sonography, *Am J Roentgenol* 155:307, 1990.

SELECTED BIBLIOGRAPHY

Botash RJ, Spirit BA: Ectopic pregnancy: review and update, *Appl Radiol* January:7-12, 2000.

Bromley B and others: Small sac size in the first trimester: a predictor of poor fetal outcome, *Radiology* 178:375, 1991.

Callen P: *Ultrasonography in obstetrics and gynecology,* ed 4, Philadelphia, 2003, WB Saunders.

Cyr DR and others: Bowel migration in the normal fetus: US detection, *Radiology* 1986:161, 1986.

Cyr DR and others: Fetal rhombencephalon: normal ultrasound findings, *Radiology* 166:691, 1988.

Dubose TJ, Cunyus JA, Johnson LF: Embryonic heart rate and age, *J Diag Med Sonogr* 6:151, 1990.

Garcia CR, Barnhart KT: Diagnosing ectopic pregnancy: decision analysis comparing six strategies, *Obstet Gynecol* 97:464-470, 2001.

Guzman ER: Early prenatal diagnosis of gastroschisis with transvaginal ultrasonography, *Am J Obstet Gynecol* 162:1253, 1990.

Hill LM, Kislak S, Martin JG: Transvaginal sonographic detection of the pseudogestational sac associated with ectopic pregnancy, *Obstet Gynecol* 75:986, 1990.

Hofmann HM and others: Cervical pregnancy: case reports and current concepts in diagnosis and treatment, *Arch Gynecol Obstet* 241:63, 1987.

Jauniaux E and others: Early sonographic diagnosis of body stalk anomaly, *Prenat Diagn* 10:127, 1990.

Jirous J and others: A correlation of the uterine and ovarian blood flows with parity of nonpregnancy women having a history of recurrent spontaneous abortions, *Gynecol Obstet Invest* 52:51-54, 2001.

Johnson MP: First trimester simple hygroma, *Am J Obstet Gynecol* 168:156, 1993.

Kurjak A, Zalud I: Doppler and color flow imaging. In Nyberg DA, Hill LM, Bohm-Velez M and others, editors: *Transvaginal ultrasound,* St Louis, 1992, Mosby.

Kurtz A and others: Detection of retained products of conception following spontaneous abortion of first trimester, *J Ultrasound Med* 10:387, 1991.

Kushnir O and others: Early transvaginal sonographic diagnosis of gastroschisis, *J Clin Ultrasound* 18:194, 1990.

Laboda LA, Estroff JA, Benaceraff BR: First trimester bradycardia: a sign of impending fetal loss, *J Ultrasound Med* 8:561, 1989.

Langer JC and others: Cervical cystic hygroma in the fetus: clinical spectrum and outcome, *J Pediatr Surg* 25:58, 1990.

Lawrence A, Jurdovic D: Three-dimensional ultrasound diagnosis of interstitial pregnancy, *Ultrasound Obstet Gynecol* 14:292-293, 1999.

Neiman HL: Transvaginal ultrasound embryology, *Semin Ultrasound CT MR* 11:22, 1990.

Nelson LH, King M: Early diagnosis of holoprosencephaly, *J Ultrasound Med* 11:57, 1992.

Nyberg DA, Hill LM: Normal early intrauterine pregnancy: sonographic development and hCG correlation. In Nyberg DA and others, editors: *Transvaginal ultrasound,* St Louis, 1992, Mosby.

Nyberg DA and others: Chromosomal abnormalities in fetuses with omphalocele: significance of omphalocele contents, *J Ultrasound Med* 8:299, 1989.

Pascual MA, Ruiz J, Tresserra F and others: Cervical ectopic twin pregnancy: diagnosis and conservative treatment, *Hum Reprod* 16:584-586, 2001.

Peisner DB, Timor-Tritsch IE: The discriminatory zone of beta-hCG for vaginal probes, *J Clin Ultrasound* 18:280, 1990.

Raziel A and others: Ovarian pregnancy: a report of 20 cases in one institution, *Am J Obstet Gynecol* 163:1182, 1990.

Rempen A: Sonographic first trimester diagnosis of umbilical cord cyst, *J Clin Ultrasound* 17:53, 1989.

Rizk B and others: Heterotopic pregnancies after in vitro fertilization and embryo transfer, *Am J Obstet Gynecol* 164:161, 1991.

Seki H, Kuromaki K, Takeda S and others: Persistent subchorionic hematoma with clinical symptoms until delivery, *Int J Gynecol Obstet* 63:123-128,1998.

Sepulveda W, Aviles G, Carstens E and others: Prenatal diagnosis of solid placental masses: the value of color flow imaging, *Ultrasound Obstet Gynecol* 16:554-558, 2000.

Sieroszewski P, Suzin J, Bernaschek G and others: Evaluation of first trimester pregnancy in cases of threatened abortion by means of Doppler sonography, *Ultraschall Med* 22:208-212, 2001.

Smith K: Color flow imaging of leiomyomas and focal myometrial contractions during pregnancy, *J Diagn Med Sonogr* 9:63-67, 1993.

Su YN, Shih JC, Chiu WH and others: Cervical pregnancy: assessment with three-dimensional power Doppler imaging and successful management with selective uterine artery embolization, *Ultrasound Obstet Gynecol* 14:282-287, 1999.

Thomas CL: *Taber's cyclopedic medical dictionary,* Philadelphia, 1997, FA Davis Co.

CHAPTER 45

Sonography of the Second and Third Trimesters

Sandra L. Hagen-Ansert

OBJECTIVES

- List the guidelines for a second- and third-trimester obstetric sonography examination
- Define terminology specific to trimesters, gravidity and parity, and fetal presentation
- Describe sonographic techniques used to image specific fetal structures
- Describe fetal anatomy visualized in an obstetric sonography examination

SUGGESTED PROTOCOL FOR AN OBSTETRIC SONOGRAPHY EXAMINATION

OBSTETRIC PARAMETERS

NORMAL FETOPLACENTAL ANATOMY OF THE SECOND AND THIRD TRIMESTERS

KEY TERMS

apex – the ventricles of the heart come to a point called the *apex;* normally the apex is directed toward the left hip

breech – indicates the fetal head is toward the fundus of the uterus

ductus arteriosus – structure that carries oxygenated blood from the pulmonary artery to the descending aorta

ductus venosus – structure that carries oxygenated blood from the umbilical vein to the inferior vena cava

frontal bossing – protrusion or bulging of the forehead that results from hydrocephalus

gravidity (G) – total number of pregnancies

human chorionic gonadotropin (hCG) – hormone within the maternal urine and serum; hCG is elevated during pregnancy

menstrual age – (also known as *gestational age*) duration of pregnancy determined from the last menstrual period (LMP)

micrognathia – abnormally small chin

midline echo (the falx) – linear echoes located centrally in the fetal head that are produced by the borders of the opposing cerebral hemispheres

nomogram – written representation by graphs, diagrams, or charts of the relationship between numerical variables

normal situs – typical position of the abdominal organs with the liver and IVC on the right, stomach on the left, and the apex of the heart directed towards the left

parity (P) – number of live births

transverse fetal lie – indicates fetus is lying transversely in the uterus, horizontal, or perpendicular to the maternal sagittal axis

trimester – pregnancy is divided into three 13-week segments called *trimesters*

vertex – indicates that the fetus is positioned head down in the uterus

The second and third trimesters are the ideal time to obtain sonographic images of detailed fetal anatomy. Fetal anatomy may be accurately assessed after 18 weeks' gestation, although structures may be seen earlier in many pregnancies. Technical factors, such as fetal movement, fluid quantity, fetal position, and maternal wall thickness or obesity, may obscure the anatomy and result in less than optimal images throughout pregnancy.

To perform a complete evaluation of the fetus, the sonographer should follow a specific protocol that includes at a minimum the components recommended for a standard examination by national organizations that govern obstetrical sonography. The guidelines for obstetric scanning as outlined by the American Institute of Ultrasound in Medicine (AIUM), in collaboration with the American College of Radiology (ACR) and the American College of Obstetricians and Gynecologists (ACOG), are described in Chapter 41.

This chapter focuses on the specific fetal anatomy the sonographer needs to recognize and analyze to develop a systematic scanning protocol. A sonographer will screen many normal fetuses when performing standard antepartum obstetrical examinations during the second or third trimester of pregnancy. A systematic protocol will assure a comprehensive review of fetal anatomy in each patient. Thoroughness and experience applied to the recommended components and to additional details, such as facial features, open hands, and fetal situs, will maximize the opportunity to detect fetal anomalies.

SUGGESTED PROTOCOL FOR AN OBSTETRIC SONOGRAPHY EXAMINATION

The protocol for second- and third-trimester sonography examinations includes a biometric and anatomic survey of the fetus. The second- and third-trimester sonography examination often includes:

1. Observation of fetal viability by visualization of cardiovascular pulsations.
2. Demonstration of presentation (fetal lie).
3. Demonstration of the number of fetuses. In multiple gestations, anatomy images are obtained on each fetus, growth parameters of each fetus are obtained and compared, placenta and membrane structures are assessed, and amniotic fluid levels in each sac are documented.
4. Characterization of the quantity of amniotic fluid as normal or abnormal by subjective visualization or by quantitative estimation techniques.
5. Characterization of the placenta, including localization and relationship to the internal cervical os. Placenta previa should be excluded by examination of the cervical area.
6. Visualization of the cervix and extension of the examination to include transperineal or endovaginal imaging if the cervix appears shortened or the patient complains of regular uterine contractions.
7. Assessment of fetal age. Multiple growth parameters are evaluated. Fetal growth studies may include a serial growth analysis when serial examinations are performed at intervals that are 3 weeks apart.
8. Biometric parameters such as the following:
   - Biparietal diameter
   - Head circumference
   - Femur length
     - Humerus length
   - Abdominal circumference
     - Fetal weight
   - Head circumference to abdominal circumference ratio (used in cases in which disproportionate growth is suspected or unusual head or body contours are observed)
     - Measurement ratios related to head shape or growth
9. Evaluation of uterus, adnexa, and cervix to exclude masses that may complicate obstetric management. Maternal ovaries may not be visualized during the second and third trimesters of pregnancy.
10. Anatomic survey of fetal anatomy to exclude major congenital malformations. Targeted studies may be necessary when a fetal anomaly is suspected.
11. Standard obstetric antepartum sonography examinations should strive to evaluate the anatomic areas listed below. Targeted or repeat studies may be appropriate if anatomy is not well visualized. Technical difficulty should be reported and images should be preserved that document visualization of the following:
    - Cerebral ventricles (evaluating for ventriculomegaly)
      - Posterior fossa of the fetal head, including the cerebellum, cisterna magna, and nuchal skin fold
      - Choroid plexus
      - Midline falx and cavum septum pellucidi
    - Spine views, including the cervical, thoracic, lumbar, and sacral spine (evaluating for spinal defects)
    - Stomach (evaluating for gastrointestinal obstruction)
    - Heart views documenting four chambers and the right and left ventricular outflow tracts (evaluating for heart defects)
    - Kidneys and urinary bladder (evaluating for renal disease)
    - Umbilical cord insertion into the fetal abdomen (evaluating for an anterior abdominal wall defect)
      - Umbilical cord arteries or a section of the cord demonstrating three vessels when possible
      - Presence or absence of four extremities
    - Gender (medically indicated in high-risk pregnancies and multiple gestations)

The sonographer should establish a systematic scanning protocol encompassing all criteria of the guidelines and any additional views requested in their practice environment. An organized approach to scanning ensures completeness and reduces the risk of missing a birth defect.

OBSTETRIC PARAMETERS

The first day of the last normal menstrual period (LMP or LNMP) is the standard way to date a pregnancy in the United States. Human pregnancy lasts 266 days, plus or minus 10 days. If conception occurs on day 14 from the LNMP, the pregnancy duration from LNMP is 280 days or 40 weeks. In reality the assessment of **menstrual** or **gestational age** is often not precise. Many women do not have normal periods, conceive within 3 months of coming off birth control pills when ovulation is irregular, do not record dates, or do not realize that they are pregnant. Even with a known menstrual date, conception may occur from day 6 to day 27, which is a difference of 3 weeks in gestational age as determined by sonography. When the LMP is unknown or when the patient has irregular menstrual cycles, the estimated date of confinement (EDC), or due date, is derived by the obstetrician or clinician using clinical parameters, such as uterine size and growth, fetal heart auscultation, sonographic biometry before 26 weeks, or ovulation indications. Gestational age is an estimate of how long the patient has been pregnant, but the normal variation in length of pregnancy thwarts determination of the exact date that labor will begin.

Pregnancy can be clinically verified approximately 6 to 8 days after ovulation by the presence of **human chorionic gonadotropin (hCG)** within the maternal urine or serum. Quantitative levels of hCG and the rate at which hCG increases in early pregnancy may be predictive of obstetrical complications, such as ectopic pregnancy (low levels increasing slowly) and molar pregnancy (high levels increasing rapidly). Later in pregnancy, hCG is one of the biochemical assays used to predict the risk of aneuploidy.

TRIMESTERS

Pregnancy is divided into **trimesters,** or thirds (Box 45-1). The first trimester covers the first week of pregnancy through the twelfth week and includes the zygote and embryonic stages of pregnancy. The second trimester continues from the 13th week through the 26th week. During the second trimester, the fetus reaches its first pound at approximately 22 weeks. The third trimester commences with the 27th week and concludes at term or the 42nd week of pregnancy. A pregnancy extending beyond the 42nd week is considered a postterm or postdate gestation.

NÄGELE'S RULE

The EDC may be calculated using Nägele's rule (Box 45-2). According to this method, the EDC is derived by subtracting 3 months from the LMP and adding 7 days. For example, an LMP of 10/17 would result in an EDC of 7/24 (10/17 − 3 months = 7/17 + 7 days = 7/24). A sonographer familiar with this rule may determine EDC or LMP when the patient verbally reports only one. Commercial date wheels simplify this method to determine the due date and to assign fetal age at the time of the sonography study.

GRAVIDITY AND PARITY

Key obstetric history of the patient is summarized using gravidity (G) and parity (P). The sonographer should recognize this clinical description of the pregnant patient. **Gravidity** (G) is the number of pregnancies, including the present one. **Parity** (P) is reported using a numeric system that describes all possible pregnancy outcomes. The letter "P" followed by four numbers in sequence, P0000, is commonly used. The numbers represent, in order, full-term deliveries, premature births and stillborns, early pregnancy loss or termination, and living children. For instance, a G4P2103 describes a patient undergoing her fourth pregnancy. She has had two full-term deliveries, one premature birth, no early pregnancy losses, and three living children.

NORMAL FETOPLACENTAL ANATOMY OF THE SECOND AND THIRD TRIMESTERS

Recognizing normal fetal anatomy is essential to the performance of obstetric sonography. The task of capturing images of standard anatomic planes and organs in a small and mobile fetus poses a considerable challenge for the sonographer. The "eye" and experience required to recognize abnormal structures develops over time. Image resolution continually improves, and the detailed anatomy that must be recognized has increased as more sophisticated equipment becomes available. The obstetrical sonographer must continuously update his or her knowledge of sonographic techniques and fetal anatomy. This section describes basic fetal anatomy imaged in the second and third trimesters.

A key to developing scanning expertise is to become organized and systematic in assessing the fetus, placenta, and amniotic fluid (Box 45-3).

The sonographer should initially determine the position of the fetus in relationship to the position of the mother. In determining fetal position and in surveying the uterine

---

BOX 45-1	**TRIMESTERS**

- First trimester = 0 to 12 weeks of gestation
- Second trimester = 13 to 26 weeks of gestation
- Third trimester = 27 to 42 weeks of gestation
- Postterm pregnancy = >42 weeks of gestation

BOX 45-2	**NÄGELE'S RULE**

EDC = LMP − 3 months + 7 days
LMP = EDC + 3 months − 7 days

EDC, Estimated date of confinement; *LMP,* last menstrual period.

BOX 45-3	**SCANNING TECHNIQUES**

- Survey uterus and determine fetal number
- Observe fetal cardiac activity
- Determine fetal position(s) and placental location(s)
- Check cervix and lower uterine segment
- Survey for uterine or adnexal masses
- Assess amniotic fluid
- Perform biometric and anatomic examination of each fetus

contents, the transducer may be systematically moved superior toward the uterine fundus, maintaining a midline path. By angling the probe from side to side, fetal position, cardiac activity, the number of fetuses, the presence of uterine and placental masses, and any obvious fetal anomalies may be recognized and the amniotic fluid assessed.

It is important to remember to view cardiac activity at the beginning of each study to ensure that the fetus is alive. If a fetal demise or an obvious anomaly is initially recognized, the sonographer is better prepared to perform the study and involve the physician immediately.

After fetal position is conceptualized, the sonographer determines the left and right side of the fetus. Being continuously aware of the right and left side of the fetus is necessary to correctly assess fetal anatomy and situs. Assessment and measurement of the fetus may proceed systematically by moving from the fetal head to feet obtaining anatomy images and measurement at each level. The obstetrical sonographer also needs to be prepared to vary this systematic examination and "catch as catch can" when pertinent anatomy presents during fetal movements. The placenta, amniotic fluid, uterus, and adnexa are also examined.

FETAL PRESENTATION

Fetal position may change as a result of fetal movement until actual labor commences. In reality, however, the fetal position changes less frequently after 34 weeks. Visualizing nonvertex fetal positions after 34 weeks may be predictive of positional difficulties during labor and delivery. An atypical fetal presentation, such as face, brow, or shoulder presentation, will complicate delivery. Similarly, hyperextension of the fetal head may alter obstetric management.

The fetal lie is described in relation to the maternal long axis. Fetuses generally assume a longitudinal, transverse, or oblique lie within the uterus (Figure 45-1). If the fetus is lying perpendicular to the long axis of the mother, it is described as a **transverse fetal lie**. When the fetus lie is transverse, the sonographer typically reports the position of the fetal head (maternal right or left) and the position of the fetal spine (inferior, superior, anterior, or posterior) (Figure 45-2). When the fetal

lie is oblique, it is generally described by stating which quadrant of the uterus contains the fetal head and the direction and position of the fetal spine. If the fetus is lying longitudinal or parallel to the maternal long axis, it is described as a **vertex** (head down) presentation or **breech** (head up) presentation (Figure 45-3).

Vertex. A simple method to determine fetal presentation consists of a midline sagittal scan in the lower uterine segment. Immediately cephalad to the symphysis pubis, the maternal bladder is visualized with the cervix and lower uterine segment posterior. This view allows the sonographer to determine which fetal part is presenting and to check the relationship between the cervix and placenta. The fetal head is visualized at this level when the fetus is in a vertex or cephalic presentation. Proceeding fundally, if the fetal body is noted to follow the head, a vertex lie is confirmed (Figure 45-4). The fetal body may lie in an oblique axis to the right or left of the maternal midline. If the body is not initially recognized in the midline, the sonographer should direct the transducer from side to side to search for the abdomen. Identification of the vertebral column entering the cranium further delineates the fetal lie. The position of a fetus in vertex position may be described by stating the relationship of the fetal occiput (back of the head) to the maternal pelvis. If the occiput is adjacent to the left anterior portion of the maternal pelvis, the fetal position is left occiput anterior (LOA). If the occiput is adjacent to the left lateral portion of the maternal pelvis, it is called left occiput transverse (LOT). Similarly, fetuses may be described as left occiput posterior (LOP), occiput posterior (OP), right occiput posterior (ROP), right occiput transverse (ROT), right occiput anterior (ROA), or occiput anterior (OA). Fetuses that are OA (looking straight down) or OP (looking straight up) may present technical difficulties in measuring the fetal head and abdomen and in visualizing fetal cranial anatomy.

Breech. When the lower extremities or buttocks are found to be in the lower uterine segment and the head is visualized in the uterine fundus, a breech presentation is suspected (Figure 45-5). In fetuses near term, determination of the specific type of breech lie provides important clinical information for the obstetrician planning the safest route of delivery. Some fetuses in a breech position, such as those in a frank breech position with the thighs flexed at the hips and the lower legs extended in front of the body and up in front of the head (Figure 45-6), may be safely turned allowing vaginal delivery. Fetuses in other breech lies, such as complete breech when both the hips and lower extremities are found in the lower pelvis, need to be delivered by cesarean section. A footling breech is found when the hips are extended and one (single footling) or both feet (double footling) are the presenting parts closest to the cervix. The position of a fetus in breech position may be described by stating the relationship of the fetal sacrum (lower spine) to the maternal pelvis. If the sacrum is adjacent to the left anterior portion of the maternal pelvis, the fetal position is left sacrum anterior (LSA). If the sacrum is adjacent to the left lateral portion of the maternal pelvis, it is called left

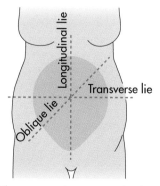

Figure 45-1   These vectors demonstrate the three major possible axes that a fetus may occupy. Fetal lie does not necessarily indicate whether the vertex or the breech is closest to the cervix.

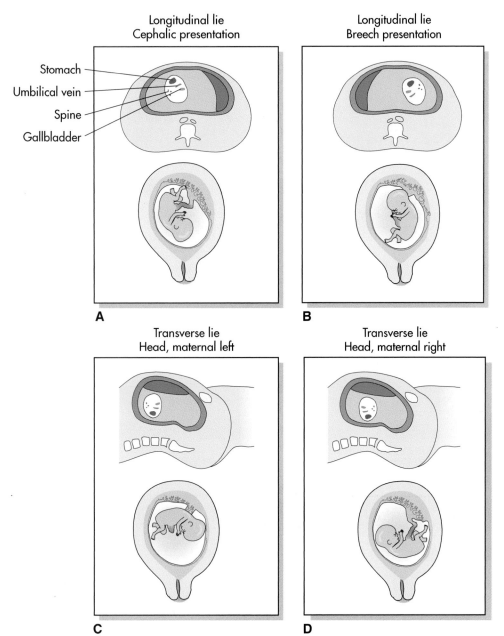

Figure 45-2 Knowledge of the plane of section across the maternal abdomen (longitudinal or transverse) and the position of the fetal spine and left-side (stomach) and right-side (gallbladder) structures, can be used to determine fetal lie and presenting part. **A,** This transverse scan of the gravid uterus demonstrates the fetal spine on the maternal right with the fetus lying with its right side down (stomach anterior, gallbladder posterior). Because these images are viewed looking up from the patient's feet, the fetus must be in longitudinal lie and cephalic presentation. **B,** When the gravid uterus is scanned transversely and the fetal spine is on the maternal left with the right side down, the fetus is in a longitudinal lie and breech presentation. **C,** When a longitudinal plane of section demonstrates the fetal body to be transected transversely and the fetal spine is nearest the uterine fundus with the fetal left side down, the fetus is in a transverse lie with the fetal head on the maternal left. **D,** When a longitudinal plane of section demonstrates the fetal body to be transected transversely and the fetal spine is nearest the lower uterine segment with the fetal left side down, the fetus is in a transverse lie with the fetal head on the maternal right. Although real-time scanning of the gravid uterus quickly allows the observer to determine fetal lie and presenting part, this maneuver of identifying specific right- and left-side structures within the fetal body forces one to determine fetal position accurately and identify normal and pathologic fetal anatomy.

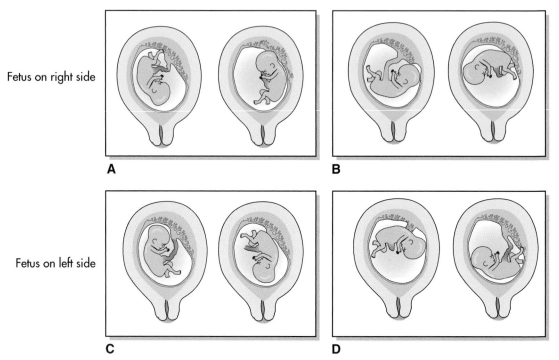

Figure 45-3   Various fetal positions and the method used to differentiate the left side from the right side. **A,** Fetus lying on the right side; whether the head is up or down, the left side of the fetus is up or closer to the transducer. **B,** Fetus lying on right side in a transverse lie; left side is closer to the transducer. **C,** Fetus lying on the left side; whether the head is up or down, the right side is up or closer to the transducer. **D,** Fetus lying on left side in a transverse lie; the right side is closer to the transducer.

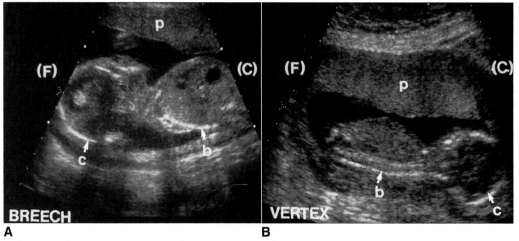

Figure 45-4   **A,** A breech presentation. The body *(b)* is closest in proximity to the direction of the cervix (C) (right of image), and the cranium *(c)* is directed toward the uterine fundus *(F)*. *p,* Placenta. **B,** A vertex presentation. The cranium *(c)* is closest in proximity to the direction of the cervix (C) (to the right of image), and the body *(b)* is directed toward the uterine fundus, *(F)*. *p,* Placenta.

sacrum transverse (LST). Similarly, fetuses may be described as left sacrum posterior (LSP), sacrum posterior (SP), right sacrum posterior (RSP), right sacrum transverse (RST), right sacrum anterior (RSA), or sacrum anterior (SA). When a fetus is in breech presentation, the shape of the head may appear elongated or "dolichocephalic," especially in the third trimester.

Transverse. When a transverse cross-section of the fetal head or body is noted in the sagittal plane, a transverse lie is suspected (Figure 45-7). By rotating the transducer perpendicular to the maternal axis, the long axis of the fetus may be observed. When a fetus remains in transverse lie late in pregnancy, it is important to screen for a mass or placenta previa in the lower uterine segment that is

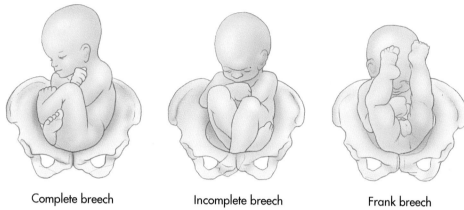

Complete breech   Incomplete breech   Frank breech

Figure 45-5   Three possible breech presentations. The complete breech demonstrates flexion of the hips and knees. The incomplete breech demonstrates intermediate deflexion of one hip and knee (single or double footling). The frank breech shows flexion of the hips and extension of both knees.

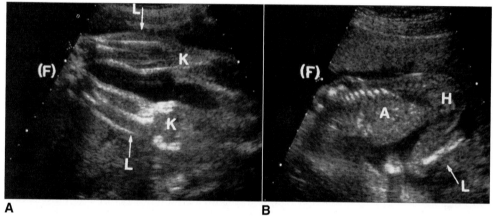

Figure 45-6   **A,** A fetus in a frank breech presentation with both legs extended upward toward the uterine fundus *(F). K,* Knee; *L,* lower leg. **B,** Complete breech presentation with one leg flexed at the hips, with the lower leg *(L)* and foot positioned under the hips *(H).* The other leg was in a similar position. *A,* Abdomen; *(F),* fundus.

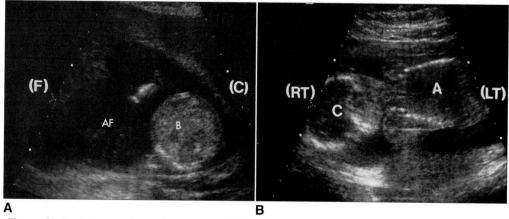

Figure 45-7   **A,** A scan obtained in an 18-week fetus using a sagittal scanning plane reveals the fetal body in a transverse position rather than a sagittal or coronal orientation (compare with Figure 45-4). *AF,* Amniotic fluid; *B,* body; *(C)* toward cervix; *(F),* fundus. **B,** In the same fetus, by rotating the transducer 90 degrees, the abdomen may be connected to the head to reveal the transverse lie with the head oriented to the maternal right side *(RT)* and the abdomen *(A)* to the maternal left side *(LT).*

preventing the fetus from moving into a vertex or breech position.

Situs. In addition to determining fetal lie, the right and left sides of the fetus need to be conceptualized to ensure **normal situs** (positioning) of fetal organs. Some sonographers memorize this relationship. For example, if the fetus is in a vertex presentation with the fetal spine toward the maternal right side, the right side of the fetus is down and the left side is up. It is more helpful, however, to practice maintaining a mental picture of the fetal body and position throughout the examination, which allows recognition of the fetal right and left sides.

A sonographer may also differentiate the right from left sides by identifying anatomic landmarks after an initial orientation is verified. For example, if the sonographer initially verifies that the fetal stomach lies on the fetal left side, later in the examination the fetal right and left may be determined in relation to the stomach. The gallbladder on the right side and the **apex** of the heart pointing toward the fetal left side may be verified by their relationship to the stomach. The fetal aorta lies slightly to the left of midline, anterior to the spine, and the inferior vena cava is to the right of midline and slightly more anterior to the aorta.

Effective obstetric scanning is founded on the operator's ability to visualize fetal position.

THE CRANIUM

The sonographer must be adept at recognizing the normal appearances and developmental changes of the fetal brain throughout pregnancy. It is imperative to identify neuroanatomy at specific levels where measurements are obtained, such as a biparietal diameter or posterior fossa, and to screen for malformations in brain development (see Chapter 21). The experienced obstetrical sonographer will understand developmental changes, recognize normal anatomic variations, and develop an ability to detect malformations. The standard antepartum obstetrical examination guidelines require the sonographer to image and record the choroid plexus, the lateral ventricles, the cerebellum, the cisterna magna, the cavum septum pellucidi, and the midline falx.

Several important principles must be understood when viewing the fetal brain. First, brain tissue, a solid structure, may appear hypoechoic or cystic because of the low density of the tissue. Brain tissue does not exhibit typical solid appearances because of the small size of the reflective interfaces; echoes are not generated unless the reflectors are large enough to cause reflections. The water content of the fetal brain is high, contributing to the cystic appearances of various brain structures. Second, as the brain develops, structures change their sonographic appearances. For example, the choroid plexuses seem large early in pregnancy, but as the brain grows, these structures appear small in relationship to the entire brain.

By the 12th week of gestation, the cranial bones ossify. By 18 weeks of gestation, the texture characteristics of each brain structure have been determined. From this point on in the pregnancy, the appearance of each brain structure should remain the same.

In general, two types of brain tissue are highly echogenic: the dura (pachymeninx) and the pia arachnoid (leptomeninx), which covers the inner and outer brain surfaces. The appearance of the brain structures largely depends on the amount of pia arachnoid tissue and cerebrospinal fluid (CSF) making up a specific structure. For example, a subarachnoid space contains a large amount of CSF and will appear cystic. In contrast, an area that contains both CSF and pia arachnoid has both echo-free and echogenic appearances. Pia arachnoid tissue appears echogenic.

In evaluating the cranium, the long axis of the fetus is determined. The transducer is aligned in a longitudinal or sagittal position over the fetus and then specifically positioned over the fetal head. Rotation of the transducer perpendicular to the sagittal plane generates transverse sections of the brain. Brain anatomy and measurements are assessed in these transverse scanning planes (occipitotransverse position) (Figure 45-8).

The first step in surveying the brain is to check the contour or outline of the skull bones. This is accomplished by sweeping the transducer through the cranium from the highest level (roof) in the brain to the skull base. The cranium appears as a circle at the highest levels and as an oval at the ventricular, peduncular, and basal levels. Check for any irregularities in the contour of the skull bones. Keep in mind that extracranial masses (e.g., cephaloceles) distort the normal configuration of the skull table; therefore, exclusion, of cranial masses should be routinely attempted.

When the fetal cranium is difficult to view, search deep in the pelvis because it may be low in the late third trimester of pregnancy, limiting study of brain anatomy and growth. Maternal bladder filling or tilting of the patient into Trendelenburg's position (maternal head directed down) may free the head from the pelvis. In some cases, especially when a brain anomaly is suspected, use of an endovaginal probe or transperineal scanning may define the skull and brain. In all cases, at a minimum, the outline of the cranium should be visible; if it is not, cranial absence (anencephaly) or deformity should be considered.

Optimal studies of the fetal brain may not be possible when the fetal head is in an occipitoposterior position (looking up) or when the head is in an occipitoanterior position (looking down).

The next step in the fetal profile is to assess the development of the brain. Although all fetal brain structures are not visible prenatally, commonly recognized neuroanatomic structures are described.

In a transverse plane, at the most cephalad level within the skull (Figure 45-9), the contour of the skull should be round or oval (depending on exact level) and should have a smooth surface (excluding a cephalocele in which the meninges, brain, or both herniate from the skull). At this level, the interhemispheric fissure (IHF), or falx cerebri, is observed as a membrane separating the brain into two equal hemispheres. The IHF is an important landmark to visualize because its presence implies that separation of the cerebrum has occurred. This excludes the severe anomaly alobar holoprosencephaly, in which there is only a single ventricle and an absent IHF.

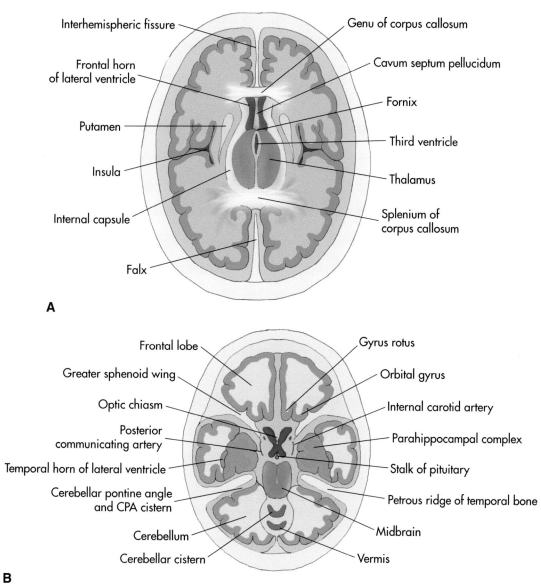

A

Interhemispheric fissure

Frontal horn of lateral ventricle

Putamen

Insula

Internal capsule

Falx

Genu of corpus callosum

Cavum septum pellucidum

Fornix

Third ventricle

Thalamus

Splenium of corpus callosum

B

Frontal lobe

Greater sphenoid wing

Optic chiasm

Posterior communicating artery

Temporal horn of lateral ventricle

Cerebellar pontine angle and CPA cistern

Cerebellum

Cerebellar cistern

Gyrus rotus

Orbital gyrus

Internal carotid artery

Parahippocampal complex

Stalk of pituitary

Petrous ridge of temporal bone

Midbrain

Vermis

Figure 45-8 **A,** Transverse view of the fetal intracranial anatomy taken at the midsection of the fetal head. **B,** Transverse view inferior to **(A)** taken at the level of the cerebellum and vermis.

Lateral and running parallel to the IHF, two linear echoes representing deep venous structures (white-matter tracts) are viewed (see Figure 45-9). It is important to recognize that the white-matter tracts are positioned above the level of the lateral ventricles.

The fetal ventricular system consists of two paired lateral ventricles, a midline third ventricle, and a fourth ventricle adjacent to the cerebellum. The ventricular system contains cerebral spinal fluid (CSF), which coats the brain and spinal cord. CSF is produced by the choroid plexus tissue within the lateral ventricles. Choroid plexus is located within the roofs of each ventricle except at the frontal ventricular horns. This sponge-like material is echogenic and very prominent in early pregnancy. Occasionally, small cysts—which are engorged spongelike cavities—may be seen in normal pregnancies. As the cerebral hemispheres grow, the ventricular system and the choroid plexus appear to occupy a much smaller portion of the cranium.

From the lateral ventricles, the fluid travels to the third ventricle through the foramen of Monro. From the third ventricle, the fluid travels through the aqueduct of Sylvius (within the third ventricle) to the fourth ventricle. When the fluid reaches the fourth ventricle, it flows into the cerebral and spinal subarachnoid spaces from the interventricular foramina and foramen of Luschka. CSF then enters the venous system (e.g., cranial venous sinuses).

The fetal ventricles are important to assess because ventriculomegaly or hydrocephalus (dilated ventricular system) is a sign of central nervous system abnormalities. Ventriculomegaly is observed in fetuses with central nervous system disorders and may be the first clue that such a problem exists. Aqueductal stenosis at the level of the aqueduct of Sylvius is

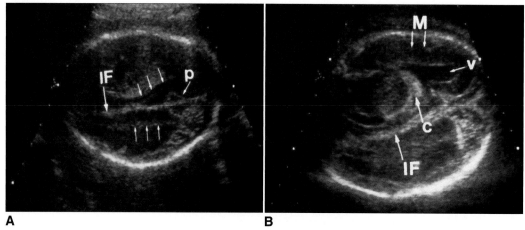

Figure 45-9 **A,** Transverse cross-section revealing white-matter tracts *(arrows)* coursing parallel to the interhemispheric fissure *(IF)* at 26 weeks of gestation. *p,* Peduncles. **B,** The choroid plexus *(c)* is located in the proximal or near hemisphere within the ventricular cavity *(v).* Note the homogeneous appearance of the brain tissue. *M,* Mantle.

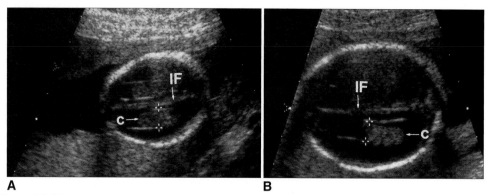

Figure 45-10 **A,** Transverse view demonstrating ventricular atrial diameter of 6 mm *(calipers)* at 16 weeks of gestation representing a normal-size ventricle. *c,* Choroid plexus; *IF,* interhemispheric fissure. **B,** In a 19-week gestation the atrial diameter of 6 mm corresponds to a normal-size ventricle.

the most common type of fetal hydrocephaly and will result in excess fluid in the lateral and third ventricles. Dilation of the entire system, including the fourth ventricle, is associated with spinal defects.

The lateral ventricles are viewed at a level just below the white-matter tracts (Figure 45-10). The lumen of the ventricles may be recognized by the bright reflection of their borders and the presence of the large choroid plexuses, which normally fill the cavity of the ventricles early in gestation. The lateral borders of the ventricular chambers (LVBs) are represented as echogenic lines coursing parallel to the IHF. The LVB is more easily imaged in the distal hemisphere, as opposed to the proximal or nearest ventricle, because of reverberation artifacts in the near field. The ventricular cavity is represented sonographically as an echo-free space, filled with choroid plexus and housed between the medial ventricular border and LVB (Figure 45-11).

As a general rule in early pregnancy (approximately 12 to 22 weeks), the LVB appears to be large in relation to the developing cranial hemispheres. Later in pregnancy, the LVB assumes a more medial position (Figure 45-12).

The choroid plexus is tear-shaped. The glomus, or body, of the choroid plexus marks the site at which the size of the ventricle may be assessed. The glomus should fill the entire ventricle. If the glomus appears to float or dangle within the cavity, measurements of ventricular size are recommended to exclude abnormally enlarged or dilated ventricles (ventriculomegaly). Atrial diameter measurements are clinically practical because the size of the ventricular atria remains the same throughout gestation.

When measuring the size of the ventricle, locate the glomus and measure directly across the posterior portion, measuring perpendicular to the long axis of the ventricle rather than the falx, while placing the calipers at the junction of the ventricular wall and lumen or cavity of the ventricle (see Figure 45-10). The normal ventricle measures 6.5 mm. Any ventricle measuring greater than 10 mm is considered outside of the normal error ranges and is therefore abnormal, warranting further consultation and prenatal testing.

The texture of the choroid plexus should be assessed to exclude the formation of cysts. It is thought that CSF may

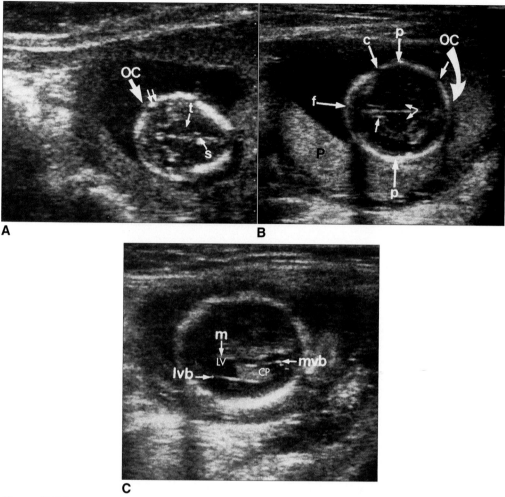

Figure 45-11   **A,** Cranial anatomy at the level of the thalamus *(t)* in a 14-week gestation. Note the contour of the bony calvarium *(double arrows).* *OC,* Occiput; *s,* cavum septum pellucidum. **B,** Cranial anatomy at the same level in an 18-week gestation. *Curved arrow,* Thalamus; *single arrow,* cavum septum pellucidum; *c,* coronal suture; *f,* frontal bone; *OC,* occiput; *P,* placenta; *p,* parietal bones. **C,** Cerebral ventricles at 19 weeks of gestation. The midline echo from the interhemispheric fissure *(m)* is noted. The medial ventricular border *(mvb)* and lateral ventricular border *(lvb)* are identified. The ventricular cavity *(LV)* and echogenic choroid plexus *(CP)* are demonstrated.

become trapped during development within the neuroepithelial folds and result in the formation of a choroid plexus cyst. This commonly represents a normal variation in fetal development, but these cysts are known to be associated with chromosomal anomalies such as trisomy 18.

Moving the transducer in a more caudal direction identifies the echogenic **midline echo** complex (at the level of **the falx** cerebri). This is the widest transverse diameter of the skull and is therefore the proper level at which to measure the biparietal diameter and to assess the development of the midline brain structures (see Figure 45-12). Along the midline echo, the paired thalamus lies on either side and resembles a heart with the apex projected toward the fetal occiput. This orientation aids in deciding which direction the face is positioned.

Between the thalamic structures lies the cavity of the third ventricle (see Figure 45-12). In the same scanning plane, the box-shaped cavum septum pellucidi (CSP) is observed in front of the thalamus. The CSP is the space between the leaves of the septum pellucidum. By viewing the CSP, an anomaly known as complete agenesis of the corpus callosum may be excluded because the presence of the CSP signifies normal development of the frontal midline.

The frontal horns of the ventricles may be seen as two diverging echo-free structures within the frontal lobes of the brain and are prominent in the presence of ventricular dilation. The corpus callosum is ill-defined sonographically and represented as the band of tissue between the frontal ventricular horns.

The ambient cisterns are pulsatile structures vascularized by the posterior cerebral artery bordering the thalamus posteriorly. When scanning laterally in the brain, the temporal lobe is visible along with evidence of the insula (i.e., sylvian cistern complex). The insula appears to pulsate because of blood

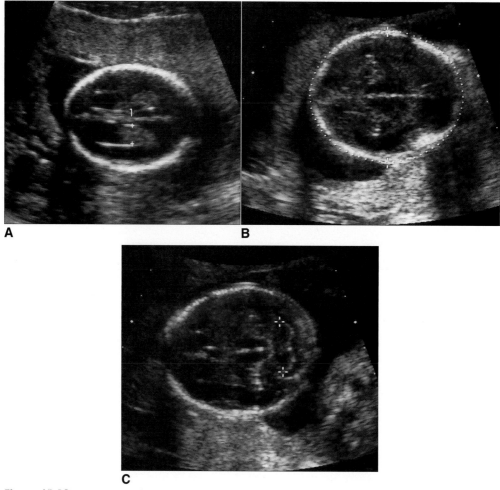

Figure 45-12   A, Transverse view at the level of the ventricles. The width of the lateral ventricle is measured from medial to lateral edges *(1).* **B,** Transverse view slightly inferior to the level of the ventricles, near the thalamus (hypoechoic "heart" structure in the center of the skull). This is the level at which the biparietal diameter and head circumference are measured. **C,** Transverse view inferior to the level of **B;** the cerebellum is demarcated by the calipers.

circulation through the middle cerebral artery, which courses through the insula (see Figure 45-12). The subarachnoid spaces may be seen projecting from the inner skull table.

The sonographer should be careful when studying anatomy in the proximal (near) cranial hemisphere because reverberation artifacts often preclude evaluation of the brain. Interpretation of the normalcy of the brain should, in general, be based on the anatomy seen in the distal hemisphere because most brain anomalies represent symmetric processes. In most cases, the defect is present bilaterally, even though the anatomy may not be adequately discerned. The sonographer may be able to achieve better visualization by angling cephalad or by endovaginal or transperineal scanning.

As the transducer is moved caudally, the heart-shaped cerebral peduncles are imaged (Figure 45-13). Although similar to the thalamus in shape, they are smaller. Pulsations from the basilar artery are observed between the lobes of the peduncles at the interpeduncular cistern. The circle of Willis may be seen anterior to the midbrain and appears as a triangular region that is highly pulsatile as a result of the midline-positioned anterior

cerebral artery and lateral convergence of the middle cerebral arteries. The suprasellar cistern may be recognized in the center of the circle of Willis.

The cerebellum is located in back of the cerebral peduncles within the posterior fossa. The cerebellar hemispheres are joined together by the cerebellar vermis (Figure 45-14). It is important to recognize the usual configuration of the cerebellum because distortion may represent findings suggestive of an open spina bifida. The "banana sign" is the sonographic term that describes the Arnold-Chiari malformation in which the cerebellum may be small or displaced downward into the foramen magnum. Measurements of cerebellar width allow assessment of fetal age and permit necessary follow-up in fetuses with spinal defects and other anomalies of the cerebellum.

The cisterna magna (a posterior fossa cistern filled with CSF) lies directly behind the cerebellum (Figure 45-15). This area should be evaluated routinely when in the cerebellar plane because a normal-appearing cisterna magna may exclude almost all open spinal defects. The cisterna magna is almost always effaced (thinned out) or obliterated in fetuses with the

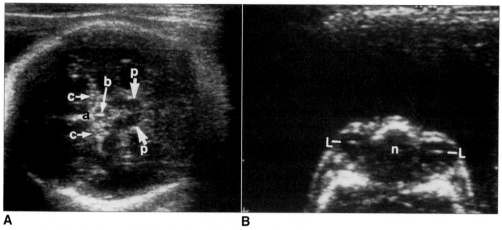

Figure 45-13   A, Circle of Willis *(c)* identified anterior to the cerebral peduncles *(p).* Arterial pulsations may be observed from the basilar artery *(b)* and anterior cerebral artery *(a)* in real-time imaging. The middle cerebral artery pulsations may be seen at the lateral margins of the circle of Willis. **B,** The lenses *(L)* of the eyes are noted when the fetus is looking upward (occipitoposterior position). The nasal cavities are identified *(n).*

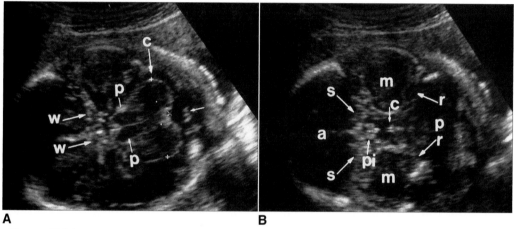

Figure 45-14   A, Anatomic depiction at the cerebellar level in a 25-week fetus showing the cerebral peduncles *(p)* positioned anteriorly to the cerebellum *(c).* The circle of Willis *(w)* is outlined. The dural folds that connect the bottom of the falx cerebelli are seen within the cisterna magna *(arrow).* **B,** In the same fetus, at a level slightly below the cerebellar level, the anterior *(a)*, middle *(m)*, and posterior fossae are shown. Note the sphenoid bones *(s)* and petrous ridges *(r). c,* Suprasellar cistern; *pi,* piarachnoid tissue in the basilar cistern.

Arnold-Chiari malformation (cranial changes associated with spina bifida). The cranial change occurs because tethering of the spinal cord resulting from spina bifida pulls brain tissue downward, obliterating the cisterna magna. In patients at low risk of spinal defect, confirmation of a normal posterior fossa suggests the absence of spina bifida. Because evaluation of the fetal spine remains challenging in excluding small spinal defects, cranial findings associated with this disorder may be very helpful in screening for these lesions.

Enlargement of the cisterna magna may indicate a space-occupying cyst, such as a Dandy-Walker malformation or other abnormalities of the posterior fossa. Enlargement is often a normal variant.

The normal cisterna magna measures 3 to 11 mm, with an average size of 5 to 6 mm. Measurements of cisterna magna size are obtained by measuring from the vermis to the inner skull table of the occipital bone. Within the cisterna magna space, linear echoes, which are paired, may be observed posteriorly. These echogenic structures represent dural folds that attach the falx cerebelli (see Figure 45-14).

In the second trimester, thickness of the nuchal skin fold is measured in a plane containing the cavum septi pellucidi, the cerebellum, and the cisterna magna. Values of skin thickness of 5 millimeters or less up to 20 weeks' gestational age are normal. Fetuses with thickened nuchal skin are at increased risk for aneuploidy.

When scanning inferior to or below the cerebellar plane, the orbits may be visualized. It is important to note that both fetal orbits (and eyes) are present and that the spacing between both orbits appears normal. If there are questions or the face appears abnormal, measurements need to be performed. Table 45-1 summarizes the measurements of orbital width that aid

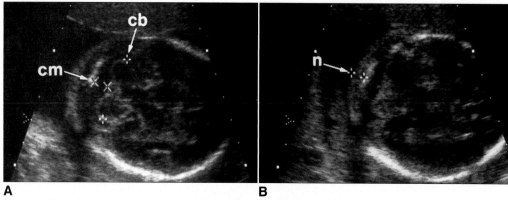

Figure 45-15 **A,** Depiction of a normal cerebellum *(cb)* and cisterna magna *(cm)* in a 24-week fetus. The cerebellum measures 26 mm, and the cisterna magna measures 5 mm in diameter. **B,** In the same fetus, at the same level, the skin behind the neck is measured. A normal nuchal skin fold *(n)* of 5 mm is shown. This measurement is unreliable after 20 weeks of gestation.

TABLE 45-1	PREDICTED BIPARIETAL DIAMETER (BPD) AND WEEKS OF GESTATION FROM THE INNER AND OUTER ORBITAL DISTANCES						
BPD (cm)	Gestation	(wk)	IOD (cm)	BPD (cm)	OOD (cm)	Gestation	(wk)
1.9	11.6	0.5	1.3	5.8	24.3	1.6	4.1
2.0	11.6	0.5	1.4	5.9	24.3	1.6	4.2
2.1	12.1	0.6	1.5	6.0	24.7	1.6	4.3
2.2	12.6	0.6	1.6	6.1	25.2	1.6	4.3
2.3	12.6	0.6	1.7	6.2	25.2	1.6	4.4
2.4	13.1	0.7	1.7	6.3	25.7	1.7	4.4
2.5	13.6	0.7	1.8	6.4	26.2	1.7	4.5
2.6	13.6	0.7	1.9	6.5	26.2	1.7	4.5
2.7	14.1	0.8	2.0	6.6	26.7	1.7	4.6
2.8	14.6	0.8	2.1	6.7	27.2	1.7	4.6
2.9	14.6	0.8	2.1	6.8	27.6	1.7	4.7
3.0	15.0	0.9	2.2	6.9	28.1	1.7	4.7
3.1	15.5	0.9	2.3	7.0	28.6	1.8	4.8
3.2	15.5	0.9	2.4	7.1	29.1	1.8	4.8
3.3	16.0	1.0	2.5	7.3	29.6	1.8	4.9
3.4	16.5	1.0	2.5	7.4	30.0	1.8	5.0
3.5	16.5	1.0	2.6	7.5	30.6	1.8	5.0
3.6	17.0	1.0	2.7	7.6	31.0	1.8	5.1
3.7	17.5	1.1	2.7	7.7	31.5	1.8	5.1
3.8	17.9	1.1	2.8	7.8	32.0	1.8	5.2
4.0	18.4	1.2	3.0	7.9	32.5	1.9	5.2
4.2	18.9	1.2	3.1	8.0	33.0	1.9	5.3
4.3	19.4	1.2	3.2	8.2	33.5	1.9	5.4
4.4	19.4	1.3	3.2	8.3	34.0	1.9	5.4
4.5	19.9	1.3	3.3	8.4	34.4	1.9	5.4
4.6	20.4	1.3	3.4	8.5	35.0	1.9	5.5
4.7	20.4	1.3	3.4	8.6	35.4	1.9	5.5
4.8	20.9	1.4	3.5	8.8	35.9	1.9	5.6
4.9	21.3	1.4	3.6	8.9	36.4	1.9	5.6
5.0	21.3	1.4	3.6	9.0	36.9	1.9	5.7
5.1	21.8	1.4	3.7	9.1	37.3	1.9	5.7
5.2	22.3	1.4	3.8	9.2	37.8	1.9	5.8
5.3	22.3	1.5	3.8	9.3	38.3	1.9	5.8
5.4	22.8	1.5	3.9	9.4	38.8	1.9	5.8
5.5	23.3	1.5	4.0	9.6	39.3	1.9	5.9
5.6	23.3	1.5	4.0	9.7	39.8	1.9	5.9
5.7	23.8	1.5	4.1				

Modified from Mayden KL and others: Orbital diameters: A new parameter for prenatal diagnosis and dating, *Am J Obstet Gynecol* 144:289, 1982.

in gestational age assignment and in detecting abnormalities of spacing. There are conditions in which eyes may be missing (anophthalmia), fused or closely spaced (hypotelorism), or abnormally widened (hypertelorism).

The fetal orbits are observed and measured in two planes when the fetal head is in an occipitotransverse position (fetal cranium on the side): (1) a coronal scan posterior to the glabella-alveolar line (Figure 45-16) and (2) a transverse scan at a level below the biparietal diameter (along the orbitomeatal line) (Figure 45-17). In these views the individual orbital rings, nasal structures, and maxillary processes can be identified. When the fetus is in an occipitoposterior position (fetal orbits directed up), orbital distances can also be determined. In this view, the orbital rings, lens, and nasal structures may be demonstrated (Figure 45-18). Measurements of the inner orbital distance (IOD) should be made from the medial border of the orbit to the opposite medial border, and the outer orbital

(or binocular) distance (OOD) is measured from the lateral border of one orbit to the opposite lateral wall (see Figures 45-16 to 45-18). **Nomograms** for orbital distance spacing have been published.

At the base of the skull, the anterior, middle, and posterior cranial fossae are observed (see Figure 45-14). The sphenoid bones create a V-shaped appearance as they separate the anterior fossa from the middle fossa, with the petrous bones further dividing the fossa posteriorly. At the junction of the sphenoid wings and petrous bones lies the sella turcica (site of the pituitary gland).

THE FACE

The architecture and morphology of the fetal face are easily appreciated after the first trimester of pregnancy. By understanding the normal appearance of the developing face, the sonographer may recognize when it is deformed. Viewing facial

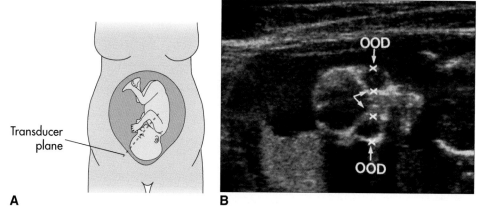

Figure 45-16   **A,** Frontal view demonstrating a fetus in a vertex presentation with the fetal cranium in an occipitotransverse position. The transducer is placed along the coronal plane (approximately 2 cm posterior to the glabella-alveolar line). **B,** Sonogram demonstrating the orbits in the coronal view. The outer orbital diameter *(OOD)* and inner orbital diameter (IOD) *(angled arrows)* are viewed. The IOD is measured from the medial border of the orbit to the opposite medial border *(angled arrows)*. The *OOD* is measured from the outermost lateral border of the orbit to the opposite lateral border.

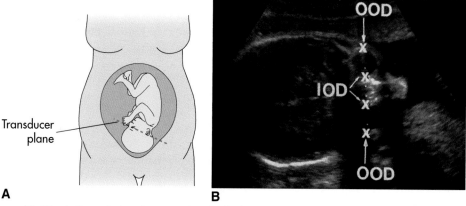

Figure 45-17   **A,** Frontal view demonstrating the fetal cranium in an occipitotransverse position. The transducer is placed along the orbitomeatal line (approximately 2 to 3 cm below the level of the biparietal diameter). **B,** Sonogram demonstrating the orbits in the occipitotransverse position. *OOD,* Outer orbital diameter; *IOD,* inner orbital diameter.

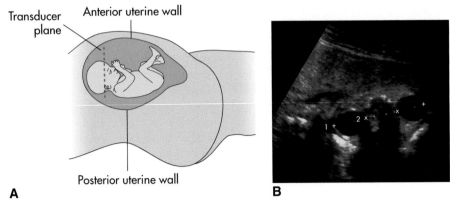

Figure 45-18 **A,** Side view demonstrating the fetus in an occipitoposterior position. The transducer is placed in a plane that transects the occiput, orbits, and nasal processes. **B,** Sonogram of the orbits in an occipitoposterior position.

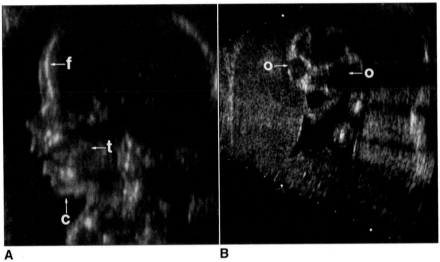

Figure 45-19 **A,** Sagittal view in a 23-week fetus showing the contour of the face in profile. Note the smooth surface of the frontal bone *(f)*, the appearance of the nose and upper and lower lips, tongue *(t)*, and chin *(c)*. **B,** Coronal facial view in an 18-week fetus, revealing a wide-open mouth. Note the nasal bones between the orbits *(o)*.

behaviors produces an enlightening scanning session because fetal yawning, swallowing, and eye movements may be observed. These behaviors may provide insightful clues to fetal well-being.

The fetal face may be recognized even in the first trimester of pregnancy and the gestational age at which the nasal bone first appears may contribute to aneuploidy risk determination. Facial morphology becomes more apparent in the second trimester, but visualization is heavily dependent on fetal positioning, adequate amounts of amniotic fluid, and excellent acoustic windows. The incorporation of three-dimensional ultrasound imaging has enhanced images of facial details and created patient demand for "fetal portraits."

Anatomic Landmarks of the Facial Profile. Views of the fetal forehead and facial profile are achieved by imaging the facial profile (Figure 45-19). In this view, the contour of the frontal bone, the nose, the upper and lower lips, and the chin may be assessed. Profile views of the face are useful in determining the relationship of the nose to the lips, in excluding forehead malformations (e.g., anterior cephaloceles, abnormal slopes, or **frontal bossing** [as seen in some forms of skeletal dysplasias]), and in assessing the formation of the chin (to exclude an abnormally small chin [**micrognathia**]). In a normally proportioned face, the segments containing the forehead, the eyes and nose, and the mouth and chin each form approximately one third of the profile.

Anatomic Landmarks of the Coronal Facial View. By placing the transducer in a coronal scanning plane, sectioning through the face reveals both orbital rings, the parietal bones, ethmoid bones, nasal septum, zygomatic bone, maxillae, and mandible (Figure 45-20). Scans obtained in an anterior plane over the orbits demonstrate the eyelids and, when directed posterior to this plane, the orbital lens. The eyeglobes, hyaloid artery, and vitreous matter have been sonographically identified.

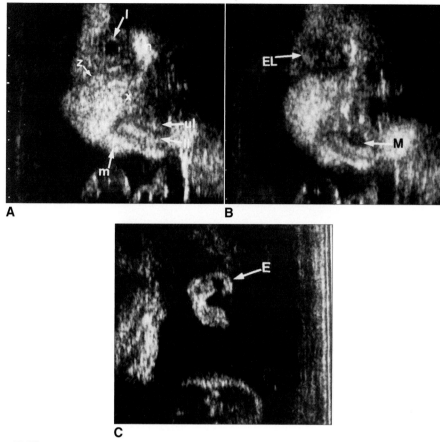

Figure 45-20 **A,** Coronal view showing facial features. *l,* Lens; *ll,* lower lip; *m,* mandible; *n,* nasal bones; *ul,* upper lip; *x,* maxilla; *z,* zygomatic bone. **B,** In the same fetus the eyelids *(EL)* and mouth *(M)* are shown. **C,** In the same fetus the ear *(E)* is shown.

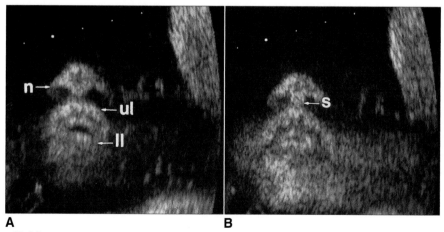

Figure 45-21 **A,** Axial view through the upper *(ul)* and lower lip *(ll)* in a fetus with an open mouth. Note the nares *(n)* and nasal septum. This is the view used to check for a cleft of the upper lip. **B,** In the same fetus, same anatomy viewed with a closed mouth. *s,* Nasal septum.

The oral cavity and tongue are frequently outlined during fetal swallowing (see Figure 45-19). Tangential views of the face help differentiate the nostrils, nares, nasal septum, maxillae, and mandible (Figure 45-21). This view is helpful in the diagnosis of craniofacial anomalies, such as cleft lip.

Sonographers should strive to diagnose cleft lip in utero, as prenatal classes for parents of these children are associated with faster weight gain, quicker surgical intervention, and better outcomes postnatally. It is important to recognize normal facial landmarks that may mimic defects as well.

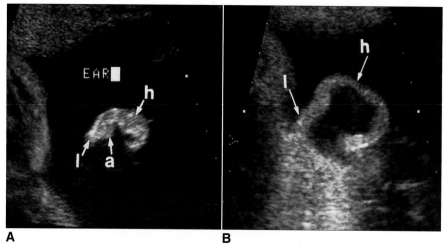

Figure 45-22   A, The external ear observed in a 26-week fetus showing the helix *(h)*, lobule *(l)*, and antitragicus *(a)*. **B,** At 36 weeks of gestation, the lobule *(l)* and helix *(h)* are observed.

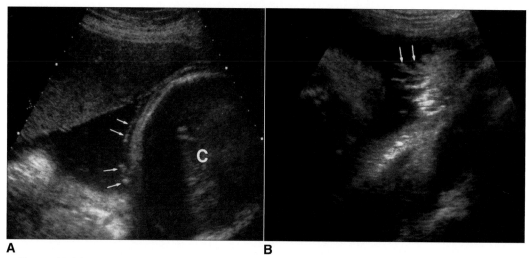

Figure 45-23   A, Fetal hair *(arrows)* observed as a series of dots around the periphery of the fetal cranium in a 39-week fetus. *C,* Cranium. **B,** Long hair *(arrows)* observed in a 34-week fetus.

The fetal ears may be defined in the second trimester as lateral protuberances emerging from the parietal bones. Later in pregnancy, the components of the external ear, helix, lobule, and antitragicus (small muscle in the pinna of the ear) may be seen (Figure 45-22). The semicircular canals and internal auditory meatus have been sonographically recognized.

Fetal hair is often observed along the periphery of the skull and must not be included in the biparietal diameter measurement (Figure 45-23).

THE VERTEBRAL COLUMN

The standard antepartum obstetrical examination guidelines require the sonographer to image and record the cervical, thoracic, lumbar, and sacral spine. The anatomy of the vertebral column should be assessed in all fetuses referred for obstetric evaluation. A gross anatomic survey of the spine should be attempted to exclude major spinal malformations (e.g., meningomyelocele).

The longitudinal fetal spine is studied in coronal, sagittal, and transverse scanning planes. There are three ossification points in each vertebra. When scanning in the coronal and sagittal planes, only two ossification points are typically seen. In a sagittal section, the spine appears as two curvilinear lines extending from the cervical spine to the sacrum. The normal fetal spine tapers near the sacrum and widens near the base of the skull (Figures 45-24 through 45-26). This double line appearance of the spine is referred to as the "railway sign" and is generated by echoes from the posterior and anterior laminae and spinal cord.

When the scanning plane crosses both laminae and equal amounts of tissue are noted on either side of the spinal echoes, the transverse processes and vertebral bodies are delineated. This is the scanning plane in which to screen for spinal defects.

In a transverse plane, all three ossification points are visible. The three are spaced equidistant and the spinal column appears as a closed circle, indicating closure of the neural

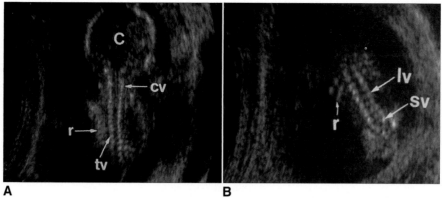

Figure 45-24 **A,** Coronal view of the fetal spine in a 15-week fetus outlining the cervical vertebrae *(cv)* and cranium *(C)*. The thoracic vertebrae *(tv)* are visualized distally. The rib *(r)* aids in localizing the thorax. **B,** In the same fetus a coronal plane outlines the lumbar *(lv)* and sacral vertebrae *(sv)*. *r,* Rib.

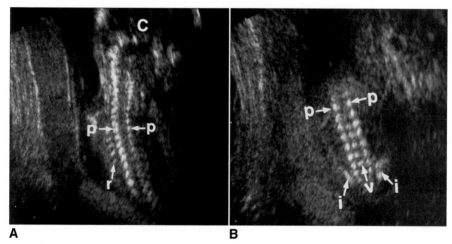

Figure 45-25 **A,** Coronal view of the spine in a 19-week fetus, demonstrating the parallel nature of the posterior elements, or laminae *(p)*, of the cervical and thoracic vertebrae. *C,* Cranium; *r,* rib. **B,** In the same fetus the lumbosacral vertebrae are observed in the coronal plane. The posterior elements *(p)*, or laminae, and vertebral body *(v)* are noted. In fetuses with spina bifida, widening across the posterior elements may be found (see Chapter 49). *i,* Iliac crest.

tube. Three echoes form a circle that represents the center of the vertebral body and the posterior elements (laminae or pedicles) (Figure 45-27). These elements should be identified in the normal fetus, whereas the pedicles appear splayed in a V-, C-, or U-shaped configuration in a fetus with a spinal defect.

When evaluating the spine, it is imperative for the sonographer to align the transducer in a perpendicular axis to the spinal elements. Incorrect angles may falsely indicate an abnormality. The spinal muscles and posterior skin border are viewed posterior to the circular ring of the ossification centers (see Figure 45-27). It is important to note the integrity of the skin surface because this membrane is absent in fetuses with open spina bifida. Inspection of the spine is often impossible when the fetus is lying with the spine posterior or against the uterine wall. Optimal viewing of the spine occurs when the fetus is lying on its side in a transverse direction with its back a slight

distance from the uterine wall. Often the sonographer will need to ask the mother to turn to either side in an effort to encourage the fetus to change positions so that a better image may be obtained.

THE THORAX

Although the fetus is unable to breathe air in utero, the lungs are important landmarks to visualize within the thoracic cavity. The lungs serve as lateral borders for the heart and are therefore helpful in assessing the relationship and position of the heart in the chest. Fetal breathing movements are also observed at this level. Like all fetal organs, the lungs are subject to abnormal development. Lung size, texture, and location should be assessed routinely to exclude a lung mass.

The fluid-filled fetal lungs are observed as solid, homogeneous masses of tissue bordered medially by the heart, inferiorly by the diaphragm, and laterally by the rib cage

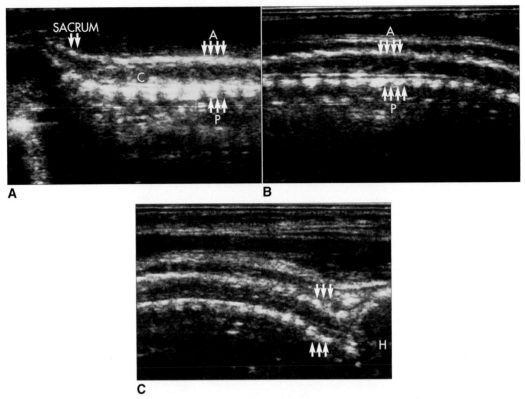

Figure 45-26 Longitudinal sections of the lumbosacral (**A**), thoracic (**B**), and cervical (**C**) spine in a 37-week fetus displaying the anterior (*A*) and posterior (*P*) elements, or laminae. Note the tapering of the spine at the sacrum (**A**) and the widening at the entrance into the base of the skull (**C**, *H* [head]). Between the posterior elements lies the spinal canal (**A**, *C*) and cord (may be seen as a linear echo within the spinal canal).

(Figure 45-28). The heart occupies a midline position within the chest; its displacement warrants further study to exclude a possible mass of the lung or a subdiaphragmatic hernia that may alter the position of the heart.

In sagittal views, lung tissue is present superior to the diaphragm and lateral to the heart (see Figure 45-28). Investigators have attempted to define textural variations of the lung in comparison to the liver. Fetal lung tissue appears more echogenic than the liver as pregnancy progresses.

The ribs, scapulae, and clavicles are bony landmarks of the chest cavity. Because these structures are composed of bone, acoustic shadowing occurs posteriorly. Portions of the rib cage may be identified when sections are obtained through the posterior aspects of the spine and rib cage (Figure 45-29). Oblique sectioning of the ribs reveals the total length of the ribs and floating ribs. On sagittal planes the echogenic rib interspersed with the intercostal space creates the typical "washboard" appearance of the rib cage (see Figure 45-29). Sound waves strike the rib and are reflected upward, leaving the characteristic void of echoes posterior to the bony element, whereas sound waves pass through the intercostal space.

On a transverse cross section through the chest and upper abdomen, the curvature of the rib may be appreciated below the skin. It is important to differentiate the rib from the skin wall, especially when measuring the abdominal circumference.

The entire rib cage is impractical to routinely examine, but study of the ribs is warranted in fetuses at risk for congenital rib anomalies (e.g., rib fractures found in osteogenesis imperfecta).

The clavicles are observed in coronal sections through the upper thorax (Figure 45-30). The clavicular length may aid in determining gestational age. In this same view the spinal elements, esophagus, and carotid arteries may be seen. The clavicles may also be demonstrated as echogenic dots superior to the ribs. Measurements of the clavicles may be useful in predicting congenital clavicular anomalies.

The scapula may be recognized on sagittal sections as an echogenic linear echo adjacent to the rib shadows, whereas on transverse sections it is viewed medial to the humeral head (see Figure 45-30). Oblique views demonstrate the entire length of the scapula. The sternum may be seen in axial sections as a bony sequence of echoes beneath the anterior chest wall.

THE HEART

The standard antepartum obstetrical examination guidelines require the sonographer to image and record a four-chamber view of the fetal heart. The reader is referred to Chapter 29 for more detailed fetal cardiac anatomy. Many major anomalies of the fetal heart are excluded when cardiac anatomy appears normal in the four-chamber view of the heart. These views

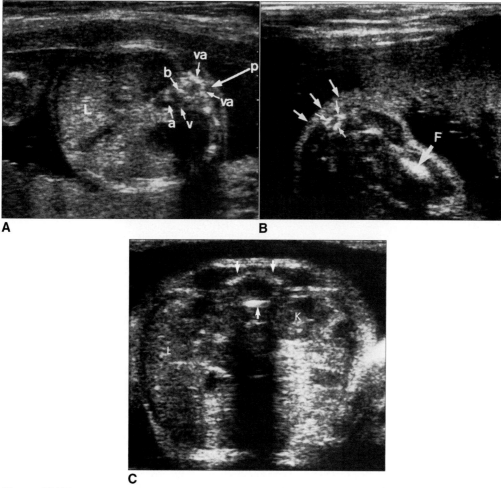

Figure 45-27 **A,** Transverse scans of the vertebral column showing the echogenic ring produced by the vertebral body and posterior elements, or laminae. Thoracic vertebrae with typical landmarks. *L,* Liver; *a,* aorta; *b,* body; *p,* posterior vertebral muscles; *v,* vena cava; *va,* vertebral arch or posterior elements. **B,** Sacral vertebra outlined *(small arrows).* Note the intact posterior skin wall in this normal fetus *(large arrows). F,* Femur. **C,** Transverse view through the spine at kidney level *(K)* demonstrating the closed-circle appearance *(arrows)* of the spine created by the intact vertebral arch. *L,* Liver.

further reduce the risk of cardiovascular anomalies. The heart lies more transversely in the fetus than in the adult because the lungs are not inflated. The apex of the heart is directed toward the left anterior chest with the right ventricle closest to the chest wall and the left atrium closest to the spine. The four chambers may be seen in a view taken with the beam perpendicular to the septum or in a view with the beam perpendicular to the valves (Figure 45-31). The four-chamber view may be obtained by angling cephalad after obtaining a transverse view of the fetal abdomen that displays the stomach. In our chamber views of the heart, it is important to assess the following:

- Cardiac position, situs, and axis. The apex of the heart should point to the fetal left side.
- Presence of the right ventricle (the ventricle found when a line is drawn from the spine to the anterior chest wall) and left ventricle.
- Equal-sized ventricles. By the end of pregnancy, the right ventricle may be larger than the left ventricle because it is

the chamber that pumps blood through the ductus arteriosus to the descending aorta and to the placenta.
- Presence of equal-sized right and left atria, with the foramen ovale opening toward the left atrium as blood is shunted from the right atrium, bypassing the lungs.
- An interventricular septum that appears uninterrupted. The septum appears wider toward the ventricles and thins as it courses cephalad within the heart.
- Normal placement of the tricuspid and mitral valves. The tricuspid valve inserts lower, or closer to the apex, than the mitral valve. Both valves should open during diastole and close during systole.
- Normal rhythm and rate (120 to 160 beats per minute).

Guidelines recommend that the standard antepartum obstetric examination include views of the ventricular outflow tracts when it is technically feasible. These views (Figure 45-32) can document that the aortic and the pulmonic outflow tracts are similar in size and appropriate in size for

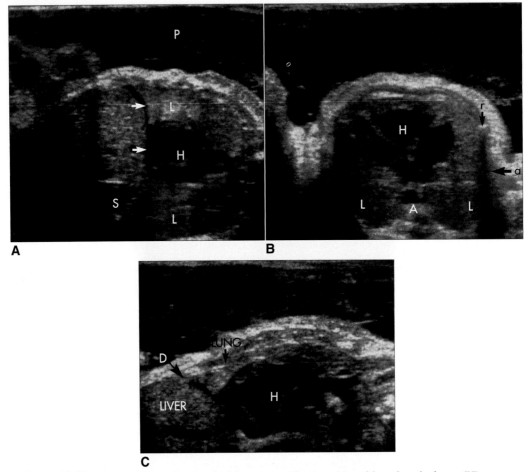

Figure 45-28 **A,** Sagittal scan showing the homogeneous lungs positioned lateral to the heart *(H)* and superior to the diaphragm *(arrows)*. Note the normal placement of the stomach *(S)* inferior to the diaphragm. *L,* Lungs; *P,* placenta. **B,** In same fetus a transverse section demonstrates the position of the lungs *(L)* in relationship to the heart *(H)*. Note the apex of the heart to the left side of the chest. The base of the heart is in the midline and anterior to the aorta *(A)*. Displacement or shifting of the heart should alert the sonographer to search for a mass of the lungs, heart, or diaphragm. Note the rib *(r)* and resultant acoustic shadow *(a)*. **C,** In the late third trimester of pregnancy, the lung tissue can be observed and compared with the liver texture. *D,* Diaphragm; *H,* heart.

gestational age, that the anterior wall of the aorta is contiguous with the ventricular septum (excludes overriding aorta), and that the great vessels are in normal alignment. These views may also provide additional images of the cardiac septum.

In fetuses at high risk for a cardiac anomaly, targeted fetal echocardiography is recommended to further evaluate the outflow tracts, pulmonic valve and veins, and other complex cardiac relationships beyond the scope of a standard obstetrical examination. (For further discussion of normal cardiac anatomy, physiology, and targeted echocardiography, see Chapters 29 and 30.)

THE DIAPHRAGM AND THORACIC VESSELS

The diaphragm is the muscle that separates the thorax and abdomen and is commonly viewed in the longitudinal plane. The diaphragm lies inferior to the heart and lungs and superior to the liver, stomach, and spleen (Figure 45-33). The diaphragm curves gently towards the thorax. If the diaphragm

extends outward toward the abdomen, it may be a sign of increased pressure in the thorax as a result of a thoracic mass or effusion. Sonographically, it appears as a sonolucent liner structure separating the thorax from the abdomen.

The diaphragm may be more obvious on the right side because of the strong liver interface, but attempts to observe an intact left diaphragm are encouraged because diaphragmatic defects occur on both sides of the diaphragm. The stomach should be viewed inferior to the diaphragm, which generally excludes a left-side diaphragmatic hernia.

Vascular structures may be observed within the thoracic cavity and neck. Vessels emanating from the heart are visible within the fetal neck. The carotid arteries (lateral to the esophagus) and the jugular veins (lateral to the carotid arteries) are frequently noted when the fetal neck is extended (Figure 45-34).

The trachea may be identified as a midline structure in both sagittal and transverse planes. The esophagus and oropharynx

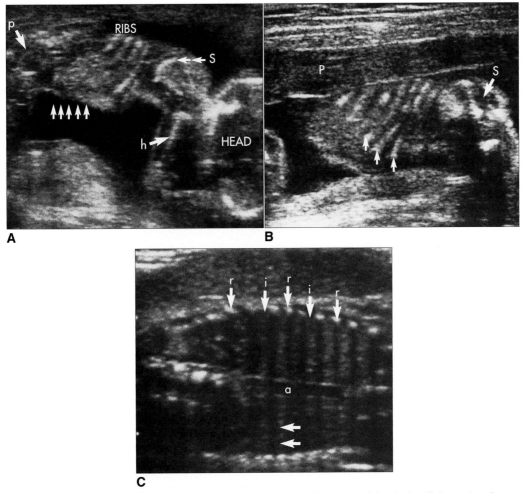

Figure 45-29 **A,** Sagittal view showing the rib cage, scapula *(S)*, anterior abdominal wall *(arrows)*, and humerus *(h)* in a fetus in a back-up position. *p,* Pelvis. **B,** Tangential view depicting the length of the ribs *(arrows)*. *P,* Placenta; *S,* shoulder. **C,** Sagittal view of the rib cage. Note that the sound waves are unable to pass through the bony rib, resulting in a shadow of echoes *(arrows)* posterior to the ribs *(r)*. Sound passes through the intercostal space *(i)*. *a,* Aorta.

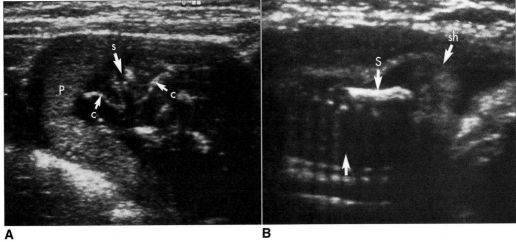

Figure 45-30 **A,** Coronal section of upper thoracic cavity showing the clavicles *(c)* and spine *(s)*. *P,* Placenta. **B,** Sagittal section demonstrating the scapula *(S)* in relationship to the shoulder *(sh)* and ribs *(arrow)*.

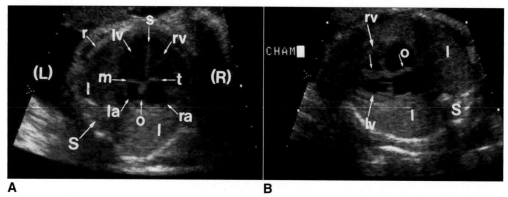

Figure 45-31 **A,** The four-chambered heart view is demonstrated in a 31-week fetus with the spine in the 7 o'clock position. The fetal right side is down and the left side is up. Structures observed are the right *(rv)* and left *(lv)* ventricles; the interventricular septum *(s)*, dividing the two ventricular chambers; and the left *(la)* and right *(ra)* atria. The foramen ovale *(o)*, which allows blood to shunt from the right to left atrium, permits the majority of blood to bypass the lungs. The flap of the foramen ovale is positioned within the left atrium. The atrioventricular valves (mitral and tricuspid) are viewed in systole (closed position). The tricuspid valve allows blood to move from the right atrium to the right ventricle *(rv)*, and the mitral valve *(m)* regulates blood flow from the left atrium to the left ventricle *(lv)*. Note the normal central position of the heart bordered by the lungs *(l)*. The apex of the heart is pointed to the fetal left side *(L)*. When a line is drawn from the spine *(S)* to the anterior chest wall, the right ventricle is found. *R,* Fetal right side; *r,* rib. **B,** In a 30-week fetus, the heart is observed in the 5 o'clock position. The fetal left side is down. The lungs *(l)* are viewed bordering the heart laterally. The muscularity of the interventricular septum *(arrow)* is observed along with the foramen ovale *(o)*, separating the atrial chambers. *lv,* Left ventricle; *rv,* right ventricle; *S,* spine.

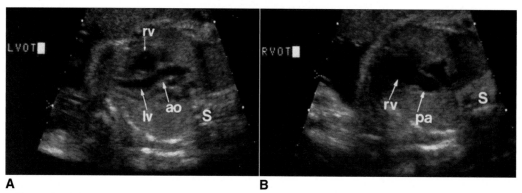

Figure 45-32 **A,** The left ventricular outflow tract *(LVOT)* is observed as the aorta *(ao)* exits the left ventricle *(lv)*. *rv,* Right ventricle; *S,* spine. **B,** The right ventricular outflow tract *(RVOT)* is observed as the pulmonary artery *(pa)* exits the right ventricle. The *LVOT* and *RVOT* should course perpendicularly to each other. *S,* Spine.

help determine the location of the carotid arteries and are outlined when amniotic fluid is swallowed by the fetus (Figure 45-35).

The aorta, inferior vena cava, and superior vena cava are routinely observed. The aorta is recognized on sagittal planes as it exits the left ventricle and forms the aortic arch (see Figure 45-33). The vessels branching cephalad into the brain may be observed in the cooperative fetus as they arise from the superior wall of the aortic arch. The innominate artery, left common carotid artery, and left subclavian artery may be identified (Figure 45-36).

As the vessels course posteriorly, the thoracic aorta and descending aorta are observed coursing into the bifurcation

of the common iliac arteries (Figure 45-37). The sonographer should recognize the characteristic arterial pulsations from the aorta and its branches. Further divisions of the aorta may be observed as the sonographer views the common iliac vessels, internal iliac vessels, and umbilical arteries (diverging laterally around the bladder) (see Figure 45-40). The external iliac arteries are observed as they enter the femoral arteries. The aorta is observed in a transverse plane to the left of the spine.

The inferior vena cava is identified coursing to the right and parallel with the aorta. Transversely, the inferior vena cava is seen anterior and to the right of the spine. It is important to note that the inferior vena cava appears anterior to the aorta

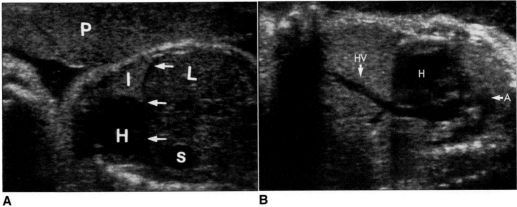

Figure 45-33 **A,** Sagittal scan showing the diaphragm *(arrows)* separating the thoracic and abdominal cavities. *H,* Heart; *L,* liver; *l,* lung; *P,* placenta; *s,* stomach. **B,** Sagittal view showing a hepatic vessel *(HV)* coursing through the liver before joining the inferior vena cava as it passes through the diaphragm and empties into the right atrium. Note the aortic arch, *(A)* exiting the heart *(H)* superiorly.

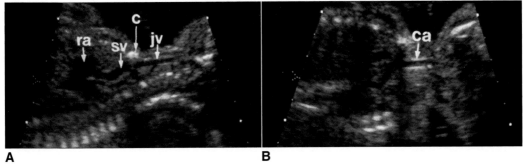

Figure 45-34 **A,** The jugular vein *(jv)* is observed laterally as it empties into the superior vena cava *(sv)* with drainage into the right atrium *(ra)* in a 25-week fetus; *c,* clavicle. This sagittal position is helpful in looking for neck masses such as a goiter (enlarged thyroid gland). **B,** A carotid artery *(ca)* is observed in a more medial location coursing cephalad into the brain.

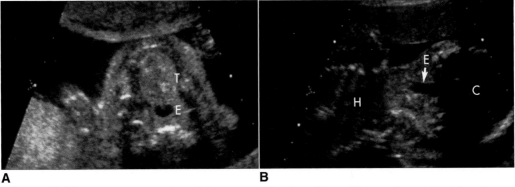

Figure 45-35 **A,** Cross section through the tongue *(T)* and esophagus *(E)* or oropharynx in a 24-week fetus. Recent swallowing of amniotic fluid by the fetus allows visualization of these structures. **B,** Fluid-filled esophagus *(E)* or oropharynx seen in a longitudinal view. The bolus of swallowed amniotic fluid will travel to the stomach. *C,* Cranium; *H,* heart.

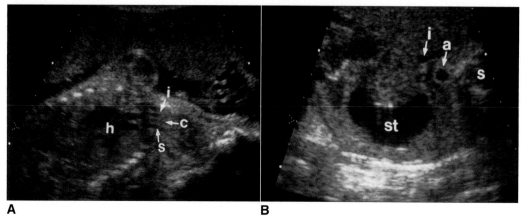

A   **B**

Figure 45-36 **A,** The aortic arch branches are shown in a 35-week fetus with an extended neck. *c,* Left common carotid artery; *h,* heart; *i,* innominate artery; *s,* left subclavian artery. **B,** Aorta *(a)* visualized to the left of the spine *(s)* in a transverse cross section. *i,* Inferior vena cava; *st,* stomach.

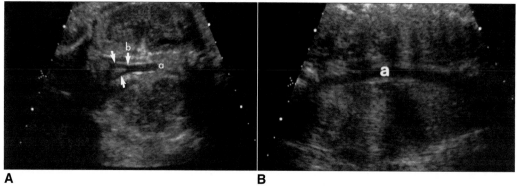

A   **B**

Figure 45-37 **A,** The bifurcation *(b)* of the aorta *(a)* into the common iliac arteries *(arrows)* is viewed in a 32-week fetus. **B,** In the same fetus a sagittal plane shows the abdominal portion of the aorta *(a).*

within the chest as the vena cava enters anteriorly at the junction of the right atrium.

The hepatic veins may be imaged in sagittal planes or in cephalad-directed transverse planes. The right, left, and middle hepatic vessels are often delineated and followed as they drain into the inferior vena cava (Figure 45-38).

Differentiation of a hepatic and portal vessel may be possible by evaluating the thickness of the vessel wall. In general, the walls of the portal vessels are more echogenic than those of hepatic vessels.

Divisions of the inferior vena cava (i.e., renal veins, hepatic veins, and iliac veins) may be observed. The superior vena cava may be outlined entering the right atrium from above the heart. By following the superior vena cava into the neck, the jugular veins may be observed.

FETAL CIRCULATION

Fetal oxygenation occurs in the placenta where small fetal vessels on the surface of the villi are bathed by maternal blood within the intervillous spaces. Fetal basal metabolic rate and temperature are higher, causing fetal blood levels of essential nutrients to be relatively low compared with maternal blood. Oxygen and nutrients from maternal blood cross by simple diffusion to fetal vessels. Concentrations of waste products, such as urea and creatinine, are higher in fetal blood, and these products diffuse into the maternal circulation.

Fetal circulation differs from postnatal circulation. Fetal circulation bypasses the lungs because the fetal lungs do not oxygenate blood. The ductus arteriosus shunts blood away from the lungs. Fetal circulation shunts oxygenated blood arriving from the placenta away from the abdomen directly to the heart and then to the brain. The hepatobiliary system serves the important function of shunting oxygen-rich blood arriving from the placenta directly to the heart through the ductus venosus (Figure 45-39).

Oxygenated blood from the placenta flows through the umbilical vein, within the umbilical cord, to the fetal cord insertion, where it enters the abdomen (Figure 45-40). From the umbilicus, the umbilical vein courses cephalad along the falciform ligament to the liver, where it connects with the left portal vein (Figure 45-41). The left portal vein courses posteriorly to meet the right anterior and right posterior portal veins (Figure 45-42). This blood then filters into the liver sinusoids, returning to the inferior vena cava by drainage into the hepatic veins.

A special vascular connection, the **ductus venosus,** carries oxygen-rich blood from the umbilical vein directly to the

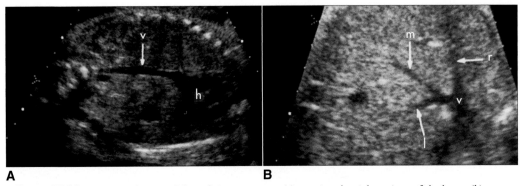

Figure 45-38   **A,** Sagittal view of the inferior vena cava *(v)* entering the right atrium of the heart *(h)*. **B,** The left *(l)*, middle *(m)*, and right *(r)* hepatic veins are shown emptying into the inferior vena cava *(v)*.

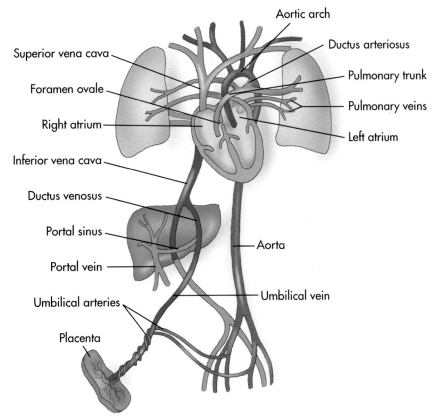

Figure 45-39   Fetoplacental circulation.

inferior vena cava, which empties directly into the right atrium. This blood bypasses the liver. Inferior vena cava blood flows from the right atrium through the left atrium by way of the foramen ovale. This blood bypasses the lungs. Less oxygenated blood from the superior vena cava and a small portion of blood from the inferior vena cava empty into the right atrium and into the right ventricle. Both ventricles pump blood into the systemic circulation at the same time. Blood ejected from the left ventricle flows to the ascending aorta and to the fetal brain. From the right ventricle, the blood courses from the pulmonary artery into the **ductus arteriosus** and through the descending aorta to provide oxygenated blood to the abdominal organs. Deoxygenated blood

exits the fetus through the umbilical arteries, which arise from the fetal iliac arteries. Only 5% to 10% of the blood actually circulates to the lungs. After birth the foramen ovale, the ductus venosus, and the ductus arteriosus close; fetal circulation converts to this pattern as seen throughout the rest of life.

THE HEPATOBILIARY SYSTEM AND UPPER ABDOMEN
The fetal hepatobiliary system includes the liver, portal venous system, hepatic veins and arteries, gallbladder, and bile ducts. The circulation of fetal blood through the ductus venosus in the hepatobiliary system is unique to intrauterine life. The ductus venosus blood flow is a direct link to the fetal heart,

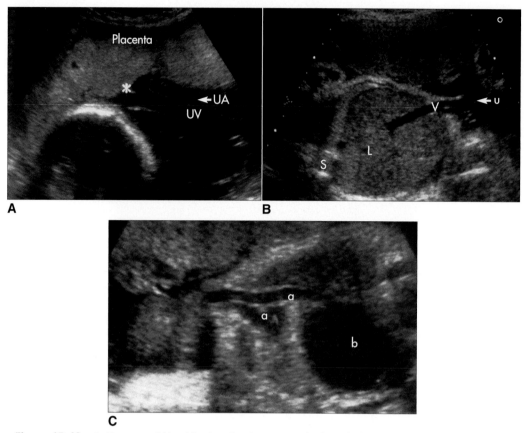

Figure 45-40 **A,** Oxygenated blood leaving the placenta travels through the umbilical vein *(UV)* to the fetal umbilicus. *UA,* Umbilical artery; *asterisk,* placental cord insertion. **B,** The umbilical vein *(v)* after entering at the umbilicus *(u)* courses cephalad and into the liver *(L). S,* Spine. **C,** The umbilical arteries *(a)* enter the umbilicus and course laterally around the bladder *(b)* to meet the common iliac arteries.

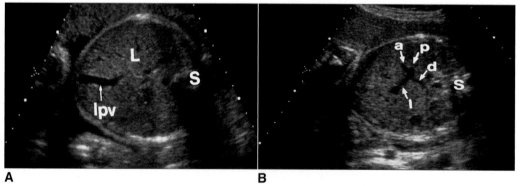

Figure 45-41 **A,** Transverse section of the liver in a 31-week fetus outlining the course of the left portal vein *(lpv)* at its entrance into the liver *(L)* from the fetal umbilical cord insertion. The left portal vein ascends upward and into the liver tissue. *S,* Spine. **B,** The left portal vein *(l)* is shown to bifurcate into the portal sinus, right anterior *(a)* and right posterior *(p)* portal veins. The ductus venosus *(d)* is observed before its drainage into the inferior vena cava. *S,* Spine.

and fetal heart failure may be diagnosed by Doppler analysis of flow through the ductus venosus.

The liver is a large organ filling most of the upper abdomen. The left lobe of the liver is larger than the right lobe because of the large quantity of oxygenated blood flowing through the left lobe. The liver appears pebble-gray and is discerned by its corresponding portal and hepatic vessels. The liver borders may be seen by viewing the diaphragm at the cephalad margin and the small bowel distally in the sagittal plane (Figure 45-43). The fetal liver is the main storage site for glucose and is very sensitive to disturbances in growth; therefore, this is the site at which abdominal measurements reflect liver size. It is

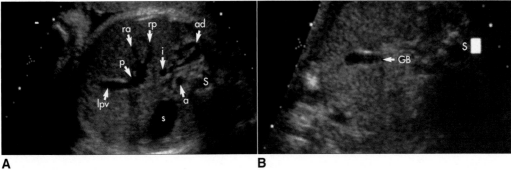

Figure 45-42 **A,** Transverse section of the liver and related structures in a 32-week fetus showing the left portal vein *(lpv)* coursing into the portal sinus *(p)*. The blood then moves into the right anterior *(ra)* and right posterior *(rp)* portal veins and ductus venosus (see Figure 28-41, *B*). The right adrenal gland *(ad)*, fluid-filled stomach *(s)*, aorta *(a)*, and inferior vena cava *(i)* are shown. **B,** The gallbladder *(GB)* is viewed in the right upper quadrant of the abdomen in a 32-week fetus. The teardrop shape of the gallbladder should be distinguished from the left portal vein. *S,* Spine.

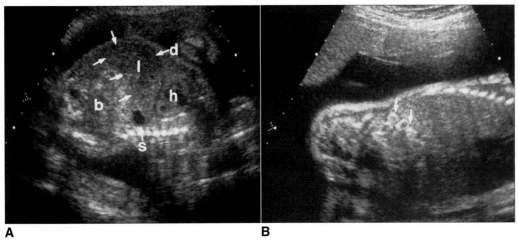

Figure 45-43 **A,** Liver *(l, arrows)* bordered by the diaphragm *(d)* superiorly and bowel inferiorly in a 29-week fetus. *b,* bowel; *h,* heart; *s,* stomach. **B,** Small bowel *(arrows)* pictured as small fluid-filled rings.

important to check for any collection of fluid around the liver margins because this indicates ascites (fluid retention resulting from anemia, heart failure, or congenital anomalies). Masses of the liver are uncommon, but may be detected.

The fetal gallbladder appears as a cone-shaped or teardrop-shaped cystic structure located in the right upper abdomen just below the left portal vein (see Figure 45-42). The gallbladder should not be misinterpreted as the left portal vein. The left portal vein is a midline vessel that appears more tubular and can be traced back to the umbilical insertion.

The fetal pancreas may be seen posterior to the stomach and anterior to the splenic vein when the fetus is lying with the spine down.

The spleen may be observed by scanning transversely and posteriorly to the left of the stomach (Figure 45-44). Recognition of the spleen is helpful when assessing the sensitized pregnancy (anti-D) to check for enlargement resulting from increased blood production (hematopoiesis) or to screen for anomalies of the spleen, such as duplication defects.

THE GASTROINTESTINAL SYSTEM

The fetal gastrointestinal tract comprises the esophagus, stomach, and small and large intestines (colon). Guidelines for the standard antepartum obstetrical examination require the sonographer to image and document the stomach. The esophagus may be recognized after fetal ingestion of amniotic fluid, which may be traced during swallowing into the oral cavity, through the hypopharynx, and as it travels downward toward the stomach (see Figure 45-35).

The stomach becomes apparent as early as the 11th week of gestation because swallowed amniotic fluid fills the stomach cavity. The full stomach should be seen in all fetuses beyond the 16th week of gestation. Some conditions prohibit normal filling of the stomach, such as diminished amounts of amniotic fluid (fetuses with rupture of the membranes) or blockage that prevents the stomach from filling (esophageal atresia). On occasion, the stomach has emptied into the small bowel before scanning and is not observed. Repeat studies to confirm the presence of the stomach are warranted. Enlargement of the

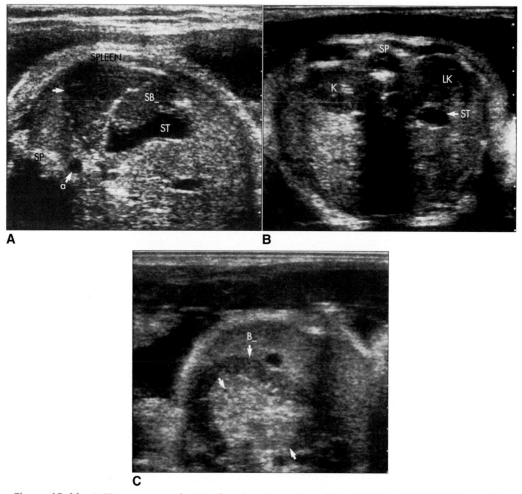

Figure 45-44 **A,** Transverse scan showing the spleen *(arrows)*, small bowel *(SB)*, and fluid-filled stomach *(ST)*. *a,* Aorta; *SP,* spine shadow. **B,** Transverse section showing the right kidney *(K)* and stomach *(ST)* anterior to the left kidney *(LK)* in a fetus in a spine-up position *(SP)*. **C,** Transverse view of the transverse colon *(B)* and small bowel *(arrows)* in a fetus in a spine-down position.

stomach may occur when a fetus ingests a large quantity of amniotic fluid (non–insulin-dependent diabetic pregnancies) or when a congenital anomaly prohibits normal passage of fluid through the bowel (duodenal atresia).

A normal bowel may be distinguished prenatally by observing characteristic sonographic patterns for each segment. Beyond 20 weeks of gestation, small bowel may be differentiated from large bowel. Small bowel appears to occupy a central position within the lower abdomen, with a cluster appearance of the bowel loops. Peristalsis and even fluid-filled small bowel loops may be observed (see Figures 45-43 and 45-44).

The large intestine with the ascending, transverse, and descending colon and rectum are identified by their peripheral locations in the lower pelvis (see Figure 45-44). The large bowel typically contains meconium particles and may measure up to 20 mm in the preterm fetus and even larger near the time of birth or in the postdate fetus.

THE URINARY SYSTEM

Guidelines for the standard antepartum obstetrical examination require the sonographer to image and document the kidneys and the bladder. The urinary system of the fetus is composed of the kidneys, adrenal glands, ureters, and bladder.

The kidneys are located on either side of the spine in the posterior abdomen and are apparent as early as the 15th week of pregnancy. The appearance of the developing kidney changes with advancing gestational age. In the second trimester of pregnancy, the kidneys appear as ovoid retroperitoneal structures that lack distinctive borders. The pelvocaliceal center may be difficult to define in early pregnancy, whereas with continued maturation of the kidneys the borders become more defined, and the renal pelvis becomes more distinct (Figure 45-45). The renal pelvis appears as an echo-free area in the center of the kidney.

The normal renal pelvis appears to contain a small amount of fluid. This most often represents a normal finding during pregnancy. A renal pelvis that measures greater than 10 mm beyond 20 weeks of gestation is considered abnormal. It is common to see extra fluid within the renal pelvis in fetuses with extra amounts of amniotic fluid and when the mother has a full bladder. There has been some association of renal pelvis dilation and chromosomal abnormalities.

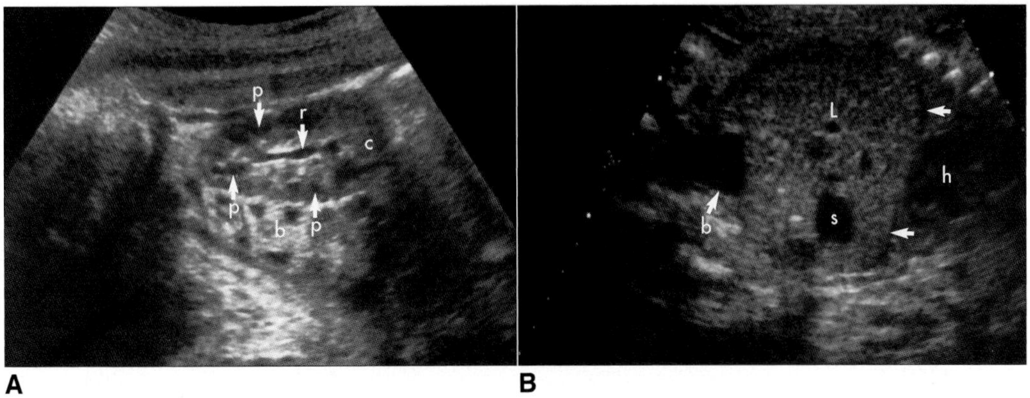

Figure 45-45 **A,** Longitudinal view of the kidney in a 35-week fetus showing the renal cortex *(c)*, pelvis, and pyramids *(p)*. The kidney is marginated by the renal capsule, which is highly visible later in pregnancy because of perirenal fat. *b,* Bowel; *r,* renal pelvis. **B,** Sagittal view of the fluid-filled bladder *(b)* in the pelvis. Note the more cephalic location of the stomach *(s)* in the upper abdomen. *h,* heart; *L,* liver; diaphragm *(arrows).*

By the third trimester of pregnancy, internal renal anatomy becomes clear with observation of the renal pyramids (lining up in sequence in anterior and posterior rows), the cortex or medulla, and renal margins (perirenal and sinus fat at this age allows clear visualization) (see Figures 45-44 and 45-45).

The kidneys appear as elliptic structures when scanning in the longitudinal axis and appear circular in their retroperitoneal locations adjacent to the spine in transverse views. Commonly, in a transverse position, the bottom or distal kidney may be shadowed by the acoustic spine. The distal kidney may be imaged by rotating to the sagittal plane. With the fetus in the spine-up or spine-down position, the kidneys are observed lateral to the spine (Figure 45-46).

The length, width, thickness, and volume of the kidney have been determined for different gestational ages. This information is useful when a renal malformation is suspected.

The fetal adrenal glands are most frequently observed in a transverse plane just above the kidneys. The adrenals are seen as early as the 20th week of pregnancy and by 23 weeks assume a rice-grain appearance (Figure 45-47). The center of the adrenal gland appears as a central echogenic line surrounded by tissue that is less echogenic. The central midline interface widens after the 35th week of gestation. The transverse aorta may be used to locate the left adrenal gland because of its close proximity to the anterior surface of the gland. Likewise, the inferior vena cava is helpful in isolating the right adrenal gland. Occasionally the adrenal glands may be identified in sagittal planes, although rib shadowing may interfere with their recognition.

It is important to realize that adrenal glands may normally appear large in utero and should not be confused with the kidneys. The texture of the adrenal gland is similar to that of the kidney; often when a kidney is missing (agenesis), the adrenal is mistaken for the kidney. Nomograms for normal adrenal size are available. Visualization of the renal arteries with color Doppler may be helpful to confirm the presence of kidneys.

At 1 mm, the normal fetal ureter is too small to be recognized. Dilated or obstructed ureters (hydroureter) are readily apparent.

The urinary bladder is visualized in either transverse or sagittal sections through the anterior lower pelvis (see Figures 45-40 and 45-45). The bladder is located in midline and appears as a round, fluid-filled cavity. The size of the bladder varies, depending on the amount of the urine contained within the bladder cavity. A fetus generally voids at least once an hour, so failure to see the bladder should prompt the investigator to recheck for bladder filling.

The bladder should be visualized in all normal fetuses. The fetal bladder is an important indicator of renal function. When the bladder and amniotic fluid appear normal, one may assume that at least one kidney is functioning. If one fails to identify the urinary bladder in the presence of oligohydramnios (severe lack of amniotic fluid), one should suspect a renal abnormality or premature rupture of the membranes (the bladder may not be full because of decreased ingestion of fluid).

The fetal bladder size may appear increased in pregnancies complicated by polyhydramnios (large quantities of amniotic fluid).

THE GENITALIA

Guidelines for the standard antepartum obstetric examination require the sonographer to image and document the stomach, the kidneys, the bladder, the umbilical cord insertion site, and the number of vessels in the umbilical cord. Documentation of gender is not medically necessary in most pregnancies. Identification of the male and female genitalia is possible provided the fetal legs are abducted and a sufficient quantity of amniotic fluid is present. Providing information regarding gender identification is clinically important when a fetus is at risk for a gender-linked disorder (e.g., aqueductal stenosis or hemophilia) and in multiple gestations. Information regarding the gender of the fetus may have significant emotional impact; therefore, guidelines should be established within each depart-

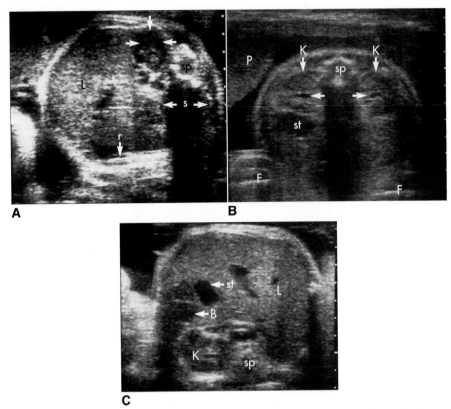

Figure 45-46 **A,** When the fetus is lying on its side, the upper kidney *(arrows)* is observed adjacent to the spine *(sp)*. The kidney on the bottom is shadowed *(s)* by the spine. *L,* Liver; *r,* rib. **B,** Kidneys *(K)* observed in a spine-up position *(sp)*. Note the renal pelvises *(arrows)*, which are filled with urine—a normal pregnancy finding. The stomach *(st)* is found anterior to the left kidney. Note the spine shadow. *F,* Femurs; *P,* placenta. **C,** When the fetus is lying with the spine *(sp)* down, the kidneys are viewed. The left kidney *(K)* is visible posterior to the bowel *(B)* and the stomach *(st)*. The right kidney is located slightly below this level. *L,* Liver.

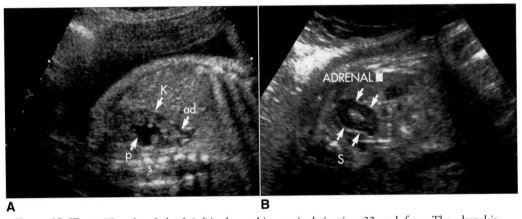

Figure 45-47 **A,** The adrenal gland *(ad)* is observed in a sagittal view in a 32-week fetus. The adrenal is located above the kidney *(K)* in this spine-down *(s)* position. The texture of the adrenal gland is similar to that of the kidney; often, when a kidney is missing (agenesis), the adrenal is mistaken for the kidney. *p,* Renal pelvis. **B,** The rice-grain appearance of the adrenal gland *(arrows)* is depicted in this transverse plane in a 36-week fetus. Note the dense central interface. *S,* Stomach.

ment regarding whether this information should be given. Only those investigators with proven gender detection skills should attempt to provide this information and only with consent of the patient.

When attempting to localize the genitalia, the sonographer should follow the long axis of the fetus toward the hips. The bladder is a helpful landmark within the pelvis by which to identify the anteriorly located genital organs. Tangential scanning planes directed between the thighs are useful in defining the genitalia. The gender of the fetus may be appreciated as early as 12 to 16 weeks of gestation, although clear delineation may not be possible until the 20th to 22nd week. When the fetus is in a breech position, gender may be impossible to determine.

The female genitalia may be seen in a transverse plane. The thighs and labia are identified ventral to the bladder, whereas in tangential projections, the entire labial folds, and often the labia minora, are visible (Figure 45-48). In scans of the perineum obtained parallel to the femurs, the shape of the genitalia appears rhomboid (Figure 45-49). Keep in mind that the labia may appear edematous and swollen. This normal finding should not be confused with the scrotum.

The scrotum and penis are fairly easy to recognize in either scanning plane (Figure 45-50). The male genitalia may be differentiated as early as the 12th week of pregnancy. The scrotal sac is seen as a mass of soft tissue between the hips, with the scrotal septum and testicles. Fluid around the testicles (hydrocele) is a common benign finding during intrauterine life.

THE UPPER AND LOWER EXTREMITIES

Guidelines for the standard antepartum obstetric examination require the sonographer to verify the presence or absence of legs and arms. The fetal limbs are accessible to both anatomic and biometric surveillance. Bones of the upper and lower appendicular skeleton have been described extensively, and many nomograms detailing normal growth patterns for each limb have been generated.

Fetal long-bone measurements help assess fetal age and growth and allow detection of skeletal dysplasias and various congenital limb malformations. The sonographer must attempt to not only measure fetal limb bones but also survey the anatomic configurations of the individual bones whenever

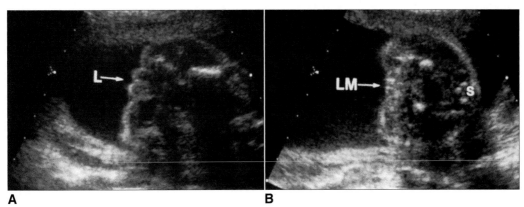

Figure 45-48   A, Female genitalia viewed axially in a 23-week fetus showing the typical appearance of the labia majora *(L).* **B,** In the same fetus, the labia minora *(LM)* are represented as linear structures between the labia majora. *s,* Spine.

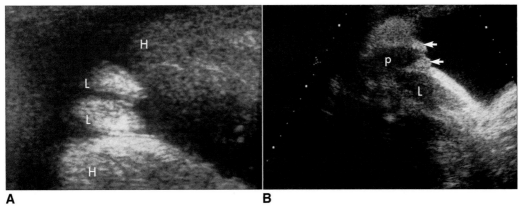

Figure 45-49   A, The labia majora *(L)* are imaged in a sagittal plane. *H,* Hips. **B,** The rhomboid-shaped perineum *(p)* is shown in a plane that runs parallel to the femur *(L).* The labia *(arrows)* are observed in a more frontal plane.

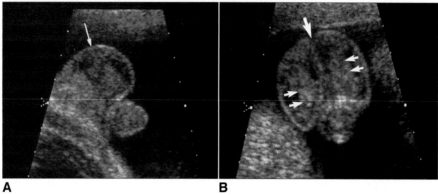

Figure 45-50 **A,** Male genitalia in a 40-week fetus showing the scrotum *(arrow)* and phallus. **B,** Coronal view of the male genitalia outlining descended testicles *(double arrows)* within the scrotum. Note the scrotal septum *(thick arrow)* and phallus.

possible for evidence of bowing, fractures, or demineralization, as seen in several common forms of skeletal dysplasias.

The upper extremity consists of the humerus, elbow, radius, ulna, wrist, metacarpals, and phalanges.

The humerus is found in a sagittal plane by moving the probe laterally away from the ribs and scapula. The long axis of the humerus should be seen lateral to the scapular echo. The cartilaginous humeral head is noted, as is the cartilage at the elbow (Figure 45-51). The shaft of the humerus should be seen, along with its characteristic acoustic shadow. Keep in mind that only the first echo interface of the bone is represented. The remainder of the bone is shadowed; therefore, the width of the bone is actually larger than what may be appreciated. The muscles and skin may be noted. Epiphyseal ossification centers may be apparent around the 39th week of pregnancy. In transverse planes, the humerus appears as a solitary bone surrounded by muscle and skin.

By tracing the humerus to the elbow, the radius and ulna are imaged (see Figures 45-51 and 45-52). In transverse sections, two bones are seen as echogenic dots, whereas in a sagittal plane the long axis of each is identified. The laterally positioned ulna projects deeper into the elbow, which is helpful in differentiating this bone from the medially located radius. When the transducer is moved downward, the wrist and hand are observed.

Coronally the hands and fingers may be viewed when opened. When the fingers are viewed in the sagittal plane, individual phalanges, interphalangeal joints, metacarpals, and digits may be observed (Figures 45-53 and 45-54). See also Figures 45-51 and 45-52. Hand movement may be studied to assess fetal tone for one component of the biophysical profile. Individual fingers may be assessed and counted. This is more commonly attempted if an anomaly is suspected, as in chromosome disorders, such as trisomy 18, in which clenching of the hands is common.

Adequate amounts of amniotic fluid are essential to evaluate the hands or feet. With oligohydramnios, the extremities may be difficult to localize.

Nomograms have been generated to determine the normal lengths of the humerus, radius, and ulna for age assessment.

These values are also beneficial in diagnosing abnormal developmental growth of the extremities, as seen in certain skeletal dysplasias.

Like the upper extremity, the bones of the lower extremity are accessible for dating conception and for detecting limb anomalies.

The femur is the most widely measured long bone and can be found by moving the transducer along the fetal body down to the fetal bladder. At this junction, the iliac wings are noted. By moving the transducer inferior to the iliac crests, the femoral echo comes into view. With the transducer centered over the femoral echo, one should rotate the probe until the shaft (diaphysis) of the femur is observed. In this view the cartilaginous femoral head, muscles, and occasionally the femoral artery are noted (Figure 45-55).

The distal femoral epiphysis is seen within the cartilage at the knee (see Figure 45-55), and this signifies a gestational age beyond 33 to 35 weeks of gestation. At the tibial end, the proximal tibial epiphyseal center is found after the 35th week of pregnancy (Figure 45-56). Medially the tibia and laterally positioned fibula (see Figure 45-56) are noted. The tibia is larger than the fibula.

The ankle, calcaneus, and foot are viewed at the most distal point (Figure 45-57). The diagnosis of clubfeet may be suspected when persistent and abnormal flexion of the ankle is seen. Individual metatarsals and toes are frequently seen (see Figure 45-57). Like the hands, the fetal feet may have malformations, such as extra digits, overlapping, and splaying.

THE UMBILICAL CORD

Guidelines for the standard antepartum obstetric examination require the sonographer to image and document the umbilical cord insertion site and the number of vessels in the umbilical cord. The normal human umbilical cord contains an umbilical vein and two umbilical arteries (Figure 45-58). The umbilical vein transports oxygenated blood from the placenta, whereas the paired umbilical arteries return deoxygenated blood from the iliac arteries of the fetus to the placenta for purification. The umbilical cord is identified at the cord

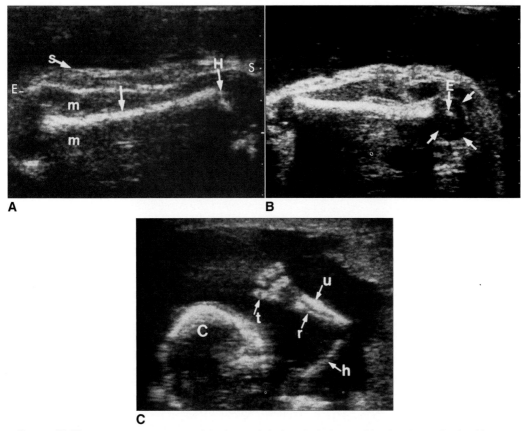

Figure 45-51 **A,** Longitudinal scan of the humeral shaft with the humeral head *(H)* near the shoulder *(s)*. Note the muscles *(m)* lateral to the bones and the skin interface *(S)*. *E,* Elbow. **B,** Similar section of a humerus in a 39-week fetus identifying the proximal humeral epiphysis *(E)* within the humeral cartilage *(arrows)*. **C,** Sagittal image of the fetal humerus. *C,* Cranium; *h,* hand with thumb; *t,* thumb; *r,* radius; *u,* ulna.

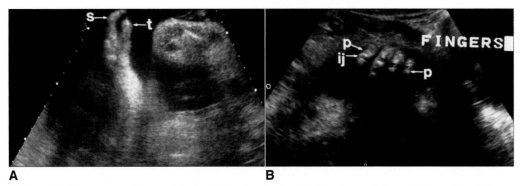

Figure 45-52 **A,** Lateral view of the hand showing the thumb *(t)* and second finger *(s)* in a 36-week fetus. **B,** Curvature of the hand in a 30-week fetus showing the phalanges *(p)* of the second through fifth fingers. The thumb is not imaged in this view because it is located slightly lower. Note the interphalangeal joints *(ij)* between the phalanges.

insertion into the placenta and at the junction of the cord into the fetal umbilicus. The arteries spiral with the larger umbilical vein, which is surrounded by Wharton's jelly (material that supports the cord) (Figure 45-59). Absent cord twists may be associated with a poor pregnancy outcome. The cord is easily imaged in both sagittal and transverse sections. The

umbilical vein diameter increases throughout gestation, reaching a maximum diameter of 0.9 cm by 30 weeks of gestation.

Identification of the placental insertion of the cord is important in choosing a site for amniocentesis and in the selection of the appropriate site for cordocentesis. Rarely

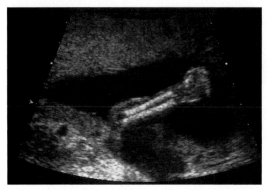

Figure 45-53 Long section of the forearm; the radius is shorter than the ulna (seen along the posterior forearm). The closed fist is shown with the thumb closest to the anterior surface.

the umbilical insertion is atypically located (velamentous insertion).

The insertion of the cord into the fetal umbilicus should be routinely scrutinized in all fetuses because anterior abdominal wall defects are present at this level. Use of color Doppler imaging at this location may demonstrate two umbilical arteries traveling on either side of the fetal bladder toward the iliacs. This image confirms two arteries and aids in three-vessel identification (Figure 45-60).

EXTRAFETAL EVALUATION

After the fetus has been studied, evaluation of the placenta, amniotic fluid, and extrauterine areas is recommended. As mentioned previously, the uterus and ovaries should be scrutinized for large masses, such as fibroids or ovarian masses that may alter pregnancy management. This evaluation may be accomplished by surveying the lateral borders of the uterus

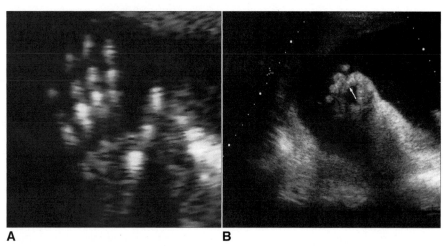

A   **B**

Figure 45-54 **A,** An open hand is shown in a 24-week fetus. **B,** A closed hand is viewed in a 38-week fetus with the thumb crossing in front of the palm of the hand *(arrow)*, with the second through fifth digits identified above the thumb.

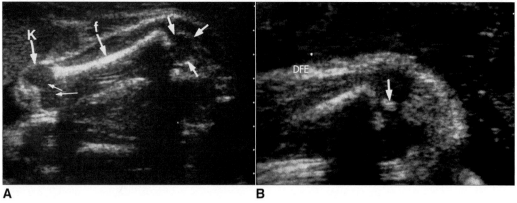

A   **B**

Figure 45-55 **A,** Longitudinal section showing the femoral shaft *(f)*, with the femoral cartilage *(thick arrows)* and epiphyseal cartilage *(thin arrows)* shown at the knee *(K)*. **B,** The distal femoral epiphysis *(arrow)* is clearly shown within the epiphyseal cartilage at the knee in a 42-week fetus. *DFE,* Distal femoral epiphysis.

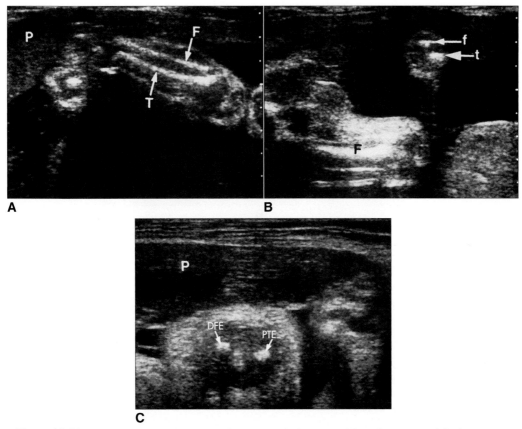

Figure 45-56 **A,** Sagittal view of the medially positioned tibia *(T)* and laterally positioned fibula *(F). P,* Placenta. **B,** In the same fetus, a transverse cross section reveals the two bones. *F,* Fibula; *f,* opposite femur; *t,* tibia. **C,** View of the knee in a 42-week fetus showing both the distal femoral epiphysis (DFE) and proximal tibial epiphysis (PTE). *P,* Placenta.

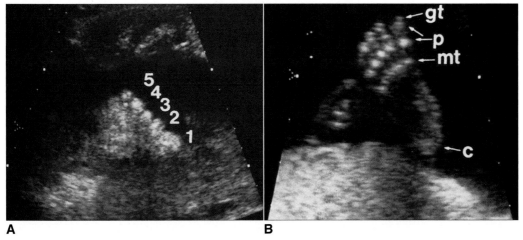

Figure 45-57 **A,** Five toes *(1* to *5)* viewed on end in a 38-week fetus. Note the continuity and shape of each toe. Extra toes, webbing, or clefts are considered abnormal. **B,** Plantar foot view in a 20-week fetus showing five toes and ossified metatarsals *(mt)* and phalanges *(p). c,* Calcaneus; *gt,* great toe.

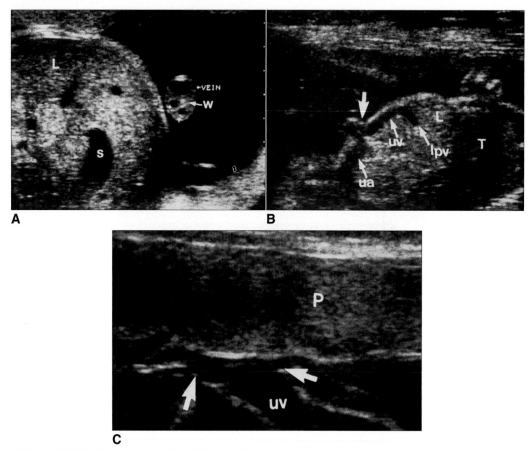

Figure 45-58 **A,** A three-vessel umbilical cord is shown in a transverse plane represented as paired umbilical arteries *(small arrows)* and a single larger umbilical vein. The vessels are supported by the gelatinous Wharton's jelly *(w)*. A cross section of the liver *(L)* and stomach *(s)* is in view. **B,** Fetal insertion of the umbilical cord into the umbilicus in a sagittal plane *(large arrow)*. The umbilical vein *(uv)* courses superiorly to enter the liver *(L)* and becomes the left portal vein *(lpv)*, whereas the umbilical arteries *(ua)* course posteriorly to join the hypogastric arteries. *T,* Thoracic cavity. **C,** Placental insertion of the umbilical cord showing the umbilical vein *(uv)* at this junction *(arrows)*. *P,* Anterior placenta.

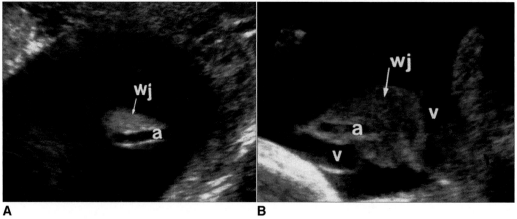

Figure 45-59 **A,** Wharton's jelly *(wj)* observed in a 30-week fetus. One of the umbilical arteries *(a)* is in view. **B,** Wharton's jelly is present adjacent to one of the umbilical arteries *(a)*, and the single umbilical vein *(v)* is observed in a 35-week fetus. Wharton's jelly is an important structure to recognize in performing cordocentesis procedures when the needle is directed into the cord vessels.

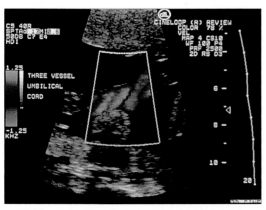

Figure 45-60   Color Doppler image showing the cord insertion into the fetal abdomen.

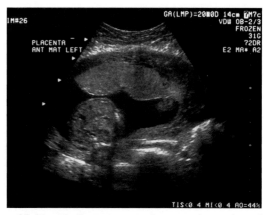

Figure 45-61   The homogeneous placenta is shown along the anterior wall of the uterus. The fetal abdomen is seen in cross section.

from the cervix to the fundus along both lateral margins following both sagittal and transverse axes.

The Placenta. The major role of the placenta is to permit the exchange of oxygenated maternal blood (rich in oxygen and nutrients) with deoxygenated fetal blood. Maternal vessels coursing posterior to the placenta circulate blood into the placenta, whereas blood from the fetus reaches this point through the umbilical cord.

The substance of the placenta assumes a relatively homogeneous pebble-gray appearance during the first part of pregnancy and is easily recognized with its characteristically smooth borders (Figure 45-61). The thickness of the placenta varies with gestational age, with a minimum diameter of 15 mm in fetuses greater than 23 weeks. The size of the placenta rarely exceeds 50 mm in the normal fetus. The sonographer must maintain a perpendicular measurement of the placental width in relation to the myometrial wall when evaluating the width of the placenta.

The position of the placenta is readily apparent on most obstetric ultrasound studies. The placenta may be located within the fundus of the uterus along the anterior, lateral, or posterior uterine walls (Figure 45-62), or it may be dangerously implanted over or near the cervix. The sonographer should attempt to carefully define the entire length of the placenta and document both upper and lower margins of this organ.

Occasionally the placenta originates in the fundus and proceeds along the anterior wall (fundal anterior placenta) or along the posterior uterine wall (fundal posterior placenta). When the placenta appears to lie on both anterior and posterior uterine walls, check for a laterally positioned placenta. By moving the transducer laterally, one should be able to define the lateral placenta.

The Amniotic Fluid. Amniotic fluid serves several important functions during intrauterine life. It allows the fetus to move freely within the amniotic cavity while maintaining intrauterine pressure and protecting the developing fetus from injury.

Amniotic fluid is produced by the umbilical cord and membranes, lungs, skin, and kidneys. Fetal urination into the amniotic sac accounts for nearly the total volume of amniotic fluid by the second half of pregnancy, so the quantity of fluid is directly related to kidney function. A fetus lacking kidneys or with malformed kidneys produces little or no amniotic fluid. The amount of amniotic fluid is regulated not only by the production of amniotic fluid but also by removal of fluid by swallowing, by fluid exchange within the lungs, and by the membranes and cord. Normal lung development is critically dependent on the exchange of amniotic fluid within the lungs. Inadequate lung development may occur when severe oligohydramnios is present, placing the fetus at high risk for developing small or hypoplastic lungs.

The volume of amniotic fluid increases to the 34th week of gestation and then slowly diminishes. The investigator must be aware of the relative differences in amniotic fluid volume throughout pregnancy. During the second and early third trimesters of pregnancy, amniotic fluid appears to surround the fetus and should be readily apparent (Figure 45-63). From 20 to 30 weeks of gestation, amniotic fluid may appear somewhat generous, although this typically represents a normal amniotic fluid variant. By the end of pregnancy, amniotic fluid is scanty, and isolated fluid pockets may be the only visible areas of fluid. Subjective observation of amniotic fluid volumes throughout pregnancy helps the sonographer determine the norm and extremes of amniotic fluid.

Several semiquantitative methods of estimating amniotic fluid volume have been developed. Measurement of the deepest vertical pocket of fluid in each of the four quadrants of the uterus and measurement of the single deepest pocket in the sac are two such methods.

Amniotic fluid generally appears echo-free, although occasionally fluid particles (particulate matter) may be seen. Vernix caseosa (fatty material found on fetal skin and in amniotic fluid late in pregnancy) may be seen within the amniotic fluid.

In accordance with the guidelines for obstetric scanning, every obstetric examination should include a thorough evaluation of amniotic fluid volume. When extremes in amniotic

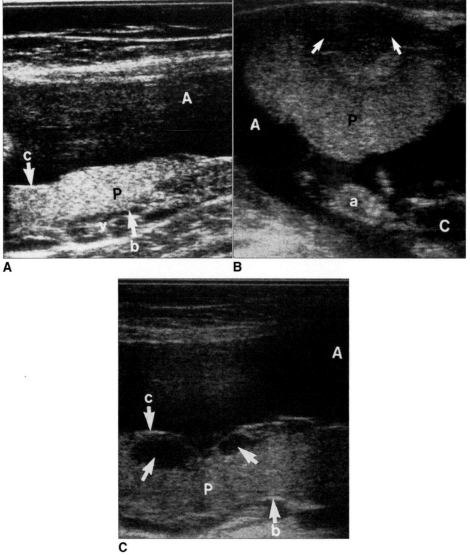

Figure 45-62 **A,** Posterior placenta *(P)* at 21 weeks of gestation showing the chorionic plate *(c),* adjacent to the amniotic cavity *(A),* and the basal plate *(b),* closest to the maternal (endometrial) vessels *(v).* **B,** Anterior placenta *(P)* at 14 weeks of gestation with evidence of a Braxton-Hicks contraction *(arrows).* *A,* Amniotic fluid; *C,* fetal cranium; *a,* fetal abdomen. **C,** Posterior placenta *(P)* at 26 weeks of gestation showing several subchorionic cystic spaces *(arrows)* that represent blood vessels or fibrin deposits. *A,* Amniotic fluid; *b,* basal plate; *c ,* chorionic plate.

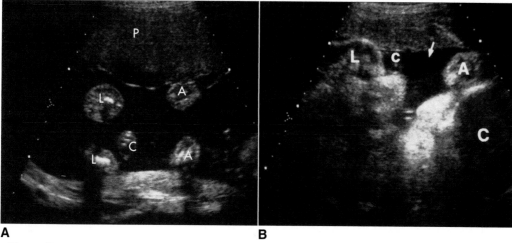

Figure 45-63 **A,** Amniotic fluid in a 20-week pregnancy outlining the legs *(L)* and arms *(A)*. This is a typical appearance of the abundance of amniotic fluid during this period of pregnancy. *C,* Umbilical cord; *P,* placenta. **B,** Amniotic fluid *(arrow)* in a 35-week pregnancy demonstrating an amniotic fluid pocket *(arrow)* surrounded by fetal parts and the placenta. The amount of amniotic fluid compared with the fetus and placenta is less at this stage of pregnancy. *A,* Arm; *C,* cranium; *c,* umbilical cord; *L,* leg.

fluid volume (hydramnios or oligohydramnios) are found, targeted studies for the exclusion of fetal anomalies are recommended.

ACKNOWLEDGMENT

The author would like to acknowledge the work of Kara L. Mayden Argo on a previous edition of this book.

SELECTED BIBLIOGRAPHY

Benson DM and others: Ultrasonic tissue characterization of fetal lung, liver and placenta for the purpose of assessing fetal maturity, *J Ultrasound Med* 2:489, 1983.

Birnholz JC: Ultrasonic fetal ophthalmology, *Early Hum Dev* 12:199, 1985.

Bowie JD and others: The changing sonographic appearance of fetal kidneys during pregnancy, *J Ultrasound Med* 2:505, 1983.

Callen PW, editor: *Ultrasonography obstetrics and gynecology,* ed 4, Philadelphia, 2003, WB Saunders.

Cardoza JD, Goldstein RB, Filly RA: Exclusion of fetal ventriculomegaly with a single measurement: the width of the lateral ventricular atrium, *Radiology* 169:711, 1988.

Chinn DH and others: Ultrasonic identification of fetal lower extremities epiphyseal ossification centers, *Radiology* 147:815, 1983.

Cicero S and others: Integrated ultrasound and biochemical screening for trisomy 21 using fetal nuchal translucency, absent fetal nasal bone, fre B-hCG and PAPP-A at 11 to 14 weeks, *Prenat Diagn* 23:306-310, 2003.

Ellis JW: Disorders of the placenta, umbilical cord, and amniotic fluid. In Ellis JW, Beckmann CRB, editors: *A clinical manual of obstetrics,* Norwalk, Conn, 1983, Appleton-Century-Crofts.

Filly RA: *The fetal neural axis: a practical approach for identifying anomalous development,* Chicago, 1992, The Society of Radiologists in Ultrasound.

Finberg HJ: Avoiding ambiguity in the sonographic determination of the direction of umbilical cord twists, *J Ultrasound Med* 11:185, 1992.

Fiske CE, Filly RA: Ultrasound evaluation of the normal and abnormal fetal neural axis, *Radiol Clin North Am* 20:285, 1982.

Gray D, Crane J, Rudolff M: Origin of midtrimester vertebral ossification centers as determined by sonographic waterbath studies of a dissected fetal spine. Paper presented at the annual meeting of the American Institute of Ultrasound in Medicine, Las Vegas, 1986.

Grignon A and others: Urinary tract dilatation in utero: classification and clinical applications, *Radiology* 160:645, 1986.

Guyton AC: Pregnancy and lactation. In Guyton AC, editor: *Textbook of medical physiology,* Philadelphia, 1981, WB Saunders.

Hoddick WK and others: Minimal fetal renal pyelectasis, *J Ultrasound Med* 4:85, 1985.

Isaacson G, Mintz MC, Crelin ES: Fetal head and neck. In Isaacson G, Mintz MC, Crelin ES, editors: *Atlas of fetal sectional anatomy,* New York, 1986, Springer-Verlag.

Jeanty P, Romero R, editors: How does a normal abdomen look? In *Obstetrical ultrasound,* New York, 1984, McGraw-Hill.

Jeanty P, Dramaix-Wilmet MS, Elkasan N: Measurement of the fetal kidney growth on ultrasound, *Radiology* 144:159, 1982.

Jeanty P, Dramaix-Wilmet MS, VanGansbeke D: Fetal ocular biometry by ultrasound, *Radiology* 143:513, 1982.

Jeanty P, Kirkpatrick C, Dramaix-Wilmet MS: Fetal limb growth, *Radiology* 140:165, 1981.

Jeanty P, Romero R, Hobbins JC: Vascular anatomy of the fetus, *J Ultrasound Med* 3:113, 1984.

Jeanty P and others: Normal ultrasonic size and characteristics of the fetal adrenal glands, *Prenatal Diagnosis* 4:21, 1984.

Jeanty P and others: Facial anatomy of the fetus, *J Ultrasound Med* 5:607, 1986.

Mahony BS and others: The fetal cisterna magna, *Radiology* 153:773, 1984.

Mahony BS and others: Epiphyseal ossification centers in the assessment of fetal maturity: sonographic correlation with the amniocentesis lung profile, *Radiology* 159:521, 1986.

Mayden KL: The umbilical vein diameter in Rh isoimmunization, *Med Ultrasound* 4:119, 1980.

Mayden KL and others: Orbital diameters: a new parameter for prenatal diagnosis and dating, *Am J Obstet Gynecol* 144:289, 1982.

Merz E: *Ultrasound in obstetrics and gynecology, vol 1: obstetrics,* New York, 2005, Thieme.

Nicolaides KH and others: *The 11-14 week scan: the diagnosis of fetal anomalies,* London, 1999 Partenon Publishing Group.

Nicolaides KH, Campbell S, Gabbe SG: Ultrasound screening for spina bifida: cranial and cerebellar signs, *Lancet* 2:72, 1986.

Nyberg DA, Mahony BS, Pretorius DH, editors: *Diagnostic ultrasound of fetal anomalies: text and atlas,* St Louis, 2004, Mosby.

Nyberg DA and others: Fetal bowel: normal sonographic findings, *J Ultrasound Med* 6:3, 1987.

O'Rahilly R, Muller F: *Human embryology and teratology,* New York, 1992, Wiley-Liss.

Pretorius DH and others: Linear echoes in the fetal cisterna magna, *J Ultrasound Med* 11:125, 1992.

Schmidt W and others: Sonographic measurements of the fetal spleen: clinical implications, *J Ultrasound Med* 4:667, 1985.

Sonek JD and others: Nasal bone length throughout gestation: normal ranges based on 3537 fetal ultrasound measurements, *Ultrasound Obstet Gynecol* 21:152-155, 2003.

CHAPTER 46

Obstetric Measurements and Gestational Age

Terry J. DuBose and Sandra L. Hagen-Ansert

OBJECTIVES

- List gestational sac growth and measurements
- Describe how to perform a crown-rump measurement
- Calculate the biparietal diameter, head circumference, abdominal circumference, and extremity measurements
- Assess fetal parameter measurements and fetal growth
- Describe when other measurements should be used to provide additional clinical information
- Evaluate fetal growth series for IUGR and growth disturbances

---

KEY TERMS

abdominal circumference (AC) – measurement at the level of the stomach, left portal vein, and left umbilical vein

age range analysis (ARA) – fetal parameter's size and proportionality expressed as age

anophthalmos – absence of one (cyclops) or both eyes

average age (AA) – average of multiple fetal parameters' ages

"banana" sign – refers to the shape of the cerebellum when a spinal defect is present (cerebellum is pulled downward into the foramen magnum)

binocular distance (BD) – measurement that includes both fetal orbits at the same time to predict gestational age

biparietal diameter (BPD) – fetal transverse cranial diameter at the level of the thalamus and cavum septum pellucidum

brachycephaly – fetal head is relatively wide in the transverse diameter and shortened in the anteroposterior diameter

Chiari malformations – associated with spinal defects

chorionic sac – see gestational sac

crown-rump length (CRL) – most accurate measurement for determining gestational age; made in the first trimester

dolichocephaly – fetal head is relatively narrow in the transverse plane and elongated in the anteroposterior plane

embryonic heart rate (EHR) – the heart rate before the early 9th week of gestation (after the LMP)

femur length (FL) – measurement of the femoral diaphysis

gestational sac – structure that is normally found within the uterus and contains the developing embryo

gestational sac diameter – used in the first trimester to estimate appropriate gestational age with menstrual dates

growth-adjusted sonar age (GASA) – the method whereby the fetus is categorized into small, average, or large growth percentile

humeral length – measurement from the humeral head to the distal end of the humerus

hypertelorism – condition in which the orbits are spaced far apart

hypotelorism – condition in which the orbits are close together

intrauterine growth restriction (IUGR) – condition in which the fetus is not growing as fast as normal, usually considered being malnourished or abnormal

last menstrual period (LMP) – the first day of the LMP is used as the start date for human pregnancies

"lemon" sign – occurs with spina bifida; frontal bones collapse inward

microphthalmos – small eyes

oxycephaly, acrocephaly – the condition of having a malformed cranial vault with a high or peaked appearance and a vertical index above 77. It is caused by premature closure of the coronal, sagittal, and lambdoidal sutures.

platycephaly – flattening of the skull
small for gestational age (SGA) – a normal but small fetus
spina bifida – failure of the vertebrae to close

Reliably assessing gestational age and the growth of the fetus has long posed a challenge to all who care for pregnant women. Although not without value, clinical parameters lack the necessary consistency to provide for optimal perinatal care. With recent advances in diagnostic sonography, fetal age and growth can now be assessed with high accuracy.

The definition of menstrual age versus fetal age is important to establish in clinical obstetrics. *Fetal age* begins at the time of conception and is also known as *conceptional age.* Conceptional age is restricted to pregnancies in which the actual date of conception is known, as found in patients with in vitro fertilization or artificial insemination. If conceptual age is already known, the menstrual age may be found by adding 14 days to the conceptual age.

Obstetricians date pregnancies in menstrual weeks, which are calculated from the first day of the **last** normal **menstrual period (LMP).** This method is called *menstrual age* or *gestational age.* The student of sonography must understand that the gestational ages are estimated from measurements of fetal parameters, and are not the actual age of the parameters. The estimated ages are no more accurate than the measurements taken, and all parameters in a fetus will not result in the same fetal age because fetuses have different proportions; some are long or short and fat or thin.

It is clinically important to know the menstrual age of a patient because this information is used for the following reasons:

- In early pregnancy to schedule invasive procedures (chorionic villus sampling and genetic amniocentesis)
- To interpret maternal serum alpha-fetoprotein screening
- To plan date of delivery
- To evaluate fetal growth

Before the use of sonographic determination of fetal growth, menstrual age was calculated by three factors: (1) the menstrual history, (2) physical examination of the fundal height of the uterus, and (3) postnatal physical examination of the neonate. This process was not always reliable if the patient could not recall the date of her last period or if other factors, such as oligomenorrhea, implantation bleeding, use of oral contraceptives, or irregular menstrual cycle, were present.

GESTATIONAL AGE ASSESSMENT: FIRST TRIMESTER

GESTATIONAL SAC DIAMETER

Endovaginal (transvaginal) sonography enables visualization and evaluation of intrauterine pregnancies earlier than was previously thought possible. The earliest sonographic finding of an intrauterine pregnancy is thickening of the decidua. Sonographically, this appears as an echogenic, thickening filling of the fundal region of the endometrial cavity occurring

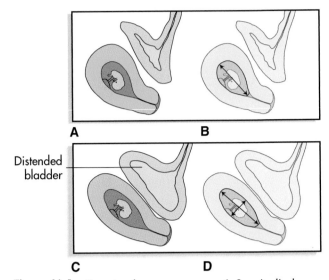

Figure 46-1   Gestational sac measurement. **A,** Longitudinal. **B,** The sac length should be measured from inner to inner borders. **C,** Transverse. **D,** The width of the sac should be measured along the inner to inner borders.

> **BOX 46-1   GESTATIONAL SAC MEASUREMENTS**
>
> - A distended urinary bladder has an effect on gestational sac measurement; it changes its shape from round to ovoid or teardrop.
> - If the sac is round, measure one diameter inner to inner.
> - If the sac is ovoid, make two measurements inner to inner: one transverse and the other perpendicular to the length.

at approximately 3 to 4 weeks of gestation (Box 46-1, Figure 46-1).

At approximately 4 weeks of menstrual age, a small hypoechoic area appears in the fundus or midportion of the uterus, known as the *double decidual sac sign.* As the sac embeds further into the uterus, it is surrounded by an echogenic rim and is seen within the choriodecidual tissue. This is known as the ***chorionic*** or ***gestational sac.***

At 5 weeks, the average of the three perpendicular internal diameters of the gestational sac, calculated as the mean of the anteroposterior diameter, the transverse diameter, and the longitudinal diameter, can provide an adequate estimation of menstrual age. A gestational sac should be seen within the uterine cavity when the beta human chorionic gonadotropin (beta hCG) is above 500 mIU/ml (second international standard). This becomes especially important when evaluating a pregnancy for ectopic implantation.

The sac grows rapidly in the first 10 weeks, with an average increase of 1 mm per day. According to one report, a gestational sac growing less than 0.7 mm per day is associated with impending early pregnancy loss.[16] Even the most experienced sonographer may incorporate a measuring error; therefore, the

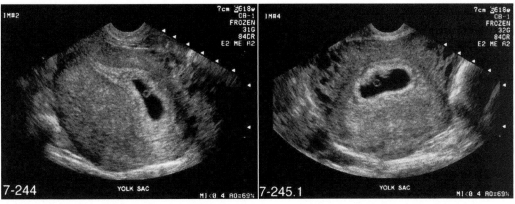

Figure 46-2   Sagittal and coronal images of a yolk sac in a 4-week gestation as seen with endovaginal ultrasound. The small gestational sac is well seen within the endometrial cavity of the uterus.

BOX 46-2   **ENDOVAGINAL SONOGRAPHIC LANDMARKS FOR EARLY PREGNANCIES**

- 500 mIU/mL beta-hCG = gestational sac seen
- > 8-mm gestational sac = yolk sac seen
- > 16-mm gestational sac = embryo seen
- < 6-mm yolk sac = normal
- > 8-mm yolk sac = abnormal
- > 7-mm fetal pole = positive cardiac activity

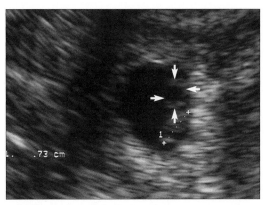

Figure 46-3   Endovaginal ultrasound measuring an early crown-rump length (CRL) *(crosses)*. The yolk sac is noted and outlined *(arrows)*. The CRL is consistent with 6.5 weeks.

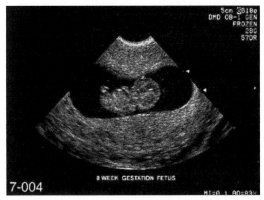

Figure 46-4   Endovaginal image of an 8-week gestation showing a developing embryo.

beta-hCG test in conjunction with a sonographic evaluation is suggested in a sequential time frame.

When the gestational sac exceeds 8 mm in mean internal diameter, a yolk sac should be seen (Figure 46-2). The yolk sac is identified as a small, spherical structure with an anechoic center within the gestational sac. It provides early transfer of nutrients from the trophoblast to the embryo. It also aids in the early formation of the primitive gut and vitelline arteries and veins and in the production of the primordial germ cells. Yolk sac size has not been correlated with gestational age determination. Normal yolk sac size should be less than 6 mm. Yolk sacs greater than 8 mm have been associated with poor pregnancy outcome, as have solid, echogenic yolk sacs. Box 46-2 lists sonographic landmarks for early pregnancy.

When the mean **gestational sac diameter** exceeds 16 mm, an embryo with definite cardiac activity should be well visualized with endovaginal scanning. This usually occurs by the 6th menstrual week (Figures 46-3 and 46-4), but may be as early as the 5th LMP week with endovaginal sonography. For the transabdominal scanning approach, the maternal urinary bladder must be filled to create an acoustic window. With this technique, the sac shape can vary secondary to bladder compression, maternal bowel gas, or myomas and should not be misinterpreted as abnormal.

Assessing gestational age using a single gestational sac diameter or even up to three averaged diameters yields an accuracy of only ±2 to 3 weeks in 90% of cases.[11] Accordingly, gestational sac diameter has not been widely used as a determinant

of gestational age after more accurate embryonic parameters can be measured (see Chapter 43).

CROWN-RUMP LENGTH

With endovaginal sonography, embryonic echoes can be identified as early as 38 to 39 days of menstrual age (Box 46-3, Figure 46-5). The **crown-rump length (CRL)** is usually 1 to 2

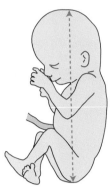

Figure 46-5   The crown-rump length should be measured along the long axis of the embryo from the top of the head to the bottom of the trunk.

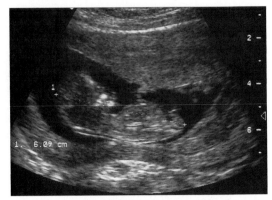

Figure 46-6   Transabdominal ultrasound demonstrating the proper landmarks for an accurate crown-rump length (CRL) measurement. The calipers should be placed at the top of the fetal head and the bottom of the fetal rump, excluding the legs or yolk sac. The CRL is consistent with a gestation of 12 weeks and 3 days.

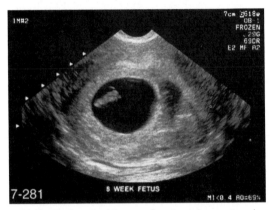

Figure 46-7   Endovaginal image of an 8-week gestation that shows a large gestational sac with a small, undeveloped embryo. No cardiac activity was identified.

> **BOX 46-3   CROWN-RUMP LENGTH (CRL)**
>
> - By endovaginal ultrasound the CRL can be measured from 6 to 12 gestational weeks.
> - Measurements should be made along the long axis of the embryo from the top of the head (crown) to the bottom of the trunk (rump).
> - This is the most accurate fetal age measurement.

mm at this stage. The embryo is usually located adjacent to the yolk sac. A CRL is the most accurate sonographic technique for establishing gestational age in the first trimester. The reason for this high accuracy is the excellent correlation between fetal length and age in early pregnancy because pathologic disorders minimally affect the growth of the embryo during this time.

The embryo can be measured easily with real-time dynamic imaging. For transabdominal imaging, the mother's bladder should be full to create an acoustic window. The measurement should be taken from the top of the fetal head to the outer fetal rump, excluding the fetal limbs or yolk sac. The accuracy is ±5 days with a 95% confidence level (Figure 46-6).[19] The average of at least three separate measurements of the CRL should be obtained to determine gestational age.

Cardiac activity should be seen when the CRL exceeds 7 mm, but may be seen by endovaginal sonography once the CRL reaches 2 mm. It is generally accepted to follow patients with small CRL and no fetal heartbeat over a few days. In general the CRL should increase at a rate of 8 mm per day. Occasionally an embryo is seen with no visible cardiac activity and a small CRL for menstrual age. It is advisable to wait a week and rescan to see if the patient spontaneously aborts the products of conception or if she needs medical intervention, such as a dilation and curettage procedure. Infrequently an appropriate fetal CRL and positive cardiac activity are seen after the week's wait (Figure 46-7). Why this happens is not known, but it has been observed by experienced sonographers.

Absence of an embryo by 7 to 8 weeks of gestation is consistent with an embryonic demise or an anembryonic preg-

nancy. If a nomogram is not readily available to identify gestational age, a convenient formula is gestational age in weeks = CRL in cm + 6. After the 12th week, a CRL is no longer considered accurate because of flexion and extension of the active fetus; therefore, other biometric parameters should be used.

EMBRYONIC HEART RATE

The embryonic heart rate accelerates linearly during the first month of beating between the 5th and 9th gestational weeks (Figure 46-8). This linear acceleration correlates well with the embryonic age before the CRL reaches 2.5 cm or before approximately 9.2 LMP weeks. The mean rate of acceleration is 3.3 beats per minute per day, 10 beats per minute every 3 days, or approximately 100 beats per minute between the start of beating until the early 9th week (Box 46-4). The embryonic age in days can be estimated with the following formula:

$$\text{LMP Age in Days} = \text{EHR} \times 0.3 + 6 \text{ days}$$

The result of the above estimation will be within ±6 days in 95% of normal pregnancies. If the age estimated by the CRL leads the age by EHR by more than 1 week, it may be prog-

Heart rate and age

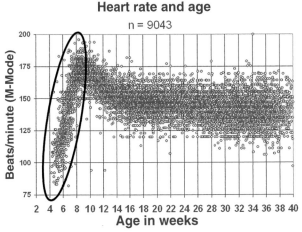

Figure 46-8   Scatter plot of 9043 embryofetal heart rates calculated by M-mode throughout gestation. Notice the rapid, linear acceleration in the first month from the early 5th week until the early 9th week. The peak heart rate of 175 beats per minute (mean, ±25) comes at 9.2 LMP weeks.

BOX 46-4   EMBRYONIC HEART RATE (EHR)

- By endovaginal ultrasound, the EHR can be measured by M-mode from the early 5th to early 9th gestational weeks when the CRL is less than 25 mm.
- The most accurate EHR measurements can be obtained by enlarging the 2-D image and using a fast sweep speed for the M-mode tracing. Measure from repeating distinct points on the M-mode.
- The EHR age will be accurate to within ±6 days. An EHR age that trails the CRL age by more than 6 days may be associated with impending first-trimester failure and warrants follow-up.
- The normal EHR accelerates linearly at 3.3 beats per minute per day, which is approximately 10 beats every 3 days, or 100 beats in the first month of beating.

---

nostic for first-trimester failure and warrants follow-up. Because the heart rate is accelerating so rapidly during the embryonic period, accurate M-mode measurements are desirable. The greatest accuracy can be achieved by magnifying the embryo as much as possible and using a fast M-mode tracing to stretch out the heartbeats for more precise cursor placement. The cursors should be carefully placed on identifiable, repeating locations of the M-mode tracing (Figure 46-9).

GESTATIONAL AGE ASSESSMENT: SECOND AND THIRD TRIMESTERS

FETAL MEASUREMENTS

In the second trimester, the gestational age parameters extend to the biparietal diameter, head circumference, abdominal circumference, femur length, and other parameters that may be used. It is critical for the sonographer to know precisely what

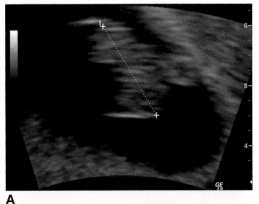

A

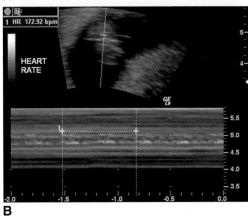

B

Figure 46-9   A, Endovaginal image measuring the CRL at 17.4 mm or 8.1 weeks. **B,** EHR of the same embryo measured by M-mode to be 173 beats per minute, which calculates to 8.3 weeks. The two-tenths difference in the ages is equal to 34 hours, or less than 2 days' difference, and is normal. (EHR age in days = $173 \times 0.3 + 6 = 57.9$ days = 8.27 weeks. (Courtesy Jyl Rogers.)

landmarks are necessary to determine these measurements. Proper gain settings, instrumentation, and fetal lie will all influence the accuracy of measurements used to estimate the gestational age.

Biparietal Diameter. In the second trimester, the **biparietal diameter (BPD)** was the first and is the most widely accepted means of measuring the fetal head and estimating fetal age. As the pregnancy enters the third trimester, an accurate measurement of fetal age becomes more difficult to obtain because the fetus begins to drop into the pelvic outlet cavity. The reproducibility of the BPD is ±1 mm (±2 standard deviations). When dating a pregnancy between 17 and 26 weeks of gestation, the predictive value is ±11 days in 95% of the population.[19] After 26 weeks, the correlation of BPD with gestational age decreases because of the increased biologic variability. The predictive value decreases to ±3 weeks in the third trimester. The growth of the fetal skull slows from 3 mm per week in the second trimester to 1.8 mm per week in the third trimester.

When measuring the BPD, it is important to determine the landmarks accurately (Box 46-5, Figures 46-10 and 46-11). The fetal head should be imaged in a transverse axial section,

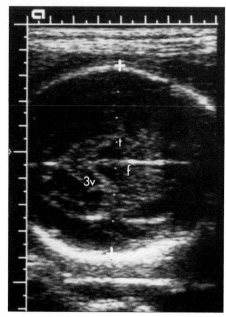

Figure 46-10 The biparietal diameter of the fetal head is made at the transverse level of the midbrain at the level of the falx *(f)*, cavum septi pellucidi, and thalamic nuclei *(t)*. *3v*, Third ventricle.

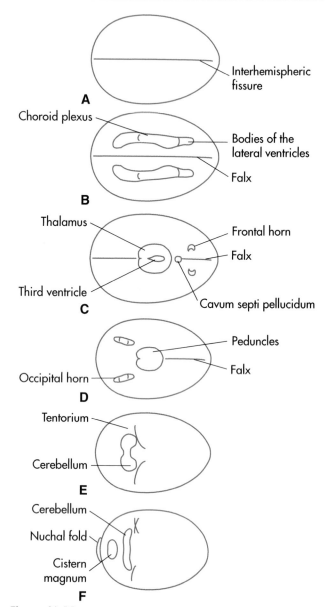

Figure 46-11 Progression of the fetal head anatomy in the transaxial plane from the level of the **A,** interhemispheric fissure; **B,** choroid plexus, falx, and bodies of the lateral ventricles; **C,** falx, thalamus, third ventricle, cavum septi pellucidum, frontal horns; **D,** falx, peduncles, occipital horns; **E,** tentorium, cerebellum; and **F,** cerebellum, cistern magnum, nuchal fold.

> **BOX 46-5 MEASURING THE BIPARIETAL DIAMETER**
>
> - Obtain biparietal leading edge–to–leading edge diameter (BPD) of the fetal head at the transverse level of the midbrain: falx, cavum septi pellucidi, and thalamic nuclei.
> - Make sure the head is symmetric and oval.
> - Measure from outer to inner margins of the skull.
> - In the third trimester, the BPD is not as accurate in predicting fetal age; may approach ±3 to 3.5 weeks.

ideally with the fetus in a direct occiput transverse position. The BPD should be measured perpendicular to the fetal skull at the level of the thalamus and the cavum septi pellucidi. Intracranial landmarks should include the falx cerebri anteriorly and posteriorly, the cavum septi pellucidi anteriorly in the midline, and the choroid plexus in the atrium of each lateral ventricle (Figure 46-12). With real-time sonography, one can identify the middle cerebral artery pulsating in the insula.

The head shape should be ovoid, not round (brachycephaly), because this can lead to overestimation of gestational age, just as a flattened or compressed head (dolichocephaly) can lead to underestimation of gestational age. The calipers should be placed from the leading edge of the parietal bone to the leading edge of the opposite parietal bone, or "outer edge to inner edge." The parietal bones should measure less than 3 mm each. On the outer edge of the fetal head, the soft tissue should not be included; measuring should begin from the skull bone, excluding the scalp. Gain settings should not be set too high because this can produce a false thickening and incorrect

measurement. A reference curve should be applicable to the local population. BPD should not be used to date a pregnancy in cases of severe ventriculomegaly, which may alter the head size and produce macrocephaly, or when microcephaly or skull-altering head lesions are present. In these cases, other biometric parameters should be used.

If the fetus is too large for an accurate CRL, but too early for a BPD with the proper landmarks identified, an approximation of the BPD can be obtained by incorporating the following landmarks: a smooth, symmetric head; visible choroid plexuses; and a well-defined midline echo that is an equal distance from both parietal bones (Figure 46-13).

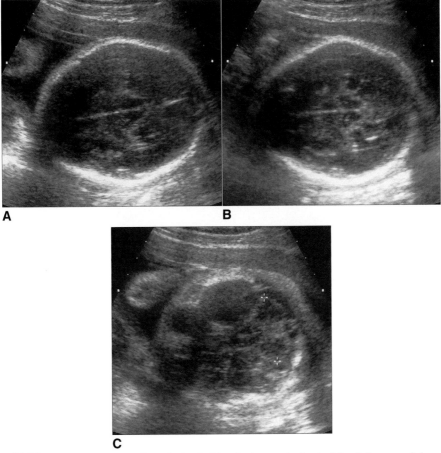

Figure 46-12   Transverse section through the fetal head taken at the level of the thalamus and the cavum septum pellucidi. **A,** The biparietal diameter (BPD) is measured from the outer border of the proximal skull to the inner border of the distal skull, or leading edge to leading edge. **B,** The head should be oval in shape because too round or too flat of a head leads to overestimation or underestimation of fetal age. **C,** Inferior angulation from the BPD shows the posterior fossa with the cerebellum *(cross bars).*

One technique to adjust for the biologic variability of fetal head growth uses the fetus as its own control. Two separate BPD measurements are obtained, the first between 20 and 26 weeks and the second between 31 and 33 weeks. The growth interval was compared with average growth. This technique has been termed **growth-adjusted sonar age (GASA).**[18] The fetus is then categorized into a small, average, or large growth percentile. The developers of this method claim the use of GASA reduces the range in gestational age from ±11 days to ±3 days in 90% of fetuses and to ±5 days in approximately 97% of fetuses.[18] Although GASA compensates for the biologic variability in the individual fetus, it does not take into consideration other factors, such as **dolichocephaly, brachycephaly,** and **oxycephaly** caused by molding, variations in head shape, or the standard error of measurement.

Head Circumference. Prenatal compression of the fetal skull is common. It occurs more often in fetal malpresentation, such as breech, or in conditions of intrauterine crowding, such as multiple pregnancies. The fetal skull can also be compressed in vertex presentations without any obvious reason or as a

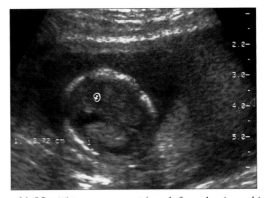

Figure 46-13   This represents a 14-week fetus that is too big for a crown-rump length measurement, yet too small to distinguish the proper biparietal landmarks in the fetal head. At this gestational age, it is acceptable to measure the fetal head at the level of the choroid plexus, which is echogenic and fills most of the head at this time. The same measurement criteria of outer border to inner border should be used.

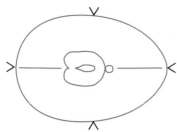

Figure 46-14   Head circumference should be taken at the level of the biparietal diameter; the calipers should be placed along the outer margin of the skull to obtain the measurement.

BOX 46-6   TRANSVERSE HEAD CIRCUMFERENCE (HC) MEASUREMENT

- Use the transverse plane at the level of the BPD to calculate head circumference (HC).
- Place area calipers along the outer margin of the skull to obtain circumference.
- Accurate to ±2 to 3 weeks.

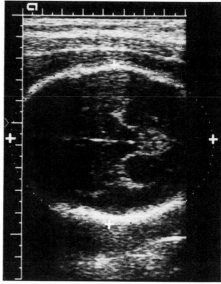

Figure 46-15   Transverse section of a fetal head demonstrating the ellipse method of measuring fetal head circumference (HC). The biparietal diameter and HC measurements can be taken from the same frozen image because the same anatomic landmarks are used. The calipers should be placed outside the entire perimeter of the fetal skull *(dotted line)*. This measurement is not affected by head shape.

result of an associated uterine abnormality, such as leiomyoma. The transverse head circumference (HC) is less affected than BPD by head compression; therefore, the HC is a valuable tool in assessing gestational age (Box 46-6, Figure 46-14).

The HC measurement is taken in the transverse plane at the level of the BPD and can be calculated from the same frozen image. Most modern ultrasound equipment has built-in electronic calipers that open to the outline of the fetal head. If this feature is not available, the measurement can be obtained with a light pen, map reader, or electronic planimeter or by manually measuring with the electronic calipers. To measure the widest transverse diameter of the skull manually, the BPD level should be measured with the calipers on the outer border of each side (D1). The length of the occipital frontal diameter (OFD) should then be measured (D2). This is done by measuring from the outer border of the occiput to the outer border of the frontal bone (Figure 46-15). To obtain an accurate HC measurement, 60% to 70% of the skull outline should be displayed on the screen. HC can then be calculated by the following formula:

$$HC = \frac{D1 + D2 \times \pi}{2}$$

Therefore:

$$HC = (D1 + D2) \times 1.57$$

Vertical Cranial Diameter, Coronal View, and 3-D BPD Correction. The coronal view of the fetal head is useful for viewing anatomy and assessing the degree of head molding and biologic changes in shape. Modern three-dimensional sonographic equipment can produce perpendicular orthogonal planes, which makes it relatively easy to perform this assess-

---

BOX 46-7   CORONAL HEAD CIRCUMFERENCE (CHC) MEASUREMENT

- Use the plane perpendicular to the transverse head circumference (HC). This plane should include the thalamus and brain stem.
- Place area calipers at the midedge of the skull to delineate the coronal triangle; the base of the triangle is tangential to the circles around the hippocampal gyri.

The height of the triangle is the vertical cranial diameter (VCD). The average of the BPD, OFD, and VCD is the 3-D-BPD correction for fetal skull molding.

- The 3-D-BPD is accurate to ±1 to 2 weeks.

---

ment of overall head shape; however, the coronal view is also easily acquired with standard two-dimensional machines. The proper coronal view should be perpendicular to the standard transverse head circumference (HC) view passing through the thalamus. Box 46-7 and Figure 46-16 demonstrate orthogonal planes of the fetal head.

The primary observation is that the coronal section of the fetal skull will be a perfect circle in normally shaped heads. In the presence of dolichocephaly, the vertical cranial diameter (VCD) may be exaggerated, resulting in some degree of oxycephaly, while brachycephaly will often be associated with platycephaly because the VCD is compressed or shortened. The VCD is the height of an isosceles triangle, the base of which is an imaginary line tangential to the caudal edges of the circles around the bilateral hippocampal gyri, and the VCD

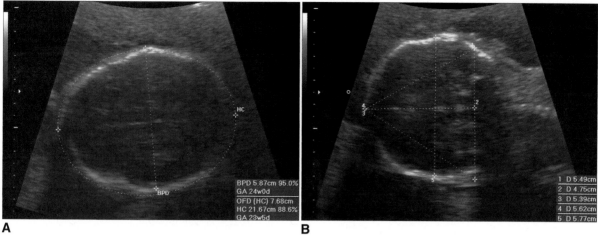

Figure 46-16 **A,** Transverse head circumference (HC) measured outer perimeter, and BPD measured leading edge to leading edge. BPD = 58.7 mm = 24.0 weeks; HC = 216.7 mm = 23.7 weeks. AA = 22.8. **B,** In the same fetus, coronal head circumference (CHC) showing the coronal triangle and vertical cranial diameter (VCD) as the height of the triangle. The 3-D-BPD correction = (58.7 + 76.8 + 47.5)/3 = 61.0 mm ≈ 24.3 weeks. This is a normally shaped fetal skull.

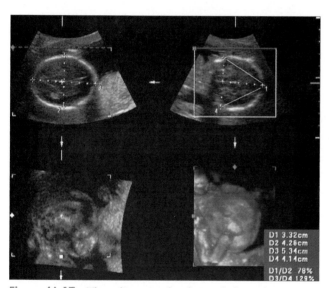

Figure 46-17 Three-dimensional orthogonal planes showing the transverse and coronal head circumferences. The sagittal plane (lower left) and 3-D surface rendering are less useful in this case.

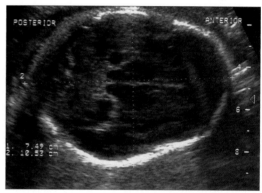

Figure 46-18 This represents a biparietal diameter (BPD) with dolichocephaly. The head is elongated in the anteroposterior diameter and falsely shortened in the transverse diameter. The BPD is mean for 29 weeks and the head circumference is mean for 30.3 weeks, but the actual gestational age is 32 weeks.

will lie along the midline from the middle of the triangle base to the cranial vertex (see Figure 46-16). The coronal view of the normal fetal skull will be a perfect circle, and the coronal triangle will be equal laterally. New 3-D orthogonal perpendicular planes will make these assessments easier (Figure 46-17).

In cases where the coronal skull is not a perfect circle, a 3-D BPD correction can be obtained by averaging the OFD, BPD, and VCD. In the presence of molding, this 3-D BPD correction will be the equivalent to the BPD for a normally shaped head at the same gestational age.

The student of sonography must realize that as the profession enters the era of true 3-D imaging modalities, all parameter measurements may not be the same from all researchers

and on all machines. Already the fetal cranium alone has had proposed 3-D measurements using outer, mid, and inner bone cursor placement. When using the ultrasound machine's measurement and age calculation packages, the operator is responsible for understanding the proper measurement end points used in that machine's software.

Cephalic Index. Two frequently noted alterations in head shape are **dolichocephaly** and **brachycephaly.** In dolichocephaly, the head is shortened in the transverse plane (BPD) and elongated in the anteroposterior plane (OFD) (Figure 46-18). In brachycephaly the head is elongated in the transverse diameter (BPD) and shortened in the anteroposterior diameter (OFD) (Figure 46-19). One can underestimate gestational age from a dolichocephalic head or overestimate with brachycephaly. Because of these variations in fetal head shape, a

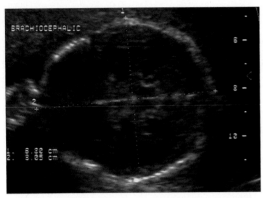

Figure 46-19 This biparietal diameter (BPD) is consistent with brachycephaly. The fetal head is falsely wider in the transverse diameter, yet shortened in the anteroposterior plane. The BPD overestimates the gestational age, but the head circumference (HC) remains relatively unaffected. The BPD is mean for 26.7 weeks, and the HC is mean for 24.9 weeks, but the actual gestational age is 23.5 weeks.

cephalic index (CI) has been devised to determine the normality of the fetal head shape:

$$CI = BPD/OFD \times 100$$

A normal cephalic index is 80% ±1 standard deviation. The range of normal CI is 75% to 85% (±1 SD ≈ 68% of the population). A CI of greater than 85% suggests brachycephaly and of less than 75% suggests dolichocephaly. In one case report, the CI changed from a high normal of 83% to a significantly abnormal index of 63% during a $2^{1}/_{2}$-week period.[8] This change would normally take approximately 7 weeks. Fetal death resulted. The authors of the report concluded that an abnormal CI may be an early indication of impending fetal death.

BPD and transverse head circumference do not account for changes in the vertical cranial diameter (VCD). The VCD is a relatively dynamic parameter because pressure on the vertex of the cranium as the fetus stretches and pushes the head against the uterine wall or maternal pubic bone will compress the VCD and exaggerate the BPD and HC in compensation, often resulting in a CI indicating brachycephaly. Conversely, if the BPD is compressed in dolichocephaly, the VCD will increase to compensate.[9,12] Unfortunately, this fact has been ignored for the most part, but as true 3-D sonography becomes available, these measurements will come into use.[5]

Abdominal Circumference. The first description of the use of the fetal **abdominal circumference (AC)** in predicting fetal weight was in 1975.[2] The AC is very useful in monitoring normal fetal growth and detecting fetal growth disturbances, such as **intrauterine growth restriction (IUGR)** and macrosomia. It is more useful as a growth parameter than in predicting gestational age.

The fetal abdomen should be measured in a transverse plane at the level of the liver where the umbilical vein branches into

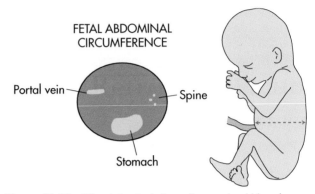

Figure 46-20 The abdominal circumference should be taken from a round transverse image at the level of the umbilical vein as it joins the left portal vein within the liver.

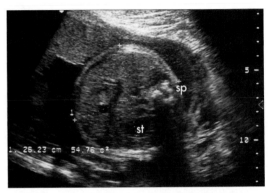

Figure 46-21 Transverse section of a fetal abdominal circumference (AC) at 30.3 weeks. The measurement should be taken at the level where the umbilical vein branches into the left portal sinus and forms a J shape. The fetal stomach *(st)* would be seen on the left at this level. One set of calipers should measure the distance from the fetal spine *(sp)* to the anterior abdominal wall. The other set should be placed perpendicular, measuring the widest transverse diameter. When tracing or using an ellipse to measure the AC, the calipers should be placed along the external perimeter of the fetus to include the skin.

BOX 46-8

MEASURING THE ABDOMINAL CIRCUMFERENCE (AC)

- The AC should be taken from a round transverse image with the umbilical portion of the left portal vein midline within the liver.
- The outer margin of the abdominal wall should be measured.
- The abdominal wall measurement is the least accurate.

---

the left portal sinus (Box 46-8, Figures 46-20 and 46-21). In this plane, the left portal vein and the right portal vein form a *J* shape. The stomach bubble may be seen at this level on the left side of the fetal abdomen. The abdomen should be more circular than oval because an oval shape indicates an oblique cut resulting in a false estimation of size. Fetal kidneys usually should not be seen when the proper plane is imaged. The AC may change shape with fetal breathing activity, transducer compression, or intrauterine crowding (as in multiple pregnancies or oligohydramnios) or secondary to fetal position, as in a breech presentation. When discrepancies do occur in AC measurements, multiple measurements should be taken and averaged to ensure accuracy. This is also true for other fetal measurements.

The AC can be measured with the same instruments used to measure the HC. The calipers should be placed along the external perimeter of the fetal abdomen to include subcutaneous soft tissue. The following formula can be used to calculate the AC:

$$AC = \frac{D1 + D2 \times \pi}{2}$$

Therefore,

$$AC = D1 + D2 \times 1.57$$

In this equation, D1 is the diameter from the skin line behind the fetal spine to the outer skin line of the anterior abdominal wall and D2 is the transverse diameter perpendicular to D1. Unlike in the fetal head, there is no consistent relationship between the anteroposterior and transverse diameters. Sonographers must be sure to measure the AC at the skin line and not to the more obvious rib, spine, and peritoneal echoes.

Of the four basic gestational age measurements, AC has the largest reported variability and is more affected by growth disturbances than the other basic parameters. Later in gestation, the AC correlates more closely with fetal weight than with age.

BONE LENGTHS

Femur. The most widely measured and easily obtainable of all fetal long bones is the femur. It usually lies at 30 to 70 degrees to the long axis of the fetal body. **Femur length (FL)** is about as accurate as BPD in determining gestational age.

Femur length is an especially useful parameter that can be used to date a pregnancy when a fetal head cannot be measured because of position or when there is a fetal head anomaly (Box 46-9).

The technique for measuring with real-time sonography is fairly simple. First, the lie of the fetus should be determined and the fetal body followed in a transverse section until the fetal bladder and iliac crests are identified. The iliac crests are echogenic and oblique to the fetal bladder. The transducer is moved slightly and rotated to visualize the full length of the femur. The ends of the femur should be distinct and blunt, not pointed, and an acoustic shadow should be cast because of the absorption of the sound waves into the bone (Figure 46-22).

Sonographers measure the femoral diaphysis, which is the calcified portion from end to end. The femoral head is not taken into account even when it is visible. After 32 weeks, the distal femoral epiphysis is seen, but it is not included in the femur length measurement. Often an echo from the near side of the cartilaginous distal femoral condyles will be seen, called the "distal femoral point" (DFP), and should not be included in the measure of the diaphysis.

Overestimating the length of the femur by high gain settings or by including the femoral head or distal epiphysis in the measurement is possible. Underestimation can result from using incorrect plane orientation and not obtaining the full length of the bone.

In any routine obstetric evaluation, the femur is usually the only long bone measured, but if there is a 2-week or greater difference between femur length and all the other biometric parameters, all fetal long bones should be measured and a targeted examination of the fetal anatomy should be performed. Three studies found an association between shortened femur and humerus lengths and trisomy.[1,10,17] Dwarfism is also a possibility. Constitutional hereditary growth factors should also be considered. Other bone lengths are sometimes valuable in assessing gestational age.

> **BOX 46-9   FEMUR MEASUREMENT**
>
> - Hyperechoic linear structure represents the ossified portion of the femoral diaphysis and corresponds to femoral length measurement from the greater trochanter to the femoral condyles. These are imaged as rounded hypoechoic masses at each end of the diaphysis called the epiphyseal cartilages; they should not be included in the femoral length measurement. Do not include the distal femoral point (DFP).
> - The normal femur has a straight lateral border and a curved medial border.
> - Femur length may be used with the same accuracy as BPD to predict gestational age.
> - Femur length may indicate skeletal dysplasias or intrauterine growth restriction.

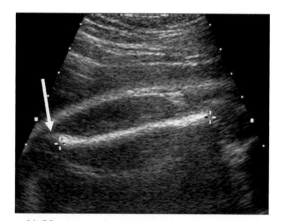

Figure 46-22 Longitudinal section through a fetal femur at 31.0 weeks. The longest section of bone should be obtained. The calipers should be placed from the major trochanter to the external condyle, excluding the DFP *(arrow)*. Note the shadow cast posterior to the bone, appropriately demonstrating the absorption of the sound waves into the fetal bone.

Distal Femoral and Proximal Tibial Epiphyseal Ossification Centers. One report has correlated the distal femoral epiphyseal ossification (DFE) and the proximal tibial epiphyseal ossification (PTE) with advanced gestational age.[3] The DFE and PTE appear as a high-amplitude echo that is separate but adjacent to the femur or the tibia. The authors of the report found that the DFE can be identified in gestations greater than 33 weeks, and that the PTE is identified in gestations greater than 35 weeks. It is not necessary to measure these ossifications; they are either present or absent. These assessments can be helpful when other growth parameters are compromised because of congenital anomalies or when differentiating an incorrectly dated fetus from a fetus that is small for gestational age (SGA), or one with intrauterine growth restriction (IUGR).

Tibia and Fibula. The tibia and fibula can be measured by first identifying the femur, then following it down until the two parallel bones can be identified. The tibia can be identified because the tibial plateau is larger than the fine, tapering fibula. The tibia is located medial to the fibula (Box 46-10, Figure 46-23).

Humerus. Humeral length is sometimes more difficult to measure than femur length. The humerus is usually found very close to the fetal abdomen, but can exhibit a wide range of motion. The "up side" humerus, or the humerus closest to the transducer, falls in the near-field zone, where detail is not always focused and the acoustic shadow is less clear. The opposite, or "down side," humerus may be obscured because of the overlying fetal spine or fetal ribs (Box 46-11, Figure 46-24). The cartilaginous humeral head surface is also acoustically shiny and may produce specular reflections that should not be included in the measurement of the humeral diaphysis. These specular reflections from the cartilaginous head of the humerus are called the proximal humeral point (PHP) as a corollary to the DFP of the femur. Both the DFP and the PHP, when observed, will always be on the side of the acoustically shiny cartilage proximal to the transducer.

Radius and Ulna. The radius and ulna can be recognized by following the humerus down until two parallel bones are visualized and then rotating the transducer slightly until the full length of the bones is identified. The forearms are very commonly found near the fetal face. The ulna can be distinguished from the radius because it penetrates much deeper into the elbow (Box 46-12, Figure 46-25). The ulna is larger and anatomically medial.

BOX 46-10   TIBIA AND FIBULA MEASUREMENTS

- Tibia is longer than the fibula.
- Fibula is lateral to the tibia and thinner.
- Measure length point to point.

BOX 46-11   HUMERUS MEASUREMENT

- Image fetal spine in upper thoracic—lower cervical region.
- Identify scapula, then rotate transducer until long axis of humerus is seen.
- Only humeral shaft (diaphysis) is ossified and is measured; do not include the proximal humeral point (PHP).

BOX 46-12   RADIUS AND ULNA MEASUREMENTS

- The ulna is longer than the radius proximally; distally they are the same.
- Measure length from point to point.

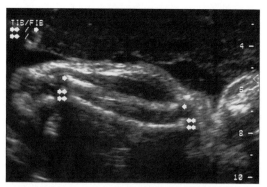

Figure 46-23 The tibia and fibula are demonstrated here at 21 weeks. The tibia can be distinguished from the fibula because the tibia is larger *(multiple arrows)* than the small tapering fibula *(single arrow)*.

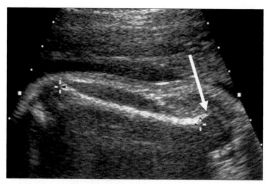

Figure 46-24 Longitudinal section through a fetal humerus at 32.4 weeks. The calipers should be placed at the most distal ends of the bone, excluding the PHP *(arrow)*. The anterior, or "up side," humerus is measured here; the humeral head can be observed with the specular echoes of the PHP and exhibiting acoustic enhancement beyond the head.

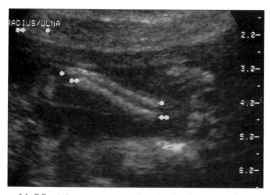

Figure 46-25 This represents a longitudinal section through the radius *(two arrows)* and ulna *(one arrow)* at 20.3 weeks of gestation. The calipers should be placed at the most distal portion of each individual bone. The ulna can be distinguished from the radius because the ulna is larger and penetrates much deeper into the elbow.

Using Multiple Parameters

No single parameter is perfect in predicting gestational age, and estimates of fetal age may improve significantly when two or more parameters are used. However, use of multiple parameters in estimating fetal age is appropriate only when the fetus is growing normally or in growth assessment time-series studies. Congenital anomalies of the head, abdomen, skeleton, and functional disturbances must be taken into consideration before using multiple parameters. In a normal population, the various ages estimated from the parameters of the fetal cranium exhibit about half the variation ($\pm 0.05\%$ of age) as do the ages from the fetal torso and extremity parameters ($\pm 0.10\%$ of age).

A birth weight table was developed based on measurements from a group of neonates who had accurate gestational dating using prenatal first-trimester sonography to improve the accuracy of neonatal birth weight percentiles.[4] Prenatally, weight tables are used in conjunction with sonographically estimated fetal weight to help guide obstetric management decisions, especially those concerning the timing of delivery. Fetal weight estimation is a useful parameter in following IUGR fetuses.

A study compared 3-D ultrasound birth weight predictions with 2-D methods and found a significant correlation existed between thigh volume and birth weight at term gestation.[13] Thigh volumes that included the soft tissue mass may represent important markers for fetal growth. The 3-D ultrasound may be an important predictor of growth-restricted fetuses, and the volume measurements may be able to be applied to each fetus to monitor growth.

One author used the technique of averaging the BPD, HC, AC, and FL to determine gestational age.[6] The value of using multiple parameters is that as fetuses individuate, some are longer or shorter, fatter or thinner, and an average age (AA) of multiple fetal parameters will result in the best estimation of age. In addition, any of the measurements may be technically incorrect and it is very unlikely that all of the measurements are overestimated or underestimated.

Age Range Analysis

An extension of the **average age (AA)** of multiple fetal parameters is the **age range analysis (ARA).** The concept of average ages is based upon the fact that not all fetal parameters grow at the same rate; therefore, a fetus with an average age of 30 weeks may have an estimated femoral age of 31 weeks, whereas the AC could measure to be 29 weeks. This fetus would be relatively long and thin, but may be normal. By studying large populations using multiple fetal parameter ages, two different groups found that for the same fetus at a given time in gestation, the range of ages of all parameters should be about $\pm 8\%$ to $\pm 10\%$ (± 2 SD) of the average age of all the parameters.[7] This means that the range of ages for a fetus with an average age of 20 weeks for all parameters should fall between 18 and 22 weeks, using the $\pm 10\%$, which is easiest to calculate. Moreover, at 30 weeks all parameter ages should fall between 27 and 33 weeks in normal fetuses (95% of the population). The ARA is a simple way of assessing proportionalities of fetal parameters.

Table 46-1 can be used to calculate the ARA for a fetus and to record time-series growth studies to assess for growth disturbances and parameter proportions. The location of a parameter in the normal distribution in standard deviations may be estimated using the Z score formula in this table.

In cases of IUGR growth disturbances, the fetal AA by sonography will lag behind the LMP age. As the case is followed in serial studies, the differences between the sonographic AA and LMP ages will increase as the IUGR becomes more pronounced later in gestation. In cases of normal but small for gestational age (SGA) fetuses, the sonographic AA may lag to some degree behind the LMP age, but the differences of the ages should not increase with time in gestation.

Other Parameters

Numerous other nomograms have been used to correlate almost every aspect of fetal anatomy with gestational age. Among the most interesting of these parameters are the orbits, the cerebellum, and the fetal epiphyseal ossification centers. In general, it can be stated that parameters that normally grow to larger sizes at term will have a more rapid growth trajectory and will generally produce the most accurate fetal age estimates.

Orbits. Another parameter useful in predicting gestational age is the fetal orbit measurements. The orbital diameter (OD), **binocular distance (BD),** and interocular distance (IOD) can be measured. Gestational age can best be predicted from the BD. This measure is more strongly related to the BPD and gestational age than are the other orbital parameters. The fetal orbits should be measured in a plane slightly more caudal than the BPD. The orbits are accessible in every head position except the occipitoanterior position (i.e., face looking down). All measurements should be taken from outer border to outer border (Box 46-13, Figure 46-26). The OD measures a single fetal orbit. The BD includes both fetal orbits at the same time, whereas the IOD measures the length between the two orbits. One view states that (1) both eyes should have the same diameter, (2) the largest diameter of the eyes should be used, and (3) the image should be symmetric. Care should be taken not

TABLE 46-1 FETAL AGE AND AGE-RANGE ANALYSIS*—BASIC BABY ©

LMP Week	E/FHR b/m	GSD mm	CRL mm	BPD mm	3D-BPD mm	OFD mm	VCD mm	CV mm³	THC* mm	Hadlock HC** mm	CHC mm	CERB mm	BD mm	FSL mm	Fem mm	Hum mm	ADA mm	AC mm	LMP WEEK	ARA Time-line
41				100	96	123	66	482	349	356	260			74	79	70	120	376	41	
40				97	96	119	70	451	339	350	264		60	73	77	67	118	371	40	
39				95	93	116	66	421	331	344	252		58	71	76	67	116	365	39	
38				93	91	116	66	397	328	340	249	51	60	69	73	65	114	359	38	
37				91	90	113	65	376	320	330	244	50	59	67	73	63	110	342	37	
36				89	88	111	64	351	314	324	240	47	59	65	71	62	103	325	36	
35				87	86	109	63	329	307	316	234	43	57	63	68	60	99	310	35	
34				85	84	106	62	307	299	309	230	41	55	61	66	58	95	299	34	
33				83	82	104	60	289	294	303	224	40	52	59	64	56	92	289	33	
32				80	80	101	58	260	285	294	217	39	51	56	62	55	89	281	32	
31				78	78	98	57	243	277	285	212	37	50	54	59	53	85	268	31	
30				75	75	95	55	220	268	277	205	36	48	52	57	51	81	253	30	
29				73	73	93	55	204	260	269	200	34	46	49	55	50	77	243	29	
28				71	71	89	52	181	251	260	192	32	46	47	53	48	74	231	28	
27				68	68	86	51	166	242	251	187	30	44	45	50	46	71	'221	27	
26				65	66	83	49	146	233	241	178	28	43	43	48	44	68	212	26	
25				62	63	79	47	127	221	231	171	27	41	41	46	43	65	205	25	
24				59	60	76	45	110	211	221	163	25	40	39	43	40	61	191	24	
23				56	56	71	42	93	199	210	154	24	38	37	40	38	58	181	23	
22				53	53	67	40	78	188	199	146	22	36	34	37	36	54	170	22	
21				49	50	62	38	65	175	188	137	21	34	32	35	34	51	160	21	
20				46	47	59	35	54	165	175	129	19	32	30	32	31	47	149	20	
19			130	44	44	55	33	44	155	163	121	19	30	28	29	29	44	138	19	
18			121	40	40	50	31	35	142	149	112	18	28	25	26	26	40	126	18	
17			113	37	37	46	29	28	131	135	104	17	25	22	23	23	36	113	17	
16			104	34	34	42	25	20	118	121	93	15	23	20	20	20	33	103	16	
15			92	30	30	37	23	14	105	105	83	14	21	17	16	16	29	91	15	
14	150		83	27	26	33	20	10	93	90	73	12	17	15	13	13	25	78	14	
13	152		71	23	23	28	17	6	81		63	10	15	13	10	10	21	68	13	
12	159		58	20	20	24	14	3.8	69		54		13	11	7	7	18	57	12	
11	163		46	16	17	20	13	2.4	56		47		13		6	5	15	48	11	

Embryonic Period

LMP Week	E/FHR b/m	GSD mm	CRL mm	BPD mm	3D-BPD mm	OFD mm	VCD mm	CV mm³	THC* mm	Hadlock HC** mm	CHC mm	CERB mm	BD mm	FSL mm	Fem mm	Hum mm	ADA mm	AC mm	LMP WEEK
10	167	53	37	13	13	17	9	1.2	42		45		9		4	4	13	40	10
9	185	44	25	11	11	13	8	0.7	31		30					10		30	9
8	165	34	17	7	7	9	5	0.2	19		19						7	22	8
7	142	26	10	5															7
6	114	18	5															6	
5	98	11	2															5	
4		4																4	

Growth Series Dating

Exams:	Date	LMP age	Ave. Age	Age Range
1st				
2nd				
3rd				
4th				

*Transverse HC mid-skull bones' edges' ellipse. Table values from single population (n = 9000+), excepting Hadlock, et al outer HC. DuBose: FETAL SONOGRAPHY, Chapter 7 Size/Age Analysis; W. B. Saunders Co. 1996. This table is a manual version of BASIC BABY© fetal size/age analysis software. Copyright 1994, 2004, T. J. DuBose. This table may be used without modification. It may not be used in computer programs except by permission.

**Adapted from Hadlock, Deter, Harrist & Park: Fetal head circumference: Relation to menstrual age. AJR 138:649, 1982 (Outer skull perimeter).

TABLE 46-1	FETAL AGE AND AGE RANGE ANALYSIS*—BASIC BABY ©—cont'd		
Parameter	Symbols	Parameter Name	Measurements in mm
GSD	G	Gestational sac diameter	Mean of two diameters
CRL	R	Crown-rump length	Top of head to rump; do not include legs
E/FHR	E	Embryofetal heart rate	M-mode beats per minute
BPD	B	Biparietal diameter	Leading edge to leading edge (outer to inner)
BPD 3-D	3	3-D BPD correction	Average (OFD + BPD + VCD)/3 = BPD
OFD	O	Occipitofrontal diameter	Middle of frontal to middle of occipital bones
VCD	V	Vertical cranial diameter	Height of coronal triangle in fetal head
THC	T	Transverse head circumference	THC = (OFD + BPD) × 1.57
CV	V	Cranial volume	CV = OFD × BPD × VCD × 0.555
CHC	C	Coronal head circumference	CHC = (VCD + BPD) × 1.57
CERB	c	Cerebellar transverse diameter	Transverse cerebellar diameter
BD	b	Binocular diameter	Outer-to-outer edges of the binocular globes
FSL	S	Fractional spine length	Seven thoracolumbar vertebral bodies and spaces
Fem	F	Femur length	Length of femoral diaphysis
Hum	H	Humerus length	Length of humeral diaphysis
AC	a	Abdominal circumference	AC = d1 + d2 × 1.57
ADA	D	Abdominal diameter average	Average transverse and AP diameters (d1+d1)/2
Ave. Age	AA	Average age in LMP weeks	Average of multiple parameter's ages
LMP	M	Last menstrual period age	May be estimated from 1st sonographic study
Range	[ ]	Range of ages	Range normally is less than 20% of ave. age
Instructions:			
To perform age range analysis (ARA) for each examination:			
Measure parameters and mark the parameter's sizes in the table to determine each parameter's age, and average all parameter ages; interpolate for more accuracy. Use a straight edge to place symbols in the time-line. Normal fetuses will form a cluster about the LMP age estimated from 1st sonographic examination. Use single table to track growth series for each fetus. IUGR will trail LMP age. Range should be <±10% (20%) of AA.			
ARA: To determine the relative location of any parameter in the time-line distribution, use the following formula:			
(Parameter age – AA)/(AA × 0.05) = Location in standard deviations (SD)			

BOX 46-13 ORBITAL MEASUREMENTS

- Orbital diameter increases from 13 mm at 12 weeks to 59 mm or greater at term.
- Measure outer to outer diameter.
- Measure inner to inner diameter.

to underestimate the measurement when there is oblique shadowing from the ethmoid bone. This parameter is especially useful when other fetal growth parameters are affected, such as in ventriculomegaly or skeletal dysplasia. With careful sonographic examinations, the fetus with **hypotelorism, hypertelorism, anophthalmos,** or **microphthalmos** can be diagnosed.

Cerebellum. One study found the fetal cerebellum to be a more accurate reflection of gestational age than the BPD in

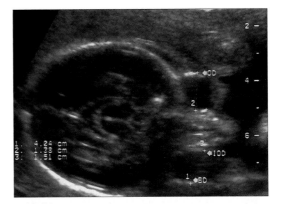

Figure 46-26 This sonogram represents a transverse section through the fetal head at the level of the orbits at 25.3 weeks. *OD* is the measure of a single fetal orbit. The binocular diameter *(BD)* is a measure of both the orbits at the same time, and the inner orbital diameter *(IOD)* is a measure of the distance between the two orbits. These measurements are especially useful when ruling out hypotelorism or hypertelorism.

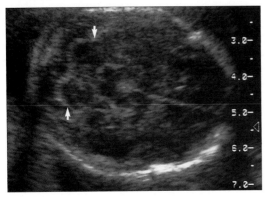

Figure 46-27   Transverse section through a fetal head demonstrating the fetal cerebellum. This image is obtained at the same anatomic level as the biparietal diameter, angling back into the posterior fossa of the fetal head. Note the classic dumbbell shape of the normal cerebellum. The widest diameter of the cerebellum should be measured *(arrows)*.

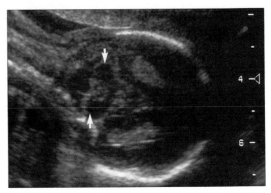

Figure 46-28   A coronal section of a fetal cerebellum, which can be used when the traditional views cannot be obtained.

The fetal cerebellum should not be used as a gestational dating parameter in the presence of a cerebellar or spinal abnormality. A more recent report states that the coronal or other views are just as accurate as long as the transverse width of the cerebellum is measured, especially in fetal heads when the traditional views are unobtainable (Figure 46-28).[20]

> ### BOX 46-14   CEREBELLAR DIMENSIONS
>
> - **Posterior fossa:** In the transaxial image of the head, obtain the BPD (cavum septi pellucidi and thalamus) and then angle the transducer inferior toward the base of the skull to image the posterior fossa.
> - Obtain the length of the cerebellum at the level of the cerebellum, vermis, and fourth ventricle.
> - Angle the transducer slightly more inferior from the cerebellum to record the cistern magnum and nuchal fold area.
> - The depth of the cisterna magna is from the posterior aspect of the cerebellum to the occipital bone measured 5 mm ± 3 mm; measurements >10 mm are abnormal.
> - The nuchal fold should measure <3 mm.

---

cases of oligohydramnios, dolichocephaly, breech presentation, or twins or in the presence of a uterine anomaly.[14] The authors of the study claim this is true because the posterior fossa is not affected by any of these conditions. The cerebellum can be measured from the level at which the BPD is obtained by angling back into the posterior fossa to include the full width of the cerebellum. The cerebellum should have a dumbbell or heart shape, depending upon the angle of the plane of view.

The widest transverse diameter of the cerebellum should be measured (Box 46-14, Figure 46-27). Authors have described the **banana** and **lemon signs** that associate an abnormally shaped cerebellum with detection of fetal **spina bifida.**[15] In the presence of spina bifida, the fetal cerebellum is displaced downward into the foramen magnum, altering its shape to appear oblong or banana shaped. The frontal bones of the fetal skull also give in to this reduced pressure, collapsing and giving the fetal head a lemon shape. This association is known as the Arnold-Chiari malformation type II.

REFERENCES

1. Benacerraf B, Neuberg D, Frigoletto FD: Humeral shortening in second trimester fetuses with Down syndrome, *Obstet Gynecol* 77:223, 1991.
2. Campbell S, Wilkin D: Ultrasonic measurement of the fetal abdominal circumference in the estimation of fetal weight, *Br J Obstet Gynecol* 82:689, 1975.
3. Chinn D and others: Ultrasonic identification of fetal lower extremity epiphyseal ossification centers, *Radiology* 147:815, 1983.
4. Doubilet PM and others: Improved birth weight table for neonates developed from gestations dated by early ultrasonography, *J Ultrasound Med* 16:241, 1997.
5. Dubose TJ: Reliability and validity of three-dimensional fetal brain volumes, *J Ultrasound Med* 21:709-711, 2002.
6. Dubose TJ, Cunyus JA, Johnson L: Embryonic heart rate and age, *J Diagn Med Sonogr* 6:151-157, 1990.
7. Dubose TJ, Poole E, Butschek C: Range of multiple fetal parameters, *J Ultrasound Med* 7:S205-206, 1988.
8. Ford K, McGahan J: Cephalic index: its possible use as a predictor of impending fetal demise, *Radiology* 143:517, 1982.
9. Goldberg BB, Kurtz AB: *Atlas of ultrasound measurements,* St Louis, 1990, Mosby.
10. Hadlock FP, Deter RL, Harris RB: Sonographic detection of abnormal fetal growth patterns, *Clin Obstet Gynecol* 27:342, 1984.
11. Hohler CW: Ultrasonic estimation of gestational age, *Clin Obstet Gynecol* 27:2, 1984.
12. Kurtz AB, Goldberg BB: Fetal head measurements. In Kurtz AB, Goldberg BB, editors: *Obstetrical measurements in ultrasound: a reference manual,* St Louis, 1988, Mosby.
13. Lee W and others: Birthweight prediction by three-dimensional ultrasonographic volumes of the fetal thigh and abdomen, *J Ultrasound Med* 16:799, 1997.
14. Mcleary R, Kuhns L, Barr M: Ultrasonography of the fetal cerebellum, *Radiology* 151:441, 1984.

15. Nicolaides KH and others: *Ultrasound screening for spina bifida: cranial and cerebellar signs,* Lancet 1:72, 1986.

16. Nyberg DA, Laing FC, Fily RA: Threatened abortion: sonographic distinction of normal and abnormal sacs, *Radiology* 158:397, 1986.

17. Rodis JF and others: Comparison of humerus length with femur length in fetuses with Down syndrome, *Am J Obstet Gynecol* 165:1051, 1992.

18. Sabbagha RE, Hughey M, Depp R: Growth-adjusted sonographic age (GASA): a simplified method, *Obstet Gynecol* 51:383, 1978.

19. Sabbagha RE, Tamura RK, Dal Campo S: Fetal dating by ultrasound, *Sem Roentgenol* 17:3, 1982.

20. Sarno AP, Rose GS, Harrington RA: Coronal transcerebellar diameter: an alternate view, *Ultrasound Obstet Gynecol* 2:158, 1992.

SELECTED BIBLIOGRAPHY

Blaas H-G K: The embryonic examination: ultrasound studies on the development of the human embryo. Tapir, Trondheim, Norway, ISBN: 82-519-1515-5, 2003.

Doubilet PM, Benson CB, Chow JS: Long-term prognosis of pregnancies complicated by slow embryonic heart rates in the early first trimester, *J Ultrasound Med* 18(8):537-541, 1999.

DuBose TJ: 3D BPD Correction, http://www.obgyn.net/us/cotm/ 0007/3d-bpd-correction.htm, accessed December 2, 2004.

DuBose TJ: Fetal biometry: vertical calvarial diameter and calvarial volume, *J Diagn Med Sonogr* 1:205-217, 1985.

DuBose TJ: *Fetal sonography,* Philadelphia, 1996, WB Saunders.

Goldstein RB, Filly RA, Simpson G: Pitfalls in femur length measurements, *J Ultrasound Med* 6:203-207, 1987.

Hadlock FP, Deter RL, Harrist RB: Sonographic detection of abnormal fetal growth pattern, *Clin Obstet Gynecol* 27:342, 1984.

Hadlock FP and others: Estimation of fetal weight with the use of head, body, and femur measurements: prospective study, *Am J Obstet Gynecol* 15:333, 1985.

Hobbins JC, Winsberg F, Berkowitz RL: *Ultrasonography in ob/gyn,* Baltimore, 1983, Williams & Wilkins.

Hurwitz SR: Yolk sac sign: sonographic appearance of the fetal yolk sac in missed abortion, *J Ultrasound Med* 5:435, 1986.

Jeanty P, Romero R: *Obstetrical ultrasound,* New York, 1984, McGraw-Hill.

Lyons E: Early pregnancy loss by endovaginal sonography. Proceedings of the State of the Art Ob/Gyn Imaging Course, San Diego convention, March 1992, American Institute of Ultrasound in Medicine.

Mayden K and others: Orbital diameters: a new parameter for prenatal diagnosis and dating, *Am J Obstet Gynecol* 144:289, 1982.

Santolaya-Forgas J, De Aleon-Luis J, D'Ancona RL and others: Evaluation of the amniotic sac and extracelomic space as seen by early ultrasound examination, *Fetal Diagn Ther* 18:262-269, 2003.

Schats R, Jansen CA, Wladimiroff JW: Embryonic heart activity: appearance and development in early human pregnancy, *Br J Obstet Gynaecol* 97(11):989-994, 1990.

Yeh M and others: Ultrasonic measurement of the femur length as an index of fetal gestational age, *Am J Obstet Gynecol* 144:519, 1982.

CHAPTER 47

Fetal Growth Assessment by Ultrasound

Sandra L. Hagen-Ansert

OBJECTIVES

- Describe how intrauterine growth restriction may be detected by ultrasound
- Differentiate between symmetric and asymmetric intrauterine growth restriction
- List which growth parameters should be used to assess intrauterine growth restriction
- Describe how to assess amniotic fluid volume
- Describe how to perform a biophysical profile on a fetus
- Discuss quantitative and qualitative Doppler measurements as applied to obstetrics
- Analyze the significance of macrosomia in a fetus

KEY TERMS

amniotic fluid index (AFI) – sum of the four quadrants of amniotic fluid

biophysical profile (BPP) – assessment of fetus to determine fetal well-being; includes evaluation of cardiac nonstress test, fetal breathing movement, gross fetal body movements, fetal tone, and amniotic fluid volume

Doppler – *the Doppler effect* is a change in the frequency of a sound wave when either the source or the listener is moving relative to one another. The difference between the received echo frequency and the frequency of the transmitted beam is the *Doppler shift. Pulsed wave Doppler* is used in most fetal examinations. This means that the transducer has the ability to send and receive Doppler signals.

estimated fetal weight (EFW) – incorporation of all fetal growth parameters (biparietal diameter, head circumference, abdominal circumference, femur and humeral length)

intrauterine growth restriction (IUGR) – decreased rate of fetal growth; may be symmetric (all growth parameters are small) or asymmetric (may be caused by placental problem; head measurements correlate with dates, body disproportionately smaller); formerly referred to as *intrauterine growth retardation*

large for gestational age (LGA) – fetus measures larger than dates (diabetic fetus)

macrosomia – birth weight greater than 4000 g or above the 90th percentile for the estimated gestational age

nonstress test (NST) – uses Doptone to record the fetal heart rate and its reactivity to the stress of uterine contraction

placental grade – technique of grading the placenta for maturity

postterm – fetus born later than the 42-week gestational period

preterm – fetus born earlier than the normal 38- to 42-week gestational period

small for gestational age (SGA) – fetus measures smaller than dates

systolic to diastolic (S/D) ratio – Doppler determination of the peak systolic velocity divided by the peak diastolic velocity

Fetal growth assessment is very important to the perinatologist and obstetric physician. Before the availability of ultrasound determination of fetal growth, physicians had to rely on their physical assessment of the neonate to determine what occurred during fetal development. The physician's assessment would determine if the fetus was born **preterm** (before 38 menstrual weeks), at term (between 38 and 42 menstrual weeks), or **postterm** (later than 42 menstrual weeks). Further classification dictated whether the fetal birth weight was **small for gestational age (SGA),** appropriate for gestational age, or **large for gestational age (LGA).** This determination allowed the clinicians to recognize the increase in perinatal morbidity and mortality for the preterm or postterm and SGA or LGA fetus.

INTRAUTERINE GROWTH RESTRICTION

Intrauterine growth restriction (IUGR) is best described as a decreased rate of fetal growth. IUGR complicates 3% to 7% of all pregnancies. It is most commonly defined as a fetal weight at or below 10% for a given gestational age. It often becomes difficult to differentiate the fetus that is constitutionally small (small for gestational age [SGA]) from one that is growth restricted. IUGR babies are at a greater risk of antepartum death, perinatal asphyxia, neonatal morbidity, and later developmental problems. Mortality is increased sixfold to tenfold, depending on the severity of the condition.

The most significant maternal factors for IUGR are the history of a previous fetus with IUGR, significant maternal hypertension or smoking, the presence of a uterine anomaly (bicornuate uterus or large leiomyoma), and significant placental hemorrhage (Box 47-1). Constitutional factors such as the gender of the infant, race of the mother, parity, body mass index, and environmental factors can affect the distribution of normal birth weight in any population.

Before abnormal growth can be diagnosed, it is necessary to accurately determine the gestational age of the pregnancy. In the prenatal period, an accurate last menstrual period or a first-trimester ultrasound can be used. If a first-trimester ultrasound was not performed, then in the second or third trimester the standard biparietal diameter (BPD), head circumference (HC), abdominal circumference (AC), and femur length (FL) should be used in conjunction with other tests of fetal well-being (e.g., biophysical profile [BPP] and fetal Doppler velocimetry).

In the postnatal period, several other body dimensions can be used. These include head circumference, crown-heel length, weight-height ratios, ponderal index (PI), and skinfold thickness. Other considerations include maternal size and race and the gender of the neonate. The standards for fetal growth have been incorporated with ultrasound computer software, and different programs exist that can be applied to a variety of geographic locations.

The reader should not confuse IUGR with the term *small for gestational age* (SGA). The SGA describes the fetus with a weight below the 10th percentile without reference to the cause. Fetal growth restriction describes a subset of the SGA fetuses with a weight below the 10th percentile as a result of pathologic process from a variety of maternal, fetal, or placental disorders. The classification of IUGR is based on the morphologic characteristics of the fetuses studied. There are two basic clarifications: symmetric and asymmetric IUGR.

Symmetric IUGR is usually the result of a first-trimester insult, such as a chromosomal abnormality or infection. This results in a fetus that is proportionately small throughout the pregnancy. Approximately 20% to 30% of all IUGR cases are symmetric. The timing of the pathologic insult is recognized as more important than the actual nature of the underlying pathologic process.

Asymmetric IUGR begins late in the second or third trimester and usually results from placental insufficiency. This fetus usually shows head sparing at the expense of abdominal and soft tissue growth. The fetal length (FL) exhibits varying degrees of compromise. An early diagnosis of IUGR and close fetal monitoring (BPP, Doppler, and fetal growth evaluation) is of significant help in managing a pregnancy suspected of IUGR. Clinical observations and appropriate actions for IUGR are shown in Box 47-2.

SYMMETRIC INTRAUTERINE GROWTH RESTRICTION

Symmetric growth restriction is characterized by a fetus that is small in all physical parameters (e.g., BPD, HC, AC, and FL). This is usually the result of a severe insult in the first trimester. The causes may include low genetic growth potential, intrauterine infection, severe maternal malnutrition, fetal

---

BOX 47-1   SIGNIFICANT MATERNAL FACTORS FOR INTRAUTERINE GROWTH RESTRICTION (IUGR)

- Previous history of fetus with IUGR
- Significant maternal hypertension
- History of tobacco use
- Presence of uterine anomaly
- Significant placental hemorrhage

BOX 47-2   CLINICAL OBSERVATIONS AND ACTIONS FOR INTRAUTERINE GROWTH RESTRICTION (IUGR)

- *Clinical signs of IUGR:* Decreased fundal height and fetal motion
- *Key IUGR sonographic markers:* Grade 3 placenta before 36 weeks or decreased placental thickness
- *Sonographer action:* Alert the physician, determine the cause (maternal history, habits, environmental exposure, viruses, diseases, drug exposure), carefully evaluate placenta and fetal anatomy with ultrasound

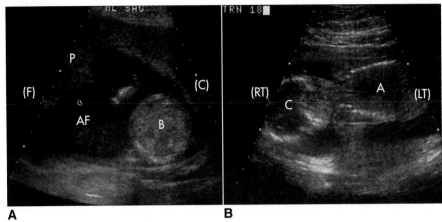

Figure 47-1   A, Second-trimester fetus with trisomy 18 shows symmetric intrauterine growth restriction. Both the head and abdomen measured well below expected growth curves. Echogenic bowel *(B)* is seen. **B,** Image shows the small cranium *(C)* and abdomen *(A)*. *F,* fundus; *C,* toward the cervix; *AF,* amniotic fluid; *(LT),* left; *P,* placenta; *(RT),* right.

alcohol syndrome, chromosomal anomaly, or severe congenital anomaly. One study demonstrated early IUGR in 9 of 11 fetuses with trisomy 13, 2 of 5 fetuses with 45 XO, and only 2 of 18 fetuses with trisomy 17.[10] Another report describes two cases of triploidy in association with early symmetric IUGR.[15] Because of the increased association of chromosomal abnormalities, prenatal testing to rule out aneuploidy should be considered (Figure 47-1).

ASYMMETRIC INTRAUTERINE GROWTH RESTRICTION

Asymmetric growth restriction is the more common form of IUGR and is usually caused by placental insufficiency. This may be the result of maternal disease, such as diabetes (classes D to F), chronic hypertension, cardiac or renal disease, abruptio placentae, multiple pregnancy, smoking, poor weight gain, drug usage, or uterine anomaly. It should be noted that IUGR fetuses have been born to mothers who have no high-risk factors; therefore, all pregnancies undergoing ultrasonic examinations should be evaluated for IUGR.

Asymmetric IUGR is characterized by an appropriate BPD and HC and a disproportionately small AC. This reinforces the brain-sparing effect, which states that the last organ to be deprived of essential nutrients is the brain. The BPD and HC may be slightly smaller, but this usually does not happen until the late third trimester.

A third type of IUGR has been described.[5] In the third type, it is proposed that fetuses with long FL (90th percentile or above) and small AC (at or below the 5th percentile) may be nutritionally deprived even though their estimated fetal weight (ETW) falls at least in the lowest 10%. The theory is that in asymmetric IUGR the fetal length is well preserved, whereas the soft tissue mass is deprived. The FL to AC ratio or PI would be abnormally low. The proponents of this theory claim this occurs in less than 1% of IUGR cases, but stress the importance of detection because these cases of IUGR have an EFW within the limits of normal.[5]

BOX 47-3   MULTIPLE PARAMETERS FOR INTRAUTERINE GROWTH RESTRICTION (IUGR)

- *BPD:* Imaged in the transverse plane using the cavum septi pellucidi, thalamic nuclei, falx cerebri, and choroid plexus as landmarks. The BPD can be misleading in cases associated with unusual head shapes. Used alone, it is a poor indicator of IUGR.
- *HC to AC ratio:* High false-positive rate for use in screening general population. The HC to AC ratio is useful in determining the type of IUGR.
- *FL to AC ratio:* Not dependent on knowing gestational age. The FL to AC ratio has a poor positive predictive value.
- *FL:* May decrease in size with symmetric IUGR.
- *AC:* Measure at level of portal-umbilical venous complex. When growth is compromised, AC is affected secondary to reduced adipose tissue and depletion of glycogen storage in liver. AC is the single most sensitive indicator of IUGR.

ULTRASOUND DIAGNOSTIC CRITERIA

The IUGR multiple parameters are shown in Box 47-3.

BIPARIETAL DIAMETER

The BPD is not a very reliable predictor of IUGR for many reasons. The first is the head-sparing theory, which is associated with asymmetric IUGR. Fetal blood is shunted away from other vital organs to nourish the fetal brain, giving the fetus an appropriate BPD (plus or minus 1 standard deviation) for the true gestational age.

The second problem is the potential alteration in fetal head shape secondary to oligohydramnios. Oligohydramnios is a decreased amount of amniotic fluid often associated with IUGR. Dolichocephaly or a falsely shortened BPD can lead to underestimation of the fetal weight, and brachycephaly or a falsely wider BPD can lead to overestimation of the EFW. The HC measurement is a more consistent parameter, but a combination of all growth parameters (BPD, HC, AC, and FL) should be used when diagnosing a fetal growth discrepancy.

ABDOMINAL CIRCUMFERENCE

Because of the variability of fetal proportion and size, the AC is a poor predictor of gestational age but is very valuable in assessing fetal size. In IUGR the fetal liver is one of the most severely affected body organs, which therefore alters the circumference of the fetal abdomen.

HEAD CIRCUMFERENCE TO ABDOMINAL CIRCUMFERENCE RATIO

The HC to AC ratio was first developed to detect IUGR in cases of uteroplacental insufficiency. The HC to AC ratio is especially useful in differentiating symmetric and asymmetric IUGR. For each gestational age, a ratio is assigned with standard deviations. In an appropriate-for-gestational-age (AGA) pregnancy, the ratio should decrease as the gestational age increases.

In the presence of IUGR and with the loss of subcutaneous tissue and fat, the ratio increases. The HC to AC ratio is at least 2 standard deviations above the mean in approximately 70% of fetuses affected with asymmetric IUGR. The HC to AC ratio is not very useful, however, in predicting symmetric IUGR, because the fetal head and fetal abdomen are equally small.

ESTIMATED FETAL WEIGHT

The most reliable **estimated fetal weight (EFW)** formulas incorporate all fetal parameters, such as BPD, HC, AC, and FL. This is important because an overall reduction in the size and mass of these parameters naturally gives a below-normal EFW. An EFW below the 10th percentile is considered by most to be IUGR.

There are numerous formulas for estimating fetal weights. One method uses the BPD and AC to derive the fetal weight, with an accuracy of plus or minus 20%. This formula does not take into consideration HC and FL, which contribute to fetal mass. It also ignores the fact that BPD can be altered slightly because of normal variations in head shape, such as brachycephaly or dolichocephaly. These variations can occur in association with oligohydramnios, which may be found with IUGR.

Another method uses three basic measurements: HC, AC, and FL. The use of the HC instead of the BPD has improved the predictive value to plus or minus 15%.

A third method defines three zones of EFW. Each zone has a different prevalence of IUGR. In zone 1 the EFW is above the lower 20% confidence limit and IUGR is ruled out. In zone 3 the EFW is below the lower 0.5% confidence limit and yields an 82% prevalence of IUGR. Patients in this zone should be delivered as soon as lung maturity can be proven. If the EFW is between zone 1 and zone 3, it falls into zone 2, which has a 24% prevalence of IUGR. Patients in this zone should have serial sonograms and fetal heart rate monitoring.

Numerous other growth curves are available, but the one chosen must be appropriate for the population of patients (e.g., sea level versus below sea level). It is also important to remember that symmetric IUGR cannot be diagnosed in a single examination. The interval growth can be plotted on a graph to show the growth sequence. Ethnicity, previous obstetric history, paternal size, fetal gender, and the results of tests of fetal well-being must be considered before IUGR, rather than a healthy SGA, can be diagnosed.

A computer-generated antenatal chart is available that can be customized for individual pregnancies, taking the mother's characteristics and birth weights from previous pregnancies into consideration. Through review of 4179 pregnancies with ultrasound-confirmed dates, one study showed that in addition to gestation and gender, maternal weight at first antenatal visit, height, ethnic group, and parity were significant determinants of birth weight in the study population.[8] Correction factors were calculated and entered into a computer program to adjust the normal birth weight percentile limits. With adjusted percentiles, the researchers found that 28% of babies that conventionally fit the criteria for SGA (less than the 10%), and 22% of those who were LGA (greater than the 90%) were in fact within normal limits for the pregnancy. Conversely, 24% and 26% of babies identified as small or large, respectively, with adjusted percentiles were missed by conventional unadjusted percentile assessment.[8]

AMNIOTIC FLUID EVALUATION

The association between IUGR and decreased amniotic fluid (oligohydramnios) is well recognized (Box 47-4). Oligohydramnios has also been associated with fetal renal anomalies, rupture of the intrauterine membranes, and postdate pregnancy. One method, developed for evaluating and quantifying amniotic fluid volume at different intervals during a pregnancy, divides the uterine cavity into four equal quadrants by two imaginary lines running perpendicular to each other. The largest vertical pocket of amniotic fluid, excluding fetal limbs or umbilical cord loops, is measured. The sum of the four quadrants is called the **amniotic fluid index (AFI).** Normal values have been calculated for each gestational age (plus or minus 2 standard deviations). Normal is 8 to 22 cm; decreased is less than 5 cm; and increased is greater than 22 cm (Figure 47-2).

BOX 47-4   **POINTS TO REMEMBER FOR INTRAUTERINE GROWTH RESTRICTION (IUGR)**

- Oligohydramnios occurs if the fetus cannot urinate.
- Polyhydramnios develops if the fetus cannot swallow.
- Amniotic fluid pocket less than 1 to 2 cm may represent IUGR.
- Not all oligohydramnios is associated with IUGR.

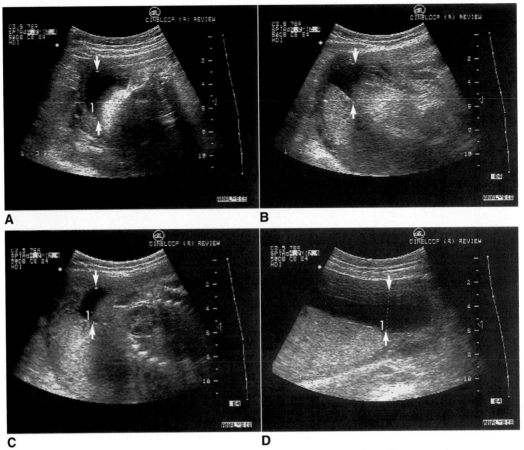

Figure 47-2   The four-quadrant technique of amniotic fluid assessment. This technique produces an amniotic fluid index (AFI). The uterus is divided into four equal parts, and the largest vertical pocket of amniotic fluid in each quadrant is measured, excluding fetal limbs or umbilical cord. The sum of the four quadrants is the AFI, which, in this case, equals 14.2 cm at 31 weeks. This is within normal limits.

Not every laboratory has adapted the AFI technique, and it is still quite acceptable to use the "eyeball technique," which is simply a subjective survey to evaluate the overall amount of amniotic fluid. Various other criteria have been described for defining oligohydramnios, such as occurring when the largest vertical pocket is less than 3 cm, less than 1 cm, or less than 0.5 cm. Whichever technique is chosen, co-workers should use it consistently. The AFI is very helpful in a busy laboratory where multiple sonographers evaluate patients and may have varying opinions on the appearance of normal, decreased, or increased amniotic fluid.

In the presence of oligohydramnios, care should be taken when evaluating fetal growth parameters because they can be compressed. Because the fetus lacks the surrounding fluid protecting it, the circumferences can actually be changed by transducer pressure on the maternal abdomen. This in turn may alter the EFW.

TESTS OF FETAL WELL-BEING

Early diagnosis and estimation of fetal well-being are the main problems in managing IUGR. Fetal breathing motion and urine production were the first functional tests to be assessed.

The fetal urine production rate was first described in 1973. The fetal bladder was measured in three dimensions, and the volume was calculated. This was repeated hourly, and the increase was calculated. Because of the time and cumbersome technique involved, this method has not been adopted for widespread use.

BIOPHYSICAL PROFILE

The **biophysical profile (BPP)** was originally described by Manning and associates in 1980.[13] Since then, numerous modifications and variations have been made by others. The BPP was adapted to form a linear relationship with the assessment of multiple fetal biophysical variables, such as the Apgar score in the newborn infant or vital signs in the adult. Five biophysical parameters were assessed individually and in combination. Each test had a high false-positive rate that was greatly reduced when all five variables were combined.

The five parameters are as follows:

1. Cardiac nonstress test (NST)
2. Observation of fetal breathing movements (FBM)
3. Gross fetal body movements (FM)
4. Fetal tone (FT)
5. Amniotic fluid volume (AFV)

The fetus has a specified time limit (30 minutes) to perform these tasks (Box 47-5). Each variable is arbitrarily assigned a score of 2 when normal and 0 when abnormal. A BPP score of 8 to 10 is considered normal. A score of 4 to 6 has no immediate significance. A score of 0 to 2 indicates either immediate delivery or extending the test to 120 minutes.

Fetal Breathing Movements. A true breathing movement is described as simultaneous inward movement of the chest wall with outward movement of the anterior abdominal wall during inspiration (Figure 47-3). An alternative area to watch for breathing is the fetal kidney movement in the longitudinal plane. Two points are given if one episode of breathing lasting 30 seconds within a 30-minute period is noted by the practitioner. If this is absent, no points are given. The fetal central nervous system initiates and regulates the frequency of fetal breathing movements; these patterns vary with sleep-wake cycles.

Fetal Body and Trunk Gross Movements. At least three definite extremity or trunk movements must be observed within the 30-minute period to score 2 points (Figure 47-4). Fewer than three movements scores zero points. The intact nervous system controls gross fetal body movements; these patterns vary with sleep-wake cycles.

Fetal Tone. Fetal tone is characterized by the presence of at least one episode of extension and immediate return to flexion of an extremity or the spine (Figure 47-5). One active extension and flexion of an open and closed hand would be a good example of positive fetal tone (Figure 47-6). Such a movement would score two points. Abnormal fetal tone is noted by a partial extension or flexion of an extremity without a quick return and would score zero points.

Amniotic Fluid Volume. Amniotic fluid volume is related to the fetal-placental unit and is not influenced by the fetal central nervous system. Premature aging of the placenta (grade III) may contribute to oligohydramnios of IUGR syndrome. Evaluation of the four-quadrant amniotic fluid volume is

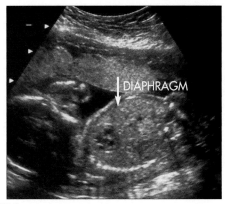

Figure 47-3 Fetal breathing may be seen as the chest wall moves inward and the anterior abdominal wall moves outward; breathing may also be seen by watching the movement of the kidney in the longitudinal plane.

BOX 47-5	BIOPHYSICAL PROFILE (BPP)

To determine the BPP, assign a value of 2 points to each of the following:

- *Fetal breathing movement (FBM):* One episode for 30 seconds continuous during a 30-minute observation.
- *Gross body movement:* At least three discrete body or limb movements in 30 minutes, unprovoked. Continuous movement for 30 minutes should be counted as one movement.
- *Fetal tone:* Active extension and flexion of at least one episode of limbs or trunk.
- *Fetal heart rate (FHR):* Also known as the nonstress test (NST). At least two episodes of fetal heart rate of 15 beats per minute and at least 15 seconds duration in a 20-minute period.
- *Amniotic fluid index (AFI):* One pocket of amniotic fluid at least 2 cm in two perpendicular planes or AFI total fluid measures of 5 to 22 cm.

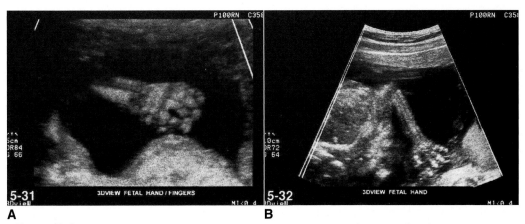

A   **B**

Figure 47-4 At least three definite extremity or trunk movements must be seen within the 30-minute period in a normal fetus. **A,** Open fetal hand and wrist. **B,** Elbow, forearm, and wrist.

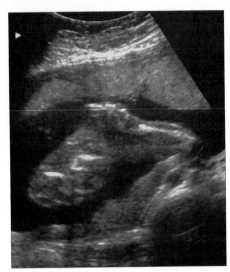

Figure 47-5 Fetal tone is characterized by the presence of at least one episode of extension and immediate return to flexion of an extremity or the spine. This view of the upper extremity is shown in flexion.

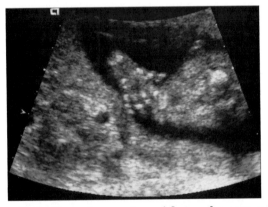

Figure 47-6 One active extension and flexion of an open and closed hand is a good example of positive fetal tone. This image shows the hand wide open, with all fingers and thumb extended.

considered normal if the pockets (quadrants) of fluid measure at least 2 cm or more in two planes and a score of two points is given. The transducer must be perpendicular to the center of the pocket of fluid in the center of the screen, and the uterine wall cannot be included as part of the fluid measurement.

Decreased amniotic fluid may represent IUGR or intrauterine stress, and serial growth parameters may need to be assessed. Fluid that is decreased near term indicates that the baby may need to be delivered earlier than planned. Decreased fluid means the blood is redistributed to the head and the heart; a decrease in blood to the kidneys causes the AFI to decrease.

Nonstress Test

The **nonstress test (NST)** is done using Doppler to record fetal heart rate and its reactivity to the stress of uterine contraction. The time expended for this portion of the examination is usually 40 minutes. Fetal motion is detected as a rapid rise on the recording of uterine activity or the patient noting fetal movements. The following conditions indicate a reactive, or normal, NST and score of two points:

- Two fetal heart rate accelerations of 15 beats per minute or more
- Accelerations lasting at least 15 seconds
- Gross fetal movements noted over 20 minutes without late decelerations

These fetal heart accelerations with fetal movements are a positive sign of fetal well-being; late reductions in rate or decelerations indicate a poor prognosis. Zero points are awarded if two fetal heart rate accelerations with gross fetal movements are not seen during a 40-minute period. Forty minutes is arbitrarily used to accommodate the fetal sleep-wake cycles.

The test is considered normal when all the variables monitored by ultrasound imaging are normal (FBM, FM, FT, AFV) without the performance of the NST.

The goal of the BPP is to find a way to predict and manage the fetus with hypoxia. One study analyzed the BPP variables based on the gradual hypoxia concept. This concept states that dynamic biophysical activities (FT, FM, FBM, and fetal heart rate reactivity) are controlled by neural activity arising in distinct anatomic sites in the brain. These become functional at different stages of development, with the later-developing centers requiring higher oxygen levels. The fetal tone center develops at 7.5 to 8.5 weeks. The fetal movement center develops at 9 weeks, and regular diaphragmatic motion develops by 20 to 21 weeks. Heart rate reactivity is the last to occur; it appears by the late second to early third trimester. This hypothesis further states that centers that develop later are more sensitive to acute hypoxia. It is therefore expected that the loss of cardiac reactivity and suppression of fetal breathing movements will occur with relatively mild hypoxia. Cessation of FM and eventually loss of FT will occur with progressively more profound hypoxemia.

Doppler Ultrasound

Obstetric **Doppler** velocimetry is one of the newest techniques to evaluate the fetal environment. Doppler is the study of reflections of blood flow. It was first described in 1842 by Christian Johann Doppler, an Austrian professor of mathematics and geometry.

There are two basic types of Doppler. The simplest technique is continuous wave (CW) Doppler. The second is pulsed wave (PW) Doppler. With CW Doppler, a single transducer has two separate piezoelectric crystals, one that continuously transmits signals and one that simultaneously receives signals. Because the crystals are either emitting or receiving sound, CW Doppler measures no specific range or depth resolution (i.e., it records all velocities along the designated line of interrogation). No intrauterine imaging is available with CW, but it may be used in conjunction with a real-time ultrasound system to locate or confirm a vessel sampling site. CW is limited to the study of superficial vessels because it cannot discriminate between signals arising from different structures along the beam path.

In pulsed wave (PW) Doppler, short bursts of ultrasound energy are emitted at regular intervals. The same piezoelectric crystal both sends and receives the signals. This allows for range or depth discrimination. The depth of the target is calculated from the elapsed time between transmission of the pulse and reception of its echoes, assuming a constant speed of sound in tissue. In PW Doppler a sonographer can electronically steer the insonating Doppler beam with the trackball or joystick on the keyboard. This permits sampling of vessels at specific anatomic locations.

In one study, CW and PW Doppler were compared using the patient as the control.[14] The systolic to diastolic (S/D or A/B) ratios were obtained from the umbilical artery and the maternal uterine arteries with both CW and PW Doppler systems. The results were comparable. Laboratories can use either a CW or PW Doppler system effectively.

Up to the present, Doppler, or real-time, ultrasound has not been associated with any ill effect to the mother or the fetus when used at the manufacturer's recommended safety level. U.S. Food and Drug Administration guidelines state that the spatial peak-temporal average intensity (SPTA, a unit used to measure ultrasound intensity) must be less than 94 milliwatts per square centimeter (mW/cm^2) in situ. Most commercial equipment uses variable acoustic outputs between 1 and 46 mW/cm^2. The power output of a given unit should be known before the unit is used on a fetus. Newer ultrasound equipment now allows the user to display this information on the screen as the examination is being performed.

Quantitative and Qualitative Measurements. Two main types of measurements can be taken from a Doppler waveform: quantitative and qualitative. Quantitative Doppler flow measurements include blood flow and velocity, whereas qualitative measurements look at the characteristics of the waveform that indirectly approximate flow and resistance to flow. Qualitative measurements include **systolic to diastolic (S/D)** ratio, resistance index (RI), and pulsatility index (Box 47-6). The S/D ratio measures peak systole to end-diastolic blood flow. The RI is calculated as systole minus diastole divided by systole. The pulsatility takes the difference between peak-systole and end-diastole and divides this by the mean of the maximum frequency over the whole cardiac cycle.

Doppler ultrasound has shown that in fetuses with asymmetric IUGR, vascular resistance increases in the aorta and umbilical artery and decreases in the fetal middle cerebral artery. This reinforces the head-sparing theory, which describes the assurance of blood flow to the fetal brain at the expense of the extremities.

Increased vascular resistance is reflected by an increased S/D ratio or pulsatility index. Some authors consider an S/D ratio of more than 3.0 in the umbilical artery after 30 weeks to be abnormal and is demonstrated by increased resistance in the fetal circulation.[19] The maternal uterine artery S/D ratio should be below 2.6 (Figures 47-7 and 47-8). A ratio above 2.6 suggests increased vascular resistance and indicates a decreased maternal blood supply to the uterus.

In the umbilical circulation, extreme cases of elevated resistance causing absent or reverse end-diastolic flow velocity waveforms are associated with high rates of morbidity and mortality. One report demonstrated that an SGA fetus with an

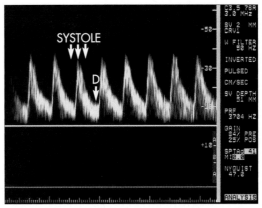

Figure 47-7 Typical umbilical artery Doppler waveform representing a normal systolic to diastolic ratio. The ratio measures peak-systolic to end-diastolic flow. The calipers should be placed at the top of the systolic peak and at the bottom of the diastolic trough. Note the normal amount of diastolic flow. *D,* Diastole.

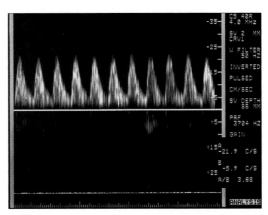

Figure 47-8 Umbilical artery Doppler waveform demonstrating increased vascular resistance (less diastolic flow) in the fetal umbilical circulation. The systolic to diastolic (S/D) ratio is 3.8. Some authors consider an S/D ratio of more than 3.0 after 30 weeks of gestation to be abnormal.

BOX 47-6   DOPPLER MEASUREMENTS

Resistive Index (RI) = maximum systolic velocity – diastolic velocity/systolic velocity

Systolic/Diastolic Ratio (S/D) = maximum systolic velocity/diastolic velocity

Pulsatility Index (PI) = maximum systolic velocity – diastolic velocity/mean velocity

Acceleration time (ACC) = time from beginning of systole to peak systole

Deceleration time (DCC) = time from peak systole to end diastole

increased umbilical artery S/D ratio is at much higher risk for poor perinatal outcome than a small fetus with a normal S/D ratio (Figures 47-9 and 47-10).[22]

In one series a growth-restricted fetus with an abnormal S/D ratio was found to be at risk for early delivery, reduced birth weight, decreased amniotic fluid at birth, admission to the neonatal intensive care unit, neonatal complications associated with IUGR, and a prolonged hospital stay.[2] Other authors have reported similar results.[17,22]

Abnormal umbilical artery S/D velocity waveforms have been shown to improve with the patient on bed rest in the left lateral position. The patients were closely monitored with serial Doppler, BPP, and fetal growth evaluation. Of 128 pregnant women, 66 (51.5%) reverted to normal flow in 4.5 weeks, ±1.5 weeks. Another group (48.5%) exhibited persistent abnormal flow.[20] None of the improved group exhibited fetal distress or perinatal mortality, whereas in the abnormal flow group 24% experienced fetal distress and 13% experienced perinatal mor-

tality. The report of the study proposes that a subset of patients with abnormal Doppler velocimetry improves with bed rest and has a better perinatal outcome, whereas patients with persistent abnormal flow are at risk for poor perinatal outcome.

In conclusion, the best method of solving the puzzle of whether a fetus has IUGR or is constitutionally small is to combine an evaluation of all parameters. A normal umbilical artery, maternal uterine artery, and fetal middle cerebral artery help in evaluating the fetus that is well and normal but just small, rather than small secondary to IUGR. The practitioner also must consider the family history of birth weights and ethnicity. For example, it is almost invalid to use the standard EFW growth curves when plotting the fetal growth of a constitutionally small ethnic group, such as Asians. A fetus could be labeled as SGA, although its size might be totally appropriate for its heritage. Use of all the fetal surveillance tests (i.e., EFW, AFI, placental grading, BPP, NST) may allow better evaluation of the in utero environment.

MACROSOMIA

Macrosomia has classically been defined as a birth weight of 4000 g or greater or above the 90th percentile for estimated gestational age. With respect to delivery, however, any fetus that is too large for the pelvis through which it must pass is macrosomic. Macrosomia has shown to be 1.2 to 2 times more frequent than normal in women who are multiparous, are 35 years or older, have a prepregnancy weight of more than 70 kg (154 lb), have a PI in the upper 10%, have pregnancy weight gain of 20 kg (44 lb) or greater, have a postdate pregnancy, or have a history of delivering an LGA fetus.

Macrosomia is also a common result of poorly controlled maternal diabetes mellitus. The frequency of macrosomia in the offspring of mothers with diabetes ranges from 25% to 45%. It is widely accepted that increased levels of glucose and other substrates result in fetal hyperinsulinemia, which promotes accelerated somatic growth. Macrosomic infants of insulin-dependent diabetic mothers are usually heavy and show a characteristic pattern of organomegaly. In addition to adipose tissue, the liver, heart, and adrenals are disproportionately increased in size. Not all infants of diabetic mothers are larger than average; diabetic mothers with severe vascular disease may in fact be growth restricted.

Malformation syndromes in which fetal increase in size, with or without organomegaly, is a feature include Beckwith-Wiedemann syndrome, Marshall-Smith syndrome, Sotos' syndrome, and Weaver's syndrome.

The macrosomic fetus has an increased incidence of morbidity and mortality as a result of head and shoulder injuries and cord compression. One study found an increasing incidence of shoulder dystocia as birth weight increased.[1] The incidence was 10% in fetuses less than 4500 g and increased to 22.6% in fetuses more than 4500 g. Another study also found an increase, but the overall percentiles were less.[18] This study reported that shoulder dystocia occurred in 4.7% of study fetuses greater than 4000 g and 9.4% of fetuses greater than 4500 g.

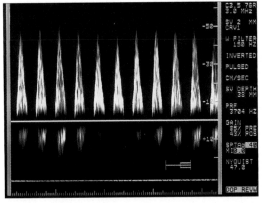

Figure 47-9 Umbilical artery waveform with absent end-diastolic velocity (AEDV). The S/D ratio cannot be measured in these cases because of the missing diastolic flow. The patient should be followed closely because AEDV has been associated with adverse perinatal outcome.

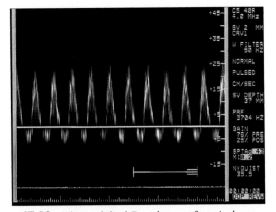

Figure 47-10 This umbilical Doppler waveform is the most severe Doppler finding and has been associated with adverse fetal outcomes. This finding is called *complete reversal of end-diastolic velocity.* Note how the diastolic flow dips below the baseline. These results should be reported immediately to the patient's physician.

Clavicular fractures, facial and brachial palsies, meconium aspiration, perinatal asphyxia, neonatal hypoglycemia, and other metabolic complications are significantly increased in macrosomic pregnancies.

Timing and mode of delivery of the potential macrosomic fetus are of great concern to the obstetrician. One study demonstrated that the incidence of macrosomia increased from 1.7% at 36 weeks to 21% at 42 weeks.[3] A retrospective study evaluated 406 women by ultrasound late in the third trimester to see if the diagnosis of LGA altered the management of labor and delivery.[12] The sonographic prediction of LGA fetuses had a sensitivity, specificity, and positive predictive value of 50%, 90%, and 52%, respectively. Although there were no significant differences in the rate of induction, use of oxytocin, or use of forceps, women with an ultrasound diagnosis of an LGA fetus more frequently received epidural anesthesia and had more cesarean deliveries than women without that diagnosis. The sonographic prediction of EFW in this series was incorrect in half of the cases, with the EFW both underestimating and overestimating the actual birth weight.

Clinical considerations of macrosomia should include the genetic constitution (e.g., familial traits) and environmental factors (e.g., maternal diabetes or prolonged pregnancy).

Two terms relating to macrosomic fetuses are *mechanical macrosomia* and *metabolic macrosomia.* Three types of mechanical macrosomia have been identified: (1) fetuses that are generally large, (2) fetuses that are generally large but with especially large shoulders, and (3) fetuses that have a normal trunk but a large head. The first type can result from genetic factors, prolonged pregnancy, or multiparity. The second type is found in the diabetic pregnancy, and the third type can be caused by genetic constitution or pathologic process, such as hydrocephalus. One type of metabolic macrosomia has been identified, which is the group of LGA fetuses based on a standard weight curve appropriate for the population being studied and a normal range extending to 2 standard deviations above the mean.[6]

BIPARIETAL DIAMETER

Accurate sonographic prediction of macrosomia would be invaluable to the obstetrician in managing and delivering a fetus with macrosomia. The detection of fetal macrosomia by BPD was first described in 1979.[4] The authors found that all fetuses that were appropriate for gestational age (AGA) at delivery had normal antenatal BPD measurements, but that 25 out of 26 fetuses with two or more BPD values above the 97th percentile were large for gestational age (LGA) at delivery.[4] Another study of the normal progression of fetal head growth in diabetic pregnancies found that, in contrast to the fetal liver, the fetal brain is not sensitive to the growth-promoting effects of insulin.[16] Most investigators believe, however, that BPD is not the optimal parameter for prediction of macrosomia.

ABDOMINAL CIRCUMFERENCE

As stated before, AC is useful as a parameter to assess fetal size. It is not very predictive of gestational age. It is probably the single most valuable biometric parameter used in assessing fetal

growth (Figure 47-11). In one series the authors were able to predict 4 of 4 macrosomic fetuses when a change in the abdominal circumference was greater than or equal to 1.2 cm per week between the 32nd and 39th weeks of pregnancy (<4000 g), 17 out of 21 (81%) of the fetuses with birth weights between 4000 and 4499 g, and 5 out of 6 (83%) of the fetuses with birth weights exceeding 4500 g.[11] When the abdominal growth was less than 1.2 cm per week (between 32 and 39 weeks), normal fetal growth was correctly identified in 89.1% of cases.

One study found that in fetuses with birth weights less than 4000 g, both the BPD and AC were within the standard deviation for the gestational age.[16] In fetuses greater than 4000 g, normal BPD values were found, but the AC values were greater than 2 standard deviations above the norm after 28 to 32 weeks.[16]

ESTIMATED FETAL WEIGHT

Sonographic estimation of fetal weight to determine macrosomia is of some value. According to one study, EFWs above the 90th percentile are considered macrosomic.[21] A significant number of false-positive and false-negative results can be expected unless the actual weight is either less than 3600 g or greater than 4500 g. The reason for this may be that currently

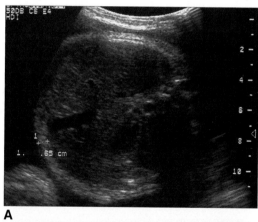

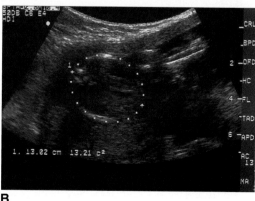

Figure 47-11 A, Transverse section through a macrosomic fetal abdomen. Note the fat rind *(calipers)* encircling the entire abdomen compared with a severely intrauterine growth-restricted fetus **(B)**, whose growth is 8 weeks behind. The fetal skin is almost transparent and difficult to differentiate from other surrounding organs.

available formulas to estimate fetal weight assume a uniform density of tissue. Because fat tissue is less dense than lean body mass, it can be hypothesized that sonographic overestimation of fetal weight, particularly in diabetic mothers, is the consequence of an elevated proportion of body fat. This results in a lower body density.

In one report, the pulsatility index (PI) and skinfold thickness were both significantly greater in infants whose sonograms overpredicted the fetal weight compared with those whose sonograms underpredicted the fetal weight.[2] The PI and skinfold thickness are indexes to directly measure fat. The study reported that estimating fetal fat would provide a correction to formulas predicting fetal weight and improve the accuracy of the estimation.

FEMUR LENGTH TO ABDOMINAL CIRCUMFERENCE

Another approach to detecting macrosomia is the femur length to abdominal circumference (FL-AC) ratio. This is a time-independent proportionality index. A study of 156 fetuses within 1 week of delivery was done using a cutoff of less than 20.5% (the 10th percentile).[9] Prenatal FL-AC values less than the 10th percentile and newborns with birth weights above the 90th percentile were classified as macrosomic, both prenatal and postnatal. The authors were only able to predict 63% of fetuses that were macrosomic, which suggests that this ratio has a limited clinical application. Current studies fail to show a significant increase in the length of the femur in the macrosomic infant.

CHEST CIRCUMFERENCE

Chest circumference has been described as a useful parameter in detecting the LGA fetus, with reported detection rates of 80% and 47% in relation to the 90th and 95th percentiles, respectively, for macrosomic fetuses.[23] The sonographic technique of the study is not used frequently. It appears that fetal chest measurements are taken just below the area where cardiac pulsations were identified at the level of the upper fetal abdomen.

MACROSOMIA INDEX

Calculating a macrosomic index can be performed by subtracting the BPD from the chest diameter. Chest circumference is measured at the level of the upper fetal abdomen. In a study involving subtraction of the BPD from the chest diameter, 87% of infants weighing more than 4000 g had a macrosomic index of 1.4 cm or greater.[7] Fetal weight less than 4000 g was predicted accurately in 92% of infants who had a macrosomic index of 1.3 or less. Although this test appears to be quite sensitive, only 61% of those with a positive result were found to be macrosomic at birth.

OTHER METHODS FOR DETECTING MACROSOMIA

In addition to the numerous biometric parameters useful for detecting macrosomia discussed, there are other ultrasound observations that can help rule out the possibility of fetal macrosomia. Mothers with diabetes may accumulate more amniotic fluid (polyhydramnios) than nondiabetic patients. The presence of polyhydramnios in the nondiabetic patient could alert the physician to the presence of undiagnosed maternal glucose intolerance. The possibility of a fetal anomaly should not be excluded; polyhydramnios has been associated with open neural tube defects.

The placentas of the macrosomic fetus can become significantly large and thick because they are not immune to the growth-enhancing effects of fetal insulin. A placental thickness greater than 5 cm is considered thick when the measurement is taken at right angles to its long axis.

REFERENCES

1. Acker DB, Sachs BP, Freidman EA: Risk factors for shoulder dystocia, *Obstet Gynecol* 66:762, 1985.
2. Bernstein I, Catalano P: Influence of fetal fat on the ultrasound estimation of fetal weight in diabetic mothers, *Obstet Gynecol* 79:561, 1992.
3. Boyd ME, Usher RH, Mclean FH: Fetal macrosomia: prediction, risks, proposed management, *Obstet Gynecol* 61:715, 1983.
4. Crane JP, Kropa MM: Prediction of intrauterine growth retardation via ultrasonically measured head/abdominal circumference ratios, *Obstet Gynecol* 54:597, 1979.
5. Dal Compo S, Sabbagha RE: Intrauterine growth retardation. In Berman M, editor: *Obstetrics and gynecology*, New York, 1991, JB Lippincott.
6. Deter RL, Hadlock FP: Use of ultrasound in the detection of macrosomia: a review, *J Clin Ultrasound* 13:519, 1985.
7. Elliott JP and others: Ultrasound prediction of fetal macrosomia in diabetic patients, *Obstet Gynecol* 60:159, 1982.
8. Gardosi J and others: Customized antenatal growth charts, *Lancet* 339:283, 1992.
9. Hadlock FP and others: Estimation of fetal weight with the use of head, body, and femur measurements: a prospective study, *Am J Obstet Gynecol* 15:333, 1985.
10. Joupilla P and others: Ultrasonic abnormalities associated with the pathology of fetal karyotype results during the early second trimester of pregnancy, *J Ultrasound Med* 7:218, 1988.
11. Landon M and others: Sonographic evaluation of fetal abdominal growth: predictor of the large-for-gestational age infant in pregnancies complicated by diabetes mellitus, *Am J Obstet Gynecol* 160:115, 1989.
12. Levine AB and others: Sonographic diagnosis of the large for gestational age fetus at term: does it make a difference? *Obstet Gynecol* 79:55, 1992.
13. Manning FA, Platt LP, Sypus L: Antepartum fetal evaluation: development of a biophysical profile, *Am J Obstet Gynecol* 136:787, 1980.
14. Mehalek K and others: Comparison of continuous wave and pulsed wave S/D ratios of umbilical and uterine arteries, *Am J Obstet Gynecol* 72:603, 1988.
15. Nicolaides KH, Rodeck CH, Goslen CM: Rapid karyotyping in non-lethal fetal malformations, *Lancet* 1:283, 1986.
16. Ogata ES and others: Serial ultrasonography to assess evolving fetal macrosomia, *JAMA* 243:2405, 1980.
17. Phelan JP and others: Amniotic fluid volume assessment with the four quadrant technique at 36-42 weeks gestation, *J Reprod Fertil* 32:540, 1987.
18. Sandmire MF, O'Halloin TJ: Shoulder dystocia: its incidence and associated risk factors, *Int J Gynecol Obstet* 26:65, 1988.
19. Schulman H and others: Umbilical velocity wave ratio in human pregnancy, *Am J Obstet Gynecol* 148:985, 1984.

20. Sengupta S and others: Perinatal outcome following improvement of abnormal umbilical artery velocimetry, *Obstet Gynecol* 78:1062, 1992.
21. Shephard MJ and others: An evaluation of two equations for predicting fetal weight by ultrasound, *AM J Obstet Gynecol* 142:47, 1982.
22. Trudinger BJ and others: Flow velocity waveforms in the material uteroplacental and fetal umbilical placental circulations, *Am J Obstet Gynecol* 152:155, 1985.
23. Wladimeroff JW, Bloemsma CA, Wallenberg HCS: Ultrasonic diagnosis of the large-for-dates infant, *Obstet Gynecol* 52:285, 1978.

SELECTED BIBLIOGRAPHY

Bracero L et al: Umbilical artery velocimetry waveform in diabetic pregnancy, *Obstet Gynecol* 68:654, 1986.

Campbell S, Thoms A: Ultrasonic measurement of the fetal head to abdominal circumference ratio in the assessment of growth retardation, *Br J Obstet Gynecol* 84:165, 1977.

Chervenak FA, Jeanty P, Hobbins JC: Current status of fetal age and growth assessment, *Clin Obstet Gynecol Pec* 10:424, 1983.

Doppler CJ: Uber das farbige Licht der Doppler-sterne, *Abhand Lungen der Koniglishen Bohmischen Gesellschaft der Wissenchaften* 2:465, 1842.

Hadlock FP, Deter RL, Harrist RB: Sonographic detection of abnormal fetal growth patterns, *Clin Obstet Gynecol* 27:342, 1984.

Hadlock FP and others: Use of the femur length/abdominal circumference ratio in detecting the macrosomic fetus, *Radiology* 154:503, 1985.

Halpern ME and others: Reliability of amniotic fluid volume estimation from ultrasonograms: intraobserver and interobserver variation before and after the establishment of criteria, *Am J Obstet Gynecol* 153:264, 1985.

Jones KL, Smith S: *Recognizable patterns of human malformation,* ed 4, Philadelphia, 1988, WB Saunders.

Landon M and others: Sonographic evaluation of fetal abdominal growth: predictor of the large-for-gestational-age infant in pregnancies complicated by diabetes mellitus, *Am J Obstet Gynecol* 160:115, 1989.

Lin CC, Santolaya-Forgas J: Current concepts of fetal growth restriction. Part I: causes, classification, and pathophysiology, *Obstet Gynecol* 92:1044-1055, 1998.

Manning FA, Hill LM, Platt LD: Qualitative amniotic fluid volume determination by ultrasound: antepartum detection of intrauterine growth retardation, *Am J Obstet Gynecol* 139:254, 1981.

Manning FA and others: Fetal assessment based on biophysical scoring, *Am J Obstet Gynecol* 162:703, 1990.

Mercer LJ and others: A survey of pregnancies complicated by decreased amniotic fluid, *Am J Obstet Gynecol* 149:355, 1984.

Ott WJ, Doyle S: Ultrasonic diagnosis of altered fetal growth by use of a normal ultrasonic fetal weight curve, *Obstet Gynecol* 63:201, 1984.

Walraven GE, Mkanje RJ, van Roosmalen J and others: Single pre-delivery symphysis-fundal height measurement as a predictor of birthweight and multiple pregnancy, *Br J Obstet Gynaecol* 102:525-529, 1995.

Xiong X, Mayes D, Demiaczuk N and others: Impact of pregnancy-induced hypertension on fetal growth, *Am J Obstet Gynecol* 180:207-213, 1999.

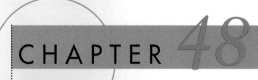

CHAPTER 48

Ultrasound and High-Risk Pregnancy

Carol Mitchell and Barbara Trampe

OBJECTIVES

- Define what is meant by a high-risk pregnancy
- List maternal factors that make a pregnancy high-risk
- List fetal factors that make a pregnancy high-risk

SCREENING TESTS

MATERNAL FACTORS IN HIGH-RISK PREGNANCY
ADVANCED MATERNAL AGE
IMMUNE AND NONIMMUNE HYDROPS
VAGINAL BLEEDING

MATERNAL DISEASES OF PREGNANCY
DIABETES
HYPERTENSION
SYSTEMIC LUPUS ERYTHEMATOSUS
OTHER MATERNAL DISEASE

ULTRASOUND IN LABOR AND DELIVERY
PREMATURE LABOR

FETAL FACTORS IN HIGH-RISK PREGNANCY
FETAL DEATH
LARGE FOR GESTATIONAL AGE
SMALL FOR GESTATIONAL AGE

MULTIPLE GESTATION PREGNANCY
DIZYGOTIC TWINS
MONOZYGOTIC TWINS
POLY-OLI SEQUENCE ("STUCK TWIN")
SCANNING MULTIPLE GESTATIONS

KEY TERMS

acardiac anomaly – a rare anomaly in monochorionic twins in which one twin develops without a heart and often without an upper half of the body

anasarca – severe generalized massive edema often seen with fetal hydrops

caudal regression syndrome – lack of development of the caudal spine and cord that may occur in the fetus of a diabetic mother

conjoined twins – occurs when the division of the egg occurs after 13 days

dizygotic – twins that arise from two separately fertilized ova

eclampsia – coma and seizures in the second- and third-trimester patient secondary to pregnancy-induced hypertension

fetus papyraceous – fetal death that occurs after the fetus has reached a certain growth that is too large to resorb into the uterus

hydrops fetalis – fluid occurring in at least two areas: pleural effusion, pericardial effusion, ascites, or skin edema

hyperemesis gravidarum – excessive vomiting that leads to dehydration and electrolyte imbalance

maternal serum alpha-fetoprotein (MSAFP) – an antigen present in the fetus; the maternal serum is tested between 15 and 22 weeks of gestation to detect abnormal levels; can also be tested directly from the amniotic fluid during amniocentesis

maternal serum quad screen – a blood test conducted during the second trimester (15 to 22 weeks) to identify pregnancies at a higher risk for chromosomal anomalies (trisomy 21 and trisomy 18) and neural tube defects

monozygotic – twins that arise from a single fertilized egg, which divides to produce two identical fetuses

nonimmune hydrops (NIH) – term that describes a group of conditions in which hydrops is present in the fetus but is not a result of fetomaternal blood group incompatibility

oligohydramnios – too little amniotic fluid; fluid measures <5 cm of the amniotic fluid index

polyhydramnios – too much amniotic fluid; fluid measures >22 cm of the amniotic fluid index

preeclampsia – (also known as pregnancy-induced hypertension [PIH]) a complication of pregnancy characterized by increasing hypertension, proteinuria, and edema

Rh blood group – system of antigens that may be found on the surface of red blood cells. When the Rh antigen is present, the blood type is Rh positive; when the Rh antigen is absent, the blood type is Rh negative. A pregnant woman who is Rh negative may become sensitized by the blood of an Rh-positive fetus. In subsequent pregnancies, if the fetus is Rh positive, the Rh antibodies produced in maternal blood may cross the placenta and destroy fetal cells, causing erythroblastosis fetalis.

Spalding's sign – overlapping of the skull bones; indicates fetal death

systemic lupus erythematosus (SLE) – inflammatory disease involving multiple organ systems; a fetus of a mother with SLE may develop heart block and pericardial effusion

twin–twin transfusion syndrome – monozygotic twin pregnancy with single placenta and arteriovenous shunt within the placenta; the donor twin becomes anemic and growth restricted with oligohydramnios; the recipient twin may develop hydrops and polyhydramnios

---

High-risk pregnancies are pregnancies that have an increased chance for an adverse outcome. At its extreme, an adverse outcome means maternal or fetal injury or death. Ultrasound plays an important role in the management of high-risk obstetric patients. It can provide a "window" through which the physician can "see" inside the uterus and look at the fetus. For example, when a mother presents with vaginal bleeding, a common obstetric complication, placental location can easily be determined. Ultrasound can also be used to determine gestational age and to monitor fetal growth. Ultrasound can detect multiple gestations early in pregnancy, providing physicians with valuable information for managing prenatal care. There are many more examples of how ultrasound can influence obstetric management of the pregnant patient. This chapter deals with the interaction between high-risk pregnancies and ultrasound.

SCREENING TESTS

Screening tests are offered to low-risk populations to identify patients whose risk is high enough to be offered diagnostic testing.

Screening for fetal anomalies can be performed in either the first or second trimester. In the first trimester, testing is performed to identify the pattern of biochemical markers associated with plasma protein A (PAPP-A) and free BhCG.[14] These lab values are used in conjunction with an ultrasound (performed between 11 and 14 weeks) to measure the nuchal translucency. Based on the patient's PAPP-A and free BhCG lab values, age, and nuchal translucency measurement, a more accurate risk calculation can be made for having a child with a chromosomal abnormality.

To offer this kind of screening, ultrasound labs must become accredited for first-trimester screening. To become accredited, sonographers and physicians performing the test must attend a specialized training course and perform 40 to 50 first-trimester nuchal translucency measurement exams, which are sent to a core lab for evaluation and monitoring.[7]

The advantage for parents with first-trimester screening is that they can evaluate their risk for having a child with a chromosomal problem much earlier in pregnancy and then decide whether to undergo invasive testing with chorionic villus sampling (CVS) or amniocentesis to obtain tissue for chromosomal analysis.

Second-trimester screening can be performed with the **maternal serum quad screen** lab value and a targeted ultrasound exam. The quad screen looks at the following serum markers: alpha-fetoprotein (AFP), human chorionic gonadotropin (hCG), unconjugated estriol (uE3), and inhibin-A. The targeted ultrasound is a detailed evaluation of all fetal anatomy that can be seen at the time of exam. Many labs prefer to perform the targeted exam between 18 and 20 weeks' gestation. This time period is chosen because it often yields the best view of fetal anatomy based on size. The targeted ultrasound exam includes, but is not limited to, the evaluation of the anatomy shown in Table 48-1.

Based on the results of the maternal serum quad screen and the targeted ultrasound, the patient's risk for having a child with a chromosomal anomaly or neural tube defect can be reassessed. Parents are counseled with this information and then can choose to have a diagnostic amniocentesis to obtain fluid for chromosomal analysis, if desired.

MATERNAL FACTORS IN HIGH-RISK PREGNANCY

ADVANCED MATERNAL AGE

By definition, advanced maternal age (AMA) refers to a patient who will be 35 or older at the time of delivery. Advanced maternal age can be an indicator for high-risk pregnancy. For example, the incidence of Down syndrome increases with age. The risk of a 35-year-old woman conceiving a fetus with Down syndrome is 1 in 385, but the risk rises to 1 in 32 at age 45.[1] Maternal age alone, however, fails to account for approximately 80% of fetuses with Down syndrome[1] because Down syndrome babies are being born to younger women without known risk factors for chromosomal abnormalities. In the United States, it is now standard practice to offer AMA women genetic counseling and invasive prenatal testing for karyotypic analysis, and the American College of Obstetrics and Gynecology (ACOG) guidelines recommend that maternal serum screening for neural tube defects and Down syndrome be offered to all women.

IMMUNE AND NONIMMUNE HYDROPS

Hydrops fetalis is a condition in which excessive fluid accumulates within the fetal body cavities. This fluid accumulation may result in **anasarca**, ascites, pericardial effusion, pleural effusion, placental edema, and polyhydramnios. There are two classifications of fetal hydrops: immune hydrops and nonimmune hydrops. Nonimmune hydrops is not related to the presence of maternal serum IgG antibody against one of the fetal blood cell antigens. By ultrasound evaluation, both types are

TABLE 48-1	TARGETED ULTRASOUND IN HIGH-RISK PREGNANCY
Anatomy	**What to Document**
Central nervous system (CNS)	• Brain • Choroid plexus • Lateral ventricle (measure at the level of the atrium) • Thalamus • Third ventricle • Cerebellum (measure) • Cisterna magna (measure) • Nuchal thickness • Biparietal diameter (BPD) • Head circumference (HC) • Spine • Longitudinal (cervical, thoracic, lumbar, sacral) • Transverse (cervical, thoracic, lumbar, sacral)
Face	• Orbits • Upper lip • Palate • Nose • Profile
Heart	• Four-chamber view • Left ventricular outflow • Right ventricular outflow • Three-vessel view • Aortic arch • Ductus arteriosus
Gastrointestinal (GI) system	• Stomach • Diaphragm • Abdominal circumference (AC)
Genitourinary (GU) system	• Kidneys • Bladder
Abdominal wall	• Cord insertion
Three-vessel cord	• Umbilical cord as it enters the abdomen, and each artery courses around the bladder
Four extremities	• Measure humerus • Measure femur • Document both hands • Document both feet
Placenta	• Location • Absence of previa
Amniotic fluid volume	• Single largest pocket until 24 weeks • Amniotic fluid index after 24 weeks
Cervix	• Screening evaluation abdominally after 16 weeks • Endovaginal evaluation of length should be greater than 3 cm

characterized by extensive accumulation of fluids in fetal tissues or body cavities.

Immune Hydrops. Blood group isoimmunization is diagnosed on routine antenatal laboratory evaluation, which tests for the presence of a variety of antibodies. Any significant antibodies are evaluated for strength of antibody response, which is reported in a titer format (i.e., 1:4, 1:16, etc.). If an antibody titer is detected, the pregnancy should be monitored.

Immune hydrops is initiated by the presence of maternal serum immunoglobulin G (IgG) antibody, which acts against one of the fetal red blood cell antigens in a process known as sensitization. An antigen is any substance that elicits an immunologic response, such as production of an antibody to that substance. In pregnancy, this can occur anytime a mother is exposed to red blood cell antigens different from her own. For example, if a father and fetus are Rh+ and a mother is Rh−, and there is a maternal-fetal hemorrhage (mixing of blood), maternal antibodies can be produced against the Rh antigen. In subsequent pregnancies, these antibodies can pass through the placenta and destroy fetal blood cells. This causes the maternal serum immunoglobulin G titer to be elevated, resulting in fetal anemia (Figure 48-1). Severe cases lead to immune hydrops. Today, this condition is rare and can be prevented if RhoGAM is given in any instance where there is the potential for mixing of the maternal and fetal circulation.

When a sensitized gravid uterus is not treated with RhoGAM, the mother develops an antibody called maternal IgG. This antibody is able to cross the maternal fetal barrier and enter the fetal circulation. It attaches to the fetal red blood cell and destroys it (hemolysis). The fetal bone marrow must then replace the destroyed red blood cells. If the bone marrow cannot keep up with the destruction, new sites are recruited to produce additional red blood cells (extramedullary poiesis). This hemolysis can result in fetal anemia, leading to congestive heart failure and edema of fetal tissue (anasarca). The severity of fetal anemia can be determined by sonographic surveillance, amniocentesis, and cordocentesis.

Sonographic surveillance. Sonographic surveillance for an isoimmunized pregnancy should include, but not be limited to, assessment for signs of hydrops. Sonographic findings of hydrops are scalp edema (Figure 48-2), pleural effusion (Figure 48-3), pericardial effusion, ascites (Figure 48-4), polyhydramnios (Figure 48-5), and thickened placenta. Hydrops can be due to fetal anemia. Another ultrasound tool available to predict fetal anemia is Doppler evaluation of the middle cerebral artery (MCA) (Figures 48-6 and 48-7). Since anemia is a condition in which there are fewer red blood cells, the viscosity of the blood is decreased. A decrease in viscosity results in a decrease in resistance to flow. This can be detected by an increase in the normal velocity of the MCA.

Amniocentesis. Amniocentesis can be used in two ways to monitor a pregnancy. The first is to obtain a sample of amniotic fluid to which direct Rh testing of the fetus can be done. The second way is to monitor the isoimmunized pregnancy with delta optical density 450 (OD450) analysis of amniotic fluid. Because hemolysis results in breakdown of red blood cells, the byproduct of this process, bilirubin, stains the amniotic fluid. Bilirubin absorbs light at the 450-nm wavelength. A spectrophotometric analysis of the fluid to check light absorption of this level indirectly measures the amount of bilirubin present in the fluid and therefore gives a measure of the degree of hemolysis. The gestational age at which the first amniocentesis is performed depends on past obstetric history and clinical presentation. Once the amniocentesis is performed and the amniotic fluid is sent for spectrophotometric analysis,

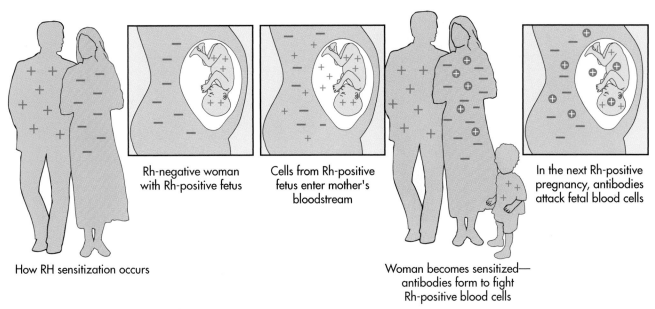

Rh-negative woman with Rh-positive fetus

Cells from Rh-positive fetus enter mother's bloodstream

In the next Rh-positive pregnancy, antibodies attack fetal blood cells

How RH sensitization occurs

Woman becomes sensitized—antibodies form to fight Rh-positive blood cells

Figure 48-1   Diagram illustrating the concept of Rh sensitization.

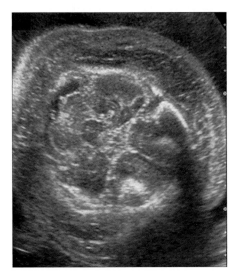

Figure 48-2   Scalp edema.

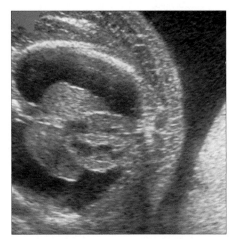

Figure 48-3   Pleural effusion.

the OD450 is categorized into three zones on the Liley curve (Figure 48-8).

1. *Low zone:* Rh-negative and mildly affected fetuses are found in the low zone. They should be followed closely and delivered at term.
2. *Midzone:* A downward trend within the midzone indicates the fetus is probably affected but will survive, and delivery should occur at 38 weeks of gestation. A horizontal or rising trend indicates that the fetus is in danger of intrauterine or neonatal death and that preterm delivery or intrauterine transfusion and preterm delivery are indicated.
3. *High zone:* Fetal death zone. The fetus in the high zone requires immediate treatment or death will result.

Cordocentesis. Cordocentesis is a procedure in which a needle is placed into the fetal umbilical vein and a blood

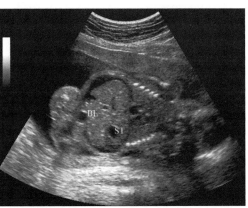

Figure 48-4   Coronal view of the fetal abdomen with ascites. *BL,* bladder; *ST,* stomach.

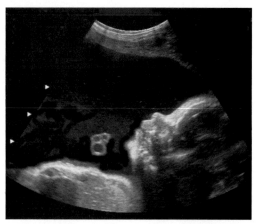

Figure 48-5 Fetal profile and polyhydramnios.

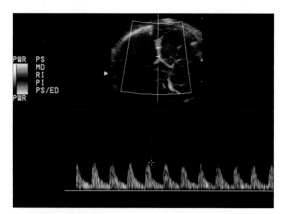

Figure 48-6 Doppler of the middle cerebral artery.

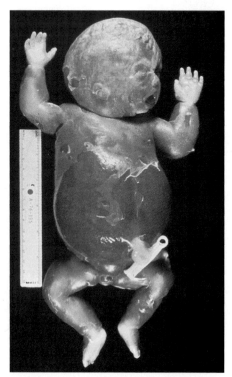

Figure 48-7 Hydropic, Rh-sensitized fetal demise. Note the edema of the extremities and protuberant abdomen.

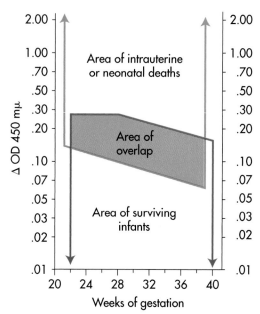

Figure 48-8 The Liley curve illustrates perinatal outcome based on *delta* OD450 values. (From Queenan JT: *Modern management of the Rh problem,* ed 2, Hagerstown, Pa, 1977, Harper & Row.)

sample obtained. The lab evaluates this sample for fetal blood type, hematocrit, and hemoglobin. If indicated, a fetal transfusion may be performed. There are two methods of transfusing a fetus.[13,14] The first, intraperitoneal, consists of using ultrasound guidance to place a needle in the peritoneal cavity of the fetus. Blood is transfused into the peritoneal space, where it is slowly absorbed by the fetus. The second method is direct intravascular transfusion via the umbilical vein (cordocentesis). Using ultrasound guidance, a fine needle is directed through the maternal abdomen toward the umbilical vein where it enters the placenta (Figure 48-9). The red blood cells are transfused directly into the umbilical vein. This method is preferred because a specimen of fetal blood can be obtained before transfusion to confirm that the fetus is truly isoimmunized. A specimen can be obtained after transfusion to document that the fetal hematocrit is adequate.

Historically the perinatal death rate for Rh-sensitized pregnancies was 25% to 35% before intrauterine transfusions were performed. With the institution of aggressive treatment and modern intensive neonatal care, the perinatal death rate has decreased significantly. The death rate depends on the severity of the disease. The more severe the disease, the greater the chance of fetal death.

Alloimmune Thrombocytopenia. In a rare circumstance, a mother may develop an immune response to fetal platelets in a manner similar to that of red blood cells. When this occurs, she develops antibodies to the fetal platelets. The result can be a fetus with a dangerously low platelet count (thrombocytopenia). Infants born with this condition are at increased risk for intracerebral hemorrhage in utero and spontaneous bleeding. Cordocentesis is performed in these cases to document fetal platelet counts before vaginal delivery is attempted.

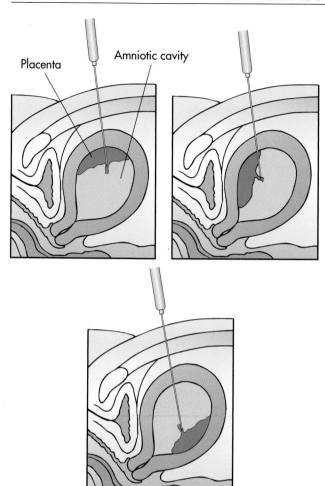

Placenta   Amniotic cavity

Figure 48-9 Possible needle paths in cordocentesis depending on placental position.

Ultrasound can also be useful to look for evidence of in utero fetal intracerebral hemorrhage.

Nonimmune Hydrops. Nonimmune hydrops (NIH) describes a group of conditions in which hydrops is present in the fetus but is not a result of fetomaternal blood group incompatibility. Numerous fetal, maternal, and placental disorders are known to cause or be associated with NIH, including cardiovascular, chromosomal, hematologic, urinary, and pulmonary problems, and twin pregnancies, malformation syndromes, and infectious diseases, specifically toxoplasmosis, rubella, cytomegalovirus, herpes simplex type I (TORCH), syphilis, congenital hepatitis, and parvovirus B19. The incidence of NIH is approximately 1 in 2500 to 1 in 3500 pregnancies, but NIH accounts for about 3% of fetal mortality.[9] The exact mechanism of how NIH occurs is unclear, although the processes described for the hydrops associated with Rh sensitization may apply to NIH.

A variety of maternal, fetal, and placental problems are known to cause or have been found in association with NIH, some of which are listed in Box 48-1. Cardiovascular lesions are the most frequent cause of NIH.[9] Congestive heart failure may result from functional cardiac problems, such as

---

BOX 48-1   DISORDERS ASSOCIATED WITH NONIMMUNE HYDROPS

CARDIOVASCULAR PROBLEMS
Tachyarrhythmia
Complex dysrhythmia
Congenital heart block
Anatomic defects
Cardiomyopathy
Myocarditis
Intracardiac tumors

CHROMOSOMAL PROBLEMS
Trisomy 21
Turner's syndrome
Other trisomies
XX/XY mosaicism
Triploidy

TWIN PREGNANCY
Twin-to-twin transfusion

HEMATOLOGIC PROBLEMS
α-Thalassemia
Arteriovenous shunts
In utero closed-space hemorrhage
Glucose-6-phosphate deficiency

URINARY PROBLEMS
Obstructive uropathies
Congenital nephrosis
Prune belly syndrome
Ureterocele

RESPIRATORY PROBLEMS
Diaphragmatic hernia
Cystic adenomatoid malformation of the lung
Tumors of the lung

GASTROINTESTINAL PROBLEMS
Jejunal atresia
Midgut volvulus
Meconium peritonitis

LIVER PROBLEMS
Hepatic vascular malformations
Biliary atresia

INFECTIOUS PROBLEMS
Cytomegalovirus
Syphilis
Herpes simplex, type I
Rubella
Toxoplasmosis

PLACENTA/UMBILICAL CORD PROBLEMS
Chorioangioma
Fetomaternal transfusion
Placental and umbilical vein thrombosis
Umbilical cord anomalies

dysrhythmias, tachycardias, and myocarditis, and from structural anomalies, such as hypoplastic left heart and other types of congenital heart disease. Obstructive vascular problems occurring outside of the heart, such as umbilical vein thrombosis, as well as pulmonary diseases, diaphragmatic hernia, and congenital cystic adenomatoid malformation (CCAM) can cause NIH. Large vascular tumors functioning as arteriovenous shunts can also result in NIH.

Severe anemia of the fetus is another well-recognized cause for NIH. Although the anemia is not caused by isoimmunization, the result is the same. Severe anemia may occur in a donor twin of a twin–twin transfusion syndrome, thalassemia, or significant fetomaternal hemorrhage. To make the diagnosis of NIH, isoimmunization is ruled out with an antibody screen.

Sonographic Findings. The fetus may appear very similar to a sensitized baby by ultrasound exam. Scalp edema, pleural, and pericardial effusions may be present along with ascites (Figures 48-10 and 48-11). Other abnormal findings may also be present, indicating the cause of the hydrops. If the hydrops is a result of a cardiac tachyarrhythmia, a heart rate in the range of 200 to 240 is common. If a diaphragmatic hernia is present, the bowel will be visible in the chest cavity.

Many times a cause for NIH cannot be determined. If a cause is found, treatment is dependent upon the cause. As an example, if hydrops results from a tachycardia, medicine can be given to the mother in an attempt to slow the fetal heart rate. Ultrasound can be useful in monitoring the progress of the fetus. Resolution of ascites and gross edema has been documented after the fetal heart was converted to a normal rhythm. If the fetus is anemic because of twin–twin transfusion, intrauterine transfusion will not solve the anemia problem because most of the fetal blood is being shunted to the recipient twin (Figure 48-12). Ultrasound can help the clinician assess how sick the fetus is by indicating the severity of the hydrops and by biophysical profile, which is discussed later in the chapter. The clinician can then make an informed choice about when to deliver the fetus.

A thorough examination of the fetus, along with fetal echocardiography, must be carried out because abnormalities of almost every organ system have been described with NIH

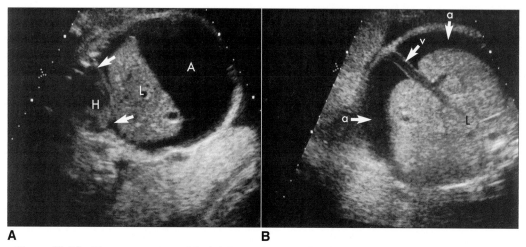

A   **B**

Figure 48-10 Transverse sections of fetal abdomen showing ascites in a fetus with nonimmune hydrops. **A,** Sagittal plane. *A,* Ascites; *H,* heart; *L,* liver. **B,** Transverse plane. *a,* ascites; *L,* liver; *v,* umbilical vein.

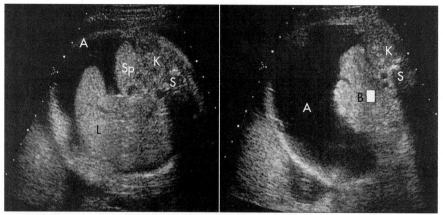

Figure 48-11 Cross section of fetal abdomen showing ascites. *A,* ascites; *B,* bowel; *K,* kidney; *L,* liver; *S,* spine.

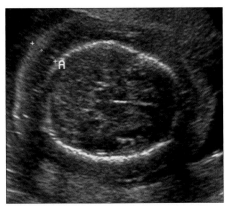

Figure 48-12 Twin–twin transfusion syndrome showing hydropic twin with scalp edema.

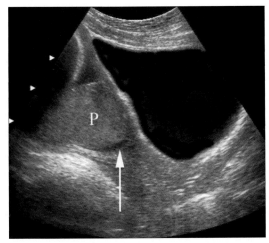

Figure 48-13 Placenta previa. Lower margin of placenta *(P)* covering cervical os *(arrow)*.

(see Box 48-1). In addition to the ultrasound examination, genetic amniocentesis for karyotype is indicated because chromosomal abnormalities have been described as causes for NIH.

VAGINAL BLEEDING

Vaginal bleeding in the second and third trimesters can be associated with placental anomalies, such as placenta previa and placenta abruption. Placenta previa is the main cause for third-trimester bleeding. In this condition, the placenta covers the internal cervical os and prohibits the delivery of the fetus (Figure 48-13). If the cervical os dilates with labor, there is a significant risk of the placenta detaching from the uterus, resulting in maternal hemorrhage and loss of oxygen and blood supply to the fetus. Endovaginal sonography is the best way to evaluate the relationship of the cervical os to the placental edge. Early in pregnancy, the placenta is often low lying, but as the uterus grows, the placenta will appear to migrate away from the cervical os. During the second half of pregnancy, if this distance is less than 2 cm, the condition may be classified as a marginal or partial placental previa. Even though the placenta may not entirely cover the internal os, the risk for blood loss

from the low-lying placental vessels remains. It is important to identify a placenta previa so that a cesarean section may be planned if the previa persists until delivery.

Vasa previa is a rare condition in which the umbilical cord is the presenting part. This condition is important to recognize because it is life threatening to the fetus. This condition is associated with a velamentous cord insertion or succenturiate lobe. Ultrasound is used to assess for vasa previa by using color Doppler to evaluate any structures in front of the cervical os to see if they are vascular. Endovaginal sonography may also assist in identifying this entity.

Placental abruption is another entity that may cause vaginal bleeding during pregnancy. Abruption is the premature separation of the placenta from the uterine wall. When evaluating for placenta abruption, the sonographer should be looking at the area between the placenta and uterine wall. Normally this area is hypoechoic and only 1 to 2 cm thick. If this area is thicker than 1 to 2 cm, it may be due to an abruption or uterine contraction. Uterine contractions typically resolve within 20 to 30 minutes and have central blood flow. Abruptions can be difficult to diagnose because acute hemorrhage has a similar echogenicity to the placenta. Thus ultrasound has a high false-negative rate in identifying abruptions. The clotted blood is hyperechoic and abruptions are easier to identify if the incident has occurred a few days before the examination. If bleeding from the abruption has been recent, the sonographer may notice a thin echolucent area between the placenta and the uterus. However, although one may be suspicious of an abruption, there may be no ultrasound signs of an abruption at all. Another way to search for an abruption is to use color flow Doppler. Blood clots from an abruption will not exhibit any color flow. The retroplacental area is hypoechoic because of a large number of blood vessels (mainly veins) located here. Therefore, when evaluating for an abruption, the sonographer should sweep with color Doppler retroplacentally looking for a flow void. If a flow void is present, one should be suspicious of abruption.

MATERNAL DISEASES OF PREGNANCY

DIABETES

Insulin-dependent diabetic mellitus (IDDM) mothers are at an increased risk for pregnancy-related complications, including early and late trimester pregnancy loss and congenital anomalies. Diabetic pregnancies may be complicated by frequent hospitalizations for glucose control, serious infections, such as pyelonephritis, and problems at the time of delivery (Box 48-2). These mothers need to be monitored frequently for adequate nutritional and fluid intake, especially if they experience hyperemesis in the first trimester.

Glucose is the primary fuel for fetal growth. If glucose levels are very high and uncontrolled (as happens in diabetes resulting from an inability to produce enough insulin), the fetus may also become macrosomic. Macrosomia is defined as a fetus whose weight is greater than the 90 percentile for gestational age. A macrosomic infant (Figure 48-14) may become too large

BOX 48-2 CONGENITAL ANOMALIES IN INFANTS OF DIABETIC MOTHERS

SKELETAL AND CENTRAL NERVOUS SYSTEM
Caudal regression syndrome
Neural tube defects, excluding anencephaly
Anencephaly with or without herniation of neural elements
Microcephaly

CARDIAC
Transposition of the great vessels with or without ventricular septal defect
Ventricular septal defect
Atrial septal defect
Coarctation of the aorta with or without ventricular septal defect
Cardiomegaly

RENAL
Hydronephrosis
Renal agenesis
Ureteral duplication

GASTROINTESTINAL
Duodenal atresia
Anorectal atresia
Small left colon syndrome

OTHER
Single umbilical artery

to fit through the mother's pelvis, making cesarean section necessary. If delivery is accomplished vaginally, however, the physician may have difficulty delivering the shoulders of the baby after the head has delivered. This is termed *shoulder dystocia.* Brachial plexus nerve injuries may result from the traction placed on the head and neck in attempts to get the remainder of the baby delivered.

Once delivered, an infant of a diabetic mother may experience problems with glucose control in the nursery, necessitating intravenous glucose administration.

Sonographic Findings. Correct dating is very important, and pregnancy dates should be confirmed with ultrasound. There is an increased risk of early fetal demise, so the presence of a fetal heart beat should be confirmed before initiating maternal diabetic protocols. There also is an increased risk of third-trimester loss and other pregnancy complications, which may necessitate the induction of labor before term when the fetal lung maturity is demonstrated. A diabetic baby delivered preterm may have respiratory distress syndrome and require placement in the high-risk nursery.

Polyhydramnios can be seen with elevated blood sugars and macrosomic fetuses. Polyhydramnios can predispose to premature labor, premature rupture of membranes, and maternal discomfort. The fetus of a diabetic mother may measure large for gestational age, making late pregnancy dating inaccurate. Increased adipose tissue may be seen on the fetus in utero (Figures 48-15 and 48-16). Monthly ultrasounds can give the clinician important information regarding fetal growth. If the estimated fetal weight is greater than 4500 g at term, the clinician will be alert to the problems of dystocia with a vaginal delivery and may prefer cesarean delivery.

Ultrasound plays a very important role in scanning for fetal anomalies. Anomalies associated with diabetes include congenital heart and neural tube defects. The most common cardiac problems in the diabetic fetus include transposition of the great arteries and tetralogy of Fallot. In diabetics who have vasculopathy, fetuses may be at risk for intrauterine growth restriction (IUGR). Sonographic findings with this condition may include small-for-gestation growth patterns and elevated S/D ratio in the umbilical artery. **Caudal regression syndrome**

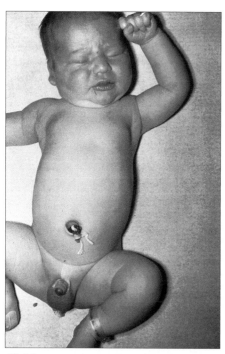

Figure 48-14 A 5280-g, (11-lb) infant of a diabetic mother.

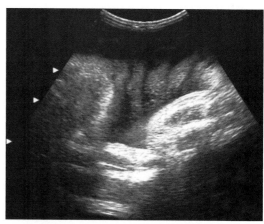

Figure 48-15 LGA infant fat rolls.

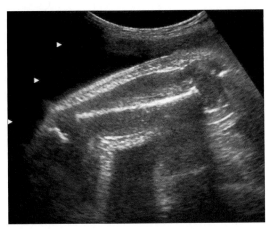

Figure 48-16   LGA fetus with adipose tissue in fetal upper arm.

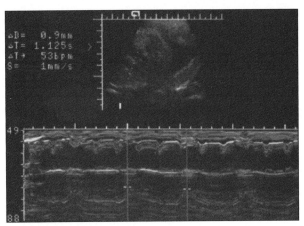

Figure 48-17   M-mode demonstrating a ventricular heart rate of 53 bpm in a fetus with complete heart block.

(lack of development of the caudal spine and cord) is seen almost exclusively in diabetic individuals.

HYPERTENSION

Hypertension is a medical complication of pregnancy, which occurs frequently in high-risk populations. Hypertension places both mother and fetus at risk. Hypertensive pregnancies may be associated with small placentas because of the effect of hypertension on blood vessels. If the placenta develops poorly, the blood supply to the fetus may be limited and growth restriction may result. Growth-restricted fetuses are at increased risk of fetal distress and death in utero.

There are various forms of hypertensive disease during pregnancy. In the past, the term *toxemia* was used to describe hypertensive disorders because it was believed that a "toxin" in the mother's bloodstream caused the hypertension. Currently, pregnancy-induced hypertension is considered to be caused by prostaglandin abnormalities.

The terminology currently used in clinical practice to describe hypertensive states during pregnancy includes: (1) pregnancy-induced hypertension (which includes preeclampsia, severe preeclampsia, and eclampsia) and (2) chronic hypertension, which was present before the woman was pregnant. Preeclampsia is a pregnancy condition in which high blood pressure develops with proteinuria (protein in the urine) or edema (swelling). If the hypertension is neglected, the patient may develop seizures that can be life threatening to both mother and fetus. Severe preeclampsia may develop in some cases and refers to the severity of hypertension and proteinuria. Severe preeclampsia generally indicates that the patient must be delivered immediately. **Eclampsia** represents the occurrence of seizures or coma in a preeclamptic patient. Chronic hypertension is diagnosed in patients in whom high blood pressure is found before 20 weeks of gestation. Chronic hypertension can result from primary essential hypertension or from secondary hypertension (renal, endocrine, or neurologic causes).

Sonographic Findings. The ultrasound team may be called on to perform serial scans for fetal growth and to monitor for the adequacy of amniotic fluid. If fetal growth is falling off the normal growth curve or oligohydramnios occurs, the obstetri-

cian may intervene and deliver the fetus, fearing that intrauterine fetal demise is imminent. Doppler ultrasound can also give the physician information regarding the fetal and maternal circulatory status that may help determine whether the pregnancy is at risk for developing intrauterine growth restriction.

SYSTEMIC LUPUS ERYTHEMATOSUS

Systemic lupus erythematosus (SLE) is a chronic autoimmune disorder that can affect almost all organ systems in the body. It is most common in women of childbearing age and may cause multiple peripartum complications. The incidence of spontaneous abortion and fetal death is 22% to 49% in patients with SLE.[3,8] The placenta is affected by the immune complex deposits and inflammatory responses in the placental vessels and may account for the increased number of spontaneous abortions, stillbirths, and intrauterine growth restricted fetuses. The fetus must be monitored to rule out congenital heart block (Figure 48-17) and pericardial effusion.

OTHER MATERNAL DISEASE

Hyperemesis. Ultrasound can be useful in the work-up of vomiting in the pregnant woman. Nausea and vomiting are common symptoms associated with pregnancy. **Hyperemesis gravidarum** exists when a pregnant woman vomits so much that she develops dehydration and electrolyte imbalance. When this occurs, hospitalization with intravenous fluid administration is usually necessary. The physician must ensure that the vomiting results strictly from pregnancy and not other disease, such as gallstones, peptic ulcers, or trophoblastic disease. Trophoblastic disease can easily be ruled out by demonstrating a viable intrauterine pregnancy. Gallstones can be ruled out by careful sonographic examination of the gallbladder.

Urinary Tract Disease. Ultrasound can also be useful in the work-up of urinary tract disease. Approximately 4% to 6% of pregnant women have asymptomatic bacteriuria. If the bacteriuria is not treated, pyelonephritis may develop. Although pyelonephritis usually presents with flank pain, fever, and white blood cells in the urine, hydronephrosis is another condition that presents with flank pain. Pregnancy is normally associated with mild hydronephrosis. The hydronephrosis may result from a combination of effects. First, progesterone has a dilatory effect on the smooth muscle of the ureter. Second, the enlarging uterus also compresses the ureters at the pelvic brim, causing a hydronephrosis or obstruction. If a woman presents with more than one episode of pyelonephritis or has continued flank pain, ultrasound examination may provide information as to the cause.

Adnexal Cysts. Physiologic ovarian cysts may be associated with early pregnancy. These cysts may be large, ranging from 8 to 10 cm, and may be associated with pelvic pain. The cyst should diminish as the pregnancy progresses. If the cyst does not resolve, surgical exploration may be necessary to rule out other ovarian pathology, including endometriomas, dermoid cysts (Figure 48-18), and even cancers. Periodic ultrasound examinations are necessary for follow-up of a cyst.

Obesity. Maternal obesity has been associated with an increased incidence of neural tube defects and may be attributed to poor maternal diet. More women who are obese start their pregnancy with chronic hypertension than do women who are of normal weight, and obese women are at an increased risk for pregnancy-induced hypertension. Likewise, obese women are at an increased risk for severe eclampsia. Multiple births and urinary tract infections have also been reported at higher incidence rates in obese women.

Uterine Fibroids. Pregnant women may periodically present with problems related to uterine fibroids. Fibroids are actually benign tumors or uterine smooth muscle that may be stimulated to excessive growth by the hormones of pregnancy, specifically estrogen. If the growth is very rapid, the fibroid may outgrow its blood supply and undergo necrosis. This in turn may cause pain and premature labor (Figure 48-19). Ultrasound examination of the uterus in a pregnant woman may detect uterine fibroids. It is important to document the size and location of these fibroids as they may obstruct a clear pathway for fetal delivery. If the placenta implants over a fibroid, it may lead to poor placental profusion in that area, which can be a cause of intrauterine growth restriction.

ULTRASOUND IN LABOR AND DELIVERY

PREMATURE LABOR

Premature labor is the onset of labor before 37 weeks of gestation (Box 48-3). Premature labor is an obstetric complication occurring in 15% to 20% of all pregnancies.[6] Premature infants are at greater risk for having problems, such as respiratory distress syndrome, intracranial hemorrhage, bowel immaturity, and feeding problems.

Potential causes of preterm labor include premature rupture of membranes, intrauterine infection, bleeding, fetal anomalies, polyhydramnios, multiple pregnancy, growth restriction, maternal illness such as diabetes or hypertension, incompetent cervix, and uterine abnormalities.

Other presumed causes include epidemiologic factors, such as socioeconomic class; maternal age, weight, and height; late prenatal care; smoking; coitus; a history of cervical injury or surgery; and a poor previous obstetric history. Another patient population at increased risk for preterm labor is patients with multiple gestation. In about 50% of cases, no cause or association can be identified as being responsible for the preterm labor.

Sonographic Findings. Ultrasound assessment of the preterm labor patient should include, but not be limited to, amniotic fluid assessment, endovaginal cervical assessment (Figure 48-20), fetal number, placental assessment, and tar-

BOX 48-3	**WARNING SIGNS OF PRETERM LABOR**

- Menstrual-like cramps (constant or intermittent)
- Low, dull backache
- Pressure (feels like baby is pushing down)
- Abdominal cramping (with or without diarrhea)
- Increase or change in vaginal discharge (contains mucus or is watery, light, or bloody)
- Fluid leaking from vagina
- Feeling unwell
- Uterine contractions

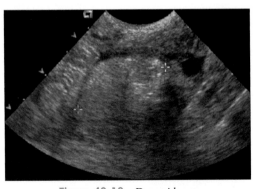

Figure 48-18   Dermoid cyst.

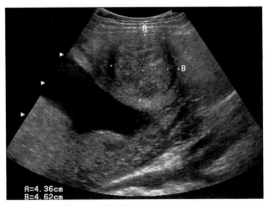

Figure 48-19   Uterine fibroid.

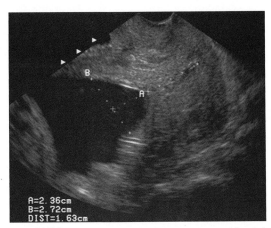

Figure 48-20 Incompetent cervix in a patient with triplets.

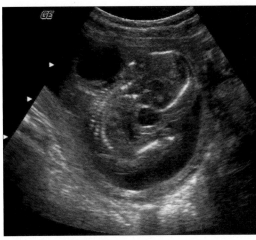

Figure 48-21 Ultrasound shows extreme curvature of the fetal spine in a fetal demise.

geted ultrasound (see Table 48-1). The sonographer should be aware of the potential causes of preterm labor and tailor the exam accordingly.

FETAL FACTORS IN HIGH-RISK PREGNANCY

FETAL DEATH

Intrauterine fetal death accounts for roughly one half of all instances of perinatal mortality. Although the cause of death cannot be determined in approximately half of the cases, known causes are infection (usually associated with premature rupture of membranes), congenital or chromosomal abnormalities, preeclampsia, placental abruption, diabetes, growth restriction, and blood group isoimmunization.

Fetal death may occur at any time during pregnancy. The incidence of pregnancy loss in the first trimester is 15 to 20 per 100 pregnancies, with most of the losses resulting from cytogenetic abnormalities.[2] As pregnancy progresses, the incidence decreases to 5 to 10 per 1000 pregnancies (one half the perinatal mortality rate), and factors other than cytogenetic play a more important role.

Clinically, first-trimester pregnancy loss may be diagnosed when the patient presents to her physician with vaginal bleeding, cramping, or passage of tissue. Ultrasound examination may reveal a blighted ovum or a fetus with no heart motion. As the pregnancy progresses into the second trimester, pregnancy landmarks become important in determining whether the pregnancy is proceeding normally. Fetal heart tones should be heard with Doppler at approximately 10 to 12 weeks of gestation. At 20 weeks of gestation, the uterine fundal height should have risen to the umbilicus, and the uterus should measure approximately 20 cm above the symphysis pubis. The mother should also perceive fetal movements on a daily basis beginning between 16 and 20 weeks of gestation. Failure to achieve any one of these landmarks may prompt the clinician to obtain an ultrasound examination.

As the pregnancy progresses, the clinician will follow the pregnant woman at regular intervals, listening to fetal heart tones and measuring the uterine fundal height at each visit.

The mother will be questioned about fetal movements. The absence of a fetal heart rate usually prompts the clinician to obtain an ultrasound examination. Cessation of fetal movements should prompt an immediate search for fetal heart tones. If none is present, ultrasound examination will confirm or rule out intrauterine fetal demise.

Sonographic Findings. Sonographic findings that are associated with fetal death are (1) absent heartbeat, (2) absent fetal movement, (3) overlap of skull bones **(Spalding's sign),** (4) an exaggerated curvature of the fetal spine (Figure 48-21), and (5) gas in the fetal abdomen. A brief ultrasound examination of the fetus for structural anomalies should be performed and biometry obtained to determine estimated weight for delivery.

LARGE FOR GESTATIONAL AGE

When a fetus is measuring large for gestational age, one is asked to evaluate for fetal macrosomia. Macrosomia is accelerated growth in utero and is defined as an estimated birth weight greater than 4000 grams. Risk factors for having a fetus with macrosomia are multiparity, AMA (>35), maternal height greater than 169 cm, prepregnant weight greater than 70 kilograms, and postdates of 1 week or longer.

SMALL FOR GESTATIONAL AGE

Small for gestational age can be due to chromosomal anomalies, intrauterine infection (Figure 48-22), genetics, and placental insufficiency (Figures 48-23 and 48-24). If chromosomal anomalies are the cause for the fetus measuring small, often the growth is symmetrically affected. Therefore, all of the fetal measurements will be smaller than expected for gestational age.

MULTIPLE GESTATION PREGNANCY

Ultrasound is an extremely valuable tool in the assessment of multiple gestation pregnancies. It may be used to monitor the growth of the fetuses and for guidance of diagnostic and therapeutic procedures. The mother with a multiple gestation is at increased risk for obstetric complications, such as

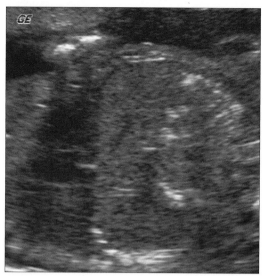

Figure 48-22 Note liver calcifications in a pregnancy affected with CMV.

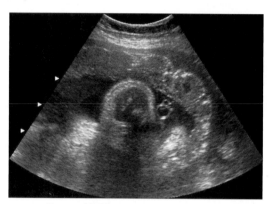

Figure 48-23 Placental calcifications.

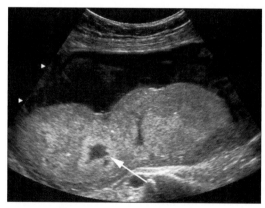

Figure 48-24 Placental infarct.

> **BOX 48-4   CAUSE OF TWINNING**
>
> - All dizygotic pregnancies are dichorionic/diamniotic
> - 25% of monozygotic pregnancies are monochorionic (one placenta)
> - In dichorionic pregnancies (whether dizygotic or monozygotic), two layers of amnion and two layers of chorion separate the fetuses

Before ultrasound was used routinely, as many as 60% of twins were not diagnosed before delivery.[11] With routine use of ultrasound, most multiple gestations are diagnosed before the onset of labor. During the first trimester, multiple pregnancy can be identified by visualizing more than one gestational sac within the uterus. A firm diagnosis cannot be made unless a fetal pole can be seen within each sac, regardless of the number of sacs that are seen.

In the second and third trimesters, several clinical findings may prompt an ultrasound examination. The patient's uterus may be larger on examination than expected for dates. **Maternal serum alpha-fetoprotein (MSAFP)** screening is performed routinely to detect neural tube defects. Twin pregnancies, by virtue of having two fetuses rather than one, are associated with elevations of MSAFP. Therefore, a patient with elevated MSAFP may present for a scan to rule out neural tube defects and be found to be carrying twins. The physician may detect two fetal heartbeats or palpate two heads, prompting an ultrasound examination. Finally, the twins may be unsuspected and found serendipitously.

Once a multiple gestation has been identified, a targeted ultrasound examination should be performed specifically looking for fetal anomalies. To understand why this is so, the cause of twinning must be reviewed (Box 48-4).

In each multiple gestation evaluated by ultrasound, the sonographer needs to evaluate placentation type. This refers to the number of chorions (chorionicity) and amnions (amnionicity). In a twin pregnancy, this depends on the number of zygotes and, in monozygotic twinning, the timing of zygotic division (Figures 48-25, 48-26, and 48-27).

DIZYGOTIC TWINS

There are two types of twins: dizygotic (fraternal) and monozygotic (identical). **Dizygotic** twins arise from two separately fertilized ova. Each ovum implants separately in the uterus and develops its own placenta, chorion, and amniotic sac (diamniotic, dichorionic). The placentas may implant in different parts of the uterus and be distinctly separate or may implant adjacent to each other and fuse. Although the placentas may be fused, their blood circulations remain distinct and separate from each other.

MONOZYGOTIC TWINS

Monozygotic twins (identical) arise from a single fertilized egg that divides, resulting in two genetically identical fetuses.

preeclampsia, third-trimester bleeding, and prolapsed cord. The fetuses are at increased risk of premature delivery and congenital anomalies. As a result, a twin has a five times greater chance of perinatal death than a singleton fetus.[10] Physicians follow multiple gestations closely with ultrasound.

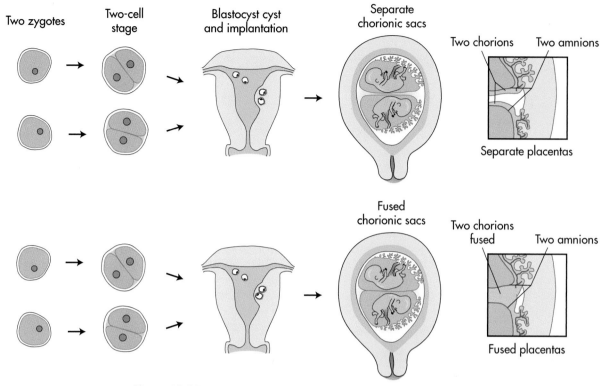

Figure 48-25   The dichorionicity and diamnionicity of dizygotic twins.

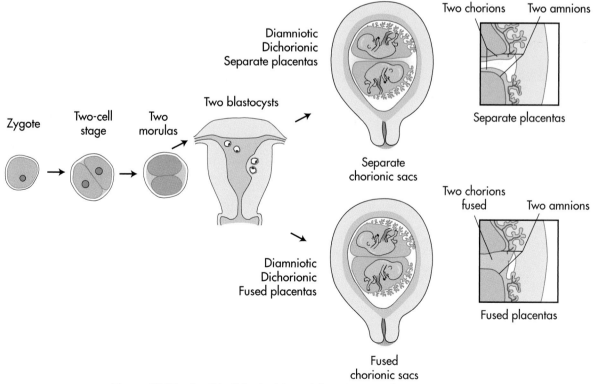

Figure 48-26   Possible dichorionicity and diamnionicity of monozygotic twins.

Depending on whether the fertilized egg divides early or late, there may be one or two placentas, chorions, and amniotic sacs. If the division occurs early (0 to 4 days postconception), there will be two amnions and two chorions (dichorionic, diamniotic). If the division occurs at 4 to 8 days, there will be one chorion and two amniotic sacs (monochorionic, diamniotic) (Figures 48-28 and 48-29). If the division occurs after 8 days, two fetuses will be present but only one chorion and one amnion (monochorionic, monoamniotic) (Figures 48-30, 48-31, and 48-32). If the division occurs after 13 days, the division may be incomplete and conjoined twins may result. The twins may be joined at a variety of sites, including head, thorax, abdomen, and pelvis (Figures 48-33, 48-34, and 48-35). Monozygotic twins present a very high-risk situation. Besides being associated with an increased incidence of fetal anomalies, if there is only one amniotic sac, the twins may entangle their umbilical cords, cutting off their blood supply. In these monochorionic diamniotic pregnancies, only the two layers of amnion separate the twins. Because the circulations

of the monozygotic twins communicate through a single placenta, they are at increased risk for a syndrome known as **twin–twin transfusion syndrome,** which will be discussed later.

Other obstacles to imaging twins include the phenomenon of the vanishing and appearing twin. One twin may die in utero and the other one continue to grow. One ultrasound study showed that 70% of pregnancies that began with twins ended with a singleton (Figure 48-36).[4] Many of these losses occur very early and are never detected. Others are detected early when the patient presents with vaginal bleeding in the second trimester and two sacs are visualized—one with a healthy fetus and one with a demise (Figure 48-37). If the demise occurs very early, complete resorption of both embryo and gestational sac or early placenta may occur. This phenomenon is sometimes referred to as the "vanishing" twin because, once reabsorbed, the products of conception of this twin will no longer be seen on ultrasound.[5] If the fetus dies after reaching a size too large for resorption, the fetus is markedly flattened from loss of fluid and most of the soft tissue. This is termed **fetus papyraceous** (Figure 48-38).

Just as a twin may appear to vanish, one may also "appear." The appearing twin is seen when ultrasound exams are performed very early in gestation (5 to 6 weeks) and the gestation sacs are undercounted. Undercounting can occur as a result of a discrepancy in gestational sac size, the locations of sacs, if the patient is scanned before yolk sacs are seen, monochorionic and monoamniotic gestation without crown-rump lengths, and failure of the operator to identify a second gestational sac.

As stated previously, multiple gestations have a high rate of anomalies, and a careful search must be performed to rule out birth defects. It is also important for the sonographer to understand what abnormalities are unique to multiple gestations they should be screening for. Several abnormalities that are

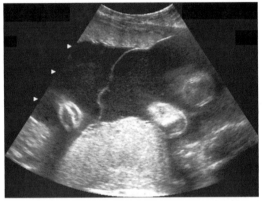

Figure 48-27 A dichorionic, diamniotic twin gestation.

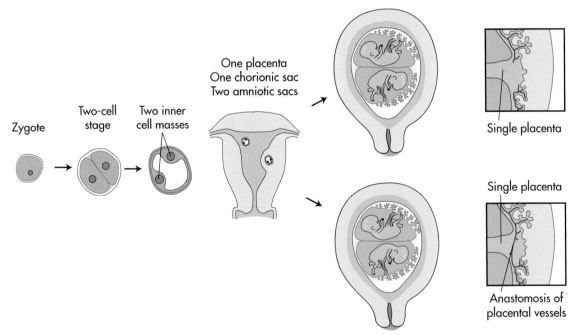

Figure 48-28 A monochorionic, diamniotic monozygotic twin gestation.

specific to multiple gestations are poly-oli sequence, acardiac anomaly, and conjoined twins.

POLY-OLI SEQUENCE ("STUCK TWIN")

Poly-oli sequence, also known as "stuck twin" syndrome, is characterized by a diamniotic pregnancy with polyhydramnios in one sac and severe oligohydramnios and a smaller twin in the other sac (Figure 48-39). This syndrome usually manifests between 16 to 26 weeks' gestation. The majority involve monochorionic gestations.[13] Stuck twin syndrome may result because of fetal anomaly in one sac resulting in polyhydramnios; compressing the blood flow in the normal twin's placenta, resulting in oligohydramnios; placental insufficiency in one placenta; and twin-twin transfusion syndrome. When oligohydramnios exists in one sac and polyhydramnios in the other, the small twin may appear stuck in position within the uterus, hence the term "stuck twin." In the event that twin–twin transfusion exists, the growth of the twins will be discordant, with the donor twin falling off the growth curve (Figure 48-40).

Twin-twin transfusion syndrome exists when there is an arteriovenous shunt within the placenta. The arterial blood of one twin is pumped into the venous system of the other twin. As a result, the donor twin becomes anemic and growth restricted. This twin has less blood flow through its kidneys, urinates less, and develops **oligohydramnios.** The recipient twin, however, gets too much blood flow. The twin may be normal or large in size. This fetus has excess blood flow

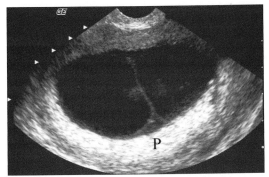

Figure 48-29   A monochorionic, diamniotic twin gestation. *P,* placenta.

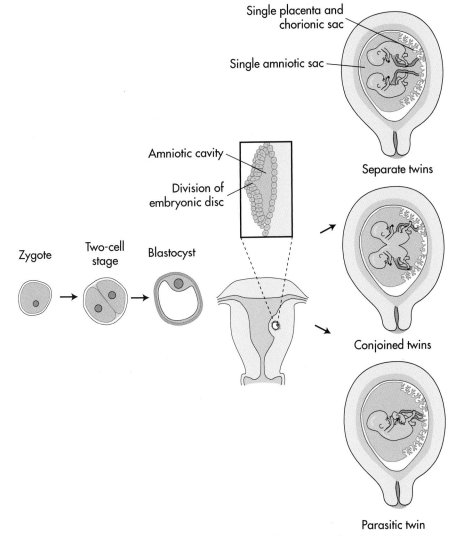

Figure 48-30   A monochorionic, monoamniotic monozygotic twin gestation.

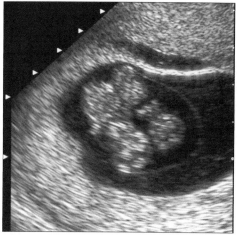

Figure 48-31 A monochorionic, monoamniotic twin gestation.

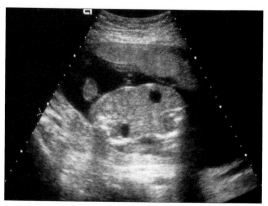

Figure 48-34 Ultrasound image demonstrating a set of conjoined twins connected at the abdomen. Note the stomach bubbles visualized on each twin.

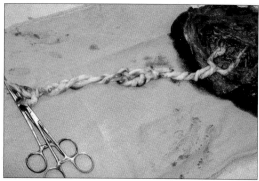

Figure 48-32 Gross illustration of a monochorionic, monoamniotic placenta demonstrating two amniotic cords tangled.

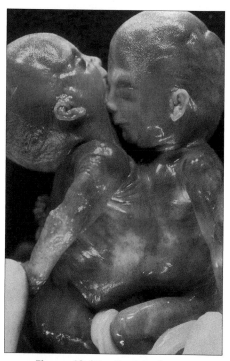

Figure 48-35 Conjoined twins.

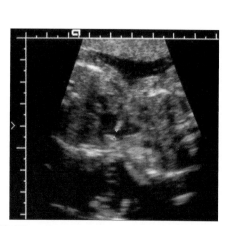

Figure 48-33 Ultrasound image demonstrating a set of conjoined twins connected at the thorax. Note that they share a single four-chamber heart.

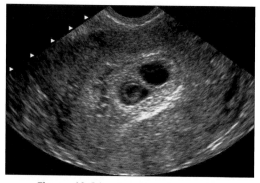

Figure 48-36 An early twin gestation.

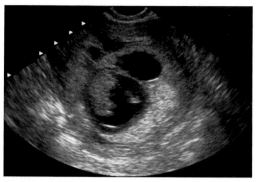

Figure 48-37   This ultrasound image is of the same patient shown in Figure 48-36 further along. Note the vanishing twin phenomenon.

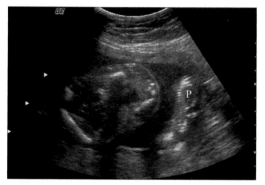

Figure 48-38   Ultrasound image demonstrating the demise of one twin resulting in a fetus papyraceous, *P.*

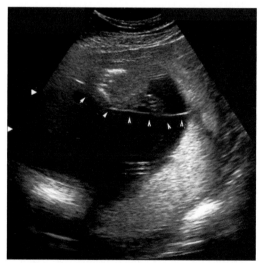

Figure 48-39   "Stuck twin." Arrowheads are pointing to the amnion surrounding the stuck twin.

through its kidneys and urinates too much, leading to **poly-hydramnios.** This twin may even go into heart failure and become hydropic.

If twin–twin transfusion exists, both twins are at risk of dying, the smaller one because its nutritional and oxygen-rich

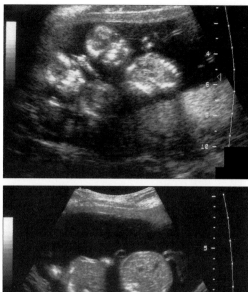

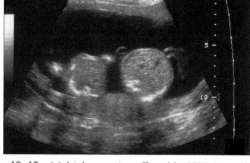

Figure 48-40   Multiple gestation affected by TTS. Note the size discrepancy between the two fetuses.

blood supply is severely restricted and the larger one because of heart failure. Depending on the gestational age, the obstetrical specialist may be forced to deliver the fetuses early if it appears that one or both of the twins are at risk of dying in utero. Fetal surveillance is increased when growth discordance, oligohydramnios, or polyhydramnios is discovered. Treatments for stuck twin syndrome include serial amniocentesis, selective feticide, umbilical cord ligation of one twin, and laser occlusion of anastomosing placental vessels.

Acardiac anomaly is another abnormality unique to twin gestations. By definition, acardiac anomaly is a rare anomaly occurring in monochorionic twins, in which one twin develops without a heart and often with absence of the upper half of the body (Figure 48-41). It is proposed that this occurs as a result of an artery to artery connection in the placenta, which leads to perfusion of the abnormal twin via the co-twin (trap phenomenon). The reversed direction of blood flow in the abnormal twin alters the hemodynamic properties necessary for normal cardiac formation. On ultrasound, one will see a monochorionic twin gestation with one normal fetus and one fetus with an absent heart. The abnormal twin also has other anomalies, such as absent head, absent organs in the thorax and abdomen, and absent or abnormal limbs.

Conjoined twins is another anomaly unique to twin gestations. Conjoined twins occur from incomplete division of the embryo after 13 days from conception. Five types of conjoined twins have been described: thoracopagus (joined at the thorax), omphalopagus (joined at the anterior wall), craniopagus (joined at the cranium, syncephalus, conjoined twins with

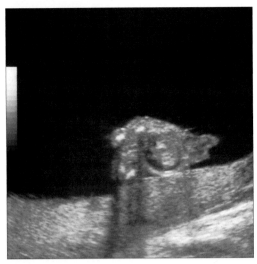

Figure 48-41   An acardiac, acephalic twin gestation.

one head), pygopagus (joined at the ischial region), and ischiopagus (attached at the buttocks).[5] On ultrasound, one will see a monochorionic, monoamniotic gestation with two fetuses connected.

SCANNING MULTIPLE GESTATIONS

Multiple gestations have many potential risks. Therefore, the sonographer must do a complete job of scanning the fetuses. In addition to the anatomy listed in Table 48-1, the ultrasound report should include the following information:

1. Number of sacs
2. Number and location of placentas
3. Gender of the fetuses
4. Biometric data
5. Presence of anomalies

Furthermore, the fetal gestational sacs should be assigned a label (typically an alphabetical letter) to consistently identify them in following exams. The sac and fetus directly over the internal os is labeled *A*. Sacs above that should be additionally identified by their placental location or additional identifying informations, such as left or right side of the uterus. This will be important in future exams to consistently evaluate the growth of each fetus against its own previous growth, not that of another sibling.

During the first trimester, the sonographer must be careful to analyze the uterine contents for the presence of multiple gestations. One article reports that multiple gestations were initially undercounted in early pregnancies under 6 weeks performed with endovaginal ultrasound.[5] The report states that an important role of first-trimester sonography is to determine pregnancy number (i.e., whether the pregnancy is singleton, twin, or higher-order multiple gestation).[5] After 6 weeks of gestational age, determining pregnancy number is easily accomplished by counting embryos in the uterus. Before 6 weeks, the embryo is not consistently visualized and the sonographer must count the gestational sacs and small yolk sacs. The article reported that the frequency of undercounting multiple gesta-

tions on a 5.0- to 5.9-week sonogram was highest for monochorionic twins (86%), followed by higher-order gestations (16%), and last by dichorionic twins (11%).[5] The authors of the report reasoned that some of the gestational sacs may differ in size or the yolk sac may be too small to adequately image so early. This may account for the "vanishing twin" or "appearing twin" phenomenon.

When scanning multiple gestations, the sonographer should always attempt to determine whether there are one or two amniotic sacs by locating the membrane that separates the sacs. If two sacs are seen, the pregnancy is known to be diamniotic, but sonography will not be able to indicate whether the twins are identical. As mentioned before, both monozygotic and dizygotic twins may have two amniotic sacs. A scan for the same sex increases the chance of any possible monozygotic detection.

Documentation of a membrane separating the fetuses confirms the presence of a diamniotic pregnancy. The membrane, composed of amnion with or without chorion, exhibits a characteristic appearance that permits distinction from other membranes of pregnancy. In a twin pregnancy with two separate placentas, the membrane extends between the fetuses obliquely across the uterus from the edge of the placenta to the contralateral edge of the other placenta. If only one placental site exists, the membrane extends between the fetuses away from the central portion of the placental site. The fetus may touch the membrane, but does not cross it, and the membrane does not adhere to entrap the fetus. The membrane has no free edge within the amniotic fluid. These features distinguish the normal membrane separating twins from other membranes or membranelike structures within the amniotic fluid (i.e., uterine synechiae, partial uterine septations, or amniotic bands).

Failure to image the membrane separating the twin fetuses does not reliably predict the presence of a monoamniotic pregnancy. If only one placenta is seen and a membrane cannot be visualized, other features may assist in the prediction of amnionicity, chorionicity, and zygosity. A male and female fetus is dizygotic, diamniotic, and dichorionic. A twin pregnancy with intertwined umbilical cords, conjoined twins, or greater than three vessels in the umbilical cord is found in a monozygotic pregnancy that is monoamniotic and monochorionic.

The location of the placenta should be determined. An attempt also should be made to determine the number of placentas. Occasionally, clearly separate placentas may be identified. If two placentas are implanted immediately adjacent to each other and fuse, it may be difficult to determine whether there are one or two placentas. The placentas appear to be one large placenta. The body of the placenta should be scanned to determine whether a line of separation can be seen.

The twins should each then be scanned for corroboration of dates and size, measuring parameters that include biparietal diameter (BPD), head circumference (HC), abdominal circumference (AC), and femur length (FL). Be sure to use the specialized charts for multiple gestations to determine gestational age.

Dolichocephaly can be common in twin pregnancies as a result of crowding. In dolichocephaly, the BPD is shortened and the occipitofrontal diameter (OFD) is lengthened because of compression. Therefore, the BPD underestimates gestational age with dolichocephaly. The sonographer should always determine the cephalic index (CI) (CI = BPD/OFD × 100). CI of less than 75% suggests dolichocephaly. The normal CI is 75% to 85%.

Because the growth of twins is similar to that of singletons early in pregnancy, singleton growth charts are generally used. It is important to keep in mind that a fetus from a multiple gestation is usually smaller than a singleton fetus. It is known that twins are smaller in size at birth than singleton fetuses of comparable gestational age. Of concern is the ability to detect growth restriction in one or both fetuses. When attempting to determine whether only one twin is growth restricted, differences between the measurements of the two twins must be examined. A difference in estimated fetal weight of more than 20%, a difference in BPD of 6 mm, a difference in AC of 20 mm, and a difference in femur length of 5 mm have been reported as predictors of discordance of growth between twins.[11]

The gender of the fetuses is important to determine. If there is growth discordance between the twins but one is a male and one is a female, then twin–twin transfusion cannot exist. If both twins are of the same sex, however, and growth discordance exists, twin–twin transfusion syndrome may be a possibility.

Umbilical cord Doppler may be useful for fetal surveillance. During the fetal cardiac cycle, there is umbilical blood flow during both the pumping (systole) and filling (diastole) phases of the heartbeat. No flow (absent end-diastolic flow) or reverse flow during diastole (reverse end-diastolic flow) (Figure 48-42) is a sign of fetal jeopardy and may prompt the obstetrician to do further fetal well-being testing or even deliver the fetuses.

One report suggests that most cases of twin–twin transfusion syndrome are identified in the second semester.[12] Abnormal Doppler studies in twin pregnancies should prompt a search for other findings seen in this syndrome, such as polyhydramnios, stuck twin, or hydrops. When Doppler flow patterns are abnormal, careful follow-up should be used to determine if shunting exists.

The multifetal pregnancy reduction method has been used on pregnancies with greater than four fetuses to improve the survival chances of the remaining fetuses. The procedure is performed toward the end of the first trimester by ultrasonographically guided injection of potassium chloride into the thoraxes of the fetuses to be aborted. Information on how the fetal reduction can result in the death of a twin pregnancy is not yet evident.

ACKNOWLEDGMENT

The authors acknowledge the contribution of Sandra L. Hagen-Ansert, Kara L. Mayden-Argo, and Laura J. Zuidema to this chapter in previous editions of this book.

REFERENCES

1. Beckman CRB, Ling FW, Laube DW and others: Embryology, anatomy, and reproductive gynecology. In *Obstetrics and gynecology,* ed 4, Philadelphia, 2002, Lippincott, Williams & Wilkins.
2. Boue J, Boue A, Lazar P: Retrospective and prospective epidemiological studies of 1500 karyotyped spontaneous human abortions, *Teratology* 12:11, 1975.
3. Classen SR, Paulson PR, Zacharias SR: Systemic lupus erythematosus: perinatal and neonatal implications, *J Obstet Gynecol Neonat Nurs* 27:493, 1998.
4. Doubilet PM, Benson CB: Appearing twin: undercounting of multiple gestations on early first trimester sonograms, *J Ultrasound Med* 17:199, 1998.
5. Doubilet PM: Sonography of multiple gestations. Syllabus update in ob/gyn ultrasound vol II, Laurel, Md, June 1-3, 1997, American Institute of Ultrasound in Medicine.
6. Gravett M: Causes of preterm delivery, *Sem Perinatol* 8:246, 1984.
7. Greene N: Fetal medicine foundation assessment and certification for the 11-14 week scan, Cedar Sinai Medical Center, South San Vicente Blvd, Suite 1004, Los Angeles, CA 90048 (course syllabus).
8. Harvey CJ, Verklan T: Systemic lupus erythematosus: obstetric and neonatal complications, *NAACOG Clin Issues Perinat Women Health Nurs* 1:177, 1990.
9. Holzgreve W and others: Investigation of nonimmune hydrops fetalis, *Am J Obstet Gynecol* 150:805, 1984.
10. Mari G, Adrignolo A, Abuhamad AZ and others: Diagnosis of fetal anemia with Doppler ultrasound in the pregnancy complicated by maternal blood group immunization, *Ultrasound Obstet Gynecol* 5:400, 1995.
11. Newton ER, Cetrulo SL: Management of twin gestation. In Cetrulo CL, Sbaria AJ, editors: *The problem-oriented medical record for high risk obstetrics,* New York, 1984, Plenum.
12. Pretorius DH and others: Doppler ultrasound of twin transfusion syndrome, *J Ultrasound Med* 7:117, 1988.
13. Reisner DP, Mahony BS, Petty CN and others: Stuck twin syndrome: outcome in thirty-seven consecutive cases, *Am J Obstet Gynecol* 169:991-995, 1996.
14. Wald N, Hackshaw A: Combining ultrasound and biochemistry in first-trimester screening for Down's syndrome, *Prenat Diagn* 17:821-829, 1997.

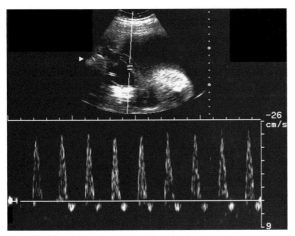

Figure 48-42 Reversal of diastolic flow in a twin gestation with TTS.

SELECTED BIBLIOGRAPHY

Beckman CRB, Ling FW, Laube DW and others: *Obstetrics and gynecology,* ed 4, Philadelphia, 2002, Lippincott, Williams & Wilkins.

Benson CM and others: Multifetal pregnancy reduction of both fetuses of a monochorionic pair by intrathoracic potassium chloride injection of one fetus, *J Ultrasound Med* 17:447, 1998.

Chinn DH: Ultrasound evaluation of hydrops fetalis. In Callan PW, editor: *Ultrasonography in obstetrics and gynecology,* ed 3, Philadelphia, 2000, WB Saunders.

Daffos F, Capella-Pavlovsky M, Forestier F: A new procedure for fetal blood sampling in utero: preliminary results of fifty three cases, *Am J Obstet Gynecol* 146:985, 1983.

Doubilet PM, Benson CB, Callen PW: Ultrasound evaluation of fetal growth. In Callen PW, editor: *Ultrasonography in obstetrics and gynecology,* ed 4, Philadelphia, 2000, WB Saunders.

Harman C: Ultrasound in the management of the alloimmunized pregnancy. In Fleischer AC and others: *Sonography in obstetrics & gynecology: principles and practice,* ed 6, New York, 2001, McGraw-Hill.

Harris RD, Alexander RD, editors: Ultrasound of the placenta. In Callen PW, editor: *Ultrasonography in obstetrics and gynecology,* ed 4, Philadelphia, 2000, WB Saunders.

Liley AW: Liquor amnii analysis in management of pregnancy complicated by rhesus sensitization, *Am J Obstet Gynecol* 82:1359, 1961.

Mahony BS, Filly RA, Callen PW: Amnionicity and chorionicity in twin pregnancies: prediction using ultrasound, *Radiology* 155:205, 1985.

Morin KH: Perinatal outcomes of obese women: a review of the literature, *J Obstet Gynecol Neonat Nurs* 27:431, 1998.

Nelson L, Melone P, King M: Diagnosis of vasa previa with transvaginal and color flow Doppler ultrasound, *Obstet Gynecol* 76:506, 1990.

Nolen G, Chenoweth-Mitchell CK, Barry-Kiefer C and others: Prenatal diagnosis of acardiac parabiotic twinning, *J Diagn Med Sonography* 14(5):207-209, 1998.

Reece EA and others: Diabetes mellitus in pregnancy and the assessment of umbilical artery waveforms using pulsed Doppler ultrasonography, *J Ultrasound Med* 13:73, 1994.

Reece EA, Hobbin JC: Diabetic embryopathy: pathogenesis, prenatal diagnosis and prevention, *Obstet Gynecol Surv* 41:325, 1986.

Rumwell C, McPharlin M: Vascular technology: an illustrated review, ed 3, Pasadena, Calif, 2004, Davies Publishing.

Sanders RC: Possible fetal anomalies. In Sanders RC, Miner NS, editors: Clinical sonography: a practical guide, ed 3, Philadelphia, 1997, Lippincott, Williams & Wilkins.

Spellacy WN: Cesarean section: update 1983, *Postgrad Obstet Gynecol* 3:1, 1983.

Trampe BS, Pryde PG, Stewart KS and others: Color Doppler ultrasonography for distinguishing myomas from uterine contractions in pregnancy, *J Reprod Med* 46(9):791-794, 2001.

Vyas S, Nicolaides KH, Campbell S: Doppler examination of the middle cerebral artery in anemic fetuses, *Am J Obstet Gynecol* 162:1066, 1990.

CHAPTER 49

Prenatal Diagnosis of Congenital Anomalies

Charlotte G. Henningsen

KEY TERMS

alpha-fetoprotein (AFP) – protein manufactured by the fetus, which can be studied in amniotic fluid and maternal serum. Elevations of alpha-fetoprotein may indicate fetal anomalies (neural tube, abdominal wall, gastrointestinal), multiple gestations, or incorrect patient dates. Decreased levels may be associated with chromosomal abnormalities.

amniocentesis – transabdominal removal of amniotic fluid from the amniotic cavity using ultrasound. Amniotic fluid studies are performed to determine fetal karyotype, lung maturity, and Rh condition.

cystic hygroma – dilation of jugular lymph sacs (may occur in axilla or groin) because of improper drainage of the lymphatic system into the venous system. Large, septated hygromas are frequently associated with Turner's and Down syndromes, congestive heart failure, and death of the fetus in utero; isolated hygromas may occur as solitary lesions at birth. May be part of a general fatal condition, lymphangiectasis, or a benign focal process.

hypertelorism – abnormally wide-spaced orbits usually found in conjunction with congenital anomalies and mental retardation

hypoplasia – underdevelopment of a tissue, organ, or body

hypotelorism – abnormally closely spaced orbits; association with holoprosencephaly, chromosomal, central nervous system disorders, and cleft palate

intrauterine growth restriction (IUGR) – a decreased rate of fetal growth, usually a fetal weight below the 10th percentile for a given gestational age

micrognathia – abnormally small chin; commonly associated with other fetal anomalies

omphalocele – anterior abdominal wall defect in which abdominal organs (liver, bowel, stomach) are atypically located within the umbilical cord; highly associated with cardiac, central nervous system, renal, and chromosomal anomalies

polydactyly – anomalies of the hands or feet in which there is an addition of a digit; may be found in association with certain skeletal dysplasias

TORCH – an acronym originally coined from the first letters of Toxoplasmosis, Rubella, Cytomegalovirus, and Herpesvirus type 2. *O* stands for other transplacental infections.

ALPHA-FETOPROTEIN AND CHROMOSOMAL DISORDERS

A major congenital anomaly is found in 3 of every 100 births, and an additional 10% to 15% of births are complicated by minor birth defects. Since prenatal ultrasound has become the investigative tool for the obstetrician to access the developing fetus, it is likely that the fetus with an anomaly will be subjected to ultrasound at some time during pregnancy. The role of the sonographer is to screen for the unsuspected anomaly and to study the fetus at risk for an anomaly. The benefits of the examination are greatest when the sonographer is adept at detecting congenital anomalies and understands the cause, progression, and prognosis of the common congenital anomalies.

When a fetal anomaly is found antenatally, a multidisciplinary team approach to managing the fetus, mother, and family is preferable because the fetus may need special monitoring (e.g., serial ultrasound), delivery, postnatal care, and surgery. This multidisciplinary team includes the perinatologist (maternal-fetal medicine specialist), neonatologist (specialist for critically ill infants), sonologist, perinatal sonographer, pediatric surgeon, other pediatric specialists, geneticist, obstetrician, perinatal and pediatric social workers, and other support personnel. Consultation with specialists is recommended when diagnosis is uncertain. Once an anomaly is found, these specialists can work as a team to optimize clinical management, to prepare the patient and family for possible surgery, to provide the patient and family with emotional support, and to plan for delivery. Most fetuses with major birth defects are delivered in perinatal regional centers where the specialized physicians, nurses, equipment, treatment, and postnatal surgery are available.

This chapter discusses chorionic villus sampling, amniocentesis, maternal serum alpha-fetoprotein (MSAFP), other similar testing, and basic medical genetics. Included is a discussion of common chromosomal abnormalities.

GENETIC TESTING

CHORIONIC VILLUS SAMPLING

Chorionic villus sampling (CVS) is an ultrasound directed biopsy of the placenta or chorionic villi (chorion frondosum). The chorion frondosum is the active trophoblastic tissue that becomes the placenta. Because the chorionic villi are fetal in origin, chromosomal abnormalities may be detected when cells from the villi are grown and analyzed. Other conditions, such as biochemical or metabolic disorders, thalassemia, and sickle cell disease (hemoglobinopathies), may also be diagnosed using chorionic villi.[33]

CVS is an alternative test used to obtain a fetal karyotype by the culturing of fetal cells similar to amniocentesis. The advantage of CVS includes the following: (1) it is performed early in pregnancy (10 to 12 weeks), (2) results are available within 1 week, and (3) earlier results allow more options for parents.

CVS is performed transcervically or transabdominally (Figure 49-1). Ultrasound performed before the actual procedure should aid in the following ways: (1) Determine the relationship between the lie of the uterus and cervix and path of the catheter. Bladder fullness influences this relationship. Filling or emptying of the bladder may be necessary to facilitate the catheter route. (2) Assess the fetus in terms of life, normal morphology, and age. (3) Identify uterine masses or potential problems that may interfere with passage of the catheter.

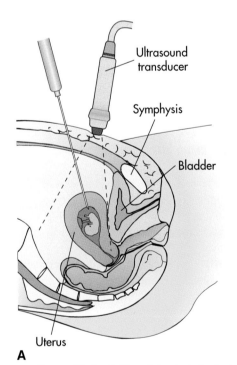
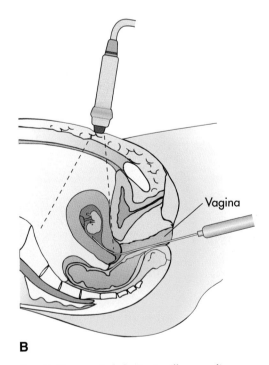

Figure 49-1 **A,** Transabdominal chorionic villus sampling. **B,** Transcervical chorionic villus sampling.

Endovaginal CVS is performed in the dorsolithotomy position (pelvic examination position). The sonographer aids the obstetrician in determining the correct route to pass the catheter through the cervix to the placenta. A guiding stylet is initially introduced to check uterine and placental position. A flexible catheter is then introduced and directed into the placental tissue (Figure 49-2). The placental cells are aspirated through the catheter. The villi are collected in media-prepared syringes and immediately transported to the cytogenetics technician for analysis. Additional retrievals often are necessary. The sonographer should monitor the fetal heart rate and check for procedural bleeding.

The transabdominal CVS approach entails using a special apparatus attached to the needle hub to permit adequate suction to withdraw the villi. The procedure is performed in a manner similar to amniocentesis (see discussion of amniocentesis).

The risk of fetal loss because of CVS is approximately 0.05% to 1.0%.[15] There has been some association with limb reduction defects when CVS is performed before 8 weeks of gestation.[15] Rh$_o$(D) immune globulin (RhoGAM) should be administered to Rh-negative unsensitized women to prevent sensitization problems in subsequent pregnancies.

EMBRYOSCOPY

Embryoscopy is a specialized prenatal test that permits the direct viewing of the developing embryo using a transcervical endoscope inserted into the extracoelomic cavity during the first trimester of pregnancy. With this method, fetal anomalies may be detected or samples of blood aspirated and checked for various blood disorders. Investigators are optimistic that this technique will permit gene therapy in the future.[25]

AMNIOCENTESIS

Amniocentesis was first used as a technique to relieve polyhydramnios, to predict Rh isoimmunization, and to document fetal lung maturity.[28] In the mid-1960s, amniocentesis was used to study fetal cells from amniotic fluid that allowed the analysis of fetal chromosomes (Figure 49-3). Normal and abnormal chromosomal patterns (Figures 49-4 and 49-5) could be identified.[12]

Amniocentesis is a test offered to expectant patients who are at risk for a chromosomal abnormality or biochemical disorder that may be prenatally detectable. Advanced maternal age is a common reason for performing amniocentesis. All pregnant women are at risk for having a child with a chromosomal defect, but the risk is greater in a woman of advanced maternal age. The risk of having a fetus with Down syndrome is 1 in 365 in a woman who is 35 years of age, whereas the risk for a woman who is 21 years of age is only about 1 in 2000. The risk of having a fetus with any chromosomal anomaly is 1 in 180 in the woman who is 35 years of age versus 1 in 500 for the woman who is 21 years of age.

Other indications for genetic amniocentesis include a history of a balance rearrangement in a parent or previous child with a chromosomal abnormality, a history of an unexplained abnormal AFP level or an abnormal triple screen, and a fetus with a congenital anomaly.

Amniocentesis for genetic reasons is ideally performed between 15 and 18 weeks of gestation. Amniocentesis may be done as early as 12 weeks, but may lead to the development of fetal scoliosis or clubfoot secondary to the reduced amount of amniotic fluid. The rate of miscarriage in early amniocentesis is not clearly defined. Some studies have shown that the loss rate is similar to midtrimester amniocentesis, whereas others have shown a higher loss rate.[15] The fetal loss rate of midtrimester amniocentesis is reported as 8.0% in the United States.[6] Amniocentesis performed beyond 20 weeks of gestation is possible, but may be associated with poor cell growth.

The amniocentesis procedure should include a fetal survey to exclude congenital anomalies. A fetal examination should be performed, and targeted areas of anatomy should be documented to exclude the physical features that would suggest a chromosomal anomaly (e.g., hand clenching, **hypoplasia** of

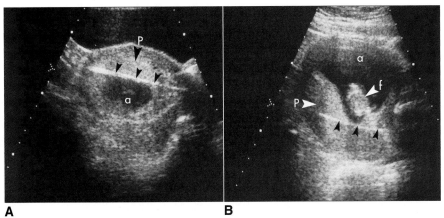

A   **B**

Figure 49-2   A, Transcervical chorionic villus sampling at 10 weeks of gestation demonstrating the placement of the sampling catheter *(arrowheads)* within an anterior placenta *(P)* or chorion frondosum. *a,* Amniotic cavity. **B,** Transcervical chorionic villus sampling at 11 weeks of gestation showing the placement of the sampling catheter *(arrowheads)* within a posterior placenta *(P)*. Note the fetal abdomen *(f)* within the amniotic cavity *(a)*.

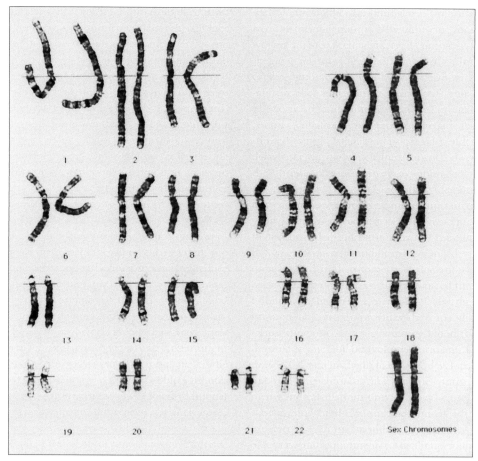

Figure 49-3 Normal karyotype demonstrating 46 chromosomes in a female fetus (46, XX).

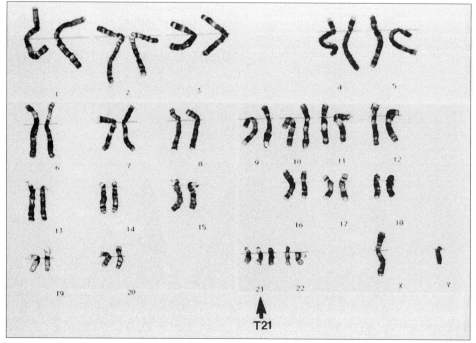

Figure 49-4 Karyotype of trisomy 21 (Down syndrome) in a male fetus (47, XY, 21). Note the extra chromosome at the twenty-first position *(arrow)*. Note the sex chromosomes indicating a male fetus.

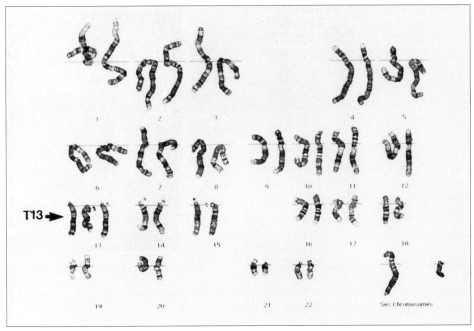

Figure 49-5   Karyotype of trisomy 13 (47, XY 13) *(arrow)* male fetus.

the fifth middle phalanx, choroid plexus cysts, ventriculomegaly, thickened nuchal fold, cardiac anomalies, omphalocele, spina bifida, or foot anomalies).

The sonographer will also assist the physician in the amniocentesis procedure. The optimal collection site for amniotic fluid should be away from the fetus, away from the central portion of the placenta, away from the umbilical cord, and near the maternal midline to avoid the maternal uterine vessels.

TECHNIQUE OF GENETIC AMNIOCENTESIS

Ultrasound-monitored amniocentesis is a technique that allows the continuous monitoring of the needle during the amniocentesis procedure.[19] Using this technique, the maternal skin is prepared with a povidone-iodine solution.

The transducer is placed in a sterile cover or sterile glove to allow monitoring on the sterile field during the procedure. Sterile coupling gel may be applied to the maternal skin to ensure good transmission of the sound beam. The amniocentesis site is rescanned to confirm the amniotic pocket, and then the site and pathway for the introduction of the needle are determined. The distance to the amniotic fluid may be measured with electronic calipers, which may be useful in obese patients in whom a longer needle may be necessary. In many instances, a new site is chosen as a result of fetal movement or a myometrial contraction in the proposed site, and the transducer is moved to a new sterile area. On successful identification of the amniocentesis site, a finger is placed between the transducer and the skin to produce an acoustic shadow. The needle is then inserted under continuous ultrasound observation (Figure 49-6). Inserting the needle in a plane perpendicular to the transducer will allow for a bright reflection of the needle tip, so that it can be easily observed (Figure 49-7) at the edge of the uterine wall and then as it punctures the uterine cavity. When incorrectly directed, the needle may be repositioned.

Amniotic fluid is aspirated through a syringe connected to the needle hub. The first few milliliters of fluid should be discarded to avoid contamination. Between 20 and 30 ml of amniotic fluid will be collected for chromosomal analysis and AFP evaluation. In advanced pregnancies, additional amniotic fluid may be required. When amniocentesis is performed because of a known fetal anomaly, acetylcholinesterase and viral studies (**TORCH** titers) may be ordered. Following aspiration of amniotic fluid, the needle is removed from the uterus under sonographic guidance.

After the amniocentesis has been completed, fetal cardiac activity should be identified and documented. If the placenta has been traversed, the site should be monitored for bleeding. The use of videotaping can allow for continuous recording and documentation of the fetal examination and the amniocentesis and postamniocentesis ultrasound evaluation.

The continuous monitoring with ultrasound during amniocentesis is invaluable in cases of oligohydramnios, anterior placental position, and premature rupture of membranes. Ultrasound imaging can help achieve a successful amniocentesis when only small pockets of fluid are available.

GENETIC AMNIOCENTESIS AND MULTIPLE GESTATIONS

Amniocentesis in multiple gestations warrants special consideration. Preliminary sonographic examination for each fetus should be performed to include a survey of fetal anatomy and growth profiles. Determination of whether the pregnancy is monozygotic or dizygotic should be made. The amount of amniotic fluid within each sac should be assessed, and it should be determined if there are multiple sacs.

The amniocentesis technique for multiple gestations is similar to the singleton method, except that each fetal sac is entered. To be certain that amniotic fluid is obtained from each sac, indigo carmine dye can be injected into the first sac. The

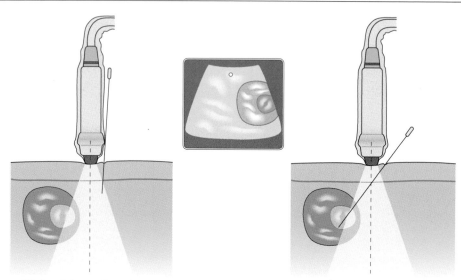

Figure 49-6 If the needle is inserted parallel to the transducer, only the tip will be represented. If the needle is inserted at an angle with the transducer, the beam will intersect the needle, but it will not demonstrate its tip, which could be in a harmful position. Notice that in both cases the image on the screen is the same. Angling the needle is a dangerous procedure that should be avoided.

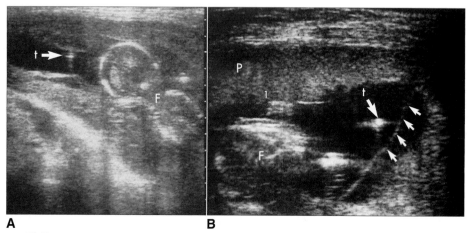

A   **B**

Figure 49-7 **A,** Genetic amniocentesis at 15.6 weeks of gestation using direct visualization method. The needle tip *(t)* is identified within the amniotic cavity. *F,* Fetus. **B,** Genetic amniocentesis at 16 weeks of gestation in a twin pregnancy. The needle tip *(t)* is identified within the sac above the amniotic membrane *(arrows)*. *F,* Fetus; *P,* placenta. *1,* Umbilical cord insertion into placenta.

presence of clear amniotic fluid indicates that the second sac has been penetrated when the second pass is made. If dye-stained fluid is visible, it indicates that the first sac has been penetrated a second time. Documentation of each amniocentesis and meticulous labeling of fluid samples are recommended. It is desirable to avoid the placenta in patients who are Rh-negative. In all Rh-negative patients, RhoGAM is administered within 72 hours of the procedure.

CORDOCENTESIS

Cordocentesis is another method in which chromosomes are analyzed. Fetal blood is obtained through needle aspiration of the umbilical cord. Karyotype results can be processed within 2 to 3 days. This rapid assessment may be beneficial for

patients with an equivocal amniocentesis result or when a fetal anomaly is detected later in pregnancy.

MATERNAL SERUM MARKERS

ALPHA-FETOPROTEIN

Alpha-fetoprotein (AFP) is the major protein in fetal serum and is produced by the yolk sac in early gestation and later by the fetal liver. AFP is found in the fetal spine, gastrointestinal tract, liver, and kidneys. This protein is transported into the amniotic fluid by fetal urination and reaches maternal circulation or blood through the fetal membranes (Figure 49-8). AFP may be measured in the maternal serum (MSAFP) or from amniotic fluid (AFAFP).

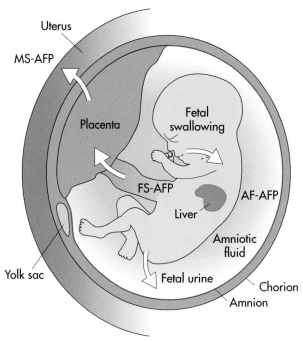

Figure 49-8 Schematic drawing showing the production and distribution of alpha-fetoprotein (AFP) into its three components: fetal tissues, amniotic fluid, and maternal serum. *AF-AFP,* Amniotic fluid AFP; *FS-AFP,* fetal serum AFT; *MS-AFP,* maternal serum AFP.

AFP levels are considered abnormal when elevated or low. Neural tube defects, such as anencephaly and open spina bifida, are common reasons for high AFP levels. In both instances, AFP leaks from the defect to enter the amniotic fluid and then diffuses into the maternal bloodstream (see Figure 49-8). AFP elevations will not be found when there is closed spina bifida (occulta) because there is no opening to allow leakage.

Monitoring of AFP is a screening test for neural tube defects and other conditions (Box 49-1). MSAFP screening detects approximately 88% of anencephalics and 79% of open spina bifida cases when 2.5 multiples of the median (MOM) are used.[32]

MSAFP levels increase with advancing gestational age and peak from 15 to 18 weeks of gestation (the ideal sampling time). AFAFP, in contrast, decreases with fetal age. A common reason for elevations is incorrect dates. Because AFP levels vary with gestational age, if the fetus is older or younger than expected, AFP levels will be reported as increased or decreased.

Other reasons for elevations are acrania and encephalocele (which may occur in association with Meckel-Gruber syndrome), with AFP leakage from the exposed membranes and tissue. The concentration of AFP correlates with the size of the defect. AFP levels tend to be significantly higher in fetuses with anencephaly than with spina bifida because more tissue is exposed. It is important to remember that approximately 20% of spina bifida lesions are covered by skin, so AFP elevations will not be detected in serum or amniotic fluid. Sacrococcygeal teratomas are also known to be associated with high AFP levels.

Two common abdominal wall defects, omphalocele and gastroschisis, produce elevations of AFP. With an **omphalo-cele,** AFP leaks through the membrane encasing the herniated bowel or liver. In gastroschisis, AFP diffuses directly into the serum and amniotic fluid from the herniated bowel, which lacks a covering membrane; thus AFP levels are higher in a fetus with gastroschisis than in a fetus with an omphalocele.

Other abdominal wall defects cause leakage in the same manner. Bladder or cloacal exstrophy, ectopia cordis (herniation of the heart out of the chest), limb-body wall complex, and amniotic band syndrome are examples of other anomalies that may present with an elevated AFP level.

It is expected that the AFP level in a twin pregnancy will be twice that of a singleton pregnancy because two fetuses make twice the AFP. In multiple gestations in which there is death of a co-twin (fetus papyraceus) or when one twin is an acardiac twin, AFP may be higher than normal.

Obstructions of the gastrointestinal tract may cause reduced clearance of AFP. This may explain elevations with anomalies, such as an annular pancreas, esophageal atresia, and duodenal atresia.

A fetus with a kidney lesion may produce increased AFP. In congenital nephrosis, extremely high levels of AFP are excreted by the kidneys. Polycystic kidneys and urinary tract obstruction may also lead to higher levels of AFP because there is abnormal clearance or filtration of AFP because of kidney maldevelopment and urinary tract leakage.

Placental lesions, such as chorioangiomas, hemangiomas, and hematomas, are known to be responsible for AFP elevations.[13] Placental problems in general may explain the prevalence of growth restriction, fetal death, and abruption in patients with unexplained AFP elevations.

In heart failure, faulty diffusion of AFP may lead to an abnormal AFP increase when hydrops, ascites, or lymphangiectasia are present. Severely sensitized fetuses with Rh isoimmunization may have heart failure because of severe anemia. In the fetus with a **cystic hygroma,** obstructed lymph sacs lead to AFP diffusion through the hygroma into the bloodstream and amniotic fluid.

Liver disease in the mother or fetus may cause high AFP levels. Hepatitis, maternal herpes virus and resultant fetal liver necrosis, skin lesions, hepatocellular carcinoma, and fetal liver tumors (hamartomas) are rare causes of elevated AFP.

Other causes include chromosomal abnormalities associated with fetal anomalies or placental problems that permit the abnormal passage of AFP. Fetuses with trisomy 13 or trisomy 18 may also have renal anomalies, neural tube defects, ventral wall defects, or skin lesions that cause elevations in the AFP level. Fetuses with Turner's syndrome often present with cystic hygromas. In triploidy, abnormal placental molar degeneration leads to increased AFP diffusion.

Cystic adenomatoid malformations cause rises in AFP because of excessive leakage from the lungs. Pilonidal cysts of the back and various skin disorders and tumors, such as epignathus and intracranial lesions, are also associated with high AFP levels. Rarely the fetus manufactures excessive amounts of AFP as a hereditary condition.

Fetal death is a frequent cause of a high MSAFP level. Pregnancies complicated by oligohydramnios may have higher

BOX 49-1

REASONS FOR ELEVATIONS OF ALPHA-FETOPROTEIN AND ACETYLCHOLINESTERASE

Neural Tube Defects
Anencephaly
Exencephaly (acrania)
Encephalocele (including Meckel-Gruber syndrome)
Spina bifida
Sacrococcygeal teratoma

Abdominal Wall Defects
Omphalocele
Gastroschisis
Limb-body wall complex
Amniotic band syndrome
Bladder or cloacal exstrophy
Ectopia cordis

Multiple Gestation
Twin with a co-twin death
Acardiac twin
Fetus papyraceous

Gastrointestinal Obstruction
Annular pancreas
Duodenal atresia
Esophageal atresia

Renal Anomalies
Congenital nephrosis
Hydronephrosis
Polycystic kidney disease (including Meckel-Gruber syndrome)
Urinary tract obstruction
Prune belly syndrome
Urethral atresia

Placental and Cord Abnormalities
Chorioangioma
Placental or cord hematoma
Umbilical cord hemangioma
Hydatidiform mole

Fetal Heart Failure
Hydrops and/or ascites
Lymphangiectasia
Rh isoimmunization

Neck Masses
Cystic hygroma
Noonan's syndrome (with hygroma)

Liver Disease
Hepatitis
Maternal herpes virus (fetal liver necrosis and skin lesions)
Hepatocellular carcinoma
Hamartoma of liver

Miscellaneous Causes
Incorrect dates
Fetal demise
Oligohydramnios
Unexplained
Hereditary overproduction of alpha-fetoprotein
Blood in amniotic fluid
Chromosome abnormalities (trisomies 18 and 13, Turner's syndrome, triploidy)
Cystadenomatoid malformation
Epignathus
Intracranial tumor
Pilonidal cyst
Skin defects
Hydrocephalus
Congenital heart defects
Viral infections (cytomegalovirus [CMV], parvovirus)

Modified from Milunsky A, editor: *Genetic disorders and the fetus: diagnosis, prevention and treatment,* ed 3, Baltimore, 1992, Johns Hopkins University Press; Nyberg DA, Mahony BS, Pretorius DH, editors: *Diagnostic ultrasound of fetal anomalies, text and atlas,* St Louis, 1990, Mosby.

concentrations of AFP because there is less amniotic fluid to diffuse the protein.

Contamination of an amniotic fluid specimen by blood may also falsely increase the level of AFP.

In utero viral infections (cytomegalovirus and parvovirus) are reported to permit excessive AFP leakage because the maternal-fetal surface may be irritated and disrupted by inflammation.

Unexplained elevations in MSAFP suggest that the pregnancy is at increased risk for complications and poor outcomes, including low birth weight and stillbirth.[13] Preeclampsia, hypertension, and abruptio placentae are other third-trimester complications associated with these elevations.

Mothers with elevated MSAFP values and normal AFAFP values are potentially at risk for other fetal anomalies unrelated to neural tube defects. Hydrocephalus, without a spinal defect

(increased cerebrospinal fluid allows increased diffusion), and congenital heart disease (probable altered perfusion of blood flow through placenta) are reported in conjunction with unexplained, nonneural tube defect problems.

Low AFP levels have been found with chromosomal abnormalities, such as trisomy 21, trisomy 18, and trisomy 13 (Box 49-2). Other causes include incorrect patient dates (fetus younger than expected), fetal death, hydatidiform moles, spontaneous abortion, and a nonpregnant state. In some cases, the cause may remain unknown.

Amniocentesis may be offered when MSAFP levels are elevated and ultrasound reveals no obvious explanation. Amniotic fluid tests usually include karyotyping for chromosomal abnormalities, AFAFP levels, and acetylcholinesterase. AFAFP is more specific for detecting levels of AFP. Acetylcholinesterase is specific for detecting an open neural tube.[13] Beyond 20 weeks

BOX
49-2   **COMMON SONOGRAPHIC FEATURES OF CHROMOSOMAL ANOMALIES**

Trisomy 21	Trisomy 18	Trisomy 13	Triploidy	Turner's Syndrome
Nuchal thickness	Heart defects	Holoprosencephaly	Hydatidiform placental	Cystic hygroma
Heart defects	Choroid plexus cysts	Heart defects	degeneration	Heart defects
Duodenal atresia	Clenched hands	Cleft lip and palate	Heart defects	Hydrops
Shortened femurs	Micrognathia	Omphalocele	Renal anomalies	Renal anomalies
Mild pyelectasis	Talipes	Polydactyly	Omphalocele	
Mild ventriculomegaly	Renal anomalies	Talipes	Cranial defects	
Echogenic bowel	Cleft lip and palate	Echogenic chordae	Facial defects	
	Omphalocele	tendineae		
	CDH	Renal anomalies		
	Cerebellar hypoplasia	Meningomyelocele		
		Micrognathia		

of gestation, acetylcholinesterase is the preferred test because AFP analysis is no longer sensitive.

When AFP is elevated (greater than 3 MOM) and the cranium (ventricles and cisterna magna) and spine appear normal, the risk of the fetus actually having a small spinal defect is approximately halved. The overall risk of miscarriage from an amniocentesis is 1 in 200, so it is important to weigh the risk of complication with the possible yield of identifying an abnormality.

Prenatal scanning and amniocentesis are used to evaluate the fetus with a low AFP value to exclude any physical features that may suggest a chromosomal abnormality. Such findings might include choroid plexus cysts, hand anomalies, or cardiac defects.

QUADRUPLE SCREEN

Another biochemical screening test used in the early second trimester is known as the quadruple screen. Formally known as the triple test or triple screen, this biochemical screening test combines three serum markers: AFP, human chorionic gonadotropin (hCG), and unconjugated estriol. This blood test improved the detection rate for trisomy 21 over MSAFP testing alone. Biochemical screening in trisomy 21 fetuses reveals high hCG levels and decreased AFP and estriol levels.[18] Additionally, biochemical screening may suggest trisomy 18 when hCG, AFP, and estriol levels are all decreased. The quadruple screen added another maternal serum marker, dimeric inhibin A, improving the sensitivity in detecting Down fetuses.[9] The risk for a neural tube defect or chromosomal problem is calculated for each mother. A patient may elect to undergo ultrasound with or without amniocentesis based on the risk for chromosomal or neural tube defects.

PREGNANCY-ASSOCIATED PLASMA PROTEIN A

A first-trimester serum marker used to detect anomalies is pregnancy-associated plasma protein A (PAPP-A). PAPP-A is a glycoprotein derived from the trophoblastic tissue that is then diffused into the maternal circulation. PAPP-A levels increase in maternal serum throughout pregnancy. PAPP-A levels have been found to be decreased in pregnancies affected by aneuploidy.[34]

FREE BETA HUMAN CHORIONIC GONADOTROPIN

Free beta-hCG is also a glycoprotein derived from the placenta that can be assessed in maternal serum in the first trimester to evaluate for increased risk of Down syndrome. Free beta-hCG and PAPP-A are being evaluated in combination with nuchal translucency measurements in the first trimester as a sensitivity screening tool for Down syndrome.[21]

MEDICAL GENETICS

A normal karyotype consists of 46 chromosomes, 22 pairs of autosomes, and a pair of sex chromosomes (see Figure 49-3). Aneuploidy is an abnormality of the number of chromosomes. One of the most common aneuploid conditions is Down syndrome, in which an individual has an extra chromosome number 21 (see Figure 49-4). The cause of trisomy is usually nondisjunction, the failure of normal chromosomal division at the time of meiosis. The cause of nondisjunction is unknown, although there is strong association with maternal age.[31]

A chromosomal disorder is caused by too much or too little chromosome material. A dominant disorder is a condition caused by a single defective gene (autosomal dominant). It is usually inherited from one parent (who is also affected), but may arise as a new mutation (spontaneous gene change). An inherited dominant disorder carries a 50% chance that each time pregnancy occurs, the fetus will have the condition. An example of an autosomal-dominant condition is osteogenesis imperfecta (types 1 and 4).

A recessive disorder (autosomal recessive) is caused by a pair of defective genes, one inherited from each parent. With each pregnancy, the parents have a 25% chance of having a fetus with the disorder. An example of an autosomal recessive condition is infantile polycystic kidney disease.

X-linked disorders are inherited by boys from their mothers. Affected males do not transmit the disorder to their sons, but all of their daughters will be carriers for the disorder. The sons of female carriers each have a 50% chance of being affected, and the daughters each have a 50% chance of being a carrier. Whereas an X-linked gene is located on the female sex chromosome (the X), an autosomal gene is located on one of the numbered chromosomes.[31] An example of an X-linked condition occurring in male fetuses is aqueductal stenosis. Aqueductal stenosis, however, may also occur in females.

A multifactorial condition is an abnormal event that arises because of the interaction of one or more genes and environmental factors. Anencephaly is an example of a multifactorial disorder.

Mosaicism is the occurrence of a gene mutation or chromosomal abnormality in a portion of an individual's cells. It is difficult to predict the types of problems that will occur when mosaicism is found.

CHROMOSOMAL ABNORMALITIES

Chromosomal abnormalities are found in 1 of every 180 live births.[22] There is a high prevalence of chromosomal abnormalities in patients referred for second-trimester amniocentesis because of advanced maternal age, abnormal AFP, abnormal quadruple screen (hCG, AFP, estriol, and inhibin A), or ultrasound detection of multiple fetal anomalies. It is important to become familiar with and to search for the physical features (see Box 49-2) that would suggest trisomies 13, 18, and 21, triploidy, and Turner's syndrome.

NUCHAL TRANSLUCENCY

An abnormal fluid collection behind the fetal neck has been strongly associated with aneuploidy.[23] This nuchal translucency (NT) has been reported as a late first-trimester finding identified between 10 and 14 weeks of gestation.[23] An NT of 3 mm or greater has been used in earlier literature to define an abnormal thickness. Current literature suggests that the NT increases with gestational age, so the NT measurement should be compared with the gestational age or crown-rump length to determine risk for aneuploidy.[29] A thickened NT is associated with chromosomal abnormalities, such as trisomies 13, 18, 21; triploidy; and Turner's syndrome (Figure 49-9).[23] This first-trimester; finding is not a precursor to the development of a cystic hygroma or second-trimester edema.[23]

Sonographic Findings. Endovaginal technique is recommended, and scanning in two planes perpendicular to each other can help to prevent error. Care should be taken to avoid confusing amnion ·with a nuchal translucency. The translucency should be oriented perpendicular to the ultrasound beam, and the measurement should be taken from inside the fetal neck to inside the nuchal membrane.

Nuchal translucency is viewed as an early, noninvasive means of assessing the risk of aneuploidy. A measurement of 3 mm increases the risk of aneuploidy four times, and nuchal translucencies of 4 mm and greater carry an even greater risk. There has also been documentation of resolution of this abnormality with a normal outcome. Even in fetuses with normal chromosomes, an increased nuchal translucency has been associated with an increased incidence of structural defects, such as cardiac, diaphragmatic, renal, and abdominal wall anomalies. In addition to the increased risk of chromosomal abnormality and other anomalies, an increased nuchal translucency has also been associated with spontaneous miscarriage and perinatal death.[23]

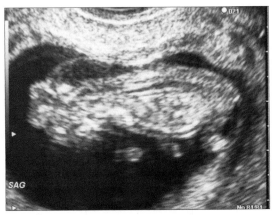

Figure 49-9   This fetus with trisomy 13 presented with a thickened and septated nuchal translucency and anencephaly in the late first trimester of pregnancy. (Courtesy Joseph Blazina, RDMS, OB/Gyn & Associates, Kissimmee, Fla.)

TRISOMY 21

Trisomy 21, also known as Down syndrome, occurs in 1 in 660 births.[10] It is one of the most common chromosomal disorders and is characterized by an extra chromosome number 21.[17] There is an association with advanced maternal age; however, this anomaly may affect infants born to women of all ages. Trisomy 21 is associated with an abnormal quadruple screen.

Infants with trisomy 21 may present with a variety of physical features (Figure 49-10) including brachycephaly; epicanthal folds (a fold of skin that covers the inner corner of the eye); a flattened nasal bridge; round, small ears; broad neck with extra skin (nuchal fold); and a protruding tongue.[4] Other anomalies that have been associated with Down syndrome include heart defects (septal defects, endocardial cushion defect, tetralogy of Fallot), duodenal atresia, esophageal atresia, anorectal atresia, and omphalocele (Figure 49-11). Cystic hygroma, nonimmune hydrops, and hydrothorax may also be observed. Skeletal anomalies may be present, including shortened extremities, space between the first and second toes, hypoplasia of the middle fifth phalanx (Figure 49-12), and clinodactyly of the fifth finger (inward curving).[3] A single palmar (hand) crease is found in approximately 30% of affected infants.[20]

The prognosis for survival depends on associated anomalies, with heart anomalies a major cause of mortality in infancy. Mental retardation is always present, with IQ ranges between 25 and 50 in childhood.[23] In addition to heart failure, alimentary defects can also be life threatening. Respiratory problems, eye problems, and premature aging are common.

Sonographic Findings. Ultrasound diagnosis of trisomy 21 is limited because of the subtleness and infrequency of some of the phenotypic expressions.[4] Anomalies that may be identified with Down syndrome include the following:

- Nuchal fold of 6 mm or greater (Figure 49-13).
- Extremity anomalies (hypoplasia of the middle phalanx or clinodactyly of the fifth finger; space between first and second toes)

- Shortened femur or short humerus
- Duodenal atresia (Figure 49-14)
- Heart defects (Figure 49-15) (present in approximately 30% to 40%)
- **Intrauterine growth restriction (IUGR)**
- Mild pyelectasis (4 mm in anteroposterior diameter)
- Echogenic bowel (Figure 49-16)
- Mild ventriculomegaly (Figure 49-17)

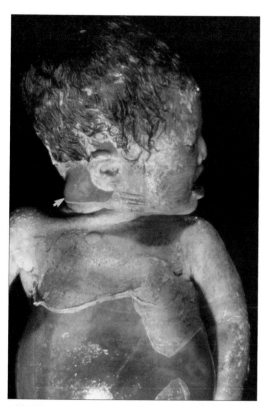

Figure 49-10   Postmortem photograph of a neonate with trisomy 21 (Down syndrome). Duodenal atresia was found. Note the nuchal thickening *(arrow)*.

- Echogenic intracardiac focus (tip of mitral valve apparatus)
- Absence of the nasal bone between 11 and 14 weeks

TRISOMY 18

Trisomy 18, also known as Edwards' syndrome, is the second most common chromosomal trisomy, occurring in 1 of 8000 live births.[5] This karyotype demonstrates an extra chromosome 18. Trisomy 18 is associated with an abnormal quadruple screen.

Physical features that have been identified in fetuses with trisomy 18 (Figure 49-18) include cardiac anomalies, which are present in the majority of fetuses with this chromosomal anomaly. Cranial anomalies that have been identified are dolichocephaly, microcephaly, hydrocephalus, agenesis of the corpus callosum, cerebellar hypoplasia, a strawberry-shaped head, and choroid plexus cysts (Figure 49-19). Facial abnormalities include low-set ears, **micrognathia,** and cleft lip (Figure 49-20) and palate. Abnormal extremities identified with trisomy 18 include persistently clenched hands, talipes, rocker-bottom feet, and radial aplasia (Figure 49-21). Other anomalies associated with Edwards' syndrome include omphalocele, congenital diaphragmatic hernia (Figure 49-22), neural tube defects, cystic hygroma, and renal anomalies.

The fetus with trisomy 18 will often spontaneously abort. Infants are profoundly retarded. It is considered a lethal anomaly, with 90% of infants dying within the first year of life.[2]

Sonographic Findings. Sonographic features of trisomy 18 are evident in 80% of affected fetuses,[2] and, in addition to the features listed above, may also include polyhydramnios, IUGR, single umbilical artery, and nonimmune hydrops.

TRISOMY 13

Trisomy 13, also known as Patau's syndrome, occurs in 1:10,000 live births.[11] It is the result of an extra chromosome 13. This extremely severe anomaly consists of multiple anomalies, many of which involve the brain.

The physical features (Figure 49-23) characteristic of trisomy 13 include holoprosencephaly (Figure 49-24), which

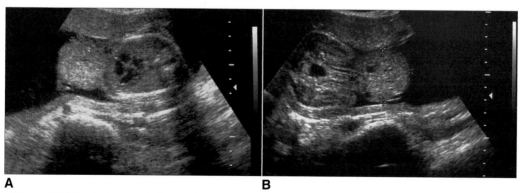

A   **B**

Figure 49-11   **A,** A 22-week fetus with tetralogy of Fallot (ventricular septal defect [VSD], overriding aorta, pulmonary stenosis, right ventricular hypertrophy). Only the VSD is appreciated in this four-chamber view. **B,** Omphalocele in same fetus. These findings together are highly suggestive of a chromosomal anomaly.

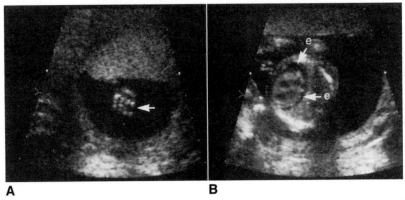

A   **B**

Figure 49-12 **A,** Absent fifth middle phalanx *(arrow)* in a chromosomally normal fetus. **B,** In the same fetus, pericardial effusion *(e)* is observed. Other anomalies were right atrial hypertrophy and outflow abnormalities.

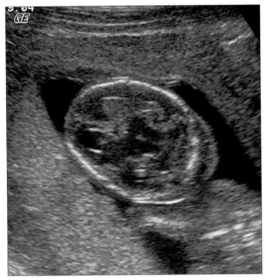

Figure 49-13 A thickened nuchal fold is seen in a fetus with trisomy 21. (From Henningsen C: *Clinical guide to ultrasonography,* St Louis, 2004, Mosby.)

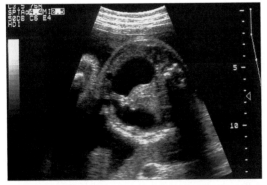

Figure 49-14 The double bubble sign is identified in this case of duodenal atresia. This is a significant finding associated with trisomy 21.

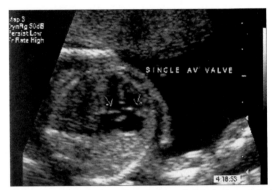

Figure 49-15 This endocardial cushion defect (atrioventricular canal) presented with an atrial septal defect, ventricular septal defect, and common valve. (Courtesy Ginny Goreczky, RDMS, Maternal Fetal Center at Florida Hospital, Orlando, Fla.)

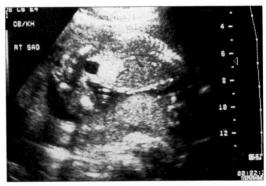

Figure 49-16 Echogenic bowel, bowel with the same echogenicity as fetal bone, is a subtle finding associated with trisomy 21.

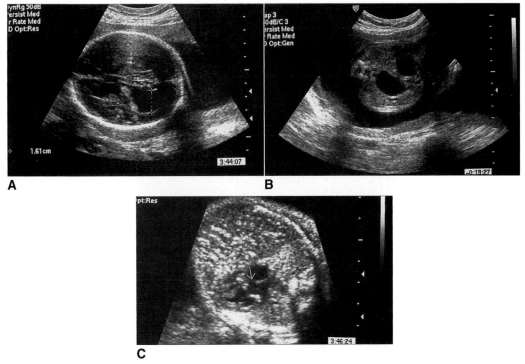

Figure 49-17   A female with fetus presented at 26 weeks of gestation with an uncertain last menstrual period. Ultrasound revealed ventriculomegaly **(A)** and duodenal atresia **(B). C,** Subsequent ultrasound examination also identified an atrial septal defect. There was fetal demise in utero at 35 weeks of gestation.

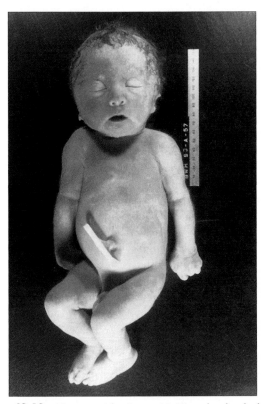

Figure 49-18   Neonate with trisomy 18. Note the clenched hands and rocker-bottom feet. Prenatal ultrasound revealed a supratentorial cyst confirmed after autopsy.

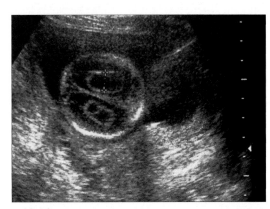

Figure 49-19   Bilateral choroid plexus cysts were identified in a pregnancy referred for triple screen suggestive of trisomy 18. Amniocentesis confirmed Edwards' syndrome.

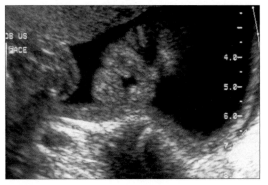

Figure 49-20   Cleft lip and palate are associated with aneuploidy. A median cleft, as in this example, and bilateral clefts carry a greater risk than a unilateral cleft. (From Henningsen C: *Clinical guide to ultrasonography,* St Louis, 2004, Mosby.)

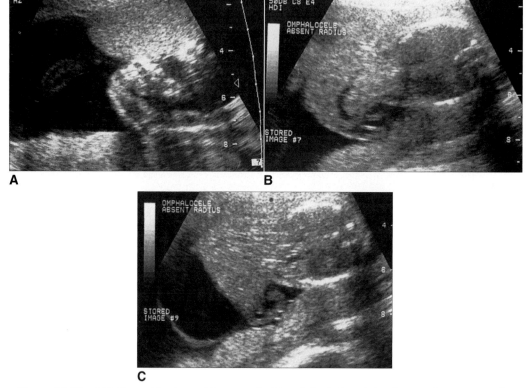

Figure 49-21 This fetus with trisomy 18 presented with radial aplasia and the ultrasound appearance of a clubbed hand (**A**) and an omphalocele (**B**). **C,** Note the ascites present in the defect.

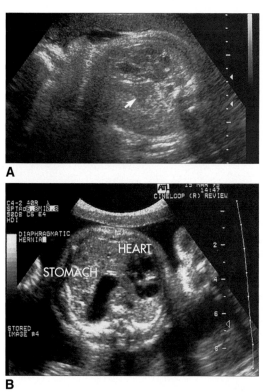

Figure 49-22 Congenital diaphragmatic hernia (CDH) is associated with aneuploidy. **A,** This is an unusual presentation of CDH in that the stomach was not identified in the thorax, even though it was a left-side defect. Note the malposition of the heart. There is the bowel adjacent to the heart. Karyotype revealed normal chromosomes. The baby died shortly after birth because of respiratory complications. **B,** A common ultrasound presentation of CDH with the stomach evident within the thorax. Note the displacement of the heart. (Courtesy of Ginny Goreczky, RDMS, Maternal Fetal Center at Florida Hospital, Orlando, Fla.)

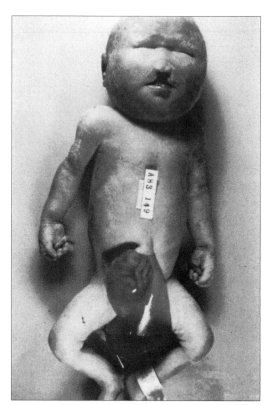

Figure 49-23 Neonate with trisomy 13. Note the hypotelorism, bilateral cleft lip and palate, bowel-filled omphalocele, and polydactyly of the hands. (From Nyberg DA, Mahony BS, Pretorius DH, editors: *Diagnostic ultrasound of fetal anomalies: text and atlas,* St Louis, 1990, Mosby.)

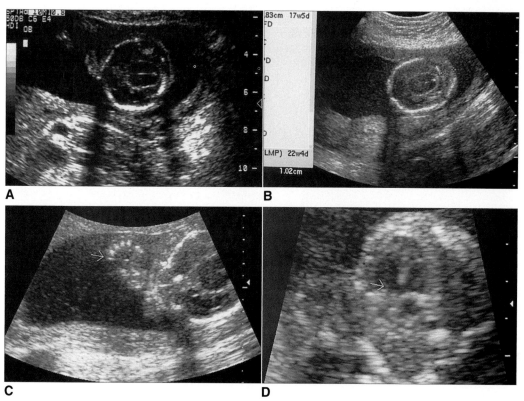

Figure 49-24   This pregnancy presented at 18 weeks and 4 days. Multiple anomalies were identified consistent with alobar holoprosencephaly. Amniocentesis confirmed trisomy 13. Ultrasound findings included a proboscis (**A**), fused thalamus and thickened nuchal fold (**B**), polydactyly (**C**), and a ventricular septal defect (**D**). A single umbilical artery and cyclopia were also evident.

is a common finding in fetuses with trisomy 13.[6] Other cranial anomalies include agenesis of the corpus callosum and microcephaly. Facial anomalies may be associated with the presence of holoprosencephaly and include **hypotelorism,** proboscis, cyclopia (Figure 49-25), and nose with a single nostril. Cleft lip and palate, microphthalmia, and micrognathia may also be present. Heart defects are present in 90% of fetuses and may include ventricular septal defect, atrial septal defect, and hypoplastic left heart.[6] Other anomalies associated with trisomy 13 include omphalocele, renal anomalies (Figure 49-26), and meningomyelocele. Associated limb anomalies (Figure 49-27) include **polydactyly,** talipes, rocker-bottom feet, and overlapping fingers. Cystic hygroma and echogenic chordae tendineae (Figure 49-28) may also be identified.

The prognosis for trisomy 13 is extremely poor, with 80% of infants dying within the first month. It is considered a lethal anomaly. Survivors are profoundly retarded, with multiple deficits and problems.[7]

Sonographic Findings. Sonographic features are evident in 90% of fetuses with trisomy 13.[3] In addition to the features listed above, trisomy 13 may also be associated with IUGR. Trisomy 13 and Meckel-Gruber syndrome (encephalocele, cystic kidneys, polydactyly) may have a similar sonographic appearance.

TRIPLOIDY

Triploidy is the result of a complete extra set of chromosomes. It often occurs as the result of an ova being fertilized by two sperm. It is estimated to occur in approximately 1% of conceptions, although most fetuses will spontaneously abort in the first trimester.[18] Only 1 in 5000 will continue to 16 to 20 weeks of gestation.[26]

Physical features of triploidy include heart defects, renal anomalies, omphalocele, and meningomyelocele. Cranial defects associated with triploidy include holoprosencephaly, agenesis of the corpus callosum, hydrocephalus, and Dandy-Walker malformation. Facial anomalies may be present and include low-set ears, **hypertelorism,** cleft lip and palate, and micrognathia. Cryptorchidism, ambiguous genitalia, syndactyly, and talipes may also be observed.

Triploidy is considered a lethal condition, with those surviving the gestational period dying shortly after birth. A mosaic form of triploidy may be compatible with survival, although these infants are affected with mental retardation.

Sonographic Findings. Sonographic features of triploidy include the above findings in addition to severe IUGR and placental changes (hydatidiform degeneration). Oligohydramnios is often present and may hamper adequate visualization of the fetus.

TURNER'S SYNDROME

Turner's syndrome (45 X) is a genetic abnormality marked by the absence of the X or Y chromosome. It is not associated with advanced maternal age. It occurs in 1 of every 2000 to 5000 live births.[24] Patients may present with an elevated MSAFP when a cystic hygroma is present.

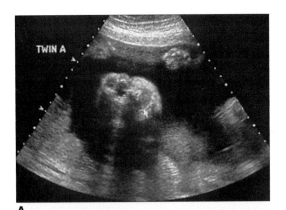

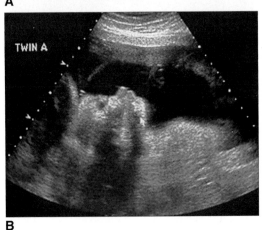

Figure 49-25 The facial anomalies associated with trisomy 13 include cyclopia **(A)**. The nose was also absent **(B).** (From Henningsen C: *Clinical guide to ultrasonography*, St Louis, 2004, Mosby.)

Cystic hygroma (Figure 49-29) is one of the most pathognomonic findings for this disorder. Other physical features include cardiac anomalies, of which coarctation of the aorta is the most common.[30] General lymphedema and hydrops may also be present. Renal anomalies, such as horseshoe kidney, renal agenesis, hydronephrosis, and hypoplastic kidney, may coexist. Short femurs are also associated with Turner's syndrome.[33]

Most fetuses with Turner's syndrome will spontaneously abort. The prognosis is especially grave when the fetus presents with a large cystic hygroma and edema or hydrops (Figure 49-30). If the hygroma is isolated, it may regress in utero. The prognosis after birth depends on the severity of associated anomalies. Female infants who survive will have immature sexual development, amenorrhea, short stature, a webbed neck, cubitus valgus (abnormal elbow angle), and a shield chest with widely spaced nipples. They may also have poor hearing, and hormone replacement is necessary for sexual development. Turner's syndrome children usually have normal intelligence.

Sonographic Findings. The previously listed ultrasound findings for Turner's syndrome may also include oligohydramnios, especially when severe renal anomalies are present.

ACKNOWLEDGMENT

I would like to acknowledge the sonographers Ginny, Maria, Lucy, and Jamie in the Maternal Fetal Center, Orlando, Fla., for continually sharing their interesting cases with me, so that I am able to share a piece of their knowledge. I would also like to thank the perinatologists, Drs. Fuentes and Busowski, for allowing me to continue to expand my skills and knowledge under their mentoring. I would also like to thank the sonographers in the Florida Hospital radiology ultrasound department who also contributed to my teaching file. Finally, I would like to recognize Beck Hutchinson, librarian, and the Florida Hospital College of Health Sciences library staff for their expertise in searching for and acquiring the research materials necessary for this project.

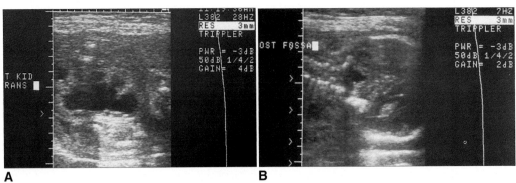

Figure 49-26 A fetus with trisomy 13 presents with hydronephrosis **(A)** and Dandy-Walker malformation **(B).**

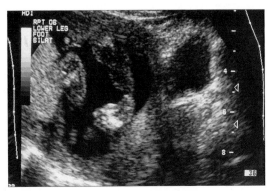

Figure 49-27 Limb anomalies associated with aneuploidy include talipes (clubfoot).

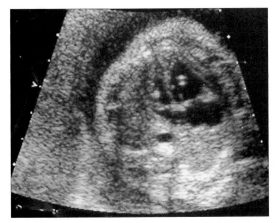

Figure 49-28 An isolated echogenic foci may be insignificant. When in the right ventricle or bilateral as seen in this image, aneuploidy should be considered. Chromosomal analysis revealed trisomy 13. (From Henningsen C: *Clinical guide to ultrasonography*, St Louis, 2004, Mosby.)

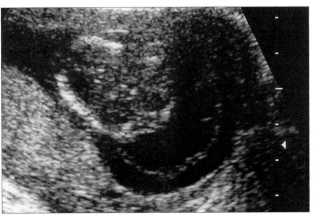

Figure 49-29 A cystic hygroma was identified in a fetus with Turner's syndrome.

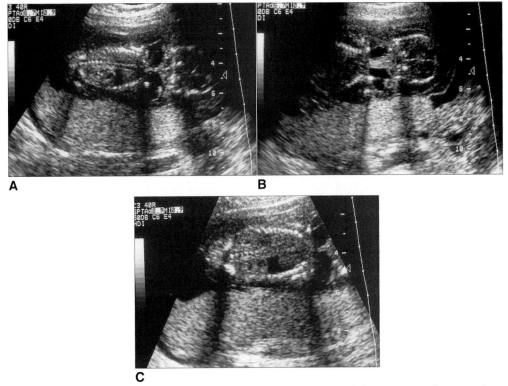

A **B**

C

Figure 49-30 Turner's syndrome. **A,** Cystic hygroma is noted in the nuchal region. **B,** Hydrops was also evident. Note the significant edema around the fetal head and the pleural effusions **(C).** Turner's syndrome with hydrops carries a grave prognosis.

REFERENCES

1. Al-Kouatly HB, Chasen ST, Streltzoff J and others: The clinical significance of fetal echogenic bowel, *Am J Obstet Gynecol* 185:1035-1038, 2001.

2. Benacerraf BR, Harlow BL, Frigoletto FD: Hypoplasia of the middle phalanx of the fifth digit: a feature of the second trimester fetus with Down syndrome, *J Ultrasound Med* 9:389, 1990.

3. Benacerraf BR: *Ultrasound of fetal syndromes,* Philadelphia, 1998, Churchill Livingstone.

4. Bilardo C: Second trimester ultrasound markers for fetal aneuploidy, *Early Hum Dev* 47(suppl):S31, 1996.

5. Brumfield CG, Wenstrom KD, Owen J and others: Ultrasound findings and multiple marker screening in trisomy 18, *Obstet Gynecol* 95:51-54, 2000.

6. Callen PW: *Ultrasonography in obstetrics and gynecology,* ed 4, Philadelphia, 2000, WB Saunders.

7. Carter PE, Pearn JH, Bell J and others: Survival in trisomy 13: life tables for use in genetic counseling and clinical pediatrics, *Clin Genetics* 27:59, 1985.

8. Cicero S, Curcio P, Papageorghiou A: Absence of nasal bone in fetuses with trisomy 21 at 11-14 weeks of gestation: an observational study, *The Lancet* 358:1665-1667, 2001.

9. Devieve F, Bouckaert A, Hubinont C and others: Multiple screening for fetal Down's syndrome with the classic triple test, dimeric inhibin A and ultrasound, *Gynecol Obstet Invest* 49:221-226, 2000.

10. Durbin SA: The use of ultrasound to identify fetuses with Down syndrome: case study and review, *JDMS* 15:107-111, 1999.

11. Eubanks SR, Kuller JA, Amjadi D and others: Prenatal diagnosis of mosaic trisomy 13: a case report, *Prenat Diagn* 18:971-974, 1998.

12. Golbus MS and others: Prenatal genetic diagnosis in 3000 amniocenteses, *N Engl J Med* 300:157, 1979.

13. Goldstein RB, Caponigro M: The role of sonography in the evaluation of pregnant women with high maternal serum alpha-fetoprotein, *Applied Radiology* 30:9-18, 2001.

14. Haddow JE and others: Prenatal screening for Down's syndrome with use of maternal serum markers, *N Engl J Med* 327:588, 1992.

15. Himes P: Early pregnancy prenatal diagnostic testing: risks associated with chorionic villus sampling and early amniocentesis and screening options, *J Perinat Neonat Nurs* 13:1-13, 1999.

16. Huggon IC, Cook AC, Simpson JM and others: Isolated echogenic foci in the fetal heart as a marker of chromosomal abnormality, *Ultrasound Obstet Gynecol* 17:11-16, 2001.

17. Itoh H and others: Nuchal-fold thickening in Down syndrome fetuses: transient appearance and spontaneous resolution in the second trimester, *J Perinat Med* 21:139, 1993.

18. Jauniaux E and others: Prenatal diagnosis of triploidy during the second trimester of pregnancy, *Obstet Gynecol* 88:983, 1996.

19. Jeanty P and others: How to improve your amniocentesis technique, *Am J Obstet Gynecol* 146:593, 1983.

20. Jeanty P: Prenatal detection of simian crease, *J Ultrasound Med* 9:131, 1990.

21. Michailidis GD, Spencer K, Economides DL: The use of nuchal translucency measurement and second trimester biochemical markers in screening for Down's syndrome, *Br J Obstet Gynaecol* 108:1047-1052, 2001.

22. Nyberg DA, Mahony BS, Pretorius DH, editors: *Diagnostic ultrasound of fetal anomalies: text and atlas,* St Louis, 1990, Mosby.

23. Pandya PP and others: Chromosomal defects and outcome in 1015 fetuses with increased nuchal translucency, *Ultrasound Obstet Gynecol* 5:15, 1995.

24. Parker KL, Wyatt DT, Blethen SL and others: Screening girls with Turner syndrome: the national cooperative growth study experience, *J Pediatrics* 143:133-135, 2003.

25. Reece EA and others: Embryoscopy: a closer look at first-trimester diagnosis and treatment, *Am J Obstet Gynecol* 166:775, 1992.

26. Rijhsinghani A and others: Risk of preeclampsia in second trimester triploid pregnancies, *Obstet Gynecol* 90:884, 1997.

27. Sanders RC and others: *Structural fetal abnormalities: the total picture,* St Louis, 1996, Mosby.

28. Scrimgeour JB: Amniocentesis: technique and complications. In Emery AEH, editor: *Antenatal diagnosis of genetic disease,* Baltimore, 1973, Williams & Wilkins.

29. Souter VL, Nyberg DA: Sonographic screening for fetal aneuploidy, *J Ultrasound Med* 20:775-790, 2001.

30. Surerus E, Huggon IC, Allan LD: Turner's syndrome in fetal life, *Ultrasound Obstet Gynecol* 22:264-267, 2003.

31. Toriello HV: General principles of human genetics, *Clin Commun Disord* 2:1, 1992.

32. United Kingdom collaborative study on alpha-fetoprotein in relation to neural tube defects: maternal serum alpha-fetoprotein measurement in antenatal screen for anencephaly and spina bifida in early pregnancy, *Lancet* 1:1323, 1977.

33. Williamson R and others: Direct gene analysis of chorionic villi: a possible technique for first trimester antenatal diagnosis of haemoglobinopathies, *Lancet* 2:1125, 1981.

34. Zimmermann R and others: Serum parameters and nuchal translucency in first trimester screening for fetal chromosomal abnormalities, *Br J Obstet Gynaecol* 103:1009, 1996.

CHAPTER 50

Sonographic 3-D and 4-D Evaluation of Fetal Anomalies

Darleen Cioffi-Ragan

OBJECTIVES

- List the applications of 3-D and 4-D ultrasound
- Describe three advantages of using 3-D ultrasound over 2-D ultrasound
- Discuss clinical opportunities that are useful to image with 3-D ultrasound

---

SCANNING PROCEDURES AND INSTRUMENTATION
TRANSDUCERS

3-D IMAGING METHODS
PLANAR RECONSTRUCTION
VOLUME RENDERING

MODES OF OPERATION
SURFACE MODE
TRANSPARENT MODE

OTHER APPLICATIONS

KEYS TO SUCCESSFUL 3-D IMAGING

KEY TERMS

four-dimensional (4-D) ultrasound – ability to reconstruct the 3-D image and see it in real time

free hand – system that uses a smooth sweeping motion in a single plane of acquisition

multiplanar imaging – ability to collect data from axial, coronal, and sagittal planes for reconstruction into 3-D format

planar reconstruction – movement of the intersection point (point of rotation) of the three orthogonal image planes

throughout the 3-D volume and rotating the image planes; the sonographer or physician has the liberty to generate anatomic views from an infinite number of perspectives.

region of interest (ROI) – region of interest

surface mode – in the surface-light mode there are brighter image intensity values to structures that are closer to the viewer and darker image intensity values to structures that are further from the viewer

three-dimensional (3-D) ultrasound – permits collection and review of data obtained from a volume of tissue in multiple imaging planes and rendering of surface features

transparent mode – sometimes called x-ray mode, is best for viewing a relatively low-contrast block of soft tissue

volume rendering – the volume is evaluated by rotating the volume data to a standard orientation and then scrolling through parallel planes. The data may be rotated to assess oblique planes.

Two-dimensional (2-D) ultrasound has proved itself to be a unique imaging modality, being a noninvasive, nonradiating, and relatively inexpensive technology with excellent capabilities for soft tissue imaging. It is well recognized that advances in diagnostic ultrasound have given physicians, sonologists, and sonographers the necessary tools to diagnose fetal anomalies early in pregnancy and in the early stages of complex diseases. The improved resolution of the two-dimensional (2-D) ultrasound, Doppler, power Doppler, color Doppler, and harmonics has revolutionized fetal diagnosis.

Three-dimensional (3-D) ultrasound now brings the added benefits of volume acquisition and display, widely known from computed tomography (CT), magnetic resonance imaging (MRI), and positron emission tomography (PET). **Three-dimensional (3-D) ultrasound** permits collection and review of data obtained from a volume of tissue in **multiplanar imaging** and rendering of surface features. Three-dimensional ultrasound has created a new understanding of anatomy and pathology and is currently finding many clinical applications for abdominal, breast, cardiac, fetal, gynecologic, vascular, and other clinical modalities. Newer advances in technology have also made it possible for information to be acquired quickly during real-time imaging of anatomic structures. This acquisition in real time is called **four-dimensional (4-D) ultrasound.** One ultrasound equipment manufacturer recently developed a new software fetal cardiac program called STIC. This software allows the sonographer or sonologist to acquire a volume of the fetal heart in real time looking at the four-chamber heart and outflow tracts.

This chapter will focus on the current technology and examples of 3-D and 4-D imaging found in the clinical setting to help the sonologist or sonographer achieve quality diagnostic 3-D volume data sets that can be used to evaluate multiple anomalies seen during a diagnostic scan.

SCANNING PROCEDURES AND INSTRUMENTATION

The basic features of 3-D ultrasound provide representation of the structure, texture, and form of a specific area of interest. Box 50-1 lists the steps necessary to obtain the 3-D image. First, echo data must process along an ultrasound beam. Second, the ultrasound beam must move over the area of interest. Third, translation and rotation of the axis from the ultrasound beam and the time of the reflected sound waves create the 3-D data set, which is converted into distance information by the assumption of the speed of sound within the volume of interest. The next step is the storage of the data and the gap-filling procedure. Finally the visualization of the data is obtained.

All of the 2-D ultrasound modalities can be used in 3-D ultrasound reconstruction as long as the software is available to create the volumetric image. The 3-D system requires images of high quality with good signal-to-noise characteristics and images with minimal refraction, absorption, and shadowing artifacts. The image quality from the rendered 3-D data set will be only as good as the 2-D image of the ultrasound machine.

TRANSDUCERS

The scanning movement of the transducer can be either manual or automatic. There are systems that incorporate one or both techniques. Three-dimensional transducers that are fully automated will contain the mechanism necessary to acquire the data set. The automated transducer movement is more accurate than hand-controlled transducers because the mechanics and/or electronics of the transducer control the beam. Therefore the 3-D data set is superior and correlates exactly to the position; this is standard in 2-D ultrasound. The 3-D system does not skip over any area of information in the region of interest. Steered phased array and/or curved/linear array transducers can be used with the 3-D mechanism. There are different types of transducers to optimize different clinical applications. The transducer used most often has an electronic array in a single direction that is mechanically swept in the orthogonal direction.

The system that uses both automatic and manual techniques has a hand-held B-mode transducer with the ability to "sweep" in a single plane of acquisition. This method is called **free-hand.** Free-hand will not provide volume data that is suitable for distance and volume measurements. Free-hand scanning needs a smooth sweeping motion in the acquisition plane. There is an electromagnetic position sensor placed on the ultrasound transducer. Sensors like these are used for flight simulation, virtual reality applications, scientific visualization, biomechanics research, and computer animation.

The manually controlled system involves a single transducer that is moved by hand for position detection to produce a single line of ultrasound information. This method has little or no value.

3-D IMAGING METHODS

There are two different methods of 3-D imaging: the planar reconstruction method and the volume-rendering method. These two methods depend on a series of separately acquired images where the spatial relationships of the images are exactly known. Computer software is used to render new views from the 3-D data set. A wide acoustic window with uniform sound transmission features is helpful. Acquisition can take as long as several seconds with some systems. Any movement by the patient (mother or fetus) or by the examiner will produce misregistration artifacts, and the volume will need to be repeated.

PLANAR RECONSTRUCTION

The first method of 3-D imaging is **planar reconstruction.** The best way to explain planar reconstruction is with a broad overview of conventional 2-D endovaginal scanning in the first trimester. In the first trimester, an endovaginal transducer is restricted because of the limited range of motion that a sonographer can use to acquire the necessary images for diagnosis and the decreased acoustic window. This is especially true with first-trimester scanning for the nuchal translucency. It is also true with fetal nasal bone scanning techniques in the evaluation of aneuploidy in conjunction with the maternal serum in the first and early second trimesters. Although it is true that there are fewer acoustic window limitations with 2-D transabdominal scanning, maternal habitus and a tipped uterus can affect the image quality and diagnosis.

With planar reconstruction, the area of interest is no longer confined to the original acoustic window after a 3-D data set is obtained and investigated with the specialized computer software that generates an orthogonal image. By moving the intersection point (point of rotation) of the three orthogonal

---

BOX 50-1   STEPS TO PRODUCE A 3-D IMAGE

- Echo data must process along an ultrasound beam
- Ultrasound beam must move over the area of interest
- Translation and rotation of the axis from the ultrasound beam and time of reflected sound waves create 3-D data set; information converted into distance
- Storage of the data and gap-filling procedure
- Visualization of data

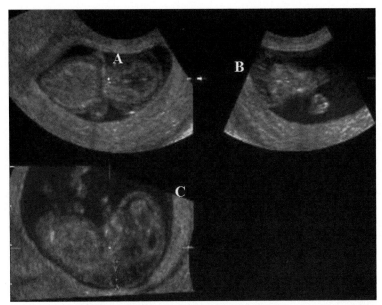

Figure 50-1   Planar reconstruction method of a 3-D image of an abnormal nuchal translucency in a 12-week fetus with a cystic hygroma. **A,** Coronal image of the fetus. **B,** Axial image of the fetus. **C,** Rendered midsagittal image of the fetus. The white dot is the center of rotation.

image planes throughout the 3-D volume and rotating the image planes, the sonographer or physician can generate anatomic views from an infinite number of perspectives. This allows the sonographer or physician to investigate anatomic relationships in ways that are not available with conventional 2-D imaging.

The sonographer or physician can maintain orientation within the 3-D volume set. The relationships of the orthogonal planes are illustrated in Figure 50-1, which shows a volume data set acquired in the coronal plane through the neck and head of a 12-week fetus with cystic hygroma. Figure 50-1, *A* is one of the original coronal cuts through the neck and head. The white dot on this image represents the center of rotation for the orthogonal set of images and represents the common point of intersection of these planes. The computer will automatically reconstruct the axial plane of the fetal neck (Figure 50-1, *B*). The third reconstructed image (Figure 50-1, *C*) is the nuchal translucency presented in the sagittal plane. Therefore the nuchal translucency can be imaged and measured in the sagittal plane when the fetus is in an axial or coronal plane after the planar reconstruction from the 3-D acquisition (Figure 50-2).

Three-dimensional technique can be masterful in obtaining a difficult nuchal translucency thickness in the first trimester. The measurement is made in the true midsagittal plane with the fetus in a neutral position. The fetus must be away from the uterine wall and the amnion to obtain a diagnostic measurement. Often the fetus is not in the correct position to obtain the nuchal translucency. By placing the image plane of the transducer at right angles to the long axis of the fetus, serial coronal images (see Figure 50-1, *A*) from crown to rump are stored as the 3-D volume. The nuchal translucency view will be demonstrated in the sagittal plane (see Figure 50-1, *C*). The

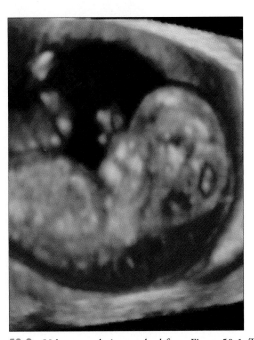

Figure 50-2   Volume rendering method from Figure 50-1. The septations can be seen within the cystic hygroma. This fetus had a normal amnio, normal fetal echo, and normal course after delivery.

third reconstructed view is the axial view (see Figure 50-1, *B*), showing the jaw and neck of the fetus in a cross section. The cystic hygroma is seen in Figure 50-2, which is the 3-D volume rendered image with internal echoes and possible septations. The neck can be measured at this level if necessary.

Figure 50-3 is another first-trimester fetus with a cystic hygroma. This patient elected to have a chorionic villus sampling (CVS) at the time of the scan. The diagnosis was Turner's

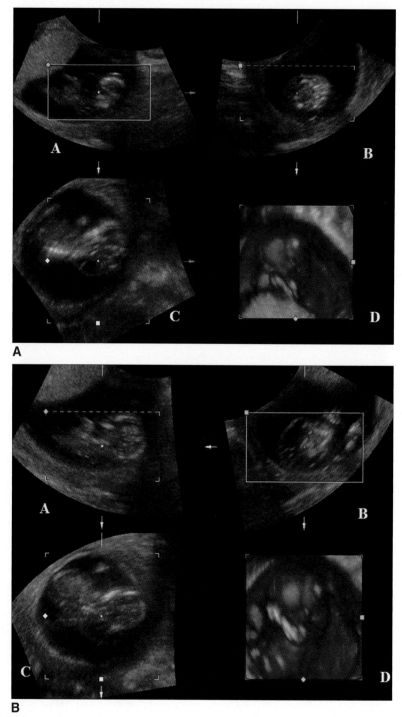

Figure 50-3 **A** and **B** show a fetus with a cystic hygroma. This fetus had a chorionic villus sampling and was diagnosed with Turner's syndrome.

syndrome. A fetus with Turner's syndrome has only 45 chromosomes, and the second X chromosome is absent. Turner's syndrome is associated with short stature, ovarian dysgenesis with sexual infantilism and infertility, and a pattern of structural abnormalities, including a webbed neck, peripheral lymphedema at birth, congenital heart defects (particularly left-sided obstructive lesions, such as bicuspid aortic valve and coarctation of the aorta), and structural renal abnormalities. In

the first trimester of pregnancy, Turner's syndrome is one of the most common causes of a thick nuchal translucency or lymphedema, hydrops, and cystic hygroma.

Figure 50-4 shows a nuchal translucency of a normal fetus in the coronal plane. Figure 50-4, *A* represents the fetal face to the left of the screen in the coronal plane. Figure 50-4, *B* is an axial image with the fetal spine to the left. Figure 50-4, *C* is a midsagittal image with the fetus in a prone presentation.

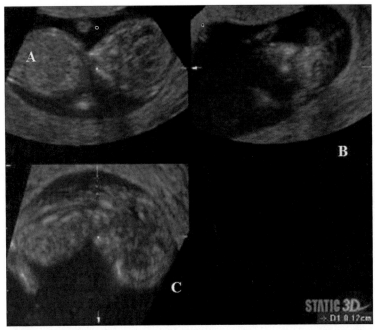

Figure 50-4   Planar reconstruction method of a 3-D image of a normal nuchal translucency of a 12-week fetus. **A,** Coronal image of the fetus. **B,** Axial image of the fetus. **C,** Rendered midsagittal image of the fetus. The white dot is the center of rotation. Measurements can be made from the midsagittal image **(C).**

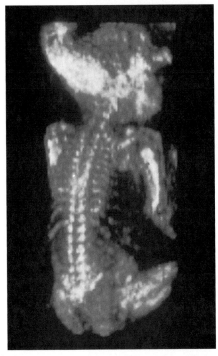

Figure 50-5   Three-dimensional reconstruction of a normal fetal spine using surface mode and x-ray mode to bring out the bony detail.

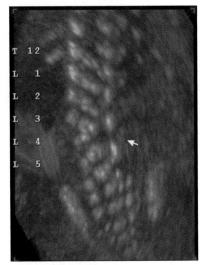

Figure 50-6   Volume rendering of coronal view of the lumbar spine in a fetus with a hemivertebra. The 4th vertebral body *(arrow)* is affected on this second-trimester fetus. The fetus also had a multicystic dysplastic kidney.

The nuchal translucency measurement can still be made on this image.

Planar reconstruction is an excellent diagnostic tool in the evaluation of neural tube defects in the second and third trimesters. The level of the neural tube defect can be determined by the volume data set. The orthogonal image planes can be oriented to demonstrate a coronal view where the 12th rib is visualized, and the vertebral bodies are identified (Figures 50-5 and 50-6). This allows confident identification of the 12th thoracic vertebra and the first lumbar vertebra. By counting the vertebral bodies from this level, they can be labeled in the sagittal plane or in the coronal plane, as seen in Figure 50-6. Three-dimensional ultrasound can greatly increase the capacity to localize the level of pathology. By contrast, 2-D ultrasound can identify the area only as cervical, thoracic, lumbar, or sacral spine.

VOLUME RENDERING

The other 3-D imaging method is the **volume rendering** method (Figure 50-7). This method is an extension of the planar reconstruction method because additional image processing techniques are applied to a **region of interest (ROI)** within the 3-D volume data set. The goal is to produce 3-D images of structures that reach over a limited depth of field and are contained within the ROI box. These structures do not reside within a flat 2-D plane and cannot be viewed with the simple planar reconstruction method. The planar reconstruction method is required to find the beginning orientation for the 3-D volume rendering method and then to refine that process.

The volume rendering method places greater constraints on the physical conditions from which 3-D images can be generated successfully. Figure 50-8 demonstrates a volume render-

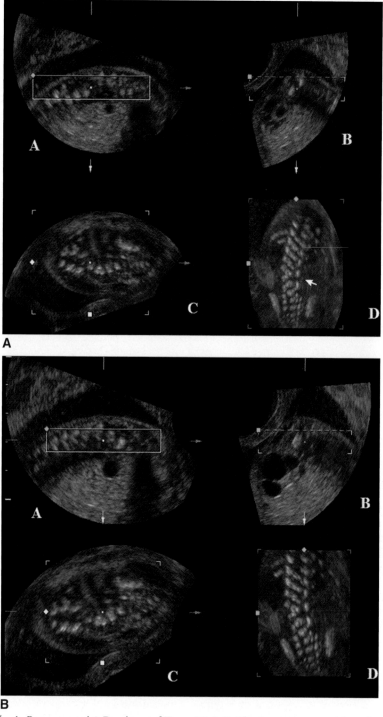

Figure 50-7 **A,** Reconstructed 3-D volume of Figure 50-6. **B,** The image was moved into the white dot (center of rotation) to demonstrate the large multicystic dysplastic kidney.

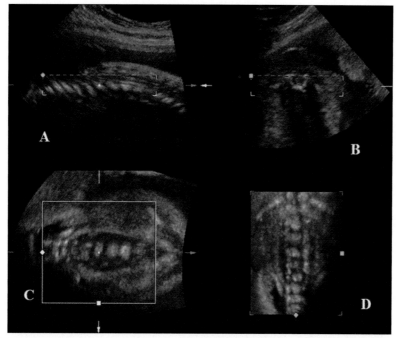

Figure 50-8   Volume rendering method in a fetus with spinal dysraphism and intact myelomeningocele. **A,** Sagittal image of the lumbar and sacral spine. **B,** Axial image of the lumbar spine. A large cystic collection containing the cerebral spinal fluid is seen above the spinal defect in images **A** and **B. C,** Coronal image of the lumbar and sacral spine. Notice the widening of the lumbar and sacral spine. There is an open neural tube defect of the fourth lumbar vertebrae. **D,** The volume rendered image.

ing method of a 3-D image of the normal first-trimester fetus with a normal nuchal translucency measurement. The 3-D volume shows the fetus in a midsagittal plane in an upright position. The umbilical cord is well demonstrated in Figure 50-9.

MODES OF OPERATION

The two modes of operation in 3-D imaging are called *surface* and *transparent*. Some manufacturers may have different terminology for these processing modes. These modes require the presence of high-contrast boundaries, such as a bone–soft tissue interface or a fluid–soft tissue interface. The image shown in Figure 50-10 is from an older Voluson 530D. It demonstrates a good fluid-soft tissue interface for the 3-D volume. The reconstruction used the surface mode to demonstrate the 3-D image of the fetal face.

SURFACE MODE

The **surface mode** needs a clear fluid interface that is stretched from the ROI box render start line to the surface as shown in Figure 50-11. A thick layer of amniotic fluid needs to outline the fetal face. A clear demonstration of the facial profile can help to define abnormalities, such as a cleft lip and palate, as seen in Figure 50-12. A fetus with polyhydramnios due to cleft lip and palate cannot swallow efficiently but can provide a layer of amniotic fluid to evaluate the facial abnormality (Figure 50-13). Structures, such as the umbilical cord, extremities, or image artifacts, can lie within the fluid path. Figure 50-14 is a

3-D volume rendering of a fetus with a known cleft lip. The fetus was scanned to evaluate for cleft palate. Figure 50-14, *A* demonstrates the fetal profile with an excellent amount of amniotic fluid outlining the fetus. Figure 50-14, *B* demonstrates a coronal of the fetal nose and cleft lip and a cross section of a fetal extremity. The 3-D reconstruction demonstrates the fetal face with the cleft lip partially obscured by the fetal arm. Multiple 3-D images were acquired before the diagnosis of cleft lip, and the palate was confirmed (Figure 50-15). Fetal extremities, the umbilical cord, or image artifacts can make the conditions under which a surface rendering of a fetal structure will be accomplished less than optimal.

Normal or increased amniotic fluid means a more successful 3-D image. Using a threshold to eliminate low-level echoes in a 3-D volume data set sometimes will improve the appearance of the 3-D rendering. There is a cutting tool to remove the unwanted adjacent structures, but this step can be time consuming and tedious. Figure 50-16 is a 3-D volume rendering of the fetal face with an excellent image of a cleft lip and extension into the palate using surface mode with a combination of surface-texture and surface-light processing techniques.

Gray values are assigned to the surface-texture mode in the 3-D surface rendering that are the same as the gray values of the original scan. In the surface-light mode, there are brighter image intensity values to structures that are closer to the viewer and darker image intensity values to structures that are further from the viewer. The best surface rendering is created when a combination of the surface-texture and surface-light features is

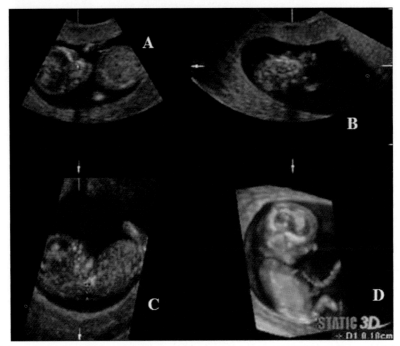

Figure 50-9   A volume rendered method of a 3-D image of a normal nuchal translucency of the fetus. **A,** Coronal image of the fetus. **B,** Axial image of the fetus. **C,** Rendered midsagittal image of the fetus. **D,** 3-D surface rendering of the midsagittal plane of the fetus. The umbilical cord is clearly seen.

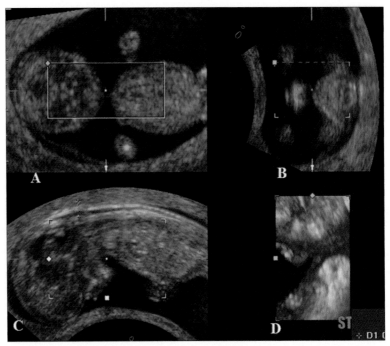

Figure 50-10   Volume rendering method of Figure 50-9. **A,** Coronal image of the fetus. **B,** Axial image of the fetus. **C,** Prone midsagittal image of the fetus with a measurement of the nuchal translucency. **D,** 3-D surface rendering of the partial fetal profile.

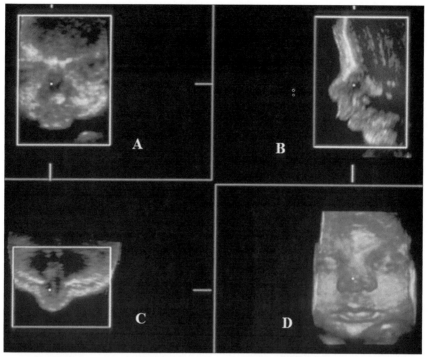

Figure 50-11 Volume rendering method of a normal fetal face in the third trimester.

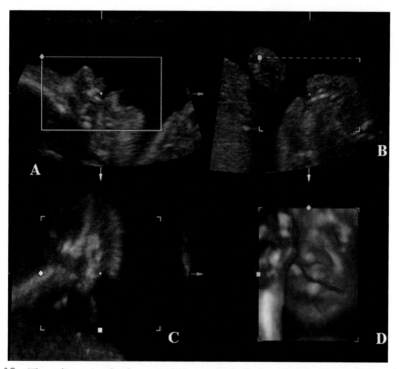

Figure 50-12 Three-dimensional volume rendering method of a late second-trimester fetus with a known cleft lip. **A,** Profile image of the fetal face. **B,** Coronal image of the fetal nose and lips; cross section of a fetal extremity. **C,** Axial image of the fetal face. **D,** 3-D volume shows the cleft lip with the fetal arm partially obscuring the face.

employed, as seen in Figure 50-17. Here a normal first-trimester fetus clearly appears to be sucking its thumb.

Selecting the correct surface rendering technique that will demonstrate a realistic image of the fetus's physical features can be an art and a science. Mastering this technique could take many hours in the early days of 3-D ultrasound. Today, however, with all the advances in ultrasound and 3-D, the time involved with 3-D reconstruction has been drastically reduced. This makes the procedure clinically relevant in a busy ultrasound department.

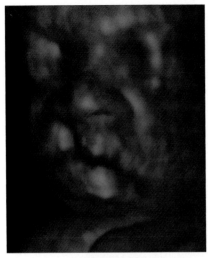

Figure 50-13 Three-dimensional volume rendering of the fetal face as seen in Figure 50-12. The fetus has finally moved its arm after several acquisitions, now showing only a cleft lip and not a cleft palate. The surface mode combination of surface-light and surface-texture was used to obtain the final 3-D image.

TRANSPARENT MODE

The **transparent mode** can look through a block of tissue, as illustrated by the ROI volume. There are different features rendered, depending on the processing criteria chosen. The transparent mode, sometimes called x-ray mode, is best for viewing a relatively low-contrast block of soft tissue. The transparent mode will exhibit a mean value of all the gray values encountered along an outlined ray within the ROI box volume. This mode is limited in obstetric imaging, and it is not very useful. The transparent mode also could be used in Figure 50-18 to look closer at the internal skeletal features of the clenched fetal fingers.

OTHER APPLICATIONS

Three-dimensional ultrasound is an excellent diagnostic tool for evaluation of fetal anomalies throughout pregnancy. With 3-D imaging, it is easier to demonstrate the fetal anomalies of the extremities to the parents by showing the relationship of the fetal hands and feet relative to the long bones (Figure 50-19). Three-dimensional ultrasound can also be used to present the fetal deformity to the parents in a more comprehensive way. However, sonographers should not point out or discuss fetal anomalies with the parents before the physician has consulted with the patient.

Figure 50-20 is a 3-D volume rendering method of a twin gestation in the third trimester. Investigation is currently being conducted to evaluate placental blood flow in twin gestations to further help in the diagnosis of intrauterine growth restriction (IUGR). Investigations have found that there is less blood flow in the twin versus the singleton gestation.

Three-dimensional ultrasound has changed the way that hysterosonography (HSG) is being diagnosed by the gynecol-

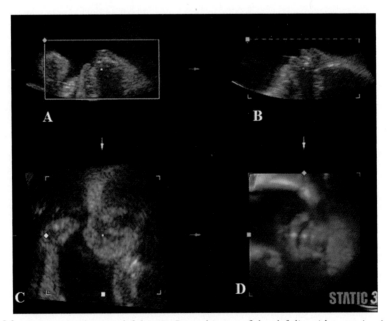

Figure 50-14 Fetus with a known cleft lip. **A,** Coronal image of the cleft lip with extension into the palate. **B,** Sagittal image of the fetal lips. **C,** Axial image of the fetal face. **D,** Volume rendered image needs to be rotated to demonstrate the cleft palate.

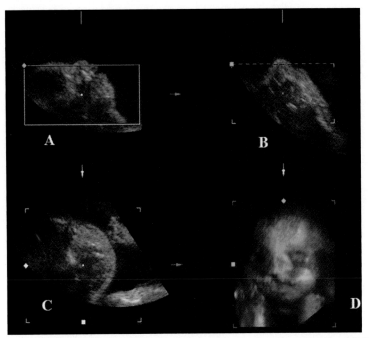

Figure 50-15   The same fetus as shown in Figure 50-14 was imaged to determine if a cleft lip and palate were present. After multiple acquisitions and slight movement of the fetus, the diagnosis of cleft palate and lip was made.

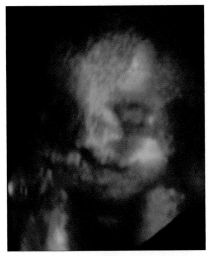

Figure 50-16   This fetus is younger in gestational age than the fetus in Figure 50-12, so the fetal face has less body fat and decreased resolution is present.

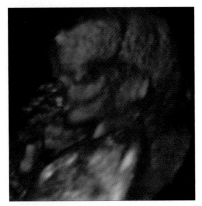

Figure 50-17   Three-dimensional image of a 13-week fetus. The image is a surface mode using a combination of surface-light and surface-texture. The fetus appears to be sucking its thumb. This 3-D volume-rendered reconstruction has excellent resolution demonstrating the fetal fingers and profile with sutures of the fetal skull well seen.

ogist. The 3-D sweep can be made quickly instead of rotating the transducer during the infusion of saline. Figure 50-21 shows a hysterosonography study of a patient with an irregular menstrual cycle. The physician made the diagnosis of a polyp, and surgery confirmed that diagnosis.

As investigators continue to learn more about the value of 3-D and 4-D ultrasound in the clinical setting, the routine use of 3-D and 4-D ultrasound to evaluate the fetus for anomalies, such as cleft palate, fetal spine, fetal extremities, fetal congenital heart defects, and multiple gynecological abnormalities is becoming more common. Already surgeons are requesting

3-D and 4-D ultrasound to aid in the localization of a mass before surgery.

KEYS TO SUCCESSFUL 3-D IMAGING

Acquiring a beautiful fetal face in the third trimester is determined by fetal position (location), amniotic fluid, the position of the placenta, and a high quality 2-D image of the fetal profile. The following technique has proven to be very effective:

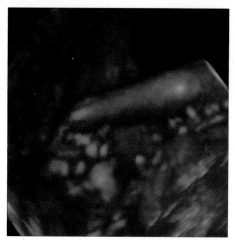

Figure 50-18 Second-trimester fetus with arthrogryposis (fixation of a joint in a flexed or contracted position). This is the volume-rendered method demonstrating the clenched hand.

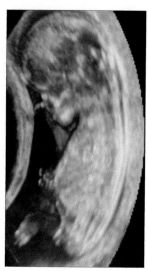

Figure 50-19 This is a 3-D profile view of the second-trimester fetus. The detail is not seen as well because at this stage the fetus does not have the fat/muscle tissue development as is seen in the late third-trimester fetus.

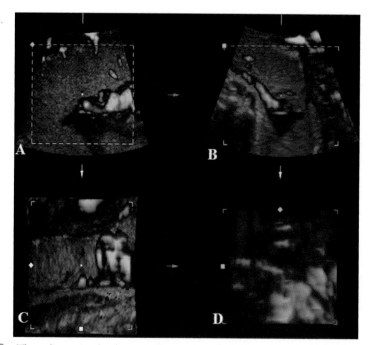

Figure 50-20 Three-dimensional volume-rendering method demonstrating power Doppler of a placenta in a twin gestation in the third trimester, evaluating blood flow to the placenta to determine if intrauterine growth restriction is present.

1. Once the fetus is in a midsagittal plane (profile) for a 3-D acquisition, place the region of interest (ROI) box on the fetal profile with the render start line (dotted green line) above the profile with a layer of amniotic fluid and decrease the size of the ROI box close to the fetal structures.

2. Next make a 3-D sweep and use the X, Y, and Z controls to rotate the image. The Voluson 730MT has mix and TH low knobs above the keyboard, which can adjust the image for better resolution. (The 3-D and 4-D ultrasound machines have come a long way in a short period of time. The acquisition and reconstruction time has been greatly reduced, and the resolution of the image has been improved.)

3. An early learning experience for the sonographer beginning 3-D and 4-D ultrasound is to try a sweep at 90 degrees to the area of interest and use the different controls to optimize the volume rendered image.

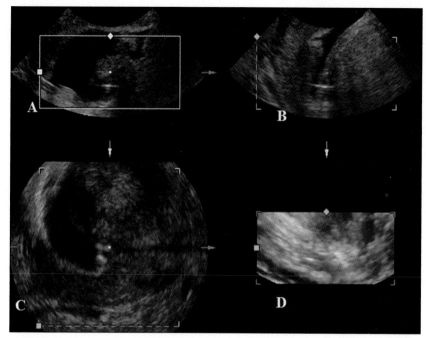

Figure 50-21   Hysterosonography and 3-D ultrasound helped to make the diagnosis of a large, irregular-shaped mass (polyp) in the endometrial cavity.

4. Three-dimensional ultrasound should be used to complement the conventional 2-D scan and provide the sonographer or sonologist with a more confident diagnosis.

SELECTED BIBLIOGRAPHY

Callen PW: *Ultrasonography in obstetrics and gynecology,* ed 4, Philadelphia, 2000, WB Saunders.

Cioffi-Ragan D: The comparison of conventional transabdominal and transvaginal ultrasound and 3-D transvaginal ultrasound in the evaluation of first trimester nuchal translucency, *J Diagn Med Sonogr* July/August, 2002.

Lee W: 3D fetal ultrasonography, *Clin Obstet Gynecol* 46(4):850-867, 2003.

Lee W, Kalache K, Chaiworapongsa T and others: Three-dimensional power Doppler ultrasonography during pregnancy, *J Ultrasound Med* 22(1):91-97, 2003.

Nelson T: Three-dimensional imaging, *Ultrasound Med Biol* 26:S35-S38, 2000.

Raatz Stephenson S: Sonographic signs of fetal neural tube and central nervous system defects, *J Diagn Med Sonogr* 19(6):347-357, 2003.

Thieme G, Manco-Johnson M, Cioffi-Ragan D: In Obstetrics, 3-D imaging solves clinical problems, *Diagn Imaging* March, 2000.

Thieme G, Manco-Johnson M, Cioffi-Ragan D: *Three-dimensional neonatal neurosonography, clinical applications of 3D sonography,* New York, 2000, The Parthenon Publishing Group.

Wiesauer F: *Methodology of three-dimensional ultrasound, clinical applications of 3D sonography,* New York, 2000, The Parthenon Publishing Group.

CHAPTER 51

The Placenta

Sandra L. Hagen-Ansert

OBJECTIVES

- Describe embryogenesis of the placenta
- List the functions of the placenta
- List and describe imaging techniques and sonographic findings for the placenta
- Identify the placental position and describe its importance
- Describe the sonographic findings and clinical significance of placental pathologies
- Recognize placental abruption on ultrasound
- Recognize the placenta in multiple gestation

KEY TERMS

abruptio placentae – premature detachment of the placenta from the maternal wall

basal plate – the maternal surface of the placenta that lies contiguous with the deciduas basalis

battledore placenta – cord insertion into the margin of the placenta

Braxton Hicks contractions – spontaneous painless uterine contractions described originally as a sign of pregnancy. They occur from the first trimester to the end of pregnancy.

chorion frondosum – the portion of the chorion that develops into the fetal portion of the placenta

chorionic plate – part of the chorionic membrane that covers the placenta

chorionic villi – vascular projections from the chorion

circummarginate placenta – a placental condition in which the chorionic plate of the placenta is smaller than the basal plate, with a flat interface between the fetal membranes and the placenta

circumvallate placenta – a placental condition in which chorionic plate of the placenta is smaller than the basal plate; the margin is raised with a rolled edge

decidua basalis – the part of the decidua that unites with the chorion to form the placenta

decidua capsularis – the part of the decidua that surrounds the chorionic sac

ductus venosus – connection that is patent during fetal life from the left portal vein to the systemic veins (inferior vena cava)

ligamentum venosum – transformation of the ductus venosus in fetal life to closure in neonatal life

lower uterine segment (LUS) – lowest segment of the uterus at the junction of the internal os and cervix

molar pregnancy – also known as gestational trophoblastic disease; abnormal proliferation of trophoblastic cells in the first trimester

placenta accreta – growth of the chorionic villi superficially into the myometrium

placenta increta – growth of the chorionic villi deep into the myometrium

placenta percreta – growth of the chorionic villi through the myometrium

placenta previa – placenta completely covers the lower uterine segment (internal os)

placental migration – the placenta is attached to the uterine wall. As the uterus enlarges, the placenta "moves" with it. Therefore a low-lying placenta may move out of the uterine segment in the second trimester

succenturiate placenta – one or more accessory lobes connected to the body of the placenta by blood vessels

vasa previa – occurs when the intramembranous vessels course across the cervical os

Wharton's jelly – mucoid connective tissue that surrounds the vessels within the umbilical cord

---

The development of the placenta has always been of interest to anatomists, researchers, obstetricians, and sonographers. Combined studies using endovaginal sonography, hysteroscopy, chorionic villus sampling, and hysterectomy specimens from the first trimester of pregnancy have indicated the absence of continuous blood flow in the intervillous space before 12 weeks of gestation.[2]

The major role of the placenta is to permit the exchange of oxygenated maternal blood (rich in oxygen and nutrients) with deoxygenated fetal blood. Maternal vessels coursing posterior to the placenta circulate blood into the placenta, whereas blood from the fetus reaches this point through the umbilical cord. The placenta is effectively studied by antenatal ultrasound. Valuable information regarding placental configuration, location, maturity, pathology, and maturation irregularities may be assessed.

The anatomic components of the placenta are discernible from as early as the 7th to 8th week of gestation. By the end of the first trimester, sonography can determine the location and position of the placenta and identify specific components of the placenta.

EMBRYOGENESIS

The transformation of endometrial cells into glycogen and lipoid cells characterizes the decidual reaction. This occurs in response to ovarian hormones (estrogen and progesterone).

BOX 51-1 DECIDUAL CHANGES

- **Decidua basalis:** The decidual reaction that occurs between the blastocyst and the myometrium
- **Decidua capsularis:** The decidual reaction occurring over the blastocyst closest to the endometrial cavity
- **Decidua vera (parietalis):** A reaction changes in the endometrium opposite the site of implantation

---

BOX 51-2 FETAL CHORION

- **Chorion frondosum:** The fetal trophoblastic tissue that, together with the decidua, forms the area for maternal and fetal circulation
- **Chorion laeve:** The chorion around the gestational sac on the opposite side of implantation
- **Chorionic plate:** The fetal surface of the placenta
- **Basal plate:** The maternal surface of the placenta

After fertilization, the development of the placenta is seen in the changes in the decidua (Box 51-1).

The chorion, amnion, yolk sac, and allantois constitute the embryonic or fetal membranes. These membranes develop from the zygote. Implantation of the blastocyst occurs 6 to 7 days after fertilization. Enlargement of trophoblasts helps to anchor the blastocyst to the endometrial lining, or *decidua*. The placenta has two components: the maternal portion, the **decidua basalis**, formed by the endometrial surface (Figure 51-1), and the fetal portion, which develops from the **chorion frondosum**.

The fetal chorion is the fusion of the trophoblast and extraembryonic mesenchyme. There are two types of trophoblastic cells: the syncytiotrophoblast is the outer layer of multinuclear cells, and the cytotrophoblast is the inner layer of mononuclear cells (Box 51-2).

The major functioning unit of the placenta is the chorionic villus (Figure 51-2). Within the chorionic villus are the intervillous spaces. The maternal blood enters the intervillous spaces. As the embryo and membranes grow, the **decidua capsularis** is stretched. The **chorionic villi** on the associated part of the chorionic sac gradually atrophy and disappear (smooth chorion or chorion laeve). The chorionic villi related to the decidua basalis increase rapidly in size and complexity (villous chorion or chorion frondosum).

The maternal surface of the placenta, which lies contiguous with the decidua basalis, is termed the **basal plate**. The fetal surface, which is contiguous with the surrounding chorion, is termed the **chorionic plate**. The cotyledons are cobblestone in appearance and composed of several mainstem villi and their branches. They are covered with a thin layer of the decidua basalis.

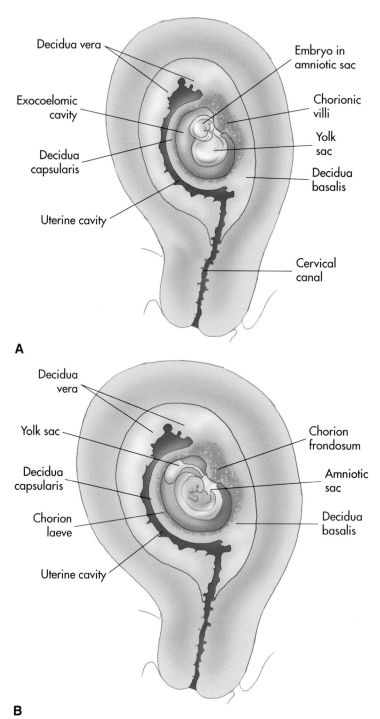

Figure 51-1 **A,** The placenta has two components: the fetal portion, developed from the chorion frondosum (chorionic plate), and a maternal portion, the decidua basalis, formed by the endometrial surface. **B,** The chorionic villi gradually atrophy and disappear (chorion laeve). The chorionic villi in the decidua basalis increase rapidly in size and complexity.

Before birth, the fetal membranes and placenta perform the following functions and activities: protection, nutrition, respiration, and excretion (Box 51-3). At birth, or *parturition,* they are separated from the fetus and cast from the uterus as the afterbirth.

FETAL-PLACENTAL-UTERINE CIRCULATION

The fetal-umbilical circulation originates with deoxygenated blood pumped by the fetal heart through the ductus arteriosus and into the descending aorta. The fetal blood continues to circulate through the hypogastric arteries to the umbilical

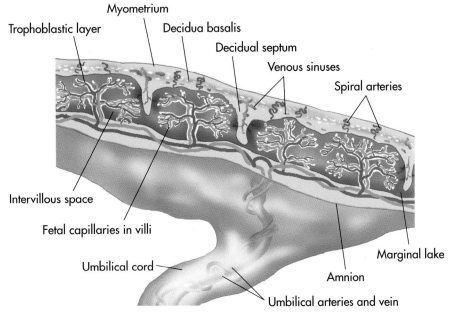

Figure 51-2   The major functioning unit of the placenta is the chorionic villus. The spiral arteries, venous sinuses, and uterine arteries line the periphery of the placenta.

FUNCTIONS OF THE PLACENTA

RESPIRATION
Oxygen in maternal blood diffuses across the placental membrane into fetal blood by diffusion. Carbon dioxide passes in the opposite direction. The placenta acts as "fetal lungs."

NUTRITION
Water, inorganic salts, carbohydrates, fats, proteins, and vitamins pass from maternal blood through the placental membrane into fetal blood.

EXCRETION
Waste products cross membrane from fetal blood and enter maternal blood. Excreted by mother's kidneys.

PROTECTION
Some microorganisms cross placental border.

STORAGE
Carbohydrates, proteins, calcium, and iron are stored in placenta and released into fetal circulation.

HORMONE PRODUCTION
Produced by syncytiotrophoblast of placenta: human chorionic gonadotropin, estrogens, progesterone.

---

arteries and into the umbilical cord. By term, approximately 40% of the fetal cardiac output is directed through the umbilical circulation.

The umbilical arteries divide within the placenta into multiple tiny capillary branches that course through the tertiary villi. A well-developed vascular network is directed to the umbilical cord.

Oxygenated maternal blood is brought to the placenta through 80 to 100 end branches of the uterine arteries—the spiral arteries. Maternal blood enters the intervillous space near the central part of each placental lobule where it flows around and over the surface of the villi. Color and power Doppler will demonstrate the placenta as a very vascular structure.

Maternal blood returns through a network of basilar, subchorial, interlobular, and marginal veins. A very thin layer normally separates the fetal blood from the maternal blood. This layer is composed of the capillary wall, the trophoblastic basement membrane, and a thin rim of cytoplasm of the syncytiotrophoblast. The circuit of blood is completed in the fetus through the liver and back to the heart.

The fetal placenta is anchored to the maternal placenta by the cytotrophoblastic shell and anchoring villi. It provides a large area where materials may be exchanged across the placental membrane and interposed between fetal and maternal circulation. It has been demonstrated that the embryo favors an environment low in oxygen during early development and that oxygen levels in placental tissue are low in the early first trimester.[1]

The placenta is dedicated to the survival of the fetus. Even when exposed to a poor maternal environment (e.g., when the mother is malnourished, diseased, or smokes or takes cocaine), the placenta can often compensate by becoming more efficient. Unfortunately, there are limits to the placenta's ability to cope with external stresses. Eventually, if multiple or severe enough, these stresses can lead to placental damage, fetal damage, and even intrauterine demise and pregnancy loss.

The maternal placental circulation may be reduced by a variety of conditions that decrease uterine blood flow, such as

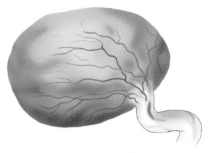

Figure 51-3 A battledore placenta refers to the insertion of the umbilical cord at the margin of the placenta.

severe hypotension, renal disease, or placental infarction. Placental defects can cause intrauterine fetal growth restriction (IUGR). The net effect is that there is a reduction of flow between the fetal and maternal blood.

Placental Membrane. The placental membrane is often called a barrier because there are a few compounds, endogenous and exogenous, that are unable to cross the placental membranes in detectable amounts.

CORDAL ATTACHMENTS

The attachment of the cord is usually near the center of the placenta. Abnormal cordal attachments to the placenta are battledore and velamentous placenta. A **battledore placenta** refers to the insertion of the umbilical cord at the margin of the placenta (Figure 51-3). It usually has no clinical significance unless the cord is forcefully torn away from the uterus during delivery. The velamentous placenta refers to a membranous insertion of the cord. In a small number of cases (less than 2%), it may be associated with significant fetal hemorrhage, especially if the membrane carrying the vessels is positioned across the internal os (vasa previa).

YOLK SAC

The secondary yolk sac forms after the regression of the primary yolk sac on the ventral surface of the embryonic disk at 28 menstrual days. The yolk sac has a role in the transfer of nutrients to the embryo during the 2nd and 3rd weeks, whereas the uteroplacental circulation is developing. It is connected to the midgut by a narrow yolk stalk. Before 5 menstrual weeks, the amniotic sac and secondary yolk sac have been pressed together with the embryonic disk between them. This structure is suspended within the chorionic cavity. The yolk sac becomes displaced from the embryo and lies between the amnion and the chorion (see Figure 51-1). By 9 weeks, the yolk sac has diminished to less than 5 mm in diameter.

IMPLANTATION OF THE PLACENTA

Normally the placenta will implant on the anterior, fundal, or posterior wall of the uterus. Occasionally the placenta will implant low in the uterus, resulting in a condition called **placenta previa.**

MEMBRANES

The fetal membranes consist of the chorion, amnion, allantois, and yolk sac. The chorion originates from the trophoblastic cells and remains in contact with the trophoblasts throughout pregnancy. The amnion develops at the 28th menstrual day and is attached to the margins of the embryonic disk. As the embryo grows and folds ventrally, the junction of the amnion is reduced to a small area on the ventral surface of the embryo to form the umbilicus.

Expansion of the amniotic cavity occurs with the production of amniotic fluid. By 16 weeks, the amnion fuses with the chorion and can no longer be seen on ultrasound as two separate membranes. If the separation extends beyond 16 weeks, it may be associated with polyhydramnios or prior amniocentesis. Hemorrhage may also have this appearance.

The secondary yolk sac forms after regression of the primary yolk sac at 28 menstrual days on the ventral surface of the embryonic disk. Before 5 menstrual weeks, the amniotic sac and secondary yolk sac have been pressed together with the embryonic disk between. This structure is suspended within another balloon (the chorion cavity) by the connecting stalk. The yolk sac becomes displaced from the embryo and lies between the amnion and the chorion (see Figure 51-1).

THE AMNIOTIC SAC AND AMNIOTIC FLUID

The amnion forms a sac that contains amniotic fluid. The sac encloses the embryo and forms the epithelial covering of the umbilical cord. Most of the amniotic fluid comes from the maternal blood by diffusion across the amnion from the decidua parietalis and intervillous spaces of the placenta.

In the first trimester, the fetus begins to excrete urine into the sac to fill the amniotic cavity. The fetus swallows this fluid, and the cycle continues throughout the pregnancy. The amniotic fluid serves as a protective buffer for the embryo and fetus. In addition, the fluid provides room for the fetal movements to occur and assists in regulating fetal body temperature.

THE PLACENTA AS ENDOCRINE GLAND

The chorionic villi are the functional endocrine units of the placenta. A central core with abundant capillaries is surrounded by an inner layer (cytotrophoblast) and an outer layer (syncytiotrophoblast). The inner layer produces neuropeptides, and the outer layer produces the protein hormone human chorionic gonadotropin (hCG) and human placental lactogen (hPL), along with the sex steroids estrogen and progesterone.

After the 7th week of gestation, most progesterone is produced by the syncytiotrophoblast from maternally derived cholesterol precursors. Progesterone production is exclusively a maternal-placental interaction, with no contribution from the fetus. The production of placental estrogen involves an intricate pathway requiring maternal, placental, and fetal contributions.

The function of the hCG is to maintain the corpus luteum in early pregnancy. It is elevated shortly after conception and peaks at 8 to 10 weeks. The hPL is responsible for the promotion of lipolysis and an antiinsulin action that serves to direct nutrients to the fetus.

THE UMBILICAL CORD

The umbilical cord forms during the first 5 weeks of gestation. The cord is surrounded by a mucoid connective tissue called **Wharton's jelly.** The intestines grow at a faster rate than the abdomen and herniate into the proximal umbilical cord at approximately 7 weeks and remain there until approximately 10 weeks of gestational age. The insertion of the cord into the ventral abdominal wall is an important sonographic anatomic landmark because scrutiny of this area will reveal abdominal wall defects, such as omphalocele, gastroschisis, or limb-body wall complex.

The normal umbilical cord has one large vein and two smaller arteries. One umbilical artery is found in approximately 1% of all singleton births and 7% of twin gestations. It is seen more commonly in diabetic mothers and is associated with low birth weight infants. Congenital malformations (genitourinary, cardiovascular, facial, and musculoskeletal) are seen in 25% to 50% of infants with one umbilical artery.

SONOGRAPHY OF THE UMBILICAL CORD

The vessels of the cord may be followed with real-time ultrasound as they leave the placenta to enter the fetal abdomen and travel toward the liver and iliac arteries (Figure 51-4). From the left portal vein, the umbilical blood flows either through the **ductus venosus** to the systemic veins (inferior vena cava or hepatic veins), bypassing the liver, or through the right portal sinus to the right portal vein (Figure 51-5).

Sonographically the ductus venous appears as a thin intrahepatic channel with echogenic walls. It lies in the groove between the left lobe and the caudate lobe. The ductus venosus is patent during fetal life until shortly after birth, when transformation of the ductus into the **ligamentum venosum** occurs (beginning in the 2nd week after birth).

The umbilical arteries may be followed caudal from the cord insertion, in their normal path adjacent to the fetal bladder, to the iliac arteries. On ultrasound, the sonographer may look at the cord in a transverse plane to see the large

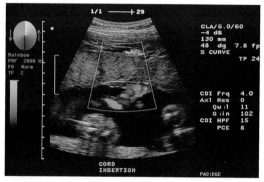

Figure 51-4   Color Doppler may demonstrate the umbilical cord as it exits the placenta.

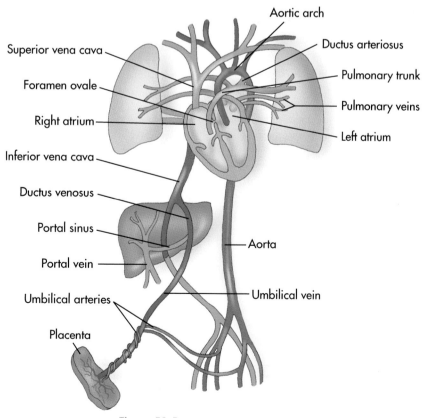

Figure 51-5   Fetal circulation diagram.

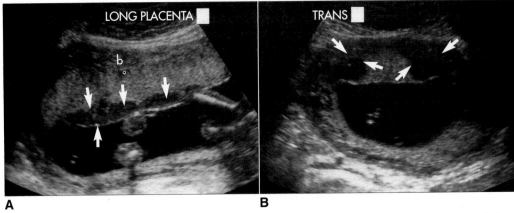

Figure 51-6   A, Longitudinal image of the placenta demonstrates the smooth homogeneous texture of the organ. Areas of echolucencies *(arrows)* are shown along the inner margin of the chorionic plate *(arrow)*. The basal surface *(b)* of the placenta is well seen along the myometrial surface of the uterus. **B,** Transverse image of the placenta as it lies along the anterior uterine wall. Echolucencies are seen representing the intervillous lakes *(arrows)*.

umbilical vein and two smaller arteries. Another approach to viewing the umbilical arteries is to image the fetal bladder in a transverse or coronal plane. The umbilical arteries will run along the lateral margins of the fetal bladder and are well seen with color flow Doppler. In the postpartum stage, the umbilical arteries become the superior vesical arteries.

SONOGRAPHIC EVALUATION OF THE NORMAL PLACENTA

Two surfaces of the placenta merit special attention because they are important in assessing normal placental anatomy and evaluating placental abruption.

The fetal surface of the placenta (portion of the placenta nearest the amniotic cavity) is represented by the echogenic chorionic plate, which courses along the placental tissue and is found at the junction with the amniotic fluid. This linear echogenicity is further enhanced by the strong interface of the amnion covering the chorionic plate (Figure 51-6).

The second surface is the basal plate or maternal portion of the placenta, which lies at the junction of the myometrium and the substance of the placenta (see Figure 51-6). Maternal blood vessels from the endometrium (endometrial veins) run behind the basal plate and are often confused with placental abruption. This represents the normal vascularity of this region. The endometrial veins are more apparent when the placenta is located in the fundus or posteriorly within the uterine cavity.

The placenta is identified on sonography as early as 8 menstrual weeks. The substance of the placenta assumes a relatively homogeneous pebble-gray appearance between 8 and 20 weeks of pregnancy and is easily recognized with its characteristically smooth borders. The thickness of the placenta varies with gestational age, with a diameter of less than 2 to 3 cm in fetuses greater than 23 weeks. The size of the placenta corresponds to the gestational age and rarely exceeds 45 to 50 mm in the

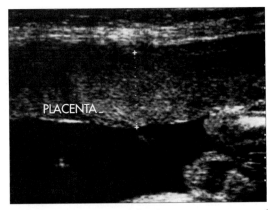

Figure 51-7   The thickness of the placenta measures more than 7 cm in this Rh-sensitized pregnancy. Calipers should be placed perpendicular to the placental borders.

normal fetus (Figure 51-7). After 20 weeks' gestation, the intraplacental sonolucencies (e.g., venous lakes or intervillous thrombi) and placental calcification may begin to appear. Enlarged placentas may also be associated with Rh sensitization, diabetes of pregnancy, or congenital anomalies. The sonographer must maintain a perpendicular measurement of the placental surface in relation to the myometrial wall when evaluating the thickness of the placenta.

Several sonolucent areas within the placenta may confuse the sonographer unfamiliar with the wide range of placental variants. Cystic structures representing large fetal vessels are commonly observed coursing behind the chorionic plate and between the amnion and chorion layers (Figure 51-8). Real-time observation of blood flow or color Doppler (Figure 51-9) helps to differentiate these vessels. Deposits of fibrin may also be found in the intervillous space posterior to the chorionic plate, and blood flow will not be seen in fibrinous areas. A heterogeneous placenta may be more commonly observed in

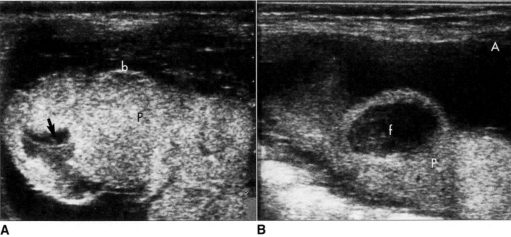

Figure 51-8 **A,** Subchorionic cystic area of the placenta at 29 weeks of gestation. Blood flow was obvious under real-time imaging *(arrow). b,* Basal plate; *P,* placenta. **B,** Subchorionic cystic area at 24 weeks of gestation, with internal echoes, representative of blood flow *(f)*. Color Doppler imaging may aid in detecting areas of blood flow. *A,* Amniotic fluid; *P,* placenta.

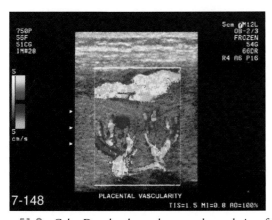

Figure 51-9 Color Doppler shows the normal vascularity of the marginal lakes, capillaries, and basal area of the placenta.

women with elevated maternal serum alpha-fetoprotein or a history of first-trimester bleeding.

Sonolucent regions may also be seen within the placental substance in the center of the placental lobes (cotyledons), which have been referred to as placental lakes. These areas may change dramatically in the course of the ultrasound examination. Blood flow should be identified within these areas with color Doppler. Placental veins may also be seen within the mass of the placenta.

The placenta is separated from the myometrium by a subplacental venous complex. These veins (basilar and marginal) can become very prominent, especially for lateral and posterior placentas, and should not be confused for a retroplacental or marginal hemorrhage. The myometrium is a thin, hypoechoic layer posterior to the basilar veins. The basilar veins and the myometrium measure as much as 9 to 10 mm in average thickness. The placenta increases in size and volume with gestational age; however, the maximum thickness does not exceed 4 cm.

PLACENTAL POSITION

The position of the placenta is readily apparent on most obstetric ultrasound studies. The placenta may be located in the mid to fundal site of the uterus, along the anterior, lateral, or posterior uterine walls (Figure 51-10). Occasionally the placenta may be dangerously implanted over or near the cervix (placenta previa) (Figure 51-11). The location of a placenta can change dramatically with an overdistended urinary bladder or the development of focal uterine contractions. **Braxton Hicks contractions** (normal contractions of pregnancy) should not be confused for placental pathology. The appearance of these contractions may distort the uterine contour; if such contractions occur, the suspicious area may be rescanned after 15 to 20 minutes to see if the uterine contour has returned to normal. These factors may also contribute to a false-positive impression of placenta previa.

Specific names are given to the placenta by its point of origin (i.e., fundus of the uterus along the anterior wall *[fundal anterior placenta]* or along the posterior uterine wall *[fundal posterior placenta]*). In early pregnancy, the chorion frondosum (primitive placenta) appears to completely surround the chorionic cavity *(circumferential placenta)*.

The sonographer should always describe the position of the placenta. The placenta should be scanned longitudinally to see whether it extends into the lower segment. If it does, a transverse scan should be obtained to determine whether the placenta is located centrally or whether it lies to one side of the cervix. Oblique scans may be necessary to visualize the relationship of the placenta to the cervix.

For the sonographer to visualize the internal os of the cervix, the patient should have a full bladder. In this way the relationship of the placenta to the internal os can be visualized (Figure 51-12). In theory, this works well. In practice, it is not always easy for the sonographer to view the internal os with the patient's bladder full. An overfilled bladder may push the internal os up, making it appear higher than it actually is. This may give the false impression of a previa. Emptying the bladder

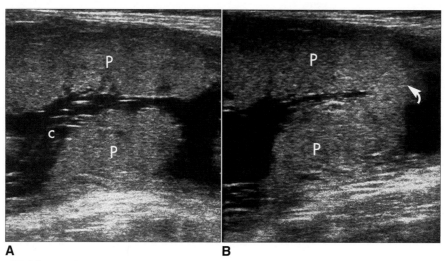

Figure 51-10   A, Placenta *(P)* appears to be located on both anterior and posterior uterine walls. *c,* Umbilical cord. **B,** By scanning laterally, the placenta is seen to communicate *(arrow),* representing a lateral placenta rather than a succenturiate lobed placenta.

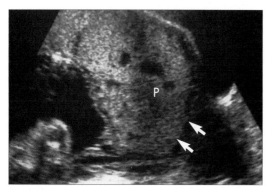

Figure 51-11   Placenta previa. *Arrows* point to the placenta *(P)* implanted over the cervical os.

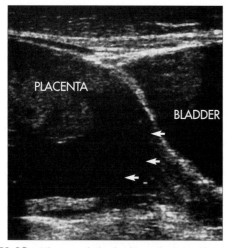

Figure 51-12   Ultrasound clearly shows the internal os of the cervix *(arrows).* The placenta is implanted away from the os.

reduces the pressure on the lower uterine segment and allows the cervix to assume a more normal position. The placenta may in fact not be a previa at all.

If a patient is actively bleeding or in active labor, the sonographer may not have time to wait for the patient to fill her bladder. If the fetal head is low in the pelvis, diagnosis of a posterior placenta previa may be difficult because the fetal skull bones block transmission of the ultrasound at a critical point. If the fetal head can be elevated out of the pelvis, it may be possible to distinguish between a posterior low-lying position and a posterior previa position. Other methods to demonstrate the os include tilting the patient in a slight Trendelenburg's position (head lower than body) to relieve pressure of the uterus on the **lower uterine segment (LUS)** or using the endovaginal or transperineal approach. The current standard of practice is that endovaginal or transperitoneal scanning should be performed any time there are questions regarding placental previa, or a low-lying or incompetent cervix.

Describing the location of the placenta has clinical importance. A previa noted on a scan alerts the obstetrician that no pelvic examination should be performed on the patient. A finger inadvertently pushed through an unknown previa can result in an amount of bleeding that frightens not only the patient but also the physician. If a placenta is noted to be a low-lying presentation early in pregnancy, the placenta location can be followed with consecutive scans to see whether this location persists.

When the placenta appears to lie on both anterior and posterior uterine walls, check for a laterally positioned placenta. When the placenta does not appear to communicate, a **succenturiate placenta** should be considered. This is a condition in which there are additional placental lobes joined to the main placenta by blood vessels. There is a risk that these connecting blood vessels may rupture or that an extra lobe may be inadvertently left in the uterus after delivery; therefore the clinician should be notified of this condition.

The concept that the placenta changes its position within the uterine cavity has been termed *placental migration,* implying that the placenta actually moves and relocates. It may be that the placenta actually does not move, but the position appears changed because of the physiologic enlargement of the uterus and development of the lower uterine segment. Other theories postulate that the low blood supply in the lower uterine segment causes the placenta in the region to atrophy and disappear, whereas the areas of rich blood supply toward the fundus of the uterus cause the placenta in that region to hypertrophy.

Although the majority of placentas that are considered previas in the early second trimester convert to fundal or low-lying placentas by the third trimester, there are exceptions. If the placenta is a complete previa in the early second trimester, it is unlikely to change its position drastically. A placenta previa should not be diagnosed before 20 weeks' gestation. In all likelihood, when the third trimester arrives, such a placenta will remain a complete previa.

DOPPLER EVALUATION OF THE PLACENTA

The normal trophoblastic invasion of spiral arteries produces a low-resistance Doppler pattern. The Doppler signals of the uterine arteries are variable depending on the gestational age and location of the placenta. In the first trimester, the flow velocity waveform shows a notched appearance in diastole. This notch usually disappears with increasing gestational age and trophoblastic invasion. The lowest resistance is seen on the side of the placenta. Before 20 weeks, the uterine artery Doppler typically shows a high-flow, low-resistance pattern, particularly for the uterine artery on the same side as the placenta (Figure 51-13). The quantitative measures of impedance to flow, such as the resistive index and pulsatility index, fall with gestational age.

Abnormal trophoblastic invasion of the spiral arteries of the maternal uteroplacental circulation is associated with a range of pregnancy complications, including IUGR, preeclampsia, and placental abruption.

EVALUATION OF THE PLACENTA AFTER DELIVERY

The normal term placenta has several characteristics at delivery. It measures about 15 to 20 cm in diameter, is discoid in shape, weighs about 600 g, and measures less than 4 cm in thickness. The clinician ascertains that the placenta has been delivered intact to prevent complications of postpartum hemorrhage or infection. Membranes of the amnion and chorion are inspected for color and consistency, with attention to meconium staining or signs of infection. The length of the umbilical cord is noted (and measured in the pathology laboratory). Short cords of less than 30 cm may result in traction during labor and delivery, leading to tearing of the cord, abruption, or inversion of the uterus. Long cords are more likely to prolapse, become twisted around the fetus, or tie in true knots.

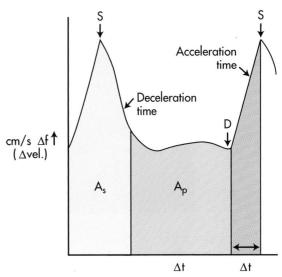

Figure 51-13   Waveform analysis. Before 20 weeks, the uterine artery Doppler typically shows a high-flow, low-resistance pattern, particularly for the uterine artery on the same side as the placenta. The quantitative measures of impedance to flow, such as the resistive index and pulsatility index, fall with gestational age.

FIBRIN DEPOSITION

Fibrin is a protein derived from fibrinogen. It is found throughout the placenta but is most pronounced in the floor of the placenta (in the septa) and increases continuously throughout pregnancy. Fibrin deposits on the villi may increase their mechanical stability; the deposits may be the result of eddies in the turbulent flow (more flow equals increased fibrin deposits). Fibrin may also be attributed to the regulation of intervillous circulation.

Sonographic Findings. On ultrasound examination, this fibrin deposition (subchorionic) appears as hypoechoic area beneath the chorionic plate of the placenta (Figure 51-14). Differential consideration of fibrin deposition includes a venous lake or a subchorionic hematoma. A venous lake shows increased flow with color flow Doppler. It may be difficult to distinguish fibrin deposits from a hematoma on ultrasound.

ABNORMALITIES OF THE PLACENTA

The major pathologic processes seen in the placenta that can adversely affect pregnancy outcome include intrauterine bacterial infections, decreased blood flow to the placenta from the mother, and immunologic attack of the placenta by the mother's immune system. Intrauterine infections (most commonly the result of migration of vaginal bacteria through the cervix into the uterine cavity) can lead to severe fetal hypoxia as a result of villous edema (fluid build up within the placenta itself). Both chronic and acute decreases in blood flow to the placenta can cause severe fetal damage and even death.

In addition to supplying the fetus with nutrition, the placenta is a barrier between the mother and fetus, protecting the fetus from immune rejection by the mother, a pathologic process that can lead to intrauterine growth restriction or even

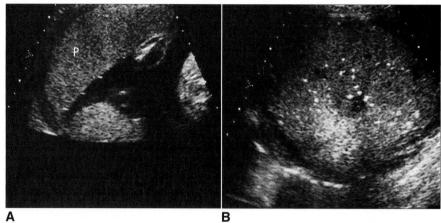

A   **B**

Figure 51-14 **A,** Fundal, anterior placenta at 20 weeks of gestation. Note the smooth homogeneous echo pattern characteristic of this early grade. There are no calcifications within the placenta *(P)* or along the basal plate. **B,** Fundal placenta at 39 weeks of gestation, showing the characteristic echogenic densities within the placental substance.

TABLE 51-1 LESIONS OF THE PLACENTA		
Lesion Significance	Incidence: Cause	Clinical Findings
Intervillous thrombosis	36%: Bleeding from fetal vessels	Fetal-maternal hemorrhage
Massive perivillous fibrin deposition	22%: Pooling and stasis of blood in intervillous space	None
Infarct	25%: Thrombosis of maternal vessel or retroplacental bleed and associated condition	Depends on extent
Subchorionic fibrin	20%: Pooling and stasis of blood in subchorionic space	None
Hydatidiform change	<1%: Complete mole	Predisposes to choriocarcinoma
	<1%: Partial mole	Associated with symptoms of preeclampsia
Chorioangioma	1%: Vascular malformation	Usually none; depends on size

demise. In addition to these major pathologic categories, many other insults, such as placental separation, cord accidents, trauma, and viral and parasitic infections, can adversely affect pregnancy outcome by affecting the function of the placenta (Table 51-1).

PLACENTOMEGALY

Placentomegaly is an enlarged placenta weighing more than 600 g. On ultrasound examination, the placenta thickness measures more than 5 cm. Maternal diabetes and Rh incompatibility are primary causes for placentomegaly (Box 51-4).

PLACENTA PREVIA

Placenta previa is the implantation of the placenta in the lower uterine segment in advance of the fetus. The placenta normally implants in the body of the uterus; however, in 1 of 200 pregnancies, the placenta implants over or near to the internal os of the cervix. This condition is called placenta previa.

The placenta may be considered (1) a complete or total previa, (2) a partial previa, (3) a marginal previa, or (4) low-lying (Figure 51-15). With complete previa, the cervical internal os is completely covered by placental tissue; this occurrence has been found in 20% of patients with previa. The previa may be symmetric or asymmetric. The majority of patients present

> **BOX 51-4 PLACENTAL SIZE AND CAUSES**
>
> **PLACENTOMEGALY**
> Maternal diabetes
> Maternal anemia
> α-Thalassemia
> Rh sensitivity
> Fetomaternal hemorrhage
> Chronic intrauterine infections
> Twin-twin transfusion syndrome
> Congenital neoplasms
> Fetal malformations
>
> **SMALL PLACENTA**
> Intrauterine growth restriction
> Intrauterine infection
> Chromosomal abnormality

with some form of previa. A partial previa only partially covers the internal os. A marginal previa does not cover the os, but its edge comes to the margin of the os. Although a low-lying placenta is implanted in the lower uterine segment, its edge does not reach the internal os.

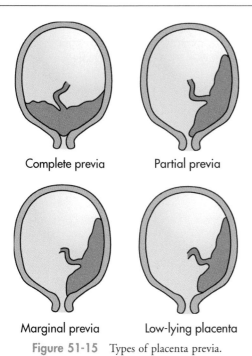

Complete previa   Partial previa

Marginal previa   Low-lying placenta

Figure 51-15 Types of placenta previa.

A pregnancy complicated by placenta previa is at high risk because of the risk of a life-threatening hemorrhage. As the pregnancy progresses into the third trimester, two very important changes occur. First, the lower uterine segment is developing (i.e., thinning and elongating in preparation for labor). As the lower uterine segment develops, the placental attachment to the lower uterine wall may be disrupted, resulting in bleeding. Second, the cervix softens and some dilation can occur before the onset of labor. Cervical dilation may also disrupt the attachment of a placenta located over or near the cervical os.

Before 20 weeks' gestation, "complete previa" may be noted in about 5% of second-trimester pregnancies, with 90% resolving by term as the placenta migrates with the growth of the uterus. Asymptomatic partial previas are seen in as many as 45% of early second-trimester pregnancies, with over 95% resolving before delivery.

Multiple factors are associated with placenta previa: advanced maternal age, smoking, cocaine use, prior placental previa, multiparity, and prior cesarean section or uterine surgery. Complications of placenta previa include premature delivery, life-threatening maternal hemorrhage, increased risk of placenta accreta, increased risk of postpartum hemorrhage, and IUGR.

Clinically the patient may present with painless, bright-red, vaginal bleeding in the third trimester. About 25% of patients will present with bleeding during the first 30 weeks. As many as 20% are associated with uterine premature contractions. Abnormal lie (either transverse or breech) is associated with placenta previa.

When a patient presents with third-trimester bleeding, diagnosis is imperative because the treatment will be different based on the clinical diagnosis. If the clinical diagnosis is

a large placental abruption, the obstetrician will deliver the fetus or it may die. If the diagnosis is placenta previa, the fetus is preterm, and the mother is not bleeding heavily, the clinical management may be conservative, with transfusion and close observation until the point where the fetus is mature or the pregnancy must be terminated because of bleeding.

When the time for delivery arrives, if the placenta completely covers the os, the fetus will have to be delivered by cesarean section. If the placenta only partially covers the os, it is possible that the fetus may deliver vaginally. The pressure of the fetus as it passes through the cervix and birth canal may compress the part of the placenta that has been disrupted and stop the bleeding (Box 51-5).

Sonographic Findings. The sonographer must be cautious in examining the lower uterine segment in relation to the location of the placenta. The maternal urinary bladder may be used as a landmark to identify the location of the internal cervical os (see Figure 51-12). The sonographer should be cautious of misinterpreting a low-lying placenta covering the internal os secondary to an overdistended bladder. The patient should be asked to empty her bladder, and the lower uterine segment should be rescanned to see the lower segment of the placenta in relation to the os. Any further question of low-lying placenta or placenta previa should be scanned endovaginally or transperineally, as that is the current standard of practice.

Although ultrasound allows easy localization of the placenta, the diagnosis of previa is difficult at times. Early in pregnancy, while the uterus is small, the relative endometrial surface covered by the placenta is large. As the pregnancy progresses, however, the amount of endometrial surface the placenta covers decreases. Therefore placentas can appear as previas early in pregnancy and may be marginal. As the lower uterine segment develops, however, and the placenta decreases relative to the uterus in size, there may be an increase in distance between the lower edge of the placenta and the internal os (Figure 51-16). The relationship of the placenta changes as pregnancy progresses, and a large number of low-lying placentas become fundal placentas by term.

Focal uterine contractions may also be misleading and a pitfall in diagnosing previa. The lower uterine segment should be scanned early in the ultrasound examination. If a contraction occurs, the sonographer may go on with the normal examination and reexamine the lower uterine segment in 20 minutes.

If the fetus is vertex and in the last trimester of pregnancy, the sonographer should examine the fetal head in relationship to the posterior wall of the uterus and the mother's sacrum. A distance of less than 1.5 cm indicates there will not be enough room for the placenta to be between the fetal head and posterior uterine wall.

The transperineal/translabial approach is also useful in evaluating the lower uterine segment when the definition of the placenta needs to be clarified. The endovaginal transducer is ideal for this approach. (The transducer should be prepared as for an endovaginal examination, with a protective covering.) The transducer is placed along the maternal labia to demonstrate the maternal bladder, the internal os (directed in a vertical orientation), the lower uterine segment, the fetal head, and the placenta (if previa). Longitudinal and transverse scans are carefully made to delineate the relation of the placenta to the cervical os.

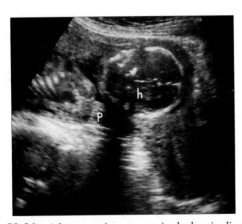

Figure 51-16   A lower uterine segment in the longitudinal plane shows the placental tissue *(P)* lying between the maternal sacrum and the fetal head *(h).*

Another approach to further define the lower uterine segment in the question of placental position is the endovaginal approach with the probe inserted only into the lower vagina. Color Doppler is useful to identify the increased placental flow.

VASA PREVIA

Vasa previa is a potentially life-threatening fetal complication of the placenta that occurs when large fetal vessels run in the fetal membranes across the cervical os, placing them at risk of rupture and life-threatening hemorrhage. Its occurrence is found in 1 in 2500 deliveries. The two most common occurrences of vasa previa are (1) when there is velamentous insertion of the umbilical cord into placental membranes, which course over the cervix, or (2) when a succenturiate lobe is present, and the connecting vessels course over the cervix. When delivery is eminent, the unsupported fetal vessels are prone to rupture as the cervix dilates, which can result in exsanguination of the fetus. The vessels may not tear; however, hypoxia may result during delivery as the fetal parts compress these vascular structures.

Sonographic Findings. Vasa previa is diagnosed with sonography when the implanted fetal umbilical vessels are seen to cover the cervix. Color Doppler and endovaginal sonography allow visualization of these vascular structures as they cover the cervical os. Care should be taken not to mistake marginal veins of a low-lying placenta or placental previa for a vasa previa.

PLACENTAL ACCRETA, INCRETA, AND PERCRETA

Placenta accreta is the abnormal adherence of all or part of the placenta with partial or complete absence of the decidua basalis (Figure 51-17). Chorionic villi grow into the myometrium, and the placental villi are anchored to muscle fibers rather than to the intervening decidual cells. Placenta accreta occurs in approximately 1 in 2500 deliveries.

Placenta increta is the further extension of the placenta through the myometrium. **Placenta percreta** is penetration of

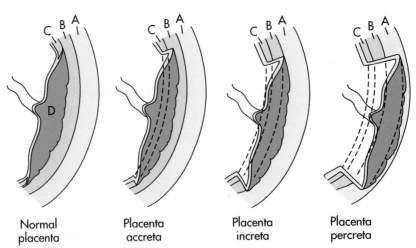

| Normal placenta | Placenta accreta | Placenta increta | Placenta percreta |

Figure 51-17   Classification of placenta accreta, increta, and percreta. **A,** Myometrium. **B,** Decidua basalis. **C,** Decidua spongiosa. **D,** Placenta. (Redrawn with permission from Newton M: Other complications of labor. In Danforth DN, editor: *Obstetrics and gynecology,* ed 5, New York, 1986, Harper & Row.)

TABLE 51-2	PLACENTA ACCRETA, PLACENTA INCRETA, AND PLACENTA PERCRETA	
Type of Bleeding	Invasion of Chorionic Villi Has Occurred	Blood Loss
Placenta accreta	Superficially into myometrium	Mild
Placenta increta	Deep into myometrium	Moderate
Placenta percreta	Through the myometrium	Severe

Data from http://telpath2.med.utah.edu/WebPath/PLACHTML/PLACO70.html

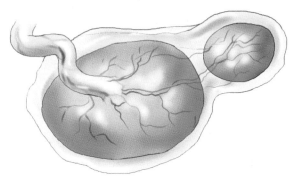

Figure 51-18 A succenturiate placenta is the presence of one or more accessory lobes connected to the body of the placenta by blood vessels.

the uterine serosa. These conditions result from the underdeveloped decidualization of the endometrium.

The risk of placenta accreta increases in patients with placenta previa and uterine scar from previous cesarean section. The risk of increta is 10% to 25% in women with one previous cesarean section when the placenta is implanted over the scar and exceeds 50% in women with placenta previa and multiple cesarean deliveries (Table 51-2).

Placenta increta results from underdeveloped decidualization of the endometrium. The association of placenta previa reflects the thin, poorly formed deciduas of the lower uterine segment that offers little resistance to deeper invasion by the trophoblast. The previous cesarean scar permits the trophoblastic invasion.

Sonographic Findings. There is a high maternal mortality and morbidity associated with placenta increta/percreta, so accurate prenatal diagnosis is critical. The primary sonographic finding typically presents as a placenta previa in the anterior location in women with as a previous history of cesarean deliveries.

The placenta is thick and heterogeneous with focal outpouching. The normal interface between the placenta and myometrium is obscured. The uterine vessels in the abnormal placental insertion site are prominent and rapidly fill with high velocity flow as seen with color Doppler. After delivery, the normal placental separation is identified by the cessation of blood flow between the basal placenta and myometrium, whereas the persistence of flow with color Doppler may suggest placenta accreta.

The sonographer should evaluate the placenta previa to look for the absence of hypoechoic subplacenta venous channels and myometrium beneath the placenta. In placenta percreta, the placental vessels extend within the urinary bladder wall. The perineal scanning approach may help the sonographer further define the lower uterine segment and the vascularity of the placenta in relationship to the maternal bladder.

SUCCENTURIATE PLACENTA

The succenturiate placenta is the presence of one or more accessory lobes connected to the body of the placenta by blood vessels (Figure 51-18). Succenturiate placenta occurs in 3% to 6% of pregnancies.

Normally the placenta is oval with a shape that varies somewhat depending on its site of implantation and areas of atrophy. When the placenta develops a secondary lobe or several other smaller lobes, these are called succenturiate lobes. These lobes have a tendency to develop infarcts and necrosis (50% of deliveries). They may create a "placenta previa" or be retained in utero after delivery.

The retention of the succenturiate lobe at delivery may result in postpartum hemorrhage and infection. Rarely, rupture of the connecting vessels may occur during delivery, causing fetal hemorrhage and demise.

Sonographic Findings. The sonographer should look for a discrete lobe that has "placenta texture" but is separate from the main body of the placenta. With color flow Doppler, vascular bands are seen connecting the lobes. The succenturiate placenta varies in appearance; it may be as large as the main lobe of the placenta and appear as two placentas. In 33% of bilobed placentas, the umbilical cord is attached to the main lobe of the placenta.

CIRCUMVALLATE/CIRCUMMARGINATE PLACENTA

A **circumvallate/circummarginate placenta** is the attachment of the placental membranes to the fetal surface of the placenta rather than to the underlying villous placental margin (Figure 51-19). This abnormality occurs in 1% to 2% of pregnancies. It results in placental villi around the border of the placenta that are not covered by the chorionic plate. A circumvallate placenta is diagnosed when the placental margin is folded, thickened, or elevated with underlying fibrin and hemorrhage. It is associated with premature rupture of the membranes, premature labor, hemorrhage, and placental abruption.

PLACENTAL HEMORRHAGE

Hemorrhage may occur within or around the placenta and is more commonly seen than a placental abruption. Placental hemorrhage refers to bleeding from the placenta from any cause. The locations of placental hemorrhage include retroplacental, subchorionic, subchorial, subamniotic, and intraplacental sites. A hemorrhage seen in the first trimester does not carry the same risk as hemorrhage in the third trimester. These lesions are more likely to resolve spontaneously.

Sonographic Findings. The sonographic appearance of placental hemorrhage varies greatly with the location, size, and

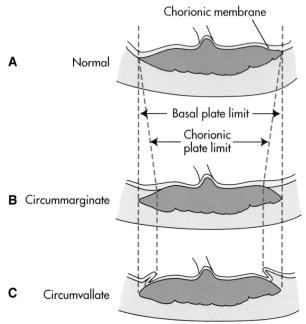

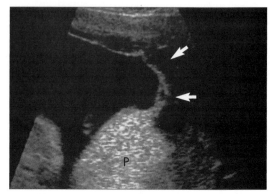

Figure 51-20 Ultrasound showing an abruption. *Arrows* point to the echolucent collection of blood lateral to the edge of the placenta. *P,* Placenta.

Figure 51-19 Comparison of extrachorial placentas with a normal placenta **(A).** The transition of membranous to villous chorion is at the placental edge. **B,** Circummarginate placenta. The transition of membranous to villous chorion occurs central to the edge of the placenta, but the chorionic surface remains smooth. **C,** Circumvallate placenta. The chorionic membrane is folding. (Redrawn with permission from Spirt BA, Kagan EH: Sonography of the placenta, *Semin Ultrasound* 1:293, 1980.)

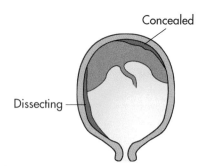

Figure 51-21 Types of placental abruption.

age of onset of the hemorrhage. Upon examination of the placenta, the sonographer will notice an abnormality in the texture and size of the placenta. If a hemorrhage is present, the echogenicity depends on the age of the hemorrhage; the acute bleed is medium level echogenic to isoechoic and may be more difficult to separate from the placenta, whereas the subacute and chronic bleed becomes more hyperechoic. The bleed may be retroplacental or subchorionic. Careful analysis should be made from the normal villus attachment of the placenta to the uterine wall to detect an abnormal collection of blood secondary to hemorrhage (Figure 51-20).

PLACENTAL ABRUPTION

Abruptio placentae or placental abruption refers to the separation of a normally implanted placenta before term delivery. Placental abruption is a premature placental detachment and occurs in 1 in 120 pregnancies. Bleeding in the decidua basalis occurs with separation (Figure 51-21). The mortality rate ranges from 20% to 60% and accounts for 15% to 25% of perinatal deaths. Clinically the patient may present with any of the following signs: preterm labor, vaginal bleeding, abdominal pain, fetal distress or demise, and uterine irritability. The detection of acute abruptions is not as sensitive with ultrasound because the medium level echogenicity makes them isoechoic to placental tissue, thus making it more difficult to be detected. Abruptio placentae may be further classified as

retroplacental or marginal. With abruption, bleeding into the deciduas basalis is apparent. The expanding hematomas can compress and elevate the overlying placenta, causing hypoxia and even fetal death.

Maternal hypertension is seen in 50% of severe abruptions and is considered a risk factor. Hypertension is chronic in half of these cases; in the other half, it is pregnancy induced. Other risk factors for abruption include a previous history of abruption, perinatal death, short umbilical cord, premature delivery, fibroids, trauma, placenta previa, and cocaine and other drugs. The recurrence of placental abruption ranges from 5% to 16% in subsequent pregnancies.

RETROPLACENTAL ABRUPTION

Retroplacental abruption results from the rupture of spiral arteries and is a "high-pressure" bleed. It is associated with hypertension and vascular disease. If the blood remains retroplacental, the patient has no visible bleeding (Figure 51-22). Sonographic findings show thickening of the placenta and occasional retroperitoneal clot.

MARGINAL ABRUPTION

Marginal abruption results from tears of the marginal veins and represents a "low-pressure" bleed. It is associated with cigarette smoking. The hemorrhage dissects beneath the placental membranes and is associated with little placental detachment.

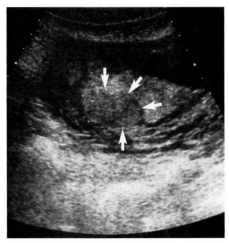

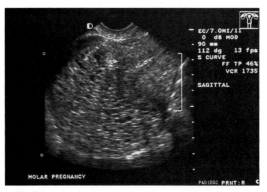

Figure 51-24   The hydatidiform mole is seen on ultrasound as multiple tiny vesicles throughout the uterine cavity.

Figure 51-22   Transverse image of a retroplacental abruption. The texture of the placenta is inhomogeneous *(arrows).*

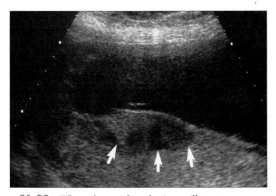

Figure 51-23   Thrombus within the intervillous spaces occurs in one third of the pregnancies. The inhomogeneity of the placenta is seen with sonolucent areas within the texture of the placenta *(arrows).*

A subchorionic hemorrhage accumulates at the site separate from the placenta.

INTERVILLOUS THROMBOSIS

The presence of thrombus within the intervillous spaces occurs in one third of pregnancies. It results from intraplacental hemorrhage caused by breaks in the villous capillaries. Usually there is little risk to the fetus, although the condition is associated with Rh sensitivity and elevated alpha-fetoprotein levels from a fetal-maternal hemorrhage.

Sonographic Findings. On ultrasound examination, sonolucencies are seen within the homogeneous texture of the placenta. These sonolucencies increase with advanced gestational age and indicate maturity of the placenta (Figure 51-23).

PLACENTA INFARCTS

Placental infarction is a focal discrete lesion caused by ischemic necrosis. Infarcts are common, are found in 25% of pregnancies, and are usually small with no clinical significance. Large infarcts may reflect underlying maternal vascular disease. Infarcts within the placenta evolve through acute, subacute, and chronic stages. The majority of infarcts are hypoechoic in the acute stage and ultrasound may be unable to distinguish them from intraplacental hemorrhages. Calcification may occur over time. Maternal floor infarction is a complication of the third trimester in which large amounts of fibrin are deposited in and around the maternal plate, with extension into the intervillous space and entrapment of chorionic villi.

PLACENTAL TUMORS

GESTATIONAL TROPHOBLASTIC DISEASE

Gestational trophoblastic disease is commonly known as **molar pregnancy** and is found in 1 in 1200 pregnancies. There are three groups of molar pregnancy: (1) complete mole (may develop into choriocarcinoma), (2) partial or incomplete mole, and (3) coexistent mole and fetus. Clinical symptoms include extreme nausea and vomiting (from elevated levels of hCG), vaginal bleeding, uterine size larger than dates, and preeclampsia. In this group, 15% to 25% will develop malignant gestational trophoblastic disease (choriocarcinoma). This disease is covered more thoroughly in Chapter 44.

Sonographic Findings. The sonogram shows uterine size larger than dates, no identifiable fetal parts, and an inhomogeneous texture with various-sized cystic structures within the placenta, which represents the multiple vesicular changes throughout the placenta (Figure 51-24). The size of the cysts varies with the gestational age. Bilateral theca lutein cysts are seen in the ovaries secondary to the hyperstimulation of the elevated hCG.

A partial mole carries little malignant potential. It is associated with an abnormal fetus or fetal tissue. On ultrasound examination, a reduced amount of amniotic fluid is noted without defined fetal parts. The placenta is thick with multiple intraplacental cystic spaces.

A coexistent mole and fetus is very rare; the mole may result from a hydatidiform degeneration of twin fetuses. This condition is more likely when two placentas are present. The abnormal placenta is hyperechoic with multiple small cysts. The coexisting fetus is alive with a normal placenta.

Differential considerations that should be considered when a molar pregnancy is suspected include intraplacental or periplacental hemorrhage, degenerating uterine leiomyomas, demise of a co-twin, or prominent maternal venous lakes.

CHORIOANGIOMA

A chorioangioma is a benign tumor of the placenta. Second to trophoblastic disease, chorioangioma is the most common "tumor" of the placenta, occurring in 1% of pregnancies. The tumor is usually small and consists of a benign proliferation of fetal vessels; the majority are capillary hemangiomas that arise beneath the chorionic plate (Figure 51-25). Large tumors can act as arteriovenous malformations shunting blood from the fetus, thus causing complications to the fetus. Complications include polyhydramnios, fetal hydrops, fetal cardiomegaly, IUGR, and fetal demise. The maternal serum alpha-fetoprotein may be elevated in the amniotic fluid or maternal serum, especially from vascular tumors. Premature labor is another complication of large chorioangiomas and is thought to be related to polyhydramnios.

Sonographic Findings. Ultrasound examination shows a circumscribed solid (hyperechoic or hypoechoic) or complex mass that protrudes from the fetal surface of the placenta. It may be located near the umbilical cord insertion site. The sonographer should look for polyhydramnios and fetal hydrops. Excessive amniotic fluid occurs as a result of transudation through the wall of abnormal tumor vessels. The differential consideration is a hematoma. Both the chorioangioma and hematoma may be associated with bleeding and elevated MSAFP. Color Doppler is helpful as flow is seen in the tumor, not in the hematoma.

Differential considerations for solid placental masses include partial hydatidiform mole, teratoma, and maternal tumor metastatic to the placenta.

THE PLACENTA IN MULTIPLE GESTATION

Depending on when during gestation the twinning event occurred, monozygotic twins are associated with all three types of membranes: dichorionic/diamniotic (di/di), monochorionic/diamniotic (mo/di), or monochorionic/monoamniotic (mo/mo). If the membranes are di/di, the pregnancy is probably dizygotic (97% chance), with only a 3% chance it is a monozygotic pregnancy. The diamniotic/dichorionic/two placentas can also occur in monozygotic pregnancies when the division occurs during the first 4 days of gestation. If the membranes are mo/di or mo/mo, they are from a monozygotic pregnancy (Box 51-6).

Sonographic Findings. The sonographer should be able to carefully scan the uterus to determine the site and number of the placentas to differentiate the type of multiple gestation present. Refer to Chapter 48 for further discussion of multiple gestations (Figure 51-26).

BOX 51-6 MULTIPLE GESTATION PREGNANCIES AND PLACENTAS

DIZYGOTIC (FRATERNAL TWINS)
Derived from two zygotes
Diamniotic/dichorionic/two placentas
Occurs during first 4 days of gestation

MONOZYGOTIC (IDENTICAL TWINS)
Derived from one zygote
Diamniotic/dichorionic/two placentas
Monochorionic/diamniotic/one placenta
Occurs during 1st week of gestation
Monochorionic/monoamniotic/one placenta
Occurs during 2nd week of gestation

RISKS INVOLVED
Monochorionic
Placental vascular anastomosis

Monoamniotic
Entanglement of umbilical cord

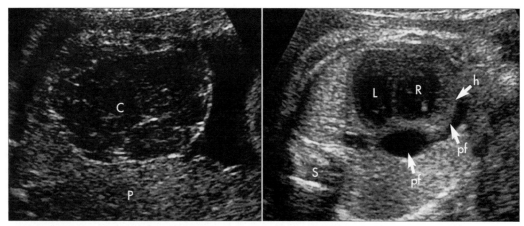

Figure 51-25 Chorioangioma *(C)* of the placenta of a fetus on the left side with dilation and hypertrophy *(h)* of the right cardiac ventricle *(R)* shown on the right side. Pleural fluid *(pf)* is shown. *L,* Left ventricle; *P,* placenta; *S,* spine.

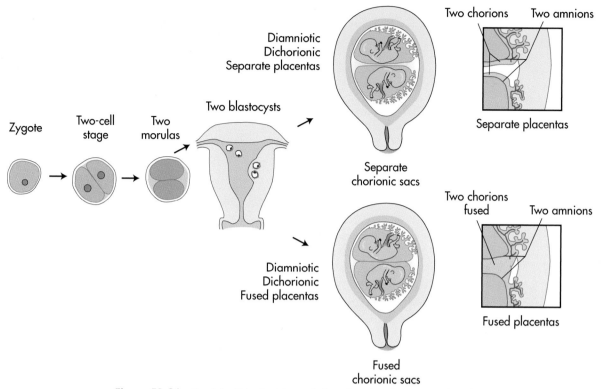

Figure 51-26   Possible dichorionicity and diamnionicity of monozygotic twins.

REFERENCES

1. Jaffe R, Jauniaux E, Hustin J: Maternal circulation in the first-trimester human placenta: myth or reality? *Am J Obstet Gynecol* 176:695, 1997.
2. Jauniaux E, Campbell S: Ultrasonographic assessment of placental abnormalities, *Am J Obstet Gynecol* 163:1650, 1990.

SELECTED BIBLIOGRAPHY

Acharya G, Wilsgaard T, Berntsen GKR and others: Reference ranges for serial measurements of umbilical artery Doppler indices in the second half of pregnancy, *Am J Obstet Gyne* 192:3, 2005.

Ananth CV, Smulian JC, Vintzileos AM: The association of placenta previa with history of cesarean delivery and abortion: a meta-analysis, *Am J Obstet Gynecol* 177:1071, 1997.

Ball RH, Buchmeier SE, Longnecker M: Clinical significance of sonographically detected uterine synechiae in pregnant patients, *J Ultrasound Med* 16:465, 1997.

Barton SM: Placental abruption. In Frederickson H, Wilkins-Haug L, editors: *Ob-gyn secrets,* St Louis, 1991, Mosby.

Benirschke K, Kaufmann P: *Pathology of the human placenta,* ed 2, New York, 1990, Springer-Verlag.

Callen P: *Ultrasonography in obstetrics & gynecology,* ed 4, Philadelphia, 2000, WB Saunders.

Gabbe S: *Obstetrics: normal and problem pregnancies,* ed 4, Philadelphia, 2002, Churchill Livingstone.

Grannum PT, Berkowitz RD, Hobbins JC: The ultrasonic changes in the maturing placenta and their relation to fetal pulmonic maturity, *Am J Obstet Gynecol* 133:915, 1979.

Hertzberg BS and others: Diagnosis of placenta previa during the third trimester: role of transperineal sonography, *Am J Radiol* 159:83, 1992.

Hobbins JC, Winsberg F, Berkowitz RL: The placenta. In Hobbins JC, Winsberg F, and Berkowitz RL, editors: *Ultrasonography in obstetrics and gynecology,* ed 2, Baltimore, 1983, Williams & Wilkins.

Jurkovic D and others: Transvaginal color Doppler assessment of the uteroplacental circulation in early pregnancy, *Obstet Gynecol* 77:365, 1991.

King DL: Placental migration demonstrated by ultrasonography, *Radiology* 109:167, 1973.

Klaisle D: The placenta. In Frederickson H, Wilkins-Haug L, editors: *Ob-gyn secrets,* St Louis, 1991, Mosby.

Kliman HJ: Behind every healthy baby is a healthy placenta, http://info.med.yale.edu/obgyn/kliman/Placenta/behind.html, accessed 1998.

Miller DA, Chollet JA, Goodwin TM: Clinical risk factors for placenta previa-placenta accreta, *Am J Obstet Gynecol* 177:210, 1997.

Nyberg D, MaGahan JP, Pretorius D and others: *Diagnostic ultrasound of fetal anomalies,* Philadelphia, 2003, Lippincott, Williams & Wilkins.

Sistrom CL, Ferguson JE: Abnormal membranes in obstetrical ultrasound: incidence and significance of amniotic sheets and circumvallate placenta, *Ultrasound Obstet Gynecol* 3:249, 1993.

Trierweiler MW: Abnormal placentation. In Frederickson H, Wilkins-Haug L, editors: *Ob-gyn secrets,* St Louis, 1991, Mosby.

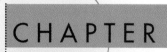

The Umbilical Cord

Sandra L. Hagen-Ansert

KEY TERMS

allantoic duct – elongated duct that contributes to the development of the umbilical cord and placenta during the first trimester

battledore placenta – marginal or eccentric insertion of the umbilical cord into the placenta

ductus venosus – the smaller, shorter, and posterior of the two branches into which the umbilical vein divides after entering the abdomen. It empties into the inferior vena cava

false knots of the umbilical cord – occurs when blood vessels are longer than the cord; they fold on themselves and produce nodulations on the surface of the cord

gastroschisis – anomaly in which part of the bowel remains outside the abdominal wall without a membrane

hemangioma of the cord – vascular tumor within the umbilical cord

membranous or **velamentous insertion of the cord** – cord inserts into the membranes before it enters the placenta

nuchal cord – occurs when the cord is wrapped around the fetal neck

omphalocele – failure of the bowel, stomach, and liver to return to the abdominal cavity; completely covered by a peritoneal-amniotic membrane

omphalomesenteric cyst – cystic lesion of the umbilical cord

single umbilical artery – high association of congenital anomalies with single umbilical artery

superior vesical arteries – after birth, the umbilical arteries become the superior vesical arteries

true knots of the umbilical cord – formed when a loop of cord is slipped over the fetal head or shoulders during delivery

umbilical herniation – failure of the anterior abdominal wall to close completely at the level of the umbilicus

vasa previa – occurs when the umbilical cord vessels cross the internal os of the cervix

Wharton's jelly – myxomatous connective tissue that surrounds the umbilical vessels and varies in size

yolk stalk – umbilical duct connecting the yolk sac with the embryo

---

DEVELOPMENT AND ANATOMY OF THE UMBILICAL CORD

The umbilical cord is the essential link for oxygen and important nutrients among the fetus, the placenta, and the mother. The amnion covers the cord and blends with the fetal skin at the umbilicus. The umbilical cord comprises two arteries and one vein surrounded by gelatinous stroma. The vascular connections within the cord serve a reverse function in the fetus; the vein carries oxygenated blood to the fetus, whereas the arteries bring venous blood back to the placenta.

Visualization of the umbilical cord with sonography can be made from the 8th gestational week until term. The amniotic membrane covers the fetal surface of the placenta and the multiple vessels that branch from the umbilical vein and arteries. The cord should normally insert into the center of the placenta.

EMBRYOLOGICAL DEVELOPMENT

The umbilical cord forms during the first 5 weeks of gestation (7 menstrual weeks) as a fusion of the omphalomesenteric **(yolk stalk)** and **allantoic ducts.** An outpouching from the urinary bladder forms the urachus, which projects into the connecting stalk to form the allantois. The allantoic vessels become the definitive umbilical vessels. The umbilical cord acquires its epithelial lining as a result of the enlargement of the amniotic cavity and the result of envelopment of the cord by amniotic membrane. The intestines grow at a faster rate than the abdomen and herniate into the proximal umbilical cord at approximately 7 weeks and remain there until approximately 10 weeks. The insertion of the umbilical cord into the ventral abdominal wall is an important sonographic anatomic landmark because scrutiny of this area will reveal abdominal wall defects, such as omphalocele, gastroschisis, or limb-body wall complex.

NORMAL ANATOMY

The umbilical cord is covered by the amniotic membrane. The cord includes two umbilical arteries and one umbilical vein (Figure 52-1) and is surrounded by a homogeneous substance called Wharton's jelly. **Wharton's jelly** is a myxomatous connective tissue that varies in size and may be imaged with high-frequency ultrasound transducers. The diameter of the cord usually measures 1 to 2 cm (variations in cord diameter are usually attributed to Wharton's jelly). The normal length of the cord is 40 to 60 cm; it is difficult to assess the length reliably with ultrasound.

The umbilical arteries arise from the fetal internal iliac arteries, course alongside the fetal bladder, and exit the umbilicus to

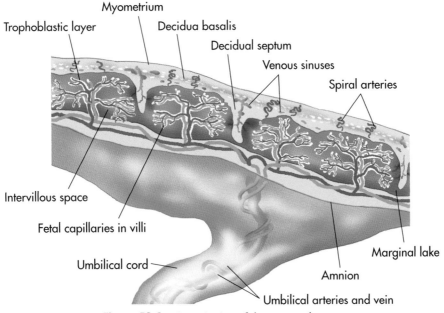

Figure 52-1 Organization of the mature placenta.

form part of the umbilical cord. The paired umbilical arteries course along the entire length of the cord in a helicoidal fashion surrounding the umbilical vein. The umbilical arteries branch along the chorionic plate of the placenta.

The umbilical vein is formed by the confluence of the chorionic veins of the placenta, with its primary purpose to transport oxygenated blood back to the fetus. The umbilical vein enters the umbilicus and joins the left portal vein as it courses through the liver. The intraabdominal portions of the umbilical vessels degenerate after birth; the umbilical arteries become the lateral ligaments of the bladder, and the umbilical vein becomes the round ligament of the liver.

SONOGRAPHIC EVALUATION OF THE UMBILICAL CORD

The umbilical cord has one large vein and two smaller arteries (Figure 52-2). The umbilical vein transports oxygenated blood from the placenta, and the paired umbilical arteries return deoxygenated blood from the fetus to the placenta for purification. The umbilical cord is identified at the cord insertion into the placenta and at the junction of the cord into the fetal umbilicus. The arteries spiral with the larger umbilical vein (Figure 52-3), which is surrounded by Wharton's jelly (Figure 52-4). Absent cord twists may be associated with decreased fetal movement and a poor pregnancy outcome.

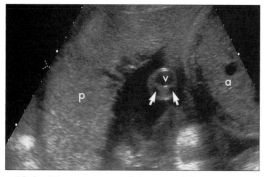

Figure 52-2 Transverse view of the normal three-vessel cord. The umbilical vein *(v)* is the largest vessel, with two smaller arteries *(arrows)* spiraling around the vein. *a,* Abdomen; *p,* placenta.

The umbilical vein diameter increases throughout gestation, reaching a maximum diameter of 0.9 cm by 30 weeks of gestation. The umbilical cord has been found to be significantly larger in fetuses of mothers with gestational diabetes than in the normal population; the increase in width is attributed mainly to an increase in Wharton's jelly content.[4]

In the second and third trimesters, the two arteries and the vein can be clearly seen. The number of umbilical arteries can be clearly seen and should be documented. The three vessels of the cord may be followed with real-time ultrasound as they enter the abdomen and travel toward the liver and iliac arteries (Figure 52-5). From the left portal vein, the umbilical blood flows either through the **ductus venosus** to the systemic veins (inferior vena cava or hepatics) bypassing the liver or through the right portal sinus to the right portal vein. The ductus venosus forms the conduit between the portal system and the systemic veins.

Sonographically the ductus venous appears as a thin intrahepatic channel with echogenic walls. It lies in the groove between the left lobe and the caudate lobe. The ductus venosus is patent during fetal life until shortly after birth, when transformation of the ductus into the *ligamentum venosum* occurs (beginning in the 2nd week after birth).

The umbilical arteries may be followed caudally from the cord insertion, in their normal path adjacent to the fetal bladder, to the iliac arteries. On ultrasound, the sonographer may look at the cord in a transverse plane to see the one large umbilical vein and two smaller umbilical arteries. Another sonographic approach to see the arteries is to look lateral to the fetal bladder in a transverse or coronal plane. The umbilical arteries run along the lateral margin of the fetal bladder and are well imaged with color flow Doppler. In the postpartum stage, the umbilical arteries become the **superior vesical arteries.**

ABNORMAL UMBILICAL CORD (LENGTH AND WIDTH)

Although the umbilical cord varies normally in length and width, researchers have found specific problems associated with a cord that varies from standard dimensions. In the first

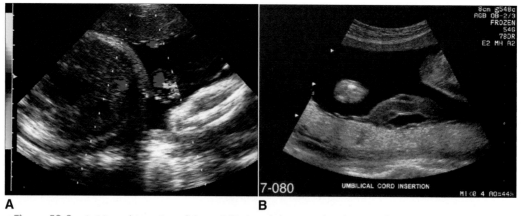

A   **B**

Figure 52-3 A, Normal insertion of the umbilical cord shown with color Doppler as it inserts into the fetal abdomen. **B,** The umbilical cord may be seen as it exits the placental surface.

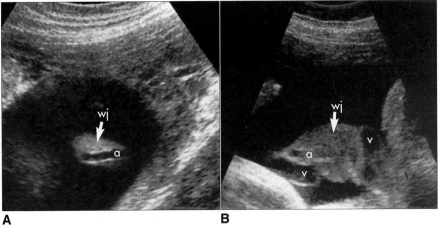

A   **B**

Figure 52-4   **A,** Wharton's jelly *(wj)* observed in a 30-week fetus. One of the umbilical arteries *(a)* is in view. **B,** Wharton's jelly *(wj)* is present adjacent to one of the umbilical arteries *(a)* and the single umbilical vein *(v)* is observed in a 35-week fetus. Wharton's jelly is an important structure to recognize when performing cordocentesis procedures in which the needle is directed into the cord vessels.

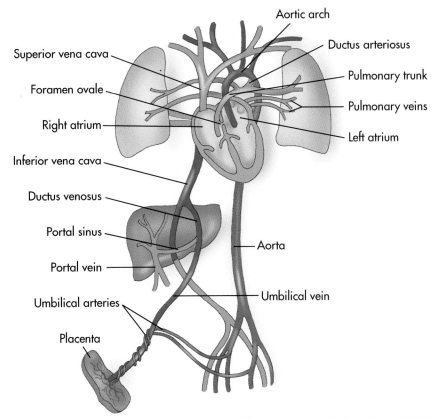

Figure 52-5   The umbilical vein leaves the placenta to deliver nutrients to the fetus. From the left portal vein, the umbilical blood flows either through the ductus venosus to the inferior vena cava or hepatics or through the right portal sinus to the right portal vein. The iliac arteries drain into the umbilical arteries.

trimester, the length is approximately the same as the crown-rump length. The normal length of the cord measures 40 to 60 cm and is difficult to assess reliably with ultrasound (Figure 52-6).

A short umbilical cord measures less than 35 cm in length. This condition is associated with or predisposed to the following:

- Oligohydramnios
- Restricted space (as in multiple gestations)
- Intrinsic fetal anomaly
- Tethering of the fetus by an amniotic band
- Inadequate fetal descent
- Cord compression
- Fetal distress

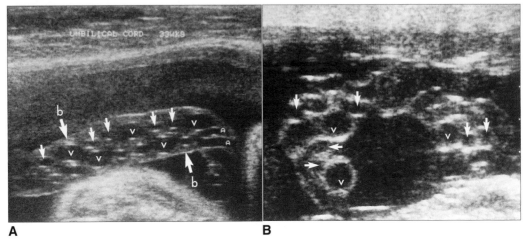

Figure 52-6 A, The umbilical cord is shown in a sagittal plane in a 33-week fetus, outlining the cord borders *(b),* the umbilical vein *(v),* and the arteries *(arrows).* The spirals of the cord vessels and Wharton's jelly are outlined. Abnormal cord twists may indicate a higher risk for stillbirth. **B,** Cross sections of the umbilical cord. *Arrows,* Umbilical arteries; *v,* umbilical vein.

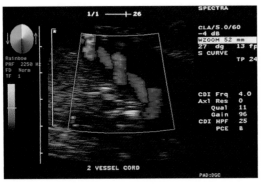

Figure 52-7 As the cord is held vertically, vessels along the anterior surface spiral downward from high left to low right, angled like the left side of the letter *V,* to indicate a left helix.

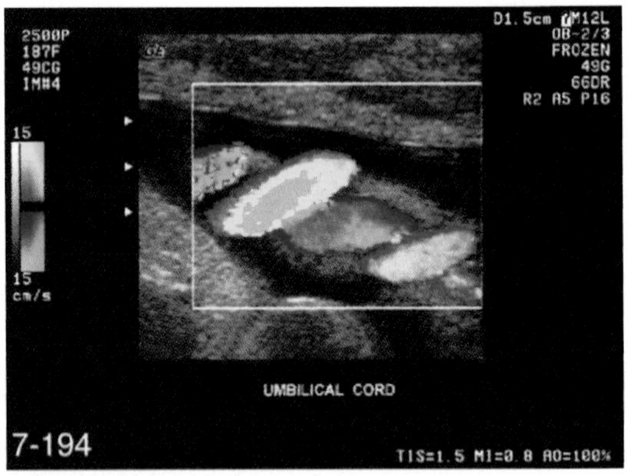

Figure 52-8 This two-vessel cord has a right twist; the fetus has multiple congenital anomalies.

Coiling of the umbilical cord is normal and is related to fetal activity. The normal cord may coil as many as 40 times, usually to the left and near the fetal insertion site. The helical twisting of the cord can be easily determined by gross pathologic inspection. With the cord held vertically, vessels along the anterior surface that spiral downward from high left to low right, angled like the left side of the letter V, indicate a left helix (Figure 52-7). The incidence of a "left" twist of the cord is found in 7:1 pregnancies. The significance of this is that a fetus with a "right" twist in the cord has a higher incidence of fetal anomalies than one with a "left" twist (Figure 52-8).

The absence of cord twisting is an indirect sign of decreased fetal movement (Figure 52-9). This event occurs in a small (4.3%) number of deliveries; however, it may lead to increased mortality and morbidity. Other obstetric problems seen with a short umbilical cord include preterm delivery, decreased heart rate during delivery, meconium staining secondary to fetal distress, and fetal anomalies. If the cord is completely atretic, the fetus is attached directly to the placenta at the umbilicus and an omphalocele is always present.

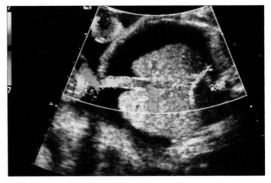

Figure 52-9 This hydropic fetus showed decreased movement over 24 hours. The cord is shown without its usual twisting and coiling, indicating decreased fetal movement.

It has been theorized that the length of the umbilical cord is determined partly by the amount of amniotic fluid present in the first and second trimesters, and fetal mobility. Therefore the presence of oligohydramnios, amniotic bands, or limitation of fetal movement for any reason may impede umbilical cord growth.

A long umbilical cord measures greater than 80 cm and may be associated with or predisposed to the following:

- Polyhydramnios
- Nuchal cord (occurs in 25% of deliveries)
- True cord knots (occur in 0.5% of deliveries); may be difficult to distinguish from "false" cord knot or redundancy of cord; true knots cause vascular compromise and fetal demise
- Umbilical cord compression, cord presentation, and prolapse of the cord lead to fetal distress
- Umbilical cord stricture or torsion resulting from excessive fetal motion

The diameter of the umbilical cord has been measured from 2.6 to 6.0 cm. Variations in cord diameter are usually attributed to diffuse accumulation of Wharton's jelly. This condition has been associated with maternal diabetes, edema secondary to fetal hydrops, Rh incompatibility, and fetal demise.

UMBILICAL CORD MASSES

Umbilical cord masses are not very common in the fetus. Many of the "masses" seen on ultrasound may be attributed to focal accumulation of Wharton's jelly and may be isolated or associated with an omphalocele or cyst. A cystic mass in the cord is usually omphalomesenteric or allantoic in origin. These are generally small (less than 2 cm), tend to be near the fetal end of the cord, and resolve by the second trimester. Cysts that persist beyond the first trimester usually are associated with other fetal anomalies and aneuploidy.

Other masses associated with the umbilical cord include:

- Omphalocele (cord runs through the middle of this mass as it protrudes from the umbilicus)
- Gastroschisis (mass usually found to the right of this cord)
- Umbilical herniation
- Teratoma of the umbilical cord
- Aneurysm of the cord
- Varix of the cord (may be intraabdominal)

- Hematoma of the cord (usually iatrogenic-cordocentesis or amniocentesis)
- True knot of the cord
- Angioma of the cord (well-circumscribed echogenic mass that may cause increased cardiac failure and hydrops; alpha-fetoprotein level is increased; associated with a cyst caused by transudation of fluid from a hemangioma)
- Thrombosis of cord secondary to compression or kinking, focal cord mass, true cord knots, velamentous cord insertion, cord entanglement in monoamniotic twins (commonly seen with fetal demise)

OMPHALOCELE

Omphalocele occurs 1 in 5000 births and results from failure of the intestines to return to the abdomen. The hernia may consist of a single loop of bowel or it may contain most of the intestines (Figure 52-10). The covering for the hernia sac is epithelium from the umbilical cord.

GASTROSCHISIS

Gastroschisis is usually a right paraumbilical defect involving all layers of the abdominal wall, usually measuring 2 to 4 cm. The small bowel always eviscerates through the defect (Figure 52-11). The loops of bowel are never covered by a membrane; thus they are directly exposed to amniotic fluid and elevated alpha-fetoprotein levels. Other organs that may eviscerate are large bowel, stomach, a portion of the gastrointestinal system and, rarely, liver.

UMBILICAL HERNIATION

Umbilical herniation occurs when the intestines return normally to the abdominal cavity and then herniate either prenatally or postnatally through an inadequately closed umbilicus (Figure 52-12).

OMPHALOMESENTERIC CYST

Omphalomesenteric cyst is a cystic lesion of the umbilical cord caused by persistence and dilation of a segment of the omphalomesenteric duct lined by epithelium of gastrointestinal

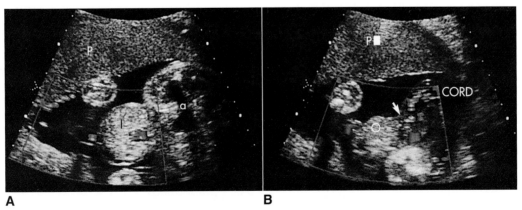

A   **B**

Figure 52-10   **A,** Image of a liver-filled omphalocele in a 26-week fetus showing hepatic vessel flow within the herniated liver. *a,* Abdomen; *P,* placenta. **B,** In the same fetus, color enhancement aids in the confirmation of the cord vessels entering the base of the omphalocele *(O, arrow); P,* placenta. No other anomalies were found and the karyotype was normal.

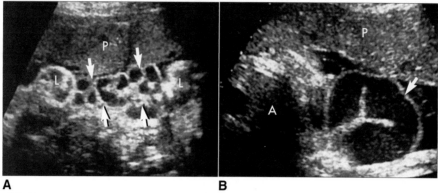

Figure 52-11 **A,** Gastroschisis showing herniated bowel *(arrows)* in the amniotic cavity. Cesarean section was performed at 36 weeks of gestation because of a nonreactive nonstress test with variable decelerations and absent breathing. A small-for-gestational age infant with a left-side gastroschisis was delivered. *L,* Limbs; *P,* placenta. **B,** Isolated bowel segment *(arrow)* observed in another fetus with gastroschisis at 29 weeks of gestation. Bowel dilation (29 mm) and obstruction (meconium ileus) are shown. Note the haustral markings within the obstructed bowel. *A,* Abdomen; *P,* placenta.

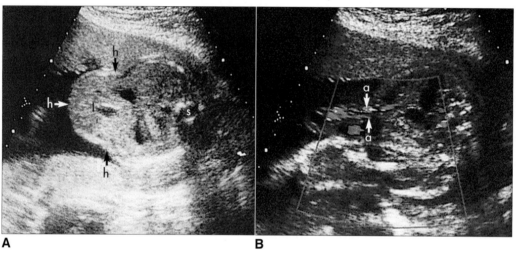

Figure 52-12 **A,** Umbilical hernia *(h, arrows)* observed in a fetus with Carpenter's syndrome (acrocephalopoly-syndactyly). *l,* Liver; *s,* spine. **B,** In the same fetus, at the cord insertion level using color imaging, the umbilical arteries are observed entering the abdomen *(a)* in a normal location. This excludes the diagnosis of omphalocele.

origin. During the third week of early development, the omphalomesenteric duct joins the embryonic gut and the yolk sac. This is closed by the 16th week of gestation; however, in some cases small vestigial remnants of the duct may be found in normal umbilical cords (Figure 52-13). The omphalomesenteric cyst is found closer to the fetal cord insertion and may vary in size (up to 6 cm). This condition affects females over males with a ratio of 5:3. In addition, there may be an associated condition of Meckel's diverticulum.

HEMANGIOMA OF THE CORD

A **hemangioma of the cord** arises from the transepithelial cells of the vessels of the umbilical cord. Pathologically, this angiomatous nodule is surrounded by edema and myxomatous degeneration of Wharton's jelly. The sites of origin are the main vessels of the umbilical cord, and it may involve more than one

vessel. This condition is rare; however, when found near the placental end of the cord the size varies from small to large (up to 15 cm). The fetus may develop nonimmune hydrops.

HEMATOMA OF THE CORD

Trauma to the umbilical vessels may occasionally cause extravasation of blood into Wharton's jelly. This occurs usually near the fetal insertion of the cord. The umbilical vein is most frequently involved. If the blood clot is new, the mass is hyperechoic on ultrasound; if the clot is old, the mass is hypoechoic and septated. Complications have been reported as high as 47% to 52% with fetal mortality.

THROMBOSIS OF THE UMBILICAL VESSELS

Thrombosis of the umbilical vessels is occlusion of one or more vessels of the umbilical cord; primarily it occurs in the umbil-

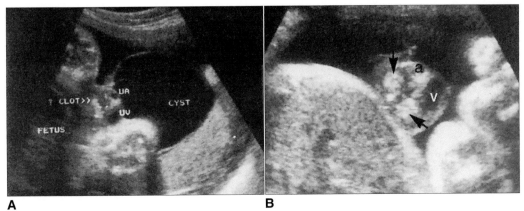

Figure 52-13 **A,** Omphalomesenteric cyst observed in a 34-week fetus. Clot formation was found within one artery. A single umbilical artery *(UA)* was viewed in proximal sections of the cord close to the cyst, and three vessels were noted distally. *UV,* Umbilical vein. **B,** In the same fetus, clot is observed *(arrows).* At birth, a 10-cm, serous-filled cyst consistent with omphalomesenteric cyst was confirmed. The cyst weighed 1 lb.

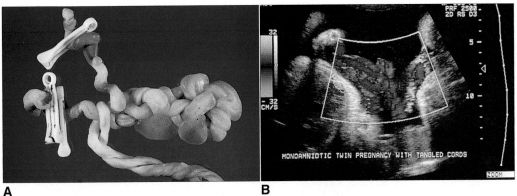

Figure 52-14 **A,** Pathologic specimen of an umbilical cord with multiple knots. **B,** Ultrasound image of a monoamniotic twin pregnancy showing multiple knots and tangles within the cord. Doppler flow shows decreased velocity in the blood flow.

ical vein. The incidence is higher in infants of diabetic mothers than in nondiabetic mothers. Thrombosis may be primary or secondary to torsion, knotting, looping, compressions, or hematoma. The sonographer should look for aneurysmal dilation of the cord and the presence of fetal hydrops. Other maternal factors are phlebitis and arteritis. The prognosis is poor in the fetus with umbilical vein thrombosis.

UMBILICAL CORD KNOTS

TRUE KNOTS OF THE CORD

True knots of the umbilical cord have been associated with long cords, polyhydramnios, intrauterine growth restriction, and monoamniotic twins. The knots may be single or multiple, with increased incidence of congenital anomalies (Figure 52-14). The mortality rate is 8% to 11%. In these cases there is a flattening or dissipation of Wharton's jelly, venous congestion distal to the knot, and vascular thrombi within the cord.

The knot may be formed when a loop of cord is slipped over the infant's head or shoulders during delivery. Usually the

umbilical vessels are protected by Wharton's jelly and are not constricted enough to cause fetal anoxia in this condition.

Color Doppler is useful to record absence of blood flow within the umbilical cord. When Doppler is used to image a false knot, flow is not completely constricted but may appear to show constriction secondary to fetal activity and tension on the cord as the fetus moves.

FALSE KNOTS OF THE CORD

False knots of the umbilical cord are seen when the blood vessels are longer than the cord. Often they are folded on themselves and produce nodulations on the surface of the cord (Figure 52-15).

NUCHAL CORD

Nuchal cord is the most common cord entanglement in the fetus. Multiple coils around the fetal neck have been reported (Figure 52-16).[2] A single loop of cord has been seen in more than 20% of deliveries; two loops have been found in 2.5%. Trouble begins as the fetus descends into the birth canal during delivery and the coils tighten to sufficiently reduce the flow of blood through the cord. Fetal heart deceleration, meconium-stained amniotic fluid, and babies requiring resuscitation are seen more frequently when there is a cord entanglement.

UMBILICAL CORD INSERTION ABNORMALITIES

MARGINAL INSERTION OF THE CORD (BATTLEDORE PLACENTA)

The differential proliferation of placenta villi may result in eccentric insertion of the umbilical cord into the placenta. The cord implants into the edge of the placenta (**battledore placenta**) instead of into the middle of the placenta (Figure 52-17). This is significant when the cord is inserted near the internal os because labor may cause the cord to prolapse or be compressed during contractions. The marginal insertion occurs in 2% to 10% of singleton births, 20% of twins, and 18% of pregnancies with a single umbilical artery.

MEMBRANOUS OR VELAMENTOUS INSERTION OF THE CORD

Membranous or **velamentous insertion of the cord** occurs when the cord inserts into the membranes before it enters the placenta rather than inserting directly into the placenta (Figure 52-18). This condition occurs in 1% of singleton births, 12% of twins, and 9% of pregnancies with a single umbilical artery. There is an increased risk of thrombosis, cord rupture during delivery, or vasa previa.

One theory states that velamentous insertion occurs when most of the placental tissue grows laterally, leaving the initially centrally located cord in an area that becomes atretic. Another theory shows a defect in the implantation of the cord that occurs in the site of the trophoblast in front of the decidua capsularis instead of the area of trophoblast that forms the placental mass. The implantation occurs in the chorion laeve where the umbilical vessels lie on the membranous surface.

Velamentous umbilical cord insertion is associated with higher risk of low birth weight, small for gestational age, preterm delivery, low Apgar scores, and abnormal intrapartum fetal heart rate pattern.

Associated anomalies occur in less than 10% of pregnancies with velamentous insertion of the cord. These anomalies include esophageal atresia, obstructive uropathies, congenital hip dislocation, spina bifida, ventricular septal defect, and cleft palate. There has been an increased risk reported for intrauterine growth restriction and premature birth.

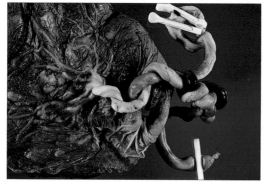

Figure 52-15   Pathologic specimen of a double placenta with a false knot.

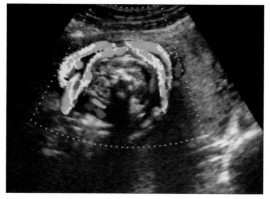

Figure 52-16   Nuchal cord is well demonstrated by color Doppler as it wraps multiple times around the fetal neck.

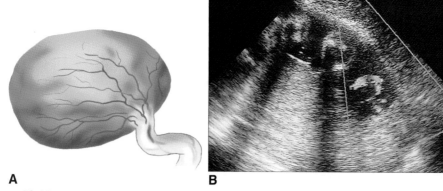

A   **B**

Figure 52-17   **A,** Battledore placenta with insertion of cord at the margin of the placenta. **B,** Color Doppler shows the marginal insertion of the cord into the edge of the placenta instead of into the middle of the placenta.

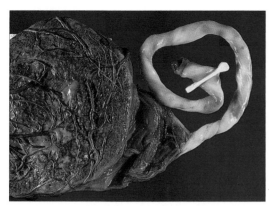

Figure 52-18 Pathologic specimen of the membranous insertion of the cord into the membranes of the placenta.

VASA PREVIA AND PROLAPSE OF THE CORD

Prolapse of the umbilical cord occurs when the cord lies below the presenting part. This condition may exist whenever the presenting part does not fit closely and fails to fill the pelvic inlet; further risk is incurred if the membranes rupture early. Compression of the cord reduces or cuts off the blood supply to the fetus and may result in fetal demise. Abnormal fetal presentation occurs in nearly half of the prolapse cord cases. A slightly higher risk is incurred when the fetus is in a transverse or breech presentation.

Vasa previa is defined as the presence of umbilical cord vessels crossing the internal os of the cervix. The mortality may be high, ranging from 60% to 70% for vaginal delivery and is caused from rupture of the vessels and fetal exsanguination. Color Doppler is the best method of detection in the ultrasound examination. Vasa previa may be due to many factors including velamentous insertion of the cord, succenturiate lobe of the placenta, or low-lying placenta with marginal insertion of the cord near the internal os.

CORD PRESENTATION AND PROLAPSE

Cord presentation and prolapse of the umbilical cord through the cervix into the vagina occurs in 0.5% of deliveries. An occult prolapse occurs when the cord lies alongside the presenting part. The perinatal mortality rate of 25% to 60% is due to cord compression during vaginal delivery. Conditions predisposing to cord presentation and prolapse are as follows:

- Abnormal fetal presentation
- Nonengagement of the fetus because of prematurity
- Long umbilical cord
- Abnormal bony pelvic inlet
- Leiomyomas
- Polyhydramnios
- Vasa previa
- Velamentous insertion of the cord
- Marginal insertion of the cord in a low-lying placenta
- Incompetent cervix with premature rupture of the membranes

PREMATURITY

Two factors contribute to failure of the fetus to fill the pelvic inlet cavity: small presenting part and increased frequency of abnormal presentations in premature labor. Fetal mortality is high in the premature population secondary to birth trauma and anoxia.

MULTIPLE PREGNANCY

Multiple pregnancy factors include failure of adequate adaptation of the presenting part to the pelvis, higher incidence of abnormal presentation, polyhydramnios, and premature rupture of the membranes of the second twin when it is unengaged.

OBSTETRIC PROCEDURES

One third of cord prolapse problems are produced during obstetric procedures:

- Artificial rupture of membranes
- Disengaging the head
- Flexion of an extended head
- Version and extraction

SINGLE UMBILICAL ARTERY

A **single umbilical artery** occurs in 0.08% to 1.9% of singleton births and 3.5% of twin pregnancies; it is more frequent in miscarriages and autopsy series (Figures 52-19 and 52-20). Reports have found single umbilical artery in 18% of pregnancies with marginal insertion of the cord and in 9% with membranous insertion of the cord. The probable cause is atrophy of one of the umbilical arteries in the early development stage. The left umbilical artery is absent a slightly higher percentage of time than the right.

Single umbilical artery has been associated with the following:[1]

- Congenital anomalies in 20% to 50% of cases
- Increased incidence of intrauterine growth restriction (small placenta) (Figure 52-21)
- Increased perinatal mortality
- Increased incidence of chromosomal abnormalities (trisomies 18, 13, and 21; Turner's syndrome; and triploidy)

Infants with single umbilical arteries have associated anomalies that affect other organ systems, such as the following:

- Musculoskeletal (23%)
- Genitourinary (20%)
- Cardiovascular (19%)
- Gastrointestinal (10%)
- Central nervous system (8%)

Multiple studies have investigated normal measurements of the vessels within the umbilical cord. A three-vessel cord showing artery to artery difference of more than 50% was defined as hypoplastic umbilical artery. A study of 100 pregnancies found that between 20 and 36 gestational weeks all pregnancies with a single umbilical artery had a transverse umbilical artery diameter of greater than 4 mm, and all

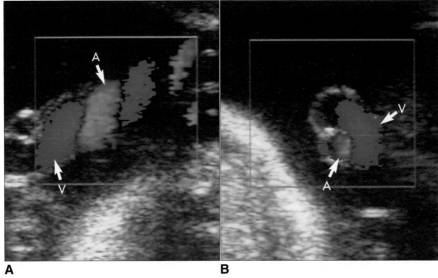

Figure 52-19 Color flow imaging of a single umbilical artery in sagittal **(A)** and transverse **(B)** images. The single umbilical artery *(A, blue)* and umbilical vein *(V, red)* are shown. The fetus had posterior urethral valve syndrome.

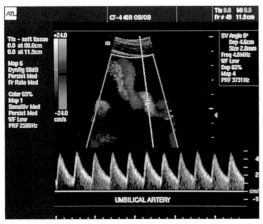

Figure 52-20 Color Doppler shows normal umbilical artery flow in a fetus with a two-vessel cord.

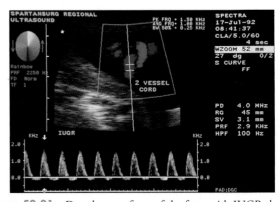

Figure 52-21 Doppler waveform of the fetus with IUGR shows no diastolic flow and prominent systolic flow in the Doppler waveform.

pregnancies with two umbilical arteries had a transverse umbilical arterial diameter of less than 4 mm. In another study the diameter of the umbilical artery was greater than 50% of that of the umbilical vein in the fetus with a single umbilical artery.[3]

The sonographic detection of a single umbilical artery (SUA) should prompt the investigation of further fetal anomalies. The incidence of associated anomalies has been reported to range from 25% to 50%. The major anomalies have included cardiac defects, skeletal abnormalities, abdominal wall defects, diaphragmatic hernia, holoprosencephaly, and hydrocephalus. The diagnosis of an SUA in the second and third trimesters has increased with the routine visualization of the number of vessels within the cord. A characteristic sonographic finding of the two-vessel cord is the disconcordance of the two vessels on cross section. Once the transducer is rotated to record the long axis view, the two-vessel cord appears straight and noncoiled, although occasionally the single artery

may loop around the vein. Visualization with color of the umbilical artery alongside the bladder may be further confirmation that only one artery is present.

Another variation that may be seen is discordant size between the two arterial vessels, with one being more hypoplastic than the other. Discordant blood flow would be seen in the umbilical artery Doppler. The resistive index is almost always higher in the smaller artery, and there may be absent end-diastolic flow.

Variations in the number of umbilical arteries have also been reported. More than three vessels in the cord have been documented in conjoined twins.

VARIX OF THE UMBILICAL VEIN

Aneurysm and varix are focal dilation of the umbilical vessels affecting the umbilical artery and vein, respectively. Focal dilation of the umbilical vein is nearly always intraabdominal, but extrahepatic in location. A varix on sonography appears as a dilated intraabdominal, extrahepatic portion of the umbilical vein. Color Doppler shows continuity with the umbilical vein. Usually the prognosis is a normal outcome in a fetus with a varix of the umbilical vein.

PERSISTENT INTRAHEPATIC RIGHT PORTAL VEIN

Persistence of right portal vein rather than normal left-sided portal vein is called persistent intrahepatic right portal vein. The development of the venous drainage is somewhat complex. At 5 to 6 weeks' gestational age, there are paired umbilical veins that carry blood from the placenta to the primitive heart. The veins join an anastomotic venous network formed by the omphalo-mesenteric veins in the developing liver to establish the umbilical-portal venous connection. By 6 weeks, the right umbilical vein regresses, and the left umbilical vein enlarges to accommodate the increasing flow. The umbilical vein now enters the left portal vein directly. The right umbilical vein usually regresses at 6 weeks' gestation and is not seen by sonography.

Persistence of the right umbilical vein is rare and may be related to an involution of the left umbilical vein. If it persists, the right umbilical vein enters the right lobe of the liver to join the right portal vein. At least 50% of these cases have other fetal anomalies. On sonography, the umbilical vein curves toward the left-sided stomach rather than toward the liver.

REFERENCES

1. Dudiak CM and others: Sonography of the umbilical cord, *Radiographics* 15:1035, 1995.
2. Heinonen S and others: Perinatal diagnostic evaluation of velamentous umbilical cord insertion, *Obstet Gynecol* 87:112, 1996.
3. Sepulveda W and others: Umbilical vein to artery ratio in fetuses with single umbilical artery, *Ultrasound Obstet Gynecol* 8:5, 1996.
4. Weissman A and others: Sonographic measurements of the umbilical cord in pregnancies complicated by gestational diabetes, *J Ultrasound Med* 16:691, 1997.

SELECTED BIBLIOGRAPHY

Bellotti M, Pennati G, DeGasperi C and others: Simultaneous measurements of umbilical venous, fetal hepatic, and ductus venosus blood flow in growth-restricted human fetuses, *Am J Obstet Gynecol* 190(5):1347-1358, 2004.

Bellver J, Lara C, Rossal LP and others: First-trimester reversed end-diastolic flow in the umbilical artery is not always an ominous sign, *Ultrasound Obstet Gynecol* 22(6):652-655, 2003.

Bornemeier S and others: Sonographic evaluation of the two-vessel umbilical cord: a comparison between umbilical arteries adjacent to the bladder and cross sections of the umbilical cord, *J Diag Med Sonogr* 12:260, 1996.

Callen P: *Ultrasonography in obstetrics & gynecology,* ed 3, Philadelphia, 1994, WB Saunders.

Chow JS and others: Frequency and nature of structural anomalies in fetuses with single umbilical arteries, *J Ultrasound Med* 17:765, 1998.

Cromi A, Ghezzi F, Duerig P and others: Sonographic atypical vascular coiling of the umbilical cord, *Prenatal Diagn* 25(1):1-6, 2005.

Ellis JW: Disorders of the placenta, umbilical cord, and amniotic fluid. In Ellis JW, Beckmann CRB, editors: *A clinical manual of obstetrics,* Norwalk, Conn, 1983, Appleton-Century Crofts.

Finberg HJ: Avoiding ambiguity in the sonographic determination of the direction of umbilical cord twists, *J Ultrasound Med* 11:185, 1992.

Fitzgerald MJT and others: *Human embryology,* Philadelphia, 1994, Bailliere Tindall.

Killiedag EB, Killieday H, Bagis T and others: Large pseudocyst of the umbilical cord associated with patent urachus, *J Obstet Gynaecol Res* 30(6):444-447, 2004.

Marino T: Ultrasound abnormalities of the amniotic fluid, membranes, umbilical cord, and placenta, *Obstet Gynecol Clin North Am* 31(1):177-200, 2004.

Moore KL: *Before we are born: basic embryology and birth defects,* ed 3, Philadelphia, 1989, WB Saunders.

Moore KL: *Essentials of human embryology,* Toronto, 1988, BC Decker.

Nyberg DA and others: *Diagnostic ultrasound of fetal anomalies,* St Louis, 1990, Mosby.

Oxorn H: *Human labor & birth,* ed 5, New York, 1986, Appleton Century Crofts.

Oyelese Y, Chavez MR, Yeo L and others: Three-dimensional sonographic diagnosis of vasa previa, *Ultrasound Obstet Gynecol* 24(2):211-215, 2004.

Persutte WH, Lenke RR: Transverse umbilical arterial diameter: technique for the prenatal diagnosis of single umbilical artery, *J Ultrasound Med* 13:763, 1994.

Petrikovsky B and others: Prenatal diagnosis and clinical significance of hypoplastic umbilical artery, *Prenatal Diagn* 16:938, 1996.

Predanic M, Perni SC, Chasen ST, and others: Assessment of umbilical cord coiling during the routine fetal sonographic anatomic survey in the second trimester, *J Ultrasound Med* 24(2):185-191, 2005.

Predanic M, Perni SC, Chasen ST and others: Fetal aneuploidy and umbilical cord thickness measured between 14 and 23 weeks' gestational age, *J Ultrasound Med* 23(9):1177-1183, 2004.

Prucka S, Clemens M, Craven C and others: Single umbilical artery: what does it mean for the fetus? A case-control analysis of pathologically ascertained cases, *Genet Med* 6(1):54-57, 2004.

Raio L, Ghezzi F, Cromi A and others: Sonographic morphology and hyaluronan content of umbilical cords of healthy and Down syndrome fetuses in early gestation, *Early Hum Dev* 77(1-2):1-12, 2004.

Ramon Y, Cajal CL, Martinez RO: Prenatal diagnosis of true knot of the umbilical cord, *Ultrasound Obstet Gynecol* 23(1):99-100, 2004.

Rembouskos G, Cicero S, Longo D and others: Single umbilical artery at 11-14 weeks' gestation: relation to chromosomal defects, *Ultrasound Obstet Gynecol* 22(6):567-570, 2003.

Romero R and others: *Prenatal diagnosis of congenital anomalies,* Norwalk, Conn, 1988, Appleton & Lange.

Sauerbrei EE and others: *A practical guide to ultrasound in obstetrics and gynecology,* ed 2, Philadelphia, 1998, Lippincott Raven.

Viora E, Sciarrone A, Bastonero S and others: Anomalies of the fetal venous system: a report of 26 cases and review of the literature, *Fetal Diagn Ther* 19(5):440-447, 2004.

CHAPTER 53

Amniotic Fluid and Membranes: Polyhydramnios and Oligohydramnios

Sandra L. Hagen-Ansert

KEY TERMS

amniotic band syndrome – multiple fibrous strands of amnion that develop in utero that may entangle fetal parts to cause amputations or malformations of the fetus

amniotic cavity – forms early in gestation and surrounds the embryo; amniotic fluid fills the cavity to protect the embryo and fetus

amniotic fluid – produced by the umbilical cord and membranes, the fetal lung, skin, and kidney

amniotic fluid index (AFI) – the uterus is divided into four quadrants; each "quadrant" is evaluated with the transducer perpendicular to the table in the deepest vertical pocket without fetal parts; the four quadrants are added together to determine the amniotic fluid index

chorion frondosum – the portion of the chorion that develops into the fetal portion of the placenta

keratinization – the process of keratin formation that takes place within the keratinocytes as they progress upward through the layers of the epidermis of skin to the surface stratum corneum.

maximum vertical pocket – another method (used more often in multiple-gestation pregnancy) to determine the amount of amniotic fluid; pocket less than 2 cm may indicate oligohydramnios; greater than 8 cm indicates polyhydramnios

oligohydramnios – too little amniotic fluid; associated with intrauterine growth restriction, renal anomalies, premature rupture of membranes, postdate pregnancy, and other factors

placental insufficiency – inability of placenta to adequately provide adequate blood/nutrient supply to the fetus to underlying maternal disease, such as hypertension or diabetes or caused by extensive placenta abruption

polyhydramnios – too much amniotic fluid; associated with central nervous system disorder, gastrointestinal anomalies, fetal hydrops, skeletal anomalies, renal disorders, and other factors

subjective assessment – sonographer surveys uterine cavity to determine visual assessment of amniotic fluid present

synechiae – scars within the uterus secondary to previous gynecologic surgery.

vernix caseosa – fatty material found on fetal skin and in amniotic fluid late in pregnancy

---

Amniotic fluid plays a vital role in fetal growth and serves several important functions during intrauterine life. **Amniotic fluid** allows the fetus to move freely within the amniotic cavity while maintaining intrauterine temperature and protecting the developing fetus from injury. Abnormalities of the fluid may interfere with the normal fetal development and cause structural abnormalities or may represent an indirect sign of an underlying anomaly, such as neural tube defect or gastrointestinal disorder. This chapter will focus on the production and sonographic patterns of amniotic fluid, the assessment and disorders of amniotic fluid volume, and the use of amniotic fluid volume in the diagnosis of fetal disorders.

DERIVATION AND CHARACTERISTICS OF AMNIOTIC FLUID

The **amniotic cavity** forms early in fetal life and is filled with amniotic fluid that completely surrounds and protects the embryo and later, the fetus. The amnion can be visualized with endovaginal sonography in the early first trimester between 4 and 5 weeks' gestation (Figure 53-1). The membrane appears as a thin membrane separating the amniotic cavity (which contains the fetus) from the extraembryonic coelom and the secondary yolk sac (Figure 53-2).

Amniotic fluid is produced by the umbilical cord, the membranes, lungs, skin, and kidneys. The amount of amniotic fluid present at any one time reflects a balance between amniotic fluid production and amniotic fluid removal. The mechanisms of amniotic fluid production and consumption, and the composition and volume of amniotic fluid, depend on gestational age. Early in gestation, the major source of amniotic fluid is the amniotic membrane, a thin membrane lined by a single layer of epithelial cells. During this stage of development, water crosses the membrane freely, and the production of amniotic fluid is accomplished by active transport of electrolytes and other solutes by the amnion, with passive diffusion of water following in response to osmotic pressure changes.

As the fetus and placenta mature, amniotic fluid production and consumption change to include movement of fluid across the chorion frondosum and fetal skin, fetal urine output and fetal swallowing, and gastrointestinal absorption. The **chorion frondosum,** the portion of the chorion that develops

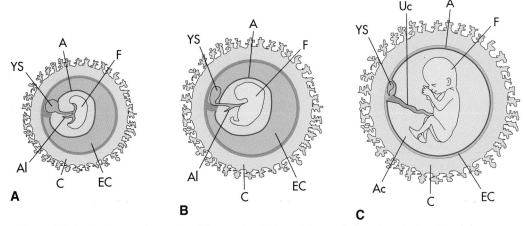

Figure 53-1   **A,** Four-week gestation. The amnion is formed from cells found on the interior of the developing cell mass that is to become the fetus and placenta. *F,* Fetus; *YS,* yolk sac; *C,* chorion; *Al,* allantois; *A,* amnion; *EC,* extraembryonic coelom. **B,** Six-week gestation. **C,** Eight-week gestation. *Ac,* Amniotic cavity; *Uc,* umbilical cord.

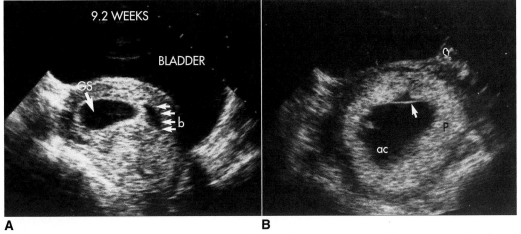

Figure 53-2   **A,** Sagittal scan through the uterine fundus demonstrating a normal-appearing gestational sac *(GS)* at 9.2 weeks with evidence of an implantation bleeding site *(b) (arrows).* **B,** Transverse scan demonstrating the amnion *(arrow)* dividing the amniotic cavity *(ac)* and chorionic cavity. *P,* Placenta.

into the fetal portion of the placenta, is a site where water is exchanged freely between fetal blood and amniotic fluid across the amnion. Fetal skin is also permeable to water and some solutes to permit a direct exchange between the fetus and amniotic fluid until **keratinization** occurs at 24 to 26 weeks.

Fetal production of urine and the ability to swallow begins between 8 and 11 weeks of gestation and becomes the major pathway for amniotic fluid production and consumption. The fetus swallows amniotic fluid, which is absorbed by the digestive tract. The fetus also produces urine, which is passed into the surrounding amniotic fluid. Fetal urination into the amniotic sac accounts for nearly the total volume of amniotic fluid by the second half of pregnancy, so the quantity of fluid is directly related to kidney function. A fetus with malformed kidneys or renal agenesis produces little or no amniotic fluid (Box 53-1).

The amount of amniotic fluid is regulated not only by the production of fluid but also by removal of the fluid by swallowing, by fluid exchange within the lungs, and by the membranes and cord (Figure 53-3). Normal lung development depends critically on the exchange of amniotic fluid within the lungs. Inadequate lung development may occur when severe oligohydramnios is present, placing the fetus at high risk for developing small or hypoplastic lungs.

Amniotic fluid has the following six functions:

1. Acts as a cushion to protect the fetus
2. Allows embryonic and fetal movements
3. Prevents adherence of the amnion to the embryo
4. Allows symmetric growth
5. Maintains a constant temperature
6. Acts as a reservoir to fetal metabolites before their excretion by the maternal system

NORMAL AMNIOTIC FLUID VOLUME

The volume of amniotic fluid increases progressively until about 33 weeks of gestation, with the average increment per week of 25 ml from the 11th to the 15th week and 50 ml from the 15th to 28th week of gestation. In the last trimester, the mean amniotic fluid volume does not change significantly. The sonographer must be aware of the relative differences in amniotic fluid volume throughout pregnancy. During the second and early third trimester of pregnancy, amniotic fluid appears

to surround the fetus and should be readily apparent (Figure 53-4). From 20 to 30 weeks of gestation, amniotic fluid may appear somewhat generous, although this typically represents a normal amniotic fluid variant (Figure 53-5). By the end of pregnancy, the amniotic fluid is scanty, and isolated fluid pockets may be the only visible areas of fluid. Toward the end of the pregnancy, between 38 to 43 weeks of gestation, there is a general decline in the amniotic fluid.

Subjective observation of amniotic fluid volumes throughout pregnancy helps the sonographer determine the norm and extremes of amniotic fluid. The amniotic fluid index aids in estimating the amount of amniotic fluid present in the uterine cavity. The amount of fluid volume correlates with fetal and placental weight. The small-for-age fetus has decreased amniotic fluid; the large-for-age fetus has increased volume of fluid.

Amniotic fluid generally appears echo-free, although occasionally fluid particles (particulate matter) may be seen (see Figure 53-4). **Vernix caseosa** (fatty material found on fetal skin late in pregnancy and in amniotic fluid late in pregnancy) may be seen within the amniotic fluid.

In accordance with the guidelines for obstetric scanning, every obstetric examination should include a thorough evaluation of amniotic fluid volume. When extremes in amniotic fluid volume (hydramnios or oligohydramnios) are found, targeted studies for the exclusion of fetal anomalies are recommended.

ASSESSMENT OF ABNORMAL AMNIOTIC FLUID VOLUME

There are several ways to assess the amount of amniotic fluid throughout the pregnancy. The gold standard for determination of amniotic fluid volume is a dye-dilution technique, which requires amniocentesis, instillation of a dye, and then repeat measurement of the dye after diffusion throughout the

---

> **BOX 53-1 AMNIOTIC FLUID VOLUME REGULATION**
>
> - Amniotic fluid volume increases rapidly during first trimester
> - Fetus swallows fluid; reabsorbed by gastrointestinal tract; recirculates through kidneys
> - Increased amniotic fluid production in first trimester
> - By 20 weeks' gestation, amniotic fluid volume increases by 10 ml/day
> - Amount of fluid produced by fetal urination slightly exceeds amount removed by fetal swallowing; >40% of fluid increase originates from other sources

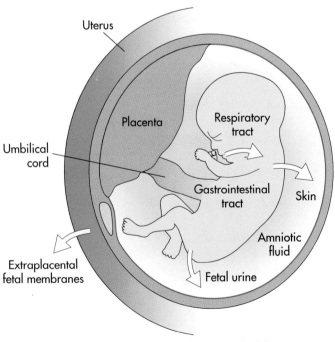

Figure 53-3 Schematic drawing of amniotic fluid formation.

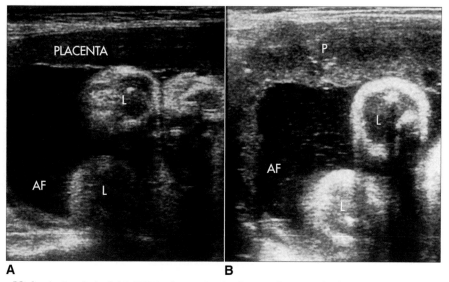

Figure 53-4 **A,** Amniotic fluid *(AF)* in the uterine fundus revealing an echo-free fluid appearance. *L,* limbs. **B,** At 38 weeks of gestation, the amniotic fluid is mixed with particulate matter or vernix. *P,* Placenta.

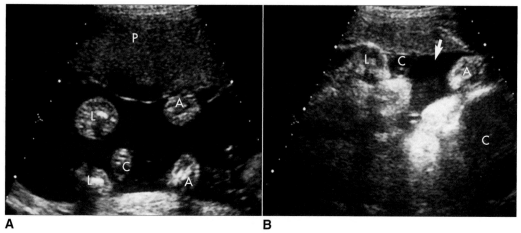

Figure 53-5 **A,** Amniotic fluid in a 20-week pregnancy outlining the legs *(L)* and arms *(A)*. This is a typical appearance of the abundance of amniotic fluid during this period of pregnancy. *C,* Umbilical cord; *P,* placenta. **B,** Amniotic fluid *(arrow)* in a 35-week pregnancy demonstrating an amniotic fluid pocket *(arrow)* surrounded by fetal parts and the placenta. The amount of amniotic fluid compared with the fetus and placenta is less at this stage of pregnancy. *A,* Arms; *C,* cranium; *L,* legs.

amniotic fluid. This method is not practical to use on a routine clinical basis and therefore other methods have been developed. These methods include both subjective and semiquantitative measurements. This assessment of fluid volume becomes important in the second and third trimesters to help determine fetal well-being. Fluid may be classified as normal, polyhydramnios, or oligohydramnios. There are several methods to achieve this measurement, including the subjective visual assessment, the semiquantitative four-quadrant assessment, and measurement of the single deepest pocket of fluid.

Subjective Assessment. Subjective assessment is performed as the sonographer initially scans "through" the entire uterus to determine the visual "eye-ball" assessment of the fluid present, the lie of the fetus, and the position of the placenta

(Figure 53-6). When amniotic fluid is assessed subjectively, decreased amniotic fluid is identified by an overall sense of crowding of the fetus and obvious lack of amniotic fluid and/or inability to identify any significant pockets of fluid in any sector of the uterus. Excessive fluid is defined subjectively when there is an obvious excess of fluid and when a transverse sonogram done at various levels of the uterine cavity identifies a fluid pocket in which one can comfortably place a cross section of the fetal trunk.

This subjective assessment is more successful in the hands of experienced sonographers than in the hands of a beginner. Generally this method will lead the sonographer to perform a more semiquantitative method to document the amniotic fluid volume. A more definitive determination of amniotic fluid volume comes with the four-quadrant method.

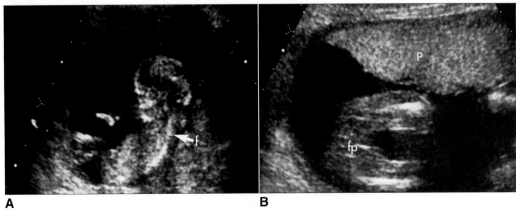

A   **B**

Figure 53-6   **A,** Amniotic fluid around a 13-week fetus in a sitting position. Note the hand in front of the fetal chest. Amniotic fluid appears in black. *f,* Fetus. **B,** Amniotic fluid around an 18-week fetus. The fetus appears to be surrounded by amniotic fluid (black areas). *P,* Placenta; *fp,* fetal pelvis.

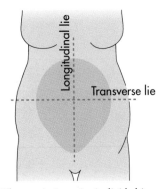

Figure 53-7   The amniotic cavity is divided into quadrants by two imaginary lines perpendicular to each other. The largest pocket of fluid is measured in each quadrant.

Four-Quadrant Assessment. This method is used most frequently for evaluating and quantifying amniotic fluid volume at different intervals during a pregnancy. With this method, the uterine cavity is divided into four equal quadrants by two imaginary lines perpendicular to each other (Figure 53-7). The largest vertical pocket of amniotic fluid, excluding fetal limbs or umbilical cord loops, is measured. The sum of the four quadrants is called the **amniotic fluid index (AFI).**

Normal values have been calculated for each gestational age (plus or minus 2 standard deviations). The values are relatively stable after 20 weeks until the end of the third trimester. Subjective assessment of normal amniotic fluid correlates with AFI of 10 to 20 cm; borderline values of 5 to 10 cm indicate low fluid; and values of 20 to 24 cm indicate increased fluid (Figure 53-8). The AFI peaks late in the third trimester of pregnancy, with a rapid decline near term. Oligohydramnios correlates with an AFI of less than 5 cm with the largest vertical pocket measuring 2 cm or less, while polyhydramnios correlates with an AFI of greater than 24 cm and the largest vertical pocket of 8 cm or more.

The sonographer must be careful to hold the transducer perpendicular to the table (not the curved skin surface) when determining these pockets of fluid. Also, care must be taken not to include the thickness of the maternal uterine wall in the measurement. As the gain is adjusted slightly, the uterine wall may be determined. Also the use of color helps the sonographer separate the umbilical cord loops from areas within the pockets of fluid. The transducer should be moved until the cord loops and/or fetal limbs are not within the pocket.

Single Pocket Assessment. Clinicians have described other criteria to define the presence of abnormal fluid volumes (Figure 53-9). The **maximum vertical pocket** (i.e., fluid should measure greater than 1 cm "rule") assessment of amniotic fluid is done by identifying the largest pocket of amniotic fluid (Figure 53-10). The depth of the pocket is measured at right angles to the uterine contour and placed into three categories: (1) less than 2 cm, indicating oligohydramnios; (2) 2 to 8 cm, indicating normal amniotic fluid; and (3) greater than 8 cm, indicating polyhydramnios. As a general rule, the approximation of the AFI may be determined by multiplying the largest pocket of amniotic fluid times three.

The two-diameter pocket determination uses the largest pocket of amniotic fluid. The horizontal and vertical dimensions of the maximum vertical pocket are multiplied together to obtain a single volume. A two-diameter pocket of 15 cm to 50 cm is considered normal.

Three-Dimensional Determination. The clinical usefulness of three-dimensional ultrasound offers a promise of more accurately quantifying the volume of amniotic fluid. The ability to obtain precise measurements of amniotic fluid volume minus the fetal volume continues to be a challenge for sonographers in obstetrical sonography.

The Preferred Method. Of all the techniques used to assess amniotic fluid volumes, the AFI is the only technique that is both valid and reproducible. The AFI is very helpful in a busy laboratory where multiple sonographers evaluate patients and may have varying subjective opinions of what normal, decreased, or increased amniotic fluid looks like.

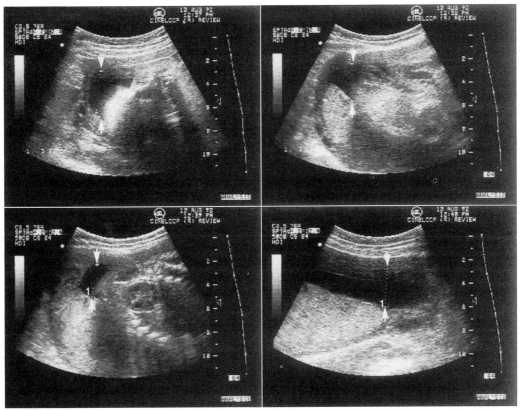

Figure 53-8 The four-quadrant technique of amniotic fluid assessment. This technique produces an amniotic fluid index (AFI). The uterus is divided into four equal parts, and the largest vertical pocket of amniotic fluid in each quadrant is measured, excluding fetal limbs or umbilical cord. The sum of the four quadrants is the AFI, which equals 14.2 cm at 31 weeks. This is within normal limits.

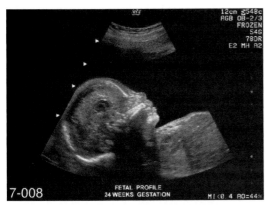

Figure 53-9 Longitudinal view of the fetal profile at 24 weeks of gestation. The amniotic fluid enables the facial detail to be well imaged. A single vertical pocket is measured perpendicular to the floor.

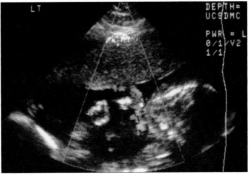

Figure 53-10 The sonographer must use color Doppler to make sure the umbilical cord is not in the way when making a single vertical measurement.

Amniotic fluid volume should be one component of a composite of fetal assessment techniques, including measurements such as fetal abdominal trunk circumferences, Doppler flow studies, and other fetal biophysical activities.

Amniotic Fluid in Twin Pregnancies. In twin pregnancies, it is important to assess each sac independently when per-

forming amniotic fluid determinations. Twin pregnancies have a slightly lower median AFI value than singleton pregnancies. The two-dimensional pocket measurement appears to be a better predictor of oligohydramnios than the AFI or the largest vertical pocket.

ABNORMAL AMNIOTIC FLUID VOLUME

Abnormal volumes of amniotic fluid may suggest that the fetus has a congenital anomaly. Amniotic fluid volume should be assessed to detect abnormally increased (polyhydramnios) or decreased (oligohydramnios) amniotic fluid volumes.

Polyhydramnios. Polyhydramnios (also known as *hydramnios*) is defined as an amniotic fluid volume of greater than 2000 ml. The incidence of polyhydramnios in pregnancy is found to range from 0.4% to 3.3%. In addition, the finding of polyhydramnios is associated with increased perinatal mortality and morbidity and maternal complications. By clinical definition, polyhydramnios is an excessive amount of fluid that causes the uterine size to be larger than expected for gestational dates. Often the patient will come for an ultrasound with the clinical finding of uterus larger than dates (rule out multiple gestation, molar pregnancy, or fetal size greater than dates).

Cause of polyhydramnios. The amniotic fluid compartment is in a dynamic equilibrium with the fetal and maternal compartments. In polyhydramnios the equilibrium shifts so that the net transfer of water is into the amniotic space. Many factors are involved in the regulation of amniotic fluid volume (e.g., swallowing, urination, uterine-placental blood flow, fetal respiratory movements, and fetal membrane physiology).

Polyhydramnios is often associated with central nervous system disorders and/or gastrointestinal problems. Central nervous system disorders cause depressed swallowing. With gastrointestinal abnormalities, often a blockage (atresia) of the esophagus, stomach, duodenum, or small bowel results in ineffective swallowing. Fetal hydrops, skeletal anomalies, and some renal disorders (usually unilateral) may also be associated with hydramnios. Many congenital anomalies are found in association with hydramnios (Box 53-2).

Increased amniotic fluid volume produces uterine stretching and enlargement that may lead to preterm labor and various other maternal symptoms. In addition, the acute onset of hydramnios may be painful, compress other organs or vascular structures, cause hydronephrosis of the kidneys, or produce shortness of breath from compression of the organs on the diaphragm.

Often polyhydramnios may be diagnosed sonographically before it is clinically suspected. Chronic hydramnios characteristically develops between the 28th week of gestation and term. Acute polyhydramnios may develop over a few days or chronically over weeks. Acute polyhydramnios occurs in the second trimester and accounts for only 2% of the cases. Usually the cause of acute polyhydramnios is twin–twin transfusion syndrome; however, other congenital anomalies may be responsible. Other forms of polyhydramnios that cannot be explained by congenital anomalies are considered idiopathic.

Once polyhydramnios has been diagnosed, the prognosis for pregnancy is guarded. There is an increased perinatal mortality and morbidity, as well as an increased maternal morbidity and mortality. The mother has an increased risk of developing pregnancy-induced hypertension, preterm labor, or postpartum hemorrhage. Other conditions associated with increased amniotic fluid volume include maternal diabetes mellitus, fetal macrosomia, and Rh isoimmunization. Diabetes mellitus is associated with an increased frequency of hydramnios and rep-resents the most common maternal cause of elevated amniotic fluid volume, especially when poorly controlled.

Sonographic Findings. Serial sonographic examinations are indicated to monitor the progression of amniotic fluid. Since amniotic fluid production is a dynamic process, changing maternal, fetal, or placenta conditions may dramatically affect the volume index.

The visual criteria for polyhydramnios includes an obvious discrepancy between the size of the fetus, size of the uterus, and the amount of amniotic fluid. During the second trimester, the amniotic fluid completely surrounds the fetus; however, as the pregnancy progresses, the fetal parts consume the majority of the uterine space and therefore the amount of amniotic fluid appears to be less than in the first and second trimesters (Figure 53-11). Serial scans may be necessary when the amniotic fluid appears to be more generous than normal at a particular gestational age.

A semiquantitative assessment may be done with the single pocket measurement or with the determination of the amniotic fluid index. Polyhydramnios may be further defined as mild when the single largest pocket is greater than 8 cm; moderate, greater than 12 cm; and severe, greater than 16 cm. The AFI index may also be further qualified as mild polyhydramnios, greater than 20 cm; moderate, greater than 24 cm; and severe, greater than 25 cm.

Sonographic signs of polyhydramnios are as follows:

- Appearance of a freely floating fetus within the swollen amniotic cavity (the fetus commonly will be seen lying on his or her back, freely moving in the amniotic fluid)
- Accentuated fetal anatomy as increased amniotic fluid improves image resolution
- AFI equal to or greater than 20 cm

Oligohydramnios. Oligohydramnios is an overall reduction in the amount of amniotic fluid resulting in fetal crowding and decreased fetal movement. The incidence of oligohydramnios is estimated to be between 0.5% to 5.5% of all pregnancies, depending on the population tested and the criteria used for diagnosis. Criteria for oligohydramnios are based on subjective experience and estimations of the AFI. Oligohydramnios may be defined as a single pocket of fluid with a depth of less than 2 cm or an AFI of less than 5 cm. A gray zone for decreased fluid ranges from 5 to 9 cm when a four-quadrant approach is used.

Cause of oligohydramnios. The development of oligohydramnios may be attributed to one of five causes: congenital anomalies, intrauterine growth restriction, postterm pregnancies, ruptured membranes, and iatrogenesis. Causes of oligohydramnios are outlined in Box 53-3. Second-trimester oligohydramnios is associated with a poor prognosis, especially if maternal serum alpha-fetoprotein level is concurrently elevated.

Fetal anomalies associated with oligohydramnios. The prevalence of congenital anomalies in the fetus with oligohydramnios is based on the size of the high-risk population. Oligohydramnios has also been associated with fetal renal anomalies (i.e., renal agenesis, bladder outlet obstruction,

BOX 53-2 CONGENITAL ANOMALIES ASSOCIATED WITH POLYHYDRAMNIOS

GASTROINTESTINAL SYSTEM
Esophageal atresia and/or tracheoesophageal fistula
Duodenal atresia
Jejunoileal atresia
Gastroschisis
Omphalocele
Diaphragmatic hernia
Meckel's diverticulum
Congenital megacolon
Meconium peritonitis
Annular pancreas
Pancreatic cyst

HEAD AND NECK
Cystic hygroma
Goiter
Cleft palate
Epignathus

RESPIRATORY SYSTEM
Cystic adenomatoid malformation
Congenital hydrothorax
Extralobar sequestration
Primary pulmonary hypoplasia
Congenital pulmonary lymphangiectasia
Pulmonary cyst
Asphyxiating thoracic dystrophy

CARDIOVASCULAR SYSTEM
Arrhythmias
Coarctation of the aorta
Myxomas and hemangiomas
Ectopia cordis
Cardiac tumors
Heart anomalies with hydrops

CENTRAL NERVOUS SYSTEM
Anencephaly
Hydrocephaly
Microcephaly
Iniencephaly
Hydranencephaly
Holoprosencephaly
Encephalocele
Spina bifida
Dandy-Walker malformation

GENITOURINARY SYSTEM
Ureteropelvic junction obstruction
Posterior urethral valves
Urethral stenosis
Multicystic kidney disease
Large ovarian cyst
Mesoblastic nephroma
Bartter syndrome
Megacystis microcolon hypoperistalsis syndrome

SKELETAL SYSTEM
Thanatophoric dwarf
Camptomelic dwarf
Osteogenesis imperfecta
Heterozygous achondroplasia
Arthrogryposis multiplex
Klippel-Feil syndrome
Nager acrofacial dysostosis
Achondrogenesis

CONGENITAL INFECTIONS
Cytomegalovirus
Toxoplasmosis
Listeriosis
Congenital hepatitis

MISCELLANEOUS
Sacrococcygeal teratoma
Cranial teratoma
Cervical teratoma
Congenital sarcoma
Placental chorioangioma
Cavernous hemangioma
Metastatic neuroblastoma
Myotonic dystrophy
Fetal acetaminophen toxicity
Retroperitoneal fibrosis
Multisystem anomalies
Pena-Shokeir syndrome
Cutaneous vascular hemarthrosis
Twin reversed arterial perfusion sequence/acardiac anomaly

From Nyberg DA, Mahony BS, Pretorius DH: *Diagnostic ultrasound of fetal anomalies: text and atlas,* St Louis, 1990, Mosby.

multicystic dysplastic kidneys, and infantile polycystic kidney disease). Oligohydramnios may cause fetal deformations, such as clubbing of the hands or feet, pulmonary hypoplasia, hip displacement, and phenotypical features of Potter's sequence. Other congenital malformations associated with oligohydramnios include central nervous system disorders, skeletal anomalies, and cardiovascular anomalies.

Intrauterine growth restriction. The association between intrauterine growth restriction (IUGR) and decreased amniotic fluid (oligohydramnios) is well recognized. Fetal hypox-emia may produce growth restriction and oligohydramnios. There is a fourfold increased risk of growth delay when oligo-hydramnios is present. Doppler evaluation of the growth-restricted fetus shows abnormal umbilical flow in patients with oligohydramnios. **Placental insufficiency** may cause IUGR associated with oligohydramnios. The placental insufficiency produces a redistribution of fetal blood flow away from the kidneys and toward the brain to counterattack the hypoxia. This results in decreased urine output, which decreases fluid volume.

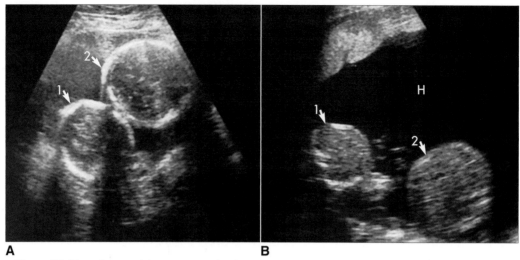

A   B

Figure 53-11   Ultrasound demonstrating the discordant growth of twins in the case of a twin–twin transfusion syndrome. **A,** The difference in the size of the heads of the twins *(1, 2)*. **B,** The difference in the size of the abdominal circumferences *(1, 2)*. *H,* Hydramnios.

Postterm pregnancies. The postterm pregnancy is defined as a gestational age of 42 weeks or more. Oligohydramnios is a common complication of postdate pregnancies (remember the decrease in amniotic fluid production near the end of pregnancy), and it is associated with diminished placental function. It is also associated with arterial redistribution of fetal blood flow with the brain-sparing effect.

Ruptured membranes. Premature rupture of the membranes occurs in approximately 10% of all pregnancies. Oligohydramnios may be observed as a consequence of first-trimester chorionic villus sampling. Persistent oligohydramnios in the second trimester carries a poor prognosis regardless of the cause. Severe oligohydramnios with a single pocket measurement of less than 1 cm lasting 14 days after a spontaneous premature rupture of the membranes at less than 25 weeks' gestation is associated with an extremely high mortality rate.

Iatrogenic causes. Iatrogenic causes of oligohydramnios include medications, insensible fluid loss, maternal intravas-

cular fluid depletion, and prior procedures such as chorionic villus sampling. Medications associated with oligohydramnios include nonsteroidal antiinflammatory drugs, angiotensin-converting enzyme inhibitors, calcium channel blockers, and nitrous oxide. The nonsteroidal drugs are prostaglandin synthetase inhibitors that inhibit renal vascular flow and decrease glomerular filtration. The angiotensin-converting enzyme inhibitors reduce fetal blood pressure and decrease renal perfusion.

Prognosis. The development of oligohydramnios may cause potential complications, such as fetal demise, pulmonary hypoplasia, and various skeletal and facial deformities from the compression of the fetus on the uterine wall. The fetus that presents with oligohydramnios in the second trimester has a higher prevalence of structural malformations than the fetus that presents in the third trimester.

Maternal hydration has been shown to improve amniotic fluid for patients with oligohydramnios and in women with normal amniotic fluid volumes. If fetal anomalies or premature ruptured membranes are present, maternal hydration will have little effect. A study was performed to see if maternal hydration would increase the AFI in women with low AFIs. The control group was instructed to drink their normal amount of fluid; the hydration group was instructed to drink 2 L of water in addition to their usual amount of fluid 2 to 4 hours before the posttreatment AFI was determined. The mean posttreatment AFI was significantly greater in the hydration group. The findings suggested that maternal oral hydration increased the amniotic fluid volume in women with decreased fluid levels.

Sonographic Findings. Poor scanning resolution is common in pregnancies complicated by oligohydramnios, and limited anatomy surveys are expected (Figure 53-12). If the intrauterine membranes are not ruptured and oligohydramnios is present before 28 weeks of gestation, careful evaluation of the fetal renal system should be made by the

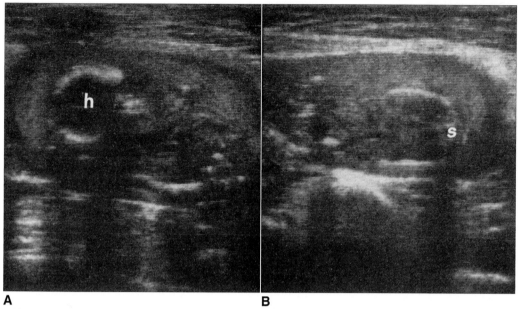

Figure 53-12   Premature rupture of membranes at 16 weeks of gestation with marked oligohydramnios. *h,* Head; *s,* spine.

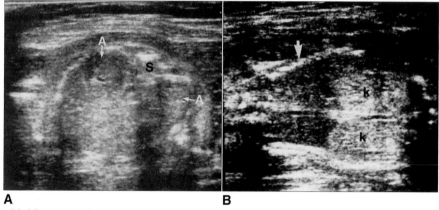

Figure 53-13   **A,** Renal agenesis in a 29-week fetus showing enlarged adrenal glands *(A)* occupying the renal spaces. Oligohydramnios and an absent bladder confirmed the diagnosis. *S,* Spine. **B,** Infantile polycystic kidney disease shown with enlarged and dense kidneys *(k).* Note the enhanced transmission of sound through the kidneys because of the dilated cystic tubules. Oligohydramnios and absent bladder were coexisting findings.

sonographer to rule out renal agenesis, infantile polycystic disease, or posterior urethral valve syndrome (Figure 53-13). If the oligohydramnios is severe in a fetus with posterior urethral valves, the prognosis is not good (Figure 53-14). Identification of the renal area may be difficult to assess in the presence of severe oligohydramnios, and the use of color Doppler to demarcate the renal arteries may be helpful for the sonographer to determine if the kidneys are present or not.

Evaluation of the blood flow in the umbilical cord, the placenta, and the cerebral vascular system with color and Doppler techniques is critical to determine the presence or absence of intrauterine growth retardation.

In the presence of oligohydramnios, care should be taken when evaluating the fetal growth parameters because the fetal head and abdomen can be compressed when the fluid level is low. Because the fetus lacks the surrounding fluid protecting it, the circumferences can actually be inaccurately measured by increased transducer pressure on the maternal abdomen. This pressure, in turn, may alter the estimated fetal weight by erroneous measurements. On the other hand, prolonged severe oligohydramnios may cause fetal anomalies secondary to pressure on the fetus by the uterine wall. Such anomalies include pulmonary hypoplasia, abnormal facial features, and abnormal limb development.

When oligohydramnios is suspected, the sonographer should also examine the fetus with endovaginal sonography to better define fetal anatomy in efforts to detect the anomaly causing the oligohydramnios.

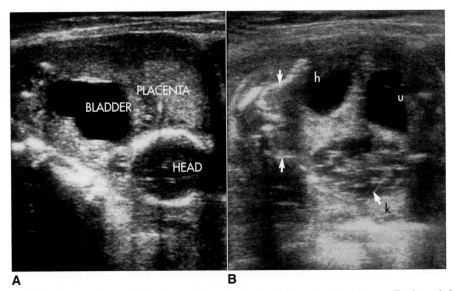

Figure 53-14 **A,** Posterior urethral valve syndrome in a 17-week fetus showing abnormally distended bladder with a keyhole urethra. Note the significant lack of amniotic fluid. **B,** In the same fetus at 21 weeks of gestation, a small thoracic cavity *(arrows)*, hydronephrosis *(h)*, hydroureter *(u)*, and enlargement and mild hydronephrosis of the contralateral kidney *(k)* are noted.

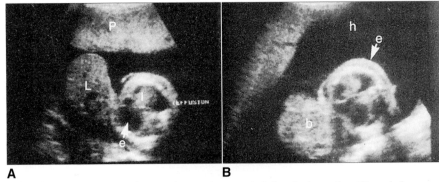

Figure 53-15 **A** and **B,** Gastroschisis with secondary amniotic bands shown in a 28-week fetus. Eviscerated liver *(L)* and bowel *(b)* are documented. Bilateral pleural effusions *(arrows)* and soft tissue edema *(e)* in **B** are apparent. Note the hydramnios *(h)*. *l,* Lung; *P,* placenta.

Cord compression by the fetus is another potential cause for fetal asphyxia leading to oligohydramnios. Often the sonographer may see signs of mild cord compression throughout the routine scan, with cardiac decompensation or changes in Doppler flow patterns. Slight rotations of the mother during the examination may stimulate the fetus to roll away from the cord, restoring blood flow. If this cord compression becomes a chronic problem, fetal well-being may be affected.

AMNIOTIC BAND SYNDROME

The **amniotic band syndrome** is a common, nonrecurrent cause of various fetal malformations involving the limbs, craniofacial region, and trunk. Various congenital malformation syndromes are thought to be caused by compression of the fetus by "amniotic bands," which results in developmental abnormalities or fetal death. Amniotic band syndrome may represent a milder form of limb-body wall complex and may be predicted by amniotic bands (fibrous tissue strands) that

entangle or amputate fetal parts (Figures 53-15 to 53-17). Facial clefts, asymmetric encephaloceles, constriction or amputation defects of the extremities, and clubfoot deformities are common findings.

The site where the amniotic band cuts across the fetus is usually evident after birth. The most widely accepted theory for the formation of amniotic bands is that rupture of the amnion leads to subsequent entanglement of various embryonic or fetal parts by fibrous mesodermic bands, which emanate from the chorionic side of the amnion. Entrapment of fetal parts by the bands may cause lymphedema, amputations, or slash defects in nonembryologic distributions. The amnion, which is contiguous with the fetal skin at the umbilicus, is thought to protect the fetus from contact with the chorion. When disruption of the amnion occurs, the fetus may adhere to and fuse with the chorion, with subsequent maldevelopment of the subjacent fetal tissue. This theory suggests that when gastroschisis results in exteriorization of

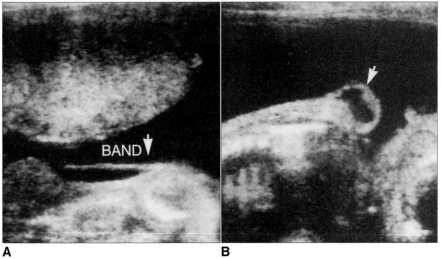

A   **B**

Figure 53-16   In the fetus depicted in Figure 53-15, multiple amniotic bands (**A,** *band*) were found adhering to the abdomen, with attachment to the shoulder (**B,** *arrow*). Normal chromosomes were found by amniocentesis. Amniotic fluid alpha-fetoprotein was extremely elevated (175 MOM) with positive acetylcholinesterase. The fetus was delivered at 28 weeks of gestation because of worsening hydrops. No resuscitative measures were undertaken. Autopsy findings revealed a right paraumbilical gastroschisis with eventration of the liver and intestine. Intestinal malrotation and small bowel obstruction were found. Moderate fetal hydrops with bilateral pleural effusions and pulmonary hypoplasia were noted. An amniotic band or peritoneal band extended from the liver to the thumb. The defect was consistent with a gastroschisis occurring early in embryogenesis because of the intestinal malrotation with secondary amniotic band rupture.

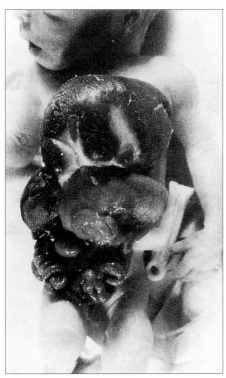

Figure 53-17   The neonate shown in Figures 53-15 and 53-16 with gastroschisis and secondary amniotic band rupture.

the liver, the amniotic band syndrome should be strongly considered.

   Sonographic Findings. The sonographer may observe these bands as the real-time obstetric study is performed to observe where the band is attached to the uterine wall and what, if any, constriction is placed on the fetus. Careful observation with real-time scanning will allow the sonographer to observe if the fetus is free from the band or if movement is restricted. Uterine sheets (synechiae) should not be confused with amniotic bands.

AMNIOTIC SHEETS AND SYNECHIAE

Amniotic sheets are believed to be caused by uterine scars, or **synechiae,** from previous instrumentation used in the uterus (usually curettage), cesarean section, or episodes of endometritis. When a pregnancy begins to grow in the uterine cavity, the expanding membranes encounter the scar and wrap around it. The flat portion of the sheet consists of apposed layers of chorion and amnion. The free edge of the sheet is defined by the course of the synechia itself, which may produce a bulbous appearance. Amniotic sheets arise because of redundant amnion-chorion, which may in turn be related to bleeding and subchorionic hemorrhages.

   Sonographic Findings. Sonographic findings in patients with amniotic sheets may show a fine echo-dense line in the uterine cavity separated from the uterine wall by an echolucent space. The membrane may completely surround the fetus, or the membrane may be freely mobile in the amniotic cavity. Amniotic sheets do not place the fetus at risk for destructive structural malformations.

Amniotic sheets are present in 0.6% of patients having screening obstetric ultrasound examinations. Care should be taken to separate the diagnosis of amniotic sheets from amniotic bands or the circumvallate placenta. In the circumvallate placenta, the chorion and attached amnion form a raised ridge of tissue at the junction of the chorion and the basal plate. Beyond this ridge the normal vessels on the fetal surface are absent; after delivery, these redundant membranes are described as being adherent to the fetal surface rather than projecting from it.

Both the circumvallate placenta and amniotic sheets appear as a thick membrane projecting into the amniotic fluid. Circumvallate placental membranes originate from the edge of the fetal surface of the placenta, whereas amniotic sheets attach to the uterine wall itself.

SELECTED BIBLIOGRAPHY

Ball RH, Buchmeier SE, Longnecker M: Clinical significance of sonographically detected uterine synechiae in pregnant patients, *J Ultrasound Med* 16:465, 1997.

Banks EH, Miller DA: Perinatal risks associated with borderline amniotic fluid index, *Am J Obstet Gynceol* 180:1461-1463, 1999.

Bianco A, Rosen T, Kucznski E and others: Measurement of the amniotic fluid index with and without colon Doppler, *J Perinat Med* 27:245-249, 1999.

Blakelock R, Upadhyay V, Kimble R and others: Is a normally functioning gastrointestinal tract necessary for normal growth in late gestation? *Pediatr Surg Int* 13:17-20, 1998.

Borgida AF, Mills A, Feldman DM and others: Outcome of pregnancies complicated by ruptured membranes after genetic amniocentesis, *Am J Obstet Gynecol* 183:937-939, 2000.

Brace RA: Physiology of amniotic fluid volume regulation, *Clin Obstet Gynecol* 40:280-289, 1997.

Croom CS, Banias BB, Ramos-Santos E: Do semiquantitative amniotic fluid indexes reflect actual volume? *Am J Obstet Gynecol* 167:995-999, 1992.

Dildy GA, Lira N, Noise JF Jr and others: Amniotic fluid volume assessment: comparison of ultrasonographic estimates versus direct measurements with a dye-dilution technique in human pregnancy, *Am J Obstet Gynecol* 167:986-994, 1992.

Elias S, Simpson JL, editors: *Maternal serum screening for fetal genetic disorders,* New York, 1992, Churchill Livingstone.

Gramellini D, Chiaie D, Piantelli G and others: Sonographic assessment of amniotic fluid volume between 11 and 24 weeks of gestation: construction of reference intervals related to gestational age, *Ultrasound Obstet Gynecol* 17:410-415, 2001.

Grover J, Mentakis A, Ross MG: Three-dimensional method for determination of amniotic fluid volume in intrauterine pockets, *Obstet Gynecol* 90:1007-1010, 1997.

Hill LM, Krohn M, Lazebnik N and others: The amniotic fluid index in normal twin pregnancies, *Am J Obstet Gynecol* 182:950-954, 2000.

Hill LM, Lazebnik N, Many A: Effect of indomethacin on individual amniotic fluid indices in multiple gestations, *J Ultrasound Med* 15:395-399, 1996.

Horsager R, Nathan I, Leveno KJ: Correlation of measured amniotic fluid volume and sonographic predictions of oligohydramnios, *Obstet Gynecol* 83:955-958, 1994.

Hsich TT, Hung TH, Chen KC and others: Perinatal outcome of oligohydramnios without associated premature rupture of membranes and fetal anomalies, *Gynecol Obstet Invest* 45:232-236, 1998.

Kilpatrick SJ and others: Maternal hydration increases amniotic fluid index, *Obstet Gynecol* 78:1098, 1991.

Magann EF, Nolan TE, Hess LW and others: Measurement of amniotic fluid volume: accuracy of ultrasonography technique, *Am J Obstet Gynecol* 167:1533-1537, 1992.

Magann EF, Martin JN Jr: Amniotic fluid assessment in singleton and twin pregnancies, *Obstet Gynecol Clin North Am* 26:579-593, 1999.

Magann EF, Chauhan SP, Whitworth NS and others: Determination of amniotic fluid volume in twin pregnancies: ultrasonographic evaluation versus operator estimation, *Am J Obstet Gynecol* 182:1606-1609, 2000.

Magann EF, Sanderson M, Martin JN and others: The amniotic fluid index, single deepest pocket, and two-diameter pocket in normal human pregnancy, *Am J Obstet Gynceol* 182:1581-1588, 2000.

Mahony BS and others: The amniotic band syndrome: antenatal sonographic diagnosis and potential pitfalls, *Obstet Gynecol* 152:63, 1985.

Manning FA, Harman CR, Morrison I and others: Fetal assessment based on fetal biophysical profile scoring IV. An analysis of perinatal morbidity and mortality, *Am J Obstet Gynecol* 162:703-709, 1990.

Moore KL, editor: *The developing human: clinically oriented embryology,* ed 4, Philadelphia, 1988, WB Saunders.

Moore TR, Cayle JE: The amniotic fluid index in normal human pregnancy, *Am J Obstet Gynceol* 162:1168-1173, 1990.

Nyberg DA, McGahan JP, Pretorius DH, editors: *Diagnostic ultrasound of fetal anomalies,* Philadelphia, 2003, Lippincott, Williams & Wilkins.

Peipert JF, Donnenfeld AE: Oligohydramnios: a review, *Obstet Gynecol Surv* 46:325, 1991.

Phelan JP and others: Amniotic fluid volume assessment with the four-quadrant technique at 36-42 weeks' gestation, *J Reprod Med* 32:540, 1987.

Potter EL: Bilateral absence of ureters and kidneys: a report of 50 cases, *Obstet Gynecol* 25:3, 1965.

Seeds JW, Cefalo RC, Herbert WN: Amniotic band syndrome, *Am J Obstet Gynecol* 144:243, 1982.

Selam B, Koksal R, Ozcan T: Fetal arterial and venous Doppler parameters in the interpretation of oligohydramnios in post-term pregnancies, *Ultrasound Obstet Gynecol* 15:403-406, 2000.

Sistrom CL, Ferguson JE: Abnormal membranes in obstetrical ultrasound: incidence and significance of amniotic sheets and circumvallate placenta, *Ultrasound Obstet Gynecol* 3:249, 1993.

Thompson O, Brown R, Gunnarson G and others: Prevalence of polyhydramnios in the third trimester in a population screened by first and second trimester ultrasonography, *J Perinat Med* 26:371-377, 1998.

Torpin R: *Fetal malformations caused by amnion rupture during gestation,* Springfield, Ill, 1968, Charles C Thomas.

Weissman A, Itskovitz-Eldor J, Jakobi P: Sonographic measurement of amniotic fluid volume in the first trimester of pregnancy, *J Ultrasound Med* 15:771-774, 1996.

Williams K: Amniotic fluid assessment, *Obstet Gynecol Surv* 48:795, 1993.

CHAPTER 54

The Fetal Face and Neck

Diana M. Strickland and Sandra L. Hagen-Ansert

KEY TERMS

anophthalmia – absent eyes

arhinia – absence of the nose

Beckwith-Wiedemann syndrome – group of disorders having in common the coexistence of an omphalocele, macroglossia, and visceromegaly

branchial cleft cyst – a cystic defect that arises from the primitive branchial apparatus

cephalocele – protrusion of the brain from the cranial cavity

craniosynostoses – premature closure of the cranial sutures

dacryocystocele – cystic dilation of the lacrimal sac at the nasocanthal angle

epignathus – teratoma located in the oropharynx

exophthalmia – abnormal protrusion of the eyeball

fetal cystic hygroma – malformation of the lymphatic system that leads to single or multiloculated lymph-filled cavities around the neck

fetal goiter (thyromegaly) – enlargement of the thyroid gland

hemifacial microsomia – abnormal smallness of one side of the face

holoprosencephaly – congenital defect caused by an extra chromosome, which causes a deficiency in the forebrain

hypertelorism – eyes too far apart

hypotelorism – eyes too close together

macroglossia – hypertrophied tongue

microcephaly – head smaller than the body

micrognathia – small chin

microphthalmia – small eyes

nuchal lucency – increased thickness in the nuchal fold area in the back of the neck associated with trisomy 21

oculodentodigital dysplasia – underdevelopment of the eyes, fingers, and mouth

otocephaly – underdevelopment of the jaw that causes the ears to be located close together toward the front of the neck

phenylketonuria (PKU) – hereditary disease caused by failure to oxidize an amino acid (phenylalanine) to tyrosine, because of a defective enzyme; if PKU is not treated early, mental retardation can develop

Pierre Robin syndrome – micrognathia and abnormal smallness of the tongue usually with a cleft palate

proboscis – a cylindrical protuberance of the face that in cyclopia or ethmocephaly represents the nose

strabismus – eye disorder in which optic axes cannot be directed to the same object

teratoma – solid tumor

Treacher Collins syndrome – underdevelopment of the jaw and cheek bone and abnormal ears

trigonocephaly – premature closure of the metopic suture

Congenital anomalies of the face affect 1 in 600 births. Cleft lip, hypotelorism, hypertelorism, and **micrognathia** are examples of facial problems that may be found by ultrasound during pregnancy. Many anomalies of the face and neck can be caused by maternal drug use (Table 54-1). As in other investigations, the detection of subtle facial malformations depends on the sonographer's skill and ability to recognize facial pathology, the position of the fetus, and the amount of amniotic fluid near the face.

TABLE 54-1	POTENTIAL FETAL MALFORMATIONS ASSOCIATED WITH MATERNAL DRUG OR CHEMICAL USE

Drug	Fetal Malformations
Acetaminophen overdose	Polyhydramnios
Acetazolamide	Sacrococcygeal teratoma
Acetylsalicylic acid	Intracranial hemorrhage, IUGR
Albuterol	Tachycardia
Alcohol (ethanol)	Microcephaly, micrognathia, cleft palate, short nose, hypoplastic philtrum, cardiac defects (VSD, ASD, double-outlet right ventricle, pulmonary atresia, dextrocardia, tetralogy of Fallot), IUGR, diaphragmatic hernia, pectus excavatum, radioulnar, synostosis, scoliosis, bifid xyphoid, NTDs
Amantadine	Cardiac defects (single ventricle with pulmonary atresia)
Aminopterin	NTDs, hydrocephalus, incomplete skull ossification, brachycephaly, micrognathia, clubfoot, syndactyly, hypoplasia of thumb and fibula, IUGR
Amitriptyline	Micrognathia, limb reduction, swelling of hands and feet, urinary retention
Amobarbital	NTDs, cardiac defects, severe limb deformities, congenital hip dislocation, polydactyly, clubfoot, cleft palate, ambiguous genitalia, soft tissue, deformity of neck
Antithyroid drugs	Goiter
Azathioprine	Cardiac defects (pulmonary valve stenosis), polydactyly
Betamethasone	Reduced head circumference
Bromides	Polydactyly, clubfoot, congenital hip dislocation
Busulfan	Pyloric stenosis, cleft palate, microphthalmia, IUGR
Caffeine	Musculoskeletal defects, hydronephrosis
Captopril	Leg reduction
Carbamazepine	NTDs, cardiac defects (atrial septal defect), nose hypoplasia, hypertelorism, cleft lip, congenital hip dislocation
Carbon monoxide	Cerebral atrophy, hydrocephalus, fetal demise
Chlordiazepoxide	Microcephaly, cardiac defects, duodenal atresia
Chloroquine	Hemihypertrophy
Chlorpheniramine	Hydrocephalus, polydactyly, congenital hip dislocation
Chlorpropamide	Microcephaly, dysmorphic hands and fingers
Clomiphene	NTDs, microcephaly, syndactyly, clubfoot, polydactyly, esophageal atresia
Cocaine	Spontaneous abortion, placental abruption, prematurity, IUGR, possible cardiac defects, skull defects, genitourinary anomalies
Codeine	Hydrocephalus, head defects, cleft palate, musculoskeletal defects, dislocated hip, pyloric stenosis, respiratory malformations
Cortisone	Hydrocephalus, cardiac defects (VSD, coarctation of aorta), clubfoot, cleft lip
Coumadin	NTDs, cardiac defects, scoliosis, skeletal deformities, nasal hypoplasia, stippled epiphyses, chondrodysplasia punctata, short phalanges, toe defects, incomplete rotation of gut, IUGR, bleeding
Cyclophosphamide	Cardiac defects, cleft palate, flattened nasal bridge, four toes on each foot, syndactyly, hypoplastic midphalanx
Cytarabine	NTDs, cardiac defects, lobster claw hand, missing digits of feet, syndactyly
Daunorubicin	NTDs, cardiac defects, syndactyly
Dextroamphetamine	NTDs, cardiac defects, IUGR
Diazepam	NTDs, cardiac defects, absence of arm, syndactyly, absence of thumbs, cleft lip/palate
Diphenhydramine	Clubfoot, cleft palate
Disulfiram	Vertebral fusion, clubfoot, radial aplasia, phocomelia, tracheoesophageal fistula
Diuretics	Respiratory malformations
Estrogens	Cardiac defects, limb reduction
Ethosuximide	Hydrocephalus, short neck, oral cleft
Fluorouracil	Radial aplasia, absent thumbs, aplasia of esophagus and duodenum, hypoplasia of lungs
Fluphenazine	Poor ossification of frontal bone, cleft palate
Haloperidol	Limb deformities
Heparin	Bleeding
Imipramine	NTDs, cleft palate, renal cysts, diaphragmatic hernia
Indomethacin	Fetal demise, hemorrhage
Isoniazid	NTDs
Lithium	NTDs, cardiac defects (VSD, Ebstein's anomaly, mitral atresia, dextrocardia)
Lysergic acid diethylamide (LSD)	NTDs, limb defects
Meclizine	Cardiac defects (hypoplastic left heart), respiratory defect
Meprobamate	Cardiac defects, limb defects
Methotrexate	Oxycephaly, absence of frontal bones, large fontanelles, micrognathia, long webbed fingers, low-set ears, IUGR, dextrocardia
Methyl mercury	Microcephaly, asymmetric head
Metronidazole	Midline facial defects
Nortriptyline	Limb reduction

TABLE 54-1 POTENTIAL FETAL MALFORMATIONS ASSOCIATED WITH MATERNAL DRUG OR CHEMICAL USE—cont'd

Drug	Fetal Malformations
Oral contraceptives	NTDs, cardiac defects, vertebral defects, limb reduction, IUGR, tracheoesophageal malformation
Paramethadione	Cardiac defects, IUGR
Phenobarbital	NTDs, digital anomalies, cleft palate, ileal atresia, IUGR, pulmonary hypoplasia
Phenothiazines	Microcephaly, syndactyly, clubfoot, omphalocele
Phenylephrine	Eye and ear abnormalities, syndactyly, clubfoot, hip dislocation, umbilical hernia
Phenylpropanolamine	Pectus excavatum, polydactyly, hip dislocation
Phenytoin (hydantoin)	Microcephaly, wide fontanelles, cardiac defects, IUGR, cleft/lip palate, hypertelorism, low-set ears, short neck, short nose, broad nasal bridge, hypoplastic distal phalanges, digital thumb, hip dislocation, rib-sternal abnormalities
Polychlorinated biphenyls	Spotted calcification in skull, fetal demise, IUGR
Primidone	Cardiac defects (VSD), webbed neck, small mandible
Procarbazine	Cerebral hemorrhage, oligodactyly
Progesterones	NTDs, hydrocephaly, cardiac defects (tetralogy of Fallot, truncus arteriosus, VSD), absent thumbs
Quinine	Hydrocephalus, cardiac defects, facial defects, vertebral anomalies, dysmelias
Retinoic acid (vitamin A)	Hydrocephalus, cerebral malformations, microcephaly, cardiac defects, limb deformities, fetal demise, cleft palate, rib abnormalities
Spermicides	Limb reduction
Sulfonamide	Limb hypoplasia, foot defects, urethral obstruction
Tetracycline	Limb hypoplasia, clubfoot
Thalidomide	Cardiac defects, spine defects, limb reduction (amelia), phocomelia, hypoplasia, duodenal stenosis or atresia, pyloric stenosis
Thioguanine	Missing digits
Tobacco	IUGR
Tolbutamide	Syndactyly, absent toes, accessory thumb
Toluene	IUGR, neonatal hyperchloremia acidosis, possible mental dysfunction, cardiac defects, dysmorphic facies
Trifluoperazine	Cardiac defects, phocomelia
Trimethadione	Microcephaly, low-set ears, broad nasal bridge, cardiac defects (ASD, VSD), IUGR, cleft lip and palate, esophageal atresia, malformed hands, clubfoot
Valproic acid	NTDs, microcephaly, wide fontanelle, cardiac defects, IUGR, cleft palate, hypoplastic nose, low-set ears, small mandible, depressed nasal bridge, polydactyly

From Nyberg DA, Mahoney BS, Pretorius DH: *Diagnostic ultrasound of fetal anomalies: text and atlas*, St Louis, 1990, Mosby.
IUGR, intrauterine growth restriction; *ASD*, atrial septal defect; *NTD*, neural tube defects; *VSD*, ventricular septal defect.

EMBRYOLOGY OF THE FETAL FACE AND NECK

In its 4th week, the embryo has characteristic external features of the head and neck area in the form of a series of branchial arches, pouches, grooves, and membranes. These structures are referred to as the *branchial apparatus* and bear a resemblance to gills.

There are six branchial arches, but only the first four are visible externally (Figure 54-1, *A*). Each of the arches is separated by branchial grooves and is composed of a core of mesenchymal cells. The mesenchyme forms the cartilages, bones, muscles, and blood vessels.

The first branchial arch is also known as the mandibular arch; it forms the jaw, zygomatic bone, ear, and temporal bone (Figure 54-1, *B*). The second branchial arch contributes to the hyoid bone.

The branchial arches consist of mesenchymal tissue derived from intraembryonic mesoderm covered by ectoderm and containing transderm. Neural crest cells migrate into the branchial arches and proliferate, resulting in swellings that demarcate each arch. The neural crest cells develop the skeletal parts of the face, and the mesoderm of each arch develops the musculature of the face and neck.

The maxillary prominences arise from the first branchial arch and grow cranially just under the eyes and the mandibular prominence, which grows inferiorly. The primitive mouth is an indentation on the surface of the ectoderm (referred to as the stomodeum) (Figure 54-2). By the 5th week of development, five prominences are identified: the frontal nasal prominence, forming the upper boundary of the stomodeum; the paired maxillary prominences of the first branchial arch, forming the lateral boundaries of the stomodeum; and the paired mandibular prominences, forming the caudal boundary.

The nasal pits are formed as the surface ectoderm thickens into the nasal placodes on each side of the frontal nasal prominence; as these placodes invaginate, the nasal pits are formed (Figure 54-3). Until 24 to 26 days of gestation, the stomodeum is separated from the pharynx by a membrane that ruptures by about the 26th day to place the primitive gut in communication with the amniotic cavity.

The maxillary prominences grow medially between the 5th and 8th weeks. This growth compresses the medial nasal

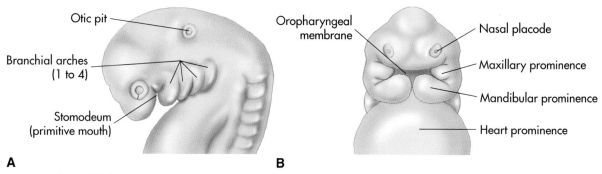

Figure 54-1   **A,** Lateral view of the embryo at 28 days shows four of the six branchial arches, otic pit, and stomodeum. **B,** Frontal view of the embryo at 24 days demonstrates the nasal placode, maxillary prominence, and mandibular prominence.

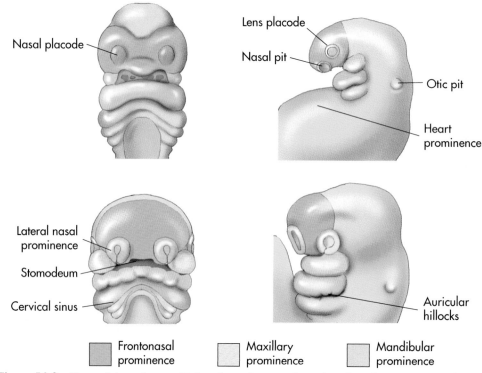

Figure 54-2   Views of the embryo at 33 days shows the stomodeum, lateral nasal prominence, and cervical sinus.

prominences together toward the midline. The two medial nasal prominences and the two maxillary prominences lateral to them fuse together to form the upper lip (Figure 54-4). The medial nasal prominences form the medial aspect of the lip, which is the origin of the labial component of the lip, the upper incisor teeth, and the anterior aspect of the primary palate. The lateral nasal prominences form the alae of the nose. The maxillary prominences and lateral nasal prominences are separated by the nasolacrimal groove. The ectoderm in the floor of this groove forms the nasolacrimal duct and lacrimal sac.

The nose is formed in three parts. The bridge of the nose originates from the frontal prominence, the two medial nasal prominences form the crest and tip of the nose, and the lateral

nasal prominences form the sides, or alae. The mandibular prominences merge at the end of the 4th to 5th week and form the lower lip, chin, and mandible.

SONOGRAPHIC EVALUATION OF THE FETAL FACE

Fetal facial evaluation is not routinely included in a basic fetal scan; however, when there is a family history of craniofacial malformation or when another congenital anomaly is found, the face should be screened for a coexisting facial malformation. Many fetuses with a facial defect also have chromosomal abnormalities. Extensive facial screening may be hindered by either bone shadowing, poor fetal position, oligohydramnios,

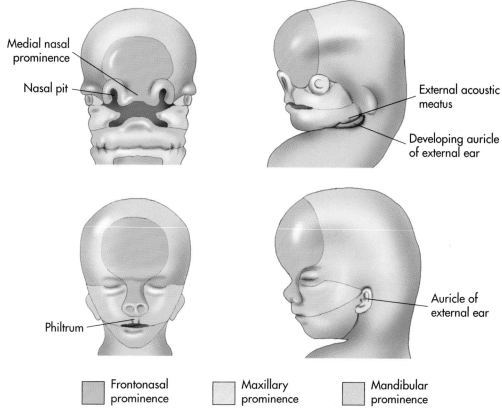

Medial nasal prominence

Nasal pit

External acoustic meatus

Developing auricle of external ear

Philtrum

Auricle of external ear

Frontonasal prominence | Maxillary prominence | Mandibular prominence

Figure 54-3 Frontal view of the embryo at 40 days shows the nasal pit and medial nasal prominence.

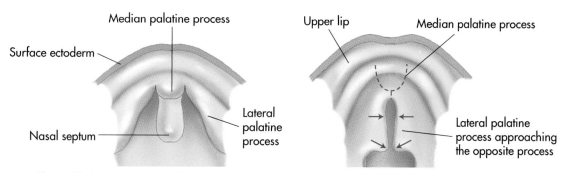

Median palatine process

Surface ectoderm

Nasal septum

Lateral palatine process

Upper lip

Median palatine process

Lateral palatine process approaching the opposite process

Figure 54-4 First trimester development of the roof of the mouth showing the formation of the upper lip and palate.

or maternal obesity. Certain facial anomalies often indicate a specific syndrome or condition (e.g., orbital fusion and a **proboscis** suggest alobar holoprosencephaly). The use of three- and four-dimensional ultrasound reconstruction has been shown in recent years to be a useful adjunct to conventional two-dimensional assessment of the fetal face (Box 54-1).

Facial anomalies are heterogeneous and occur as isolated defects or as part of a syndrome. A family history of a facial anomaly (e.g., cleft lip) may prompt a targeted study, although recurrence risks are relatively low (less than 5%). Hemangiomas and teratomas may occur anywhere on the body, and the fetal head and neck are no exception. Any mass should be investigated with Color Doppler to delineate any vascular characteristics (Figure 54-9).

ABNORMALITIES OF THE FACE AND NECK

ABNORMALITIES OF THE FACIAL PROFILE

Forehead. The fetal forehead may be appreciated by evaluation of the profile. This is achieved by a series of midsagittal scans through the face. The fetal forehead (frontal bone) appears as a curvilinear surface with differentiation of the nose, lips, and chin seen inferiorly. This view allows diagnosis of anterior **cephaloceles**, which may arise from the frontal bone or midface. Anterior cephaloceles may cause widely spaced orbits (hypertelorism) (Boxes 54-2 and 54-3).

Off-axis, or nonmidline, encephaloceles have also been reported with amniotic band syndrome. This occurs when the amnion disrupts early in the embryonic period, leaving strands of tissue within the uterus that may lead to malformation of the fetus.

Skull. Craniosynostosis (premature closure of any or all six of the cranial sutures) causes the fetal cranium to become abnormally shaped. *Clover-leaf skull* (Kleeblattschädel) appears as an unusually misshapen skull with a clover-leaf appearance in the anterior view. Clover-leaf skull has been associated with numerous skeletal dysplasias (most notably thanatophoric dysplasia) and ventriculomegaly (Figure 54-10). **Trigonocephaly** (premature closure of the metopic suture) may cause the forehead to have an elongated (tall) appearance in the sagittal plane and appear triangular shaped in the axial plane (Figure 54-11). Three-dimensional imaging has been shown to be useful in evaluating the fetal

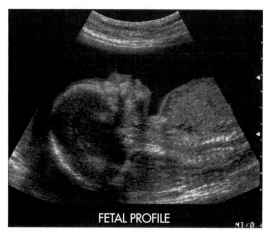

FETAL PROFILE

Figure 54-5 The fetal profile is well seen with amniotic fluid surrounding the face. This is a useful place to image the forehead, nose, lips, and chin.

BOX 54-1   SONOGRAPHIC POINTS TO REMEMBER

- Features of the fetal face can be identified at the end of the first trimester.
- The fetal profile is well imaged with endovaginal sonography beginning late first trimester to early second trimester (make sure adequate amniotic fluid surrounds the face) (Figure 54-5).
- The modified coronal view is best to image the cleft lip and palate (Figure 54-6).
- The maxilla and orbits are well imaged in a true coronal plane.
- The lens of the eye is seen as a small echogenic circle within the orbit (Figure 54-7).
- The longitudinal view demonstrates the nasal bones, soft tissue, and mandible (useful to rule out micrognathia, anterior encephalocele, or nasal bridge defects; examine upper lip) (Figure 54-8).
- Transverse view shows orbital abnormalities and intraorbital distances (useful to evaluate the maxilla, mandible, and tongue).

BOX 54-2   QUESTIONS FOR THE SONOGRAPHER EVALUATING FACIAL PROFILE

- Are the orbits normally spaced?
- Are the nose and nasal bridge clearly imaged; is a proboscis or cebocephaly present?
- Are any periorbital masses apparent?
- Is the upper lip intact?
- Is the tongue normal size?
- Is the chin abnormally small?
- Are the ears normal size and in normal position?

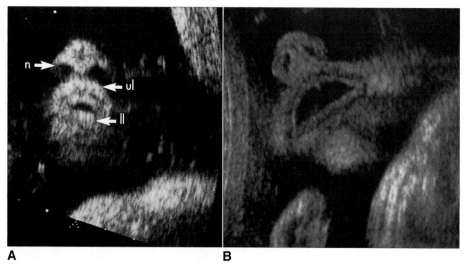

Figure 54-6 **A,** Axial view through the upper *(ul)* and lower lip *(ll)* in a fetus with an open mouth. Note the nares *(n)* and nasal septum. This is the view used to check for a cleft of the upper lip. **B,** In another fetus, the nasal septum is well seen and the vermilion (red) tissue of the lips can be differentiated.

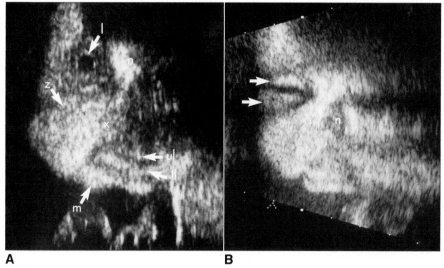

Figure 54-7 **A,** Coronal view showing facial features. Lens *(l)*, zygomatic bone *(z)*, maxilla *(x)*, upper lip *(ul)*, lower lip *(ll)*, mandible *(m)*, nasal bones *(n)*. **B,** In the same fetus, in a more anterior coronal view, the upper and lower eyelids *(arrows)* and nose *(n)* are shown.

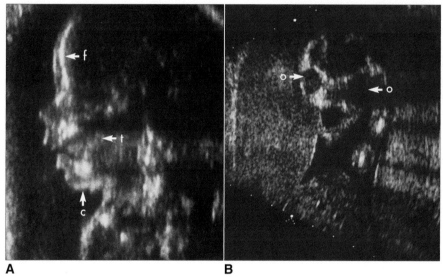

Figure 54-8 **A,** Sagittal view in a 23-week fetus showing the contour of the face in profile. Note the smooth surface of the frontal bone *(f)* and the appearance of the nose, upper and lower lips, tongue *(t)*, and chin *(c)*. **B,** Coronal facial view in an 18-week fetus revealing a wide-open mouth. Note the nasal bones between the orbits *(o)*.

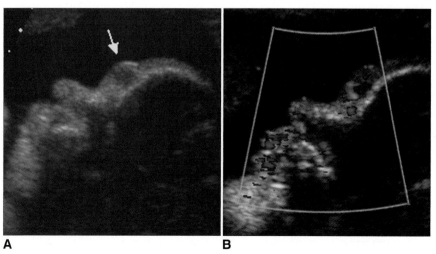

Figure 54-9 **A,** A soft tissue mass is seen overlying the fetal forehead *(arrow)*. **B,** Color Doppler demonstrates the mass to have vascular flow within, suggesting a hemangioma.

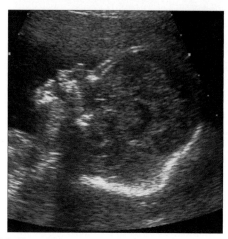

Figure 54-10 Sagittal view of a fetus with thanatophoric dysplasia with a clover-leaf skull or Kleeblattschädel.

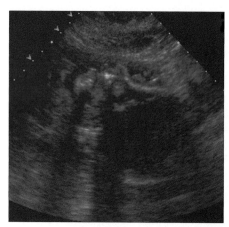

Figure 54-11 Sagittal view of a fetus with premature closure of the metopic suture, which elongated and flattened the fetal forehead.

BOX 54-3	SONOGRAPHY OF THE FACIAL PROFILE

Use midsagittal scans through the face to assess

- Curvilinear surface with differentiation of forehead, nose, lips, and chin
- Clover-leaf skull: appears as misshapened skull with clover-leaf appearance
- Frontal bossing: may appear as lemon-shaped skull or absent, depressed nasal bridge
- Strawberry-shaped cranium: bulging of frontal bones and wide occiput
- Masses of nose and upper lip: distortion of facial profile (look for cleft lip)

---

cranial sutures. *Frontal bossing* may be observed in a fetus with a lemon-shaped skull (from spina bifida) or with skeletal dysplasias. Any irregularities in the contour of the forehead should prompt the investigator to search for other malformations.

Midface hypoplasia. Midface hypoplasia, or maxillary hypoplasia with depressed or absent nasal bridge, is an underdevelopment of the middle structures of the face. The flat facies this defect produces are more easily noted with coexisting frontal bossing. Midface hypoplasia may be seen in fetuses with chromosome anomalies, such as trisomy 21; craniosynostosis syndromes, such as Apert's syndrome; and limb and skeletal abnormalities, such as achondroplasia, chondrodysplasia punctata, and asphyxiating thoracic dysplasia and others (Figure 54-12). The fetal nasal bone may be small or absent with certain chromosome anomalies, particularly trisomy 21. Recent studies have evaluated the demonstration of the presence or absence of the fetal nasal bone as a predictor of chromosome anomalies (Figure 54-13).

Frontonasal dysplasia. Frontonasal dysplasia is a median-cleft face syndrome consisting of a range of midline facial defects involving the eyes, forehead, and nose. Abnormalities include ocular hypertelorism, a variable bifid nose, broad nasal bridge, midline defect of the frontal bone, and extension of the frontal hairline to form a widow's peak. The cause of frontonasal dysplasia is unknown, and the occurrence is sporadic.

By ultrasound, the primary finding will likely be hypertelorism. If one cranial abnormality is found, the sonographer should carefully look for additional dysmorphic features (Figure 54-14).

Nuchal Area. The association of first-trimester fetal **nuchal lucency** with aneuploidy is well established and is dependent on the size and extent of the nuchal abnormality.[6] The latest studies of nuchal translucency (NT) thickness have attempted to delineate the exact role of this measurement as a screening tool for chromosome anomalies. In a review of recent studies,[3] it was shown that when fetal NT is performed in conjunction with maternal biochemical screening (maternal serum free-[beta]-human chorionic gonadotropin and pregnancy-associated plasma protein-A or PAPP-A) the detection rate of chromosome anomalies is 87%, as opposed to 76.8% with the fetal NT measurement alone. The optimal gestational age for the measurement of fetal NT is 11 weeks of gestation to 13 weeks, 6 days of gestation. The fetal crown-rump length should be within the range of 45 to 84 mm. It is important to adjust the depth and image magnification so that the head and upper torso comprise 75% of the image field. In a midline sagittal plane, care should be taken to ensure delineation of the amnion and nuchal borders by either waiting for the fetus to move or by gently bouncing the transducer on the maternal abdomen. Calipers should be placed on the borders of the nuchal translucency and not in the nuchal fluid area. A measurement greater than 3 mm is abnormal, and the thicker the fetal NT is above 3 mm, the greater the chance of the fetus being affected by a chromosome anomaly or other defects, such as congenital heart disease (Figure 54-15).

Nose and Upper Lip. Masses of the nose and upper lip may distort the facial profile and indicate a cleft lip. Tumors may disrupt the facial contour in the sagittal plane, such as an

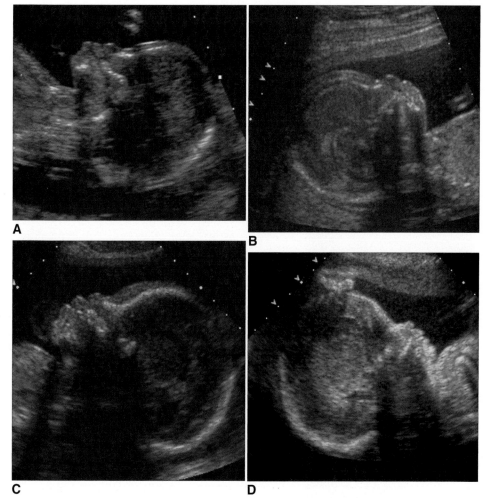

Figure 54-12 Midline sagittal views. **A,** A fetus affected by familial midface hypoplasia. **B,** A fetus with trisomy 21 (Down syndrome); note flattened facies. **C,** A fetus with a skeletal dysplasia demonstrates mild frontal bossing and midface hypoplasia. **D,** A fetus with neonatal progeroid syndrome; note smallness of facial profile compared with head. Cranial biometry was consistent with gestational age.

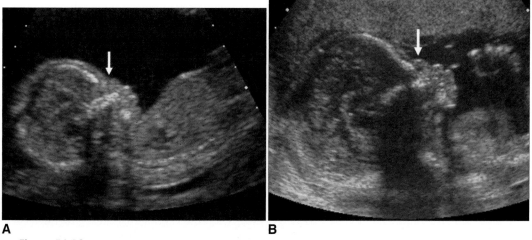

Figure 54-13 **A,** Trisomy 21 fetus with absent nasal bone *(arrow)*. **B,** Another fetus with trisomy 21 with absent nasal bone *(arrow)*.

epignathus or a teratoma. These anomalies will be discussed in more detail in later sections.

Tongue. Tongue protrusion may suggest **macroglossia** (enlarged tongue), a condition found in **Beckwith-Wiedemann syndrome** (congenital overgrowth of tissues) (Figure 54-16). Organomegaly is also a feature of this syndrome. Some glycogen storage diseases may also exhibit macroglossia and organomegaly (Figure 54-17).

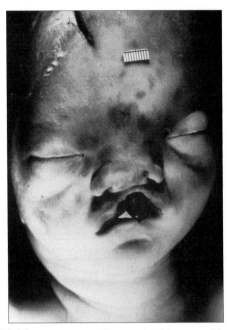

Figure 54-14 Postmortem photograph of neonate with median cleft facial syndrome (frontonasal dysplasia). Note the hypertelorism and mass of the upper lip. Other abnormalities observed prenatally include severe ventriculomegaly with a shift of the interhemispheric fissure.

Mandible. Congenital **micrognathia** should be suspected when a small chin is observed. Most cases of micrognathia are detected from the subjective appearance of a small chin when imaging the fetal profile (Figure 54-18). Several authors have proposed more objective methods of evaluation of the fetal mandible by providing quantitative data to assess the size of the mandible either by an index or according to gestational age. Mandibular width is measured in an axial plane laterally from rami to rami. Mandibular length, or AP diameter, is assessed by measuring from the mentum of the mandible to the bisection of the lateral width line (Figure 54-19). Palladini and others proposed the use of an established jaw index using the anteroposterior diameter of the mandible and the biparietal diameter (AP Diam/BPD × 100) for diagnosing micrognathia.[5] An index of 21 or less yielded a 100% positive predictive value. Lee and others believed that 3-D imaging added complimentary information to 2-D imaging of the chin and that a true midline plane could be better achieved using 3-D reconstructed images.[2] Micrognathia is associated with many conditions that can be subdivided into three groups of anomalies: chromosome anomalies, such as trisomy 18 and triploidy; skeletal dysplasias; and primary mandibular disorders, such as **Pierre Robin syndrome** and **Treacher Collins syndrome**. An abnormally small chin may be so severe that polyhydramnios occurs because of the inability of the fetus to swallow, and airway obstruction may be a complication at delivery.

Ear. The fetal ears may be imaged either in a parasagittal plane or in a coronal plane. Ear malformations are rarely predicted prenatally. Low-set ears may be appreciated in a longitudinal or coronal view when the placement of the ear appears lower than usual in many craniofacial malformations and syndromes. Ear malformation may be observed in Goldenhar's syndrome with **anophthalmia** (absent eye) and **hemifacial microsomia** (abnormal smallness of one side of the face).

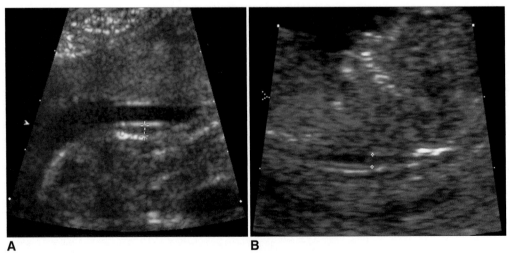

A   **B**

Figure 54-15 **A,** A 13-week, 6-day fetus. Caliper placement demonstrates the measurement of a normal fetal nuchal translucency. **B,** An 11-week, 4-day fetus. Fetal nuchal translucency measurement from an anteroposterior sagittal plane.

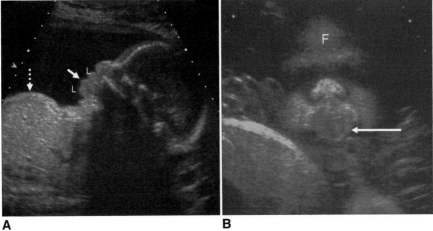

A   **B**

Figure 54-16   A, A fetus with Beckwith-Wiedemann syndrome. Note tongue protruding from mouth *(arrow)* between lips *(L)* and enlarged fetal liver *(dotted arrow).* **B,** Another fetus with Beckwith-Wiedemann syndrome. Coronal view of the fetal face demonstrates a protruding tongue suggesting macroglossia *(arrow).* The fetal liver was also enlarged in this fetus. *F,* forehead.

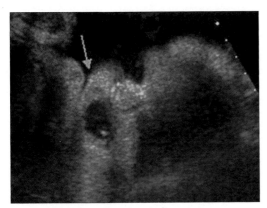

Figure 54-17   Coronal view of fetal face showing a hypoechoic mass in fetal mouth. A sublingual cyst was noted to move in and out of the fetal mouth in the sagittal plane *(arrow).*

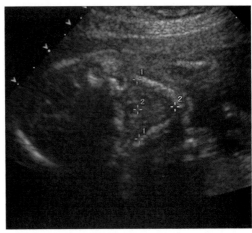

Figure 54-19   Axial view of a normal fetal mandible demonstrating the mandibular width *(1)* and the mandibular AP diameter *(2).*

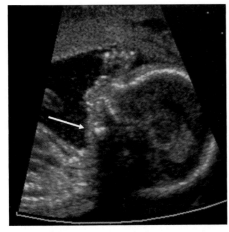

Figure 54-18   Sagittal plane of a fetus with micrognathia *(arrow).*

Small ears (Roberts' syndrome) and inadequate development of the ear (Nager acrofacial dysostosis syndrome and Treacher Collins syndrome) may be observed prenatally (Figure 54-20). **Otocephaly** is a rare anomaly where absence of the mandible causes the ears to form close together anteriorly and toward the neck.

ABNORMALITIES OF THE ORBITS

Orbital architecture has become increasingly important in the evaluation of craniofacial anomalies. The anatomy of the orbits, the use of orbital measurements in gestational age assessment, and the role of ultrasound in detecting ocular abnormalities have been investigated (Figure 54-21).

The sonographer must document the presence of both eyes and assess the overall size of the eyes to exclude **microphthalmia** (small eyes) and **anophthalmia** (absent eyes). Masses of the orbit (periorbital) and of the eye (intraocular) may be excluded with careful scanning of the eyes. Periorbital masses, such as lacrimal duct cysts **(dacryocystoceles),** dermoids, and hemangiomas, have been reported (Figure 54-22). In a laterally approached axial plane, the hyaloid artery may be observed within the fetal eye. The hyaloid artery, which regresses in the third trimester, is a branch of the primitive dorsal ophthalmic artery. It extends from the optic nerve through the vitreous cavity to the lens to aid in its development (Figure 54-23).

Endovaginal sonography has aided in early detection of ocular anomalies and other intracranial abnormalities. The fetal eyes are evaluated on endovaginal sonography in a transverse section of the fetal skull at the orbital plane. In addition, an oblique tangential section from the nasal bridge is used to detect the hypoechogenic circles lateral to the nose, in the anterior part of the orbits, representing the fetal lens. Using this method, ocular abnormalities, including **strabismus,** microphthalmia, divergence of lens, **exophthalmia,** and cataracts have been demonstrated.

Orbital distance measurements are helpful in the diagnosis of fetal conditions in which hypotelorism or hypertelorism is a feature (Figure 54-24). Both of these conditions are associated with other anomalies, and often the orbital problem aids in the diagnosis of which type of cranial anomaly or genetic syndrome is present. An anatomic and biometric evaluation of the fetal orbits should be attempted in fetuses at risk for abnormal orbital distance.

Hypotelorism. **Hypotelorism** is a condition characterized by a decreased distance between the orbits (Figures 54-25 and 54-26). It is associated with several syndromes and other anomalies, including **holoprosencephaly, microcephaly, craniosynostoses,** and **phenylketonuria (PKU).**

Obvious hypotelorism will be seen in ethmocephaly and cebocephaly or may be so severe that a single orbit is demonstrated with a fused or single eye, as seen in cyclopia (Figures 54-27 and 54-28). Measurements of orbital width may identify fetuses with hypotelorism.

Hypertelorism. **Hypertelorism** is characterized by abnormally wide-spaced orbits. Hypertelorism is found in several abnormal fetal conditions, genetic syndromes, and chromosomal anomalies. Fetuses exposed to phenytoin (Dilantin) during pregnancy may manifest signs of hypertelorism as part of the fetal phenytoin syndrome (microcephaly; growth abnormalities; cleft lip and/or palate; cardiac, genitourinary, central nervous system, and skeletal anomalies). In Pfeiffer syndrome and Apert's syndrome, hypertelorism and brachycephaly have been described as a result of abnormal closure of the cranial sutures (craniosynostosis). In both syndromes, ventriculomegaly may be present. Other conditions that manifest with hypertelorism and premature suture closure include Crouzon syndrome, cephalosyndactyly, acrocephalopolysyndactyly, and **oculodentodigital dysplasia.**

Fetal hypertelorism may be diagnosed by orbital distances that fall above normal ranges for gestational age.

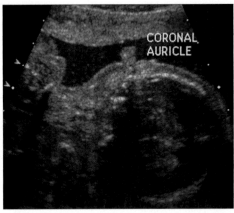

Figure 54-20 A coronal plane in a fetus with an unusual appearing ear lobe of a posteriorly rotated ear.

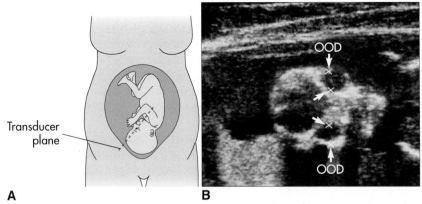

A   **B**

Figure 54-21 **A,** Frontal view demonstrating a fetus in a vertex presentation with the fetal cranium in an occipitotransverse position. The transducer is placed along the coronal plane (approximately 2 cm posterior to the glabella-alveolar line). **B,** Sonogram demonstrating the orbits in the coronal view. The outer orbital diameter *(OOD)* and inner orbital diameter (IOD) *(angled arrows)* are viewed. The IOD is measured from the medial border of the orbit to the opposite medial border *(angled arrows).* The OOD is measured from the outermost lateral border of the orbit to the opposite lateral border.

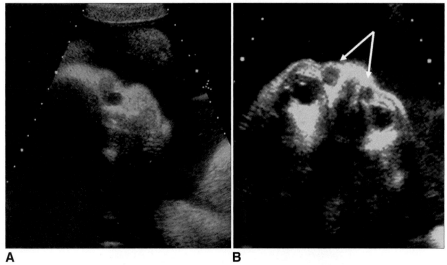

Figure 54-22 **A,** A coronal view of the fetal face reveals a small hypoechoic mass just inferomedial to the eye. **B,** In the transverse plane, bilateral lacrimal duct cysts are exhibited *(arrows)*.

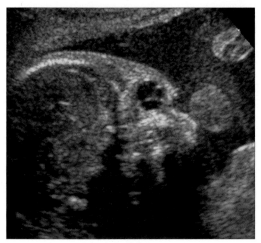

Figure 54-23 An axial view of the fetal head demonstrates the hyaloid artery seen as a linear structure within the vitreous cavity of the eye.

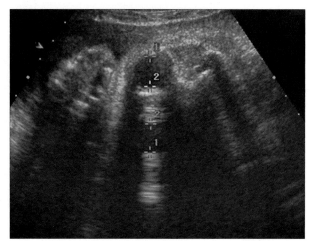

Figure 54-24 Axial image through the fetal orbits exhibits the correct placement of calipers to measure the outer-to-outer distance of the orbits *(1)*, sometimes referred to as the binocular measurement, and the inner-to-inner orbital measurement *(2)*.

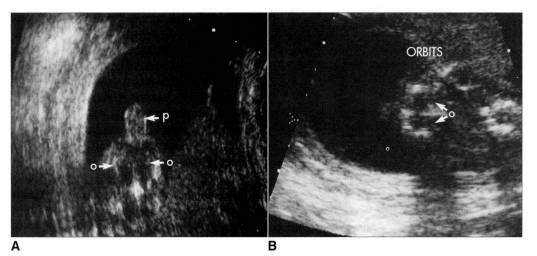

Figure 54-25 **A,** Proboscis *(p)* observed in a frontal facial view in a midline position above the closely spaced orbits *(o)* in a 20-week fetus with ethmocephaly. **B,** In the same fetus the orbits *(o)* are observed. A single eye was found with fused orbits. Trisomy 13 was found after delivery.

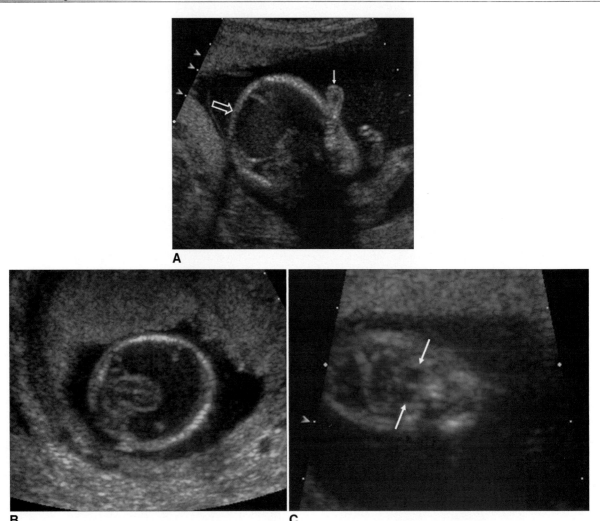

Figure 54-26 **A,** A midline sagittal view of the face in a fetus with holoprosencephaly shows a proboscis *(arrow),* and a dorsal sac (sometimes seen with holoprosencephaly) can be seen in the posterior fetal cranium *(open arrow).* **B,** An axial view of the same fetus displays the monoventricle seen with holoprosencephaly. **C,** Coronal view of the same fetus reveals hypotelorism *(arrows).*

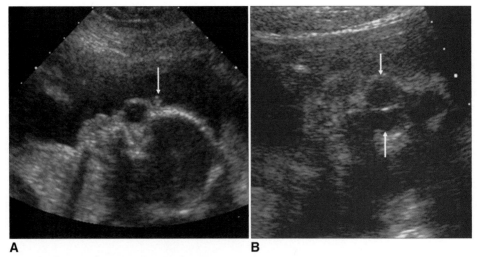

Figure 54-27 **A,** A midline sagittal plane through the face of a fetus with holoprosencephaly demonstrates cyclopia with a small proboscis *(arrow)* above the central eye. **B,** The coronal view of the same fetus shows two asymmetric sized eyes within one orbit *(arrows).*

Recognition of hypertelorism may provide evidence for a particular genetic syndrome or concurrent anomalies. Frontal cephaloceles may widen the space between the eyes (Figure 54-29). The reader is referred to comprehensive sources for a detailed list of conditions associated with hypertelorism.[4]

Frontonasal dysplasia (median cleft facial syndrome) was diagnosed in a fetus with ventriculomegaly based on the sonographic findings of hypertelorism and cleft lip (see Figure 54-14).

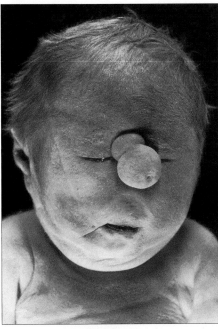

Figure 54-28 Postmortem photograph of a neonate with ethmocephaly. Note the proboscis and hypotelorism. The mouth appeared normal. A common ventricle and absent optic and ophthalmic nerves were noted. The chromosomes were consistent with trisomy 13.

ABNORMALITIES OF THE NOSE, MAXILLA, LIPS, AND PALATE

The nose, maxilla, lips, and palate may be viewed by placing the transducer in a lateral coronal plane, sagittal profile plane, and in modified tangential maxillary view or modified coronal view (inferior-superior projection) (Figure 54-30, *A*). In the lateral coronal view, the integrity of the nasal structures in relationship to the orbital rings and maxillae is studied. In a profile plane the contour of the nose, the upper and lower lips, and chin is observed. This is an important view in assessing the presence or absence of the nose, lips, and chin. Irregularities in nasal contour may indicate a particular syndrome. Tangential cuts, with the transducer angled inferiorly to superiorly through the maxilla, demonstrate the nasal septum and nostril openings, or nares (Figures 54-30 and 54-31). In holoprosencephaly, nasal anomalies range from absence of the nose (**arhinia**) to the presence of a proboscis to a single-nostril nose (cebocephaly) (Figure 54-32).

Evaluation of the nasal triad should assess (1) nostril symmetry, (2) nasal septum integrity, and (3) continuity of the upper lip to exclude cleft lip and palate. The sonographer should not mistake the normal nostrils or frenulum for a cleft. The maxilla marks the posterior border of the nose and is a landmark in assessing the fetus at risk for premaxillary protuberance as seen in Roberts' syndrome.

Lip and Palate. Cleft lip with or without cleft palate represents the most common congenital anomaly of the face. The frequency of cleft lip with or without a cleft palate shows ethnic variation. This disorder occurs in 1 per 600 births in Caucasians, in 1 per 3000 births in African-Americans, in 1 per 350 births in Asians, and in 1 per 150 to 1 per 250 births in Native Americans. Cleft lip occurs because of failure to fuse the primary and secondary palate, resulting in a cleft defect coursing anteriorly through the upper lip and alveolus. A cleft palate occurs when the lateral palatine processes fail to fuse in

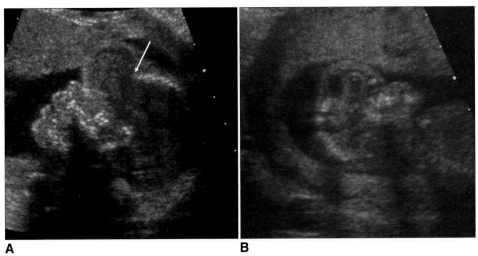

A   **B**

Figure 54-29 A, Midline sagittal view of a fetus with an anterior (frontal) encephalocele and delineation of the bony defect *(arrow).* **B,** Midline sagittal image of a large frontal encephalocele that also involved facial structures.

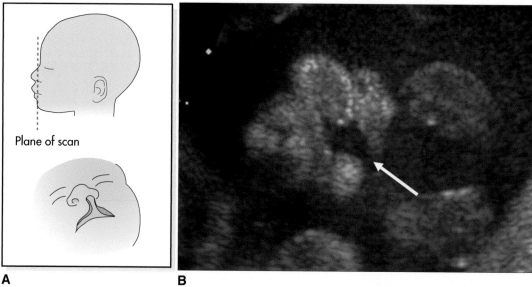

Figure 54-30   A, Facial cleft. This drawing illustrates a plane of section that visualizes clefts of the upper lip. **B,** A modified coronal plane demonstrates a unilateral cleft lip *(arrow)*. The cleft extended into the fetal nose and an associated cleft palate was present.

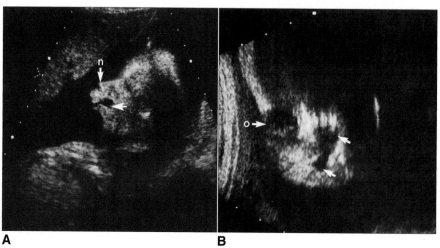

Figure 54-31   A, Unilateral cleft lip in the fetus shown in Figure 54-10, with clefting defect extending through the palate into the nasal cavity *(arrow)* in a sagittal plane in a 25-week fetus. Note the globular appearance of the tissue under the nose *(n)* (premaxillary protuberance). **B,** In the same fetus, a coronal plane illustrates the extent of the clefting *(arrows)*. Note the defect extending from the upper lip to the nasal cavity. *O,* orbit.

the midline. Cleft lip and palate occur together when both fusions are absent.

A facial cleft may involve only the upper lip or may extend to involve the alveolus, posterior hard palate, and soft palate. Clefts may be unilateral or bilateral and may occur in isolation or in association with other anatomic and karyotype abnormalities. Isolated posterior cleft palate is recognized as a distinct entity, quite separate from isolated cleft lip alone or cleft lip and palate.

Clefts of the face may occur along various facial planes. Defects range from clefting of the lip alone to involvement of the hard and soft palate, which may extend into the nose and in rare cases to the inferior border of the orbit. In rare instances, lateral clefts (may be called macrostomia if bilateral) may be observed where clefting courses laterally from the corner of the mouth and in severe cases may extend to the ear. Additionally, oblique and asymmetrical clefts may occur with amniotic band syndrome.

Isolated cleft lip may occur as a unilateral or bilateral defect and, when unilateral, commonly originates on the left side of the face. When there is a bilateral lesion, cleft palate is found in up to 85% of neonates. When unilateral, cleft palate may be seen in 70% of infants. Isolated cleft palate is a separate disorder from cleft lip associated with cleft palate. There are more than 200 facial cleft syndromes, and counseling regarding

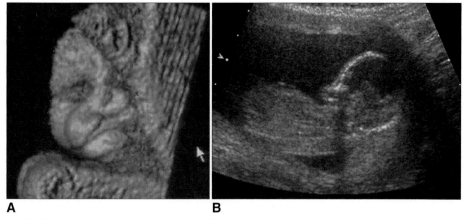

A   B

Figure 54-32 **A,** An early 3-D image of a median facial cleft seen with holoprosencephaly. **B,** Fourteen-week fetus midline sagittal view demonstrates midface anomalies, which included hypotelorism and arhinia with median facial cleft, which assisted in the early detection of holoprosencephaly.

recurrence is challenging (Figure 54-33). It has been reported that fetal breathing may be observed with color Doppler in both the nasopharynx and oropharynx when a cleft palate is present. In the presence of a normal palate, color flow should only be observed in the fetal nasopharynx when the mouth is closed (Figure 54-34).

The majority of cleft lip and/or palate occurrences are thought to have multiple causes. Causes that may be prenatally detected include a familial predisposition for a cleft or chromosomal abnormalities (trisomies 13, 18, 21; triploidy; and translocations). Other prenatally detectable clefting conditions include acrocephalopolysyndactyly, amniotic band syndrome, anencephaly, congenital cardiac disease, diastrophic dysplasia, holoprosencephaly, Kniest dysplasia, spondyloepiphyseal dysplasia congenita, Meckel-Gruber, Roberts', and multiple pterygium syndromes. A premaxillary protrusion or premaxillary mass suggests the presence of a bilateral cleft lip and palate, even when sonographically only a unilateral defect is suspected. This premaxillary mass of tissue corresponds to the abnormal anterior herniation of the hard palate and teeth caused by the defect of the alveolar ridge (Figure 54-35).

Sonographically, visualization of the hard and soft palates remains a diagnostic challenge because of considerable bony shadowing. The sonographer needs to use a systematic approach to examine the fetal face for clefts in the coronal and axial planes. The addition of 3-D and 4-D reconstruction may compliment the 2-D assessment of facial anomalies, in particular facial clefts. It has been shown to be valuable in understanding the extent of abnormalities and in helping the plastic surgeon and patient to understand the fetal defect suspected. A caution about 3-D imaging: When viewing 3-D images, patients may be able to recognize abnormalities before the doctor has had the opportunity to clarify the diagnosis and counsel them (Figure 54-36, Box 54-4).

ABNORMALITIES OF THE ORAL CAVITY

Few congenital malformations of the oral cavity exist. The normal fetus may exhibit various behavioral patterns, such as

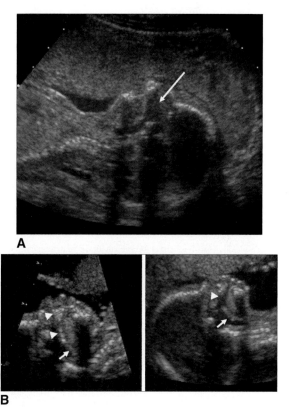

Figure 54-33 **A,** Sagittal image of a fetus with a bilateral cleft lip and palate. Fluid is seen in common oropharynx-nasopharynx area suggesting a cleft palate *(arrow)*. **B,** Midline sagittal plane of a normal palate in a 29-week fetus *(left)* and a 21-week fetus *(right)*. The hard palate can be seen adjacent to the fetal tongue *(arrowheads)*, and the fetal soft palate can be visualized between the oropharynx and nasopharynx *(arrows)*. Observation of the fetus while swallowing and moving the mouth may aid in the delineation of these structures.

swallowing, protrusion and retrusion of the tongue, and hic-coughing. An abnormal positioning of the tongue may be indicative of a mass of the oral cavity, an obstructive process, or **macroglossia** (large tongue in Beckwith-Wiedemann syndrome).

The antenatal sonographic diagnosis of epignathus has been reported.[1] An **epignathus** is a teratoma located in the oropharynx. These masses may be highly complex and contain solid, cystic, or calcified components. In fetuses with epignathus, swallowing may be impaired, resulting in hydramnios. In these cases, a small stomach may be present (Figure 54-37).

ABNORMALITIES OF THE NECK

Congenital anomalies of the neck are rare but when present may represent life-threatening disorders. Neck masses are usually large and obvious because their presence causes distor-tion of the neck contour and adjacent structures. The most common neck mass is cystic hygroma colli (lymphatic obstruction). Rarer lesions include cervical meningomyelocele, hemangiomas, teratomas, goiter, sarcoma, and metastatic adenopathy. **Branchial cleft cysts** (Figure 54-38) are prena-tally detectable.

Clinically, a fetal neck mass is cause for concern. When a large tumor exists, delivery of the infant is complicated because the tumor may cause delivery dystocia (inability to deliver the trunk once the head has been delivered) and obstruction of the airway, which may require an EXIT procedure at delivery.

A goiter observed prenatally suggests that the mother may have thyroid disease. When cystic hygroma is found, there is a high risk for Turner's syndrome (45 X). Other chromosomal defects are also associated with cystic hygroma. Cystic hygroma or lymphangiectasia may also result from heart failure (e.g., because of a cardiac malformation or abnormal cardiac function).

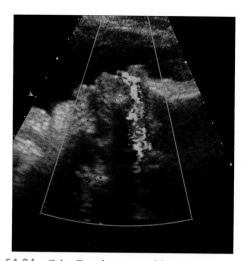

Figure 54-34 Color Doppler image of fetal breathing in a fetus with a normal palate demonstrating color only seen in the nasopharynx.

BOX 54-4 SONOGRAPHIC FINDINGS OF CLEFT LIP AND PALATE

- Median cleft lip: Caused by incomplete merging of the two medial nasal prominences in the midline
- Oblique facial cleft: Failure of maxillary prominence to merge with the lateral nasal swelling, with exposure of the nasolacrimal duct
- Complete bilateral cleft lip and palate: Large gap in upper lip on modified coronal view; nose is flattened and widened; a premaxillary mass may be present
- Unilateral complete cleft lip and palate: Incomplete fusion of maxillary prominence to the medial prominence on one side; modified coronal view
- Incomplete cleft: Nose is intact; modified coronal view of lip

---

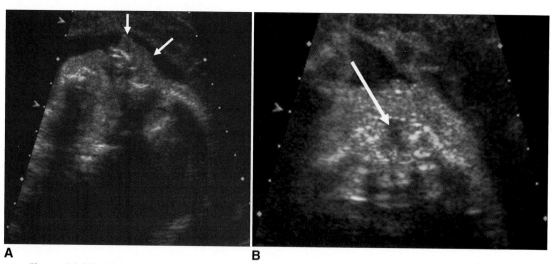

A   **B**

Figure 54-35 **A,** Sagittal image of a fetus with a cleft lip and palate. The fetal profile is distorted by a premaxillary mass *(lower arrow)*. Fetal nose *(upper arrow)*. **B,** Axial view of the maxilla in the same fetus delineates the bony defect of the maxilla *(arrow)*.

Cystic Hygroma. **Fetal cystic hygroma** results from a malformation of the lymphatic system that leads to single or multiloculated lymph-filled cavities around the neck. Normally the lymphatic vessels empty into two sacs lateral to the jugular veins (jugular lymph sacs) that communicate with the jugular veins and form the right lymphatic duct and thoracic duct. Failure of the lymphatic system to properly connect with the venous system results in distention of the jugular lymph sacs and the accumulation of lymph in fetal tissue. This abnormal collection of lymph causes distention of the lymph cavities, which may lead to fetal hydrops and even fetal death (Figure 54-39). About 70% of cystic hygromas involve the neck (usually arising from the posterior aspect of the neck bilaterally, but more rarely may arise from the anterior or lateral surface), and up to 20% involve the axillae (atypical cystic hygroma). Cystic hygromas may present as isolated small cystic cavities with or without septations. Fifty percent of cystic hygromas are associated with chromosomal anomalies and should therefore be accompanied by a thorough anatomic survey (Figure 54-40, *A, B*).

Cystic hygromas may be small and regress because alternate routes of lymph drainage may eventually develop. With this type of hygroma, webbing of the neck and swelling of the extremities may be appreciated after birth (Figure 54-40, *C*). These features are frequently seen in neonates with Turner's syndrome (45 X). These females are of short stature and are sterile because they only develop ovarian streaks. Cardiac and renal diseases are common. If the posterior neck skin appears thick without significant fluid-filled areas, this may represent a thickened nuchal fold seen with other chromosome anomalies, such as trisomy 21. This area should be measured in a suboccipital-bregmatic view (a tangential axial image that includes the anterior fontanel, or bregma, and the cerebellum) between 15 and 21 weeks. A measurement that is 6 mm is considered abnormal, and the fetus should have further prenatal genetic screening tests.

Large fetal cystic hygromas have a typical sonographic appearance. They appear as bilateral large cystic masses at the

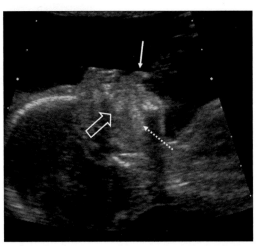

Figure 54-37 Sagittal view of a fetus with a small epignathus: external portion of the mass *(solid arrow)*, mass erupting from the maxilla *(open arrow)*, and tongue compressed against the lower jaw *(dotted arrow)*.

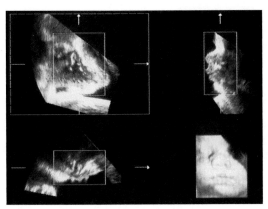

Figure 54-36 Three-dimensional reconstruction of the fetal face in a 34-week fetus. The X, Y, and Z axes are aligned to reproduce the 3-D image on the lower right.

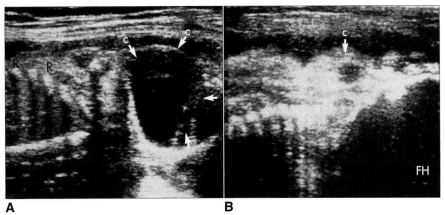

A   **B**

Figure 54-38 **A,** Brachial cleft cyst represented as a large unilateral septated cystic neck mass *(c, arrows)*. *R,* Rib. **B,** In the same fetus the brachial cleft cyst *(c)* at term had almost completely resolved. The neonate had no complications after birth. *FH,* Fetal head.

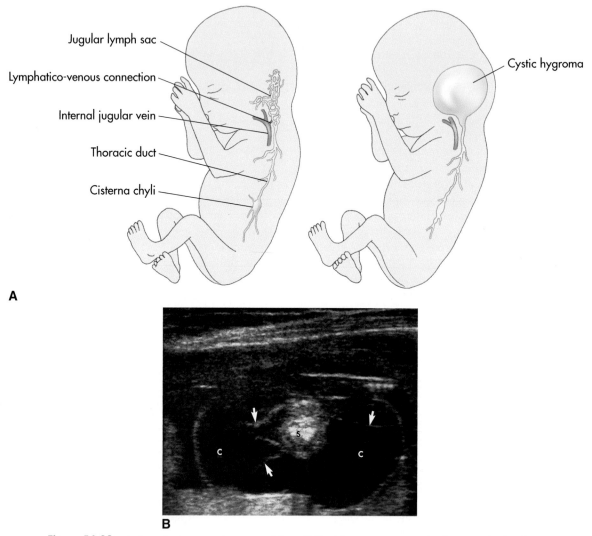

Figure 54-39   A, Lymphatic system in a normal fetus *(left)* with a patent connection between the jugular lymph sac and the internal jugular vein, and a cystic hygroma and hydrops from a failed lymphaticovenous connection *(right)*. **B,** Transverse neck view showing large posterolateral cystic masses *(c)* representing cystic hygromas in a fetus with Turner's syndrome. Note the multiple septations within the hygromas *(arrows)*. s, Cervical spine. (**A** from Chervenak FA and others: Fetal cystic hygroma: cause and natural history, *N Eng J Med* 309:822, 1985.)

posterolateral borders of the neck that may in severe cases surround the neck and head and upper trunk. Typically a dense midline septum divides the hygroma, with septations noted within the dilated lymph sacs. Because of an accumulation of lymph in the fetal tissue, fetal hydrops may result. Cystic hygroma with fetal hydrops carries 100% mortality. Pericardial or pleural effusions, edema of thoracic and abdominal skin, ascites, and limb edema are common. Heart failure commonly results in intrauterine death (Figures 54-41, 54-42, and 54-43). The differential considerations for cystic hygroma include meningomyelocele, encephalocele, nuchal edema, branchial cleft cyst, cystic teratoma, hemangiomas, and thyroglossal duct cysts (Figure 54-44).

Fetal Goiter. Whenever maternal thyroid disease is present, the fetal thyroid should be evaluated. A **fetal goiter (thy-**romegaly**)** usually appears as a symmetrical (bilobed), solid, homogeneous mass arising from the anterior fetal neck in the region of the fetal thyroid gland (Figure 54-45). The esophagus may be obstructed in the instance of a large goiter and hyperextended fetal neck, resulting in hydramnios and a small or absent stomach. When a goiter is suspected, the fetus may be either hypothyroid or hyperthyroid. Circulating maternal antibodies (i.e., thyroid stimulating immunoglobulin [TSI] and/or thyrotrophic binding inhibiting immunoglobulin [TBII]) determine whether the fetal thyroid function is inhibited (hypothyroid) or stimulated (hyperthyroid). However, if both antibodies coexist, the fetal thyroid function cannot be assessed accurately. Fetal thyroid function may then be determined by performing percutaneous umbilical blood sampling (PUBS) of the umbilical vein. If the fetus is found to be hypothyroid, then intrauterine fetal therapy may involve

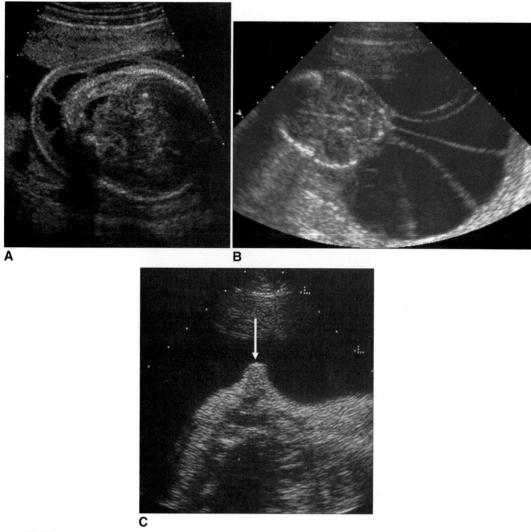

Figure 54-40 **A,** A transverse view of the neck demonstrates a small cystic hygroma. **B,** The large septated compartments seen in a fetus with a large cystic hygroma. **C,** Transverse view of the fetal neck demonstrates the remaining "webbing" from resolution of a cystic hygroma.

the weekly instillation of thyroxine via amniocentesis or may result in the increase of maternal medication (propylthiouracil [PTU]) for the hyperthyroid fetus because these drugs cross the placenta very readily. With intrauterine therapy, most fetal goiters regress and the physical exam is normal at birth. Follow-up studies of fetuses with goiter should include fetal thyroid size, signs of fetal tachycardia (if fetus is hyperthyroid), and amniotic fluid volume.

Teratoma. Neck **teratomas** are usually unilateral and usually located anteriorly. They may have complex sonographic (cystic, solid, echogenic) patterns similar to teratomas of other organs (Figure 54-46). Color Doppler may help differentiate this mass from atypical hygromas or other more cystic masses.

The neck is often difficult to assess when amniotic fluid is decreased, when the fetus is in an unfavorable position, or when the neck is in close proximity to the placenta. Nonetheless, evaluation of the neck should be routinely attempted. Box 54-5 lists the questions the sonographer should answer about fetal neck masses.

> **BOX 54-5   QUESTIONS FOR THE SONOGRAPHER EVALUATING A FETAL NECK MASS**
>
> - What is the position of mass (anterior, posterior, lateral, or midline)?
> - Is it a unilateral or bilateral lesion?
> - Is a nuchal ligament present?
> - What are the Doppler properties? (Hemangiomas have arterial and venous characteristics.)
> - Is there polyhydramnios?
> - Are there heart failure and hydrops?
> - Are there coexisting anomalies?
> - Is there hyperextension, which may suggest neck mass or iniencephaly (fusion of occiput to spine)?

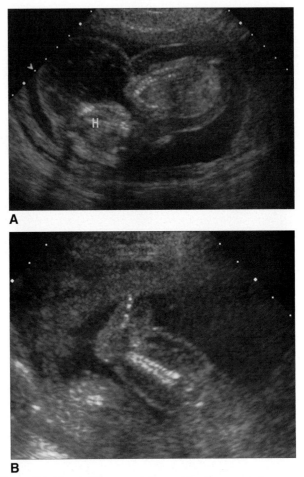

Figure 54-41 **A,** Fifteen-week fetus with a large cystic hygroma *(H)* that extends to include most of the fetal trunk. **B,** Limb edema in a fetus with cystic hygroma and generalized anasarca.

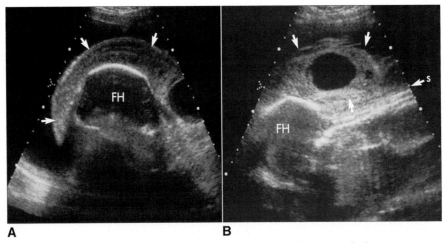

Figure 54-42 **A,** In the fetus shown in Figure 54-25, at 26 weeks of gestation, fetal movements were decreased, prompting ultrasound evaluation, which revealed a fetal demise. Note the helmetlike appearance of the scalp edema *(arrows)*. *FH,* Fetal head. **B,** In the same fetus, sagittal views revealed the posterolateral cystic hygroma *(arrows)* caused by lymphangiectasia from heart failure. *FH,* Fetal head; *s,* spine. Tetralogy of Fallot was revealed on autopsy.

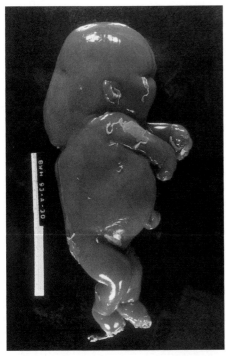

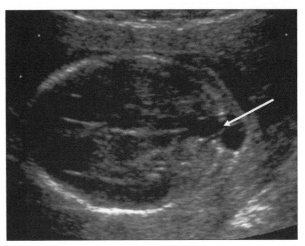

Figure 54-44   A fetus with a small encephalocele that could be mistaken for a small cystic hygroma. The identification of a bony defect suggests an encephalocele *(arrow)*.

Figure 54-43   In the neonate shown in Figure 54-24, a side view shows the posterior lateral positioning of the cystic hygromas.

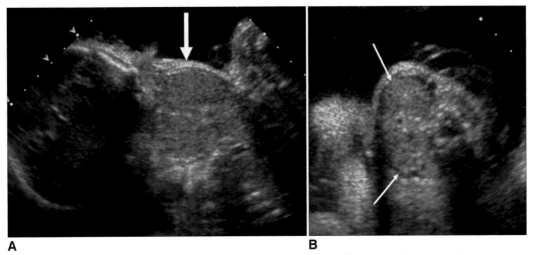

A   **B**

Figure 54-45   **A,** Axial image of the fetal neck, which reveals the bilobed enlarged fetal thyroid gland *(arrow).* **B,** A coronal view of the same fetus with the enlarged thyroid gland *(arrows).*

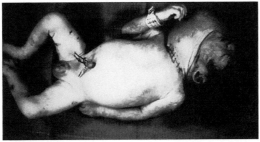

Figure 54-46   A large teratoma was found to arise from the posterior neck on this neonate. Multiple ultrasound studies demonstrated the mass to be complex in texture.

REFERENCES

1. Chung CS and others: Factors affecting risks of congenital malformations. I. Epidemiological analysis, *Birth Defects* 11:1, 1975.
2. Lee W and others: Three-dimensional ultrasonographic presentation of micrognathia, *J Ultrasound Med* 21:775, 2002.
3. Nicholaides KH: Nuchal translucency and other first-trimester sonographic markers of chromosomal abnormalities, *Am J Obstet Gynecol* 191(1):45, 2004.
4. Nyberg DA and others: Premaxillary protrusion: a sonographic clue to bilateral cleft lip and palate, *J Ultrasound Med* 12:331, 1993.
5. Palladini D and others: Objective diagnosis of micrognathia in the fetus: the jaw index, *Ultrasound Obstet Gynecol* 93(3):382, 1999.
6. Sanders RC: Ultrasonic assessment of the face and neck. In Sanders RC, editor: *The principles and practice of ultrasonography in obstetrics and gynecology*, Norwalk, Conn, 1985, Appleton-Century-Crofts.

SELECTED BIBLIOGRAPHY

Askar I and others: Lateral facial clefts (macrostomia), *Ann Plast Surg* 47(3):355, 2001.

Babcook CJ and others: Axial ultrasonographic imaging of the fetal maxilla for accurate characterization of facial clefts, *J Ultrasound Med* 16:619-625, 1997.

Benacerraf BR: *Ultrasound of fetal syndromes*, Philadelphia, 1998, Churchill Livingstone.

Benoit B: Three-dimensional ultrasonography of congenital ichthyosis, *J Ultrasound Obstet Gynecol* 13:380, 1999.

Bronshtein M and others: First and second trimester diagnosis of fetal ocular defects and associated anomalies: report of eight cases, *Obstet Gynecol* 77:443-449, 1991.

Callen DW, editor: *Ultrasonography in obstetrics and gynecology*, ed 3, Philadelphia, 1995, WB Saunders.

Chervenak FA and others: Fetal cystic hygroma: cause and natural history, *N Engl J Med* 309:822, 1985.

Chervenak FA and others: Antenatal sonographic diagnosis of epignathus, *J Ultrasound Med* 3:235, 1984.

Chervenak FA and others: Median cleft face syndrome: ultrasonic demonstration of cleft lip and hypertelorism, *Am J Obstet Gynecol* 149:94, 1984.

Chervenak FA and others: Diagnosis and management of fetal teratomas, *Obstet Gynecol* 66:666, 1985.

Chmait R and others: Prenatal evaluation of facial clefts with two-dimensional and adjunctive three-dimensional ultrasonography: a prospective trial, *Am J Obstet Gynecol* 187:946, 2002.

Cusick W and others: Fetal nasal bone length in euploid and aneuploid fetuses between 11 and 20 weeks' gestation: a prospective study, *J Ultrasound Med* 23(10):1327, 2004.

Dikkeboom CM and others: The role of three-dimensional ultrasound in visualizing the fetal cranial sutures and fontanels during the second half of pregnancy, *Ultrasound Obstet Gynecol* 24(4): 412, 2004.

Finberg HJ and others: Craniofacial damage from amniotic band syndrome subsequent to pathologic chorioamniotic separation at 10 weeks gestation, *J Ultrasound Med* 15:665-668, 1996.

Frattarelli JL and others: Prenatal diagnosis of frontonasal dysplasia (median cleft syndrome), *J Ultrasound Med* 15:81-83, 1996.

Hadi HA and others: In utero treatment of fetal goitrous hypothyroidism caused by maternal Graves' disease, *Am J Perinatol* 12(6):455, 1995.

Hadi HA and others: Prenatal diagnosis and management of fetal goiter caused by maternal Grave's disease, *Am J Perinatol* 12(4):240, 1995.

Hertzberg BS and others: Normal sonographic appearance of the fetal neck late in the first trimester: the pseudomembrane, *Radiology* 171:427-429, 1989.

Jeanty P and others: The binocular distance: a new parameter to estimated fetal age, *J Ultrasound Med* 3:241, 1984.

Jones KL: *Smith's recognizable patterns of human malformation*, ed 5, Philadelphia, 1997, WB Saunders.

Kincaid K and others: Prenatal sonographic detection of cleft lip and palate, *J Diagn Med Sonog* 6:309, 1989.

Malone FD and others: First-trimester nasal bone evaluation for aneuploidy in the general population, *Am J Obstet Gynecol* 104(6):1222, 2004.

Mayden KL and others: Orbital diameters: a new parameter for prenatal diagnosis and dating, *Am J Obstet Gynecol* 144:289, 1982.

Mittermayer C and others: Foetal facial clefts: prenatal evaluation of lip and primary palate by 2D and 3D ultrasound, *Ultraschall Med* 25(2):120, 2004.

Moore KL, editor: *The developing human: clinically oriented embryology*, ed 4, Philadelphia, 1988, WB Saunders.

Nyberg DA, Mahony BS, Pretorius DH, editors: *Diagnostic ultrasound of fetal anomalies: text and atlas*, St Louis, 1990, Mosby.

Otano L and others: Association between first trimester absence of fetal nasal bone on ultrasound and Down syndrome, *Prenat Diagn* 22(10):930, 2002.

Reynders CS and others: First trimester isolated fetal nuchal lucency: significance and outcome, *J Ultrasound Med* 16:101-105, 1997.

Rotten D and others: Two- and three-dimensional sonographic assessment of the fetal face. 2. Analysis of cleft lip, alveolus and palate, *Ultrasound Obstet Gynecol* 24(4):402, 2004.

Shipp TD and others: The ultrasonographic appearance and outcome for fetuses with masses distorting the fetal face, *J Ultrasound Med* 14:673, 1995.

Slavkin HC: Congenital craniofacial malformations: issues and perspectives, *J Prosthet Dent* 51:109, 1984.

Turner CD and others: Prenatal diagnosis of alobar holoprosencephaly at 10 weeks gestation, *J Ultrasound Obstet Gynecol* 13:360, 1999.

van der Haven I and others: The jaw index: new guide defining micrognathia in newborns, *J Cleft Palate Craniofac* 34:240, 1997.

Wong HS and others: First-trimester ultrasound diagnosis of holoprosencephaly: three case reports, *J Ultrasound Obstet Gynecol* 13:356, 1999.

The Fetal Neural Axis

Charlotte G. Henningsen

KEY TERMS

acrania – condition associated with anencephaly in which there is complete or partial absence of the cranial bones

alobar holoprosencephaly – most severe form of holoprosencephaly characterized by a single common ventricle and malformed brain; orbital anomalies range from fused orbits to hypotelorism, with frequent nasal anomalies and clefting of the lip and palate

anencephaly – neural tube defect characterized by the lack of development of the cerebral and cerebellar hemispheres and cranial vault; this abnormality is incompatible with life

anomaly – an abnormality or congenital malformation

cebocephaly – form of holoprosencephaly characterized by a common ventricle, hypotelorism, and a nose with a single nostril

cyclopia – severe form of holoprosencephaly characterized by a common ventricle, fusion of the orbits with one or two eyes present, and a proboscis (maldeveloped cylindrical nose)

cystic hygroma – an increase in size of the jugular lymphatic sacs because of abnormal development

holoprosencephaly – a range of abnormalities from abnormal cleavage of the forebrain

hydranencephaly – congenital absence of the cerebral hemispheres because of an occlusion of the carotid arteries; midbrain structures are present, and fluid replaces cerebral tissue

hydrocephalus – ventriculomegaly in the neonate; abnormal accumulation of cerebrospinal fluid within the cerebral ventricles, resulting in compression and frequently destruction of brain tissue

macrocephaly – enlargement of the fetal cranium as a result of ventriculomegaly

meningocele – open spinal defect characterized by protrusion of the spinal meninges

meningomyelocele – open spinal defect characterized by protrusion of meninges and spinal cord through the defect, usually within a meningeal sac

spina bifida – neural tube defect of the spine in which the dorsal vertebrae (vertebral arches) fail to fuse together, allowing the protrusion of meninges and/or spinal cord through the defect; two types exist: spina bifida occulta (skin-covered defect of the spine without protrusion of meninges or cord) and spina bifida cystica (open spinal defect marked by sac containing protruding meninges and/or cord)

spina bifida occulta – closed defect of the spine without protrusion of meninges or spinal cord; alpha-fetoprotein analysis will not detect these lesions

ventriculomegaly – abnormal accumulation of cerebrospinal fluid within the cerebral ventricles resulting in dilation of the ventricles; compression of developing brain tissue and brain damage may result; commonly associated with additional fetal anomalies

EMBRYOLOGY

The central nervous system (CNS) arises from the ectodermal neural plate at around 18 gestational days. The cephalic neural plate develops into the forebrain, and the caudal end forms the spinal cord. The midbrain and hindbrain then form, and the neural plate begins to fold. The cranial and caudal neuropores represent unfused regions of the neural tube that will close between 24 and 26 gestational days. The forebrain will continue to develop into the prosencephalon, the midbrain will become the mesencephalon, and the hindbrain will form the rhombencephalon.

At the end of the 3rd week, the cephalic end of the neural tube will bend into the shape of a C (cephalic flexure), with the area of the mesencephalon having a very prominent bend. The brain then folds back on itself, and by the beginning of the 5th week another prominent bend, the cervical flexure, appears between the hindbrain and the spinal cord. The brain that originally was composed of three parts has now further divided into five parts. The prosencephalon divides into the telencephalon, which becomes the cerebral hemispheres, and diencephalon, which eventually develops into the epithalamus, thalamus, hypothalamus, and infundibulum. The rhombencephalon also subdivides into the metencephalon, which ultimately becomes the cerebellum and pons, and the myelencephalon, which transforms into the medulla. The fundamental organization of the brain is represented in these five divisions that persist into adult life.

The primitive spinal cord divides into two regions. The alar plate region matures into the sensory region of the cord, and the basal plate region develops into the motor region of the cord. These regions further subdivide into specialized functions. Initially the spinal cord and vertebral column extend the length of the body. After the first trimester, the posterior portion of the body grows beyond the vertebral column and spinal cord, and the growth of the spinal cord lags behind that of the vertebral column. At birth the spinal cord terminates at the level of the third lumbar vertebra, although by adulthood the cord will end at the level of the second lumbar vertebra.

Neural function begins at 6 weeks of gestation and commences with primitive reflex movements at the level of the face and neck. By 12 weeks of gestation, sensitivity has spread across the surface of the body except at the back and top of the head. The fetus begins to have defined periods of activity and inactivity at the end of the fourth month. Between the fourth and fifth months, the fetus can grip objects and is capable of weak respiratory movements. At 6 months of gestation, the fetus displays the sucking reflex, and by about 28 weeks there have been significant changes in brain wave patterns.

Many of the congenital malformations of the CNS result from incomplete closure of the neural tube. A wide range of defects may affect the spine and/or brain. The remainder of this chapter presents anomalies of the CNS (Table 55-1).

Correctly identifying anomalies of the fetal head and spine can be a complex task. Some of the distinguishing characteristics that help define specific anomalies are listed in Table 55-2.

ANENCEPHALY

Anencephaly is the most common neural tube defect, with an overall incidence of approximately 1 in 1000 pregnancies in the United States. The incidence varies with geographic location, with a much higher prevalence in the United Kingdom. The incidence also varies with gender and race, having a female

TABLE 55-1	ANOMALIES MOST FREQUENTLY ASSOCIATED WITH VENTRICULOMEGALY
Anomaly	Distinguishing Characteristics
Spina bifida	Deformed cranium "lemon sign"; usually disappears in third trimester
	Obliteration of cisterna magna
	Open spinal defect
Cephalocele	Open cranial defect; usually occipital skull base
	Obliteration of the cisterna magna
	Occasional lemon sign
Holoprosencephaly	Absent/incomplete midline
	Single ventricular cavity
	Facial anomalies
Dandy-Walker complex	Midline posterior fossa cyst
	Defect in cerebellar vermis
Agenesis of corpus callosum	Absent cavum septi pellucidi
	Elevated third ventricle
	Interhemispheric cyst/lipoma
Arachnoid/glioependymal cyst	Intracranial cyst with regular contours displacing/compressing cortex
Porencephaly	Intracranial cyst jagged outline often communicating with lateral ventricles
Schizencephaly	Clefts in cortical mantle
Intracranial hemorrhage	Echogenic/complex mass in lateral ventricles/brain parenchyma
Microcephaly	Small head
Vascular malformations	Fluid-filled lesion with blood flow at Doppler examination
Craniostenosis	Abnormal skull shape
Lissencephaly	Absent/reduced cerebral convolutions
Infection	Intracranial/periventricular echogenicities

From Nyberg D and others: *Diagnostic imaging of fetal anomalies*, Philadelphia, 2003, Lippincott, Williams & Wilkins.

TABLE 55-2 DIFFERENTIAL CONSIDERATIONS FOR CENTRAL NERVOUS SYSTEM ANOMALIES

Anomaly	Sonographic Findings	Differential Considerations	Distinguishing Characteristics
Anencephaly	Absence of brain and cranial vault Froglike appearance Cerebrovasculosa	Microcephaly Acrania Cephalocele	No calvarium above orbits
Cephalocele	Extracranial mass Bony defect in calvarium	Cystic hygroma	Defect in skull
Dandy-Walker malformation	Posterior fossa cyst Splaying of cerebellar hemispheres	Arachnoid cyst Cerebellar hypoplasia	Cerebellar hemispheres will be splayed
Vein of Galen aneurysm	Midline cystic structure Turbulent Doppler flow	Arachnoid cyst Porencephalic cyst	Doppler flow in the cystic space
Porencephalic cyst	Cyst within brain parenchyma No mass effect Communication with ventricle	Arachnoid cyst	No mass effect Cyst communicating with ventricle
Hydranencephaly	Absence of brain tissue Fluid-filled brain Absent or partially absent falx	Hydrocephaly Holoprosencephaly	Lack of intact falx No rim of brain tissue

prevalence of 4 to 1 over males and a prevalence of white over black of 6 to 1. There is also a significant recurrence risk of 2% to 3% for subsequent pregnancies for a woman with a history of a prior pregnancy with an open neural tube defect.

Anencephaly, which means absence of the brain, is caused by failure of closure of the neural tube at the cranial end. The result is absence of the cranial vault, complete or partial absence of the forebrain, which may partially develop and then degenerate, and the presence of the brain stem, midbrain, skull base, and facial structures. The remnant brain is covered by a thick membrane called *angiomatous stroma* or *cerebrovasculosa*.

Anencephaly is a lethal disorder, with up to 50% of cases resulting in fetal demise. The remainder die at birth or shortly thereafter. Because of the severity of this disorder, early diagnosis is preferred. Prenatal diagnosis is often made with ultrasound following referral for increased maternal serum alpha-fetoprotein levels, which are extremely high with this defect because of the absent skull and exposed tissue.

The causes of neural tube defects including anencephaly are numerous. Anencephaly may result from a syndrome, such as Meckel-Gruber (i.e., cystic kidneys, occipital encephalocele and/or polydactyly (postaxial), microcephaly, microphthalmia, cleft palate, and genitourinary anomalies) or a chromosomal abnormality, such as trisomy 13. There is an increased risk in patients with diabetes mellitus, including patients whose disorders are well controlled. Environmental and dietary factors may also increase the prevalence of neural tube defects, including hyperthermia, folate and vitamin deficiencies, and teratogenic levels of zinc. Other teratogens associated with neural tube defects include valproic acid, methotrexate, and aminopterin. Another cause of neural tube defects is amniotic band syndrome, which may manifest with clefting defects.

Sonographic Findings. Anencephaly may be detected with ultrasound as early as 10 to 14 weeks of gestation, although

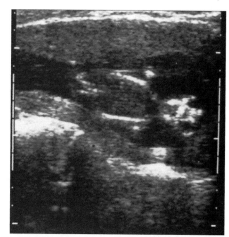

Figure 55-1 A 15-week anencephalic fetus. Note the froglike appearance.

the only sonographic feature may be acrania. The crown-rump length may be normal because the degeneration of the fetal brain is progressive, leading to a reduction in the crown-rump length with advancing gestation. Second-trimester identification of anencephaly is more obvious, with absent cerebral hemispheres evident, along with the absence of the skull.

Sonographic features of anencephaly include the following:

- Absence of the brain and cranial vault (Figure 55-1)
- Rudimentary brain tissue characterized as the cerebrovasculosa (Figure 55-2)
- Bulging fetal orbits, giving the fetus a froglike appearance (Figure 55-3)

Other sonographic findings associated with anencephaly include polyhydramnios, which is commonly seen but may not be present until after 26 weeks of gestation, although oligohydramnios may occasionally be identified. Coexisting spina bifida and/or craniorachischisis may be identified in fetuses with anencephaly. Additional anomalies include cleft lip and palate, hydronephrosis, diaphragmatic hernia, cardiac defects, omphalocele, gastrointestinal defects, and talipes.

When severe, microcephaly may be confused with anencephaly, although the presence of the cranium should aid in a definitive diagnosis. Other defects that may mimic anencephaly include acrania (brain is abnormal but present), cephalocele (brain herniation), and amniotic band syndrome (usually asymmetric cranial defects).

ACRANIA

Acrania, also known as exencephaly, is a lethal **anomaly** that manifests as absence of the cranial bones with the presence of complete, although abnormal, development of the cerebral hemispheres. This anomaly occurs at the beginning of the 4th gestational week when the mesenchymal tissue fails to migrate and does not allow bone formation over the cerebral tissue. The prevalence of acrania is rare, with only a few cases reported in the literature.[3] In addition, acrania usually progresses to

anencephaly as the brain slowly degenerates as a result of exposure to amniotic fluid.

Acrania may be confused with anencephaly, although the presence of significant brain tissue and the lack of a froglike appearance should establish the diagnosis. Other disorders that may mimic acrania include hypophosphatasia and osteogenesis imperfecta, both of which result in hypomineralization of the cranium. The identification of additional findings, such as long bone fractures, should help to distinguish these disorders from acrania. In addition to a lack of other skeletal anomalies, the lack of a calvarium allows differentiation of the cerebral hemispheres within the amniotic fluid giving the fetal head a bilobed appearance. This bilobed brain is best identified in the first trimester and has been described as a "Mickey Mouse" appearance.

Sonographic Findings. Sonographic features of acrania include the following:

- The presence of brain tissue without the presence of a calvarium (Figure 55-4)
- Disorganization of brain tissue
- Prominent sulcal markings (Figures 55-5 to 55-7)

Acrania may be associated with other anomalies, including spinal defects, cleft lip and palate, talipes, cardiac defects, and omphalocele. Acrania has also been associated with amniotic band syndrome (see Figure 55-4, *B*).

CEPHALOCELE

A cephalocele is a neural tube defect in which the meninges alone or meninges and brain herniate through a defect in the calvarium. *Encephalocele* is the term used to describe herniation of the meninges and brain through the defect; *cranial meningocele* describes the herniation of only meninges (Figure 55-8). Cephaloceles occur at a rate of 1 in 2000 live births.

Cephaloceles involve the occipital bone (Figure 55-9) and are located in the midline in 75% of cases, although they may also involve the parietal and frontal regions.

The prognosis for the infant with a cephalocele varies based on the size, location, and involvement of other brain struc-

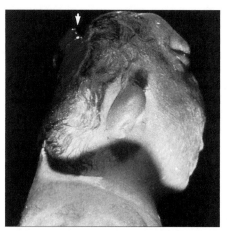

Figure 55-2   Postmortem photograph of anencephaly. The *arrow* points to the rudimentary brain (cerebrovasculosa).

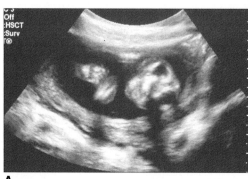
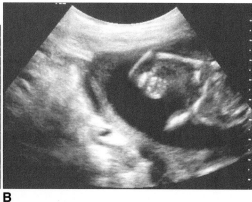

A   **B**

Figure 55-3   **A,** Anencephaly was identified in a fetus with a **(B)** radial ray defect and tetralogy of Fallot. A chromosomal anomaly was suspected. (Courtesy Ginny Goreczky, Maternal Fetal Center, Orlando, Fla.)

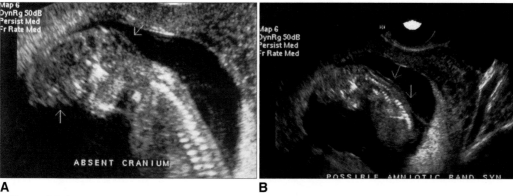

Figure 55-4 Acrania. Patient presented with an elevated maternal serum alpha-fetoprotein. Note the amnion *(arrows)* along the back of the fetus. Amniotic band syndrome was the probable cause.

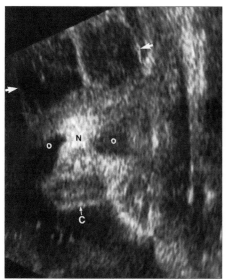

Figure 55-5 Coronal facial view showing absence of the parietal bones *(arrows)*, with highly visible brain tissue *(arrows)* representing acrania or exencephaly. *c,* Chin; *N,* nose; *o,* orbits.

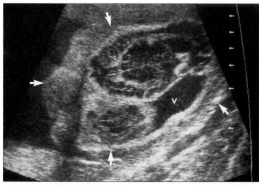

Figure 55-6 In the fetus shown in Figure 55-5, a transverse view shows the disorganized and freely floating brain tissue *(arrows)*. The brain anatomy is enhanced because of the absent skull bones. Note the herniated ventricle *(v)* and sulcal markings.

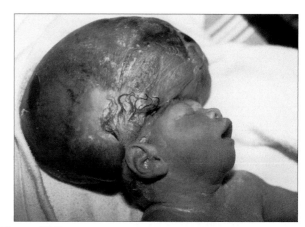

Figure 55-7 Same neonate shown in Figures 55-5 and 55-6, with acrania shortly after birth. The infant died within a few hours.

tures. The presence of brain in the defect dictates a poor prognosis. Microcephaly and other associated anomalies worsen the outcome. An infant with an isolated cranial meningocele has a 60% chance of normal mentation.

Sonographic Findings. The sonographic appearance of a cephalocele largely depends on the location, size, and involvement of brain structures. Cephaloceles containing meninges only; brain tissue only; meninges and brain tissue; and meninges, brain tissue, and lateral ventricles are referred to as meningocele, encephalocele, encephalomeningocele, and encephalomeningocystocele, respectively. According to the size of the lesion, cephaloceles are classified as occipital cephaloceles, which occur when the defect lies between the lambdoid suture and foramen magnum; parietal cephaloceles, which occur between the bregma and the lambda; and anterior cephaloceles, which lie between the anterior aspect of the ethmoid bone. Anterior cephaloceles are further classified into frontal and basal varieties. The frontal cephaloceles are always external lesions that occur near the root of the nose. Basal cephaloceles are internal lesions that occur within the nose, the pharynx, or the orbit.

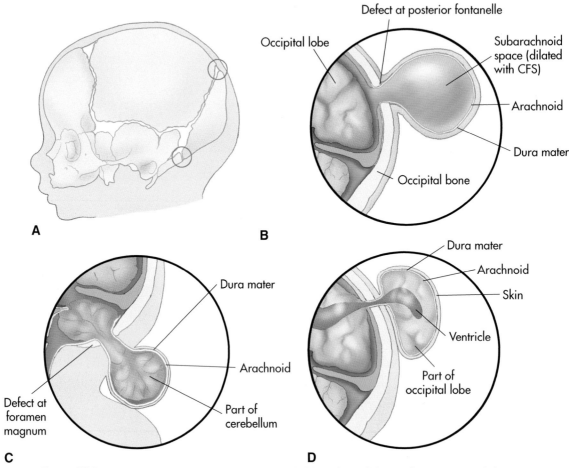

Figure 55-8 Schematic drawings illustrating cranium bifidum (bony defect in the cranium) and the various types of herniation of the brain and/or meninges. **A,** Sketch of the head of a newborn infant with a large protrusion from the occipital region of the skull. The upper circle indicates a cranial defect at the posterior fontanelle, and the lower circle indicates a cranial defect near the foramen magnum. **B,** Meningocele consisting of a protrusion of the cranial meninges that is filled with cerebrospinal fluid. **C,** Meningoencephalocele consisting of a protrusion of part of the cerebellum that is covered by meninges and skin. **D,** Meningohydroencephalocele consisting of a protrusion of part of the occipital lobe that contains part of the posterior horn of a lateral ventricle.

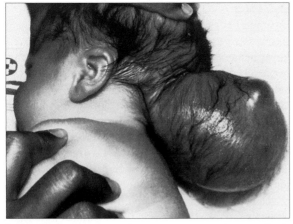

Figure 55-9 Neonate with a posterior occipital encephalocele.

Sonographic features of cephaloceles include the following:

- An extracranial mass (Figure 55-10), which may be fluid filled (cranial meningocele) or contain solid components (encephalocele)
- A bony defect in the skull
- Ventriculomegaly, which is more commonly identified with an encephalocele

Another sonographic finding associated with cephaloceles is polyhydramnios. Coexisting anomalies include microcephaly, agenesis of the corpus callosum, facial clefts, spina bifida, cardiac anomalies, and genital anomalies. Chromosomal anomalies and syndromes have been identified with cephaloceles, including trisomy 13 and Meckel-Gruber syndrome, which is an autosomal-recessive disorder characterized by encephalocele, polydactyly, and polycystic kidneys (Figure 55-11). Other syndromes linked with cephalocele include Chemke, cryptophthalmos, Knobloch, dyssegmental dysplasia, von Voss, Roberts', and Walker-Warburg. Cephaloceles located off midline are usually the result of amniotic band syndrome and may be further distinguished by associated limb anomalies and abdominal wall defects.

Cephaloceles may be confused with **cystic hygromas**, although they lack a cranial defect. Anencephaly may be difficult to distinguish from encephaloceles of significant size, and the presence of the cranial vault with encephalocele should establish the diagnosis. Frontal encephaloceles may be difficult to distinguish from a facial teratoma.

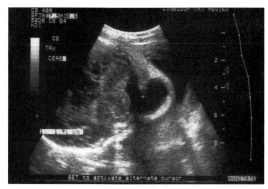

Figure 55-10   Cranial meningocele. The sac protruding from the cranium is fluid-filled.

SPINA BIFIDA

Spina bifida encompasses a wide range of vertebral defects that result from failure of neural tube closure. The meninges and neural elements may protrude through this defect. The defect may occur anywhere along the vertebral column but most commonly occurs along the lumbar and sacral regions. The incidence of this defect has declined over the last 10 years as a result of campaigning by the Public Health Service, which encourages women to increase their intake of folic acid before becoming pregnant. Decreases in the prevalence of anencephaly and encephalocele have also been noted.

The term *spina bifida* means that there is a cleft or opening in the spine (Figure 55-12). When covered with skin or hair, it is referred to as *spina bifida occulta*, an anomaly that is associated with a normal spinal cord and nerves and normal neurologic development. Spina bifida occulta is extremely difficult to detect in the fetus. Because the defect is covered by skin, the maternal serum alpha-fetoprotein level will be normal.

When the defect involves only protrusion of the meninges, it is termed a *meningocele*. More commonly the meninges and neural elements protrude through the defect. This is called a *meningomyelocele*. If the defect is very large and severe, it is termed *rachischisis*. These defects are commonly associated with increased maternal serum alpha-fetoprotein.

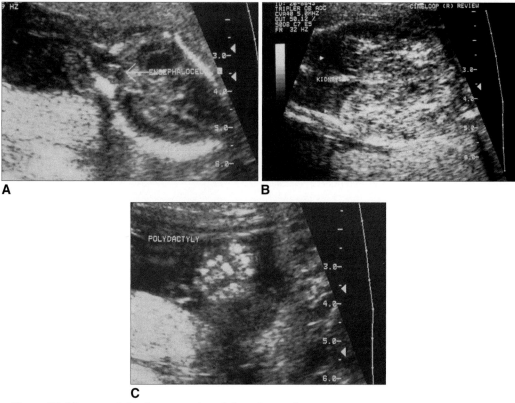

Figure 55-11   Encephalocele as part of Meckel-Gruber syndrome. **A,** Brain tissue herniating from the occipital region. **B,** Large echogenic kidneys consistent with autosomal-recessive polycystic kidney disease (ARPKD). **C,** Polydactyly was noted on the hands.

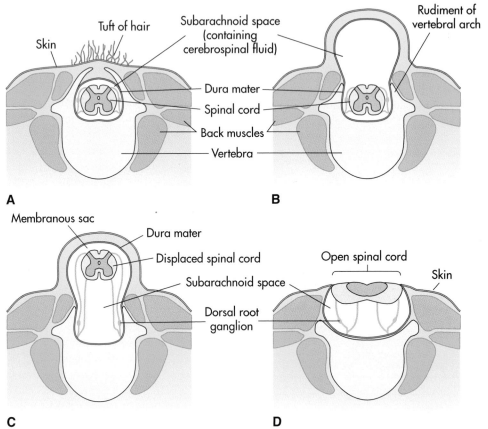

Figure 55-12 Diagrammatic sketches illustrating various types of spina bifida and the commonly associated malformations of the nervous system. **A,** Spina bifida occulta. About 10% of people have this vertebral defect in L5 and/or S1. It usually causes no back problems. **B,** Spina bifida with meningocele. **C,** Spina bifida with meningomyelocele. **D,** Spina bifida with myeloschisis. The types illustrated in **B** to **D** are often referred to collectively as *spina bifida cystica* because of the cystic sac that is associated with them.

Spina bifida is also associated with varying degrees of neurologic impairment, which may include minor anesthesia, paraparesis, or death. Fetuses with myelomeningoceles often present with the cranial defects associated with the Arnold-Chiari (type II) malformation, which is identified in 90% of patients. The Arnold-Chiari II malformation presents invariably with hydrocephalus because of the cerebellar vermis, which becomes displaced into the cervical canal. This changes the shape of the cerebellum, giving it a "banana" appearance, and leads to obliteration of the cisterna magna. In addition, caudal displacement of the cranial structures causes scalloping of the frontal bones of the skull, making the fetal head resemble a lemon.

Management of a fetus with spina bifida usually includes serial ultrasound examinations to monitor progression and extent of ventriculomegaly and to follow fetal growth. Fetuses may be delivered early for ventricular shunting, usually by cesarean section to preserve as much motor function as possible. Surgical repair of these defects is also being performed, though is still considered experimental. The benefit of surgery has been limited relative to improving lower extremity function; however, fewer children have required a shunt to decrease the sequelae of hydrocephalus. Risks incurred with this proce-

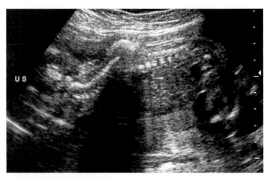

Figure 55-13 A large spinal defect at the thoracic level is seen in the fetus. The prognosis was expected to be extremely poor. (From Henningsen C: *Clinical guide to ultrasonography,* St Louis, 2004, Mosby.)

dure include premature delivery, maternal morbidity, and fetal mortality.

The prognosis for an infant with spina bifida varies greatly according to the type, size, and location of the defect. Rachischisis is invariably lethal, and higher lesions (Figure 55-13) tend to have a worse prognosis. When intervention is desired,

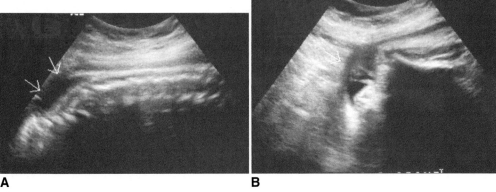

Figure 55-14   Sagittal **(A)** and transverse **(B)** views of the fetal spine *(arrows)* demonstrate this defect in the lumbar region. (Courtesy Ginny Goreczky, Maternal Fetal Center, Orlando, Fla.)

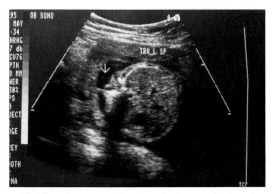

Figure 55-15   Meningomyelocele with the spinal splaying appearing as a V.

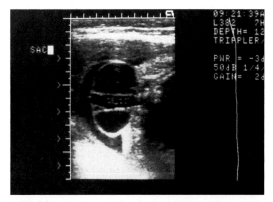

Figure 55-16   Meningomyelocele identified in a fetus with mild ventriculomegaly. Note the neural elements protruding into the sac.

surgical closure of the defect is performed to preserve existing neurologic function. In addition to management of the actual defect, attention to any hydrocephalus, urinary tract anomalies or dysfunction, and orthopedic issues may be part of the long-term care for this child.

Sonographic Findings. Sonographic examination of the fetal spine should include a methodical survey of the spine in the sagittal and transverse planes (Figure 55-14). The normal fetal spine should demonstrate the posterior ossification centers completing a spinal circle. The survey of the fetal spine may be impeded when the spine is down, when the fetus is in the breech position, when oligohydramnios is present, and when maternal obesity precludes adequate visualization.

Sonographic features of spina bifida include the following:

- Splaying of the posterior ossification centers with a V or U configuration (Figure 55-15)
- Protrusion of a saclike structure that may be anechoic (meningocele) or contain neural elements (myelomeningocele) (Figure 55-16)
- A cleft in the skin (Figure 55-17)

After a spinal defect has been identified, the level and extent of the defect, the presence or absence of neural elements contained in the protruding sac, and associated intracranial findings should be documented.

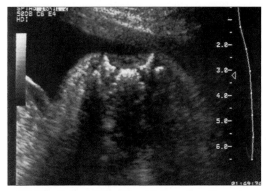

Figure 55-17   Spina bifida with a U-shaped configuration and an open cleft in the skin.

The associated sonographic cranial findings include the following:

- Flattening of the frontal bones, giving the head a "lemon" shape (Figure 55-18)
- Obliteration of the cisterna magna
- Inferior displacement of the cerebellar vermis, giving the cerebellum a rounded, "banana" shape (see Figure 55-18)
- Ventriculomegaly (Figures 55-19 and 55-20)

The "lemon sign" is not specific for spina bifida, and similar head shapes have been described with other CNS malformations, such as encephalocele, and non-CNS malformations, such as thanatophoric dysplasia. This appearance may also be indistinguishable from the "strawberry sign" described in association with trisomy 18.

Other sonographic findings associated with spina bifida include talipes, cephaloceles, cleft lip and palate, hypotelorism, heart defects, and genitourinary anomalies (Figures 55-21 and 55-22). Spina bifida has also been associated with multiple syndromes and chromosomal anomalies, including trisomy 18. Fetuses exposed to teratogens, such as valproic acid (Figure 55-23), methotrexate, and aminopterin are also at greater risk for developing spina bifida. Maternal diabetes, hyperthermia, and folic acid deficiency have also been associated with spina bifida.

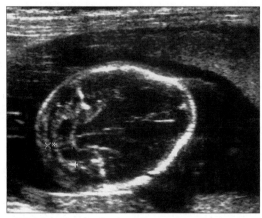

Figure 55-18 Abnormally shaped cerebellum "banana sign" *(calipers [+])* in a 21-week fetus with a lumbosacral meningomyelocele. Note the lemon-shaped frontal bones consistent with frontal bossing.

DANDY-WALKER MALFORMATION

Dandy-Walker malformation (DWM) is a defect that may have varying degrees of severity. It manifests with agenesis or hypoplasia of the cerebellar vermis with resulting dilation on the fourth ventricle. The occurrence rate is 1 in 25,000 to 35,000.

DWM is thought to occur before the 6th or 7th gestational week as the result of abnormal embryogenesis of the roof of the fourth ventricle. In its milder form, it is referred to as the Dandy-Walker variant. DWM causes 4% of cases of hydrocephalus, which is commonly identified in conjunction with this anomaly.

DWM is associated with other intracranial anomalies about 50% of the time. These include agenesis of the corpus callosum, aqueductal stenosis, microcephaly, **macrocephaly**, encephalocele, gyral malformations, and lipomas. Chromosomal anomalies that may be associated with DWM include trisomies 13, 18, and 21. DWM has been associated with several syndromes, including Meckel-Gruber syndrome, Walker-Warburg syndrome, and Aicardi's syndrome, and has been linked with congenital infections.

The prognosis for DWM depends on the presence or absence of associated anomalies. Mortality depends highly on other anomalies. Many infants with isolated DWM have a subnormal IQ, although some may have normal function.

Sonographic Findings. Sonographic survey may reveal extracranial anomalies that are also associated with DWM, including cardiac anomalies, polydactyly, facial clefts, and urinary tract anomalies.

Sonographic features of DWM include the following:

- A posterior fossa cyst that can vary considerably in size (Figure 55-24)
- Splaying of the cerebellar hemispheres as a result of the complete or partial agenesis of the cerebellar vermis
- An enlarged cisterna magna caused by the cerebellar vermis anomaly and posterior fossa cyst
- Ventriculomegaly (Figure 55-25)

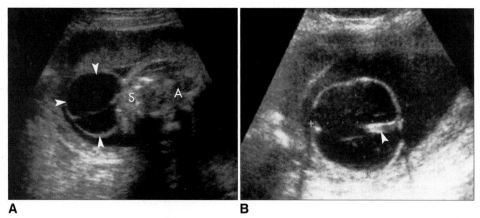

A   **B**

Figure 55-19 **A,** Lumbosacral meningomyelocele *(arrows)* shown in a 21-week fetus, detected on a basic fetal scan. *A,* Abdomen; *S,* spine. **B,** Lumbosacral meningomyelocele measuring 6 cm *(calipers)* observed in a 33-week fetus during a basic fetal scan. Note the spinal elements *(arrow)* within the meningomyelocele sac. Additional anomalies include clubbing of the feet and inward rotation of the legs. Ventriculomegaly was present, but effacement of the cisterna magna was not apparent.

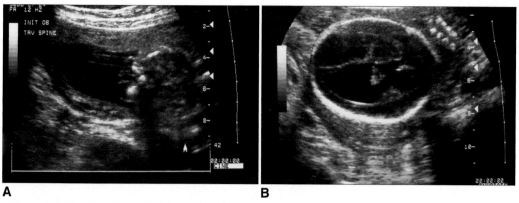

A   **B**

Figure 55-20   **A,** A fetus of 24.6 weeks of gestation with a meningomyelocele. Neural elements were identified in the sac. **B,** A significant amount of ventricular dilation was identified within the fetal head.

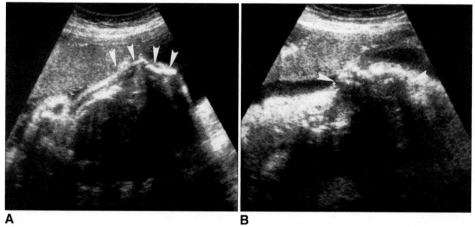

A   **B**

Figure 55-21   **A,** Thoracic meningomyelocele demonstrated with significant disruption of the bony elements *(arrows)*. **B,** In the same fetus, another view demonstrating the spinal defect. Coexisting anomalies included significant ventriculomegaly of 27 mm, unilateral renal agenesis, and single umbilical artery.

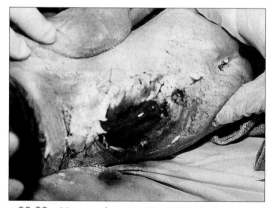

Figure 55-22   Neonate shown in Figure 55-21, demonstrating large thoracic meningomyelocele.

The differential considerations should include the arachnoid cyst, but the identification of the splayed cerebellar hemispheres may help to confirm DWM. Cerebellar hypoplasia should also be included when the cisterna magna is enlarged; however, confirming the small cerebellum may make this diagnosis of Dandy-Walker malformation.

HOLOPROSENCEPHALY

Holoprosencephaly encompasses a range of abnormalities resulting from abnormal cleavage of the prosencephalon (forebrain). The incidence is 0.6 in 1000 live births, although the incidence in embryos has been much higher (1 in 250). Holoprosencephaly has been associated with chromosomal anomalies in up to 50% of cases; however, it may also be a sporadic event or associated with syndromes, genetic factors, and teratogens. The recurrence risk has been reported as high as 13% to 14% when identified as a sporadic event.[1]

There are three forms of holoprosencephaly. The most severe form is classified as alobar, the intermediate form as semilobar, and the mildest form as lobar. Identification of the specific form depends on the degree of failed hemispheric division.

Alobar holoprosencephaly is characterized by a singular monoventricle brain tissue that is small and may have a cup, ball, or pancake configuration (Figure 55-26); fusion of the thalamus; and absence of the interhemispheric fissure, cavum septum pellucidum, corpus callosum, optic tracts, and olfactory bulbs. Semilobar holoprosencephaly (Figure 55-27)

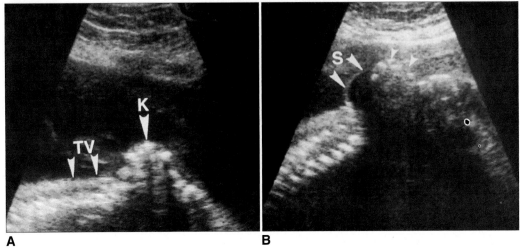

Figure 55-23 A, Meningomyelocele caused by a teratogen (valproic acid [Depakene]) in a 26-week fetus. Sagittal view showing thoracolumbar meningomyelocele with marked kyphosis *(K)* of the spinal elements. *TV,* Thoracic vertebrae. **B,** In the same fetus a meningomyelocele sac *(S)* is observed outlining the marked disruption and malalignment of the vertebrae (*small* arrowheads). This mother was given valproic acid for a seizure disorder during the first trimester of pregnancy. Valproic acid is a known teratogen that may produce neural tube defects. Elevated levels of maternal serum alpha-fetoprotein prompted the fetal study. Coexisting anomalies included ventriculomegaly, small cranium, and a unilateral clubfoot.

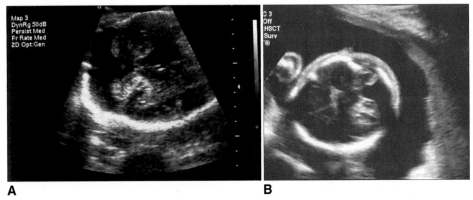

Figure 55-24 A, Dandy-Walker cyst. Note the splayed cerebellar hemispheres. (Courtesy Ginny Goreczky, Maternal Fetal Center, Florida Hospital, Orlando, Fla.) **B,** This Dandy-Walker malformation was associated with ventriculomegaly. Amniocentesis revealed normal chromosomes. (Courtesy Maria Roman, Maternal Fetal Center, Florida Hospital, Orlando, Fla.)

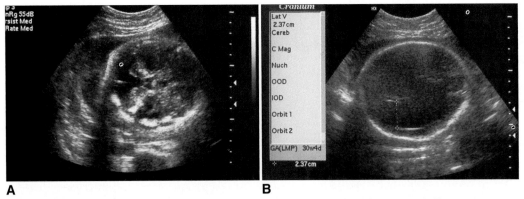

Figure 55-25 This patient had a history of elevated maternal serum alpha-fetoprotein. Follow-up in a maternal fetal center for a history of hydrocephalus revealed a Dandy-Walker malformation **(A)** and ventriculomegaly **(B).** The fetus was 30 weeks and 4 days, with a head size typical of 36 weeks of gestation.

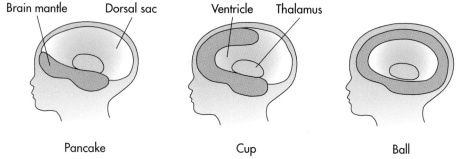

Figure 55-26 Diagram of three morphologic types of alobar holoprosencephaly (and semilobar holoprosencephaly) in sagittal view. In the pancake type, the residual brain mantle is flattened at the base of the brain. The dorsal sac is correspondingly large. The cup type has more brain mantle present, but it does not cover the monoventricle. In the ball type, the brain mantle completely covers the monoventricle, and a dorsal sac may or may not be present.

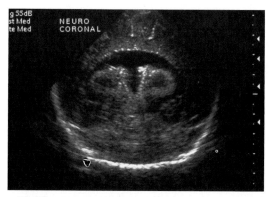

Figure 55-27 A neonatal ultrasound in a newborn revealed semilobar holoprosencephaly. There was no history of a prenatal ultrasound because of the normal course of the pregnancy. The infant only lived for a few weeks.

presents with a singular ventricular cavity with partial formation of the occipital horns, partial or complete fusion of the thalamus, a rudimentary falx and interhemispheric fissure, and absent corpus callosum, cavum septum pellucidum, and olfactory bulbs. In lobar holoprosencephaly, there is almost complete division of the ventricles with a corpus callosum that may be normal, hypoplastic, or absent, although the cavum septum pellucidum will still be absent.

The cause of holoprosencephaly varies. It is usually sporadic but has been associated with chromosomal anomalies, most specifically trisomy 13, and there have been rare familial patterns transmitted in autosomal dominant and autosomal recessive forms. Multiple syndromes have also been associated with holoprosencephaly, including Meckel-Gruber syndrome, Aicardi's syndrome, Fryns syndrome, and hydrolethalus syndrome. Teratogens reported to produce holoprosencephaly include alcohol, phenytoin, retinoic acid, maternal diabetes, and congenital infections.

The prognosis for holoprosencephaly is considered uniformly poor. In its most severe forms, fetuses die at birth or shortly thereafter. In the least severe form, survival is possible, although usually with severe mental retardation.

Sonographic Findings. Sonographic features of holoprosencephaly include the following:

- A common C-shaped ventricle that may or may not be enlarged (Figure 55-28)
- Brain tissue with a horseshoe shape as it surrounds the monoventricle
- Fusion of the thalamus with absence of the third ventricle
- Absence of the interhemispheric fissure
- A dorsal sac with expansion of the monoventricle posteriorly
- Absence of the corpus callosum
- Absence of the cavum septum pellucidum

Holoprosencephaly is often associated with facial abnormalities, especially with the most severe forms (Figure 55-29). The facial anomalies identified include **cyclopia,** hypotelorism (Figure 55-30, *A*), an absent nose, a flattened nose with a single nostril, and a proboscis (Figures 55-30, *B* and 55-31). **Cebocephaly** consists of the combination of hypotelorism with a normally placed nose with a single nostril. Ethmocephaly consists of severe hypotelorism with a proboscis superior to the eyes. In addition, facial clefts may be present, with median or bilateral clefting most commonly observed.

Other sonographic findings associated with holoprosencephaly include hydrocephaly, microcephaly, polyhydramnios, and intrauterine growth restriction (IUGR). In addition, renal cysts or dysplasia, omphalocele, cardiac defects, spina bifida, talipes, and gastrointestinal anomalies have been identified in the presence of holoprosencephaly. Chromosomal anomalies must also be considered if holoprosencephaly is present, especially trisomy 13.

AGENESIS OF THE CORPUS CALLOSUM

The corpus callosum is a fibrous tract that connects the cerebral hemispheres and aids in learning and memory. Dysgenesis of the corpus callosum describes a range of complete to partial absence of the callosal fibers that cross the midline,

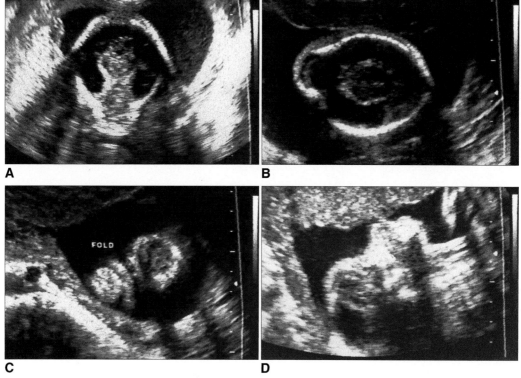

Figure 55-28 Holoprosencephaly. This patient had a history of six previous pregnancies, two of which were also affected by holoprosencephaly. This was an autosomal dominant form of holoprosencephaly. **A,** C-shaped monoventricle. **B,** An encephalocele was also noted. **C,** Imaging of the face revealed redundant skin folds at the level of the nose and hypotelorism. **D,** Note the abnormal-appearing profile.

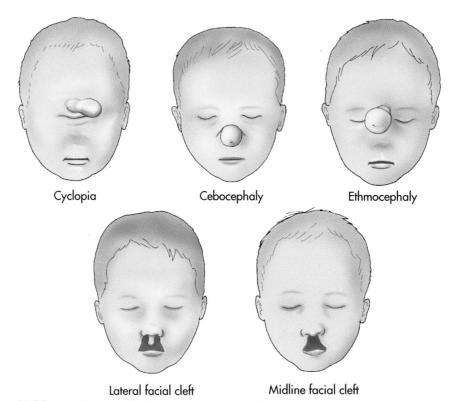

Cyclopia   Cebocephaly   Ethmocephaly

Lateral facial cleft   Midline facial cleft

Figure 55-29 Facial features of holoprosencephaly. These drawings illustrate the normal facial features in contrast with the variable facial features of holoprosencephaly. In cyclopia the proboscis projects from the lower forehead superior to one median orbit, and the nose is absent. Ethmocephaly is very similar to cyclopia, but has two narrowly placed orbits with a proboscis and absent nose. In cebocephaly a rudimentary nose with a single nostril and hypotelorism are present. Hypotelorism may occur with a median cleft lip or bilateral cleft lip.

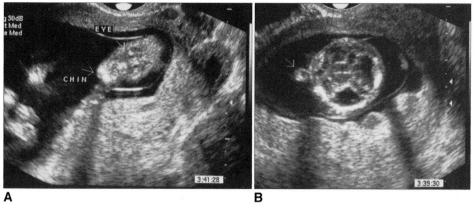

Figure 55-30 **A,** A fetus with trisomy 13 demonstrates small eyes with hypotelorism. **B,** In the same fetus, a proboscis *(arrow)* is seen above the orbits. (Courtesy Ginny Goreczky, Maternal Fetal Center, Orlando, Fla.)

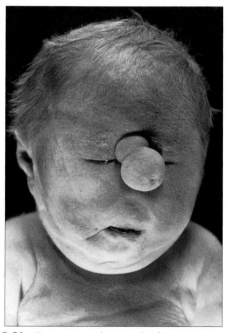

Figure 55-31   Postmortem photograph of a neonate with ethmocephaly. Note the proboscis and hypotelorism. The mouth appears normal. A common ventricle and absent optic and ophthalmic nerves were found. The chromosomes were consistent with trisomy 13.

forming a connection between the two hemispheres. The incidence is reported to be 1 to 3 in 1000 births.[2]

The corpus callosum begins to develop at 12 weeks of gestation and is not complete until 20 weeks. The cause of agenesis of the corpus callosum is somewhat unclear but is thought to involve a vascular disruption or inflammatory lesion before 12 weeks. Cases of agenesis of the corpus callosum, also known as callosal agenesis, are sporadic. It may be associated with other CNS malformations, and autosomal dominant, autosomal recessive, and X-linked syndromes have also been identified. Chromosomal anomalies that may accompany agenesis of the corpus callosum include trisomies 13 and 18.

The prognosis for agenesis of the corpus callosum depends largely on the high incidence of associated anomalies, many of which carry a poor prognosis. As an isolated event, agenesis of the corpus callosum may be asymptomatic or associated with mental retardation and/or seizures.

Sonographic Findings. Sonographic features of agenesis of the corpus callosum (Figure 55-32) include the following:

- Absence of the corpus callosum
- Elevation and dilation of the third ventricle
- Widely separated lateral ventricular frontal horns with medial indentation of the medial walls
- Dilated occipital horns (colpocephaly), giving the lateral ventricles a teardrop shape
- Absence of the cavum septum pellucidum

Other sonographic findings associated with agenesis of the corpus callosum include other CNS anomalies, such as holoprosencephaly, DWM, cranial lipoma, Arnold-Chiari malformation, septo-optic dysplasia, hydrocephaly, encephalocele, porencephaly, microcephaly, and lissencephaly. Other abnormalities associated with agenesis of the corpus callosum include cardiac malformations, diaphragmatic hernia, lung agenesis or dysplasia, and absent or dysplastic kidneys. Multiple chromosomal anomalies and syndromes have been linked with agenesis of the corpus callosum, including trisomies 13, 18, and 8 and Aicardi's syndrome.

AQUEDUCTAL STENOSIS

Aqueductal stenosis results from an obstruction, atresia, or stenosis of the aqueduct of Sylvius causing ventriculomegaly. The aqueduct of Sylvius connects the third and fourth ventricles, which explains the enlargement of the lateral ventricles and third ventricle in the presence of a normal fourth ventricle.

Aqueductal stenosis is usually a sporadic anomaly, but may also result from intrauterine infections, such as cytomegalovirus, rubella, and toxoplasmosis. Cranial masses and ventricular hemorrhage are also contributing factors of

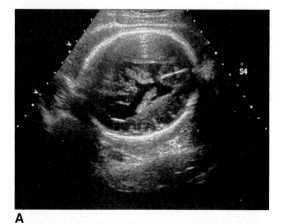

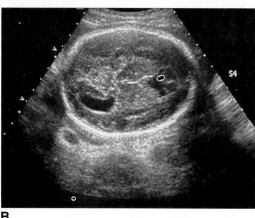

Figure 55-32 **A,** Agenesis of the corpus callosum is diagnosed in this fetus with an absent cavum septum pellucidum. **B,** The occipital horn of the lateral ventricle also appears dilated. (From Henningsen C: *Clinical guide to ultrasonography,* St Louis, 2004, Mosby.)

acquired obstruction. Primary aqueductal stenosis is usually X-linked and has an autosomal-recessive inheritance.

The prognosis for aqueductal stenosis is considered poor and varies with associated anomalies. Approximately 90% of survivors have an IQ less than 70. Infants with X-linked aqueductal stenosis are profoundly mentally retarded.

Sonographic Findings. Sonographic features of aqueductal stenosis include the following:

- Ventricular enlargement of the lateral ventricles, which may be severe (Figures 55-33 and 55-34)
- Third ventricular dilation
- Flexion and adduction of the thumb (seen in the X-linked form)

VEIN OF GALEN ANEURYSM

An aneurysm of the vein of Galen, also known as a vein of Galen malformation, is a rare arteriovenous malformation. The vein will be enlarged and communicate with normal-appearing arteries.

Vein of Galen aneurysm is considered a sporadic event and has a male predominance. It is usually an isolated anomaly, although it has been associated with congenital heart defects, **cystic hygromas,** and hydrops.

The prognosis for vein of Galen aneurysm is generally poor, especially when associated with hydrops and/or cardiac failure. When symptoms present later in older children and young adults, the prognosis is generally good.

Sonographic Findings. Sonographic features of vein of Galen aneurysm include the following:

- A cystic space that may be irregular in shape and is located midline and posterosuperior to the third ventricle
- Turbulent flow with Doppler evaluation

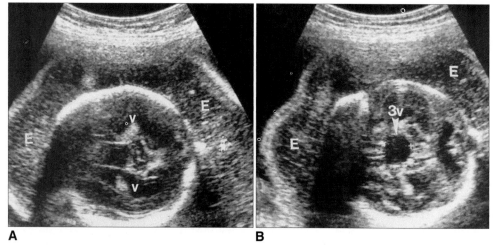

Figure 55-33 **A,** Ventricular view in a fetus with acquired aqueductal stenosis because of parvovirus infection. Dilation of the ventricular system *(v)* resulted from inflammation, causing obstruction to the flow of cerebrospinal fluid. The fetus was severely hydropic. Note the significant scalp edema *(E).* **B,** In the same fetus, third ventricle *(3v)* dilation is demonstrated. Cordocentesis was performed to find a cause for the severe nonimmune hydrops, and parvovirus was detected within the fetal blood. The fetus died shortly after birth. *E,* Scalp edema.

Other sonographic findings associated with a vein of Galen aneurysm include fetal cardiomegaly and nonimmune hydrops. Ventriculomegaly with resultant macrocephaly may also develop.

The vein of Galen aneurysm may be confused with arachnoid cysts, which are very rare and may occur anywhere within the brain. Doppler evaluation of an arachnoid cyst will reveal no blood flow within the structure. Porencephalic cysts should also be listed in the differential considerations; however, these may be distinguished by the absence of blood flow and this cyst's communication with the ventricle.

CHOROID PLEXUS CYSTS

Choroid plexus cysts are round or ovoid anechoic structures found within the choroid plexus. These cysts are common, occurring with a frequency of 0.4% to 3.6%. Choroid plexus cysts contain cerebrospinal fluid and cellular debris that has become trapped with the neuroepithelial folds.

Choroid plexus cysts are usually isolated findings without association with other anomalies. Furthermore, they will often resolve by 22 to 26 weeks of gestation. Choroid plexus cysts have been identified in association with aneuploidy, most commonly trisomies 18 and 21.

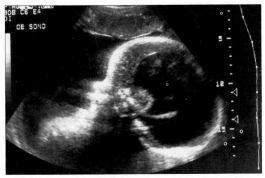

Figure 55-34   A sagittal image of a fetus with severe hydrocephaly, which was thought to result from aqueductal stenosis.

Sonographic Findings. Sonographic features of choroid plexus cysts include the following:

- Cysts within the choroid plexus ranging in size from 0.3 to 2 cm
- Unilateral or bilateral cysts (Figure 55-35)
- Solitary or multiple
- Unilocular or multilocular
- Enlargement of the ventricle with large cyst

A careful sonographic survey for anomalies that might suggest aneuploidy should follow identification of a choroid plexus cyst to include nuchal fold measurement, meticulous survey of the heart, and a survey of the feet and hands to look for abnormal posturing and polydactyly. Amniocentesis for karyotyping may be offered, especially when other factors that may increase the risk for aneuploidy are considered, including maternal age, abnormal triple screen, and other ultrasound findings.

PORENCEPHALIC CYSTS

Porencephalic cysts, also known as porencephaly, are cysts filled with cerebrospinal fluid that communicate with the ventricular system or subarachnoid space. They may result from hemorrhage, infarction, delivery trauma, or inflammatory changes in the nervous system. The affected brain parenchyma undergoes necrosis, brain tissue is resorbed, and a cystic lesion remains.

There are no known associated anomalies in fetuses with porencephalic cysts. Postnatal problems may include seizures, developmental delays, motor deficits, visual and sensory problems, and hydrocephalus.

Sonographic Findings. The sonographic features of porencephalic cysts include the following:

- A cyst within the brain parenchyma without mass effect
- Communication of the cyst with the ventricle or subarachnoid space (Figure 55-36)
- Reduction in size of the affected hemisphere, which may cause a midline shift and contralateral ventricular enlargement

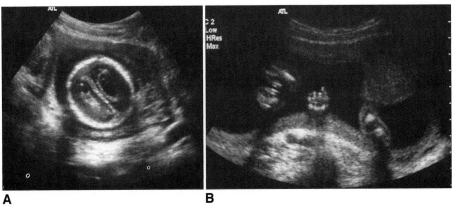

A   **B**

Figure 55-35   **A,** Bilateral choroid plexus cysts are observed in this fetus with trisomy 18. **B,** The same fetus also had a heart defect and these persistently clenched hands. (Courtesy Maria Roman, Maternal Fetal Center, Florida Hospital, Orlando, Fla.)

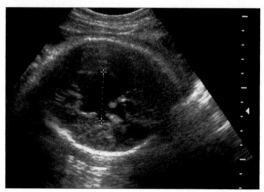

Figure 55-36   This patient was referred at 32 weeks of gestation to a fetal diagnostic center with a history of hydrocephalus seen on ultrasound examination. A porencephalic cyst was identified communicating with the lateral ventricle. Ventriculomegaly was also noted. The patient was counseled that this finding carried a poor prognosis.

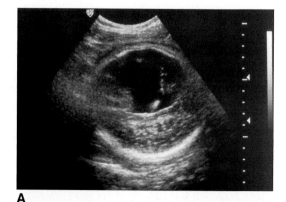

A

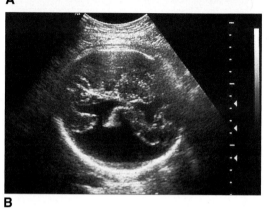

B

Figure 55-37   **A** and **B,** This patient came for an initial ultrasound at 32 weeks of gestation for late prenatal care. The ultrasound revealed hydrocephaly, and the patient was referred to a maternal-fetal center where the diagnosis of schizencephaly was made based on the cleft that extends to the calvarium. This diagnosis was confirmed at birth with computed tomography.

Porencephalic cysts may be confused with arachnoid cysts (see Figure 55-40), although the lack of a mass effect seen with porencephaly may aid in differentiating the two.

SCHIZENCEPHALY

Schizencephaly is a rare disorder characterized by clefts in the cerebral cortex. The clefts may be unilateral or bilateral, open-lip or closed-lip defects. Schizencephaly is thought to result from abnormal migration of neurons. These clefts can extend from the ventricle to the outer surface of the brain and are lined with abnormal gray matter.

The cause of schizencephaly remains unclear, although it has been linked with multiple assaults during pregnancy. Schizencephaly has been associated with congenital infections, drugs and other toxic exposures, vascular accidents, and metabolic abnormalities. There is also an association with aneuploidy.

The prognosis for patients with schizencephaly varies, with mild to severe outcomes. Open-lip lesions and bilateral clefts carry a worse prognosis. Long-term effects include blindness; motor deficits, which may include spastic quadriparesis; hemiparesis; and hypotonia. Seizures, which may be uncontrollable, mental retardation, and language impairment are also possible. Hydrocephalus may be progressive and require shunt placement.

Sonographic Findings. Sonographic features of schizencephaly include the following:

- A fluid-filled cleft in the cerebral cortex extending from the ventricle to the calvarium (Figure 55-37)
- Ventriculomegaly may be observed

Schizencephaly is associated with absence of the septum pellucidum and corpus callosum. Septo-optic dysplasia may also be present. Hydrocephaly can be seen when ventriculomegaly is present, but microcephaly has also been observed.

HYDRANENCEPHALY

Hydranencephaly is destruction of the cerebral hemispheres by occlusion of the internal carotid arteries. Brain parenchyma is destroyed and is replaced by cerebrospinal fluid. Because the posterior communicating arteries are preserved, the midbrain and cerebellum are present, and the basal ganglia, choroid plexus, and thalamus may also be spared. This rare abnormality occurs with a frequency of approximately 1 in 10,000 births.

Hydranencephaly may also be associated with polyhydramnios. No coexisting structural or chromosomal anomalies are associated.

The cause of hydranencephaly usually involves congenital infection or ischemia. Infections associated with hydranencephaly include cytomegalovirus and toxoplasmosis. Brain ischemia may result from maternal hypotension, twin-to-twin embolization, or vascular agenesis; and hydranencephaly has also been associated with cocaine abuse. It is believed that hydranencephaly may occur later in pregnancy, and that brain structures may initially be normal. The assault to the brain by infection or ischemic event subsequently destroys normal brain tissue.

The prognosis for hydranencephaly is grave (Figure 55-38), with death occurring at birth or shortly thereafter.

Sonographic Findings. Sonographic features of hydranencephaly include the following:

- Absence of normal brain tissue with almost complete replacement by cerebrospinal fluid (Figure 55-39)
- An absent or partially absent falx
- Presence of the midbrain, basal ganglia, and cerebellum
- The choroid plexus may be identified
- Macrocephaly may occur

Hydranencephaly may be confused with severe hydrocephaly, although the presence of an intact falx and surrounding rim of brain parenchyma may help to differentiate hydrocephaly from hydranencephaly. Holoprosencephaly with severe ventriculomegaly may also have a similar appearance. These three anomalies, however, have extremely poor outcomes.

VENTRICULOMEGALY (HYDROCEPHALUS)

Ventriculomegaly refers to dilation of the ventricles within the brain. **Hydrocephalus** occurs when ventriculomegaly is coupled with enlargement of the fetal head. The incidence of hydrocephalus occurs in 0.3 to 1.5 per 1000 live births. Enlargement of the ventricles occurs with obstruction of cerebrospinal fluid flow. This obstruction may be caused by a ventricular defect, such as aqueductal stenosis, and is referred to as *noncommunicating hydrocephalus.* The obstruction may be outside of the ventricular system, such as with an arachnoid cyst (Figure 55-40), and is referred to as *communicating hydrocephalus* (Figure 55-41). Rarely, ventriculomegaly results from an overproduction of cerebrospinal fluid by a choroid plexus papilloma.

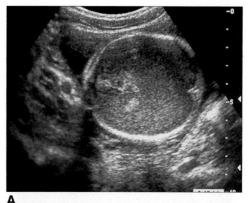

A

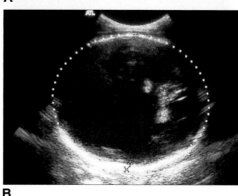

B

Figure 55-38 **A,** Hydranencephaly was suspected in this young woman with poorly controlled diabetes. The low-level echoes seen in this image of the fetal head swirled on real-time examination. **B,** Follow-up examinations revealed a grossly enlarged head with little brain tissue identified and replacement of the low-level echoes by anechoic fluid. The woman presented to labor and delivery near term with absence of movement, and fetal demise was confirmed with ultrasound. (From Henningsen C: *Clinical guide to ultrasonography,* St Louis, 2004, Mosby.)

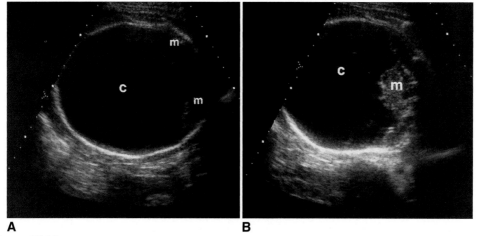

A   **B**

Figure 55-39 **A,** Hydranencephaly *(c)* in a fetus at 33 weeks of gestation showing massive collection of cerebrospinal fluid. Note the brain tissue in the occipital region *(m).* **B,** In the same fetus, hydranencephaly *(c)* and the midbrain *(m)* are observed. Other anomalies included clubfoot and cardiac defects. In utero, a computed tomography scan confirmed the diagnosis of hydranencephaly. Macrocephaly (11-cm biparietal diameter) was found by cranial measurements. Cephalocentesis (decompression of the head) was performed to allow vaginal delivery.

Physiologically, when an obstruction occurs, the ventricles dilate as the flow of cerebrospinal fluid is blocked. This increases the pressure within the ventricular system, which leads to ventricular expansion. Enlarged ventricles may exert pressure on the brain tissue, sometimes producing irreversible brain damage.

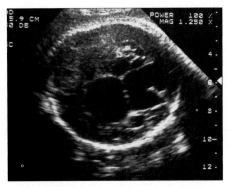

Figure 55-40   Multiple arachnoid cysts identified in this fetal head.

Hydrocephalus may be associated with an anomaly, or the cause may remain unknown. Many of the abnormalities linked with ventricular dilation were discussed earlier in this chapter and include aqueductal stenosis, arachnoid cysts, and vein of Galen aneurysms. Common causes of ventriculomegaly include spina bifida and encephaloceles. Dandy-Walker malformation, agenesis of the corpus callosum, lissencephaly, schizencephaly, and holoprosencephaly may also present with hydrocephalus. Intracranial neoplasm, such as a teratoma, may cause ventricular dilation. Ventriculomegaly may also be associated with musculoskeletal anomalies, such as thanatophoric dysplasia and achondroplasia. Ventricular enlargement has also been linked to congenital infections, such as toxoplasmosis and cytomegalovirus (Figure 55-42).

Ventriculomegaly may be a manifestation of a syndrome or chromosomal abnormality. Mild ventriculomegaly has been associated with trisomy 21, and ventriculomegaly has also been identified in trisomies 13 and 18. Other syndromes associated with ventriculomegaly include Meckel-Gruber syndrome, Apert's syndrome, Roberts' syndrome, hydrolethalus, Walker-Warburg, Smith-Lemli-Opitz syndrome, nasal-facial-digital syndrome, and Albers-Schönberg disease.

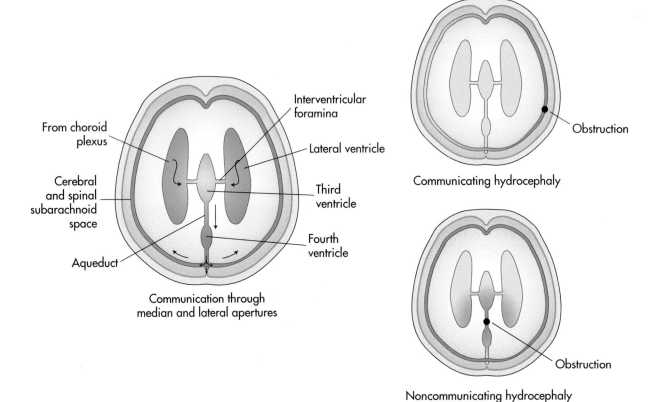

Figure 55-41   The course of the cerebrospinal fluid and its obstruction in hydrocephaly. Normally the cerebrospinal fluid from the choroid plexuses flows through the interventricular foramina to the third ventricle, aqueduct, fourth ventricle, median and lateral apertures, and spinal and cerebral subarachnoid space. It is then taken into the venous system (e.g., the cranial venous sinuses). Obstruction occurs within the ventricular system (e.g., at the aqueduct) in noncommunicating hydrocephaly (i.e., the ventricles and the subarachnoid space do not communicate). Obstruction occurs outside the ventricular system (e.g., in the cranial subarachnoid space) in communicating hydrocephaly (i.e., the ventricles and the subarachnoid space communicate).

Fetal ventriculomegaly typically progresses from the occipital horns into the temporal and then to the frontal ventricular horns. Ventriculomegaly may be quantitated by measuring the ventricular atrium across the glomus of the choroid plexus. A ventricle is considered dilated when its diameter exceeds 10 mm. The proximal ventricle may be difficult to adequately image because of reverberation artifacts from the calvarium. An effort should be made to determine if the ventricular enlargement is unilateral or bilateral; a unilateral ventriculomegaly, especially when isolated and mild, may have a good prognosis. Endovaginal technique may be used to further clarify the defect when the fetus is in a vertex position.

The mortality for fetuses with hydrocephalus is high. Outcome depends largely on the presence and severity of associated anomalies. The prognosis for survivors is generally considered poor, with only half identified to have a normal intellect. Survivors may require ventricular shunting to improve survival and intellectual outcome.

Sonographic Findings. Sonographic features of ventriculomegaly include the following:

- Lateral ventricular enlargement exceeding 10 mm (Figure 55-43)
- A "dangling choroid sign" as the gravity-dependent choroid plexus falls into the increased ventricular space (Figure 55-44)

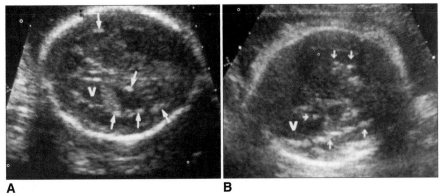

Figure 55-42   A, Periventricular calcifications *(arrows)* and ventriculomegaly *(v)* found in a 20-week fetus. An infectious cause was suspected. All testing had proven negative. **B,** In the same fetus at 30 weeks of gestation, persistent periventricular calcifications *(arrows)* with ventriculomegaly *(v)* was observed. No other anomalies or complications were present.

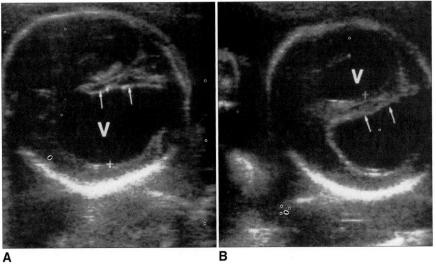

Figure 55-43   A, Ventriculomegaly observed in the distal cranial hemisphere in a 25-week twin fetus with severe growth restriction. The ventricle measured 28 mm in diameter. *Arrows,* Interhemispheric fissure. **B,** In the same fetus the proximal ventricle *(V)* is displayed measuring 17 mm in diameter. Note the asymmetry between the ventricles, suggesting a shift of the interhemispheric fissure *(arrows)* and porencephaly. The larger distal ventricle represents the actual porencephalic cyst, whereas the smaller ventricle has dilated in response to the infarction. Premature delivery occurred at 26 weeks of gestation because of chronic twin–twin transfusion syndrome in a monochorionic pregnancy. The twin, depicted in these figures, died shortly after birth. Autopsy confirmed the occurrence of the porencephalic event as an end result of the severe shunting of blood within the placental cotyledons.

- Possible dilation of the third and fourth ventricles
- Fetal head enlargement when the biparietal and head circumference measurements exceed those for the established gestational age

The fetus should also be surveyed for associated anomalies, which are present in 80% of cases of ventriculomegaly. Obstetric management may include amniocentesis to rule out chromosomal anomalies and laboratory tests to rule out congenital infections. In addition to numerous intracranial abnormalities associated with ventriculomegaly, the fetus should be surveyed for defects involving the face, heart, kidneys, abdominal wall, thorax, and limbs. In the absence of other abnormalities, fetal therapy for shunt placement may be an option. Cesarean delivery may also be necessary because of the large size of the fetal head.

Severe hydrocephaly may be confused with hydranencephaly and holoprosencephaly. Documenting a complete falx and the presence of the choroid plexus in the lateral ventricles, as well as a separate third and fourth ventricle, may help to differentiate severe ventriculomegaly from other anomalies.

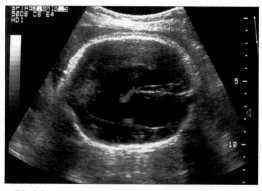

Figure 55-44 Ventriculomegaly caused by spina bifida. The anterior choroid plexus "dangles" into the posterior ventricle.

MICROCEPHALY

Microcephaly is an abnormally small head that falls 2 standard deviations below the mean. It occurs because the brain is reduced in size. Isolated microcephaly occurs in 1 per 1000 births but is more commonly caused by an associated anomaly.

Microcephaly may result from inheritance of either an autosomal-dominant or autosomal-recessive pattern. Microcephaly may also occur with chromosomal aberrations and various brain anomalies. Teratogens linked with microcephaly include congenital infections (rubella, toxoplasmosis, cytomegalovirus), maternal alcohol abuse, heroin addiction, mercury poisoning, maternal phenylketonuria, radiation, and hypoxia.

The prognosis for fetuses with microcephaly depends to a degree on the cause. About 85% of children with microcephaly are mentally retarded.

Sonographic Findings. Sonographic diagnosis of microcephaly depends on an accurate assessment of fetal age. Biparietal diameter, occipitofrontal diameter, and head circumference should be used when evaluating for microcephaly. In addition, ratios comparing the head perimeter to abdominal perimeter and the head perimeter to the femur length are also useful. Impaired cranial growth should coincide with appropriate growth of the abdominal circumference and femur length. Serial measurements for a fetus at risk for microcephalus should be performed at monthly intervals. Because microcephaly may manifest later in the pregnancy, diagnosis before 24 weeks of gestation may be impossible.

Sonographic features of microcephaly include the following:

- A small biparietal diameter (Figure 55-45)
- A small head circumference
- Abnormal head circumference/abdomen circumference and head circumference to femur length ratios

Other sonographic findings associated with microcephaly may include disorganized brain tissue and ventriculomegaly. A

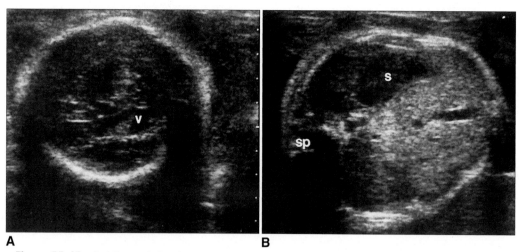

A   B

Figure 55-45 **A,** Microcephalus shown in a 32-week fetus with marked head to abdomen disproportion. Cranial diameters fell 3 to 5 standard deviations below the mean. Ventriculomegaly was observed. *v,* Lateral ventricle. **B,** In the same fetus, the cross section through the abdomen is shown. *s,* Stomach; *sp,* spine. There was a positive family history for autosomal-dominant congenital microcephalus.

may aid in estimating the size of the thoracic cavity and may predict an abnormally small chest cavity and secondary pulmonary hypoplasia. Nomograms for thoracic circumference size are available (Table 56-1). These data vary from the more recent data of Laudy and Wladimiroff, especially during the end of the last trimester.[3] Methods for measuring the lung include the length, area, and volume, using 3-D ultrasound. The right lung volume is slightly greater than the left.

When the heart position and axis vary from the normal position, the sonographer should look closely for any abnormality that may be the cause of such displacement (i.e., pleural mass or diaphragmatic hernia). Fetal echocardiography is beneficial for excluding cardiac involvement, and evaluation of an intact diaphragm is necessary to exclude diaphragmatic hernia. Abnormalities in cardiac rhythm and fetal hydrops may be present in fetuses with lung masses because of compression of venous return and cardiac failure. Pleural effusions are commonly found in conjunction with lung masses.

The lungs will not grow or develop properly when there is a small uterine cavity resulting from severe oligohydramnios, when the chest cavity is abnormally small, when the balance between tracheal and airway pressure and fluid volume is inadequate, or when the fetus is unable to practice breathing movements.

A mass within the thoracic cavity may have detrimental effects on lung development. The heart and mediastinal structures may be displaced from the normal position, and the lung may be compressed and destroyed. These effects may lead to pulmonary hypoplasia.

Pulmonary Hypoplasia. Pulmonary hypoplasia is caused by a decrease in the number of lung cells, airways, and alveoli, with a resulting decrease in organ size and weight. This reduction in lung volume results in small, inadequately developed lungs. A decreased ratio of lung weight to body weight is a consistent method of diagnosing pulmonary hypoplasia. This condition most commonly occurs from prolonged oligohydramnios or is secondary to a small thoracic cavity as a result of a structural or chromosomal abnormality.

Pulmonary hypoplasia may occur when there is an extreme reduction in amniotic fluid volume. Kidney abnormalities (bilateral renal agenesis, bilateral multicystic kidney disease, severe renal obstruction [e.g., posterior urethral valve syndrome], unilateral renal agenesis with contralateral multicystic kidney development or severe obstruction, and infantile polycystic kidney disease) result in lethal pulmonary hypoplasia. Pulmonary hypoplasia may also occur in fetuses with severe intrauterine growth restriction and early rupture of the membranes.

Masses within the thoracic cavity, including pleural effusion, diaphragmatic hernia (and eventration), cystic adenomatoid malformation of the lung, bronchopulmonary sequestration, and other large cysts and tumors of the lung and thorax, may lead to pulmonary hypoplasia. Cardiac defects,

TABLE 56-1 FETAL THORACIC CIRCUMFERENCE MEASUREMENTS*

Gestational Age (week)	No.	Predictive Percentiles								
		2.5	5	10	25	50	75	90	95	97.5
16	6	5.9	6.4	7.0	8.0	9.1	10.3	11.3	11.9	12.4
17	22	6.8	7.3	7.9	8.9	10.0	11.2	12.2	12.8	13.3
18	31	7.7	8.2	8.8	9.8	11.0	12.1	13.1	13.7	14.2
19	21	8.6	9.1	9.7	10.7	11.9	13.0	14.0	14.6	15.1
20	20	9.5	10.0	10.6	11.7	12.9	13.9	15.0	15.5	16.0
21	30	10.4	11.0	11.6	12.6	13.7	14.8	15.8	16.4	16.9
22	18	11.3	11.9	12.5	13.5	14.6	15.7	16.7	17.3	17.8
23	21	12.2	12.8	13.4	14.4	15.5	16.6	17.6	18.2	18.8
24	27	13.2	13.7	14.3	15.3	16.4	17.5	18.5	19.1	19.7
25	20	14.1	14.6	15.2	16.2	17.3	18.4	19.4	20.0	20.6
26	25	15.0	15.5	16.1	17.1	18.2	19.3	20.3	21.0	21.5
27	24	15.9	16.4	17.0	18.0	19.1	20.2	21.3	21.9	22.4
28	24	16.8	17.3	17.9	18.9	20.0	21.2	22.2	22.8	23.3
29	24	17.7	18.2	18.8	19.8	21.0	22.1	23.1	23.7	24.2
30	27	18.6	19.1	19.7	20.7	21.9	23.0	24.0	24.6	25.1
31	24	19.5	20.0	20.6	21.6	22.8	23.9	24.9	25.5	26.0
32	28	20.4	20.9	21.5	22.6	23.7	24.8	25.8	26.4	26.9
33	27	21.3	21.8	22.5	23.5	24.6	25.7	26.7	27.3	27.8
34	25	22.2	22.8	23.4	24.4	25.5	26.6	27.6	28.2	28.7
35	20	23.1	23.7	24.3	25.3	26.4	27.5	28.5	29.1	29.6
36	23	24.0	24.6	25.2	26.2	27.3	28.4	29.4	30.0	30.6
37	22	24.9	25.5	26.1	27.1	28.2	29.3	30.3	30.9	31.5
38	21	25.9	26.4	27.0	28.0	29.1	30.2	31.2	31.9	32.4
39	7	26.8	27.3	27.9	28.9	30.0	31.1	32.2	32.8	33.3
40	6	27.7	28.2	28.8	29.8	30.9	32.1	33.1	33.7	34.2

From Chitkara and others: Prenatal assessment of the fetal thorax: normal values, *Am J Obstet Gynecol* 156:1069, 1987.
*Measurements in centimeters.

some skeletal dysplasias, central nervous system disorders, and chromosomal trisomies (13, 18, and 21) may manifest with pulmonary hypoplasia. A small percentage of infants have pulmonary hypoplasia without any fetal or uterine problem.

Unilateral pulmonary agenesis or hypoplasia is a rare anomaly that is often associated with other fetal malformations. An absent lung should be considered in the differential diagnosis of every fetus with a mediastinal shift and apparent chest mass, especially when it is seen in conjunction with other defects, such as esophageal abnormalities.

The prognosis for infants with pulmonary hypoplasia is grave, with 80% dying after birth. The severity of pulmonary hypoplasia depends on when pulmonary hypoplasia occurred during pregnancy, its severity, and duration (Box 56-2). Other factors, such as pulmonary fluid dynamics, fetal breathing movements, and hormonal influences, may contribute to pulmonary hypoplasia.

Sonographic Findings. Various methods have been used to determine the presence of pulmonary hypoplasia that include thoracic measurements, various lung measurements, estimation of lung volume, Doppler studies of the pulmonary arteries, and assessment of fetal breathing activity. The sonographer may be able to check for pulmonary hypoplasia by measuring the thoracic circumference at the level of the four-chamber heart view, excluding the skin and subcutaneous tissues. A thoracic circumference below the 5th percentile suggests the possibility of pulmonary hypoplasia. The sonographer should understand that this measurement may not be helpful in conditions in which there is an intrathoracic mass that compresses lung tissue and yet the thoracic circumference remains normal (i.e., diaphragmatic hernia, pleural effusion, and cystic adenomatoid malformations). The sonographer should also look for the finding of small echogenic lungs, as they lie lateral to the cardiac chambers in the fetus with pulmonary hypoplasia.

Cystic Lung Masses. Lung cysts are echo-free masses that replace normal lung parenchyma (Figure 56-7). Lung cysts may vary in size, ranging from small isolated lesions to large cystic masses that may cause notable shifts of intrathoracic structures. Simple cysts may be surgically excised after delivery (Box 56-3).

Bronchogenic cysts. The most common lung cyst detected prenatally is the **bronchogenic cyst.** Bronchogenic cysts occur as a result of abnormal budding of the foregut and lack any communication with the trachea or bronchial tree. They typically occur within the mediastinum or lung; infrequently they are inferior to the diaphragm.

Sonographic Findings. Sonographically, bronchogenic cysts appear as small circumscribed masses without evidence of a mediastinal shift or heart failure (see Figures 56-7 and 56-8). Amniotic fluid volume is within a normal range.

Pleural Effusion (Hydrothorax). Accumulation of fluid within the pleural cavity that may appear as an isolated lesion or secondary to multiple fetal anomalies is called a **pleural effusion** or **hydrothorax** (see Figure 56-7). The most common reason for a pleural effusion is chylothorax occurring as a right-side unilateral collection of fluid secondary to a malformed thoracic duct. Hydramnios often accompanies chylothorax resulting from esophageal compression. Fetal hydrothorax can be unilateral or bilateral. When it is bilateral, it occurs about equally on the right and left sides.

Pleural effusions may result from immune (e.g., Rh hemolytic disease) or nonimmune causes or from congestive heart failure. Effusions may also occur in fetuses with chromosomal abnormalities (e.g., trisomy 21) or in the fetus with a cardiac mass. Other reasons for pleural effusions include **lymphangiectasia,** cystic adenomatoid malformations, bronchopulmonary sequestration, diaphragmatic hernia, hamartoma, atresia of the pulmonary vein, or other unknown causes.

Sonographic Findings. Sonographically, pleural effusions appear as echo-free peripheral masses on one or both sides of the fetal heart (Figure 56-9). The effusions conform to the thoracic cavity and often compress lung tissue. The lung appears to float in the fluid. Pleural fluid is rarely encountered before the 15th week of gestation, except in association with Down or Turner's syndrome. Compression of lung parenchyma may cause pulmonary hypoplasia, which often represents a life-threatening consequence for the neonate (Figure 56-10).

The presence of a pleural effusion may cause a shift of mediastinal structures, compression of the heart, and inversion of the diaphragm. The shape of the lung appears normal in the presence of a pleural effusion. Once a pleural effusion has been discovered, a careful search for lung, cardiac, and diaphragmatic lesions should be attempted. Likewise, evaluation for signs of hydrops (ascites, scalp edema, and tissue edema)

BOX 56-2   PULMONARY HYPOPLASIA

- Reduction in lung volume resulting in small, inadequately developed lungs
- Occurs from prolonged oligohydramnios or secondary to small thoracic cavity
- Look for chromosome anomalies, renal anomalies, intrauterine growth restriction, premature rupture of membranes, masses within thoracic cavity

---

BOX 56-3   CYSTIC LUNG MASSES

- *Bronchogenic cysts:* Most common; unilocular or multilocular cysts usually within mediastinum or lung; normal amniotic fluid
- *Pleural effusions:* Hydramnios accompanies chylothorax (esophageal compression); may result from immune or nonimmune causes or congestive heart failure; may occur with cardiac mass; lymphangiectasia, CAM, sequestration, hernia; compression of lung tissue; shift of mediastinal structures

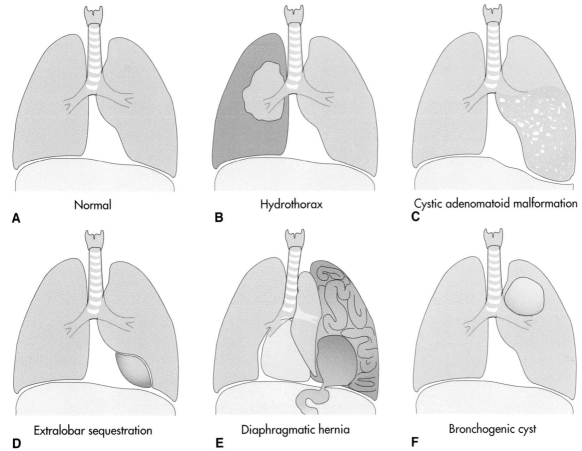

A Normal

B Hydrothorax

C Cystic adenomatoid malformation

D Extralobar sequestration

E Diaphragmatic hernia

F Bronchogenic cyst

Figure 56-7 Schematic drawings of thoracic masses and mass effect. **A,** Normal thorax. The lungs have convex margins anterolaterally. **B,** Hydrothorax. Anechoic pleural fluid displaces the lungs away from the chest wall and compresses the lungs. **C,** Cystic adenomatoid malformation. An intrapulmonary mass of variable echogenicity may shift the mediastinum and create hydrops. **D,** Bronchopulmonary extralobar sequestration. A spherical or triangular echogenic mass is evident in the inferior portion of the thorax or upper abdomen. **E,** Diaphragmatic hernia. A complex mass (usually on the left side) creates mediastinal shift. Peristalsing bowel in the thorax provides convincing evidence of the diagnosis. Displaced stomach or scaphoid abdomen is an ancillary finding. **F,** Bronchogenic cyst. If it causes bronchial compression, a simple cyst near the mediastinum or centrally in the lung may produce a mediastinal shift.

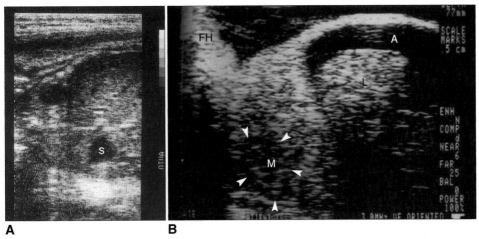

A **B**

Figure 56-8 **A,** Longitudinal section of chest revealing small cystic mass in the lung. Note the relationship of the stomach *(s)* to the cyst. A benign bronchogenic cyst was found after birth.
B, Longitudinal scan showing bulky noncystic mass *(M)* in thorax consistent with cystic adenomatoid malformation (type 3). Abdominal ascites *(A)* is present. *L,* Liver; *FH,* fetal head. (From Mayden KL and others: Cystic adenomatoid malformation in the fetus: Ultrasound evaluation, *Am J Obstet Gynecol* 148:349, 1984.)

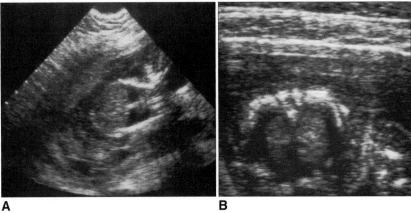

Figure 56-9 **A,** Bilateral pleural effusions in a 23-week fetus. **B,** Transverse view of bilateral pleural effusions.

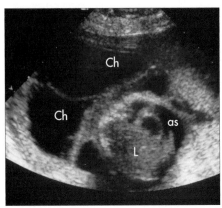

Figure 56-10 Tranverse scan of a 26-week fetus with a huge cystic hygroma *(Ch)* and fetal hydrops. Ascites *(as)* may be seen surrounding the fetal liver *(L)*. The sonographer should also look for the presence of pleural and pericardial effusion.

should be performed. Correlation with clinical parameters is warranted to exclude immunologic causes of pleural effusions.

The mortality rate for the infant with a pleural effusion approaches 50%; the prognosis is poorer with associated hydrops. When the pleural effusion is large, lung development is impaired, which may result in pulmonary hypoplasia. Some neonatologists advocate draining a large pleural collection (thoracentesis) by placing a thoracoamniotic shunt within the pleural space. This is an attempt to allow for lung growth when it is performed during the second trimester of pregnancy. Thoracentesis may be performed to determine whether the lung has the ability to reexpand once the fluid is removed, thus excluding pulmonary hypoplasia, lessening the effects of hydramnios, and obtaining a fetal karyotype using lymphocytes from the aspirated lung fluid.

Solid Lung Masses. Solid tumors of the fetal lungs have been reported by ultrasound, appearing as echo-dense masses in the lung tissue. Pulmonary sequestration and certain types of cystic adenomatoid malformations (CAMs) appear as solid lung masses (see Figure 56-7) (Box 56-4).

> **BOX 56-4 SONOGRAPHIC FINDINGS IN SEQUESTRATION**
>
> • Echogenic solid mass resembling lung tissue
> • Rarely occurs below diaphragm
> • Associated with hydrops and polyhydramnios, diaphragmatic hernia, gastrointestinal anomalies
> • Normal intraabdominal anatomy

Pulmonary sequestration. Pulmonary sequestration is a supernumerary lobe of the lung, separated from the normal tracheobronchial tree. In **pulmonary sequestration,** extra pulmonary tissue is present within the pleural lung sac (intralobar) or is connected to the inferior border of the lung within its own pleural sac (extralobar). This probably develops from a separate outpouching of the foregut or by separation of a segment of the developing lung from the tracheobronchial tree. This extra lung tissue is nonfunctional and receives its blood supply from systemic circulation. The arterial supply is usually from the thoracic aorta, with venous drainage into the vena cava.

Sonographic Findings. Sonographically, an echo-dense solid mass resembling lung tissue is observed, usually in the lower lobe of the lung (Figure 56-11). The majority of extralobar defects occur on the left side and rarely below the diaphragm. Intralobar lesions are spherical, and extralobar sequestration appears as a cone-shaped or triangular mass. These lesions may resemble a cystic adenomatoid (type II) malformation. Color Doppler may aid the sonographer in viewing this anomalous circulation. A hypoplastic lung may be observed on the affected side. Hydrops is a frequent finding. Other associated anomalies are diaphragmatic hernia and gastrointestinal and lung anomalies (pulmonary hypoplasia).

The prognosis for intralobar sequestration is very favorable, whereas extralobar sequestration carries a poor prognosis because of associated anomalies and hydrops.

Laryngeal atresia may be diagnosed when bilateral lung enlargement is observed (Figure 56-12).

Congenital cystic adenomatoid malformation. Congenital cystic adenomatoid malformation (CCAM) is a multicystic mass within the lung consisting of primitive lung tissue and abnormal bronchial and bronchiolar-like structures. CCAM is one of the bronchopulmonary foregut malformations (see Figure 56-7). CCAM results from an embryogenetic alteration in the developing lung during the first 8 to 9 gestational weeks. The lesion may involve one or more lobes of the lung or an entire lung, or, in rare cases, may be bilateral. The malformation may communicate with the bronchial tree. The cysts within the mass may be large or small with a texture that varies from solid, mixed, or cystic in appearance. Most of the lesions are unilateral without favor to either lung.

There are three forms of cystic adenomatoid malformation. In CCAM type I (macrocystic), one or more large cysts replace

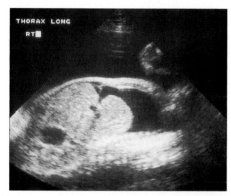

Figure 56-11 Longitudinal scan of the 23-week fetus with a right-side pulmonary sequestration. The echogenic mass is well seen in the lower lobe of the thoracic cavity. A large pleural effusion surrounds the mass.

normal lung tissue (single or multiple cysts measuring more than 2 cm and up to 10 cm) (Figure 56-13). Type II (macrocystic with a microcystic component) lesions consist of multiple small cysts (less than 1 cm) (Figure 56-14). Type II lesions are associated with fetal and/or chromosomal abnormalities in 25% of cases. These anomalies may include renal agenesis, pulmonary anomalies, and diaphragmatic hernia. Type III (microcystic) malformations are characterized as bulky, large, noncystic lesions appearing as echo-dense masses of the entire lung lobe (Figure 56-15). When there is a shift of the mediastinal structures, lung compression may occur and hydrops may develop. Hydramnios may be observed secondary to esophageal compression, preventing normal fetal swallowing.

Differentiation of the type of cystic adenomatoid malformations is imperative because prognosis varies depending on the type of lesion. Type I lesions have favorable outcomes, whereas type II and III lesions have poor prognoses.

Sonographic Findings. When a cystic or solid lung mass has been identified, the sonographer should attempt to do the following:

- Determine the number and size(s) of cystic structure(s)
- Check for presence or absence of a mediastinal shift
- Identify and assess the size of the lungs
- Look for fetal hydrops
- Exclude cardiac masses
- Search for other fetal anomalies

Based on these findings, an appropriate prognosis and management plan may be instituted (Box 56-5).

A review of the spontaneous improvement of these thoracic masses in utero indicates the following:[1]

- Sonographically detected fetal chest masses may result in pathologically proven thoracic-derived lesions or may resolve, some without sequelae

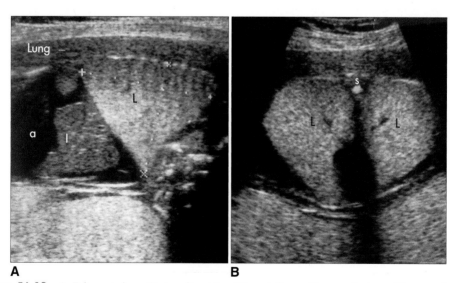

Figure 56-12 **A,** Echogenic lung *(L, in calipers)* in a 21-week fetus with severe hydrops. The opposite lung appeared similar in texture. Oligohydramnios and episodes of bradycardia were evident. *a,* Ascites; *l,* liver. **B,** In the same fetus, both echogenic lungs *(L)* are viewed. Laryngeal or tracheal agenesis was suspected. It is believed that excess lung fluid is manufactured by the abnormal lung. *s,* Spine.

- The mass lesions may change in size and echogenicity
- Sonograms of fetuses with CAM may be normal in the first and second trimester and only later show abnormalities on ultrasound
- The presence of polyhydramnios, hydrops, or notable cardiac deviation predicts poor outcome more accurately than the lesion type

Congenital bronchial atresia. Congenital bronchial atresia is a rare pulmonary anomaly that results from the focal obliteration of a segment of the bronchial lumen. It is found most commonly in the left upper lobe and appears on ultrasound as an echogenic pulmonary mass lesion. In normal fetuses, the bronchi are not visualized. If a fetal main stem or segmental bronchus can be seen on sonography, it is probably because it is fluid-filled and abnormal.

Other Complex Lung Masses. The internal components of complex lung masses are cystic and solid and appear hetero-

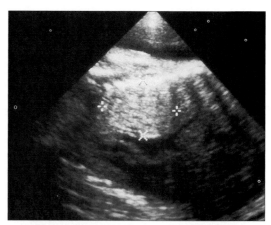

Figure 56-14 Type II cystic adenomatoid malformation shows multiple cystic areas under 1 cm in size. The mass is echogenic at the base of the thoracic cavity.

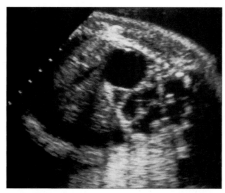

Figure 56-13 Type I cystic adenomatoid malformation showing multiple large cystic areas replacing normal lung tissue.

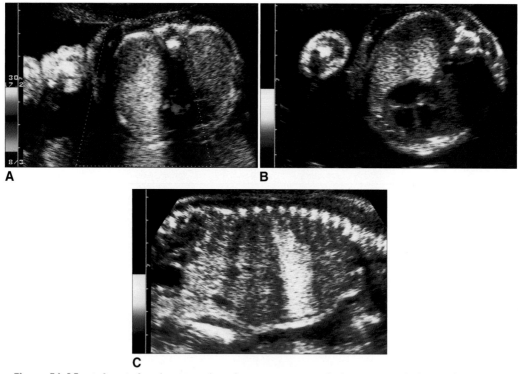

Figure 56-15 A fetus is found at 32 weeks to have asymmetry in the lung tissue, which turned out to be type III cystic adenomatoid malformation. This echogenic mass affected the right lung. **A,** Gray-scale transverse scan comparing both textures of the lung. The right lobe is clearly more echogenic. **B,** B-Color display of the cystic adenomatoid malformation as it slightly displaces the cardiac axis. **C,** Longitudinal B-color scan of the echo-dense mass just above the diaphragm in the thoracic cavity.

SONOGRAPHIC FINDINGS IN CYSTIC ADENOMATOID MALFORMATIONS

- *Type I:* Single or multiple large cysts 2 cm in diameter; good prognosis after resection of affected lung
- *Type II:* Multiple small cysts, <1 cm in diameter, echogenic; high incidence of other congenital anomalies (renal, gastrointestinal)
- *Type III:* Large, bulky, noncystic lesions producing mediastinal shift; poor prognosis
- Usually only one lobe is affected
- Associated polyhydramnios and anasarca have poor prognosis

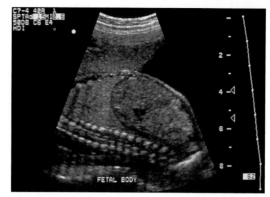

Figure 56-16 Longitudinal scan of the diaphragm as it separates the thoracic from the abdominal cavities.

geneous. At times, compressed adjacent thoracic organs further complicate determination of the type of lesion (pleural effusion surrounding lungs and heart). Congenital dilation of the bronchial tree may have both cystic and solid characteristics.

Congenital lobar emphysema is lobar overinflation of the lung without destruction of alveolar septa. It usually occurs in the upper left or middle lobe and is located within the normal pleural envelope. This condition may appear identical to microcystic CCAM, presenting as a large solid mass.

Laryngeal and tracheal atresia is an uncommon finding in utero. The sonographic findings show enlarged, bilateral, symmetrically distended echogenic fetal lungs. This is due to the fluid distention of the tiny air spaces within the lung tissue. The heart may be displaced anteriorly in the midline and may appear engulfed by the prominent lung fields. The trachea and bronchi may be fluid filled. Fetal ascites is usually present without other findings of hydrops. Polyhydramnios may be seen secondary to the esophageal compression. Oligohydramnios has also been reported as a result of cardiac compromise or diminished lung fluid efflux into the amniotic space.

ABNORMALITIES OF THE DIAPHRAGM

The diaphragm is an important muscle separating the thoracic cavity from the abdomen. The diaphragm is specifically studied in fetuses at risk for congenital defects of the diaphragm when there is a shift in the cardiac silhouette or when atypical structures are found in the fetal chest. In the normal fetus, the diaphragm should appear as a curvilinear hypoechoic structure coursing anteriorly to posteriorly (Figure 56-16). The fetal stomach and liver should be identified caudal to the diaphragm, with the lungs and heart positioned cephalad. Failure to recognize these normal relationships should prompt the sonographer to search for diaphragmatic defects.

Congenital Diaphragmatic Hernia. Congenital diaphragmatic hernia **(CDH)** is a herniation of the abdominal viscera into the chest that results from a congenital defect in the fetal diaphragm. It is a sporadic defect, occurring in 1 per 2000 to 1 per 5000 births. The muscular diaphragm forms between the 6th and 14th week of gestation as a result of a chain of events involving the fusion of four structures: (1) the septum transversum (future central tendon), (2) pleuroperitoneal mem-

branes, (3) dorsal mesentery of the esophagus (future crura), and (4) body wall. Normally the primitive diaphragm is intact by the end of the 8th menstrual week. The most posterior aspect of the diaphragm, derived from the body wall, is the part of the diaphragm that forms last and is the most commonly defective.

During the embryologic phase, when the gut is moving back into the abdominal cavity (around 10 to 12 weeks), sufficient intraabdominal pressure may be produced so that if fusion of the primitive diaphragmatic structures is incomplete, abdominal viscera can herniate into the thorax.

The diaphragmatic hernia permits the abdominal organs to enter the fetal chest (see Figures 56-7 and 56-17 to 56-19). The most common type of diaphragmatic defect (more than 90% of defects) occurs posteriorly and laterally in the diaphragm (herniation through the **foramen of Bochdalek**). This hernia is usually found on the left side of the diaphragm, and left-sided organs (stomach, spleen, and portions of the liver) enter the chest through the opening. The abnormally positioned abdominal organs shift the heart and mediastinal structures to the right side of the chest. Usually the stomach is in the chest near the heart, instead of below the diaphragm. In left-sided hernias, the sonographer should look for the stomach, portions of the small and large intestines, and the left lobe of the liver and spleen in the thoracic cavity. Peristalsis of the bowel loops within the thoracic cavity may be seen (Box 56-6).

Diaphragmatic hernias may occur anteriorly and medially in the diaphragm, through the **foramen of Morgagni,** and may communicate with the pericardial sac. In anteromedial defects, the heart may be normally positioned but surrounded by pleural fluid, while the fetal stomach may be located in its normal position in the abdomen (Figure 56-20). Thinning of the diaphragm (eventration) may give rise to sonographic characteristics similar to those of diaphragmatic hernias.

Defects on the right side of the diaphragm allow the right-side abdominal viscera (liver, gallbladder, intestines) to enter the chest. As a consequence of herniated abdominal organs, the lungs are compressed and may become hypoplastic.

The size of the diaphragmatic defects can be quite variable, ranging from small to quite large to complete absence of both

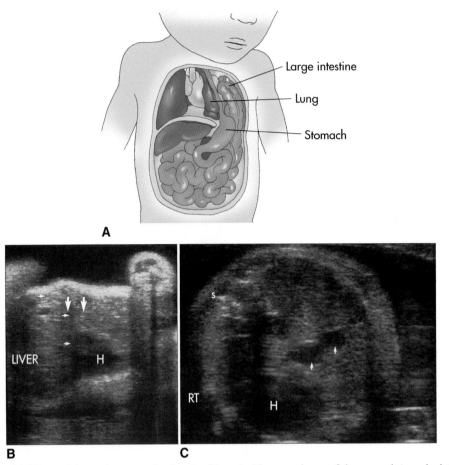

Figure 56-17   **A,** Schema demonstrating hernia of intestinal loops and part of the stomach into the left pleural cavity. The heart and mediastinum are pushed to the right, whereas the left lung is compressed. **B,** Sagittal view in a fetus with a diaphragmatic hernia. The heart *(H)* is displaced to the right side of fetal thorax by herniated bowel *(large arrows)*. Diaphragm *(small arrows)*. **C,** Transverse section in same patient showing the herniated stomach *(arrows)* at the level of the heart *(H)*. s, Spine; *RT*, right.

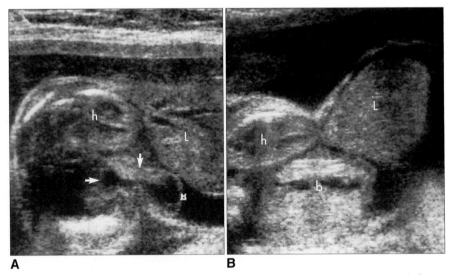

Figure 56-18   **A,** Diaphragmatic hernia in association with omphalocele shown in a 28-week fetus. Displacement of the heart *(h)* to the right chest is demonstrated. Herniated bowel *(arrowheads)* with peristalsis demonstrated by real-time imaging confirmed the diagnosis. *L,* Lung. **B,** In the same fetus the liver *(L)* is shown in close proximity to the heart *(h)* and bowel *(b)* because of the absent diaphragm.

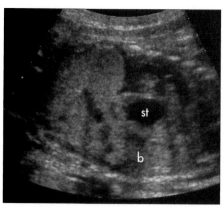

Figure 56-19   Longitudinal image of a 25-week fetus with a large left-side hernia. The stomach *(st)* and bowel *(b)* are seen within the thoracic cavity.

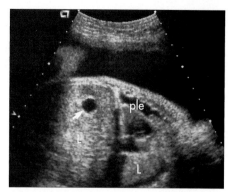

Figure 56-20   Longitudinal scan of the right-sided diaphragmatic hernia; the liver *(L)* is seen in the thoracic cavity. Pleural effusion *(ple)* is present. The gallbladder *(arrow)* is seen within the liver.

BOX 56-6   SONOGRAPHIC CRITERIA SUGGESTIVE OF A DIAPHRAGMATIC HERNIA

- Shift of the heart and mediastinal structures (right shift in left-side defects; left shift in right-side defects)
- Mass within the thoracic cavity (liver, stomach, spleen, and large bowel in left-side defects; liver, gallbladder, intestines in right-side defects)
- Small abdominal circumference resulting from herniated abdominal structures
- Obvious diaphragm defect
- Hydramnios
- More than 50% have structural anomalies or chromosomal abnormalities
- Structural defects include cardiovascular (tetralogy of Fallot and others), genitourinary (renal agenesis, cystic dysplasia, and ureteropelvic junction obstruction), central nervous system (holoprosencephaly, hydrocephalus, and spinal anomalies), clubbed feet, hemivertebrae and absent ribs, genital (ambiguous genitalia and others), and gastrointestinal (imperforate anus, annular pancreas, and absence of the gallbladder)*
- Growth restriction suggests associated anomalies
- The abdominal circumference below the 5th percentile and liver in the chest indicate poor prognosis†

*Data from Nyberg DA, Mahony BS, Pretorius DH, editors: *Diagnostic ultrasound of fetal anomalies: text and atlas,* St Louis, 1990, Mosby.
†Data from Teixeira J and others: Abdominal circumference in fetuses with congenital diaphragmatic hernia: correlation with hernia content and pregnancy outcome, *J Ultrasound Med* 16:407, 1997.

BOX 56-7   SONOGRAPHIC FEATURES OF LEFT CONGENITAL HERNIA

- Intrathoracic stomach
- Displaced cardiac apex
- Cardiomediastinal shift is critical in making the diagnosis
- Intrathoracic liver (look for portal venous flow)
- Small right lung
- Small left ventricle of heart
- Evaluate for chromosomal abnormalities

---

diaphragms. The smaller defects are difficult to diagnose in utero. Hydrops is usually not present with left-sided congenital diaphragmatic hernias unless associated fetal malformations are present. The presence of pulmonary hypoplasia and pulmonary hypertension is the real issue that results from the size of the hernia. The pulmonary arteries become hypertrophied and thickened, resulting in pulmonary hypertension that after birth leads to persistent fetal circulation. Bilateral hernias are

very unusual and more difficult to detect with sonography because the degree of cardiomediastinal shift may not be present. The heart may be slightly displaced anteriorly and superiorly and the stomach may be found in the left chest.

Sonographic Findings. On sonographic examination, a *left congenital diaphragmatic hernia* is usually found when the cardiac silhouette is displaced to the right and an ectopic stomach is in the chest. It is very important to note the cardiomediastinal shift to make the diagnosis of a hernia. The apex of the heart will be abnormally shifted, depending upon the size of the CDH defect. The small bowel and colon are commonly intrathoracic, but are often collapsed and difficult to specifically identify if peristalsis is not present. The sagittal image of the fetus may allow visualization of the diaphragm, depending on how large the defect is. The fetal lung may be small and compressed.

A portion of the liver herniates into the chest in approximately two thirds of cases, and the presence or absence of intrathoracic liver is important to note because the intrathoracic liver is associated with a poorer outcome. Color flow may be useful in demarcating the portal vasculature within the liver to ascertain whether the tissue is truly liver or not. Box 56-7 lists the sonographic features of left congenital heart.

In a *right-sided diaphragmatic hernia,* the sonographer will see the liver in the chest, a collapsed bowel may be present, and the heart deviated far to the left. The stomach alignment will be abnormal, but inferior to the diaphragm, and moved to the right. Color may help to trace the portal vasculature in the liver as it lies within the chest cavity. The gallbladder may also herniate into the thoracic cavity and appear as a solitary "cystic" mass in the lung. A small amount of ascitic fluid adjacent to the liver may be present with right-sided hernias. Pleural fluid is not usually associated with other chest masses except in sequestration. At birth, respiration may be severely compromised, which may result in death of the newborn.

The amniotic fluid may be normal unless the bowel is obstructed with resulting polyhydramnios. The placenta is normal; the abdominal circumference will be abnormally small. Careful scanning before 18 weeks of gestation is important to identify the normal contour of the diaphragm in the sagittal and coronal views. A small defect may not show abnormalities early in the gestational period.

The prognosis is poor for the fetus if the congenital diaphragmatic hernia is detected before birth; if the presence of the stomach is found in the chest, especially if it is dilated; if the left heart is underdeveloped; or if congenital heart disease is present. The primary cause of death is pulmonary hypoplasia. If the diagnosis is made before 25 weeks of gestation and the development of polyhydramnios is present, the survival rate is low.

Frequently associated abnormalities include cardiac malformations (20%), central nervous system malformations (30%), renal anomalies, vertebral defects, pulmonary hypoplasia, and facial clefts. In addition, chromosome abnormalities (trisomy 18 and 21) have also been associated with diaphragmatic hernia.

It is important to note that when a diaphragmatic hernia is present, the stomach may not be filled when there is concomitant oligohydramnios or if the fetus is swallowing abnormally. The only clue to a diaphragmatic hernia in this situation may be evidence of a solid mass in the chest. Peristalsis within the herniated intestines confirms the diagnosis. When the sonographer is unable to demonstrate the stomach bubble in the normal anatomic location after repeated observations, a search for a diaphragmatic hernia should be attempted.

Lung and mediastinal masses, in particular cystic adenomatoid malformations, may be difficult to distinguish from diaphragmatic hernias. The normally positioned peritoneal organs should aid in differentiating these two conditions.

At birth, the majority of infants with congenital diaphragmatic hernia have pulmonary hypoplasia and secondary respiratory insufficiency. There is a high mortality rate (75%) because of the increased frequency of coexisting fetal congenital anomalies. The development of the ECMO (extracorporeal membrane oxygenation) procedure has allowed such babies with severe diaphragmatic hernias a chance for survival immediately after delivery. This procedure canalizes the carotid artery (while occluding the opposite carotid artery) in an effort to bypass the pulmonary circulation to provide an opportunity for the lung tissue to mature before circulation demands are in place.

REFERENCES

1. Budorick NE and others: Spontaneous improvement of intrathoracic masses diagnosed in utero, *J Ultrasound Med* 11:653, 1992.

2. Johnson A and others: Ultrasonic ratio of fetal thoracic to abdominal circumference: an association with fetal pulmonary hypoplasia, *Am J Obstet Gynecol* 157:764, 1987.

3. Laudy JA, Wladimiroff JW: The fetal lung. 2. Pulmonary hypoplasia, *Ultrasound Obstet Gynecol* 16:482-494, 2000.

SELECTED BIBLIOGRAPHY

Bahlmann F, Merz E, Hallermann C and others: Congenital diaphragmatic hernia: ultrasonic measurement of fetal lungs to predict pulmonary hypoplasia, *Ultrasound Obstet Gynecol* 14(3):162-168, 1999.

Besinger RE, Compton AA, Hayashi RH: The presence or absence of fetal breathing movements as a predictor of outcome in preterm labor, *Am J Obstet Gynecol* 157:753, 1987.

Bootstaylor BS, Filly RA, Harrison MR and others: Prenatal sonographic predictors of liver herniation in congenital diaphragmatic hernia, *J Ultrasound Med* 14:515-520, 1995.

Bromley B, Benacerraf B: Unilateral lung hypoplasia: report of three cases, *J Ultrasound Med* 16:599, 1997.

Bromley B and others: Fetal lung masses: prenatal course and outcome, *J Ultrasound Med* 14:927, 1995.

Bunduki V, Ruano R, de Liva MM and others: Prognostic factors associated with congenital cystic adenomatoid malformation of the lung, *Prenat Diagn* 20:459-464, 2000.

Callen P: *Ultrasonography in obstetrics and gynecology*, ed 3, Philadelphia, 2003, WB Saunders.

Cass DL, Crombleholme TM, Howell LJ and others: Cystic lung lesions with systemic arterial blood supply; a hybrid of congenital cystic adenomatoid malformation and bronchopulmonary sequestration, *J Pediatr Surg* 32:986-990, 1997.

Cosmi EV, Aneschi MM, Cosmi E and others: Ultrasonographic patterns of fetal breathing movements in normal pregnancy, *Int J Gynaecol Obstet* 80(3):285-290, 2003.

D'Arcy TJ, Hughes SW, Chiu WSC and others: Estimation of fetal lung volume using enhanced 3-dimensional ultrasound: a new method and first result, *Br J Obstet Gynaecol* 103:1015-1020, 1996.

De Santis M, Masini L, Nois G and others: Congenital cystic adenomatoid malformation of the lung: antenatal ultrasound findings and fetal-neonatal outcome. Fifteen years of experience, *Fetal Diagn Ter* 15:246-250, 2000.

Enns G, Cox VA, Goldstein RB and others: Congenital diaphragmatic defects and associated syndromes, malformations, and chromosome anomalies: a retrospective study of 60 patients and literature review, *Am J Med Genet* 79:215-225, 1998.

Harrison MR, Bressack MA, Kchurg AM and others: Correction of congenital diaphragmatic hernia in utero. II. Simulated correction permits fetal lung growth with survival at birth, *Surgery* 88:260-268, 1980.

Ishikawa S, Kamata S, Usui N and others: Ultrasonographic prediction of clinical pulmonary hypoplasia: measurement of the chest/trunk-length ratio in fetuses, *Pediatr Surg Int* 19(3):172-175, 2003.

Johnson AM, Hubbard AM: Congenital anomalies of the fetal/neonatal chest, *Semin Roentgenol* 39(2):197-214, 2004.

La Torre R, Cosmi E, Anceschi MH and others: Preliminary report on a new and noninvasive method for the assessment of fetal lung maturity, *J Perinat Med* 31(5):431-434, 2003.

Laudy JA, Wladimiroff JW: The fetal lung. I. Developmental aspects, *Obstet Gynecol* 16:284-290, 2000.

Mayden KL and others: The antenatal, sonographic detection of lung masses, *Am J Obstet Gynecol* 148:349, 1984.

Merz E, Miric-Tesanic D, Bahlmann F and others: Prenatal sonographic chest and lung measurements for predicting severe pulmonary hypoplasia, *Prenat Diagn* 19:614-619, 1999.

Moore KL: *Before we are born,* ed 3, Toronto, 1989, WB Saunders.

Nyberg DA, McGahan JP, Pretorius DH and others, editors: *Diagnostic ultrasound of fetal anomalies,* Philadelphia, 2003, Lippincott, Williams & Wilkins.

Osada H, Iitsuka Y, Masua K and others: Application of lung volume measurement by three-dimensional ultrasonography for clinical assessment of fetal lung development, *J Ultrasound Med* 21(8):841-847, 2002.

Pohls UG, Rempen A: Fetal lung volumetry by three-dimensional ultrasound, *Obstet Gynecol* 11:6-12, 1998.

Reyes C, Chang IK, Waffam F, and others: Delayed repair of congenital diaphragmatic hernia with early high-frequency oscillatory ventilation during preoperative stabilization, *J Pediatr Surg* 22:1010-1016, 1998.

Rotschild A, Ling KEW, Puterman ML and others: Neonatal outcome after prolonged preterm rupture of the membranes, *Am J Obstet Gynecol* 162:46-52, 1990.

Ruano R, Benachi A, Aubry MC and others: Prenatal sonographic diagnosis of congenital hiatal hernia, *Prenat Diagn* 24(1):26-30, 2004.

Sharland GK and others: Prognosis in fetal diaphragmatic hernia, *Am J Obstet Gynecol* 166:9, 1992.

Song MS, Yoo SJ, Smallhorn JF and others: Bilateral congenital diaphragmatic hernia: diagnostic clues at fetal sonography, *Ultrasound Obstet Gynecol* 17(3):255-258, 2001.

Teixeira J and others: Abdominal circumference in fetuses with congenital diaphragmatic hernia: correlation with hernia content and pregnancy outcome, *J Ultrasound Med* 16:407, 1997.

Tekesin I, Anderer G, Hellmeyer L and others: Assessment of fetal lung development by quantitative ultrasonic tissue characterization: a methodical study, *Prenat Diagn* 24(9):671-676, 2004.

Usui N, Kamata S, Sawai S and others: Outcome predictors for infants with cystic lung disease, *J Pediatric Surg* 39(4):603-606, 2004.

Van Eyck J, van der Morren K, Wladimiroff JW: Ductus arteriosus flow velocity modulation by fetal breathing movements as a measure of fetal lung development, *Am J Obstet Gynecol* 163:558-566, 1990.

Vintzileos AM and others: Comparison of six different ultrasonographic methods for predicting lethal fetal pulmonary hypoplasia, *Am J Obstet Gynecol* 161:606, 1989.

Winters WD, Effmann EL, Nghiem HV and others: Congenital masses of the lung: changes in cross-sectional area during gestation, *J Clin Ultrasound* 25:372-377, 1997.

CHAPTER 57

The Fetal Anterior Abdominal Wall

Sandra L. Hagen-Ansert and Denise Spradley

OBJECTIVES

- Describe the embryology of the abdominal wall
- Differentiate among an omphalocele, a gastroschisis, and an umbilical hernia
- List the sonographic findings in a fetus with an omphalocele
- List the sonographic findings in a fetus with a gastroschisis
- Describe limb-body wall defects, cloacal exstrophy, and pentalogy of Cantrell

EMBRYOLOGY OF THE ABDOMINAL WALL

SONOGRAPHIC EVALUATION OF THE FETAL ABDOMINAL WALL

ABNORMALITIES OF THE ANTERIOR ABDOMINAL WALL

OMPHALOCELE
GASTROSCHISIS
AMNIOTIC BAND SYNDROME
BECKWITH-WIEDEMANN SYNDROME
BLADDER AND CLOACAL EXSTROPHY
PENTALOGY OF CANTRELL, ECTOPIC CORDIS, AND CLEFT
    STERNUM
LIMB-BODY WALL COMPLEX

KEY TERMS

amniotic band syndrome – rupture of the amnion that leads to entrapment or entanglement of the fetal parts by the "sticky" chorion

Beckwith-Wiedemann syndrome – group of disorders having in common the coexistence of an omphalocele, macroglossia, and visceromegaly

cloacal exstrophy – defect in the lower abdominal wall and anterior wall of the urinary bladder

encephalocele – protrusion of the brain through a cranial fissure

exencephaly – abnormal condition in which the brain is located outside the cranium

gastroschisis – opening in the layers of the abdominal wall with evisceration of the bowel (and occasionally the stomach and genitourinary organs, but rarely the liver)

limb-body wall complex – anomaly with large cranial defects, facial cleft, large body wall defects, and limb abnormalities

omphalocele – develops when there is a midline defect of the abdominal muscles, fascia, and skin that results in herniation of intraabdominal structures into the base of the umbilical cord

pentalogy of Cantrell – rare anomaly with five defects: omphalocele, ectopic heart, lower sternum, anterior diaphragm, and diaphragmatic pericardium

scoliosis – abnormal curvature of the spine

Ultrasound has proven to be very effective for detecting anterior abdominal wall defects in utero. These defects occur during the first trimester as the midgut elongates and migrates into the umbilical cord. The midgut usually returns into the abdominal cavity by the 11th week of gestation. When this fails to occur, an abdominal wall defect is formed. The two most common defects are omphalocele and gastroschisis. Less common defects are ectopia cordis, limb-body wall complex, and cloacal exstrophy.

EMBRYOLOGY OF THE ABDOMINAL WALL

By the end of the 5th week of development, an embryo is a flat disk consisting of three layers: ectoderm, mesoderm, and endoderm. In the 6th week a process called *folding* helps the embryo transform itself into a cylindrical shape. This transformation is a critical part of the process of closing the abdominal wall.

As the embryo folds at the cranial end, the base of the yolk sac is partially incorporated as the foregut, which later develops as the pharynx, lower respiratory system, esophagus, stomach, duodenum (proximal to the opening of the bile duct), liver, pancreas, gallbladder, and biliary duct system.

The growth of the neural tube causes the embryo to fold at the caudal end, incorporating part of the yolk sac as the hindgut, which turns into the cloaca. It also causes the connecting stalk (located at the tail) to move to the ventral surface of the embryo, incorporating the allantois into the umbilical cord. The derivatives of the hindgut are the distal part of the transverse colon, the descending colon, the sigmoid colon, the rectum, the superior portion of the anal canal, the epithelium of the urinary bladder, and most of the urethra (Figure 57-1).

The sides of the embryo fold, leading to the formation of the lateral and anterior abdominal wall. The midgut is the primordium of the small intestines (including most of the duodenum), cecum, vermiform appendix, ascending colon, and the right half to two thirds of the transverse colon. The connection of the yolk sac and body stalk will form the umbilical cord at the ventral region of the embryo. Expansion of the amniotic cavity will cover the umbilical cord by the amnion.

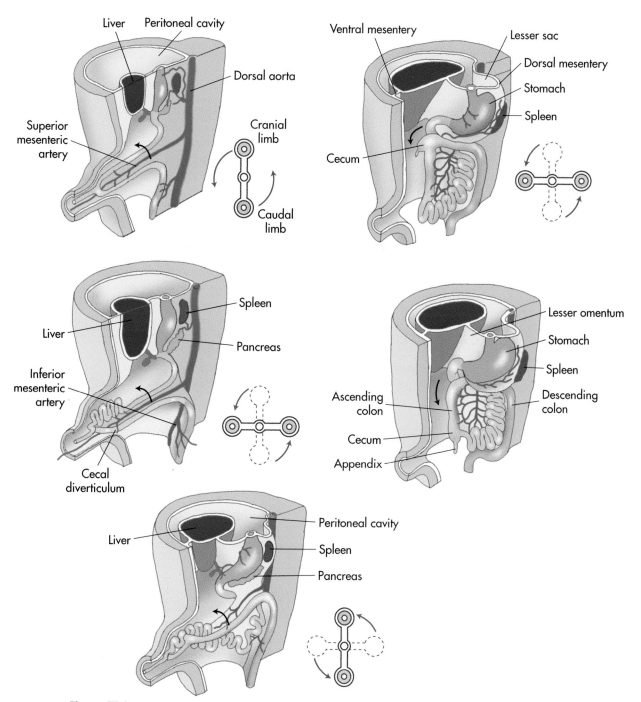

Figure 57-1   Development and rotation of the midgut from the 6th to 11th week. The midgut is the primordium of the small intestines, cecum, appendix, ascending colon, and right half to two thirds of the transverse colon. The connection of the yolk sac and body stalk will form the umbilical cord at the ventral region of the embryo.

Fusion of the midline begins during the 7th week of development and is completed by the 8th week.

The umbilical veins drain the placenta, body stalk, and the evolving abdominal wall. During the 7th week the hepatic bud enlarges, and the right umbilical vein atrophies. The proximal portion of the left umbilical vein between the subhepatic portion and the common cardinal vein also atrophies. Branches of the aorta now replace the nutritive function of the umbilical veins with respect to the developing abdominal wall. The superior mesenteric artery is formed from the right omphalomesenteric artery.

Umbilication hernia of the bowel occurs during the 8th week of development as the midgut extends to the extraembryonic coelom in the proximal portion of the umbilical cord. The midgut grows faster than the abdominal cavity at this stage because of the increased size of the liver and kidneys. Thus the herniation develops. The intestines return to the abdominal cavity by the 12th week of gestation.

SONOGRAPHIC EVALUATION OF THE FETAL ABDOMINAL WALL

It should be possible to detect abdominal wall defects in utero as the defects form early in embryologic development. It is very important to image the cord insertion site and the fetal anterior abdominal wall to evaluate for the presence or absence of such defects. If the urinary bladder and pelvis are evaluated closely, the diagnosis of bladder and cloacal exstrophy may also be made with sonography. The most common types of abdominal wall defects are gastroschisis, omphalocele, and umbilical hernia. Other types of abdominal ventral wall defects include ectopia cordia, bladder and cloacal exstrophy, amniotic band syndrome, and the limb-body wall complex. The following questions should be routinely answered:

1. Is a limiting membrane present?
2. What is the relation of the umbilical cord to the defect?
3. Which organs are eviscerated?
4. Is the bowel normal in appearance?
5. Are other fetal malformations evident?

ABNORMALITIES OF THE ANTERIOR ABDOMINAL WALL

Abdominal wall defects cause distortion of the normal contour of the ventral or anterior surface of the fetal abdomen. Table 57-1 summarizes the typical sonographic features and associated conditions of fetal abdominal wall defects.

The three most common abdominal wall defects are the **omphalocele**, umbilical hernia (a form of omphalocele), and **gastroschisis**. The incidence of omphaloceles is roughly 1 in 4000 live births. Rarer abdominal wall defects include ectopia cordis, pentalogy of Cantrell, limb-body wall complex, amnion rupture sequence, and bladder and cloacal exstrophy. Overall, gastroschisis has an incidence of 12 per 10,000, although only rarely are affected infants born to older mothers. The role of the perinatal team is to distinguish among these lesions because

---

BOX 57-1   DIFFERENTIATION OF OMPHALOCELE FROM GASTROSCHISIS

The sonographer should investigate the following to differentiate an omphalocele from a gastroschisis:

- Look for the presence of a membrane; gastroschisis does not have one.
- Look at the umbilical cord; the cord goes through the omphalocele, whereas gastroschisis is found to the right of the cord.
- Determine which organs are eviscerated.
- Determine if the bowel is normal in texture.
- Look for other anomalies because omphaloceles often occur with chromosomal abnormalities.

---

clinical management, associated anomalies, delivery, and postnatal surgical survival vary, depending on the specific type of abdominal wall defect.

Box 57-1 outlines what the sonographer should investigate to distinguish between omphalocele and gastroschisis.

OMPHALOCELE

During the 8th to 12th weeks of development, the fetal bowel normally migrates into the umbilical cord from the abdominal cavity. This normal embryologic herniation of the bowel permits the development of the intraabdominal organs and allows necessary bowel rotation. Because of the lack of space within the abdominal cavity and the large fetal liver and kidneys, the bowel is forced from the abdomen and into the extraembryonic coelom of the umbilical cord. This herniation permits the bowel to rotate around the superior mesenteric artery. These herniated loops of bowel normally return and rotate into position within the abdominal cavity by the 12th week of pregnancy. When bowel loops fail to return to the abdomen, a bowel-containing omphalocele occurs (Figure 57-2).

An omphalocele develops when there is a midline defect of the abdominal muscles, fascia, and skin that results in herniation of intraabdominal structures into the base of the umbilical cord (Figure 57-3). This herniation is covered by a membrane that consists of the amnion and peritoneum. The alpha-fetoprotein (AFP) level may be slightly elevated or within normal limits. Omphaloceles are characterized as two types: (1) those that contain the liver within the sac and (2) those that contain a variable amount of bowel without liver.

Fetuses with an omphalocele that contains only a bowel have a higher risk for chromosomal abnormalities and other anomalies (Figures 57-4 and 57-5). Bowel within the omphalocele develops because the intestine fails to return to the abdomen (primitive body stalk remains). A liver omphalocele represents a developmental defect in abdominal wall closure. This type of omphalocele affects the abdominal wall muscles, fascia, and skin. Liver omphaloceles may contain a bowel and demonstrate a relatively large abdominal wall defect in comparison with the abdominal diameter (Figures 57-6 and 57-7).

TABLE 57-1	TYPICAL FEATURES OF VENTRAL WALL DEFECTS AND ASSOCIATED CONDITIONS		
Type of Defect	Description	Sonographic Features	Other Anomalies
Gastroschisis	Paraumbilical defect	Typically only bowel is eviscerated; occasionally other organs, but almost never the liver	Associated anomalies are uncommon; high rate of bowel-related complications
Omphalocele	Midline defect, contained by membrane	Variable	High risk of other anomalies and/or aneuploidy
Extracorporeal liver		Typically large	When isolated without other detectable anomalies, risk of aneuploidy is very low; however, high rate of cardiac anomalies
Intracorporeal liver		Typically small	>50% risk of aneuploidy when detected prenatally
Beckwith-Wiedemann syndrome	Syndromic condition	Macroglossia; omphalocele; visceromegaly	Omphalocele is typically intracorporeal liver type
Pentalogy of Cantrell	Omphalocele Anterior diaphragmatic hernia Distal partial sternal defect Pericardial defect Cardiac defect	May appear only as high omphalocele; pleural effusion, even transient, is highly suggestive of diaphragmatic hernia in this situation	None
Absent sternum	Absent sternum	Dynamic heart covered by skin	Rare; usually isolated
Ectopic cordis	Thoracic defect of sternum and skin	Dynamic heart not covered by skin	Rare; high rate of cardiac and other defects; may be associated with high omphalocele
Bladder exstrophy	Eviscerated urinary bladder	Nonvisualization of urinary bladder; soft tissue mass of anterior abdominal wall may be subtle	Increased risk of fetal aneuploidy
Cloacal exstrophy	Eviscerated cloaca with two hemibladders	Nonvisualization of urinary bladder; in one variation, ileal prolapse produces "elephant trunk" appearance	Severe, complex anomaly
Limb-body wall complex	Multiple anomaly condition	Bizarre, complex defect with ventral wall defect, close attachment to placenta, cranial defects, scoliosis	100% lethal, but no risk of aneuploidy

Nyberg DA, McGahan JP, Pretorius DH and others, editors: *Diagnostic ultrasound of fetal anomalies: text and atlas,* Philadelphia, 2003, Lippincott, Williams & Wilkins.

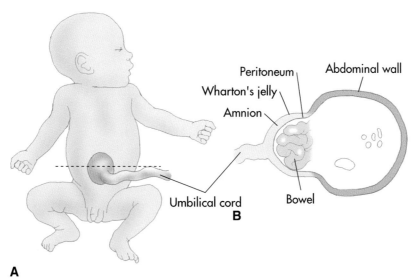

Figure 57-2   Typical features of bowel-containing omphalocele (intracorporeal liver) shown on external examination **(A)** and on cross-sectional view **(B).**

The prognosis for infants with an omphalocele varies according to the extent of the primary defect and associated structural and chromosomal abnormalities. Perinatal mortality approaches 80% when more than one fetal abnormality exists, and almost all infants die when there is a chromosomal or major heart defect. Without other anomalies, the mortality rate is approximately 10% with an isolated omphalocele.

The mode of delivery for fetuses with an omphalocele varies according to the type of omphalocele and other anomalies. The obstetrician may elect vaginal delivery when a chromosomal abnormality and other major anomalies predict no chance for survival.

Sonographic Findings. The sonographic signs of an omphalocele are as follows:

- Central abdominal wall defect with evisceration of the bowel or a combination of liver and bowel into the base of the umbilical cord. Color flow imaging may aid in viewing the continuity of the umbilical cord into the omphalocele. The stomach may be involved (Figure 57-8). Bowel omphaloceles appear echogenic and must be distinguished from umbilical hernia (covered by skin and fat).

- Membrane consisting of the peritoneum and amnion forms the omphalocele sac encasing the herniated organs.

- Umbilical hernias may be confused with liver omphaloceles; however, a normal cord insertion suggests hernia (Figure 57-9).

- Ascites may coexist with an omphalocele.

- Hydramnios is found in one third of fetuses.

- Associated anomalies (50% to 70%) include complex cardiac disease (30% to 50%) and gastrointestinal, neural tube, and genitourinary tract anomalies (polycystic kidneys with a small omphalocele may indicate trisomy 13) (Figure 57-10).

- Omphaloceles may occur concurrently with diaphragmatic hernia.

- Chromosomal anomalies occur in 35% to 60% of omphaloceles. Most common are trisomies 13 and 18. Omphaloceles may be found with trisomy 21, Turner's syndrome, and triploidy.

- When scoliosis is found, consider limb-body wall complex (or body-stalk anomaly), a lethal disorder, which also includes severe cranial defects (acrania, encephalocele), facial clefts, extensive abdominal wall defect of the chest, and abdomen and limb defects. Abnormal fusion of the amnion and chorion extends as a sheet from the cord and adheres to the fetus and placenta (Figures 57-11 and 57-12).

- Amniotic band syndrome may represent a milder form of limb-body wall complex and may be predicted by amniotic bands (fibrous tissue strands) that entangle or amputate fetal parts. Facial clefts, asymmetric encephaloceles, constriction or amputation defects of the extremities, and clubfoot deformities are common findings. Uterine sheets (synechiae) should not be confused with amniotic bands.

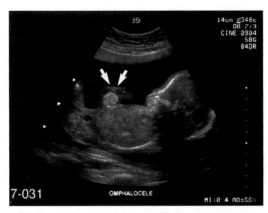

Figure 57-3 Longitudinal image of a 14-week fetus showing a small omphalocele with its covering membrane *(arrows)* projecting from the umbilical area.

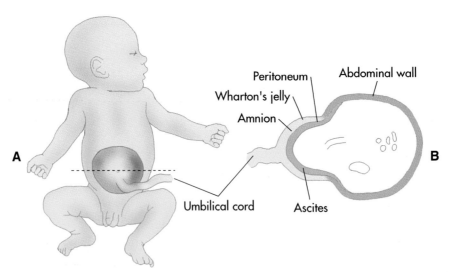

Figure 57-4 Typical features of liver-containing omphalocele shown on external examination (**A**) and on cross-sectional view (**B**).

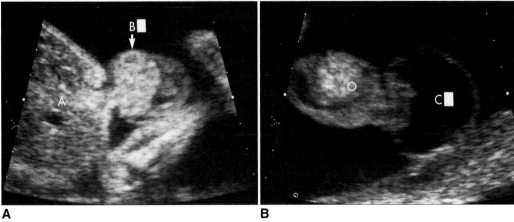

Figure 57-5   A, Bowel omphalocele *(B)* in a fetus with trisomy 18. *A,* Abdomen. **B,** In the same fetus an umbilical cord cyst *(C)* is noted coursing distally into the omphalocele *(O)*. Other anomalies observed include a strawberry-shaped cranium, hypoplastic cerebellum, nuchal fold, and esophageal atresia. Additionally, a large atrial septal defect, hypoplastic left ventricle, single umbilical artery, and hydramnios were found.

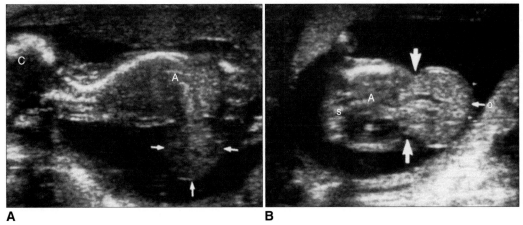

Figure 57-6   A, Sagittal scan in an 18-week fetus in a spine-up position with a mass herniating from the anterior abdominal wall representing an omphalocele *(arrows)*. *A,* Abdomen; *C,* cranium. **B,** In the same fetus, in a transverse direction, herniation of the liver into the omphalocele *(o)* is observed. Note the portal vessel within the liver. *A,* Abdomen; *large arrows,* first border of the omphalocele; *s,* spine.

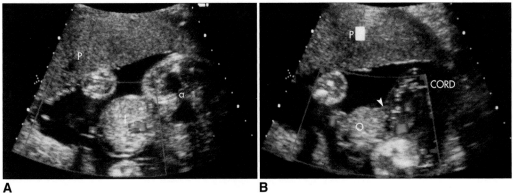

Figure 57-7   A, Color flow imaging of a liver-filled omphalocele in a 26-week fetus showing hepatic vessel flow within the herniated liver. *a,* Abdomen; *P,* placenta. **B,** In the same fetus, color enhancement aids in the confirmation of the cord vessels entering the base of the omphalocele *(O, arrow)*; *P,* placenta. No other anomalies were found, and the karyotype was normal.

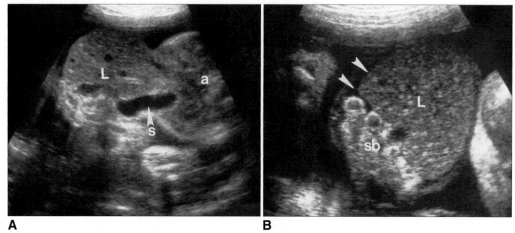

Figure 57-8 **A,** Large, liver-filled *(L)* omphalocele shown in a 27-week fetus. This omphalocele also contained a portion of the stomach *(s)* and small bowel. *a,* Abdomen. The karyotype was normal and no other sonographic anomalies were detected. **B,** In the same fetus, small bowel *(sb)* and ascites *(arrows)* are shown. Surgical repair of the omphalocele was successful after birth. *L,* Liver.

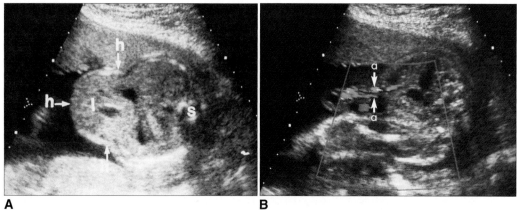

Figure 57-9 **A,** Umbilical hernia *(h; arrows)* observed in a fetus with Carpenter's syndrome (acrocephalopolysyndactyly). *l,* Liver; *s,* spine. **B,** In the same fetus, at the cord insertion level and using color imaging, the umbilical arteries are observed entering the abdomen in a normal location. This excludes the diagnosis of an omphalocele. *a,* Artery.

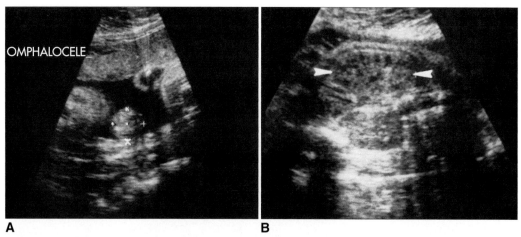

Figure 57-10 **A,** Bowel-filled omphalocele (2 mm) *(calipers)* in a 27-week fetus. **B,** In the same fetus, enlarged polycystic kidneys *(arrows)* were observed bilaterally. Oligohydramnios, an 8-mm nuchal fold, cerebellar hypoplasia, and enlarged cisterna magna with Dandy-Walker malformation and asymmetry of the heart were found. Genetic amniocentesis was declined. Intrauterine growth restriction was apparent by 33 weeks of gestation. Trisomy 13 was suspected. Neonatal karyotype after birth confirmed the diagnosis of trisomy 13 with translocation. The infant died within 1 hour of birth.

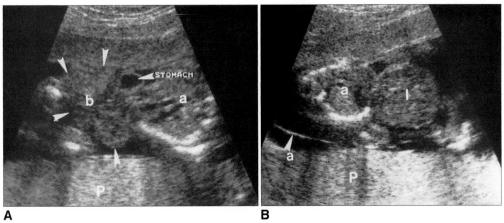

A   **B**

Figure 57-11   **A,** Early amnion rupture sequence or body stalk anomaly in a 17-week fetus revealing extensive herniation of the abdominal organs. The stomach and bowel *(b)* are eviscerated. *a,* Abdomen; *P,* placenta. **B,** In the same fetus, herniation of the liver *(l)* is noted. Note the amniotic band *(a, arrow)* outlined within the amniotic cavity. Amniocentesis reveals a chromosomally normal infant. *a,* Abdomen.

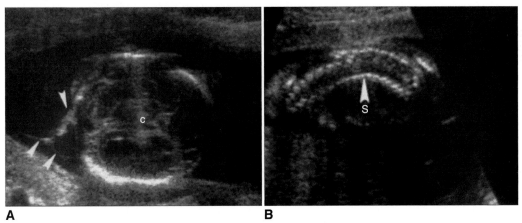

A   **B**

Figure 57-12   **A,** In the fetus depicted in Figure 57-11, amniotic bands *(arrows)* are shown adhering to the cranium *(c).* **B,** In the same fetus, scoliosis *(s)* is demonstrated. The fetus delivered prematurely at 29 weeks of gestation because of premature rupture of the membranes. Autopsy revealed posterior scalp defects with attachment of amniotic bands. Low-set ears and posteriorly rotated ears, bilateral cleft lip and palate, absent toes unilaterally, constriction ring of the thumb and first finger of one hand, and bilateral simian creases were found. The abdominal wall defect included herniation of the stomach, intestine, liver, and two spleens. A wide midline defect that was continuous with the cord was found. Scoliosis was also confirmed.

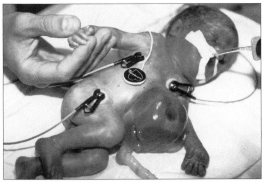

Figure 57-13   Neonate depicted in Figure 57-14 with diaphragmatic hernia and an omphalocele.

- Pentalogy of Cantrell is considered when a large omphalocele, diaphragmatic hernia, ectopia cordis (evisceration of heart), and other heart defects are observed (Figures 57-13 and 57-14).
- Consider bladder or cloacal exstrophy when a low omphalocele is observed. Other anomalies may include anal atresia, spina bifida, and lower-limb defects.
- When organomegaly and macroglossia are observed, Beckwith-Wiedemann syndrome is suspected (occurs in 12% of infants with an omphalocele).

GASTROSCHISIS

Gastroschisis is a periumbilical defect that nearly always is located to the right of the umbilicus. Gastroschisis is an opening in the layers of the abdominal wall with evisceration

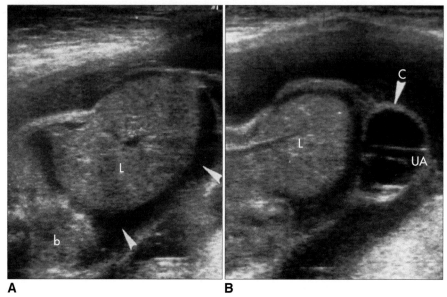

Figure 57-14   **A,** In the fetus shown in Figure 57-13, a coexisting liver-filled omphalocele *(L)* and ascites *(arrows)* are observed. Displaced bowel in chest *(b)*. **B,** In the same fetus, umbilical cord dilation *(C)* at the base of the omphalocele is demonstrated. *UA,* Umbilical artery.

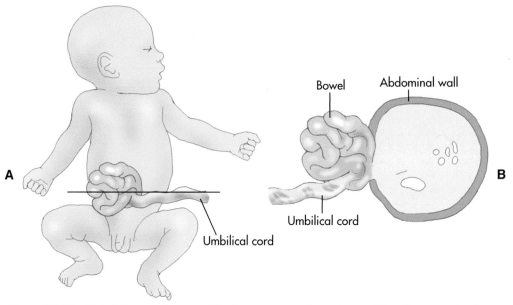

Figure 57-15   Typical features of gastroschisis shown on external examination **(A)** and cross-sectional view **(B).**

(herniation) of the bowel and, infrequently, the stomach and genitourinary organs but rarely the liver (Figure 57-15). It is thought that gastroschisis is a consequence of atrophy of the right umbilical vein or a disruption of the omphalomesenteric artery. Gastroschisis defects are usually not known to be genetically transmitted, although the recurrence risk for gastroschisis has been estimated at 3.5%.

Gastroschisis defects are small (2 to 4 cm in size) and are located next to the normal cord insertion. In the majority of cases, the defect is positioned to the right of the umbilical cord. The insertion of the umbilical cord is normal in fetuses with gastroschisis (Figures 57-16 and 57-17). Small bowel is always found in the herniation. Other organs that may be involved in the herniation include the large bowel, the stomach, occasionally portions of the genitourinary system, and rarely the liver.

Alpha-fetoprotein levels are significantly higher in gastroschisis compared with an omphalocele because of the exposed bowel. The occurrence of gastroschisis is 1.75 to 2.5 in 10,000 live births. It has been found more frequently in males.

Although coexisting anomalies are rare with gastroschisis, associated gastrointestinal problems may be of considerable medical consequence to the infant. This defect prevents the occurrence of normal bowel rotation, and intestinal atresia or

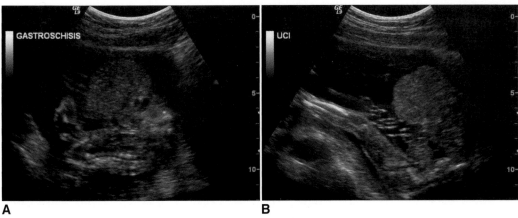

Figure 57-16 **A,** Appearance of gastroschisis in a 19-week fetus with elevation of maternal serum alpha-fetoprotein. Note the typical appearance of herniated, free-floating bowel loops. **B,** In the same fetus, a normal cord insertion is shown with herniated bowel.

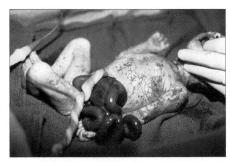

Figure 57-17 Neonate with left-side gastroschisis shown in Figure 57-19, *A.* Note the insertion of the cord to the right of the defect.

stenosis may ensue because of ischemia (compression of mesenteric vessels or bowel torsion). Ischemia may cause bowel perforation or meconium peritonitis. In several neonatal studies, over half of the infants with gastroschisis in which ischemia and gangrene of the bowel were present subsequently died.

The obstetrician usually prefers to deliver the infant by cesarean section to prevent bowel damage and contamination from a vaginal delivery. The prognosis for the infant with uncomplicated gastroschisis is excellent. Surgical repair usually occurs within hours of delivery; with extensive defects, reconstruction is performed in stages using Silastic sheets.

Sonographic Findings. The sonographer may be able to detect gastroschisis after 12 weeks of gestation. The patient usually has a notably elevated maternal serum AFP level. As the sonographer evaluates the area of umbilical cord insertion, multiple loops of the bowel (small bowel and often colon) may be seen outside the abdominal cavity in the area of the cord. The cord is normally inserted into the abdominal wall, and the defect is most always to the right of the umbilical cord insertion. The edges of the bowel are irregular and free floating without a covering membrane, as is seen with an omphalocele. Ascites is not present in the abdominal cavity.

The sonographic appearance of gastroschisis is as follows:

- Right paraumbilical defect of abdominal wall, rarely a left-side defect (Figure 57-18).
- Free-floating herniated small bowel. Large bowel, stomach, gallbladder, urinary bladder, and pelvic organs may be involved. When organs other than small or large bowel are seen, body stalk anomalies should be suspected.
- A herniated bowel may be mildly dilated with a bowel wall thickening (chemical peritonitis because of irritation by urine within amniotic fluid) (Figure 57-19). Dilation may be seen in herniated portions of the bowel and/or within the fetal abdominal cavity.
- Notably dilated bowel may suggest infarction or bowel atresia (Figure 57-20).
- Hydronephrosis, bladder deviation (Figure 57-21), and exstrophy (Figure 57-22) may be observed.
- Consider amniotic band syndrome amputations when clefting of the face and/or encephalocele is found. Severe body wall defects may be seen in gastroschisis with secondary band formation (Figures 57-23 through 57-25).

AMNIOTIC BAND SYNDROME

Amniotic band syndrome is the rupture of the amnion, which leads to entrapment or entanglement of the fetal parts by the "sticky" chorion. This may cause amputation or defects in random sites. Early entrapment by the bands may lead to severe craniofacial defects and internal malformations. Late entrapment leads to amputations or limb restrictions. The prevalence of this syndrome is low, occurring in 7.8 in 10,000 births. Anomalies associated with amniotic band syndrome include anomalies of the limbs, cranium, face, thorax, spine, abdominal wall (gastroschisis, omphalocele, bladder exstrophy), and the perineum.

BECKWITH-WIEDEMANN SYNDROME

Beckwith-Wiedemann syndrome is a rare group of disorders having in common the coexistence of an omphalocele, macroglossia, and visceromegaly. Most of the cases are

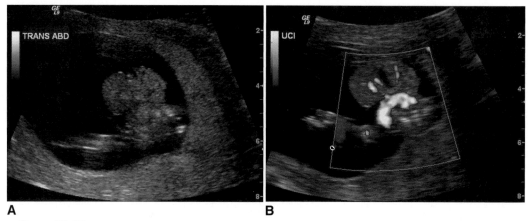

Figure 57-18 **A,** Transverse image of a 22-week fetus with moderate-sized gastroschisis. **B,** The umbilical cord is well seen with color as it enters to the right of the defect.

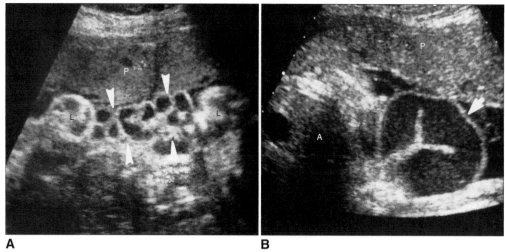

Figure 57-19 **A,** Gastroschisis showing herniated bowel *(arrows)* in the amniotic cavity. Cesarean section was performed at 36 weeks of gestation because of a nonreactive nonstress test with variable decelerations and absent breathing. A small-for-gestational age infant with left-side gastroschisis was delivered. *L,* Limb; *p,* placenta. **B,** Isolated bowel segment *(arrow)* observed in another fetus with gastroschisis at 29 weeks of gestation. Bowel dilation (29 mm) and obstruction (meconium ileus) are shown. Note the haustral markings within the obstructed bowel. *A,* Abdomen, *p,* placenta.

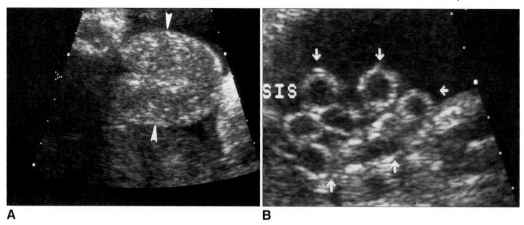

Figure 57-20 **A,** Herniated large intestine *(arrows)* with meconium at 34 weeks of gestation in a fetus with gastroschisis. Note the dilated bowel, which measured 20 mm in diameter. **B,** In the same fetus, portions of the small bowel *(arrow)* are observed with mild dilation.

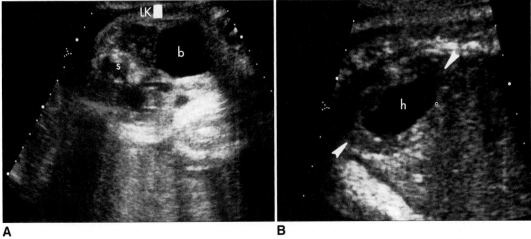

Figure 57-21   In a fetus with gastroschisis, concomitant anomalies were detected and included **(A)** deviation of the bladder **(B)** and unilateral hydronephrosis *(h, arrows). LK,* Normal left kidney; *s,* spine; *b,* bladder.

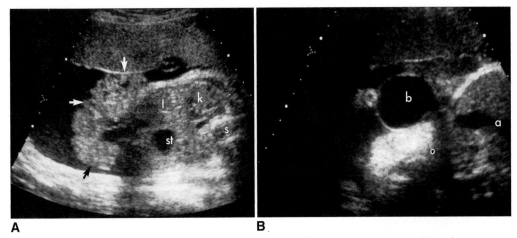

Figure 57-22   **A,** Gastroschisis *(arrows)* evident in a 34-week fetus in a transverse view. Note the intraabdominal position of the stomach *(st),* liver *(l),* and kidney *(k). s,* Spine. **B,** In the same fetus, note that the bladder *(b)* is herniated from the pelvis (exstrophy). The uterus and ovaries were also found to be herniated from the pelvis after delivery. Congenital microcolon was also found. *a,* Abdomen.

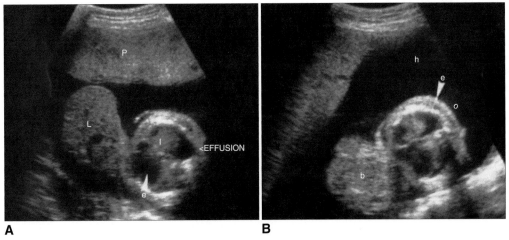

Figure 57-23   Gastroschisis with secondary amniotic bands shown in a 28-week fetus. **A,** Eviscerated liver *(L)* and bowel *(b)* are documented. Bilateral pleural effusions *(arrows)* and soft tissue edema *(e)* in **B** are apparent. Note the hydramnios *(h). l,* Lung; *P,* placenta.

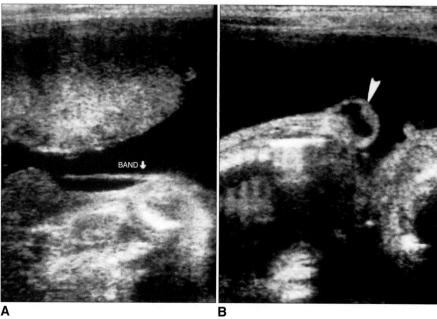

Figure 57-24   In the fetus depicted in Figures 57-23 and 57-25, multiple amniotic bands *(BAND)* **(A)** were found adhering to the abdomen with attachment to the shoulder *(arrow)* in **(B).** Normal chromosomes were found by amniocentesis. Amniotic fluid alpha-fetoprotein was extremely elevated (175 MOM) with positive acetylcholinesterase. The fetus was delivered at 28 weeks of gestation because of worsening hydrops. No resuscitative measures were undertaken. Autopsy findings revealed right paraumbilical gastroschisis with eventration of the liver and intestine. Intestinal malrotation and small-bowel obstruction were found. Moderate fetal hydrops with bilateral pleural effusions and pulmonary hypoplasia were noted. An amniotic band or peritoneal band extended from the liver to the thumb. The defect was consistent with gastroschisis occurring early in embryogenesis because of the intestinal malrotation with secondary amniotic band rupture.

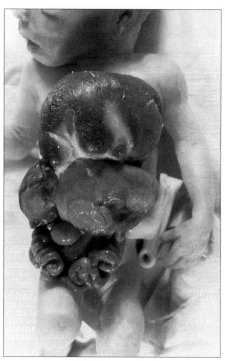

Figure 57-25   Neonate depicted in Figures 57-23 and 57-24 with gastroschisis and secondary amniotic band rupture.

sporadic. Beckwith-Wiedemann syndrome is characterized by macrosomia, macroglossia, visceromegaly, embryonic tumors (i.e., Wilms' tumor, hepatoblastoma, neuroblastoma, and rhabdomyosarcoma), an omphalocele, neonatal hypoglycemia, and ear creases. Sonographic findings usually note the presence of an omphalocele, growth acceleration, macroglossia, and visceromegaly. In the third trimester, polyhydramnios may be present.

BLADDER AND CLOACAL EXSTROPHY

Bladder exstrophy is characterized by a defect in the lower abdominal wall and anterior wall of the urinary bladder. The everted bladder becomes exposed on the lower abdominal wall. The anomaly may be mild or severe (accompanied by an omphalocele, inguinal hernia, undescended testes, and anal problems). **Cloacal exstrophy** is rare and more complex than bladder exstrophy. This condition occurs early in development with involvement of the primitive gut and persistent cloaca. It results in exstrophy of the bladder in which two hemibladders are separated by intestinal mucosa.

Sonographic Findings. With bladder exstrophy, the normal urinary bladder is not visible upon sonographic evaluation. Instead, a soft tissue mass, representing the exposed bladder mucosa, may be seen on the surface of the lower abdominal wall. In addition, an anterior abdominal wall defect may be the primary ultrasound finding of cloacal exstrophy.

PENTALOGY OF CANTRELL, ECTOPIC CORDIS, AND CLEFT STERNUM

The **pentalogy of Cantrell** is rare and is the association of a cleft distal sternum, diaphragmatic defect, midline anterior ventral wall defect, defect of the apical pericardium with communication into the peritoneum, and an internal cardiac defect. A high or superumbilical omphalocele is usually the primary finding of pentalogy of Cantrell. If the diaphragmatic defect is large enough to produce a diaphragmatic hernia, displacement of the heart and mediastinum may be observed, but the sternal and pericardial defects are not well seen. The presence of pericardial effusion may be found. Pentalogy of Cantrell may be associated with various cardiac defects, cleft lip (may also have cleft palate), encephalocele, exencephaly, and sirenomelia. In the first trimester, cystic hygroma may be present. This has also been associated with trisomies 13 and 18 and 45 X (Turner's syndrome).

In ectopia cordis, the exposed heart presents outside the chest wall through a cleft sternum. The most dramatic finding is the presence of a heart outside the thoracic cavity; a portion or all of the heart may protrude through the defect in the sternum. Anomalies most frequently associated with ectopia cordis include an omphalocele, cardiovascular malformations, and craniofacial defects.

A cleft sternum may be either partial or absent without ectopia cordis, and is typically a superior or total cleft. Dramatic pulsations of the anterior chest wall occur from the heart beating against the chest without the presence of the sternum to protect it. This condition is associated with vascular malformations, including cavernous hemangiomas and an omphalocele.

Sonographic Findings. On ultrasound examination, the heart may be seen to lie outside the normal thoracic cavity or bulge through the defective sternum. It is common to see pericardial and pleural effusions. Differential considerations include body stalk anomaly, amniotic band syndrome, and isolated ectopia cordis. The prognosis depends on many factors, including the extent of the defect and the size of the thoracic cavity that allows surgical intervention to place the heart back into the chest.

LIMB-BODY WALL COMPLEX

The **limb-body wall complex** anomaly is associated with large cranial defects (**exencephaly** or **encephalocele**); facial cleft; body wall complex defects involving the thorax, abdomen, or both; and limb defects. Other anomalies include **scoliosis** and various internal malformations. The limb-body wall complex occurs with the fusion of the amnion and chorion; the amnion does not cover the umbilical cord normally, but extends as a sheet from the margin of the cord and is continuous with both the body wall and the placenta. Left-side body wall defects are three times more common than right-side defects.

Sonographic Findings. On ultrasound examination the defects are large and involve the abdomen and thorax. The eviscerated organs form a complex, bizarre-appearing mass entangled with membranes. The umbilical cord is short and adherent to the placental membranes.

SELECTED BIBLIOGRAPHY

Arey LB: The vascular system. In Arey LB, editor: *Developmental anatomy,* ed 7, Philadelphia, 1974, WB Saunders.

Barnewolt CT: Congenital abnormalities of the gastrointestinal tract, *Semin Roentgenol* 39(2):263-281, 2004.

Bonilla-Musoles F, Machado LE, Bailao LA and others: Abdominal wall defects: two- versus three-dimensional ultrasonographic diagnosis, *J Ultrasound Med* 20(4):379-389, 2001.

Boyd PA, Bhattacarjee A, Gould S and others: Outcome of prenatally diagnosed anterior abdominal wall defects, *Arch Dis Child Fetal Neonatal Ed* 78(3):F209-213, 1998.

Callen DW, editor: *Ultrasonography in obstetrics and gynecology,* ed 4, Philadelphia, 2000, WB Saunders.

Chen CP, Lin SP, Hwu YM and others: Prenatal identification of fetal overgrowth, abdominal wall defect, and neural tube defect in pregnancies achieved by assisted reproductive technology, *Prenat Diagn* 24(5):396-398, 2004.

Davenport M, Haugen S, Greenough A and others: Closed gastroschisis: antenatal and postnatal features, *J Pediatr Surg* 36(12):1834-1837, 2001.

Fong KW, Toi A, Hornberger LK and others: Detection of fetal structural abnormalities with US during early pregnancy, *Radiographics* 24(1):157-174, 2004.

Gibbin C, Touch S, Broth RE and others: Abdominal wall defects and congenital heart disease, *Ultrasound Obstet Gynecol* 21(4):334-337, 2003.

Hossain GA, Islam SM, Mahmood S and others: Abdominal wall defect: a case report and review, *Mymensigh Med J* 12(1):64-68, 2003.

Kiliedag EB, Kilieday H, Bagis T and others: Large pseudocyst of the umbilical cord associated with patent urachus, *J Obstet Gyneacol Res* 30(6):444-447, 2004.

Langman J: Caudal part of the foregut. In Langman J, editor: *Medical embryology,* Baltimore, 1975, Williams & Wilkins.

Leon G, Chedrau P, San Miguel G: Prenatal diagnosis of Cantrell's pentalogy with conventional and three-dimensional sonography, *J Matern Fetal Neonatal Med* 12(3):209-211, 2002.

Martin RW: Screening for fetal abdominal wall defects, *Obstet Gynecol Clin North Am* 25(3):517-526, 1998.

Matsumi H, Kozuma S, Baba K and others: Three-dimensional ultrasound is useful in diagnosing the fetus with abdominal wall defect, *Ultrasound Obstet Gynecol* 8(5)356-358, 1996.

Moore KL, editor: *The developing human: clinically oriented embryology,* ed 4, Philadelphia, 1988, WB Saunders.

Nakayama DK: Management of the fetus with an abdominal wall defect. In Harrison MR, Golbus MS, Filly RA, editors: *The unborn patient: prenatal diagnosis and treatment,* Orlando, Fla, 1984, Grune & Stratton.

Nyberg DA, McGahan JP, Pretorius DH and others, editors: *Diagnostic ultrasound of fetal anomalies: text and atlas,* Philadelphia, 2003, Lippincott, Williams & Wilkins.

Ortiz VN, Villarreal DH, Gonzalez O and others: Gastroschisis: a ten year review, *Bol Assoc Med PR* 90(4-6):69-73, 1998.

Raynor BD, Richards D: Growth retardation in fetuses with gastroschisis, *J Ultrasound Med* 16:13, 1997.

Robinson JN, Abuhamad AZ: Abdominal wall and umbilical cord anomalies, *Clin Perinatol* 27(4):947-978, 2000.

Salihu HM, Boos R, Schmidt W: Omphalocele and gastroschisis, *J Obstet Gynaecol* 22(5):489-492, 2002.

Salvesen KA: Fetal abdominal wall defects—easy to diagnose—and then what? *Ultrasound Obstet Gynecol* 18(4):301-304, 2001.

Sanders RC, editor: *Clinical sonography: a practical guide,* ed 3, Boston, 1998, Little, Brown.

Smrcek JM, Germer U, Krokowski M and others: Prenatal ultrasound diagnosis and management of body stalk anomaly: analysis of nine singleton and two multiple pregnancies, *Ultrasound Obstet Gynecol* 21(4):322-328, 2003.

Stepan H, Horn LC, Bennek J and others: Congenital hernia of the abdominal wall: a differential diagnosis of fetal abdominal wall defects, *Ultrasound Obstet Gynecol* 13(3):207-209, 1999.

Tamon y Cajal CL: Umbilical vein and middle cerebral artery blood flow response to partial occlusion by external compression of the umbilical vein (pressure test), *J Matern Fetal Neonatal Med* 12 (2):104-111, 2002.

Tawil A, Comstock CH, Chang CH: Prenatal closure of abdominal defect in gastroschisis: case report and review of the literature, *Pediatr Dev Pathol* 4(6):580-584, 2001.

Wu JL, Fang KH, Yeh GP and others: Using color Doppler sonography to identify the perivesical umbilical arteries: a useful method in the prenatal diagnosis of omphalocele-exstrophy-imperforate anus-spinal defects complex, *J Ultrasound Med* 23(9):1211-1215, 2004.

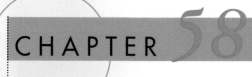
The Fetal Abdomen

Sandra L. Hagen-Ansert

KEY TERMS

anorectal atresia – complex disorder of the bowel and genitourinary tract

asplenia – no development of splenic tissue

choledochal cyst – cystic growth of the common bile duct

cholelithiasis – gallstones

cystic fibrosis – mucous buildup within the lungs and other areas of the body

duodenal atresia – complete blockage at the pyloric sphincter

duodenal stenosis – narrowing of the pyloric sphincter

esophageal atresia – congenital hypoplasia of the esophagus; usually associated with a tracheoesophageal fistula

esophageal stenosis – narrowing of the esophagus, usually in the distal third segment

gastroschisis – abnormality of the abdominal wall in which the bowel, without a covering membrane, protrudes outside of the wall

haustral folds – one of the sacculations of the colon caused by longitudinal bands that are shorter than the gut

hemopoiesis – formation of blood

Hirschsprung's disease (megacolon) – a congenital disorder in which there is abnormal innervation of the large intestine

jejunoileal atresia – blockage of the jejunum and ileal bowel segments that appears as multiple cystic structures within the fetal abdomen

Meckel's diverticulum – remnant of the proximal part of the yolk stalk

meconium ileus – small-bowel disorder marked by the presence of thick echogenic meconium in the distal ileum

omphalocele – abnormality of the abdominal wall in which bowel and liver, both covered by a membrane, protrude outside the wall

partial situs inversus – condition in which only the heart or the abdominal organs are reversed (dextrocardia or liver on the left, stomach on the right)

peristalsis – movement of the bowel

polysplenia – more than one spleen; associated with cardiac malformations

pseudoascites – sonolucent band near the fetal anterior abdominal wall from the abdominal wall muscles in the fetus over 18 weeks (does not outline the falciform ligament or bowel as ascites will)

situs inversus – heart and abdominal organs are completely reversed

VACTERL – vertebral defects, heart defects, renal and limb abnormalities

---

The fetal abdominal organs, liver, biliary system, spleen, stomach, kidneys, and colon are well formed by the second trimester. The following differences between the fetal and adult abdomen have been noted:

- The umbilical arteries and vein provide important anatomic landmarks for fetal abdominal anatomy and measurements.
- The ductus venous is patent and serves as a conduit between the portal veins and systemic veins.
- The proportions of the fetal body differ from those in the adult: the fetal abdomen is larger relative to body length, and the liver occupies a larger volume of the fetal abdomen.
- The fetal pelvic cavity is small; therefore, the urinary bladder, ovaries, and uterus lie in the abdominal cavity.
- The apron of the greater omentum is small, contains little fat, and remains unfused in the fetus. Fetal ascites may therefore separate the omental leaves.

EMBRYOLOGY OF THE DIGESTIVE SYSTEM

The primitive gut forms during the 4th week of gestation as the dorsal part of the yolk sac is incorporated into the embryo during folding. The primitive gut is divided into three sections: foregut, midgut, and hindgut.

THE FOREGUT

The derivatives of the foregut are the pharynx, lower respiratory system, esophagus, stomach, part of the duodenum, liver and biliary apparatus, and pancreas.

Esophagus. The esophagus is short in the beginning, but it rapidly lengthens as the body grows, reaching its final length by the 7th week. The *tracheoesophageal septum* partitions the trachea from the esophagus. **Esophageal atresia,** usually associated with a tracheoesophageal fistula, results from abnormal deviation of the tracheoesophageal septum in a posterior direction. When this occurs, amniotic fluid cannot pass to the intestines for absorption and hydramnios results.

Esophageal stenosis is the narrowing of the esophagus, usually in the distal third portion. This occurs from incomplete recanalization of the esophagus during the 8th week of development.

Stomach. The stomach appears as a fusiform dilation of the caudal part of the foregut (Figure 58-1). During the 5th and 6th weeks, the dorsal border (greater curvature) grows faster than the ventral border (lesser curvature). The stomach is suspended from the dorsal wall of the abdominal cavity by the dorsal mesentery or dorsal mesogastrium. The dorsal mesogastrium is carried to the left during rotation of the stomach and formation of a cavity known as the omental bursa or lesser sac of the peritoneum.

The lesser sac communicates with the main peritoneal cavity or greater peritoneal sac through a small opening, called the epiploic foramen.

Duodenum. The duodenum develops from the caudal part of the foregut and cranial part of the midgut (see Figure 58-1). The two parts grow rapidly and form a C-shaped loop that rotates to the right, where it comes to lie primarily in the retroperitoneum. The junction of the two embryonic parts of the duodenum in the adult is just distal to the entrance of the common bile duct. The duodenum is supplied by branches of the celiac trunk and the superior mesenteric artery.

During the 5th and 6th weeks, the lumen of the duodenum becomes partly or totally occluded (depending on the proliferation of its lining of epithelial cells). Normally the duodenum is recanalized by the end of the 8th week. Partial or complete failure of this process results in either **duodenal stenosis** (narrowing) or duodenal atresia (blockage). Usually the third or fourth parts of the duodenal are affected.

Liver and Biliary System. The liver, gallbladder, and biliary ducts arise as a bud from the most caudal part of the foregut in the 4th week (see Figure 58-1). The hepatic diverticulum grows between the layers of the ventral mesentery, where it rapidly enlarges and divides into two parts. The liver grows rapidly and intermingles with the vitelline and umbilical veins, divides into two parts, and fills most of the abdominal cavity. The large cranial part is the primordium of the parenchyma of the liver. The small caudal part gives rise to the gallbladder and cystic duct.

The hemopoietic cells, Kupffer cells, and connective tissue cells are derived from the mesenchyme in the septum transversum. The septum transversum is a mass of mesoderm between the pericardial cavity and the yolk stalk. It forms a major part of the diaphragm and the ventral mesentery.

Hemopoiesis (blood formation) begins during the 6th week and accounts for the large size of the liver between the 7th and 9th weeks of development. By the 12th week, bile formation by the hepatic cells has begun.

Extrahepatic biliary atresia. Blockage of the bile ducts results from their failure to recanalize following the solid stage of their development. This malformation may also result from interference with the blood supply of the ducts resulting from infection during the fetal period.

Pancreas. The pancreas develops from the dorsal and ventral pancreatic buds of the endodermal cells that arise from the caudal part of the foregut (see Figure 58-1). When the

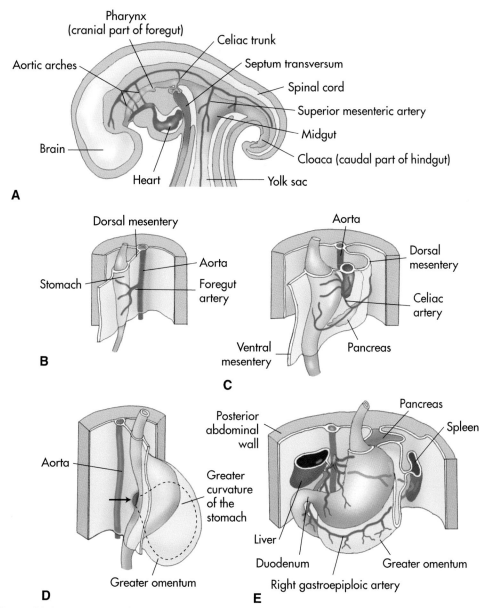

Figure 58-1 Development of the digestive system. **A,** Four weeks. **B,** Five weeks. **C,** Six weeks. **D** and **E,** Development of stomach. Seven weeks.

duodenum grows and rotates to the right, the ventral bud is carried dorsally and fuses with the dorsal bud. The ducts of the two pancreatic buds join. The combined duct becomes the main pancreatic duct that opens with the bile duct into the duodenum. The proximal part of the duct may persist as the accessory pancreatic duct.

Spleen. The spleen is a lymphatic organ that is derived from a mass of mesenchymal cells located between the layers of the dorsal mesogastrium (see Figure 58-1). The spleen is lobulated in the fetal period.

THE MIDGUT

The derivatives of the midgut are the small intestines (including most of the duodenum), the cecum and cloaca exstrophy,

the ascending colon, and most of the transverse colon. All of these structures are supplied by the superior mesenteric artery.

The midgut is suspended from the abdominal wall by an elongated dorsal mesentery. It communicates with the yolk sac via the yolk stalk. While the midgut lengthens and forms a midgut loop, it herniates outside the abdomen into the proximal part of the umbilical cord. Usually by the 10th or 11th week, this midgut herniation returns to the abdomen and undergoes further rotation resulting from the decrease in size of the liver and kidneys and the growth of the abdominal cavity.

After the intestines return to the abdominal cavity, they enlarge, lengthen, and assume their final positions. Their mesenteries are pressed against the posterior abdominal wall. At this time, the ascending colon and descending colon become retroperitoneal. Likewise the duodenum and most of the pancreas also become retroperitoneal structures. At the same time, the small intestines form a new line of attachment that extends from where the duodenum becomes retroperitoneal to the ileocecal junction. The mesentery of the transverse colon fuses with the dorsal mesogastrium to form the posterior wall of the inferior part of the omental bursa. The sigmoid colon retains its mesentery, but it is shorter than in the early fetus.

MALFORMATIONS OF THE MIDGUT

Omphalocele and Gastroschisis. Omphalocele and gastroschisis are defects that occur when the midgut fails to return to the abdominal cavity from the umbilical cord during the 10th week. In an **omphalocele,** coils of intestine protrude from the umbilicus and are covered by a transparent sac of amnion. The umbilical cord pierces the central part of the omphalocele. Conversely a **gastroschisis** is a condition in which the bowel and/or organs are free floating from the midline defect. The gastroschisis is usually located to the right of the umbilical cord. (See Chapter 57 for further discussion of omphalocele and gastroschisis.)

Umbilical Hernia. When the intestines return normally to the abdominal cavity and then herniate either prenatally or postnatally through an inadequately closed umbilicus, an umbilical hernia forms. The hernia differs from an omphalocele in that the protruding mass (omentum or loop of bowel) is covered by subcutaneous tissue and skin.

Meckel's Diverticulum. Meckel's diverticulum is the most common malformation of the midgut. A **Meckel's diverticulum** is a remnant of the proximal part of the yolk stalk that fails to degenerate and disappear during the early fetal period. It is usually a small fingerlike sac, about 5 cm long, that projects from the border of the ileum.

THE HINDGUT

The derivatives of the hindgut are the left part of the transverse colon, the descending colon, the sigmoid colon, the rectum, the superior portion of the anal canal, the epithelium of the urinary bladder, and most of the urethra. All of these structures are supplied by the inferior mesenteric artery.

SONOGRAPHIC EVALUATION OF THE ABDOMINAL CAVITY

The sonographer needs to carefully evaluate the gastrointestinal system during each routine scan. The stomach, liver and vascular structures, cord insertion, small bowel, and colon should be clearly identified by the sonographer.

GASTROINTESTINAL SYSTEM

Stomach. The stomach should be identified as a fluid-filled structure in the left upper quadrant inferior to the diaphragm. A marked variation in the size of the stomach can be seen, even within the same fetus. Most fetuses older than 14 to 16 weeks should have fluid in their stomachs (Figure 58-2). If no fluid is apparent, the stomach should be reevaluated in 20 to 30 minutes to rule out the possibility of a central nervous system problem (swallowing disorders), obstruction, oligohydramnios, or atresia. If fluid is still not noted during the sonographic evaluation, the fetus may be reexamined the following day or week to see if there has been a change in the size of the stomach. Esophageal anomalies are the least common problem for nonvisualization of the stomach.

The fluid within the stomach should be anechoic in the normal fetus. Echogenic debris may sometimes be seen along the dependent wall of the stomach that may represent vernix, protein, or intraamniotic hemorrhage. The presence of an echogenic mass in the fetal stomach in a patient who demonstrates clinical or sonographic evidence of placental abruption should raise the possibility of hematoma formation associated with an intraamniotic hemorrhage.

Esophagus. The normal esophagus can be visualized in the thorax during the second and third trimesters as two or more parallel echogenic lines ("multilayered" pattern).

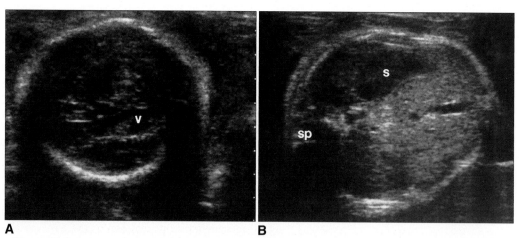

A   **B**

Figure 58-2   A 32-week fetus with microcephaly. **A,** Small head and ventricle *(v)*. **B,** Transverse image at the level of the stomach *(s)* and spine *(sp)*.

Abdominal Circumference. The abdominal circumference is measured at the level of the portal sinus and the umbilical portion of the left portal vein ("hockey stick" appearance on the sonogram) (Figure 58-3). Be careful to avoid oblique scanning of the abdomen that may lead to an incorrect diameter-circumference measurement. The abdomen should be round, not oval. The pressure of the transducer should not compress the abdominal cavity.

Umbilical Cord Insertion. In the fetus, the umbilical vein courses cephalically in the free, inferior margin of the falciform ligament. It joins the umbilical portion of the left portal vein at the caudal margin of the left intersegmental fissure of the liver (Figure 58-4). The insertion of the umbilical cord must be imaged with color because it inserts into both the fetal abdomen and the placenta. Visualization of the umbilical cord insertion site must be made to rule out the presence of an omphalocele, gastroschisis, hernia, or mass formation. After birth, the umbilical vein collapses and ultimately becomes the ligamentum teres hepatis.

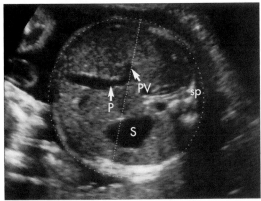

Figure 58-3   The abdominal circumference is measured from a transverse image at the level of the portal sinus *(P)* and the umbilical portion of the left portal vein *(PV)*. The stomach *(S)* is seen posterior; the spine *(sp)* is at 3 o'clock.

Bowel. Movement of the gastric musculature begins in approximately the 4th to 5th month of gestation. The sonographic appearance of the bowel varies with menstrual age. The fetus is capable of swallowing sufficient amounts of amniotic fluid to permit visualization of the stomach by 11 menstrual weeks. In the second trimester, this movement and fetal swallowing result in the delivery of increased amniotic fluid volume distally into the small bowel and colon where fluid and nutrients are reabsorbed. After the 15th to 16th week, meconium begins to accumulate in the distal part of the small intestine as a combination of desquamated cells, bile pigments, and mucoproteins.

Until the mid-second trimester, the small bowel lumen is quite difficult to demonstrate and appears as an ill-defined area of increased echogenicity in the mid to lower abdomen. The distinction of the large bowel from the small bowel is possible after 20 menstrual weeks. The region of the small bowel can be seen because it is slightly hyperechoic, compared with the liver, and may appear "masslike" in the central abdomen and pelvis (Figure 58-5). The hyperechoic appearance could be secondary to reflections from the walls of collapsed loops of the small bowel or from mesenteric fat between the loops. This hyperechoic appearance of the small bowel persists throughout the pregnancy. As the pregnancy progresses, the hyperechoic area becomes less prominent, and the small bowel is located more centrally in the abdomen than the colon. After 27 weeks, **peristalsis** of the normal small bowel is increasingly observed. The normal diameter of the small bowel lumen is less than or equal to 5 mm, with a length of 15 mm near term.

The colon is seen near the end of the second trimester as a long tubular hypoechoic structure with well-defined walls. The **haustral folds** of the colon help to differentiate it from the small bowel. In early gestation, haustral folds appear as thin linear echoes within the lumen of the colon; later, the colon diameter increases and the folds become longer and thicker. Normal measurements of the colon diameter range from 3 to 5 mm at 20 weeks to 23 mm or larger at term. The colon is more peripheral than the small bowel. Hypoechoic echoes

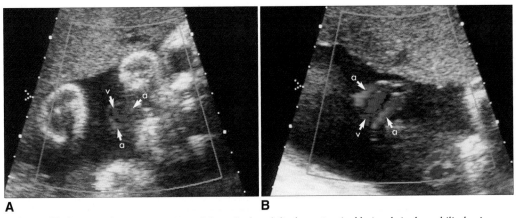

A   **B**

Figure 58-4   **A,** Color representation of the paired umbilical arteries *(a, blue)* and single umbilical vein *(v, red)* in a 30-week fetus viewed in a transverse plane. **B,** Sagittal view of the umbilical arteries *(a, blue)* and umbilical vein *(v, red)*. Color flow imaging may highlight vessels that may not be obvious because of fetal position, oligohydramnios, and congenital anomalies.

from the meconium may be seen within the lumen. The colon does not have peristalsis like the small bowel.

After 14 weeks of gestation, lipid is absorbed from the fetal colon and the remaining contents collect in the colon as meconium. The meconium within the lumen of the colon appears hypoechoic relative to the fetal liver and in comparison with the bowel wall. This is the point where the normal colon can be mistaken for an abnormally dilated small bowel or other pathologic processes, including renal cysts and pelvic masses. This pitfall is more prominent when the meconium has a more sonolucent appearance than usual (reflective of increased water content). The meconium increases slightly in echogenicity as the fetus grows nearer to term delivery.

HEPATOBILIARY SYSTEM

Liver. The fetal liver is relatively large compared with the other intraabdominal organs and occupies most of the upper abdomen in the fetus. It accounts for 10% of the total weight of the fetus at 11 weeks and 5% of the total weight at term.

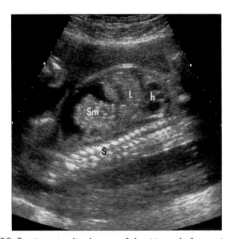

Figure 58-5 Longitudinal scan of the 23-week fetus with abdominal ascites surrounding the small bowel *(Sm). h,* Heart; *L,* liver; *S,* spine.

The hepatic veins and fissures are formed by the end of the first trimester (Figure 58-6). The left lobe of the liver is larger than the right in utero secondary to the greater supply of oxygenated blood. This of course reverses after birth.

Gallbladder. The normal gallbladder may be seen sonographically after 20 weeks of gestation. Both the gallbladder and portal-umbilical vein appear as oblong fluid-filled structures on the transverse view of the fetal abdomen through the liver (Figure 58-7). The gallbladder is distinguished by its location to the right of the portal-umbilical vein and as an oblong, more oval structure than the "tubular" intrahepatic umbilical vein.

Pancreas. The normal fetal pancreas has been seen in utero, but is more difficult to routinely recognize because of the lack of fatty tissue within the gland. It lies in the retroperitoneal cavity anterior to the superior mesenteric vessels, aorta, and inferior vena cava (Figure 58-8).

Spleen. The spleen is homogeneous in texture, similar in echogenicity to the kidney, and slightly less echogenic than the liver. It increases in size during gestation. The spleen is imaged on a transverse plane posterior and to the left of the fetal stomach.

ABNORMALITIES OF THE HEPATOBILIARY SYSTEM

Anomalies of the liver, gallbladder, pancreas, and spleen are rare. Detection of abnormal morphology is beneficial because many lesions may be undetected in the newborn period.

LIVER

The fetal liver, although involved in several congenital anomalies (diaphragmatic hernia, omphalocele), is rarely affected by isolated hepatic lesions. Liver parenchymal cysts and hemangiomas of the liver have been reported. The liver enlarges in

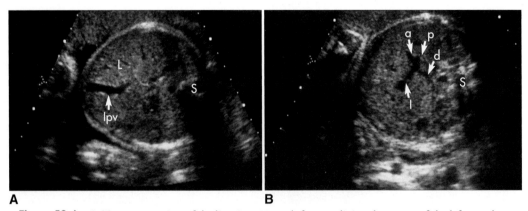

A   **B**

Figure 58-6 **A,** Transverse section of the liver in a 31-week fetus outlining the course of the left portal vein *(lpv)* at its entrance into the liver *(L)* from the fetal umbilical cord insertion. The left portal vein ascends upward and into the liver tissue *(L). S,* Spine. **B,** The left portal vein *(l)* is shown to bifurcate into the portal sinus, right anterior *(a),* and right posterior *(p)* portal veins. The ductus venosus *(d)* is observed before its drainage into the inferior vena cava. *S,* Spine.

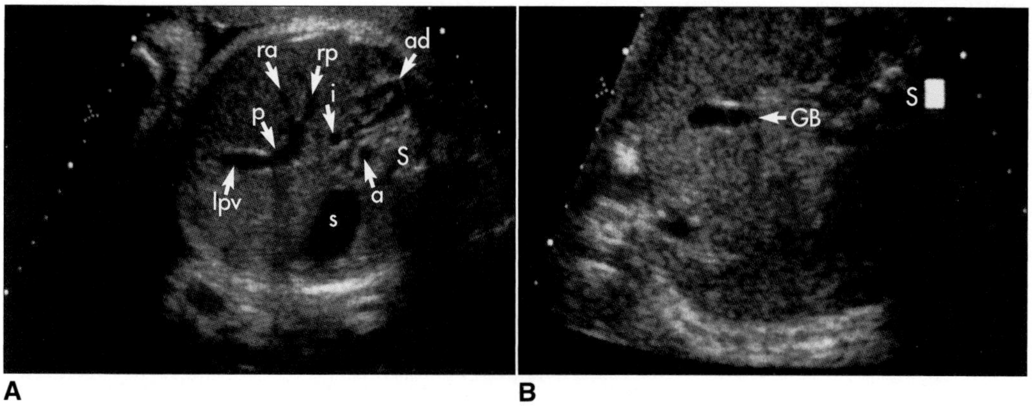

A   B

Figure 58-7 **A,** Transverse section of the liver and related structures in a 32-week fetus showing the left portal vein *(lpv)* coursing into the portal sinus *(p)*. The blood then moves into the right anterior *(ra),* and right posterior *(rp),* portal veins and ductus venosus (see Figure 58-6, *B*). The right adrenal gland *(ad),* fluid-filled stomach *(s),* aorta *(a),* and inferior vena cava *(i)* are shown. *S,* Spine. **B,** The gallbladder *(GB)* is viewed in the right upper quadrant of the abdomen in a 32-week fetus. The teardrop shape of the gallbladder should be distinguished from the left portal vein. *S,* Spine.

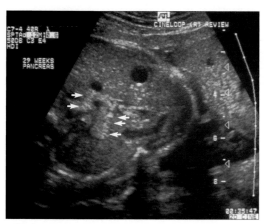

Figure 58-8 Transverse image of the fetal abdomen. The fetal spine is shown at 8 o'clock with the pancreas just anterior *(arrows)*.

fetuses with Rh-immune disease in response to increased hematopoiesis (red blood cell production in the liver).

Liver tumors, hamartoma, and hepatoblastoma are uncommon and may be observed prenatally. Other tumors seen with sonography include hepatic teratoma, adenoma, or metastases from neuroblastoma. Although a rare tumor, hemangioendothelioma is the most common, symptomatic, vascular hepatic tumor of infancy and may cause nonimmune hydrops in the fetus.

Sonographic Findings. Most of these tumors appear as hypoechoic solid masses within the liver, although cystic components have also been reported as mixed with the solid masses. About 5% of benign and malignant liver tumors are calcified.

Liver calcification may be observed as an isolated echogenic focus. This calcification is usually a benign finding; rarely, it may be a hemangioma, multiple foci secondary to infection (transplacental infections, cytomegalovirus, toxoplasmosis), or

hepatic necrosis from ischemia. If multiple calcifications are seen within the liver, other organs such as the brain and spleen may also be affected.

SITUS INVERSUS

Situs inversus may present as a total reversal of the thoracic and abdominal organs or as a partial reversal (mirror image of some organs). Partial situs inversus is a more severe disorder and may develop in two different combinations of organ reversals. In partial situs inversus, the stomach may or may not be reversed. **Asplenia** (absence of the spleen) is represented by an abnormally positioned liver and gallbladder (more midline position), and abnormal positioning of the aorta and inferior vena cava on the same side. **Polysplenia** (more than one spleen) is represented as a transposition of the liver and stomach, absence of the gallbladder, and disruption of the inferior vena cava. At least two spleens are present along the greater curvature of the stomach (which is on the right side). Heart block is common in polysplenia syndrome.

The cause of situs inversus is unclear, but it is thought to occur early in embryogenesis before normal laterality determination (before 3 weeks). Cardiac malformations are particularly common (99%) in asplenia syndrome and are seen with less frequency in polysplenia syndrome (90%). Cardiac defects include endocardial cushion defects, hypoplastic left heart (Figure 58-9), and transposition of the great vessels.

The infant with total situs inversus usually has a normal outcome. About 20% may have Kartagener's syndrome (immotile cilia, bronchiectasis). The mortality rate for **partial situs inversus** is extremely high, with death occurring in 90% to 95% with asplenia syndrome and 80% with polysplenia syndrome.

Sonographic Findings. Sonographically, the following signs may be observed:

• Total situs inversus (right-side heart axis and aorta; transposition of liver, stomach, and spleen; left-side gallbladder).

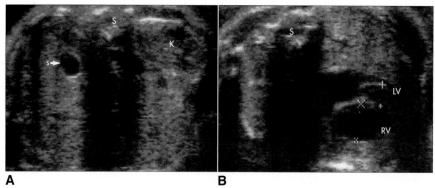

Figure 58-9 **A,** Partial situs inversus observed in a transverse spine-up position. The stomach *(s with arrow)* was found on the right side of the abdomen. *K,* Kidney; *S,* spine. **B,** In the same fetus, a hypoplastic left ventricle *(LV)* is shown. Other findings included bilateral liver, a left-side inferior vena cava, and a right-side descending aorta, right gallbladder, double inlet right ventricle *(RV)*, common atrioventricular valve, atrial septal defect, and one outflow vessel (pulmonary artery). *S,* spine.

BOX 58-1   CAUSES OF ASCITES

- Genitourinary
- Gastrointestinal
- Liver
- Cardiac
- Infections
- Metabolic storage disorders
- Idiopathic

- Partial situs inversus (right-side stomach, left-side liver). Dextrocardia with normal stomach position (see previous section).
- Other anomalies to check for include gastrointestinal, genitourinary, and neural tube defects.

PSEUDOASCITES

A sonolucent band near the fetal anterior abdominal wall is commonly identified during routine obstetric examinations in the fetus over 18 weeks of gestation. This band results from normal musculature surrounding the abdominal wall. True ascites is identified within the peritoneal recesses, whereas pseudoascites is always confined to an anterior or anterolateral aspect of the fetal abdomen. Furthermore, **pseudoascites** never outlines the falciform ligament like true ascites (Box 58-1).

GALLBLADDER

Anomalies of the gallbladder may be detected using prenatal sonographic techniques. **Cholelithiasis** (gallstones) may be identified in the fetus when calcifications are found within the gallbladder. These gallstones resolve spontaneously in utero or in the childhood period (Figure 58-10).

A **choledochal cyst** (dilation of the common bile duct) may be diagnosed when a cystic mass is identified adjacent to the

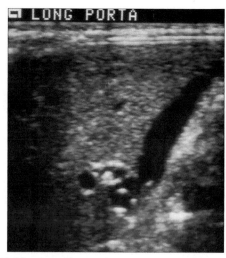

Figure 58-10 Sagittal scan of a neonate with gallstones. Small calcifications with shadowing were seen in the fetal ultrasound in the gallbladder.

fetal stomach and gallbladder (Box 58-2). Choledochal cysts may be confused with malformations of the stomach or bowel or duodenal atresia. The sonographer should remember that the gallbladder is more anterior than the duodenum and thus a cystic mass attached to the bile duct near the gallbladder would make the mass more likely a choledochal cyst. Choledochal cysts may be associated with intermittent biliary obstruction and severe biliary cirrhosis; therefore, early diagnosis is important. (See Chapter 22 for further information.)

Agenesis of the gallbladder occurs in approximately 20% of patients with biliary atresia. Absence of the gallbladder also can occur in association with polysplenia and rare multiple anomaly syndromes. The ability to visualize the fetal gallbladder routinely increases with gestational age.

PANCREAS

Pancreatic cysts are uncommon, but when present, may appear as midline cystic masses in the fetal abdomen.

BOX 58-2 **SONOGRAPHIC CRITERIA FOR CHOLEDOCHAL CYST**

- Close proximity of the cyst to the neck of the gallbladder
- An ovoid right upper quadrant cyst with an entering bile duct
- A cyst and gallbladder that enlarge as gestation progresses
- Absence of peristaltic activity in the cyst

From Schwartz and others: Choledochal cyst in a second trimester fetus, *J Diagn Med Sonogr* 1:10, 1989.

BOX 58-3 **CAUSES OF NONVISUALIZATION OF THE STOMACH**

- Esophageal atresia or tracheoesophageal fistula
- Diaphragmatic hernia
- Facial cleft
- Central nervous system disorder
- Other swallowing disorders
- Oligohydramnios from other causes

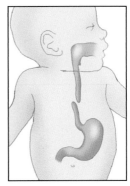

Figure 58-11 Esophageal atresia is a congenital blockage of the esophagus. The primary sonographic findings are polyhydramnios and an absence of the stomach bubble.

BOX 58-4 **ATRESIAS**

- Develop when a portion of the bowel grows and infarcts
- Occurs anywhere in the gastrointestinal tract
- Polyhydramnios evident on ultrasound

SPLEEN

Evaluation of the fetal spleen for exclusion of splenic anomalies is possible. Asplenia (absence of the spleen) may be amenable to antenatal identification, and in association with congenital heart disease the polysplenia-asplenia syndrome should be considered.

Congenital splenic cysts are rare but have been reported in utero. Enlargement of the spleen (splenomegaly) may be seen on the ultrasound examination. The spleen, like the liver, may enlarge in fetuses with Rh-immune disease. Nomograms are available to detect hepatomegaly and splenomegaly.

ABNORMALITIES OF THE GASTROINTESTINAL TRACT

The majority of gastrointestinal malformations are correctable after birth; consequently, recognition of a gastrointestinal anomaly before delivery may prevent the complications of dehydration, bowel necrosis, and respiratory difficulties that occur when these lesions are unsuspected before delivery (Box 58-3). The fetal bowel can be altered by a number of pathologic processes. A bowel obstruction results in proximal bowel dilation, which is characteristically recognized as one or more tubular structures within the fetal abdomen. Dilated bowel loops are generally sonolucent in texture but may be normal or increased in echogenicity. The most reliable criterion for diagnosing a dilated bowel is the bowel diameter, rather than the sonographic appearance. One should be careful not to mistake a dilated ureter for a dilated loop of the bowel. Most cases of bowel dilation do not become evident on sonography until after 20 weeks of gestation. Polyhydramnios commonly

accompanies obstruction of the gastrointestinal tract, and this rarely develops before 20 weeks of gestation as a result of a gastrointestinal cause.

ESOPHAGUS, STOMACH, AND DUODENUM

The normal upper esophagus may be seen after amniotic fluid is swallowed. This fluid passes from the esophagus into the fetal stomach. Obstruction of the normal swallowing sequence may occur because of an atretic or obstructive process. A membrane covering the lumen and intestinal loops enlarges above the obstruction; and bowel loops below the atresia are narrowed (stenotic). This enlargement of the bowel proximal to the obstruction is readily apparent on ultrasound. Blockage results in the back-up of amniotic fluid and hydramnios.

Esophageal atresia is a congenital blockage of the esophagus resulting from the faulty separation of the foregut into its respiratory and digestive components (Figure 58-11, Box 58-4). The most common form occurs in conjunction with a fistula, communicating between the trachea and esophagus (tracheoesophageal fistula), that allows the passage of amniotic fluid into the stomach. Gastric secretions may contribute to stomach fluid. In some instances, however, a fistula is not present and fluid will not reach the stomach; hence the stomach will not be visualized by ultrasound. The combination of polyhydramnios and an absent stomach over repeated studies may be suggestive of esophageal atresia. Esophageal atresia will not be diagnosed in the majority of cases because of a tracheoesophageal fistula.

Esophageal atresia occurs in 1 in 2500 live births. The sonographer may observe the absent stomach and hydramnios (Figure 58-12). However, in more than half of the cases, the

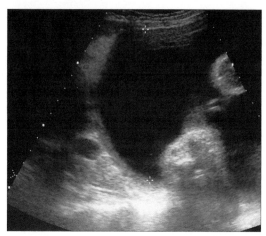

Figure 58-12 Longitudinal scan of a patient who had polyhydramnios. This quadrant of fluid measured more than 10 cm, which alone qualifies for an abnormal collection of fluid. The fetus did not show a stomach bubble and was diagnosed with esophageal atresia.

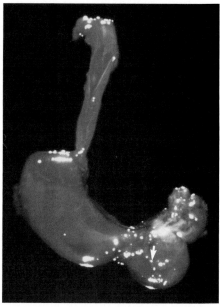

Figure 58-13 Gross specimen showing duodenal atresia from a neonate with trisomy 21 (Down syndrome). Note the narrowing at the duodenum *(arrow)*.

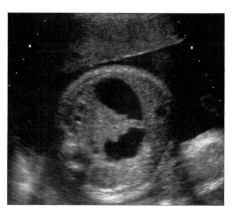

Figure 58-14 Transverse image of the fetal abdomen showing two large echo-free structures that communicated on real-time imaging. The fetus had duodenal atresia.

stomach is present because a fistula is usually present that leads to fluid filling the stomach. Hydramnios may exist from impaired reabsorption of swallowed fluid and may be associated with esophageal atresia, but it usually does not develop until the third trimester. The upper neck sign has been observed as an additional finding in a patient with esophageal atresia. A fluid-filled, blind-ending esophagus during fetal swallowing has been noted in a 22-week fetus.

Coexisting anomalies are common in 50% to 70% of fetuses with esophageal atresia. The most commonly observed anomaly is anorectal atresia (others include vertebral defects, heart defects, and renal and limb anomalies [**VACTERL**]). Growth restriction is present in 40% of the cases. Chromosomal trisomies (18 and 21) are reported in association. Survival depends on the presence of associated congenital anomalies.

Duodenal atresia is a blockage of the duodenal lumen by a membrane that prohibits the passage of swallowed amniotic fluid (Figure 58-13). Atresia or narrowing of the bowel segment below the obstruction occurs. In duodenal atresia, the amniotic fluid fails to move beyond the obstruction, and consequently, amniotic fluid backs up in the duodenum and stomach.

Sonographic Findings. Two echo-free structures (stomach and duodenum) are found in the upper fetal abdomen and they communicate. This sonographic appearance is termed the double bubble sign (Figure 58-14, Box 58-5). Hydramnios is almost always seen with duodenal atresias later in pregnancy. Most cases of duodenal atresia are found distal to the ampulla and often coexist with annular pancreas.

About 30% of fetuses with duodenal atresia have trisomy 21 (Down syndrome) (Figure 58-15). Cardiovascular anomalies are frequent, and therefore fetal echocardiography is invaluable in excluding cardiac lesions. Anomalies occur in approximately 50% of infants with duodenal atresia. Genitourinary anomalies (horseshoe kidney, ectopic kidneys) may coexist with this condition. Other gastrointestinal abnormali-

---

BOX 58-5   CAUSES OF DOUBLE BUBBLE

- Duodenal atresia
- Duodenal stenosis
- Annular pancreas
- Ladd's bands
- Proximal jejunal atresia
- Malrotation
- Diaphragmatic hernia

ties, such as imperforate anus and atresia of the small bowel, may be present. Esophageal atresia may also be found.

Symmetric growth restriction commonly occurs in fetuses with duodenal atresia. Amniotic fluid alpha-fetoprotein values are commonly elevated in fetuses with duodenal atresia caused by faulty swallowing. Infants with duodenal atresia require immediate surgery after birth to connect the stomach to the jejunum, thus bypassing the obstruction.

BOWEL

Intestinal Obstructions. Atresia or stenosis of the jejunum or ileum, or both, and small bowel atresia are slightly more common than duodenal atresia; it occurs in 1 in 3000 to 5000 live births and is thought to be secondary to a vascular accident, sporadic, or secondary to volvulus or gastroschisis. Various fetal malformations may also occur with maternal drug usage (Table 58-1). The entire length of the bowel is subject to obstruction. Blockage of the jejunum and ileal bowel segments (**jejunoileal atresia** or stenosis) appears as multiple cystic structures (more than two) proximal to the site of atresia within the fetal abdomen. Because these structures are high in

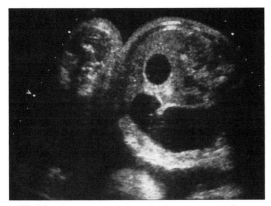

Figure 58-15 This 24-week fetus had trisomy 21. The transverse abdomen showed a very dilated stomach with communication into a smaller sac. Thirty percent of trisomy 21 pregnancies will also have duodenal atresia.

the abdomen, hydramnios may be present. The general rule is the more distal the obstruction, the less severe the hydramnios, and the later it will develop. The causes of fetal small-bowel obstruction include malrotation, atresias, volvulus, peritoneal bands, and cystic fibrosis. The dilated bowel loops may be isolated or may be associated with other anomalies, ascites, or meconium peritonitis.

Sonographic Findings. Sonographically, intestinal obstructions appear as cystic bowel loops that are discontinuous with the stomach (Figure 58-16). It is important to remember that bowel loops may be identified in the third trimester of pregnancy. One study reported that the normal fetal colon progressively increased in diameter after 23 weeks of gestation, although it never exceeded 18 mm in a preterm fetus.[1] Fetal intestinal obstruction should be suspected when clear cystic structures are found in the pelvis. In some instances, echoes within the bowel may be identified in intestinal obstructions but may also represent normal meconium patterns (see Figure 58-16). Vascular restriction may lead to obstruction secondary to a gastroschisis (Figure 58-17).

Meconium ileus. Meconium ileus is a small-bowel disorder marked by the presence of thick meconium in the distal ileum. Meconium ileus is the earliest manifestation of cystic fibrosis occurring in 10% to 15% of patients and is the third most common form of neonatal bowel obstruction after atresia and malrotation. Most cases of meconium ileus occur in newborns with cystic fibrosis. Infants with **cystic fibrosis** have multiple medical problems, including pancreatic disease and respiratory problems resulting from long-standing lung disease. Cystic fibrosis is an autosomal-recessive condition.

Meconium begins to accumulate in the fetal bowel in the second trimester, at which time it can be seen sonographically as tiny echogenic reflections within the peristaltic small bowel (Figure 58-18). Because the colon does not exhibit peristalsis in utero, the meconium remains suspended at the rectum. The anal sphincter prevents the passage of meconium (meconium plug) into the amniotic fluid unless the fetus is stressed or traumatized.

TABLE 58-1	POTENTIAL FETAL MALFORMATIONS ASSOCIATED WITH MATERNAL DRUG OR CHEMICAL USE	
Drug	Fetal Malformations	
Acetaminophen overdose	Polyhydramnios	
Clomiphene	NTDs, microcephaly, syndactyly, clubfoot, polydactyly, esophageal atresia	
Coumadin	NTDs, cardiac defects, scoliosis, skeletal deformities, nasal hypoplasia, stippled epiphyses, chondrodysplasia punctata, short phalanges, toe defects, incomplete rotation of gut, IUGR, bleeding	
Disulfiram	Vertebral fusion, clubfoot, radial aplasia, phocomelia, tracheoesophageal fistula	
Fluorouracil of lungs	Radial aplasia, absent thumbs, aplasia of esophagus and duodenum, hypoplasia	
Oral contraceptives	NTDs, cardiac defects, vertebral defects, limb reduction, IUGR, tracheoesophageal malformation	
Phenothiazines	Microcephaly, syndactyly, clubfoot, omphalocele	
Phenylephrine	Eye and ear abnormalities, syndactyly, clubfoot, hip dislocation, umbilical hernia	

From Nyberg DA, Mahony BS, Pretorius DH: *Diagnostic ultrasound of fetal anomalies: text and atlas,* St Louis, 1990, Mosby.
IUGR, Intrauterine growth restriction; *NTDs,* neural tube defects.

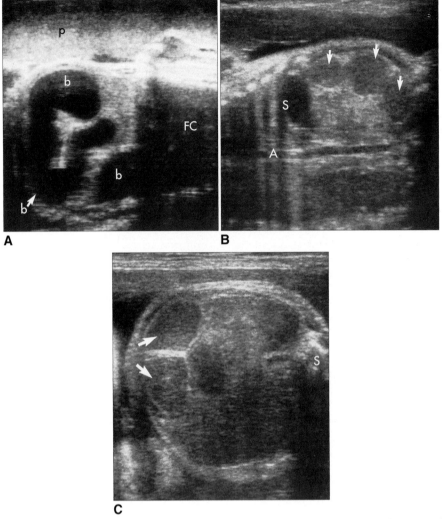

Figure 58-16 **A,** Bowel obstruction secondary to gastroschisis. Note the tubular shape of the cystic bowel loops *(b)*. *FC,* Fetal chest; *p,* placenta. **B,** Bowel obstruction in a fetus with cystic fibrosis at 36 weeks of gestation. Note that the bowel loops in this case are filled with meconium *(arrows)* rather than cystic, as in **A.** *A,* Aorta; *S,* stomach. **C,** In the fetus shown in **B,** echo-filled bowel loops are viewed in a transverse direction *(arrows)*. *S,* Spine.

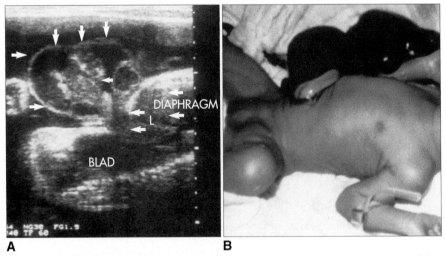

Figure 58-17 **A,** Sagittal scan demonstrating anterior abdominal wall defect with protrusion of the entire small bowel in a fetus with a gastroschisis *(arrows)*. Note the obstructed (cystic) components of small bowel. *L,* Liver. **B,** Gastroschisis defect in same patient after birth. Note the normal cord insertion.

Sonographic Findings. With meconium ileus, the ileum dilates because of impacted meconium (which appears echogenic) (Figure 58-19). Increased production of mucus by the gastrointestinal organs and electrolyte imbalance explains the overproduction of meconium (characteristic of cystic fibrosis). It is important to realize that the normal small bowel may appear echogenic during the second trimester of pregnancy. Other fetal conditions have been associated with echogenic small bowel (cytomegalovirus and trisomy 21). Meconium peritonitis may occur secondary to perforation of an obstructed bowel. An inflammatory response occurs because of leakage of the bowel contents, which may cause fibrosis of

tissue and calcifications. A pseudocyst may develop because of chronic meconium peritonitis (Box 58-6).

Other Small Bowel Obstructions. Rarer small-bowel obstructions, chloridorrhea (life-threatening diarrhea in the newborn) and megacystis-microcolon intestinal hypoperistalsis syndrome (absence of peristalsis), may be observed during pregnancy. In the latter, bladder dilation and hydronephrosis are characteristic findings in predominantly female fetuses. Amniotic fluid volume is typically normal to increased. Obstruction may also be present when gastroschisis is present (see Figure 58-17). Obstructions of the large intestine diagnosed prenatally include anorectal atresia and Hirschsprung's disease.

Anorectal atresia. Anorectal atresia presents as a complex disorder of the bowel and genitourinary tract. Imperforate anus

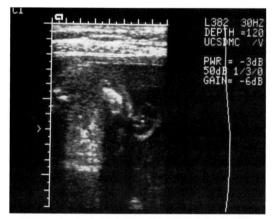

Figure 58-18 Meconium accumulates in the fetal bowel in the second trimester and is seen sonographically as echogenic reflections (notice shadowing) within the peristaltic small bowel.

> **BOX 58-6 PITFALLS IN THE DIAGNOSIS OF MECONIUM ILEUS**
>
> - Significant dilation of the meconium-filled ileum in meconium ileus can simulate colon in morphology and location, especially in the presence of the expected microcolon.
> - More proximal small bowel can retain the expected features of active peristalsis and fluid-filled contents, and the discrepancy in caliber between proximal and distal small bowel should not distract the sonologist from the diagnosis of small-bowel obstruction or meconium ileus.

From Goldstein RB, Filly RA, Callen PW: Sonographic diagnosis of meconium ileus in utero, *J Ultrasound Med* 6:663, 1987.

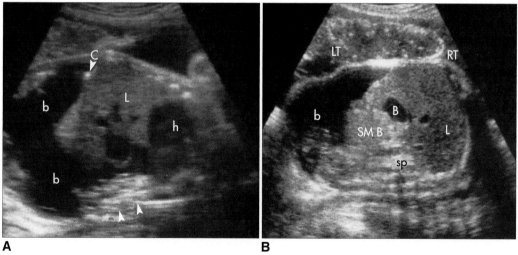

Figure 58-19 A, Meconium peritonitis secondary to bowel obstruction is shown with an irregular appearance of the bowel *(b)* in the lower pelvis extending upward toward the chest in a 30-week fetus. Calcifications *(C)* are observed in several locations. Clumping of bowel was observed *(arrows)*. Meconium peritonitis with bowel perforation was suspected. There was a moderate increase in the amniotic fluid volume by 33 weeks of gestation. *h*, Heart; *L*, liver. **B,** In the same fetus, transverse view showing bowel dilation *(b)* in a spine-down position. Note the normal-appearing small bowel *(SM B)*. *L*, Liver; *LT*, left side of abdomen; *RT*, right side of abdomen; *sp*, spine. At birth the neonate was diagnosed with meconium ileus and peritonitis necessitating an ileostomy. At 2 months of age, the infant was discharged on normal formula feedings. Cystic fibrosis was suspected.

(a finding in anorectal atresia) is a disorder that occurs when a membrane covers the anus prohibiting the expulsion of meconium. Anorectal atresia may present as part of the VACTERL association or in caudal regression. The prognosis is poor with anorectal atresia because of associated anomalies. Incontinence of both bowel and bladder is common in the infant.

Sonographic Findings. Anorectal atresia may be diagnosed sonographically by observing dilated colon and calcified meconium. Amniotic fluid is typically normal or may be decreased when there are associated renal problems.

Hirschsprung's disease. Hirschsprung's disease (megacolon) is a congenital disorder in which there is abnormal innervation of the large intestine.

Sonographic Findings. This condition is difficult to diagnose prenatally but may be suspected when dilated bowel loops are observed.

Meconium peritonitis. Meconium peritonitis is a condition that may arise when the fetus has a sterile chemical peritonitis secondary to in utero bowel perforation. Hydramnios is present in 65% of the fetuses with meconium peritonitis. A complication may result in the formation of a meconium pseudocyst as the inflammatory reaction seals the perforation.

Sonographic Findings. On ultrasound examination, calcifications are seen on the peritoneal surfaces or in the scrotum via the processus vaginalis. The ascitic fluid may also be echogenic. It is unusual to see calcification in the meconium ileus in a fetus with cystic fibrosis.

Hyperechoic bowel. Hyperechoic bowel is a subjective impression of an unusually echogenic bowel, typically seen during the second trimester. The cause of hyperechoic bowel may be due to decreased water content, alterations of meconium, or both. The decreased water content may be secondary to hypoperistalsis, given that fluid is normally resorbed by the small bowel.

Sonographic Findings. The significance of hyperechoic bowel varies with its location in the small bowel or colon, menstrual age, and degree of echogenicity (Box 58-7). The degree

of hyperechogenicity may be compared with the iliac wing of the fetus. There are three gradations of determining the degree of hyperechogenicity of the bowel:

- Grade 1: mildly echogenic and typically diffuse
- Grade 2: moderately echogenic and typically focal
- Grade 3: very echogenic, similar to that of bone structures

Ascites. True ascites in the fetal abdomen is always abnormal. In the fetus, the ascitic fluid collects between the two leaves of unfused omentum, resulting in a cystlike appearance in the abdomen (Figure 58-20). The prognosis is poor in nonimmune hydrops. Other conditions that may cause ascites to develop include bowel perforation or urinary ascites secondary to bladder rupture.

Sonographic Findings. Ascites usually outlines the falciform ligament and umbilical vein. When ascites is associated

---

BOX 58-7   CAUSES OF ECHOGENIC AREAS IN THE FETAL ABDOMEN

CALCIFICATION
Peritoneal calcification: Meconium peritonitis, hydrometrocolpos
Intraluminal meconium calcification: Anorectal atresia, small bowel atresia; rarely isolated without bowel obstruction
Parenchymal: Liver, splenic, adrenal, ovarian cyst
Cholelithiasis: gallbladder

NONCALCIFIED
Echogenic meconium
Intraabdominal extrathoracic pulmonary sequestration
Tumors
Adrenal hemorrhage

From Nyberg DA, Neilsen IR: Abdomen and gastrointestinal tract. In Nyberg DA, McGahan JP, Pretorius DH and others, editors: *Diagnostic imaging of fetal anomalies*, Philadelphia, 2003, Lippincott, Williams & Wilkins.

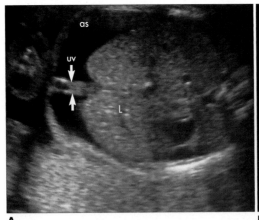
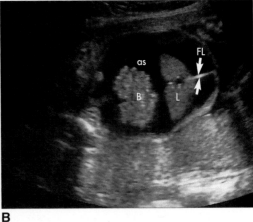

Figure 58-20   A, Fetal ascites *(as)* surrounds the umbilical vein *(uv)*. *L,* liver. **B,** Ascites *(as)* completely surrounds the liver *(L)* and falciform ligament *(FL)*. *B,* Bowel.

<table>
<tr><td>

BOX 58-8 ABDOMINAL CYSTIC MASS

It is important for the sonographic team to determine:

1. The precise location of the mass
2. The size of the mass
3. Resultant compression of other organ systems (hydronephrosis, hydroureter, fetal hydrops)

</td></tr>
</table>

with hydrops fetalis, pleural effusions, and pericardial effusion, integumentary edema will often be observed.

MISCELLANEOUS CYSTIC MASSES OF THE ABDOMEN

Cystic masses of the lower fetal abdomen may be observed prenatally (Box 58-8). As demonstrated previously, cystic dilations of many organ systems may occur during the fetal period.

When a cystic mass is discovered, attempts should be made to determine the characteristics of the mass. A description of the mass should include the components of the structure, such as (1) an echo-free versus an echo-filled mass, (2) presence or absence of septations, and (3) coexisting fetal anomalies. The sonographer should systematically investigate all abdominal organ systems to determine the anatomic origin of the mass. The hepatic system (liver, gallbladder, spleen, and pancreatic areas) should be evaluated along with the gastrointestinal system (esophagus, stomach, and intestines) and genitourinary system (kidneys, ureters, and bladder).

Occasionally, cysts arise from the urachus (dilation of remnant allantoic stalk between umbilicus and bladder), fetal ovary, or omentum. Ovarian and omental cysts are generally isolated and well circumscribed. Determination of the fetal gender is beneficial when an ovarian mass is suspected. If abdominal masses are large, they may occupy the entire lower fetal pelvis, making a specific intrauterine diagnosis impossible.

REFERENCE

1. Nyberg DA, Mahony BS, Pretorius DH, editors: *Diagnostic ultrasound of fetal anomalies: text and atlas*, St Louis, 1990, Mosby.

SELECTED BIBLIOGRAPHY

Barnewolt CE: Congenital abnormalities of the gastrointestinal tract, *Semin Roentgenol* 2004 39(2):263-281.

Bethune M, Bell R: Evaluation of the measurement of the fetal fat layer, interventricular septum, and abdominal circumference percentile in the prediction of macrosomia in pregnancies affected by gestational diabetes, *Ultrasound Obstet Gynecol* 22(6):586-590, 2003.

Boito SM, Laudy JA, Stuijk PC and others: Three-dimensional US assessment of hepatic volume, head circumference, and abdominal circumference in healthy and growth-restricted fetuses, *Radiology* 223(3):661-665, 2002.

Bronshtein M, Gover A, Zimmer EZ: Sonographic definition of the fetal situs, *Obstet Gynecol* 99(6):1129-1130, 2002.

Bustamante S, Koldovsky O: Synopsis of development of the main morphological structures of the human gastrointestinal tract. In Lebenthal E, editor: *Textbook of gastroenterology and nutrition in infancy*, New York, 1981, Raven Press.

Callen DW, editor: *Ultrasonography in obstetrics and gynecology*, ed 4, Philadelphia, 2001, WB Saunders.

Centini G, Rosignoli L, Kenanidis A and others: Prenatal diagnosis of esophageal atresia with the pouch sign, *Ultrasound Obstet Gynecol* 21(5):494-497, 2003.

Chinn DH, Filly RA, Callen PW: Ultrasonic evaluation of fetal umbilical and hepatic vascular anatomy, *Rad* 144:153, 1982.

Grand RI, Watkins JB, Torti FM: Development of the human gastrointestinal tract, *Gastroenterology* 70:790, 1976.

Gul A, Tekoglu G, Aslan H and others: Prenatal sonographic features of esophageal and ileal duplications at 18 weeks of gestation, *Prenat Diagn* 15:24(12):969-971, 2004.

Haratz-Rubinstein N, Sherer DM: Prenatal sonographic findings of congenital duplication of the cecum, *Obstet Gynecol* 101(5 Pt 2):1085-1087, 2003.

Ji EK, Lee EK, Kwon TH: Isolated echogenic foci in the left upper quadrant of the fetal abdomen: are they significant? *J Ultrasound Med* 23(4):483-488, 2004.

Kalache KD and others: The upper neck pouch sign: a prenatal sonographic marker for esophageal atresia, *Ultrasound Obstet Gynecol* 11:138, 1998.

Kamata S, Nose K, Sawai T and others: Fetal mesenchymal hamartoma of the liver: report of a case, *J Pediatr Surg* 38(4):639-641, 2003.

McEwing R, Hayward C, Furness M: Foetal cystic abdominal masses, *Australas Radiol* 47(2):101-110, 2003.

Moore KL, editor: *The developing human: clinically oriented embryology*, ed 4, Philadelphia, 1988, WB Saunders.

Parulekar SG: Sonography of the normal fetal bowel, *J Ultrasound Med* 10:211, 1991.

Pretorius DH and others: Tracheoesophageal fistula in utero (twenty-two cases), *J Ultrasound Med* 6:509, 1987.

Roberts AB, Mitchell JM, Pattison NS: Fetal liver length in normal and isoimmunized pregnancies, *Am J Obstet Gynecol* 161:42, 1989.

Sanders RC, editor: *Clinical sonography: a practical guide*, ed 3, Boston, 1998, Little, Brown.

Schmidt W and others: Sonographic measurements of the fetal spleen, *J Ultrasound Med* 4:667, 1985.

Schwartz H and others: Choledochal cyst in a second trimester fetus, *J Diagn Med Sonogr* 1:10, 1989.

Yoshizato T, Satoh S, Taguchi T and others: Intermittent "double bubble" sign in a case of congenital pyloric atresia, *Fetal Diagn Ther* 17(6):334-338, 2002.

CHAPTER 59

The Fetal Urogenital System

Sandra L. Hagen-Ansert

KEY TERMS

bicornuate uterus – duplication of the uterus (two horns and one vagina)

caliectasis – rounded calyces with renal pelvis dilation measuring greater than 10 mm in the anteroposterior direction

crossed renal ectopia – occurs when the kidney is located on the opposite side of its ureteral orifice

cryptorchidism – failure of the testes to descend into the scrotum

fetal hydronephrosis – dilated renal pelvis

hermaphroditism – condition in which both ovarian and testicular tissues are present

horseshoe kidney – forms when the inferior poles of the kidney fuse while they are in the pelvis

hydrometrocolpos – collection of fluid in the vagina and uterus

hydroureters – dilated ureters

hypospadias – abnormal congenital opening of the male urethra on the undersurface of the penis

infantile polycystic kidney disease (IPKD) – autosomal recessive disease that affects the fetal kidneys and liver; the kidneys are enlarged and echogenic on ultrasound

megacystis – the level of the urethra where the urinary tract may become obstructed

megaureter – dilation of the lower end of the ureter; the common presentation of ureterovesical junction obstruction

multicystic dysplastic kidney disease – multiple cysts replace normal renal tissue throughout the kidney; usually causes renal obstruction

ovarian cyst – may be found in the fetus; results from maternal hormone stimulation and is usually benign

pelvic kidney – occurs when the kidney does not migrate upward into the retroperitoneal space

posterior urethral valve – occurs only in male fetuses; is manifested by the presence of a valve in the posterior urethra

Potter's syndrome – characterized by renal agenesis, oligohydramnios, pulmonary hypoplasia, abnormal facies, and malformed hands and feet

prune belly syndrome – dilation of the fetal abdomen secondary to severe bilateral hydronephrosis and fetal ascites; fetus also has oligohydramnios and pulmonary hypoplasia

pyelectasis – dilated renal pelvis measuring 5 to 9 mm in the anteroposterior direction

renal agenesis – renal system fails to develop

unicornuate uterus – anomaly of the uterus in which only one horn and tube develop

urachal cyst – a small part of the lumen of the allantois that persists while the urachus forms

ureteropelvic junction – junction of the ureter entering the renal pelvis; most common site of obstruction

ureterovesical junction – junction where the ureter enters the bladder

urethral atresia – this condition causes a massively distended bladder (prune belly)

uterus didelphys – double uterus and double vagina

Prenatal ultrasound is capable of diagnosing many anomalies of the genitourinary system. In the presence of oligohydramnios, the sonographer should carefully search the renal areas and bladder to determine if an obstruction is present that may lead to the diminished production of amniotic fluid. On the other hand, abnormalities of the genitourinary system may be discovered incidentally during the complete obstetric ultrasound evaluation. If there is a maternal history of drug usage, there is an increased risk of urogenital fetal malformations as listed in Table 59-1. A complete ultrasound examination includes evaluation of both kidneys, documentation of the urinary bladder, and assessment of amniotic fluid.

EMBRYOLOGY OF THE UROGENITAL SYSTEM

Embryologically and functionally the urogenital system can be divided into two parts: the urinary system and the genital system. Both systems develop from the intermediate mesoderm, and the excretory ducts of both systems initially enter a common cavity called the cloaca.

As development proceeds, the overlapping of the two systems is particularly obvious in the male. The primitive excretory duct of the mesonephric kidney (mesonephric duct) originally serves as a urinary duct. Later the mesonephric duct is transformed into the main genital duct, the ductus deferens (vas deferens).

The ureter develops from a small ureteric bud and develops later in the adult male. The urinary and genital organs discharge their secretions through a common urogenital canal in the penis known as the *spongy urethra*.

While the embryo bends and folds in the horizontal plane during the 4th week, the intermediate mesoderm forms a longitudinal mass on both sides of the aorta called the *urogenital ridge*. Both the urinary and genital systems develop from the mesoderm in these ridges. The part of the urogenital ridge that gives rise to the urinary system is known as the nephrogenic cord or nephrogenic ridge. The part that gives rise to the genital system is known as the gonadal ridge or *genital ridge*. The urinary system develops first.

THE URINARY SYSTEM

DEVELOPMENT OF THE KIDNEYS

There are three sets of excretory organs that develop in the embryo: the pronephros, mesonephros, and metanephros. Only the third set remains as the permanent kidneys (Figure 59-1). The first pair of "kidneys," *pronephros*, are rudimentary and nonfunctional. The second pair of "kidneys," *mesonephroi*, function for a short time during the early fetal period and degenerate after they are replaced by the metanephros or permanent kidneys.

The permanent kidneys (metanephros) begin to develop early in the 5th week while the mesonephroi are still

---

TABLE 59-1	**POTENTIAL UROGENITAL FETAL MALFORMATIONS ASSOCIATED WITH MATERNAL DRUG OR CHEMICAL USE**
Drug	Fetal Malformations
Amitriptyline	Micrognathia, limb reduction, swelling of hands and feet, urinary retention
Amobarbital	NTDs, cardiac defects, severe limb deformities, congenital hip dislocation, polydactyly, clubfoot, cleft palate, ambiguous genitalia, soft tissue, deformity of neck
Caffeine	Musculoskeletal defects, hydronephrosis
Cocaine	Spontaneous abortion, placental abruption, prematurity, IUGR, possible cardiac defects, skull defects, genitourinary anomalies
Imipramine	NTDs, cleft palate, renal cysts, diaphragmatic hernia
Sulfonamide	Limb hypoplasia, foot defects, urethral obstruction

Modified from Nyberg DA, Mahony BS, Pretorius DH: *Diagnostic ultrasound of fetal anomalies: text and atlas*, St Louis, 1990, Mosby.
NTDs, Neural tube defects.

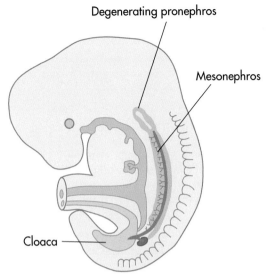

Figure 59-1 Five-week embryo showing three sets of kidneys that developed in the embryo. The pronephros is rudimentary and nonfunctional. The mesonephros functions for 2 weeks and then degenerates. The metanephros develops into the permanent kidney.

developing (Figure 59-2). Urine formation begins toward the end of the first trimester, around the 11th to 12th week and continues actively throughout fetal life. Urine is excreted into the amniotic cavity and forms a major part of the amniotic fluid. The kidneys do not need to function in utero because the placenta eliminates waste from the fetal blood. The kidneys must be able to assume their waste excretion role after birth, however.

The permanent kidneys develop from two different sources: (1) the metanephric diverticulum or ureteric bud and (2) the metanephric mesoderm (Figure 59-3). The ureteric bud gives rise to the ureter, renal pelvis, calyces, and collecting tubules. The collecting tubule is also derived from the ureteric bud. The major and minor calyces are developed from these collecting tubules.

The ends of the tubules form metanephric vesicles. The ends of these tubules are invaginated by an ingrowth of the fine blood vessels, the glomerulus, to form a double-layered cup called the glomerular capsule or Bowman's capsule. The renal corpuscle (glomerulus and capsule) and its associated tubules form a nephron. Each distal convoluted tubule contacts an arched collecting tubule, and then the tubules become confluent, forming a uriniferous tubule. Each uriniferous tubule consists of two parts: a nephron and a collecting tubule.

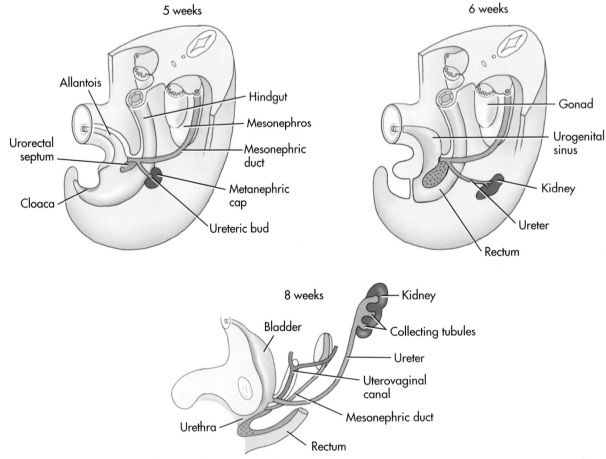

Figure 59-2 Early embryological development of the urinary system.

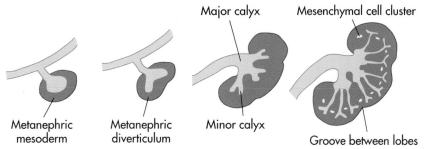

Figure 59-3   Developing kidney in weeks 5 through 8.

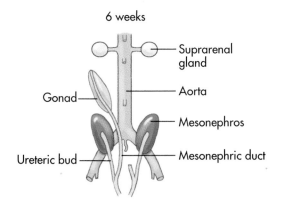

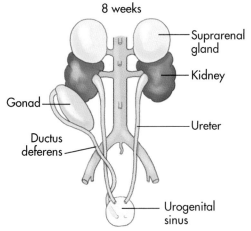

Figure 59-4   The kidneys begin in the pelvis with gradual migration into the abdomen.

The kidneys initially lie very close together in the pelvis. Gradually they migrate into the abdomen and become separated from one another (Figure 59-4). They normally complete this migration by the 9th week of gestation. In some cases, one of the kidneys may remain in the pelvic cavity while the other migrates into the posterior flank of the abdomen. With sonography, the identification of a **pelvic kidney** may be seen with adequate bladder dilation and may appear in females as a pelvic mass.

The arterial vascular supply to the kidneys comes from the arteries that arise from the aorta. Usually these vessels disap-

pear when the kidneys ascend, but some of them may persist, which accounts for the variations that can be found in the renal arteries. At least 25% of adult kidneys have two to four renal arteries.

The fetal kidneys are subdivided into lobes that may be separated by grooves. This lobulation usually diminishes by the end of the fetal period, but in some cases the lobes may still be noticeable by the end of the neonatal period. In adolescent and adult patients, persistence of the fetal lobulation and groove may be seen on ultrasound as an echogenic triangular notch along the anterior wall of the right kidney.

CONGENITAL MALFORMATIONS OF THE KIDNEYS

Complete absence of the kidneys is known as **renal agenesis.** This condition occurs when the ureteric buds fail to develop or when they degenerate before they can induce the metanephric mesoderm to form nephrons. Because the uriniferous tubules develop from two different sources, the failure of the tubules to join results in congenital polycystic disease of the kidneys.

Division of the ureteric bud at an early stage results in a double or divided kidney. The ureteral bud closest to the sinus drains the lower renal pole and enters the bladder at the trigone. The ureter drains the upper pole of the kidney as it enters the bladder in a more medial and caudal position (ectopic ureter). The lower pole is more prone to reflux and the upper pole more prone to obstruction. The hydronephrotic, nonfunctioning upper pole may cause downward displacement of the lower pole calyces.

A **horseshoe kidney** forms when the inferior poles of the kidney fuse while they are in the pelvis. This fusion may occur in 1 to 4 in 1000 births and is two to three times more common in males (Figure 59-5).

Another variation from the horseshoe kidney may result in **crossed renal ectopia** and abnormal renal position. In this case, the kidney is located on the opposite side of its ureteral orifice. Crossed renal ectopia usually affects the left kidney going toward the right and is inferior to the normal kidney. This is more common in males.

DEVELOPMENT OF THE URINARY BLADDER

The fetal urinary bladder is derived from the hindgut derivative known as the urogenital sinus (see Figure 59-2). The

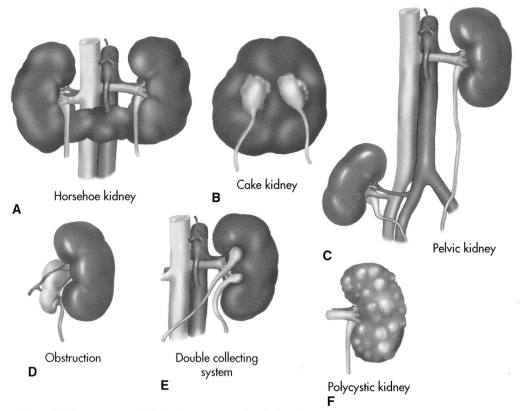

Figure 59-5 Variations of the kidney. **A,** Horseshoe kidney shown as two kidneys connected by an isthmus anterior to the aorta and inferior vena cava. **B,** "Cake" kidney that has failed to divide with a double collecting system. **C,** Pelvic kidney with one kidney in the normal retroperitoneal position. **D,** Extrarenal pelvis. **E,** Double collecting system. **F,** Polycystic kidney.

caudal ends of the mesonephric ducts open into the cloaca, and parts of them are gradually absorbed into the wall of the urinary bladder. This development causes the ureters (derived from the ureteric buds) and the mesonephric ducts to enter the bladder separately.

Although the kidneys migrate upward, the orifices of the ureters move cranially, and the primordia of the ejaculatory ducts (derived from the mesonephric ducts) move toward one another and enter the prostatic part of the urethra.

Exstrophy of the Bladder. Exstrophy of the bladder occurs primarily in males and the incidence is 1 in 50,000 births. It is characterized by the protrusion of the posterior wall of the urinary bladder, which contains the trigone of the bladder and the ureteric orifices. Exstrophy of the bladder is caused by the defective closure of the inferior part of the anterior abdominal wall during the 4th week of gestation. As a result of this defect, no muscle or connective tissue forms in the anterior abdominal wall to cover the urinary bladder, and therefore the bladder is formed external to the abdominal wall.

DEVELOPMENT OF THE URETHRA
The epithelium of the female urethra and most of the epithelium of the male urethra is derived from the endoderm of the urogenital sinus.

DEVELOPMENT OF THE PROSTATE GLAND
The prostate gland is an auxiliary genital gland that is derived from evaginations of the epithelium of the prostatic portion of the urethra that penetrates the surrounding mesenchyme. The urethral and paraurethral glands in the female are comparable with the prostate gland.

THE URACHUS
Early in development, the urinary bladder is continuous with the allantois. The allantois regresses to become a fibrous cord known as the urachus. This cord, or ligament, extends from the apex of the bladder to the umbilicus. If the lumen of the allantois persists while the urachus forms, a urachal fistula develops, which causes urine to drain from the bladder to the umbilicus. If only a small part of the lumen of the allantois persists, it is called a **urachal cyst**. If a larger portion of the lumen persists, it may cause a urachal sinus to develop that may open at the umbilicus or into the urinary bladder.

SONOGRAPHIC EVALUATION OF THE URINARY TRACT

The sonographer should be familiar with several important concepts when evaluating the fetal urinary tract. With endovaginal sonography, the fetal kidneys have been documented as early as 9 weeks' gestation. By 12 weeks' gestation, at least 86% of the fetal kidneys may be imaged. The fetal kidneys and bladder may be seen by 13 weeks of gestation. At this time period, the kidneys appear as bilateral hyperechoic structures in the paravertebral regions. The renal pelves can be seen as sonolucent areas within the central kidney. The bladder is imaged as a rounded echo-free area located centrally in the pelvis. By 25 weeks it is possible to distinguish the renal cortex from the medulla, outline the renal capsule clearly, and see a central echogenic area in the renal sinus region (Box 59-1).

BOX 59-1

SONOGRAPHIC EVALUATION OF THE URINARY TRACT

- Bladder: assess presence and size
- Kidneys: assess presence, number, position, appearance (texture)
- Collecting system: assess if normal or dilated; if dilated, look for level and cause of obstruction, whether it is unilateral or bilateral
- Fetal gender

The kidneys should be evaluated by assessing their anatomy, texture, and size. Normal anatomic structures of the kidney include the relatively homogeneous renal cortex and parenchyma, echogenic pyramids and calyces, and anechoic renal pelvis (Figure 59-6). Between 18 and 20 weeks of gestation, the kidneys are slightly hyperechoic with regard to surrounding tissues (i.e., bowel and paravertebral tissues). On coronal images, the kidneys are bordered medially by the psoas muscles and superiorly by the adrenal glands. The renal pyramids are hypoechoic structures within the renal parenchyma. The renal pelves are seen as echo-free areas medially.

Notable deviations of anatomy should alert the sonographer to investigate the urinary tract more extensively. It is important to remember that a small amount of urine may be seen in the renal pelvis in the normal fetus. On transverse images, the kidneys are circular structures and the renal pelves may be measured in their anterior-posterior diameter when the fetal spine is towards the maternal anterior wall (Figure 59-7). The upper limit of normal is 4 mm up to 33 weeks' gestation and 7 mm from 33 weeks' gestation until term.

The normal fetal ureters are usually unobserved because they measure less than 1 mm in diameter. When the ureters are pathologically dilated, they become visible as tortuous cystic masses in the midportion of the lower fetal pelvis.

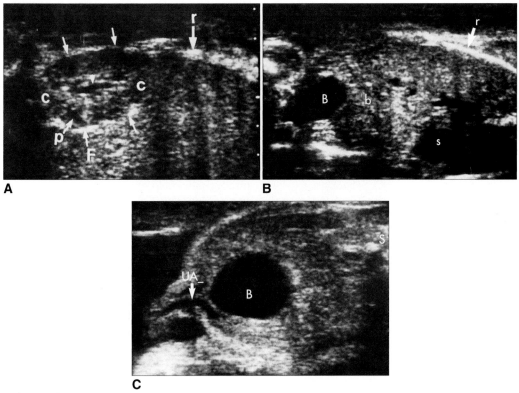

Figure 59-6 **A,** Longitudinal image of the kidney in a 37-week fetus revealing the renal cortex *(c)*, pelvis *(arrowhead)*, and pyramids *(p)*. The kidney is marginated by the capsule of the kidney *(arrows)*, which is sonographically enhanced because of perirenal fat *(F)*. *r,* Rib. **B,** Sagittal view of the fluid-filled bladder *(B)* in the pelvis. Note the more cephalic location of the stomach *(s)* in the upper abdomen. *b,* Bowel; *r,* rib. **C,** Transverse view of the bladder *(B)* with demonstration of the umbilical arteries *(UA)* as they course around the bladder after exiting the umbilical cord. *S,* Spine.

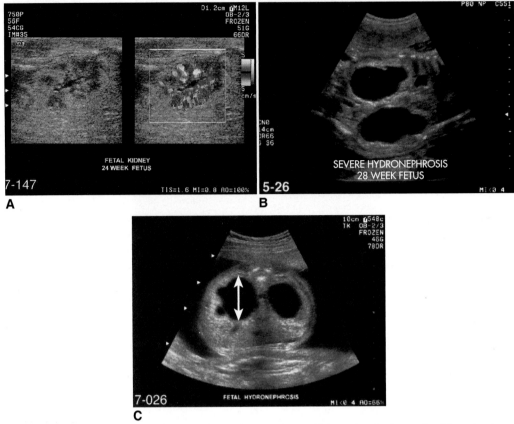

Figure 59-7   A, Sagittal view of normal fetal kidneys with a small separation in the renal pelvis measuring less than 1 to 2 mm. Color flow shows the tremendous vascularity of the renal parenchyma. Sagittal **(B)** and transverse **(C)** view of the severe hydronephrosis. The separation of the collecting system may be measured on the transverse anterior-posterior scan *(arrow).*

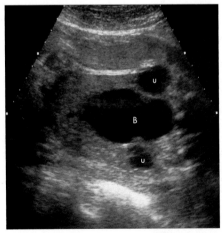

Figure 59-8   Coronal view of the fetal abdomen and pelvis demonstrates a huge urinary bladder *(B)* with extension into the ureters *(u)* in a fetus with bladder outlet obstruction.

Abnormally dilated ureters are referred to as **hydroureters** and may be traced into the kidney and bladder (Figure 59-8).

The fetal bladder is normally visualized in all fetuses. If the bladder appears too large, it should be evaluated again at the end of the study (assuming the examination takes at least 45

to 60 minutes) to see if normal emptying has occurred. The normal bladder wall measures up to 2 mm in diameter and is best measured at the level of the umbilical artery.

Failure to observe the bladder may indicate a severe renal abnormality when accompanied by oligohydramnios. The bladder wall should be thin in a normal fetus. When obstruction occurs at the level of the urethra, the bladder wall becomes hypertrophied. The presence of ureteral jets may be assessed in the fetus to rule out obstruction. Color Doppler is focused over the area of the bladder, near the base, and the presence of ureteral jets streaming into the bladder over time indicates that the ureter is not obstructed.

The urethra, like the ureters, is usually unidentifiable in the normal fetus. Dilation of the posterior urethra is highly suspicious for an obstructive process, such as posterior urethral valve syndrome, known as the "key bladder sign" on sonography, as the dilated bladder has the shape of a keyhole superior to the obstructed urethra (Figure 59-9). The **posterior urethral valve** occurs only in male fetuses and is manifested by the presence of a valve in the posterior urethra.

The sonographer should evaluate the fetal kidneys, urinary bladder, and amniotic fluid volume in a systematic approach. Both kidneys should be visualized adjacent to the spine. If a kidney is not well seen, the evaluation of the fetal pelvis should

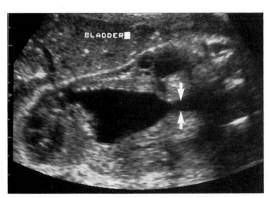

Figure 59-9 Coronal view of the dilated bladder and urethra *(arrows)* in the same patient as seen in Figure 59-8.

be made to rule out the presence of an ectopic kidney. The use of color Doppler is sometimes helpful to determine the location of the renal vessels leading into the kidney. It is possible to have unilateral renal agenesis, but the contralateral kidney is usually quite large to compensate for this abnormality.

If macroscopic cysts are present in one kidney, careful assessment of the adjacent kidney should be made. Do not confuse multicystic renal disease with hydronephrosis. The multicystic kidney shows a large central cyst with multiple small peripheral cysts to look like a pelviureteral junction obstruction, but these cysts do not communicate with one another as is seen with hydronephrosis. If a single large cyst is found, it most likely represents a simple renal cyst.

When the kidneys appear enlarged and echogenic, the sonographer should think of infantile polycystic renal disease (with oligohydramnios) or occasionally, adult polycystic disease (normal amniotic fluid volume). Enlarged echogenic kidneys may also represent a number of syndromes including Meckel-Gruber or trisomy 13.

Obstructions of the urinary system may originate anywhere along the urinary tract. The consequences of an obstruction depend on the origin of the blockage. For example, in fetuses with complete posterior urethral valve obstruction, urine is unable to pass through the urethra and into the amniotic fluid. Consequently, urine backs up in the posterior urethra, bladder, and ureters and often extends to the kidneys (hydronephrosis).

Dilation of the renal collecting system suggests either hydronephrosis or reflux. Visualization of the bladder may help to determine if obstruction is present or not. When the entire collecting system is involved, a simple hydronephrosis is usually the cause. The level of obstruction is determined by the degree of dilation of the renal pelvis and ureter. Pelviureteral junction obstruction shows dilation of the renal pelvis, whereas ureteric dilation suggests either a vesicoureteric junction obstruction or reflux. Analysis of the renal parenchyma should be made in the presence of hydronephrosis. If an echogenic cortex is present with subcapsular cysts, secondary renal dysplasia and poor function of the affected kidney may be present.

When the hydronephrosis is bilateral, the possibility of bladder outlet obstruction should be considered. The sonographer should look for dilated ureters, thickened (hypertro-phied) bladder wall, and dilation of the posterior urethra. Vesicoureteric reflux may also cause bilateral hydronephrosis.

The effect of maternal hydration on the fetus has been evaluated by many investigators. One study reported that maternal hydration influences fetal renal diameter.[1] The larger fetal renal diameters seen in the hydrated group supported physiologic theories that the effects of maternal hydration on amniotic fluid volume are partially mediated via fetal urine production. Another study showed no significant change in the degree of fetal renal pyelectasis before and after maternal hydration.[3]

The size of the fetal kidneys may be assessed by measuring the length, width, and height of the kidney (Table 59-2). The length of the kidney closely correlates with the gestational age of the fetus.

ABNORMALITIES OF THE URINARY TRACT

Renal malformations may be divided into two categories: (1) those involving congenital malformation and (2) those resulting from an obstructive process. The consequences of renal malformations vary depending on the type of lesion and extent of obstruction. Amniotic fluid volume is a significant factor in predicting outcome. Box 59-2 lists common renal abnormalities.

The recognition of urinary tract anomalies is of significant clinical concern because several fetal conditions are incompatible with life. In unilateral obstructions of the urinary tract, early delivery of the fetus is often warranted to salvage the normal kidney. Intrauterine decompression of an obstructed urinary tract (posterior urethral valve syndrome) has been performed to relieve the obstruction and allow expansion of the lungs to prevent pulmonary hypoplasia. Recognition of lethal or treatable renal anomalies is necessary to ensure appropriate clinical and therapeutic management.

Amniotic fluid is a critical marker in the assessment of renal function. The fetal kidneys begin to excrete urine after the 11th week but do not become the major contributor of fetal urine (and hence of amniotic fluid volume) until 14 to 16 weeks of pregnancy. Therefore the observation of normal amniotic fluid volume before this time will not exclude the possibility of renal agenesis (absent kidneys).

TABLE 59-2   KIDNEY DIMENSIONS: NORMAL VALUES

Age (weeks)	Kidney Thickness (mm)			Kidney Width (mm)			Kidney Length (mm)			Kidney Volume (cm³)		
	5th	50th	95th	5th	50th	95th	5th	50th	95th	5th	50th	95th
16	2	6	10	6	10	13	7	13	18	—	0.4	2.6
17	3	7	11	6	10	14	10	15	20	—	0.6	2.8
18	4	8	12	6	10	14	12	17	22	—	0.7	2.9
19	5	9	13	7	10	14	14	19	24	—	0.9	3.1
20	6	10	13	7	11	15	15	21	26	—	1.1	3.3
21	6	10	14	8	12	15	17	22	28	—	1.4	3.6
22	7	11	15	8	12	16	19	24	29	—	1.7	3.9
23	8	12	16	9	13	17	21	26	31	—	2.1	4.3
24	9	13	17	10	14	18	22	28	33	0.3	2.5	4.7
25	10	14	18	11	15	19	24	29	34	0.8	3.0	5.2
26	11	15	19	12	16	19	25	31	36	1.3	3.5	5.7
27	11	15	19	12	16	20	27	32	37	1.9	4.1	6.3
28	12	16	20	13	17	21	28	33	38	2.5	4.7	6.9
29	13	17	21	14	18	22	29	35	40	3.2	5.4	7.6
30	14	18	22	15	19	23	31	36	41	3.9	6.1	8.3
31	14	18	22	16	20	24	32	37	42	4.6	6.8	9.0
32	15	19	23	17	20	24	33	38	43	5.4	7.5	9.7
33	16	20	23	17	21	25	34	39	44	6.1	8.3	10.5
34	16	20	24	18	22	26	35	40	45	6.8	9.0	11.2
35	17	21	25	18	22	26	35	41	46	7.4	9.6	11.8
36	17	21	25	19	23	27	36	41	47	8.1	10.2	12.4
37	18	22	26	19	23	27	37	42	47	8.6	10.8	13.0
38	18	22	26	19	23	27	37	43	48	9.0	11.2	13.4
39	19	23	27	19	23	27	38	43	48	9.4	11.6	13.8
40	19	23	27	19	23	27	38	44	49	9.6	11.8	14.0

From Romero R and others: *Prenatal diagnosis of congenital anomalies,* Norwalk, Conn, 1988, Appleton and Lange.

In fetuses with severe renal disease, amniotic fluid is reduced, and in the most severe malformations it is virtually absent. When severe oligohydramnios is found, usually both kidneys or ureters and the urethra are malformed. Unilateral obstructions may yield a normal amount of amniotic fluid because the contralateral kidney produces urine. Conversely, hydramnios may be present with some renal disorders, such as mesoblastic nephroma and unilateral renal obstruction. It is important to identify the fetal bladder early in the ultrasound examination to make sure adequate fluid is present. If no bladder is seen, the sonographer should reevaluate the bladder at the end of the examination. It usually takes at least 30 minutes to fill and empty the fetal bladder.

It is important to determine whether the pathology is unilateral, which implies ureteral bud defect with good prognosis, or bilateral. When bilateral, decide if the condition is asymmetric (dissimilar abnormal patterns for each kidney) or symmetric (same abnormal pattern for both kidneys). Symmetry may imply a genetic condition, such as autosomal-recessive infantile polycystic kidney or multicystic dysplastic kidney disease.

ABNORMALITIES OF KIDNEY DEVELOPMENT

A renal malformation may represent a serious or life-threatening condition. Renal agenesis and infantile polycystic kidney disease are fetal conditions incompatible with life. When bilateral, multicystic dysplastic kidneys result in

BOX 59-3   SONOGRAPHIC FINDINGS IN RENAL AGENESIS

- Severe oligohydramnios after 13 to 15 weeks menstrual age
- Persistent absence of urine in fetal bladder (observe for period of 1 hour)
- Failure to visualize kidneys or renal arteries (use color flow to outline renal arteries)
- Abnormally small thorax

Note: Difficulties arise when oligohydramnios is present or when fetus is in breech presentation. Be careful not to mistake bowel or adrenal gland for kidneys. An empty bladder may be due to other impaired renal function problems.

immediate neonatal death. Recognition of these fetal disorders is crucial in the antenatal period. The clinician will be able to provide information distinguishing lethal conditions from those with good outcomes.

Renal Agenesis. Renal agenesis means the virtual absence of one or both of the kidneys. Box 59-3 summarizes the sonographic findings in renal agenesis. Bilateral agenesis occurs in 1 in 3000 to 1 in 10,000 births. The male to female ratio is 2.5:1. In this disease, the kidneys and bladder are not visualized sonographically (Figure 59-10). Amniotic fluid is absent

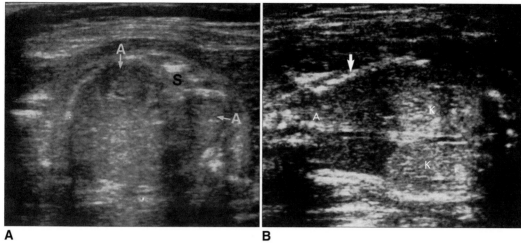

Figure 59-10 **A,** Renal agenesis in a 29-week fetus showing enlarged adrenal glands *(A)* occupying the renal spaces. Oligohydramnios and an absent bladder confirmed the diagnosis. **B,** Infantile polycystic kidney disease shown with enlarged and dense kidneys *(K)*. Note the enhanced transmission of sound through the kidneys because of the dilated cystic tubules. Oligohydramnios and absent bladder were coexisting findings.

or severely decreased (oligohydramnios) because urine is not produced. The combination of these findings is highly suggestive of this lethal disorder. It is important to remember that in the early stages of renal agenesis, amniotic fluid may be visible because it is produced from other fetal sources. In renal agenesis, the adrenal glands may be large and may mimic the kidneys.

Fetal anomalies found in association with renal agenesis include cardiac defects and musculoskeletal disorders (sirenomelia, absent radius and fibula, anomalies of the digits, sacral agenesis, diaphragmatic hernia, and cleft palate). Central nervous system anomalies include hydrocephalus, meningocele, cephalocele, holoprosencephaly, anencephaly, and microcephaly. Gastrointestinal anomalies include duodenal atresia, imperforate anus, tracheoesophageal fistula, malrotation, and omphalocele. The sonographer should understand that most of these malformations are not detected prenatally because of poor visualization resulting from anhydramnios (complete lack of amniotic fluid).

Sonographic Findings. The lower fetal pelvis should be carefully searched when the kidneys cannot be found in their normal locations. Ectopic kidneys should be considered when the kidneys are not located in their normal retroperitoneal location. Oligohydramnios usually is associated with bilateral renal agenesis. The presence of oligohydramnios does make it more difficult to image the fetal kidneys. Color Doppler may be useful in trying to delineate the renal vessels in the area of the kidneys. The presence or absence of the urinary bladder will determine if the kidneys are present or not.

Unilateral renal agenesis occurs in 1 in 500 to 1 in 1000 births and therefore is more common than bilateral disease. Unilateral agenesis may be associated with uterine anomalies in females and testicular hypoplasia, agenesis, or hypospadias in males. The contralateral kidney may be hypertrophied to compensate for the absent kidney. With a normal contralateral kidney, adequate amounts of amniotic fluid are produced and

chances for survival are excellent. The adrenal gland fills the renal fossa in the absent kidney site to produce a unilateral lying down adrenal sign without a renal artery on color Doppler.

Amniotic fluid may be normal in a fetus with bilateral renal agenesis when esophageal atresia and tracheoesophageal fistula are present.

Renal Ectopia. This occurs when the kidney lies outside of its normal position in the renal fossa, usually in the area of the pelvis (see Figure 59-5). Occasional crossed fused ectopia will occur. With ultrasound, the kidney will be absent in its normal position, with the adrenal gland filling the space of the renal fossa. Evaluation of the pelvis finds the kidney lying superior to the bladder.

Crossed Renal Ectopia. The ectopic kidney lies on the opposite side of the abdomen relative to its ureteral insertion into the bladder (see Figure 59-5). The kidneys are usually fused together and are found usually on the right side of the abdomen.

Horseshoe Kidney. The horseshoe kidney is the fusion of the lower poles of both kidneys (see Figure 59-5). Transverse images of the fetal abdomen demonstrate an abnormal lie of the kidney. If the spine is down, the connecting isthmus may be seen anterior to the aorta.

RENAL CYSTIC DISEASE

Renal cystic disease is a heterogeneous group of heritable, developmental, and acquired disorders. The Potter classification makes an attempt to cover most of the renal cystic conditions seen in the prenatal period. A number of very rare syndromes are associated with renal cystic disease as outlined in Table 59-3.

TABLE 59-3	SYNDROMES ASSOCIATED WITH CYSTIC RENAL DISEASE
Syndrome	Clinical Findings
Meckel-Gruber syndrome	Large echogenic kidneys, polydactyly, encephalocele
Patau's syndrome (trisomy 13)	Large echogenic kidneys, polydactyly, holoprosencephaly, facial clefting
Beckwith-Wiedemann syndrome	Large echogenic kidneys, macrosomia, hepatosplenomegaly, macroglossia, omphalocele
Jeune syndrome	Echogenic kidneys, dwarfism, small thorax
Short rib polydactyly syndrome	Large echogenic kidneys, dwarfism, polydactyly, small thorax
Laurence-Moon syndrome (Bardet-Biedl syndrome)	Cystic kidneys, hypotonicity, limb contractures, congenital cataracts, hypoplastic corpus callosum, heterotopias

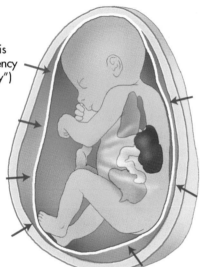

Hydroureter and megacystis
Abdominal muscle deficiency
syndrome ("prune belly")

Hydronephrosis
Type IV cystic dysplasia
Renal failure

Oligohydramnios
Potter's facies
Hypoplastic lungs
Flexion
Contraction

Figure 59-11 Schematic of Potter sequence and the consequences of fetal urethral blockage.

POTTER'S SYNDROME

Potter's syndrome occurs in 3 in 10,000 births. It is characterized by renal agenesis, oligohydramnios, pulmonary hypoplasia, abnormal facies, and malformed hands and feet (Figure 59-11). The oligohypoplastic lung complex is also seen in other genitourinary malformations, such as renal hypoplasia, cystic dysplasia, posterior urethral valves, and prune belly syndrome. Intrauterine shunting may reduce renal damage and the devastating effects of oligohydramnios. Potter's syndrome can be unilateral or bilateral.

Potter described the classifications of cystic renal anomalies:

Type 1: Autosomal recessive (AR) infantile polycystic kidney disease

Type 2: Renal agenesis, multicystic dysplastic kidneys, renal dysplasia

Type 3: Autosomal dominant (AD) polycystic kidney disease

Type 4: Renal dysplasia, obstructive kidney disease

Box 59-4 lists the sonographic findings associated with the four types of renal cystic disease.

BOX 59-4 RENAL CYSTIC DISEASE

POTTER'S TYPE I: SONOGRAPHIC FINDINGS IN INFANTILE POLYCYSTIC KIDNEY DISEASE
- Progressive renal enlargement
- Echogenic renal parenchyma
- Empty bladder and oligohydramnios

POTTER'S TYPE II: SONOGRAPHIC FINDINGS IN ADULT MULTICYSTIC DYSPLASTIC KIDNEY
- Multiple noncommunicating cysts of variable size
- No distinct renal pelvis
- No distinct renal parenchyma
- Renal size may be normal, hypoplastic, or enlarged
- Severe oligohydramnios if bilateral

POTTER'S TYPE III: SONOGRAPHIC FINDINGS IN ADULT POLYCYSTIC KIDNEY DISEASE
- Large kidneys with hyperechoic parenchyma
- Size may be asymmetric
- Genetic link

POTTER'S TYPE IV: SONOGRAPHIC FINDINGS IN OBSTRUCTIVE CYSTIC DISEASE
- Small, echogenic kidneys
- Cortical peripheral cysts
- Bilateral disease: "keyhole bladder," bilateral hydronephrosis, thick-walled bladder, severe oligohydramnios

---

Potter's Syndrome Type I: Infantile Polycystic Kidney Disease. Infantile polycystic kidney disease (IPKD) is an autosomal-recessive disorder (25% chance of recurrence) that affects the fetal kidneys and liver. This disease has varying presentations and affects 1 in 40,000 to 50,000 births. Most commonly, abnormal kidneys may be found in association with liver cysts. The most severe forms of IPKD are those found prenatally. The characteristic finding is symmetric enlargement of both kidneys secondary to renal collecting tube dilation. The kidneys are echogenic with a small or absent bladder, and oligohydramnios is found. This is associated with varying degrees of hepatic fibrosis and biliary ectasia.

In the most severe cases of IPKD, renal failure occurs with oligohydramnios and an absent urinary bladder. In some cases the kidneys are so massive that they fill the entire abdomen. In view of the high recurrence rate and dismal prognosis in severe IPKD, recognition of this defect is important. IPKD may occur as part of a genetic syndrome, such as Meckel-Gruber syndrome. The intrauterine diagnosis of IPKD should only be considered when the following characteristics are found:

- Family history of IPKD
- Bilateral enlarged kidneys
- Highly echogenic kidney texture
- Significant oligohydramnios
- Inability to identify the fetal bladder

Renal hyperplasia has also been associated with Beckwith-Wiedemann syndrome (Figure 59-12), along with omphalocele, macroglossia, gigantism, medullary dysplasia, adrenal cytomegaly, pancreatic islet-cell hyperplasia, facial nevus flammeus, and hypoglycemia.

Sonographic Findings. In this disease the collecting tubules of the kidney are microscopically dilated. By ultrasound, individual cysts are not identified; instead the kidneys are massively enlarged because of hundreds of dilated tubules (Figure 59-13). Enlargement of the kidneys may not occur until the 24th week of gestation; therefore, serial studies of at-risk fetuses are recommended. Enhanced renal tissue echogenicity is characteristic because of the multiple interfaces created by the dilated cystic tubules. Oligohydramnios and a small or absent bladder are present.

Potter's Syndrome Type II: Multicystic Dysplastic Kidney Disease. Multicystic dysplastic kidney disease is the most common form of renal cystic disease in childhood and represents one of the most common abdominal masses in the

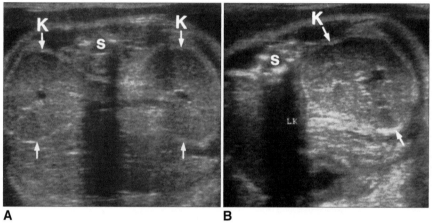

Figure 59-12   A, Bilateral renal enlargement of the kidneys *(K, arrows)* in a 32-week fetus with Beckwith-Wiedemann syndrome (congenital visceromegaly of organs, which may present with or without an omphalocele). Both kidneys occupy more than half of the abdomen. *s,* Spine. **B,** In the same fetus, a sagittal view shows an enlarged left kidney *(K, arrow).*

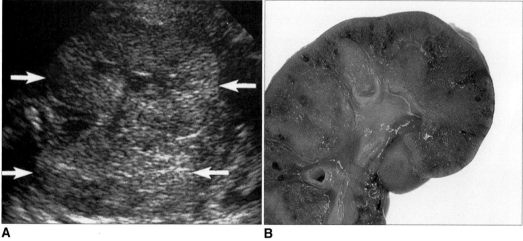

Figure 59-13   Autosomal recessive polycystic kidney disease. A, Kidneys are enlarged with increased echogenicity at 27 weeks' gestation. **B,** Gross pathology of the disease showing diffuse microscopic cysts. (From Rumack C, Wilson S, Charboneau W: Diagnostic ultrasound, ed 3, St Louis, 2005, Mosby.)

neonate. The incidence in 1 of 3000 births is found more in males than females. Although most cases are unilateral, nearly one quarter of the cases are bilateral. The multicystic dysplastic kidney disease is composed of multiple, smooth-walled, nonfunctioning, noncommunicating cysts of variable size and number. In this condition renal tissue is replaced by cysts of varying sizes that are found throughout the kidney (Figures 59-14 and 59-15). Kidney borders are difficult to define because of the distorted renal outline and absence of significant renal parenchyma. The ureter and renal pelvis may be atretic and the renal artery is hypoplastic or absent. The affected kidney is nonfunctional. When a multicystic kidney has been identified, a careful search for anomalies of the opposite kidney should be undertaken.

When both kidneys are found to be multicystic, and oligohydramnios and an absent bladder are expected, a lethal condition exists for the neonate. The prognosis for infants with multicystic kidney disease varies based on the prenatal findings. Figure 59-16 illustrates several presentations of multicystic dysplastic kidney disease. For example, when one kidney is

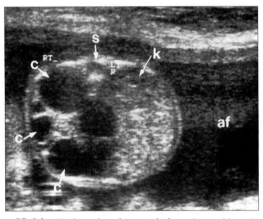

Figure 59-14   Unilateral multicystic kidney *(arrows)* in a 21-week fetus. Note the varying sizes of the cysts *(c)* and the normal contralateral kidney *(k)*. Amniotic fluid *(af)* is normal because of the functioning unaffected kidney. *RT,* Right; *s,* spine.

multicystic and the other absent, the infant will not survive. Many syndromes are associated with cysts of the kidneys.

Sonographic Findings. In the midtrimester ultrasound scan, the fetus with multicystic renal dysplasia will present with at least one kidney, demonstrating multiple cysts of varying size that may affect a part or all of the kidney. The bladder and amniotic fluid volume are usually normal. When the condition is bilateral, there is oligohydramnios and absence of the bladder. The multicystic kidneys may increase or decrease in size with gestational growth; therefore, follow-up scans are useful to monitor the process of the condition.

Potter Type III: Adult Dominant Polycystic Kidney Disease. In adult dominant polycystic kidney disease, both kidneys show cystic dilation of the nephrons. This autosomal dominant condition has an incidence of 1 in 1000 births and is the most common of the hereditary renal cystic diseases. Autosomal-dominant (adult) polycystic kidney disease may be diagnosed in a fetus when there is a family history of polycystic kidneys, liver, or both. The fetal kidneys appear large and echogenic, and rarely, cysts may be observed prenatally. Amniotic fluid volume is normal. Conversely, visualization of bilateral enlargement of the kidneys may prompt a renal and liver work-up in the parents to exclude this disorder.

Bilateral echogenic renal enlargement may be found in association with a syndrome, such as Beckwith-Wiedemann syndrome, in which visceromegaly of many organs is present (see Figure 59-12). The urinary bladder is usually present. The corticomedullary junction may appear accentuated or be indistinct.

Associated anomalies include encephalocele suggestive of Meckel-Gruber syndrome in the presence of bilateral renal cystic disease, polydactyly, and severe oligohydramnios. Multicystic kidney disease may also be associated with ureteral atresia.

Sonographic Findings. The sonographic appearance is similar to autosomal recessive polycystic renal disease in that the kidneys are symmetrically enlarged and echogenic (Figure 59-17). The bladder is usually present and amniotic fluid volume is normal. The corticomedullary junction may appear

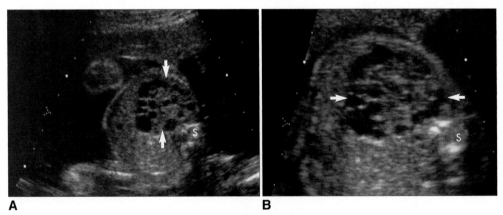

Figure 59-15   **A,** Unilateral dysplastic multicystic kidney *(arrows)* in a 25-week fetus. The contralateral kidney appeared normal with adequate amniotic fluid volume. A single umbilical artery was identified. *S,* Spine. **B,** In the same fetus, a magnified view of the dysplastic kidney *(arrows)*.

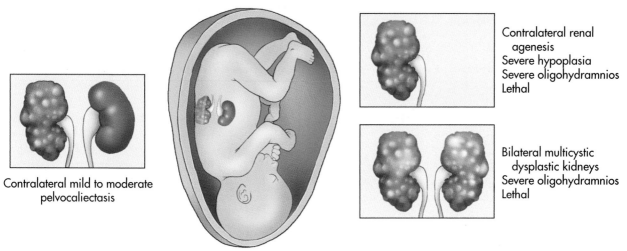

Contralateral mild to moderate
pelvocaliectasis

Contralateral renal
agenesis
Severe hypoplasia
Severe oligohydramnios
Lethal

Bilateral multicystic
dysplastic kidneys
Severe oligohydramnios
Lethal

Figure 59-16   Multicystic dysplastic kidney disease may be unilateral, bilateral, or associated with contralateral renal agenesis. Although the affected kidney typically produces very little urine, it may change in size throughout gestation. Because the contralateral kidney is the only potentially functional kidney, it must be examined carefully.

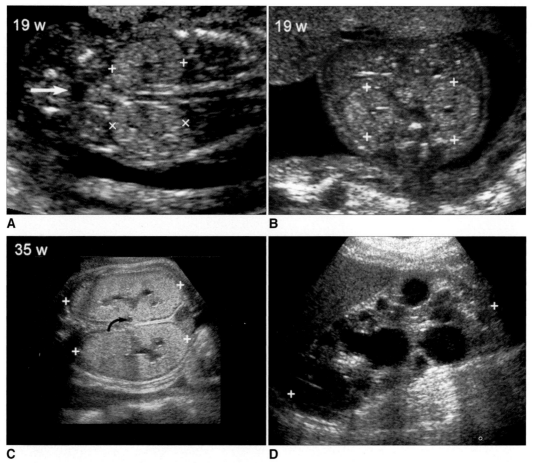

Figure 59-17   Autosomal dominant polycystic kidney disease. **A** and **B,** Coronal and transverse scans of 19-week fetus show slightly enlarged, echogenic kidneys *(cursors).* There is normal amniotic fluid volume and bladder filling *(arrow).* **C,** Coronal scan at 35 weeks shows notably enlarged kidneys *(cursors).* They measure 9 cm in length, and multiple small cortical cysts *(curved arrow)* can be seen. **D,** Maternal autosomal dominant polycystic kidney disease. Classic appearance of an enlarged kidney with multiple cystic structures. (From Rumack C, Wilson S, Charboneau W: *Diagnostic ultrasound,* ed 3, St Louis, 2005, Mosby.)

accentuated or indistinct. Occasionally, macroscopic cysts within the echogenic kidneys are seen. This condition is nearly always bilateral.

Potter Type IV: Obstructive Cystic Dysplasia. In obstructive cystic dysplasia, renal dysplasia occurs secondary to obstruction in the first or early second trimester of pregnancy. The incidence is 1 in 8000 births, although this is difficult to determine because only a small number of obstructive kidneys progress to renal dysplasia. This condition is caused by early renal obstruction. Unilateral disease can be caused by a pelvi-ureteral or vesicoureteric junction obstruction. Severe obstruction from a ureterocele can cause dysplasia in an upper pole moiety of a duplex kidney. Bilateral obstructive dysplasia is caused by severe bladder outlet obstruction, usually urethral atresia or posterior urethral valves.

Sonographic Findings. The fetal kidneys appear small and echogenic with cortical peripheral cysts. If the disease is bilateral, look for early bladder outlet obstruction ("keyhole bladder"), bilateral hydronephrosis, a thick-walled bladder, and severe oligohydramnios. The renal cortex is dysplastic and replaced with the multiple cortical cysts.

OBSTRUCTIVE URINARY TRACT ABNORMALITIES

The urinary tract may be obstructed at the junction of the ureter entering the renal pelvis **(ureteropelvic junction),** or at the junction of the ureter where it enters the bladder **(ureterovesical junction),** or at the level of the urethra **(megacystis).** The amount and degree of obstruction will depend upon the gestational age at which the obstruction began. If the obstruction is early, a multicystic kidney may develop. If the obstruction occurs in the first or second trimester, cystic dysplasia may result. Late obstruction produces hydronephrosis.

Hydronephrosis. Fetal hydronephrosis is the most common fetal anomaly. The sonographic appearance of

urinary tract obstruction varies depending on the site and extent of blockage (Box 59-5). Up to 22 weeks' gestation, the measurements of the renal pelvis are quite uniform. After 22 weeks' gestation, the obstructed kidneys produce increased real pelvic diameters and true hydronephrosis. Therefore it is important to do follow-up scans in the third trimester when dilation is suspected.

Dilation of the renal pelvis (hydronephrosis) occurs in response to a blockage of urine at some junction in the urinary system. This blocked urine is unable to pass the obstruction. Urine is continually produced and will back up into the kidney. Hydronephrosis commonly occurs when there is an obstruction in the ureter, bladder, or urethra. Hydronephrosis is generally the end result of an obstruction at a lower level in the urinary tract.

Sonographic Findings. The ultrasound appearance of hydronephrosis varies according to the severity of the underlying obstruction. The dilated renal pelvis, which often communicates with the calyces (caliectasis), is centrally located and distended with urine (Figure 59-18). The remaining renal tissue may be identified in all but the most severe cases of hydronephrosis.

BOX 59-5   SONOGRAPHIC FINDINGS IN HYDRONEPHROSIS

- Before 20 weeks, the renal pelvic diameter should measure <4 mm in diameter. Measurement of 4 mm or greater is abnormal, and fetus should be followed with serial sonograms.
- In the third trimester, an anteroposterior renal pelvic diameter greater than 8 to 10 mm is abnormal
- Rim of renal parenchyma preserved
- Calyceal distention with central pelvis communication

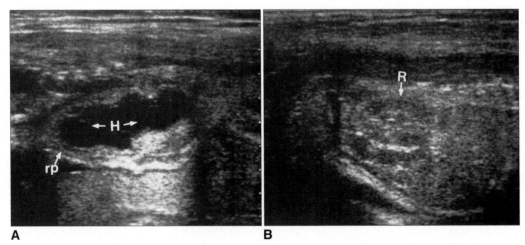

A   **B**

Figure 59-18   A, Unilateral ureteropelvic junction obstruction showing collection of urine within the renal pelvis, communicating with the renal calyces (hydronephrosis *[H]*). It is important to study the remaining renal parenchyma *(rp)* for pathologic changes. **B,** In the same fetus the contralateral kidney is normal. *R,* Renal architecture.

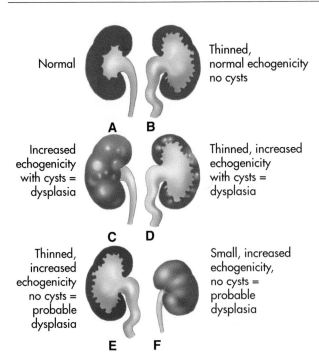

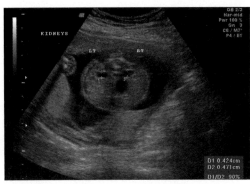

Figure 59-20 Measurement of the renal pelvic diameter is measured in the A-P direction *(cursors).*

Figure 59-19 Renal parenchymal responses to obstruction. **A,** In distal urinary tract obstruction without reflux, the kidneys may remain normal. **B,** Pyelocaliectasis may thin the renal parenchyma. **C,** Cystic dysplasia may occur with renal cysts and fibrosis (increased echogenicity) and cease to function (lack of pyelocaliectasis). **D,** Cystic dysplasia may occur with persistent pyelocaliectasis. **E,** Increased renal echogenicity with visible cysts suggests, but is not diagnostic of, dysplasia. **F,** A small, echogenic kidney without pyelocaliectasis is also suggestive, but not diagnostic, of dysplasia.

Measurements of the renal pelvis have a wide discrepancy, varying between 4 and 10 mm in the second trimester and 7 and 10 mm in the third trimester. The gray zone between 4 and 10 mm may represent a condition of vesicoureteric reflux. Dilation of the renal pelves should not be misinterpreted as an abnormal collection of urine within the renal pelvis, **pyelectasis** (5 to 9 mm), or **calyectasis,** rounded calyces with renal pelvis dilation (greater than 10 mm), which may lead to severe hydronephrosis (Figure 59-19). A renal pelvis diameter, measured in an anteroposterior direction in a transverse plane that exceeds 10 to 15 mm, is considered abnormal (Figure 59-20).

Renal dysplasia often occurs and represents cystic changes within the renal tissue. Several obstructive patterns may be observed. The sonographic team should attempt to define the severity of the cystic changes affecting the kidney.

Fetal hydronephrosis may occur as a unilateral or bilateral process. Unilateral renal hydronephrosis commonly results from an obstruction at the junction of the renal pelvis and the ureter. This is called a ureteropelvic junction obstruction.

Ureteropelvic junction obstruction. Ureteropelvic junction obstruction is the most common reason for hydronephrosis in the neonate. This obstruction occurs at the junction between the renal pelvis and ureter. Only half of these disorders are found during early childhood; therefore, early prenatal detection may improve long-term renal function. The

causes of ureteropelvic junction obstructions are abnormal bends or kinks in the ureter, adhesions, abnormal valves in the ureter, abnormal outlet shape at the ureteropelvic junction, or absence of the longitudinal muscle that is imperative to the normal excretion of urine from the kidney.

Uteropelvic junction obstruction is usually a unilateral defect, and amniotic fluid remains normal because of the normal contralateral kidney. Bilateral ureteropelvic junction obstruction is uncommon. Anomalies associated with this disorder may involve the presence of a urinoma, which presents as a large cyst that is in contact with the spine (Figure 59-21). Urinary ascites may also be a complicating feature of ureteropelvic junction obstruction.

Sonographic Findings. Sonographically, there is a collection of urine located medially within the renal pelvis that communicates with the calyces (caliectasis) (Figures 59-22 and 59-23). The ureter, bladder, and amniotic fluid are usually normal. Ureteropelvic junction obstruction may be severe.

Ureterovesical junction obstruction. Ureterovesical junction obstruction commonly presents with dilation of the lower end of the ureter **(megaureter).** Megaureter may result from a primary ureteral defect (stenotic ureteral valves or fibrosis) or occur secondary to obstruction at another level (causing reflux or backward flow of urine) (Figure 59-24).

Sonographic Findings. The affected kidney shows dilation of the renal pelvis and tortuous dilated ureter. Other defects, such as duplication of the renal collecting system, are common and may be diagnosed prenatally. When a dilated upper renal pole is observed with a normal lower pole, an obstructed duplicated collecting system may be indicated. This defect may result from an ectopic ureterocele within the bladder causing obstruction of the upper pole of the kidney.

Secondary Obstruction to Ureterocele and Ectopic Ureter. A ureterocele is a cystic dilation of the intravesical (bladder) segment of the distal ureter. An ectopic ureter is one that does not insert near the posterolateral angle of the trigone of the bladder. In females it may insert in the vagina, vestibule, or uterus; in males it may insert in the seminal vesicle, vas deferens, or ejaculatory ducts. It may also inset in the bladder in an ectopic location. Unless hydronephrosis is present, this condition is difficult to diagnose in utero.

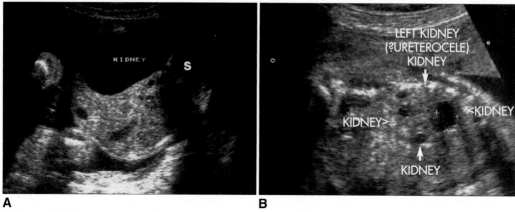

Figure 59-21   A, Massively dilated renal pelvis *(kidney)* shown in a transverse plane in a 28-week fetus. *S,* Spine. **B,** In the same fetus at 30 weeks of gestation, the renal cyst ruptured, with only a small, upper-pole cyst *(calipers)* evident. A urinoma was suspected.

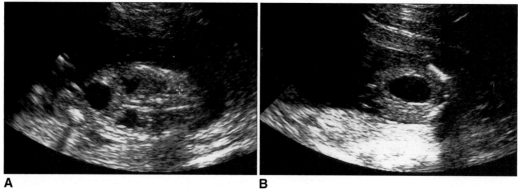

Figure 59-22   A, Coronal scan of a 20-week fetus with moderate hydronephrosis and a prominent bladder. **B,** The bladder remained dilated after 45 minutes, suggesting an outlet obstruction.

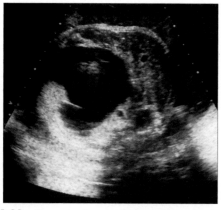

Figure 59-23   Transverse image of a fetal kidney that has severe unilateral hydronephrosis. The renal parenchyma is no longer visible.

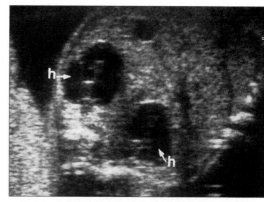

Figure 59-24   Bilateral megaureters (hydroureters) *(h)* noted in an axial pelvic view. Partial blockage to the posterior urethra was found after birth.

Posterior Urethral Valve Obstruction. Bladder outlet obstruction is produced by a membrane within the posterior urethra. Posterior urethral valve obstruction results in hydronephrosis, hydroureters, or dilation of the bladder and posterior urethra (Figures 59-25 and 59-26). Cystic dysplasia

and poor renal function are suggested when sodium, chloride, and osmolality are unusually elevated. This entity occurs only in male fetuses and is manifested by the presence of a valve(s) in the posterior urethra. As a result, urine is unable to pass through the urethra and into the amniotic fluid. This obstruc-

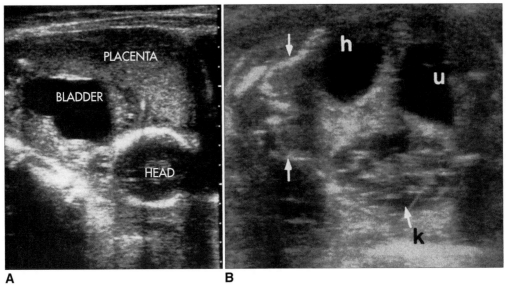

Figure 59-25 **A,** Posterior urethral valve syndrome in a 17-week fetus showing abnormally distended bladder with a keyhole urethra. Note the significant lack of amniotic fluid. **B,** In the same fetus at 21 weeks of gestation, a small thoracic cavity *(arrows)*, hydronephrosis *(h)*, hydroureter *(u)*, and enlargement and mild hydronephrosis of the contralateral kidney *(k)* are noted.

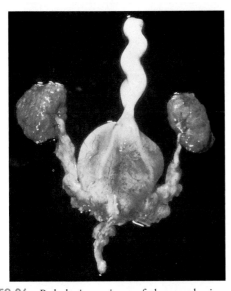

Figure 59-26 Pathologic specimen of obstructed urinary tract showing bladder enlargement, hydroureters, and bilateral hydronephrosis in posterior urethral valve syndrome.

BOX 59-6   SONOGRAPHIC FINDINGS IN POSTERIOR URETHRAL VALVE OBSTRUCTION

- Dilated bladder (thickening of the bladder wall)
- Dilated posterior urethra ("keyhole" appearance)
- Oligohydramnios
- Hydroureters
- Hydronephrosis and dysplasia
- Fetal ascites (some cases)
- Distention of fetal abdomen (urethral obstruction malformation complex/prune belly syndrome)
- Male fetus

From Hobbins JC and others: *Am J Obtet Gynecol* 148:868, 1984.

---

tion causes a back-up of urine in the bladder, ureter, and, in the most severe cases, the kidneys.

Sonographic Findings. The bladder wall is severely thickened with a dilated posterior urethra—"the keyhole sign." Bilateral hydroureter and hydronephrosis are present. Such oligohydramnios causes the lungs to be hypoplastic, and the chest circumference will be severely depressed. Severe oligohydramnios is a classic finding in the complete obstruction form (Box 59-6).

When these sonographic signs occur in the female fetus, abnormalities of the sacrum (caudal regression anomalies) and

megacystis-microcolon intestinal hypoperistalsis syndrome should be considered.

Fetal renal function may be assessed by aspirating urine from an obstructed bladder (Figures 59-27 and 59-28).

Intermittent posterior urethral valve obstruction may occur with a normal amount of amniotic fluid (Figures 59-29 and 59-30). Diminishing fluid volume and increased hydronephrosis may prompt early delivery.

Prune Belly Syndrome. Prune belly syndrome may be called the urethral obstruction malformation complex. The condition consists of cryptorchidism, agenesis of abdominal wall muscle, megaureters, and bladder outlet obstruction caused by urethral anomalies, such as atresia, stenotic valves, or diverticulum (Box 59-7).

Sonographic Findings. Sonographic findings in prune belly syndrome include oligohydramnios, mild to severe

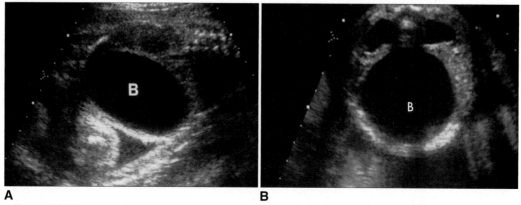

A   B

Figure 59-27   Massively enlarged bladder *(B)* in a 28-week fetus in both sagittal **(A)** and transverse **(B)** views. Bilateral hydronephrosis *(right* and *left)* is evident. Amniotic fluid volume was increased.

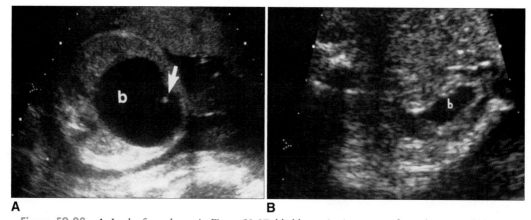

A   B

Figure 59-28   A, In the fetus shown in Figure 59-27, bladder aspiration was performed to assess kidney function. Note the needle *(arrow)* within the bladder *(b).* **B,** After urine aspiration, decompression of the bladder *(b)* occurred. Note the thickened bladder wall. Laboratory analysis of osmolality, sodium, potassium, and chloride indicates favorable renal function. Bilateral reflux was diagnosed after birth.

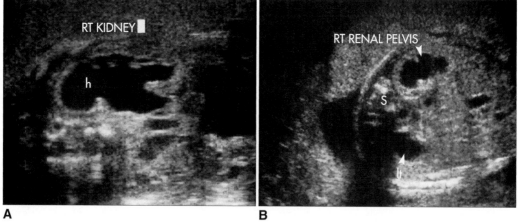

A   B

Figure 59-29   Bilateral posterior urethral valve syndrome shown in a 24-week fetus with severe hydronephrosis *(h)* of the right kidney in a male fetus in both sagittal **(A)** and transverse **(B)** views. *lt,* Left kidney; *S,* spine.

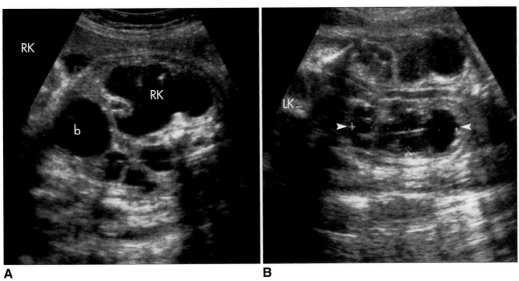

Figure 59-30   In the fetus shown in Figure 59-29, the hydronephrotic right kidney *(RK)* is shown in **(A)**, and the opposite kidney *(LK)* is shown in a coronal view **(B)**, with hydronephrosis. Amniotic fluid volume was normal. At 32 weeks of gestation, worsening hydronephrosis prompted early delivery. After birth, the right kidney did not function and the left kidney had reasonable function. The child, however, awaits a renal implant. *b,* Bladder.

> **BOX 59-7   SONOGRAPHIC FINDINGS IN PRUNE BELLY SYNDROME**
>
> - Absent abdominal musculature
> - Undescended testes
> - Large urinary bladder
> - Dilated prostatic urethra
> - Dilated and tortuous ureters
> - Kidneys can be normal, hydronephrotic, or dysplastic

bilateral hydronephrosis, fetal ascites, and hypoplastic lungs. The abdomen is extremely distended compared with the small thoracic cavity. The dilated ureters and bladder appear as numerous cystic lesions within the distended abdominal cavity. The bladder may be obstructed and massively dilated, or it may not be seen because of bladder rupture with resultant fetal ascites.

Fetal Surgery in Obstructive Uropathy. The prognosis of posterior urethral valve syndrome is invariably fatal, but in selected fetuses with documented normal renal function, placement of an indwelling bladder shunt to relieve the obstruction has improved chances for survival in some cases (Figure 59-31). This shunt drains the blocked urine into the amniotic fluid, allowing the fetal lungs to develop. When the urinary tract is completely blocked, severe oligohydramnios and the Potter sequence occur.

Other Urinary Anomalies. Rare disorders like **urethral atresia** may cause a massively dilated bladder (prune belly) (Figures 59-32 and 59-33). Duplication of the renal complexes

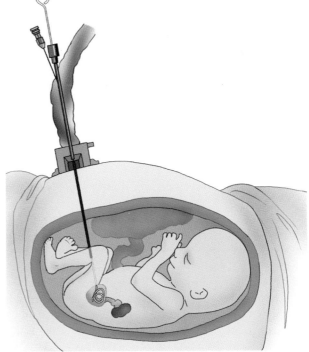

Figure 59-31   Schematic showing initial steps in a bladder shunt procedure.

and ectopic ureteroceles may be detected. Dilation of the ureters may occur as isolated lesions (primary megaureters), resulting from atresia of the distal ureter. The disorders are generally associated with adequate to increased amounts of amniotic fluid and a normal bladder. Infrequently, renal pelvis hydronephrosis may occur. The antenatal diagnosis of crossed

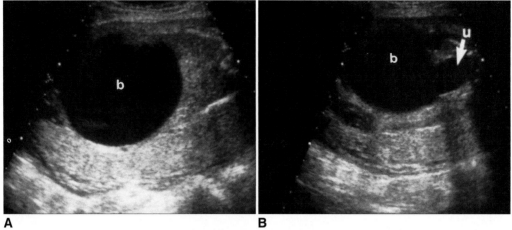

Figure 59-32 **A,** Urethral atresia shown with massively dilated bladder *(b)* in a 24-week fetus. **B,** In the same fetus, urethral dilation *(u)* is evident at a lower level. *b,* Bladder.

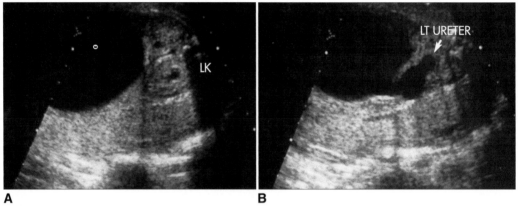

Figure 59-33 **A,** In the fetus shown in Figure 59-32, transverse views reveal a normal-appearing left kidney *(LK).* **B,** In the same fetus a left unilateral hydroureter is shown. Severe oligohydramnios was found. Spontaneous labor occurred at 32 weeks of gestation, and urethral atresia was confirmed. The infant died shortly after birth.

renal ectopia (both kidneys fused on one side) has been reported. Failure to identify a kidney should prompt the sonographer to check for this condition, as well as pelvic kidneys (located ectopically in the pelvis), unilateral renal agenesis, or horseshoe kidneys. Horseshoe kidneys are normal in location (one on each side).

Tumors of the fetal kidney are rare. Masses in the kidney should be suspected when the contour of the kidney is distorted or replaced by a mass and the pelvicaliceal echoes are absent.

The most common renal tumor is a mesoblastic nephroma, which is a hamartoma (Figure 59-34). A hamartoma is a collection of oddly arranged tissue indigenous to the area. Mesoblastic nephromas are sonographically observed as large, single, solid masses originating from the kidney. Polyhydramnios is a typical manifestation. The opposite kidney is usually normal and therefore, with surgical removal of the affected kidney, prognosis is excellent.

An adrenal tumor, neuroblastoma, may be observed prenatally above the kidney. These tumors have varying echo patterns and are associated with liver and placental metastasis. The prenatal diagnosis of nephroblastomatosis (premalignant precursor of Wilms' tumor) has been reported.[2] Bilateral renal enlargement with calcifications with shadowing was observed.

THE GENITAL SYSTEM

The sex of the fetus is determined at the time of fertilization, but there is no morphologic indication of gender until the 7th week of development (Figure 59-35). Early embryogenesis shows similar development in both sexes. The gonads are derived from the gonadal ridges and are the first parts of the genital system to undergo development. As the genital ridge enlarges and frees itself from the mesonephros by developing a mesentery, the male ridge becomes the mesorchium and the

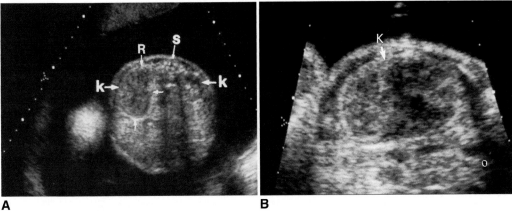

A   **B**

Figure 59-34   **A,** Mesoblastic nephroma in a 32-week fetus showing obvious enlargement of the right kidney *(k, arrows) (R)* compared with the left kidney *(k)*. Hydramnios was observed. *S, Spine.* **B,** In the same fetus the encapsulated and solid appearance of the nephroma *(K)* was observed. The nephroma was removed within a few days after birth.

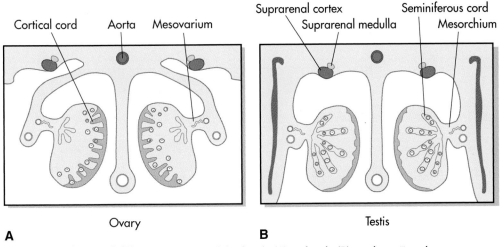

Figure 59-35   Development of the female **(A)** and male **(B)** gender at 7 weeks.

female the mesovarium. At the same time, the coelomic epithelium that covers the primitive gonads proliferates and forms the cords of cells, called primary sex cords, that grow into the mesenchyme of the developing gonads. The primordial germ cells originate in the wall of the yolk sac and migrate into the embryo and enter the primary sex cords to give rise to the ova and sperm.

DEVELOPMENT OF THE EXTERNAL GENITALIA

Although the early development of the external genitalia is similar for both sexes, distinguishing sexual characteristics begin during the 9th week and external genital organs are fully differentiated by the 12th week of gestation (Figure 59-36).

In the 4th week, a genital tubercle develops at the cranial end of the cloacal membrane. Labioscrotal swellings and urogenital folds develop on either side of this membrane. The genital tubercle elongates to form a phallus, which is similar in both sexes. The hormonal changes cause further

development of the male and female reproductive system (Figure 59-37).

Development of the Male External Genitalia. The fetal testes produce androgens that cause the masculinization of the external genitalia. The phallus elongates to form the penis (Figure 59-38). This sonographic finding is known as the "turtle sign." The urogenital folds fuse on the ventral surface of the penis to form the spongy urethra. The labioscrotal swellings grow toward the median plane and fuse to form the scrotum. The line of fusion of the labioscrotal folds is called the scrotal raphe.

Development of the Female External Genitalia. Both the urethra and vagina open into the urogenital sinus, the vestibule of the vagina. The urogenital folds become the labia minora, the labioscrotal swellings become the labia majora, and the phallus becomes the clitoris (Figure 59-39). This sonographic finding is known as the "hamburger sign."

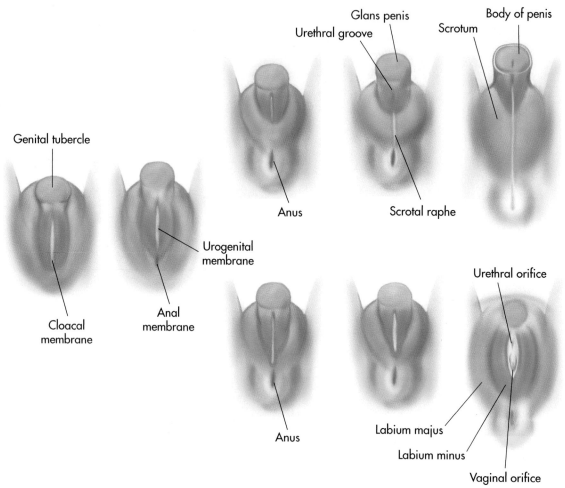

Figure 59-36   Sexual characteristics begin to develop during the 9th week and are fully differentiated by the 12th week.

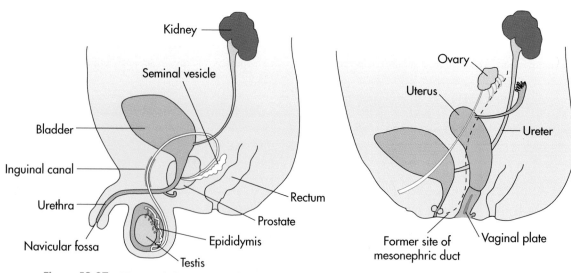

Figure 59-37   Hormonal changes cause further development of the male and female reproductive systems.

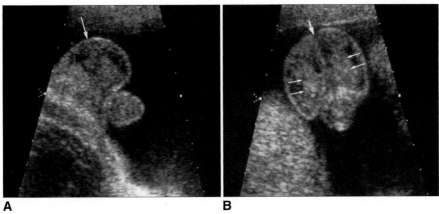

Figure 59-38 A, Male genitalia in a 40-week fetus showing the scrotum *(arrow)* and phallus. **B,** Coronal view of the male genitalia outlining descended testicles *(double arrows)* within the scrotum. Note the scrotal septum *(thick arrow)* and phallus.

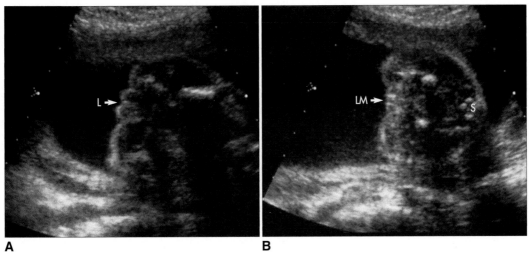

Figure 59-39 A, Female genitalia viewed axially in a 23-week fetus showing the typical appearance of the labia majora *(L).* **B,** In the same fetus the labia minora *(LM)* are represented as linear structures between the labia majora.

CONGENITAL MALFORMATIONS OF THE GENITAL SYSTEM

Although congenital malformations of the genital organs are rare, the sonographic team may be requested to determine the gender of the fetus when a gender-linked disorder is considered (i.e., hemophilia or aqueductal stenosis). Because these conditions usually occur in male fetuses, identification of male genitalia aids in counseling and diagnostic testing. Likewise the demonstration of abnormal fetal genitalia may be indicative of syndromes of the endocrine and genital systems. In the female, positive identification of the labia is as essential to the diagnosis as demonstration of the penis and scrotum is in the male.

Early determination of gender is difficult since development of the external genitalia is similar for both sexes until after the 11th week of gestation, when external genital organs become fully differentiated. The most useful scanning plane is the sagittal plane. The clitoris or penis may be seen after the first 11 weeks of gestation.

HYPOSPADIAS

Incomplete fusion of the urogenital folds may cause abnormal openings of the urethra along the ventral aspect of the penis **(hypospadias).** This disorder occurs in 1 in every 300 infants. The abnormal urethral orifice may be near the glans penis (glandular hypospadias). The other type of hypospadias is called *penile hypospadias.* This disorder results from defective closure of the urogenital folds, causing the urethra to open on the ventral surface of the body of the penis.

MALFORMATIONS OF THE UTERUS AND VAGINA

The formation of the uterus is dependent on the fusion of two paramesonephric ducts (müllerian ducts). If this fusion is incomplete, various forms of duplication of the uterus and/or vagina may occur. Complete failure of the fusion will give rise to a duplication of the entire female genital tract, **uterus didelphys** (double uterus and double vagina). Duplication of the uterus **(bicornuate uterus)** with one vagina may also occur. If only one paramesonephric duct develops, a **unicornuate uterus** (single uterine tube and horn) is formed (see Chapter 35).

HYDROCELE

Hydrocele occurs in the male fetus and is seen as an accumulation of serous fluid surrounding the testicle, resulting from a communication with the peritoneal cavity. Lesions may occur as unilateral or bilateral and are generally benign.

DESCENT OF THE GONADS

The gonads eventually descend from the abdomen to the pelvis. As this occurs, a diverticulum of the peritoneum, the processus vaginalis, protrudes through the anterior abdominal wall to form the primordium of the inguinal canal. The processus vaginalis is attached to a ligament that extends from the caudal pole of the gonad to the labioscrotal swelling.

In the male, the testes remain near the deep inguinal rings until the 28th week. They descend through the inguinal canals and enter the scrotum before birth. Failure to complete this descent results in undescended testes, **cryptorchidism.** The distal part of the processus vaginalis persists as the tunica vaginalis of the testis.

In the female, the ligament attaches to the uterus to form the ovarium ligament and the round ligament. The processus vaginalis completely obliterates.

AMBIGUOUS GENITALIA

The sonographer must be careful diagnosing ambiguous genitalia because penile and clitoral size may vary in the normal fetus. True **hermaphroditism** is a rare condition in which both ovarian and testicular tissues are present. The internal and external genitalia are variable. Most fetuses will have a normal karyotype, but some are mosaics (46,XX/46,XY). Determination of fetal gender may be critical in establishing a correct diagnosis (Figure 59-40).

Female Pseudohermaphrodites. The female fetus with pseudohermaphroditism has a 46,XX karyotype. The most common cause is congenital virilizing adrenal hyperplasia that causes masculinization of the external genitalia (enlarged clitoris, abnormalities of the urogenital sinus, and partial fusion of the labia majora).

Male Pseudohermaphrodites. The male fetus with pseudohermaphroditism has testes and a 46,XY karyotype. There is variable external and internal genitalia depending on the development of the penis and genital ducts.

OTHER PELVIC MASSES

Hydrometrocolpos. A collection of fluid in the vagina and uterus is called hydrometrocolpos. Hydrometrocolpos in conjunction with a double uterus and septated vagina (vagina divided by a septum into two components) has been described. The fluid collection may be so large that it extends into the abdominal cavity or may cause compression of the ureters and hydronephrosis of the kidneys.

Sonographic Findings. On ultrasound examination, hydrometrocolpos appears as a hypoechoic "cystlike" mass posterior to the bladder in the area of the uterus. These masses may be predominantly cystic, may contain midlevel echoes, or may have fluid-debris levels. Echoes within these masses may result from mucous secretions.

Ovarian Cyst. An **ovarian cyst** may also occur in the female fetus. The ovarian mass results from maternal hormonal stimulation and is usually benign. Differential considerations would include a mesenteric cyst, a urachal cyst, or an enteric duplication.

Sonographic Findings. The ovarian cyst often appears multiseptated and bilateral. The mass may twist on itself, which may lead to torsion, rupture, or intestinal obstruction.

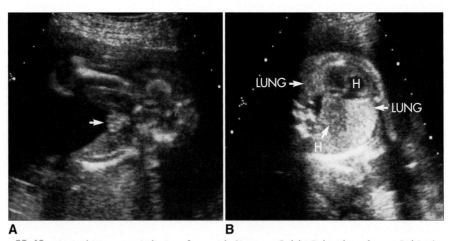

A   **B**

Figure 59-40 A, Ambiguous genitalia in a fetus with Simpson-Golabi-Behmel syndrome. Labia *(arrow)* were observed in this fetus with a male karyotype. Other multiple anomalies included an umbilical hernia, hydronephrosis, a 12-mm nuchal fold, and a right diaphragmatic hernia (shown in **B**). *H,* Heart.

REFERENCES

1. Allen KS and others: Effects of maternal hydration on fetal renal pyelectasis, *Radiology* 163:8-7, 1987.

2. Ambrosino MM and others: Prenatal diagnosis of nephroblastomatosis in two siblings, *J Ultrasound Med* 9:49, 1990.

3. Harrison MR, Golbus MS, Filly RA: Congenital hydronephrosis. In Harrison MR, Golbus MS, Filly RA, editors: *The unborn patient: prenatal diagnosis and management,* Orlando, Fla, 1984, Grune & Stratton.

SELECTED BIBLIOGRAPHY

Anderson NG and others: Detection of obstructive uropathy in the fetus: predictive value of sonographic measurements of renal pelvic diameter at various gestational ages, *Am J Roentgenol* 164:719, 1995.

Anderson NG, Allan RB, Abbott GKD: Fluctuating fetal or neonatal renal pelvis: marker of high-grade vesicoureteral reflux, *Pediatr Nephrol* 19(7):749-753, 2004.

Apocalypsa GT, Oliverira EA, Rabelo EA and others: Outcome of apparent ureteropelvic junction obstruction identified by investigation of fetal hydronephrosis, *Int Urol Nephrol* 35(4):441-448, 2003.

Babcook CJ and others: Effect of maternal hydration on mild fetal pyelectasis, *J Ultrasound Med* 17:539, 1998.

Bateman GA, Giles WK, Enland SL: Renal venous Doppler sonography in preeclampsia, *J Ultrasound Med* 23(12):1607-1611, 2004.

Berkowitz RL and others: Fetal urinary tract obstruction: what is the role of surgical intervention in utero? *Am J Obstet Gynecol* 144:367, 1982.

Birewar S, Zawada ET Jr: Early onset polycystic kidney disease: how early is early? *S D J Med* 56(11):465-468, 2003.

Bobrowski RA and others: In utero progression of isolated renal pelvis dilation, *Am J Perinatol* 14:423, 1997.

Borrelli AL, Borrelli P, Di Domenico A and others: The incidence of chromosomal anomalies in fetuses affected by mild renal pyelectasis, *Minerva Ginecol* 56(2):137-140, 2004.

Callen DW, editor: *Ultrasonography in obstetrics and gynecology,* ed 4, Philadelphia, 2000, WB Saunders.

Chitty LS, Altman DG: Charts of fetal size: kidney and renal pelvis measurements, *Prenat Diagn* 23(11):891-897, 2003.

Curtis MR and others: Prenatal ultrasound characterization of the suprarenal mass: distinction between neuroblastoma and subdiaphragmatic extralobar pulmonary sequestration, *J Ultrasound Med* 16:75, 1997.

DeVore GR: The value of color Doppler sonography in the diagnosis of renal agenesis, *J Ultrasound Med* 14:443, 1995.

Dremsek PA and others: Renal pyelectasis in fetuses and neonates: diagnostic value of renal pelvis diameter in pre- and postnatal sonographic screening, *Am J Roentgenol* 168:1017, 1997.

Eckoldt F, Heling KS, Woderich R: Posterior urethral valves: prenatal diagnostic signs and outcome, *Urol Int* 73(4):296-301, 2004.

Grignon A and others: Urinary tract dilatation in utero: classification and clinical applications, *Radiology* 160:645, 1986.

Hadlock FP and others: Sonography of fetal urinary tract anomalies, *Am J Roentgenol* 137:261, 1981.

Hayden SA and others: Posterior urethral obstruction: prenatal sonographic findings and clinical outcome in fourteen cases, *J Ultrasound Med* 7:371, 1988.

Hobbins JC and others: Antenatal diagnosis of renal anomalies with ultrasound: obstructive uropathy, *Am J Obstet Gynecol* 148:868, 1984.

Ismaili K, Ayni FE, Martin Wissing K and others: Long-term clinical outcome of infants with mild and moderate fetal pyelectasis: validation of neonatal ultrasound as a screening tool to detect significant nephrouropathies, *J Pediatr* 144(6):759-765, 2004.

John U, Kahler C, Schultz S and others: The impact of fetal renal pelvic diameter on postnatal outcome, *Prenat Diagn* 24(8):591-595, 2004.

Kohler M, Pease PW, Upadhayay V: Megacystis-microcolon-intestinal hypoperistalsis syndrome (MMIHS) in siblings: case report and review of the literature, *Eur J Pediatr Surg* 14(5):362-367, 2004.

Maizels M, Alpert SA, Houston JT and others: Fetal bladder sagittal length: a simple monitor to assess normal and enlarged fetal bladder size, and forecast outcome, *J Urol* 172(S Pt 1):1995-1999, 2004.

Mazza V, Di Monte I, Pati M and others: Sonographic biometrical range of external genitalia differentiation in the first trimester of pregnancy: analysis of 2593 cases, *Prenat Diag* 24(9):677-684, 2004.

Montemarano H and others: Bladder distention and pyelectasis in the male fetus: causes, comparisons, and contrasts, *J Ultrasound Med* 17:743, 1998.

Moore KL: *Before we are born,* ed 3, Toronto, 1989, WB Saunders.

Nyberg DA, McGahan JP, Pretorius DH and others, editors: *Diagnostic ultrasound of fetal anomalies: text and atlas,* Philadelphia, 2003, Lippincott, Williams & Wilkins.

Odibo AO, Raab E, Elovitz M and others: Prenatal mild pyelectasis: evaluating the thresholds of renal pelvic diameter associated with normal postnatal renal function, *J Ultrasound Med* 23(4):513-517, 2004.

Pinette MG, Wax JR, Blackstone J: Normal growth and development of fetal external genitalia demonstrated by sonography, *J Clin Ultrasound* 31(9):465-472, 2003.

Potter EL: Bilateral absence of ureters and kidneys: a report of 50 cases, *Obstet Gynecol* 25:3, 1965.

Romero R and others: The diagnosis of congenital renal anomalies with ultrasound. II. Infantile polycystic kidney disease, *Am J Obstet Gynecol* 150:259, 1984.

Russ PD and others: Hydrometrocolpos, uterus didelphys and septate vagina: an antenatal sonographic diagnosis, *J Ultrasound Med* 3:371, 1984.

Souzada MC, Oliverira EA, Pereira AK and others: Diagnostic accuracy of postnatal renal pelvic diameter as a predictor of uropathy: a prospective study, *Pediatr Radiol* 34(10):798-804, 2004.

Toiviainen-Salo S, Garel L, Grignon A and others: Fetal hydronephrosis: is there hope for consensus? *Pediatr Radiol* 34(7):519-529, 2004.

Vijayaraghavan SB, Nirmala AB: Complete duplication of urinary bladder and urethra: prenatal sonographic features, *Ultrasound Obstet Gynecol* 24(4):464-466, 2004.

Weinstein L, Anderson C: In utero diagnosis of Beckwith-Wiedemann syndrome by ultrasound, *Radiology* 134:474, 1980.

The Fetal Skeleton

Charlotte G. Henningsen

KEY TERMS

achondrogenesis – lethal autosomal-recessive short-limb dwarfism marked by long bone and trunk shortening, decreased echogenicity of the bones and spine, and "flipperlike" appendages

achondroplasia – a defect in the development of cartilage at the epiphyseal centers of the long bones producing short, square bones

craniosynostosis – early ossification of the calvarium with destruction of the sutures; hypertelorism frequently found in association; sonographically the fetal cranium may appear brachycephalic

heterozygous achondroplasia – short-limb dysplasia that manifests in the second trimester of pregnancy; conversion abnormality of cartilage to bone affecting the epiphyseal growth centers; extremities are notably shortened at birth, with a normal trunk and frequent enlargement of the head

homozygous achondroplasia – short-limb dwarfism affecting fetuses of achondroplastic parents

hypophosphatasia – congenital condition characterized by decreased mineralization of the bones resulting in "ribbon-like" and bowed limbs, underossified cranium, and compression of the chest; early death often occurs

osteogenesis imperfecta – metabolic disorder affecting the fetal collagen system that leads to varying forms of bone disease; intrauterine bone fractures, shortened long bones, poorly mineralized calvaria, and compression of the chest found in type II forms

polydactyly – anomalies of the hands or feet in which there is an addition of a digit; may be found in association with certain skeletal dysplasias

thanatophoric dysplasia – lethal short-limb dwarfism characterized by a notable reduction in the length of the long bones, pear-shaped chest, soft tissue redundancy, and frequently clover-leaf skull deformity and ventriculomegaly

EMBRYOLOGY OF THE FETAL SKELETON

The majority of the musculoskeletal system forms from the primitive mesoderm arising from mesenchymal cells that are the embryonic connective tissue. These cells arise from different regions of the body. The vertebral column and ribs arise from the somites, and the limbs arise from the lateral plate mesoderm. The formation of the head is more complex in that the cranial bones that form the roof and base of the skull arise from mesenchymal cells of the primitive mesoderm, but the facial bones actually arise from mesenchymal cells arising from the neural crest, which is ectodermal in origin. The skeleton initially appears as cartilaginous forms that later undergo ossification.

Limb development begins the 26th or 27th day after conception with the appearance of upper limb buds. Lower extremity development begins 2 days later. Although the stages of development for the upper and lower extremities are the same, lower extremity development continues to lag behind that of the upper extremities. Initially the limbs have a paddle shape with a ridge of thickened ectoderm, known as the apical ectodermal ridge, at the apex of each bud. Digital rays begin to differentiate from the apical ectodermal ridge around day 41 through a process of cell death of the ridge between the digits. The fingers are distinctly evident by day 49, although they are still webbed, and by the eighth week of development the fingers are longer. The development of the feet and toes is essentially complete by the ninth week, although the soles of the feet are still turned inward at this time.

Anomalies of the skeletal system often result from genetic factors, though the cause may be unknown or be the result of environmental factors, including drug or mechanical effects.

ABNORMALITIES OF THE SKELETON

Skeletal dysplasia is the term used to describe abnormal growth and density of cartilage and bone. Dwarfism occurs secondary to a skeletal dysplasia and refers to a disproportionately short stature. There are over 100 types of skeletal dysplasias, and not all of them are amenable to sonographic detection. The perinatal team may be able to isolate a skeletal dysplasia when abnormal skeletal structures are observed, such as bone shortening or hypomineralization.

Some skeletal dysplasias are incompatible with life. The lethal forms characteristically are extremely severe in their prenatal appearance, as with severe micromelia. Nonlethal skeletal dysplasias tend to manifest in a milder form. The sonographer should become familiar with the sonographic characteristics of the more common skeletal dysplasias that can be diagnosed in utero.

There are multiple anomalies of the musculoskeletal system that may be identified with ultrasound. Many of these osteochondrodysplasias have similar features, although often there are distinguishing features that can lead to a diagnosis. A list of short-limb skeletal dysplasias, ultrasound characteristics, and their distinguishing features are listed in Table 60-1.

SONOGRAPHIC EVALUATION OF SKELETAL DYSPLASIAS

The patient whose fetus is at risk for a skeletal dysplasia is commonly referred to a maternal-fetal center for genetic counseling and a targeted ultrasound. Although many skeletal dysplasias are inherited, sporadic occurrences and new mutations do occur, so it is important to screen for skeletal dysplasias as part of every obstetric ultrasound examination. The majority of prenatally diagnosed skeletal dysplasia occurs in association with polyhydramnios or other fetal anomalies or when there is a risk for recurrence.

When a skeletal dysplasia is suspected, the protocol of the obstetric ultrasound examination should be adjusted to include the following criteria:

TABLE 60-1	OSTEOCHONDRODYSPLASIA FINDINGS	
Anomaly	Sonographic Findings	Distinguishing Characteristics
Thanatophoric dysplasia	Severe micromelia Macrocephaly Cloverleaf skull Narrow thorax	Cloverleaf skull
Achondrogenesis	Severe micromelia Macrocephaly Poor ossification of spine, skull Short thorax	Decreased ossification Severity of limb shortening
Achondroplasia	Rhizomelia Macrocephaly Trident hands	Rhizomelic shortening Trident hands
Camptomelic dysplasia	Hypoplastic fibulas Long bone bowing Micrognathia Small thorax Talipes	Fibula hypoplasia Bowing affects lower extremities
Osteogenesis imperfecta (type II)	Severe micromelia Generalized hypomineralization Narrow thorax Multiple fractures	Normal head size Hypomineralization of skull Multiple fractures
Short-rib polydactyly syndrome	Micromelia Narrow thorax Facial cleft Polydactyly	Facial anomalies Polydactyly
Hypophosphatasia	Mild limb shortening Narrow thorax Limb fractures and bowing	Hypomineralization of skull Fractures

1. Assess limb shortening. All long bones should be measured. A skeletal dysplasia is suspected when limb lengths fall more than 2 standard deviations below the mean (Tables 60-2 and 60-3).

2. Assess bone contour. Thickness, abnormal bowing or curvature, fractures, and a ribbonlike appearance should be noted.

3. Estimate degree of ossification. Decreased attenuation of the bones with decreased shadowing suggests hypomineralization. Special attention should be focused toward this assessment of the cranium, spine, ribs, and long bones.

4. Evaluate the thoracic circumference and shape. A long, narrow chest or a bell-shaped chest may be indicative of specific dysplasias.

5. Survey for coexistent hand and foot anomalies, such as talipes and polydactyly.

6. Evaluate the face and profile for facial clefts, frontal bossing, micrognathia, hypertelorism, and other facial anomalies that may be associated with skeletal dysplasias.

7. Survey for other associated anomalies, such as hydrocephaly, heart defects, and nonimmune hydrops.

TABLE 60-2 LENGTH OF THE BONES OF THE LEG: NORMAL VALUES

Week No.	Tibia Percentile 5th	50th	95th	Fibula Percentile 5th	50th	95th
12	—	7	—	—	6	—
13	—	10	—	—	9	—
14	7	12	17	6	12	19
15	9	15	20	9	15	21
16	12	17	22	13	18	23
17	15	20	25	13	21	28
18	17	22	27	15	23	31
19	20	25	30	19	26	33
20	22	27	33	21	28	36
21	25	30	35	24	31	37
22	27	32	38	27	33	39
23	30	35	40	28	35	42
24	32	37	42	29	37	45
25	34	40	45	34	40	45
26	37	42	47	36	42	47
27	39	44	49	37	44	50
28	41	46	51	38	45	53
29	43	48	53	41	47	54
30	45	50	55	43	49	56
31	47	52	57	42	51	59
32	48	54	59	42	52	63
33	50	55	60	46	54	62
34	52	57	62	46	55	65
35	53	58	64	51	57	62
36	55	60	65	54	58	63
37	56	61	67	54	59	65
38	58	63	68	56	61	65
39	59	64	69	56	62	67
40	61	66	71	59	63	67
	mm	mm	mm	mm	mm	mm

From Jeanty P, Romero R, editors: *Obstetrical ultrasound,* New York, 1984, McGraw-Hill.

TABLE 60-3 LENGTH OF THE BONES OF THE ARM: NORMAL VALUES

Week No.	Ulna Percentile 5th	50th	95th	Radius Percentile 5th	50th	95th
12	—	7	—	—	7	—
13	5	10	15	6	10	14
14	8	13	18	8	13	17
15	11	16	21	11	15	20
16	13	18	23	13	18	22
17	16	21	26	14	20	26
18	19	24	29	15	22	29
19	21	26	31	20	24	29
20	24	29	34	22	27	32
21	26	31	36	24	29	33
22	28	33	38	27	31	34
23	31	36	41	26	32	39
24	33	38	43	26	34	42
25	35	40	45	31	36	41
26	37	42	47	32	37	43
27	39	44	49	33	39	45
28	41	46	51	33	40	48
29	43	48	53	36	42	47
30	44	49	54	36	43	49
31	46	51	56	38	44	50
32	48	53	58	37	45	53
33	49	54	59	41	46	51
34	51	56	61	40	47	53
35	52	57	62	41	48	54
36	53	58	63	39	48	57
37	55	60	65	45	49	53
38	56	61	66	45	49	54
39	57	62	67	45	50	54
40	58	63	68	46	50	55
	mm	mm	mm	mm	mm	mm

From Jeanty P, Romero R, editors: *Obstetrical ultrasound,* New York, 1984, McGraw-Hill.

The manifestation of skeletal dysplasias varies based on the specific dysplasia. Long bones are affected in different patterns (Figure 60-1) according to the dysplasia. Rhizomelia is shortening of the proximal bone segment (humerus and femur). Mesomelia refers to shortening of the middle segments (radius/ulna and tibia/fibula). Micromelia describes the shortening of the entire extremity. Sonographic examination of the long bones should include an assessment to define whether there is segmental shortening or micromelia, because this will aid in the diagnosis.

THANATOPHORIC DYSPLASIA

Thanatophoric dysplasia is the most common lethal skeletal dysplasia and occurs in 0.2 to 0.5 in 10,000 births (Figure 60-2). The term *thanatophoric* comes from the Greek word *thanatoos,* which means death personified. The two main subdivisions of thanatophoric dysplasia are types I and II. Type I is characterized by short, curved femurs and flat vertebral bodies. Type II is characterized by straight, short femurs, flat vertebral bodies, and a cloverleaf skull. Most cases of thanatophoric dysplasia are sporadic occurrences and the result of mutations in the fibroblast growth factor receptor 3 (FGFR3) gene. Prenatal molecular analysis can aid in making the definitive diagnosis.

The prognosis for thanatophoric dysplasia is extremely grim. It is considered a lethal anomaly, with most infants dying shortly after birth as a result of pulmonary hypoplasia, which results from the narrow thorax.

Sonographic Findings. The sonographic features of thanatophoric dysplasia include the following:

- Severe micromelia (Figure 60-3, *A* and *B*), especially of the proximal bones (rhizomelia)
- Cloverleaf deformity (Kleeblattschädel skull) occurs as a result of premature **craniosynostosis**
- Narrow thorax with shortened ribs (Figure 60-3, *C* and *D*)
- Protuberant abdomen
- Frontal bossing (bulging forehead)
- Hypertelorism (widely spaced eyes)
- Flat vertebral bodies (platyspondyly)

Other sonographic findings that may be associated with thanatophoric dysplasia include severe polyhydramnios, hydrocephalus, and nonimmune hydrops.

ACHONDROPLASIA

Achondroplasia is the most common nonlethal skeletal dysplasia and occurs in 2.53 of every 100,000 births. It results from decreased endochondral bone formation, which produces short, squat bones. It is most commonly the result of a spontaneous mutation but can also be transmitted in an autosomal fashion. Advanced paternal age increases the risk for this dysplasia.

The prognosis for achondroplasia depends on the form. **Heterozygous achondroplasia** has a good survival rate with normal intelligence and a normal lifespan. Health problems may include neurologic complications that may require orthopedic or neurologic surgical intervention. **Homozygous achondroplasia** is considered lethal (with the sonographic findings also more severe, including a narrow thorax), with most infants dying shortly after birth from respiratory complications.

Sonographic Findings. The sonographic features of achondroplasia may not be evident until after 22 weeks of gestation,

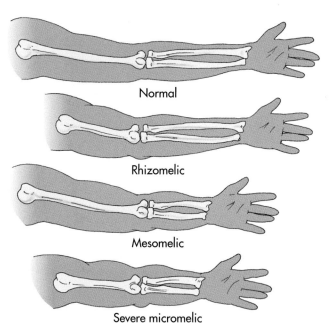

Figure 60-1 Varieties of short-limb dysplasia according to the affected bones. Rhizomelic dysplasia is characterized by shortening of the proximal long bones (humerus and femur). Mesomelic dysplasia is described as shortening of the distal extremities (radius/ulna and tibia/fibula). Severe micromelia produces shortening of both proximal and distal extremities.

Normal

Rhizomelic

Mesomelic

Severe micromelic

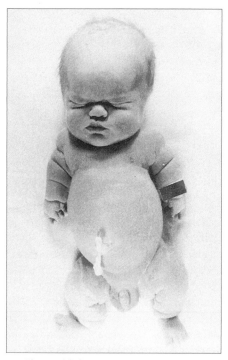

Figure 60-2 Thanatophoric neonate.

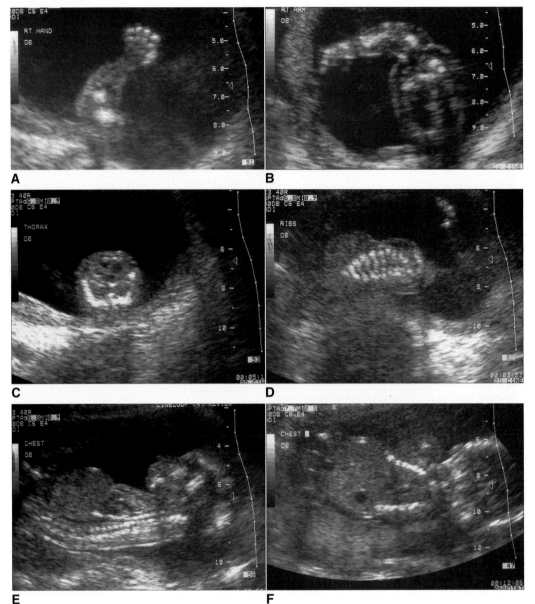

Figure 60-3 Lethal skeletal dysplasia consistent with thanatophoric dysplasia at a gestational age of 18 weeks, 1 day. **A** and **B,** The right arm demonstrates micromelia. The lower extremities were also short, with the femurs measuring a gestational age of 14 weeks. **C,** The thorax was very narrow. **D,** The ribs were short. The abdomen was protuberant (**E**) and compared with the narrow thorax (**F**) gives the appearance of a "champagne cork."

when biometry becomes abnormal. Sonographic findings include the following:

- Rhizomelia
- Macrocephaly
- Trident hands (short proximal and middle phalanges)
- A depressed nasal bridge
- Frontal bossing
- Mild ventriculomegaly may be identified

ACHONDROGENESIS

Achondrogenesis is a rare, lethal skeletal dysplasia occurring in 2.3 to 2.8 per 100,000 births. It is caused by cartilage abnormali-

ties that result in abnormal bone formation and hypomineralization. The two types of achondrogenesis are types I (Parenti-Fraccaro) and II (Langer-Saldino). Type I is considered more severe and is transmitted in an autosomal recessive mode, whereas Type II is less severe and is the result of a spontaneous mutation.

The prognosis for achondrogenesis is grim. It is a lethal abnormality with infants either being stillborn or dying shortly after birth from pulmonary hypoplasia.

Sonographic Findings. The sonographic features (Figure 60-4) of achondrogenesis include the following:

- Severe micromelia
- Decreased or absent ossification of the spine

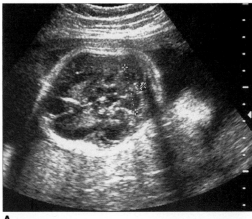

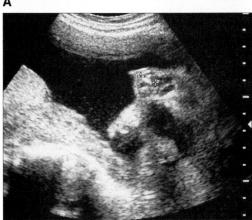

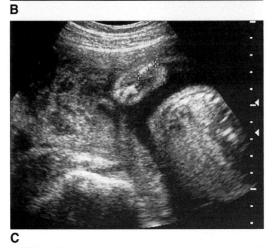

Figure 60-4 This fetus at 24 weeks' gestation presented with decreased ossification that was noted in the spine and (A) calvarium, which was compressible. Severe micromelia is evidenced in the (B) femur and (C) humerus, which measured consistent with a 13 weeks' gestation. Achondrogenesis was diagnosed following delivery, and the baby died shortly thereafter. (From Henningsen C: *Clinical guide to ultrasonography,* St Louis, 2004, Mosby.)

- Macrocephaly
- Short trunk
- Short thorax and short ribs
- Micrognathia
- Polyhydramnios
- Hydrops possibly identified

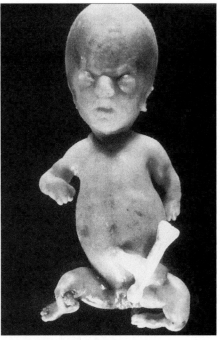

Figure 60-5 Postmortem photograph of neonate with osteogenesis imperfecta (type II).

OSTEOGENESIS IMPERFECTA

Osteogenesis imperfecta is a rare disorder of collagen production leading to brittle bones; manifestations in the teeth, skin, and ligaments; and blue sclera. There are four classifications, types I to IV. Types I and IV are the mildest forms, and it would be unlikely that a diagnosis would be made in utero. Types I and IV are transmitted in an autosomal-dominant fashion. Type III is a severe form that may be transmitted in an autosomal-dominant or autosomal-recessive manner. Type II (Figure 60-5) is considered the most severe form of osteogenesis imperfecta, having a lethal outcome. It has a prevalence of 1 in 60,000 births and is inherited in autosomal-dominant or recessive fashion or may result from a spontaneous mutation.

The prognosis for osteogenesis imperfecta depends on the type. Children with types I and IV may have multiple fractures during childhood and may be short. Type I children may also suffer with kyphoscoliosis and deafness. Because of the severity of the brittle bones and multiple fractures, osteogenesis imperfecta type III may produce significant handicaps with progressive deformities of the long bones and spine. Infants with type II usually die shortly after birth because of respiratory complications.

Sonographic Findings. The sonographic features of osteogenesis imperfecta type II include the following:

- Generalized hypomineralization of the bones, especially the calvarium (Figure 60-6)
- Multiple fractures of the long bones, ribs, and spine (Figure 60-7)
- Narrow thorax (see Figure 60-6, *A*)
- Micromelia (Figure 60-8)

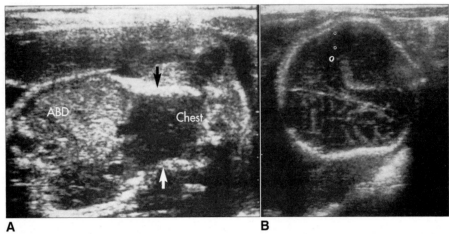

Figure 60-6   A, In the fetus shown in Figure 60-8 with osteogenesis imperfecta (type II), a small thoracic cavity *(arrows)* is shown. *ABD,* Abdomen. **B,** In the same fetus, hypomineralization of the skull is evident. Note the improved resolution of brain anatomy because of the lack of calvarial calcification.

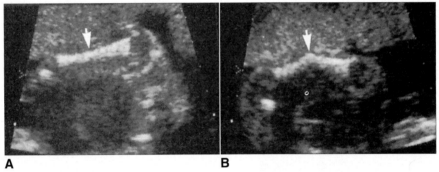

Figure 60-7   Images of both femurs in a 22-week fetus. **A,** The femur *(arrow)* is normal compared with **B,** in which a femoral fracture *(arrow)* is shown. Other long bones appeared normal in length and contour. There was hypomineralization of the spine. Osteogenesis imperfecta type I or IV is considered.

In addition to these findings, brain structures are clearly visualized because of the hypomineralization of the calvarium. The calvarium will also be compressible. The multiple fractures that have occurred during the course of pregnancy may leave the bones bowed, thickened, and sharply angulated. Polyhydramnios may also be evident.

The sonographic features of osteogenesis imperfecta type III are similar to those of type II, though it is less severe.

CONGENITAL HYPOPHOSPHATASIA

Congenital **hypophosphatasia** is a condition that presents with diffuse hypomineralization of the bone caused by an alkaline phosphatase deficiency. The occurrence rate is 1 per 100,000 births. It is an inherited condition transmitted in an autosomal-recessive manner. Congenital hypophosphatasia may have features similar to osteogenesis imperfecta and achondrogenesis. Diagnosis can be confirmed with alkaline phosphatase assay, which can be achieved through fetal blood sampling or chorionic villus sampling, or through DNA analysis.

Congenital hypophosphatasia is a lethal disorder, with death usually occurring shortly after birth as a result of respiratory complications.

Sonographic Findings. The sonographic features of congenital hypophosphatasia include the following:

- Diffuse hypomineralization of the bones
- Moderate to severe micromelia
- Extremities that may be bowed, fractured, or absent
- Poorly ossified cranium with well-visualized brain structures
- Small thoracic cavity

DIASTROPHIC DYSPLASIA

Diastrophic dysplasia is a very rare disorder characterized by micromelia, talipes, cleft palate, micrognathia, scoliosis, short stature, earlobe deformities, and hand abnormalities (Figure 60-9). It is inherited in an autosomal-recessive pattern.

The prognosis for diastrophic dysplasia is variable. There is an increase in infant mortality because of respiratory complications related to the micrognathia and kyphoscoliosis. This is not a lethal disorder, with most patients having a normal life span and normal intelligence. Adult height is usually less than 4 feet, and orthopedic abnormalities can cause significant handicaps.

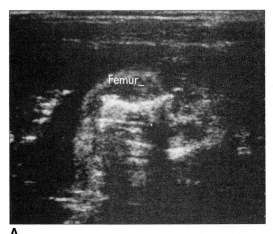

A

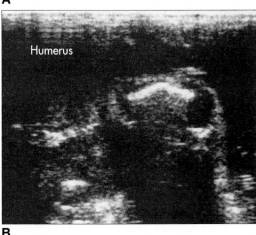

B

Figure 60-8 **A,** Marked micromelia in a 30-week fetus with osteogenesis imperfecta (type II). The femur measured 29 mm (normal for 30 weeks is 57 mm). **B,** In the same fetus, a humeral fracture is shown. Humeral length measured 27 mm (normal for 30 weeks is 51 mm).

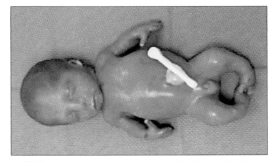

Figure 60-9 Postmortem photograph of a fetus with diastrophic dysplasia. (Courtesy Armando Fuentes, MD, Director, Maternal Fetal Center, Orlando, Fla.)

Sonographic Findings. The sonographic features of diastrophic dysplasia include the following:

- Micromelia (Figure 60-10)
- Talipes
- Fixed abducted thumb (hitchhiker thumb; see Figure 60-10, *B*)

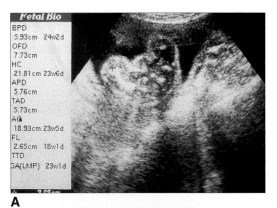

A

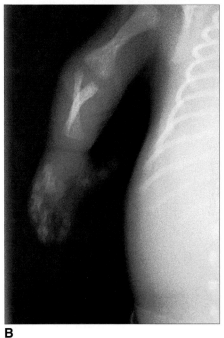

B

Figure 60-10 Diastrophic dysplasia imaged at 23 weeks and 1 day. **A,** Micromelia is demonstrated in this femur measuring 18 weeks, 1 day. The thoracic circumference was also small. **B,** Postmortem radiograph demonstrates the "hitchhiker thumb."

- Scoliosis
- Talipes (clubfoot)
- Micrognathia (small chin)
- Cleft palate

CAMPTOMELIC DYSPLASIA

Camptomelic (bent bone) dysplasia is a group of lethal skeletal dysplasias that are characterized by bowing of the long bones. This rare, short-limbed dysplasia occurs in 1 per 150,000 births. Most cases occur as a spontaneous mutation, but camptomelic dysplasia is also inherited in an autosomal-recessive pattern.

Camptomelia dysplasia is considered a lethal anomaly, with most infants dying in the neonatal period because of pulmonary hypoplasia. Infants surviving the neonatal period usually die within the first year of life and suffer with respiratory and feeding problems, are developmentally delayed, and are mentally retarded.

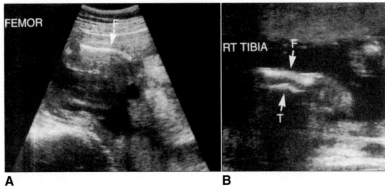

Figure 60-11 **A,** Camptomelic dysplasia and Swyer syndrome in a 20-week fetus with femoral bowing *(F)* found bilaterally. The femoral lengths were normal. **B,** In the same fetus, the tibias *(T)* were short and hypoplastic with sharp anterior bowing of the midshaft of the bone. Distal bowing was also observed. The fibulas *(F)* were hypoplastic and bowed. The upper extremities were normal in length without bowing or angulation. Bilateral hydronephrosis was observed. Examination of the neonate and radiologic findings (see Figure 60-12) confirmed the diagnosis of camptomelic dysplasia. Gonadal dysgenesis (female internal and external genitalia with a male karyotype) was consistent with Swyer syndrome. The neonate had other characteristic signs of the disorder, including tall and narrow hypomineralized ischial bones, absent pubic bone ossification, receding chin, hypoplastic cervical vertebra, elongated clavicles, hypoplastic scapulae, and flexion abnormalities of the feet.

Sonographic Findings. The sonographic features of camptomelic dysplasia include the following:

- Bowing of the long bones with the lower extremities affected most severely (Figures 60-11 and 60-12)
- Small thorax
- Hypoplastic fibulas
- Hypoplastic scapulae
- Hypertelorism
- Cleft palate
- Micrognathia
- Talipes (Figures 60-13 and 60-14)
- Hydrocephalus
- Polyhydramnios
- Hydronephrosis

ROBERTS' SYNDROME

Roberts' syndrome is a rare condition characterized by phocomelia and facial anomalies. Roberts' syndrome is an autosomal-recessive disorder; it is also known as a pseudothalidomide syndrome.

The prognosis for Roberts' syndrome is poor. Stillbirth and infant mortality are common. Survivors are growth restricted and have severe mental retardation.

Sonographic Findings. The sonographic features of Roberts' syndrome include the following:

- Phocomelia with the upper extremities more severely affected
- Bilateral cleft lip and palate
- Hypertelorism
- Microcephaly
- Cardiovascular, renal, and gastrointestinal anomalies may be identified

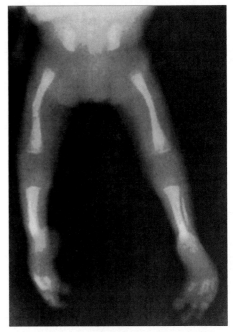

Figure 60-12 Radiograph of neonate shown in Figures 60-11, 60-13, and 60-14 with camptomelic dysplasia and Swyer syndrome. The radiograph demonstrates the lower extremity deformities, including anterior lateral bowing of the femurs at the midshaft. Both tibias are short, with sharp anterior bowing at midshaft and mild bowing at the distal ends. The fibulas are hypoplastic and bowed. Minimal ischial ossification and absent mineralization of the pubic bone are shown. Hypoplastic cervical vertebrae, normal ribs, elongated clavicles, and hypoplastic distorted scapulae are additional findings and upper extremity bones are normal.

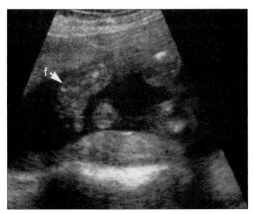

Figure 60-13   In the fetus with camptomelic dysplasia and Swyer syndrome, as shown in Figures 60-11, 60-13, and 60-14, abnormal plantar flexion of the feet is shown. The feet *(f)* are notably supinated, with curvature to the soles of the feet. The toes are plantar flexed, with the great toes separated by flexion.

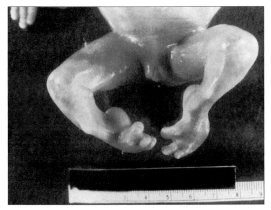

Figure 60-14   Postmortem photograph of neonate shown in Figures 60-11, 60-12, and 60-13, with camptomelic dysplasia and Swyer syndrome. Note the markedly angulated lower legs with protrusion of the tibia anteriorly at the midshaft. The fibulas were hypoplastic and bowed. The feet, as shown in Figure 60-13, are abnormally rotated with prominent heels (rocker-bottom feet).

SHORT-RIB POLYDACTYLY SYNDROME

Short-rib polydactyly syndrome is a lethal skeletal dysplasia characterized by short ribs, short limbs, and **polydactyly**. There are four types of this dysplasia, which are inherited in an autosomal-recessive manner. Type I is also known as Saldino-Noonan syndrome, type II is also known as Majewski syndrome, and type III is known as Naumoff syndrome. Type IV, Beemer-Langer dysplasia, was included in this group of short-rib dysplasias in the 1992 International Classification of Osteochondrodysplasias.

Short-rib polydactyly syndrome is considered a lethal anomaly. Most infants die shortly after birth as a result of pulmonary hypoplasia.

Sonographic Findings. Common sonographic features of short-rib polydactyly syndrome include the following:

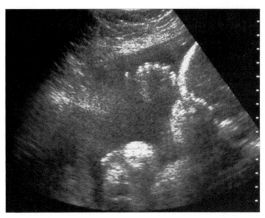

Figure 60-15   Polydactyly of the fetal hands is identified. (From Henningsen C: *Clinical guide to ultrasonography,* St Louis, 2004, Mosby.)

- Narrow thorax with short ribs
- Polydactyly (Figure 60-15)
- Micromelia
- Midline facial cleft

Other sonographic findings associated with short-rib dysplasias include anomalies of the central nervous system, cardiovascular system, and genitourinary tract. Polyhydramnios may also be identified. Saldino-Noonan and Naumoff syndromes are usually not associated with cleft lip and palate, and polydactyly may not always be present in Beemer-Langer dysplasia.

JEUNE'S SYNDROME

Jeune's syndrome, also known as asphyxiating thoracic dysplasia, is a skeletal dysplasia characterized by a very narrow thorax. The prevalence of Jeune's syndrome is 1 in 100,000 to 130,000 births, and it is inherited in an autosomal-recessive manner. Two types of Jeune's syndrome have been described, and there is a range of severity with the most severe form resulting in death because of pulmonary hypoplasia, which results from the narrow thorax.

Sonographic Findings. The sonographic features of Jeune's syndrome include the following:

- Small thorax
- Rhizomelia
- Renal dysplasia
- Polydactyly (less common)

ELLIS–VAN CREVELD SYNDROME

Ellis–van Creveld syndrome is also known as chondroectodermal dysplasia. The prevalence is 1 in 60,000 births, with an increased frequency in the Amish community. It is inherited in an autosomal-recessive pattern.

Ellis–van Creveld syndrome may present with a narrow thorax, causing pulmonary hypoplasia, and heart defects, the most common of which is the atrial septal defect (ASD). Approximately one half of these patients will die during infancy from cardiorespiratory complications. Other features identified with this syndrome include abnormal teeth, hypoplastic nails, and thin hair. Survivors have normal intellect and are short in stature.

Sonographic Findings. The sonographic features of Ellis-van Creveld include the following:

- Limb shortening
- Narrow thorax
- Polydactyly (see Figure 60-15)
- Heart defects (50% to 60%)

CAUDAL REGRESSION SYNDROME/SIRENOMELIA

Caudal regression syndrome (CRS) includes a range of malformations of the caudal end of the neural tube. Sirenomelia is an anomaly in which there is fusion of the lower extremities. Sirenomelia has been considered the extreme form of CRS, but it is currently thought to be a separate entity. The overall incidence of CRS is unknown; the incidence of sirenomelia is reported to be 1 in 60,000 births, with a male prevalence of 3 to 1.

The cause of CRS is not completely understood, although it has been associated with diabetes. Genetic factors have also been linked with this disorder. Vascular hypoperfusion is thought to be a causative factor in sirenomelia, with a single umbilical artery commonly associated that may divert blood flow to the caudal end. Sirenomelia is also associated with monozygotic twinning.

The prognosis for caudal regression syndrome depends on the severity and the associated anomalies. Neurologic and orthopedic evaluations with their interventional techniques can help to reduce and correct deformities and minimize handicaps. Sirenomelia is considered a lethal anomaly because of the severe renal anomalies that result in oligohydramnios and pulmonary hypoplasia.

Sonographic Findings. Sonographic features of caudal regression syndrome include the following:

- Sacral agenesis (Figure 60-16)
- Talipes
- Abnormal lumbar vertebrae, pelvic abnormalities, and contractures or decreased movement of the lower extremities may also be seen

Sonographic features of sirenomelia include the following:

- Variable fusion of the lower extremities (Figure 60-17)
- Bilateral renal agenesis
- Oligohydramnios
- Single umbilical artery

When severe oligohydramnios is present, a confident diagnosis with ultrasound may be difficult. Amnioinfusion and magnetic resonance imaging may be used to evaluate the severity of anomalies.

VACTERL ASSOCIATION

The VACTERL association is a group of anomalies that may occur together. In this sporadic group of anomalies, *v*ertebral defects, *a*nal atresia, *c*ardiac anomalies, *t*racheo *e*sophageal fistula, *r*enal anomalies, and *l*imb dysplasia may occur in combination. For the VACTERL association to be considered, three of these features must be identified. A single umbilical artery may also be identified. When the VACTERL association is seen with accompanying hydrocephalus, it has been termed VACTERL-H syndrome.

POSTURAL ANOMALIES

The normal development of the fetus requires movement. There are multiple events that can cause a decrease in fetal movement, including oligohydramnios, multiple gestations, and congenital uterine anomalies. Decreased movement may also be due to an abnormality of the fetal nerves, connective tissue, or musculature. These fetal conditions may not only cause a decrease or absence of fetal movement, but they may also result in abnormal contractures and postural deformities.

Arthrogryposis Multiplex Congenita. Arthrogryposis multiplex congenita is a condition marked by severe contractures of the extremities because of abnormal innervation and disorders of the muscles and connective tissue. It represents a group of disorders that may be inherited or sporadic.

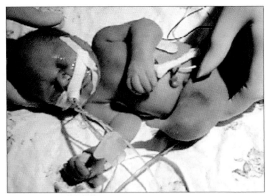

Figure 60-17   A neonate with sirenomelia. Note the fusion of the lower extremities. There was also bilateral renal agenesis, and the infant died shortly after birth. This was a twin pregnancy, and the other infant was normal. (Courtesy Armando Fuentes, MD, Director, Maternal Fetal Center, Orlando, Fla.)

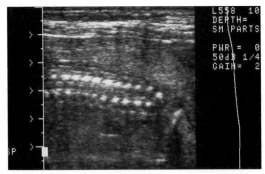

Figure 60-16   Sacral agenesis noted at 21 weeks of gestation. Note the lack of tapering usually seen in the lumbosacral area.

Sonographic Findings. The sonographic findings for arthrogryposis include the following:

- Rigid extremities
- Flexed arms
- Hyperextension of the knees
- Clinched hands
- Talipes

Polyhydramnios or oligohydramnios may accompany this anomaly, as can anomalies of the central nervous system. Other defects that may be associated include facial and renal anomalies.

Lethal Multiple Pterygium Syndrome. Lethal multiple pterygium syndrome is characterized by webbing across the joints and multiple contractures. It is usually inherited in an autosomal-recessive fashion.

Sonographic Findings. The sonographic findings for pterygium syndrome include the following:

- Limb contractures
- Webbing across joints
- Cystic hygroma

Micrognathia, hydrops, and polyhydramnios are also associated with this syndrome.

Pena-Shokeir Syndrome. Pena-Shokeir syndrome is characterized by abnormal joint contractures, facial abnormalities, polyhydramnios, intrauterine growth restriction, and pulmonary hypoplasia. This syndrome may be inherited in an autosomal-recessive manner or as a sporadic occurrence. Pena-Shokeir syndrome and trisomy 18 have similar features, so karyotyping should be offered.

Sonographic Findings. The sonographic findings of Pena-Shokeir (Figure 60-18) include the following:

- Limb abnormalities such as contractures, clinched hands, talipes, and rocker-bottom feet

- Facial abnormalities, including micrognathia and cleft palate

Polyhydramnios and hydrops may also be identified.

MISCELLANEOUS LIMB ABNORMALITIES

Hand and foot abnormalities may occur with skeletal dysplasias, as part of a chromosomal syndrome, or as an isolated event. Amputation defects may be identified as total or partial absence and may be associated with amniotic band syndrome. Congenital absence of one or more extremities (amelia) may be observed prenatally (Figure 60-19).

Hand anomalies may include missing digits, fused digits (syndactyly, Figure 60-20), or a split hand (lobster-claw deformity, Figure 60-21). Extra digits (polydactyly) may be isolated or part of a syndrome or chromosomal anomaly (Figures 60-22 to 60-24). Overlapping digits (clinodactyly) and clinched hands may also be a feature of a syndrome or chromosomal anomaly.

Radial ray defects include hypoplasia or aplasia of the radius and thumb. Radial ray defects (Figure 60-25) are associated with chromosomal anomalies, such as trisomies 13 and 18 and the VACTERL association. Numerous syndromes have also presented with an absent or hypoplastic radius and thumb, including Holt-Oram syndrome and thrombocytopenia with absent radii (TAR) syndrome (Figure 60-26).

Clubfoot, also known as talipes, describes deformities of the foot and ankle. It occurs in approximately 1 to 3 in 1000 live births. There is a male predominance, and half of the cases of clubfoot are unilateral.

The majority of cases of talipes are idiopathic and isolated findings. Talipes may be associated with chromosomal anomalies, syndromes, musculoskeletal disorders, and spina bifida. It has also been associated with exposure to tubocurarine, sodium aminopterin, and lead poisoning. Clubfoot has also been identified with oligohydramnios and in multiple gestations. Because of the numerous anomalies that may be identified, karyotyping should be offered.

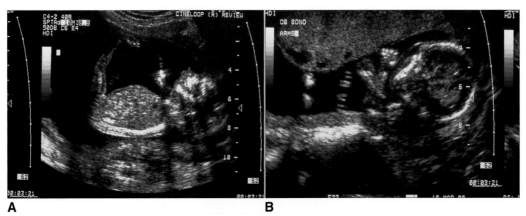

Figure 60-18 **A,** An ultrasound at 19 weeks of gestation revealed rigid legs with the knees hyperextended. **B,** The arms were contracted and crossed over the chest with hands clenched. Polyhydramnios and micrognathia were also noted. The primary diagnosis was Pena-Shokeir syndrome.

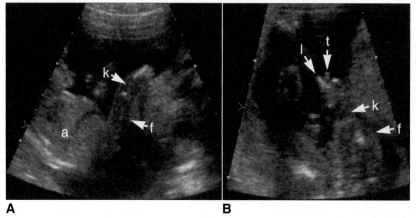

Figure 60-19 **A,** Partial amelia (absence) of the lower extremity. The femur *(f)* is observed without evidence of a lower leg or foot. *a,* Abdomen; *k,* knees. **B,** In the same fetus, magnified view of distal extremity anomaly. Note the single short bone in the lower leg *(l)* and single toe *(t)* protruding from the defect. All other extremities were of normal length and appeared anatomically normal. There were no amniotic bands observed. These findings were confirmed after birth. *f,* Femur; *k,* knee.

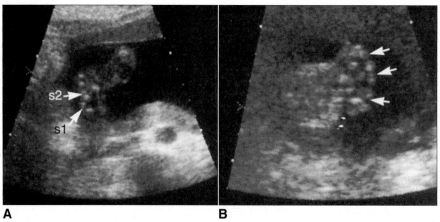

Figure 60-20 **A,** Polysyndactyly in a fetus with Carpenter's syndrome. There was webbing (syndactyly) of the first and second toes *(s1)* and of the third and fourth toes *(s2)*. Six toes were present (polydactyly). **B,** In the same fetus, scans of the toes *(arrows)* show malalignment of the phalanges. Other sonographic findings included craniosynostosis, ventriculomegaly, and umbilical hernia.

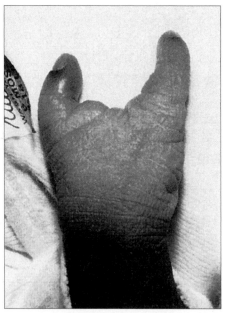

Figure 60-21 Pathologic specimen showing a split-hand deformity (ectrodactyly).

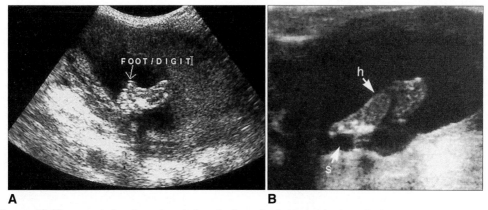

Figure 60-22 **A,** Polydactyly is identified in the foot of a fetus. **B,** The foot of a fetus with trisomy 18 was split (ectrodactyly). Note the splaying of the toes *(s)* and malalignment of the metatarsals. Coexisting anomalies included a septal cardiac defect, bilateral choroid plexus cysts, polydactyly, hydramnios, and growth restriction. Autopsy was declined. *h,* Heel. (**A** from Henningsen C: *Clinical guide to ultrasonography,* St Louis, 2004, Mosby.)

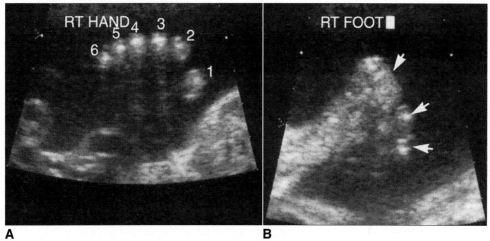

Figure 60-23 **A,** Polydactyly (six fingers) in a 26-week fetus with multiple congenital anomalies, including micromelic dwarfism and semilobar holoprosencephaly. A normal karyotype was found by amniocentesis, but genetic evaluation after birth suggested pseudotrisomy 13 (an autosomal-recessive condition). **B,** In the same fetus, duplication of the great toe *(arrows)* is shown.

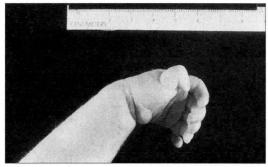

Figure 60-24 Polydactyly of a hand shown in a neonate.

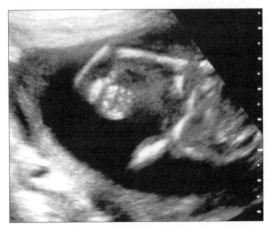

Figure 60-25 A radial ray defect in a fetus that also presented with anencephaly and tetralogy of Fallot. A chromosomal anomaly was suspected. (Courtesy Ginny Goreczky, Maternal Fetal Center, Orlando, Fla.)

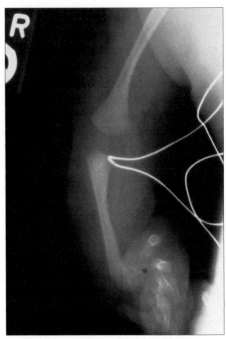

Figure 60-26 A radiograph of a neonate with thrombocytopenia with absent radii (TAR) syndrome. Note the absence of the radius in the arm and the turned-back hand.

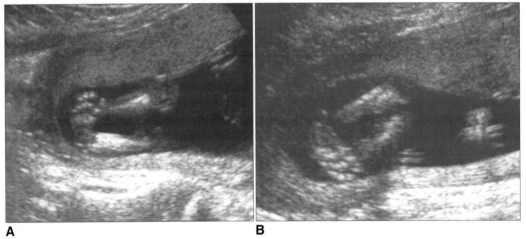

A   **B**

Figure 60-27 Bilateral talipes is identified in this fetus. The right (**A**) and left (**B**) feet are both noted to be medially inverted. The patient and her grandmother also had histories of talipes.

Clubfoot may be identified sonographically when there is persistent abnormal inversion of the foot perpendicular to the lower leg (Figure 60-27).

Rocker-bottom foot is characterized by a prominent heel and a convex sole. It has been associated with multiple syndromes and chromosomal anomalies, especially trisomy 18.

SELECTED BIBLIOGRAPHY

Bar-Hava I and others: Caution: prenatal clubfoot can be both a transient and a late-onset phenomenon, *Prenat Diagn* 17:457, 1997.

Benacerraf BR: *Ultrasound of fetal syndromes,* Philadelphia, 1998, WB Saunders.

Bonilla-Musoles F, Machado LE, Osborne NG: Multiple congenital contractures (congenital multiple arthrogryposis), *J Perinat Med* 30:99-104, 2002.

Bromley B, Shipp TD, Benacerraf B: Isolated polydactyly: prenatal diagnosis and perinatal outcome, *Prenat Diagn* 20:905-908, 2000.

Callen PW: *Ultrasonography in obstetrics and gynecology,* ed 4, Philadelphia, 2000, WB Saunders.

Carillon L, Seince N, Largilliere C: First-trimester diagnosis of sirenomelia, *Fetal Diagn Ther* 16:284-288, 2001.

Carlson BM: *Human embryology and developmental biology*, ed 2, St Louis, 1999, Mosby.

Chen C-P, Chern S-R, Shih J-C and others: Prenatal diagnosis and genetic analysis of type I and type II thanatophoric dysplasia, *Prenat Diagn* 21:89-95, 2001.

Das BB, Rajegowda BK, Bainbridge R and others: Caudal regression syndrome versus sirenomelia: a case report, *J Perinat* 22:168-170, 2002.

Den Hollander NS and others: Early transvaginal ultrasonographic diagnosis of Beemer-Langer dysplasia: a report of two cases, *Ultrasound Obstet Gynecol* 11:298, 1998.

Den Hollander NS, Robben SGF, Hoogeboom AJM: Early prenatal sonographic diagnosis and follow-up of Jeune syndrome, *Ultrasound Obstet Gynecol* 18:378-383, 2001.

Dugoff L, Thieme G, Hobbins JC: First trimester prenatal diagnosis of chondroectodermal dysplasia (Ellis-van Creveld syndrome) with ultrasound, *Ultrasound Obstet Gynecol* 17:88, 2001.

Golombeck K, Jacobs VR, von Kaisenberg C and others: Short rib-polydactyly syndrome type III: comparison of ultrasound, radiology, and pathology findings, *Fetal Diagn Ther* 16:133-138, 2001.

Guzman ER and others: Prenatal ultrasonographic demonstration of the trident hand in heterozygous achondroplasia, *J Ultrasound Med*, 13:63, 1994.

Herman TE, Seigel MJ: VACTERL-H syndrome, *J Perinat* 22:496-498, 2002.

Hertzberg BS, Kliewer MA, Paulyson-Nunez K: Lethal multiple pterygium syndrome: antenatal ultrasonographic diagnosis, *J Ultrasound Med* 19:657-660, 2000.

Keret D, Ezra E, Lokiec F and others: Efficacy of prenatal ultrasonography in confirmed club foot, *J Bone Joint Surg* 84-B:1015-1019, 2002.

Lemyre E, Azouz EM, Teebi AS and others: Achondroplasia, hypochondroplasia, and thanatophoric dysplasia: review and update, *Canadian Assoc Radiol J* 50:185-197, 1999.

Lomas FE, Dahlstrom JE, Ford JH: VACTERL with hydrocephalus: family with X-linked VACTERL-H, *Am J Med Genet* 76:74-78, 1998.

Machado LE, Bonilla-Musoles F, Osborne NG: Thanatophoric dysplasia, *Ultrasound Obstet Gynecol* 18:85-86, 2001.

McEwing RL, Alton K, Johnson J: First-trimester diagnosis of osteogenesis imperfecta type II by three-dimensional sonography, *J Ultrasound Med* 22:311-314, 2003.

Miller O, Kolon TF: Prenatal diagnosis of VACTERL association, *J Urol* 166:2389-2391, 2001.

Moore KL, Persaud TVN, Shiota K: *Color atlas of clinical embryology*, Philadelphia, 1994, WB Saunders.

Murphy JC, Neale D, Bromley B and others: Hypoechogenicity of fetal long bones: a new ultrasound marker for arthrogryposis, *Prenat Diagn* 22:1219-1222, 2002.

Ozeren S, Yuksel A, Tukel T: Prenatal sonographic diagnosis of type I achondrogenesis with a large cystic hygroma, *Ultrasound Obstet Gynecol* 13:76-75, 1999.

Paladini D, Tartaglione A, Agangi A and others: Pena-Shokeir phenotype with variable onset in three consecutive pregnancies, *Ultrasound Obstet Gynecol* 17:163-165, 2001.

Paladini D: Prenatal ultrasound diagnosis of Roberts' syndrome in a family with negative history, *Ultrasound Obstet Gynecol* 7:208, 1996.

Patel MD, Filly RA: Homozygous achondroplasia: US distinction between homozygous, heterozygous, and unaffected fetuses in the second trimester, *Radiology* 196:541, 1995.

Rijhsinghani A, Yankowitz J, Kanis AB and others: Antenatal sonographic diagnosis of club foot with particular attention to the implications and outcomes of isolated club foot, *Ultrasound Obstet Gynecol* 11:103-106, 1998.

Schiesser M, Holzgreve W, Lapaire O and others: Sirenomelia, the mermaid syndrome—detection in the first trimester, *Prenat Diagn* 23:493-495, 2003.

Shipp TD, Benacerraf BR: The significance of prenatally isolated clubfoot: is amniocentesis indicated? *Am J Ostet Gynecol* 178:600, 1998.

Sidden CR, Filly RA, Norton ME and others: A case of chondrodysplasia punctata with features of osteogenesis imperfecta type II, *J Ultrasound Med* 20:699-703, 2001.

Sirichotiyakul S, Tongsong T, Wanapirak C and others: Prenatal sonographic diagnosis of Majewski syndrome, *J Clin Ultrasound* 3:303-306, 2002.

Tongsong T, Chanprapaph P, Thongpadungroj T: Prenatal sonographic findings associated with asphyxiating thoracic dystrophy (Jeune syndrome), *J Ultrasound Med* 18:573-576, 1999.

Tongsong T, Chanprapaph P: Prenatal sonographic diagnosis of Ellis-van Creveld syndrome, *J Clin Ultrasound* 1:38-41, 2000.

Tongsong T, Pongsatha S: Early prenatal sonographic diagnosis of congenital hypophosphatasia, *Ultrasound Obstet Gynecol* 15:252-255, 2000.

Tongsong T, Sirichotiyakul S, Chanprapaph P: Prenatal diagnosis of thrombocytopenia-absent-radius (TAR) syndrome, *Ultrasound Obstet Gynecol* 15:256-258, 2002.

Tongsong T, Wanapirak C, Pongsatha S: Prenatal diagnosis of camptomelic dysplasia, *Ultrasound Obstet Gynecol* 15:428-430, 2000.

Tongsong T, Wanapirak C, Sirichotiyakul S: Prenatal sonographic diagnosis of diastrophic dwarfism, *J Clin Ultrasound* 30:103-105, 2002.

Wax JR, Carpenter M, Smith W and others: Second-trimester sonographic diagnosis of diastrophic dysplasia, *J Ultrasound Med* 22:805-808, 2003.

Won HS, Yoo HK, Lee PR and others: A case of achondrogenesis type II associated with huge cystic hygroma: prenatal diagnosis by ultrasonography, *Ultrasound Obstet Gynecol* 14:288-291, 1999.

Glossary

abdominal aortic aneurysm – permanent localized dilation of an artery, with an increase in diameter of 1.5 times its normal diameter.

abdominal circumference (AC) – measurement at the level of the stomach, left portal vein, and left umbilical vein.

abduction – to move away from the body.

abruptio placenta – premature detachment of the placenta from the maternal wall.

abscess – localized collection of pus.

absorption – process of nutrient molecules passing through wall of intestine into blood or lymph system.

acardiac anomaly – a rare anomaly in monochorionic twins in which one twin develops without a heart and often without an upper half of the body.

accessory spleen – results from the failure of fusion of separate splenic masses forming on the dorsal mesogastrium; most commonly found in the splenic hilum or along the splenic vessels or associated ligaments.

achondrogenesis – lethal autosomal-recessive short-limb dwarfism marked by long bone and trunk shortening, decreased echogenicity of the bones and spine, and "flipperlike" appendages.

achondroplasia – a defect in the development of cartilage at the epiphyseal centers of the long bones producing short, square bones.

acidic – a type of solution that contains more hydrogen ions than hydroxyl ions.

acini cells – cells that perform exocrine function.

acinus (acini) – glandular (milk producing) component of the breast lobule (see terminal ductal-lobular unit, or TDLU). Each breast contains hundreds of lobules that each contain one or a few small glands (acini) along with the surrounding stromal connective tissue elements, the small ducts, a variable amount of fat, and Cooper's ligaments. The TDLU (a terminal duct and its corresponding acinus) is the site of origin of nearly all pathologic processes of the breast.

acoustic emission – occurs when an appropriate level of acoustic energy is applied to the tissue, the microbubbles first oscillate and then rupture; the rupture of the microbubbles results in random Doppler shifts appearing as a transient mosaic of colors on a color Doppler display.

acoustic impedance – measure of a material's resistance to the propagation of sound; expressed as the product of acoustic velocity of the medium and the density of the medium ($Z = \rho c$).

acrania – condition associated with anencephaly in which there is complete or partial absence of the cranial bones.

acrocephalopolysyndactyly – congenital anomaly characterized by a peaked head and webbed fingers and toes.

acromioclavicular joint (AC) – the joint found in the shoulder that connects the clavicle to the acromion process of the scapula.

acute tubular necrosis – acute damage to the renal tubules; usually due to ischemia associated with shock.

Addison's disease – condition caused by hyposecretion of hormones from the adrenal cortex.

adduction – to move toward the body.

adenoma – tumor of the glandular tissue.

adenomyomatosis – small polypoid projections.

adenomyosis – benign invasive growth of the endometrium that may cause heavy, painful menstrual bleeding.

adenopathy – enlargement of the lymph nodes.

adenosis – disease of the glands. In the breast, overgrowth of the stromal and epithelial elements of the small glands (acini) within the breast lobule. Adenosis is one component of fibrocystic condition, recognized by characteristic histopathologic changes in a breast biopsy specimen. Adenosis can exist by itself or in conjunction with other manifestations of fibrocystic conditions, such as fibrosis (e.g., sclerosing adenosis combines adenosis with surrounding fibrosis), and is often mistaken for possible breast cancer.

adrenal hemorrhage – hemorrhage that occurs when the fetus is stressed during a difficult delivery or a hypoxic insult.

afferent arteriole – arteriole that carries blood into the glomerulus of the nephron.

alimentary canal – also known as the gastrointestinal tract; includes the mouth, pharynx, esophagus, stomach, duodenum, and small and large intestines.

alkaline – a type of solution that contains more hydroxyl ions than hydrogen ions.

allantoic duct – elongated duct that contributes to the development of the umbilical cord and placenta during the first trimester.

alobar holoprosencephaly – most severe form of holoprosencephaly, characterized by a single common ventricle and malformed brain; orbital anomalies range from fused orbits to hypotelorism, with frequent nasal anomalies and clefting of the lip and palate.

alpha-fetoprotein (AFP) – protein manufactured by the fetus, which can be studied in amniotic fluid and maternal serum. Elevations of alpha-fetoprotein may indicate fetal anomalies (neural tube, abdominal wall, gastrointestinal), multiple gestations, or incorrect patient dates. Decreased levels may be associated with chromosomal abnormalities.

amaurosis fugax – transient partial or complete loss of vision in one eye.

American College of Radiology (ACR) – a national professional organization of physicians who specialize in radiology. Agency that first began voluntary accreditation of facilities performing screening mammography and that created the BI-RADS system of reporting and classifying mammograms that was later made mandatory by federal legislation (Mammography Quality Standards Act of 1994).

amniocentesis – aspiration of a sample of amniotic fluid through the mother's abdomen for diagnosis of fetal maturity and/or disease by assay of the constituents of the fluid.

amnion – smooth membrane enclosing the fetus and amniotic fluid; it is loosely fused with the outer chorionic membrane.

amniotic band syndrome – rupture of the amnion that leads to entrapment or entanglement of the fetal parts by the "sticky" chorion.

amniotic bands – multiple fibrous strands of amnion that develop in utero that may entangle fetal parts to cause amputations or malformations of the fetus.

amniotic cavity – cavity in which the fetus exists that forms early in gestation and surrounds the embryo; amniotic fluid fills the cavity to protect the embryo and fetus.

amniotic fluid – produced by the umbilical cord and membranes, and by the fetal lung, skin, and kidneys.

amniotic fluid index (AFI) – sum of the four quadrants of amniotic fluid. The uterus is divided into four quadrants; each "quadrant" is evaluated with the transducer perpendicular to the table in the deepest vertical pocket without fetal parts; the four quadrants are added together to determine the amniotic fluid index.

amplitude – strength of the ultrasound wave measured in decibels.

ampulla of Vater – small opening in the duodenum in which the pancreatic and common bile duct enter to release secretions.

amylase – enzyme secreted by the pancreas to aid in the digestion of carbohydrates.

amyloidosis – metabolic disorder marked by amyloid deposits in organs and tissue.

anaplastic carcinoma – rare, undifferentiated carcinoma occurring in middle age.

androgen – substance that stimulates the development of male characteristics, such as the hormones testosterone and androsterone.

anechoic – without echoes; simple cyst on ultrasound should be anechoic.

anembryonic pregnancy (blighted ovum) – ovum without an embryo.

anemia – abnormal condition in which blood lacks either a normal number of red blood cells or normal concentration of hemoglobin.

anencephaly – neural tube defect characterized by the lack of development of the cerebral and cerebellar hemispheres and cranial vault; this abnormality is incompatible with life.

angle of incidence – angle at which the ultrasound beams strike the interface between two types of tissue.

angle of reflection – the amplitude of the reflected wave depends on the difference between the acoustic impedances of the two materials forming the interface.

anisotropy – the quality of comprising varying values of a given property when measured in different directions.

anomaly – an abnormality or congenital malformation.

anophthalmia – absent eyes.

anophthalmos – absence of one (cyclops) or both eyes.

anorectal atresia – complex disorder of the bowel and genitourinary tract.

anterior cerebral artery (ACA) – smaller of the two terminal branches of the internal carotid artery.

anterior communicating artery (AcoA) – a short vessel that connects the anterior cerebral arteries at the interhemispheric fissure.

anterior pararenal space – space located between the anterior surface of the renal fascia and the posterior area of the peritoneum.

anterior tibial artery – artery that begins at the popliteal artery and travels down the lateral calf in the anterior compartment to the level of the ankle.

anterior tibial veins – veins that drain blood from the dorsum of the foot and anterior compartment of the calf.

anteverted – position of the uterus when the fundus is tipped slightly forward.

antiradial – plane of imaging on ultrasound of the breast that is perpendicular to the radial plane of imaging. The radial plane of imaging uses the nipple as the center point of an imaginary clock face imposed on the breast, such that the radial 12 o'clock plane is a line extending upward toward the top of the breast. Similarly, the radial 9 o'clock plane extends straight out to the right aspect of the breast, and so on. Three-dimensional measurements of a breast mass can be recorded using sagittal transverse or radial/antiradial planes.

aorta – largest arterial structure in the body; arises from the left ventricle of the heart to supply blood to the head, upper and lower extremities, and abdominopelvic cavity by descending into the abdominal cavity to branch into iliac vessels at the level of the umbilicus.

apex of prostate – inferior region of the prostate.

apex of ventricle – the ventricles of the heart come to a point called the *apex*; normally the apex is directed toward the left hip.

aphasia – inability to communicate by speech or writing.

apical – position of the transducer located over cardiac apex (at the point of maximal impulse).

apocrine metaplasia – in the breast, an increase in the number and activity of the lining cells of the breast acini (glands). These lining cells normally secrete only a small amount of fluid in the nonlactating breast. Fluid production can often increase with apocrine metaplasia, which is one of the conditions thought to be responsible for the formation of benign fluid-filled breast cysts.

aponeurosis – band-like flat tendons connecting muscle to the bone.

appendicitis – inflammation of the appendix.

appendicolith – echogenic structure within the appendix.

aqueductal stenosis – blockage of the duct connecting the third and fourth ventricles.

arcuate arteries – arteries that lie at the bases of the medullary pyramids and appear as echogenic structures.

arcuate vessels – small vessels found along the periphery of the uterus.

arcuate arteries – small vessels found at the bases of the renal pyramids.

areola – the pigmented skin surrounding the breast nipple.

arhinia – absence of the nose.

Arnold-Chiari malformation – defect in which the cerebellum and brainstem are pulled toward the spinal cord (banana sign); frontal bossing, or "lemon head," is also evident on ultrasound.

arteries – vascular structures that carry blood away from the heart.

arteriosclerosis – thickening and hardening of arterial walls.

arteriovenous fistula – communication between an artery and vein.

ascites – accumulation of serous fluid in the peritoneal cavity.

asphyxiating thoracic dystrophy – significantly narrow diameter of the chest in a fetus.

asplenia – no development of splenic tissue.

assisted reproductive technology (ART) – technologies employed to assist the infertility patient to become pregnant. These methods include in vitro fertilization, gamete intrafallopian transfer, zygote intrafallopian transfer, and artificial insemination.

asymptomatic – without symptoms.

ataxia – impaired ability to coordinate movement, especially disturbances of gait.

atrial fibrillation – condition in which the atria beat more than 400 beats per minute and the ventricular rate is 120 to 200 beats per minute.

atrial septal defect – communication between the right and left atrium that persists after birth.

atrioventricular block – block of transmission of the electrical impulse from the atria to the ventricles (may be 2:1 or 3:1 block).

atrioventricular node – area of specialized cardiac muscle that receives the cardiac impulse from the sinoatrial node and conducts it to the atrioventricular bundles.

atrioventricular septal defect – defect that occurs when the endocardial cushion fails to fuse in the center of the heart.

atrioventricular valve – valve located between the atria and ventricle.

atrium (trigone) of the lateral ventricles – the ventricle is measured at this site (junction of the anterior, occipital, and temporal horn) on the axial view.

attenuation – reduction in the amplitude and intensity of a sound wave as it propagates through a medium; attenuation of ultrasound waves in tissue is caused by absorption and by scattering and reflection.

atypical ductal hyperplasia (ADH) – see atypical hyperplasia.

atypical hyperplasia – abnormal proliferation of cells with atypical features involving the TDLU, with an increased likelihood of evolving into breast cancer; in atypical ductal hyperplasia (ADH), the pathologist recognizes some, but not all, of the features of ductal carcinoma in situ (DCIS); atypical lobular hyperplasia (ALH) shows some, but not all, of the features of lobular carcinoma in situ (LCIS); ALH and LCIS are now grouped by some authors under the term lobular neoplasia.

atypical lobular hyperplasia (ALH) – see atypical hyperplasia; lobular neoplasia.

augmentation – increase in blood flow velocity with distal limb compression or with the release of proximal limb compression.

auscultation – procedure of listening to the heart sounds with a stethoscope.

autoimmune hemolytic anemia – anemia caused by antibodies produced by the patient's own immune system.

autonomy – self-governing or self-directing freedom and especially moral independence; the right of persons to choose and to have their choices respected.

axial plane – placement of the transducer above the ear (above the canthomeatal line).

axilla – armpit.

axillary artery – continuation of the subclavian artery.

axillary vein – vein that begins where the basilic vein joins the brachial vein in the upper arm and terminates beneath the clavicle at the outer border of the first rib.

banana sign – the shape of the cerebellum when a spinal defect is present (cerebellum is pulled downward into the foramen magnum).

bare area – area superior to the liver that is not covered by peritoneum so that the inferior vena cava may enter the chest.

Barlow maneuver – the patient lies in the supine position with the hip flexed 90 degrees and adducted. Downward and outward pressure is applied. If the hip is dislocated, the examiner will feel the femoral head move out of the acetabulum.

basal body temperature – the morning body temperature taken orally before the patient does any activity.

base – superior region of the prostate.

basilar artery – artery formed by the union of the two vertebral arteries.

basilic vein – vein that originates on the small finger side of the dorsum of the hand.

battledore placenta – marginal or eccentric insertion of the umbilical cord into the placenta.

Beckwith-Wiedemann syndrome – group of disorders having in common the coexistence of an omphalocele, macroglossia, and visceromegaly.

beneficence – quality or state of being beneficent (doing good, such as performing acts of kindness).

benign prostatic hypertrophy – enlargement of the glandular component of the prostate.

bicornuate uterus – duplication of the uterus (two horns and one vagina).

bicuspid aortic valve – two leaflets instead of the normal three leaflets with asymmetric cusps.

bile – bile pigment, old blood cells, and the by-products of phagocytosis are known together as *bile*.

bilirubin – yellow pigment in bile formed by the breakdown of red blood cells.

biophysical profile (BPP) – assessment of fetus to determine fetal well-being; includes evaluation of cardiac non-stress test, fetal breathing movement, gross fetal body movements, fetal tone, and amniotic fluid volume.

biparietal diameter (BPD) – measurement of the fetal head at the level of the thalamus and cavum septum pellucidum.

blood urea nitrogen (BUN) – laboratory measurement of the amount of nitrogenous waste, along with creatinine; waste products accumulate in the blood when kidneys malfunction.

body of the pancreas – located in the midepigastrium anterior to the superior mesenteric artery and vein, aorta, and inferior vena cava.

bowel herniation – extrusion of the bowel outside the abdominal cavity; during the first trimester normally occurs between 8 and 12 weeks.

Bowman's capsule – the cup-shaped end of a renal tubule enclosing a glomerulus; site of filtration of the kidney; contains water, salts, glucose, urea, and amino acids.

brachial artery – continuation of the axillary artery.

brachycephaly – fetal head is elongated in the transverse diameter and shortened in the anteroposterior diameter.

brainstem – comprises the midbrain, pons, and medulla oblongata.

branchial cleft cyst – remnant of embryonic development that appears as a cyst in the neck.

Braxton-Hicks contractions – spontaneous painless uterine contractions described originally as a sign of pregnancy; they occur from the first trimester to the end of pregnancy.

breast – differentiated apocrine sweat gland with a functional purpose of secreting milk during lactation.

breast cancer (breast carcinoma) – breast cancer involves two main types of cells: ductal and lobular. Ductal cancer, accounting for approximately 85% of the breast cancer cases, also includes many subtypes, such as medullary, mucinous, tubular, apocrine, or papillary types. In addition, very early or preinvasive breast cancer is generally ductal in type. This preinvasive breast cancer is also called *in situ*, *noninvasive*, or *intraductal* breast cancer. Another commonly used term for this early type of cancer is *ductal carcinoma in situ*, or *DCIS*.

breast cancer screening – screening for breast cancer involves annual screening mammography (starting at age 40), monthly breast self-examination (BSE), and self-breast examination (SBE).

Breast Imaging Reporting and Data System (BI-RADS) – trademark system created by the American College of Radiology (ACR) to standardize mammographic reporting terminology, categorize breast abnormalities according to the level of suspicion for malignancy, and facilitate outcome monitoring. This system of classification of breast imaging results has now been made a mandatory part of mammogram reports by federal legislation (Mammography Quality Standards Act of 1994).

breast self-examination (BSE) – part of breast cancer screening; every woman is encouraged to perform breast self-examination monthly starting at age 20; BSE is usually best performed at the end of menses.

breech – indicates the fetal head is toward the fundus of the uterus.

bronchogenic cyst – most common lung cyst detected prenatally.

bronchopulmonary sequestration – extrapulmonary tissue is present within the pleural lung sac (intralobar) or connected to the inferior border of the lung within its own pleural sac (extralobar).

bruit – noise caused by tissue vibration produced by turbulence.

Budd-Chiari syndrome – thrombosis of the hepatic veins.

buffer – chemical compound that can act as a weak acid or a base to combine with excess hydrogen or hydroxyl ions to neutralize the pH in blood.

bulbus cordis – primitive chamber that forms the right ventricle.

bulk modulus – amount of pressure required to compress a small volume of material a small amount.

bull's eye (target) lesion – hypoechoic mass with echogenic central core (abscess, metastasis).

bursa – a saclike structure containing thick fluid that surrounds areas subject to friction, such as the interface between bone and tendon.

calcitonin – a thyroid hormone that is important for maintaining a dense, strong bone matrix and regulating the blood calcium level.

caliectasis – rounded calyces with renal pelvis dilation measuring greater than 10 mm in the anteroposterior direction.

calyx – part of the collecting system adjacent to the pyramid that collects urine and is connected to the major calyx.

capillaries – minute vessels that connect the arterial and venous systems.

cardiac orifice – entrance of the esophagus into the stomach occurs at the cardiac orifice.

cardiomyopathy – disease of the myocardial muscle layer of the heart that causes the heart to dilate secondary to regurgitation and also affects cardiac function.

cardiosplenic syndromes – sporadic disorders characterized by symmetric development of normally asymmetric organs or organ systems.

cartilage interface sign – echogenic line on the anterior surface of the cartilage surrounding the humeral head.

cauda equina – bundle of nerve roots from the lumbar, sacral, and coccygeal spinal nerves that descend nearly vertically from the spinal cord until they reach their respective openings in the vertebral column.

caudal pancreatic artery – branch of the splenic artery that supplies the tail of the pancreas.

caudal regression syndrome – lack of development of the lower limbs (may occur in the fetus of a diabetic mother).

caudate lobe – small lobe of the liver situated on the posterosuperior surface of the left lobe; the ligamentum venosum is the anterior border.

caudate nucleus – area of the brain that forms the lateral borders of the anterior horns, anterior to the thalamus.

cavernous transformation of the portal vein – periportal collateral channels in patients with chronic portal vein obstruction.

cavum septum pellucidum – prominent structure best seen in the midline filled with cerebrospinal fluid in the premature infant.

cebocephaly – form of holoprosencephaly characterized by a common ventricle, hypotelorism, and a nose with a single nostril.

celiac axis – first major anterior artery to arise from the abdominal aorta inferior to the diaphragm; it branches into the hepatic, splenic, and left gastric arteries.

central zone – portion of the prostate that surrounds the urethra; site of benign prostatic hypertrophy.

centripetal artery – terminal intratesticular arteries arising from the capsular arteries.

cephalic vein – vein that begins on the thumb side of the dorsum of the hand.

cephalocele – protrusion of the brain from the cranial cavity.

cerebellum – area of the brain that lies posterior to the brainstem below the tentorium.

cerebral vasospasm – vasoconstriction of the arteries.

cerebrum – two equal hemispheres; largest part of the brain.

cervical polyp – hyperplastic protrusion of the epithelium of the cervix; may be broad based or pedunculated.

cervical stenosis – acquired condition with obstruction of the cervical canal.

cervix – inferior segment of the uterus; more than 3.5 cm long during normal pregnancy, decreases in length during labor.

cholangitis – inflammation of the bile duct.

cholecystectomy – removal of the gallbladder.

cholecystitis – acute or chronic inflammation of the gallbladder.

cholecystokinin – hormone secreted into the blood by the mucosa of the upper small intestine; stimulates contraction of the gallbladder and pancreatic secretion of enzymes.

choledochal cyst – cystic growth of the common bile duct that may cause obstruction.

choledocholithiasis – stones in the bile duct.

cholelithiasis – gallstones.

cholesterosis – variant of adenomyomatosis; cholesterol polyps.

choriocarcinoma – malignant invasive form of gestational trophoblastic disease.

chorion – cellular, outermost extraembryonic membrane, composed of trophoblast lined with mesoderm; it develops villi about 2 weeks after fertilization, is vascularized by allantoic vessels a week later, gives rise to the placenta, and persists until birth.

chorion frondosum – the portion of the chorion that develops into the fetal portion of the placenta.

chorionic cavity – surrounds the amniotic cavity; the yolk sac is between the chorion and amnion.

chorionic plate – that part of the chorionic membrane that covers the placenta.

chorionic villi – vascular projections from the chorion.

choroid plexus – echogenic cluster of cells important in the production of cerebrospinal fluid that lie along the atrium of the lateral ventricles.

circle of Willis – vascular network at the base of the brain.

circummarginate placenta – condition in which the chorionic plate of the placenta is smaller than the basal plate, with a flat interface between the fetal membranes and the placenta.

circumvallate placenta – condition in which the chorionic plate of the placenta is smaller than the basal plate; the margin is raised with a rolled edge.

cistern – reservoir for cerebrospinal fluid.

clapper-in-the-bell sign – hypoechoic hematoma found at the end of a completely retracted muscle fragment.

claudication – walking-induced muscular discomfort of the calf, thigh, hip, or buttock.

clinical breast examination (CBE) – examination of the breast by a health care provider; part of breast cancer screening. Every woman is encouraged to have a thorough CBE in conjunction with her routine health care assessment. Between ages 20 and 40, CBE is advised every 3 years. From age 40 on, CBE should be performed by the woman's regular health care provider annually.

cloacal exstrophy – defect in the lower abdominal wall and anterior wall of the urinary bladder.

C-loop of the duodenum – forms the lateral border of the head of the pancreas.

coagulopathy – a defect in blood-clotting mechanisms.

coarctation of the aorta – discrete or long segment narrowing in the aortic arch, usually at the level of the left subclavian artery near the insertion of the ductus arteriosus.

coccygeus muscles – muscles that form the floor of the pelvis.

collateral circulation – circulation that develops when normal venous channels become obstructed.

collateral vessels – ancillary vessels that develop when portal hypertension occurs.

color flow mapping (CFM) – ability to display blood flow in multiple colors depending on the velocity, direction of flow, and extent of turbulence.

column of Bertin – bands of cortical tissue that separate the renal pyramids; a prominent column of Bertin may mimic a renal mass on sonography.

comet tail artifact (ring-down) – posterior linear equidistant artifact created when sound reverberates between two strong reflectors, such as air bubbles, metal, and glass.

common bile duct – duct that extends from the point where the common hepatic duct meets the cystic duct; drains into the duodenum after it joins with the main pancreatic duct.

common carotid artery (CCA) – artery that rises from the aortic arch to supply blood to the head and neck.

common duct – refers to common bile or hepatic ducts when cystic duct is not seen.

common femoral arteries – arteries originating from the iliac arteries and seen in the inguinal region into the upper thigh.

common femoral vein – vein formed by the confluence of the profunda femoris and the superficial femoral vein; also receives the greater saphenous vein.

common hepatic artery – artery arising from the celiac trunk to supply the liver.

common hepatic duct – bile duct system that drains the liver into the common bile duct.

common iliac arteries – a division of the abdominal aorta at the level of the umbilicus to supply blood to the lower extremities.

common iliac vein – vein formed by the confluence of the internal and external iliac veins.

complete abortion – complete removal of all products of conception, including the placenta.

complete atrioventricular septal defect – large ventricular and atrial septal defect with a single, undivided, free-floating leaflet that stretches between both ventricles.

complete mole – trophoblastic parts without a fetus; forms when the sperm fertilizes an empty egg.

confidentiality – the nondisclosure of certain information except to another authorized person.

confluence of the splenic and portal veins – junction of the splenic and portal veins that occurs in the midabdomen and serves as the posterior border of the pancreas.

congenital bronchial atresia – pulmonary anomaly that results from the focal obliteration of a segment of the bronchial lumen.

congenital mesoblastic nephroma – most common benign renal tumor of the neonate and infant.

conjoined twins – monozygotic twins physically joined by varying degrees; condition that occurs when the division of the egg occurs after 13 days.

continuous wave probe – probe with which sound is continuously emitted from one transducer and continuously received by a second transducer.

contrast-enhanced sonography – sonography in which an agent is used to reduce or eliminate some of the current limitations of ultrasound imaging and Doppler blood flow detection.

conus medullaris – the caudal end of the spinal cord.

Cooper's ligaments – connective tissue septae that connect perpendicularly to the breast lobules and extend out to the skin; are considered to be the fibrous "skeleton" supporting the breast glandular tissue.

coronal – horizontal plane through the longitudinal axis of the body to image structures from anterior to posterior.

coronal plane – transducer is perpendicular to the anterior fontanelle in the coronal axis of the head.

corpus callosum – prominent group of nerve fibers that connect the right and left sides of the brain; found superior to the third ventricle.

corpus luteum – yellow body formed from the Graafian follicle after ovulation that produces estrogen and progesterone.

corpus luteum cyst – small endocrine structure that develops within a ruptured ovarian follicle and secretes progesterone and estrogen. It may persist until the 20th to 24th week of pregnancy.

cortex – outer parenchyma of an organ. Liver cortex is thin in the neonate, with echogenicity similar to or slightly greater than that of the normal liver parenchyma.

cran- – helmet; *cranial*: pertaining to the portion of the skull that surrounds the brain.

craniosynostoses – premature closure of the cranial sutures.

creatinine (Cr) – a product of metabolism; laboratory test measures the ability of the kidney to get rid of waste; waste products accumulate in the blood when the kidneys are malfunctioning.

cremasteric artery – small artery arising from the inferior epigastric artery (a branch of the external iliac artery), which supplies the peritesticular tissue, including the cremasteric muscle.

cremasteric muscle – an extension of the internal oblique muscle that descends to the testis with the spermatic cord; contraction of the cremasteric muscle shortens the spermatic cord and elevates the testis.

critical aortic stenosis – abnormal thickening and closure of the aortic leaflets in the second or third trimester causes the left ventricle to "balloon" from increased pressure.

Crohn's disease – inflammation of the bowel, accompanied by abscess and bowel wall thickening.

crossed renal ectopia – condition that occurs when the kidney is located on the opposite side of its ureteral orifice.

crown-rump length (CRL) – most accurate measurement for determining gestational age in the first trimester.

crus of the diaphragm – muscular structure in the upper abdomen at the level of the celiac axis.

cryptorchidism – failure of the testes to descend into the scrotum; testicles remain within the abdomen or groin and fail to descend into the scrotal sac.

crystal – special material in the ultrasound transducer that has the ability to convert electrical impulses into sound waves.

culling – process by which the spleen removes nuclei from the red blood cells as they pass through.

Cushing's syndrome – condition caused by hypersecretion of hormones from the adrenal cortex.

cycle – measurement of the vibration of the crystal in frequency per second.

cyclopia – severe form of holoprosencephaly characterized by a common ventricle, fusion of the orbits with one or two eyes present, and a proboscis (maldeveloped cylindrical nose).

cyst – fluid-filled sac of variable size.

cyst aspiration – common breast procedure (both diagnostic and interventional) that involves placing a needle through the skin of the breast into a cystic mass and pulling fluid out of the cystic mass through the needle. In the case of a palpable cyst, this procedure can be performed in a physician's office. In the case of a small, complex, or nonpalpable cyst, image guidance (usually with ultrasound) can be used to facilitate the aspiration.

cystadenocarcinoma – a malignant tumor that forms cysts.

cystadenoma – benign adenoma containing cysts.

cystic adenomatoid malformation – abnormality in the formation of the bronchial tree with secondary overgrowth of mesenchymal tissue from arrested bronchial development.

cystic duct – duct that connects the gallbladder to the common hepatic duct.

cystic fibrosis – inherited disorder of the exocrine glands; symptoms include mucus build-up within the lungs and other areas of the body.

cystic hygroma – dilation of jugular lymph sacs (may occur in axilla or groin) because of improper drainage of the lymphatic system into the venous system. Large, septated hygromas are frequently associated with Turner's syndrome, congestive heart failure, and death of the fetus in utero; isolated hygromas may occur as solitary lesions at birth.

cystic medial necrosis – weakening of the arterial wall.

dacryocystocele – cystic dilation of the lacrimal sac at the nasocanthal angle.

Dandy-Walker syndrome – displacement of the fourth ventricle, often accompanied by hydrocephalus.

dartos – layer of muscle underneath the scrotal skin.

decibel (dB) – unit used to quantitatively express the ratio of two amplitudes or intensities; decibels are not absolute units, but express one sound level or intensity in terms of another or in terms of a reference (e.g., the amplitude 10 cm from the transducer is 10 dB lower than the amplitude 5 cm from the transducer).

decidua basalis – the part of the decidua that unites with the chorion to form the placenta.

decidua capsularis – the part of the decidua that surrounds the chorionic sac.

deep femoral vein – vein that travels with the profunda femoris artery to unite with the superficial femoral vein to form the common femoral vein.

deep venous thrombosis (DVT) – blockage of the venous circulation (upper or lower) by a blood clot.

deferential artery – arises from the vesicle artery (a branch of the internal iliac artery) and supplies the vas deferens and epididymis.

DeQuervain's thyroiditis – inflammatory condition of the thyroid, sometimes occurring after a viral respiratory infection.

dermoid – benign tumor comprised of hair, muscle, teeth, and fat.

developmental displacement of the hip – abnormal condition of the hip that results in congenital hip dysplasia; includes dysplastic, subluxated, dislocatable, and dislocated hips.

diagnostic breast imaging – also called "consultative," "workup," or "problem-solving" mammography or breast imaging. This type of breast imaging examination is more intensive than routine screening mammography. Diagnostic breast imaging is usually directed toward a specific clinical symptom of possible breast cancer, or an abnormal finding on a screening mammogram. The goal of diagnostic breast imaging is to categorize the abnormality according to the level of suspicion for cancer (see Breast Imaging and Reporting System [BI-RADS]).

diamniotic – multiple pregnancy with two amniotic sacs.

diaphragmatic hernia – opening in the pleuroperitoneal membrane that develops in the first trimester.

diastematomyelia – a congenital fissure of the spinal cord, frequently associated with spina bifida cystica.

diastole – part of the cardiac cycle in which the ventricles are filling with blood; the tricuspid and mitral valves are open during this time.

dichorionic – multiple pregnancy with two chorionic sacs.

diffuse hepatocellular disease – disease that affects hepatocytes and interferes with liver function.

diffuse nontoxic goiter – condition that occurs as a compensatory enlargement of the thyroid gland resulting from thyroid hormone deficiency; also known as colloid goiter.

diplopia – double vision.

dissecting aneurysm – tear in the intima and/or media of the abdominal aorta.

dizygotic – twins that arise from two separately fertilized ova.

dolichocephaly – fetal head is shortened in the transverse plane and elongated in the anteroposterior plane.

Doppler effect – change in the frequency of a sound wave when either the source or the listener is moving relative to one another; the difference between the received echo frequency and the frequency of the transmitted beam is the Doppler shift; pulsed wave Doppler is used in most fetal examinations; this means that the transducer has the ability to send and receive Doppler signals.

Doppler sample volume – the sonographer selects the exact site to record Doppler signals and sets the sample volume (gate) at this site.

Doppler shift in frequency – change in frequency as red blood cells move from a lower-frequency sound source at rest toward a higher-frequency sound source; change in frequency.

dors- – back; *dorsal*: position toward the back of the body.

dorsal pancreatic artery – branch of the splenic artery that supplies the body of the pancreas.

dorsalis pedis artery – continuation of the anterior tibial artery on the top of the foot.

dorsiflexion – upward movement of the hand or foot.

double decidual sac sign – interface between the decidua capsularis and the echogenic, highly vascular endometrium.

double outlet right ventricle – ventricular septal defect with the overriding aorta directed more to the right ventricular outflow tract than the left (more than 50% override toward the right).

dromedary hump – normal variant that occurs on the left kidney as a bulge of the lateral border.

duct of Santorini – small accessory duct of the pancreas found in the head of the gland.

duct of Wirsung – largest duct of the pancreas that drains the tail, body, and head of the gland; it joins the common bile duct to enter the duodenum through the ampulla of Vater.

ductus arteriosus – communication between the pulmonary artery and descending aorta that closes after birth.

ductus venosus – fetal vein that connects the umbilical vein to the inferior vena cava and runs at an oblique axis through the liver.

duodenal atresia – complete blockage at the pyloric sphincter.

duodenal bulb – first part of the duodenum.

duodenal stenosis – narrowing of the pyloric sphincter.

dynamic range – ratio of the largest to smallest signals that an instrument or component of an instrument can respond to without distortion.

dysarthria – difficulty with speech because of impairment of the tongue or muscles essential to speech.

dysphagia – inability or difficulty in swallowing.

dysraphic – refers to the anomalies associated by incomplete embryologic development.

dysuria – painful or difficult urination.

Ebstein's anomaly – abnormal apical displacement of the septal leaflet of the tricuspid valve.

eclampsia – coma and seizures in the second- and third-trimester patient secondary to pregnancy-induced hypertension.

ectopia cordis – condition in which the ventral wall fails to close and the heart develops outside the thoracic cavity.

ectopic kidney – kidney located outside of the normal position, most often in the pelvic cavity.

ectopic pregnancy – pregnancy occurring outside the uterine cavity.

ectopic ureterocele – ectopic insertion and cystic dilation of distal ureter of duplicated renal collecting system; occurs more commonly in females (on left side).

efferent arteriole – arteriole that supplies the peritubular capillaries of the kidneys, which also supply the convoluted tubules.

ejaculatory ducts – ducts that connect the seminal vesicle and the vas deferens to the urethra at the verumontanum.

electrocardiography – study of the heart's electrical activity.

embryo – conceptus to the end of the ninth week of gestation.

embryo transfer – a technique that follows IVF in which the fertilized ova are injected into the uterus through the cervix.

embryologic age (conceptual age) – age since the date of conception.

embryonic period – time between 6 and 12 weeks.

encephalocele – protrusion of the brain through a cranial fissure.

endocardium – inner layer of the heart wall.

endocrine – process of cells that secrete into the blood or lymph circulation that has a specific effect on tissues in another part of the body.

endometrial carcinoma – condition that presents with abnormal thickening of the endometrial cavity; usually presents with irregular bleeding in perimenopausal and postmenopausal women.

endometrial hyperplasia – condition that results from estrogen stimulation to the endometrium without the influence of progestin; frequent cause of bleeding (especially in post-menopausal women).

endometrial polyp – pedunculated or sessile well-defined mass attached to the endometrial cavity.

endometrioma – localized tumor of endometriosis most frequently found in the ovary, cul-de-sac, rectovaginal septum, and peritoneal surface of the posterior wall of the uterus.

endometriosis – condition that occurs when functioning endometrial tissue invades sites outside the uterus.

endometritis – infection within the endometrium of the uterus.

endometrium – inner lining of the uterine cavity that appears echogenic to hypoechoic on ultrasound, depending on the menstrual cycle.

epicardium – outer layer of the heart wall.

epididymal cyst – cyst filled with clear, serous fluid located in the epididymis.

epididymis – anatomic structure that lies posterior and lateral to the testes in which the spermatozoa accumulate.

epididymitis – infection and inflammation of the epididymis.

epigastric – above the umbilicus and between the costal margins.

epigastrium – area between the right and left hypochondrium that contains part of the liver, duodenum, and pancreas.

epignathus – teratoma located in the oropharynx.

epineurium – the covering of a nerve that consists of connective tissue.

epiploic foramen – opening to the lesser sac.

epitheliosis – overgrowth of cells lining the small ducts of the terminal ductal-lobular unit; one of the common components of most varieties of fibrocystic condition.

erythroblastosis fetalis – hemolytic disease marked by anemia, enlargement of liver and spleen, and hydrops fetalis.

erythrocyte – red blood cell.

erythropoiesis – production of red blood cells.

esophageal atresia – congenital hypoplasia of the esophagus; usually associated with a tracheoesophageal fistula.

esophageal stenosis – narrowing of the esophagus, usually in the distal third segment.

estimated fetal weight (EFW) – estimation based on incorporation of all fetal growth parameters (biparietal diameter, head circumference, abdominal circumference, femur and humeral length).

estrogen – the female hormone produced by the ovary.

ethics – discipline dealing with what is good and bad and with moral duty and obligation.

euthyroid – refers to a normal functioning thyroid gland.

exencephaly – abnormal condition in which the brain is located outside the cranium.

exocrine – process of secreting outwardly through a duct to the surface of an organ or tissue or into a vessel.

exophthalmia – abnormal protrusion of the eyeball.

exstrophy of the bladder – protrusion of the posterior wall of the urinary bladder, which contains the trigone of the bladder and the ureteric orifices.

external carotid artery (ECA) – smaller of the two terminal branches of the common carotid artery.

external iliac vein – vein that drains the pelvis along with the internal iliac vein.

extracorporeal shock-wave lithotripsy – a device that breaks up kidney stones; the shock waves are focused on the stones, disintegrating them and permitting their passage in the urine.

extrahepatic – outside the liver.

falciform ligament – ligament that attaches the liver to the anterior abdominal wall and undersurface of the diaphragm.

false knots of the umbilical cord – condition that occurs when blood vessels are longer than the cord; they fold on themselves and produce nodulations on the surface of the cord.

false pelvis – portion of the pelvic cavity that is above the pelvic brim, bounded posteriorly by the lumbar vertebrae, laterally by the iliac fossae and iliacus muscles, and anteriorly by the lower anterior abdominal wall.

falx cerebri (interhemispheric fissure) – echogenic fibrous structure separating the cerebral hemispheres.

fascia lata – deep fascia of the thigh.

fasciculi – term describing a small bundle of muscles, nerves, and tendons.

febrile – has a fever.

fecalith – calculus that may form around fecal material associated with appendicitis.

femoral triangle – description of a region at the front of the upper thigh, just below the inguinal ligament.

femoral veins – upper part of the venous drainage system of the lower extremity that empties into the inferior vena cava at the level of the diaphragm.

femur length (FL) – measurement from the femoral head to the distal end of the femur.

fetal cystic hygroma – malformation of the lymphatic system that leads to single or multiloculated lymph-filled cavities around the neck.

fetal goiter (thyromegaly) – enlargement of the thyroid gland.

fetal hydronephrosis – dilated renal pelvis.

fetus papyraceous – fetal death that occurs after the fetus has reached a certain growth that is too large to resorb into the uterus.

fever – elevation of normal body temperature (above 98.6° F).

fibroadenoma – most common benign solid tumor of the breast, consisting predominantly of fibrous and epithelial (adenomatous) tissue elements. These masses tend to develop in young women (even teenagers), tend to run in families, and can be multiple. The usual appearance of a fibroadenoma is a benign-appearing mammographic mass (round, oval, or gently lobular and well circumscribed) with a correlating sonographic mass that is well defined and demonstrates homogeneous echogenicity.

fibrocystic condition (FCC) – also called *fibrocystic change* or *fibrocystic breast*, this condition represents many different tissue processes within the breast that are all basically normal processes that over time can get exaggerated to the point of causing symptoms or mammographic changes that raise concern for breast cancer. The main fibrocystic tissue processes are adenosis, epitheliosis, and fibrosis. These processes can cause symptoms such as breast lumps and pain. These processes can cause mammographic changes such as cysts, microcalcifications, distortion, and mass-like densities. Pathologic changes of fibrocystic condition include apocrine metaplasia, microcystic adenosis, blunt ductal adenosis, epithelial ductal hyperplasia, lobular hyperplasia, and sclerosing adenosis. Only a few fibrocystic tissue processes are associated with an increased risk of subsequent development of breast cancer. These include atypical ductal hyperplasia and lobular neoplasia (formerly called lobular carcinoma in situ).

filum terminale – slender tapering terminal section of the spinal cord.

fine needle aspiration – the use of a fine-gauge needle to obtain cells from a mass.

first generation agents – agents containing room air (i.e., Albunex).

focal nodular hyperplasia – liver tumors with an abundance of Kupffer cells; sonographically, they are isoechoic to the surrounding normal liver tissue.

focal zone – the region over which the effective width of the sound beam is within some measure of its width at the focal distance.

focused assessment with sonography for trauma – limited examination of the abdomen or pelvis to evaluate free fluid or pericardial fluid.

follicle-stimulating hormone (FSH) – hormone produced in the pituitary that influences the ovaries.

follicular carcinoma – occurs as a solitary mass within the thyroid gland.

follicular cyst – benign cyst within the ovary that may occur and disappear on a cyclic basis.

fontanelle – soft space between the bones; the space is usually large enough to accommodate the ultrasound transducer until the age of 12 months.

foramen of Bochdalek – type of diaphragmatic defect that occurs posterior and lateral in the diaphragm; usually found in the left side.

foramen of Morgagni – diaphragmatic hernia that occurs anterior and medial in the diaphragm and may communicate with the pericardial sac.

foramen ovale – opening between the free edge of the septum secundum and the dorsal wall of the atrium; also termed *fossae ovale*.

four chamber – view that transects the heart approximately parallel with dorsal and ventral surfaces of body.

four-dimensional (4-D) ultrasound – ability to reconstruct the 3-D image and see it in real time.

frame rate – rate at which images are updated on the display; dependent on frequency of the transducer and depth selection.

frank dislocation – the hip is laterally and posteriorly displaced to the extent that the femoral head has no contact with the acetabulum and the normal "U" configuration cannot be obtained on ultrasound.

free hand – system that uses a smooth sweeping motion in a single plane of acquisition.

fremitus – refers to vibrations produced by phonation and felt through the chest wall during palpation; a technique used in conjunction with power Doppler to identify the margins of a lesion.

frequency – number of cycles per second that a periodic event or function undergoes; number of cycles completed per unit of time; the frequency of a sound wave is determined by the number of oscillations per second of the vibrating source.

frontal bossing – slight indentation of the frontal bones of the skull; also known as "lemon head."

functional cyst – cyst resulting from the normal function of the ovary.

fusiform dilation – enlargement with tapering at both ends.

gain – measure of the strength of the ultrasound signal; can be expressed as a simple ratio or in decibels; overall gain amplifies all signals by a constant factor regardless of the depth.

Galeazzi sign – the knee is lower in position on the affected side when the patient is supine and the knees are flexed. On physical examination, the knee is lower in position on the affected side of the neonate with DDH when the patient is supine and the knees are flexed.

gallbladder – storage pouch for bile.

gamete intrafallopian transfer (GIFT) – a human fertilization technique in which male and female gametes are injected through a laparoscope into the fimbriated ends of the fallopian tubes. Recently, this has been performed under ultrasound guidance.

Gartner's duct cyst – small cyst within the vagina.

gastrin – endocrine hormone released from the stomach (stimulates secretion of gastric acid).

gastrocnemius veins – paired veins that lie in the medial and lateral gastrocnemius muscles and terminate into the popliteal vein.

gastroduodenal artery – branch of the common hepatic artery that supplies the stomach and duodenum.

gastrophrenic ligament – ligament that helps support the greater curvature of the stomach.

gastroschisis – congenital fissure that remains open in the wall of the abdomen just to the right of the umbilical cord; bowel and other organs may protrude outside the abdomen from this opening.

gastrosplenic ligament – one of the ligaments between the stomach and spleen that helps hold the spleen in place.

Gaucher's disease – one of the storage diseases in which fat and proteins are deposited abnormally in the body.

germinal matrix – fragile periventricular tissue (includes the caudate nucleus) that easily bleeds in the premature infant.

Gerota's fascia – another term for the renal fascia; the kidney is covered by the renal capsule, perirenal fat, Gerota's fascia, and pararenal fat.

gestational age – age of embryo since the date of conception.

gestational sac – structure that is normally within the uterus that contains the developing embryo.

gestational sac diameter – measurement used in the first trimester to estimate appropriate gestational age with menstrual dates.

gestational trophoblastic disease – trophoblastic tissue that has overtaken the pregnancy and has propagated throughout the uterine cavity; these tumors arise from the placental chorionic villi.

glomerulus – part of the filtration process in the kidney.

glucagon – hormone that stimulates the liver to convert glycogen to glucose; produced by alpha cells.

goiter – any enlargement of the thyroid, focal or diffuse, regardless of cause.

gonadotropin – a hormonal substance that stimulates the function of the testes and ovaries.

Graves' disease – syndrome characterized by a diffuse toxic goiter, ophthalmopathy, and cutaneous manifestations.

gravidity – total number of pregnancies.

gray scale – B-mode scanning technique that permits the brightness of the B-mode dots to be displayed in various shades of gray to represent different echo amplitudes.

grayscale harmonic imaging – allows detection of contrast-enhanced blood flow and organs with grayscale ultrasound; in the harmonic-imaging mode, the echoes from the oscillating microbubbles have a higher signal-to-noise ratio than found in conventional ultrasound; regions with microbubbles (e.g., blood vessels and organ parenchyma) are better visualized.

greater omentum – double fold of the peritoneum attached to the duodenum, stomach, and large intestine; helps support the greater curve of the stomach; known as the "fatty apron."

greater sac – primary compartment of the peritoneal cavity; extends across the anterior abdomen from the diaphragm to the pelvis.

greater saphenous vein – originates on the dorsum of the foot and ascends anterior to the medial malleolus and along the anteromedial side of the calf and thigh; joins the common femoral vein in the proximal thigh.

growth-adjusted sonar age (GASA) – method whereby the fetus is categorized into small, average, or large growth percentile.

gutters – most dependent areas in the flanks of the abdomen and pelvis where fluid collections may accumulate.

Guyon's canal or tunnel – a fibrous tunnel that contains the ulnar artery and vein, ulnar nerve, and some fatty tissue.

gynecomastia – hypertrophy of residual ductal elements that persist behind the nipple in the male, causing a palpable, tender lump. There is generally no lobular (glandular) tissue in the male. A breast mass resulting from gynecomastia must be distinguished from male breast cancer.

harmonic imaging – in the HI mode, the ultrasound system is configured to receive only echoes at the second harmonic frequency, which is twice the transmit frequency.

Hartmann's pouch – small part of the gallbladder that lies near the cystic duct where stones may collect.

Hashimoto's thyroiditis – chronic inflammation of the thyroid (goiter).

haustra – normal segmentation of the wall of the colon.

head of the pancreas – portion of the pancreas that lies in the C-loop of the duodenum; the gastroduodenal artery is the anterolateral border and the common bile duct is the posterolateral border.

Heister's valves – tiny valves found within the cystic duct.

hemangioma of the cord – vascular tumor within the umbilical cord.

hematocele – blood within the sac surrounding the testes.

hematochezia – passage of bloody stools.

hematocrit – the percent of the total blood volume containing the red blood cells, white blood cells, and the platelets.

hematometrocolpos – blood-filled vagina and uterus.

hematopoiesis – blood-cell production.

hemifacial microsomia – abnormal smallness of one side of the face.

hemiparesis – unilateral partial or complete paralysis.

hemoglobin – oxygen-binding protein found in red blood cells.

hemolytic anemia – anemia resulting from hemolysis of red blood cells.

hemoperitoneum – collection of bloody fluid in the abdomen or pelvis secondary to trauma or surgical procedure.

hemopoiesis – formation of blood.

hemorrhage – collection of blood.

hemosiderin – pigment released from hemoglobin process.

hepatic artery (HA) – common hepatic artery arises from the celiac trunk and courses to the right of the abdomen and branches into the gastroduodenal artery and proper HA.

hepatic flexure – point at which the ascending colon arises from the right lower quadrant to bend at this point to form the transverse colon.

hepatic veins – largest tributaries that drain the liver and empty into the inferior vena cava at the level of the diaphragm.

hepatocellular carcinoma – a common liver malignancy related to cirrhosis; the carcinoma may present as a solitary massive tumor, multiple nodules throughout the liver, or diffuse infiltrative masses in the liver; HCC can be very invasive.

hepatofugal – flow away from the liver.

hepatopetal – flow toward the liver.

hermaphroditism – condition in which both ovarian and testicular tissues are present.

hertz (Hz) – unit for frequency, equal to 1 cycle per second.

heterotopic pregnancy – simultaneous intrauterine and extrauterine pregnancy.

heterozygous achondroplasia – short-limb dysplasia that manifests in the second trimester of pregnancy; conversion abnormality of cartilage to bone affecting the epiphyseal growth centers; extremities are markedly shortened at birth with a normal trunk and frequent enlargement of the head.

hilus – area of kidney where vessels, ureter, and lymphatics enter and exit.

hip joint – formed by the articulation of the head of the femur with the acetabulum of the hip bone.

Hirschsprung's disease – congenital megacolon.

holoprosencephaly – congenital defect caused by an extra chromosome which causes a deficiency in the forebrain.

homeo- – same.

homeostasis – maintenance of a stable internal environment.

homozygous achondroplasia – short-limb dwarfism affecting fetuses of achondroplastic parents.

horseshoe kidney – congenital malformation in which both kidneys are joined together, most commonly at the lower poles.

human chorionic gonadotropin (hCG) – hormone within the maternal urine and serum; hCG is elevated during pregnancy; laboratory test that indicates pregnancy when values are elevated.

humeral length – measurement from the humeral head to the distal end of the humerus.

hydatidiform mole – benign form of gestational trophoblastic disease in which there is partial or complete conversion of the chorionic villi into grapelike vesicles; villia are avascular and there is trophoblastic proliferation; condition may result in malignant trophoblastic disease.

hydranencephaly – congenital absence of the cerebral hemispheres because of an occlusion of the carotid arteries; midbrain structures are present, and fluid replaces cerebral tissue.

hydrocele – fluid within the sac surrounding the testes.

hydrocephalus – ventriculomegaly in the neonate; abnormal accumulation of cerebrospinal fluid within the cerebral ventricles, resulting in compression and frequently destruction of brain tissue.

hydrocolpos – fluid-filled vagina.

hydrometrocolpos – collection of fluid in the vagina and uterus.

hydromyelia – dilation of the central canal of the spinal cord.

hydronephrosis – dilation of the renal collecting system.

hydrops – massive enlargement of the gallbladder.

hydrops fetalis – fluid occurring in at least two areas in the fetus: pleural effusion, pericardial effusion, ascites, or skin edema.

hydrosalpinx – fluid within the fallopian tube.

hydroureters – dilated ureters.

hyperechoic – echo texture that is more echogenic than the surrounding tissue. Hyperechoic masses in the breast are nearly always benign.

hyperemesis gravidarum – excessive vomiting that leads to dehydration and electrolyte imbalance.

hyperglycemia – uncontrolled increase in glucose levels in the blood.

hyperlipidemia – congenital condition in which there are elevated fat levels that may cause pancreatitis.

hyperplasia – enlargement of the adrenal glands.

hypertelorism – abnormally wide-spaced orbits usually found in conjunction with congenital anomalies and mental retardation.

hypertension – elevation of maternal blood pressure that may put fetus at risk.

hyperthyroidism – overactive thyroid gland.

hypertrophic pyloric stenosis (HPS) – thickened muscle in the pylorus that prevents food from entering the duodenum; occurs more frequently in males.

hyperventilation – deficiency of carbon dioxide.

hypochondrium – area of the duodenum in the upper zone on both sides of the epigastric region beneath the cartilages of the lower ribs.

hypoechoic – echo texture that is less echogenic than the surrounding tissue. Most solid breast masses (including cancer) are hypoechoic.

hypoglycemia – deficiency of glucose in the blood.

hypophosphatasia – congenital condition characterized by decreased mineralization of the bones resulting in "ribbonlike" and bowed limbs, underossified cranium, and compression of the chest; early death often occurs.

hypoplastic left heart – underdevelopment of the mitral valve, left ventricle, and aorta.

hypoplastic right heart – underdevelopment of the tricuspid valve, right ventricle, and pulmonary artery.

hypospadias – abnormal congenital opening of the male urethra on the undersurface of the penis.

hypotelorism – abnormally closely spaced orbits; association with holoprosencephaly, chromosomal and central nervous system disorders, and cleft palate.

hypotension – low blood pressure.

hypothyroidism – underactive thyroid gland.

hypoventilation – abnormal condition of the respiratory system of insufficient ventilation resulting in an excess of carbon dioxide.

iliac arteries – arteries that originate from the bifurcation of the aorta at the level of the umbilicus.

iliacus muscles – paired muscles that form the lateral wall of the pelvis.

ileus – dilated loops of bowel without peristalsis; associated with various abdominal problems, including pancreatitis, sickle cell crisis, and bowel obstruction.

incarcerated hernia – confinement of a part of the bowel; the visceral contents cannot be reduced.

incompetent cervix – cervix dilation that can result in the membranes bulging and rupturing so that fetus drops out; occurs silently in the second trimester.

incomplete abortion – retained products of conception.

incomplete atrioventricular septal defect – membranous septal defect, abnormal tricuspid valve, primum atrial septal defect, and cleft mitral valve.

induced acoustic emission – After the injection of the tissue-specific UCA Sonazoid, the reflectivity of the contrast-containing tissue increases; when the right level of acoustic energy is applied to tissue, the contrast microbubbles eventually rupture, resulting in random Doppler shifts; these shifts appear as a transient mosaic of colors on the color Doppler display; masses that have destroyed or replaced normal Kupffer cells will be displayed as color-free areas.

infantile polycystic kidney disease – autosomal recessive disease that affects the fetal kidneys and liver; the kidneys are enlarged and echogenic on ultrasound.

inferior mesenteric artery (IMA) – artery that arises from the anterior aortic wall at the level of the third or fourth lumbar vertebra to supply the left transverse colon, descending colon, sigmoid colon, and part of the rectum.

inferior mesenteric vein – vein that drains the left third of the colon and upper colon and joins the splenic vein.

inferior vena cava – largest venous abdominal vessel, formed by the union of the common iliac veins; supplies the right atrium of the heart along the posterior lateral wall.

infiltrating (invasive) ductal carcinoma – cancer of the ductal epithelium; most common general category of breast cancer, accounting for around approximately 85% of all breast cancers. This cancer usually arises in the terminal duct in the TDLU. If the cancerous cells remain within the duct without invading the breast tissue beyond the duct wall, this is ductal carcinoma in situ (DCIS). If the cancerous cells invade breast tissue (i.e., invasive ductal carcinoma or IDC), the cancer may spread into the regional lymph nodes and beyond. Of the many subtypes of IDC, the most common is infiltrating ductal carcinoma, not otherwise specified (IDC-NOS).

infiltrating (invasive) lobular carcinoma (ILC) – cancer of the lobular epithelium of the breast, arises at the level of the TDLU; accounts for 12% to 15% of all breast cancers.

informed consent – consent to surgery by a patient or to participation in a medical procedure or experiment by a subject after achieving an understanding of what is involved.

infracristal septal defect – defects found below the crista supraventricularis ridge in the membranous or muscular area.

inguinal ligament – ligament between the anterior superior iliac spine and the pubic tubercle.

innominate artery – first branch artery from the aortic arch.

innominate veins – veins that follow these courses: on the right, courses vertically downwards to join the left innominate vein below the first rib to form the superior vena cava; on the left, courses from left chest beneath the sternum to join the right innominate vein; the left innominate vein is longer than the right.

insulin – hormone that allows circulating glucose to enter tissue cells; failure to produce insulin results in diabetes mellitus.

interface – surface forming the boundary between media having different properties.

internal carotid artery – larger of the two terminal branches of the common carotid artery that arises from the common carotid artery to supply the anterior brain and meninges.

internal os – inner surface of the cervical os.

international normalized ratio – a method developed to standardize prothrombin time (PT) results among laboratories by accounting for the different thromboplastin reagents used to determine PT.

interstitial pregnancy – pregnancy occurring in the cornu of the uterus.

intertubercular plane – lowest horizontal line joins the tubercles on the iliac crests.

intrahepatic – within the liver.

intramural leiomyoma – most common type of leiomyoma; deforms the myometrium.

intraperitoneal – within the peritoneal cavity.

intrauterine contraceptive device (IUD, IUCD) – device inserted into the endometrial cavity to prevent pregnancy.

intrauterine growth restriction (IUGR) – decreased rate of fetal growth, usually a fetal weight below the tenth percentile for a given gestational age; may be symmetric (all growth parameters are small) or asymmetric (maybe caused by placental problem; head measurements correlate with dates; body disproportionately smaller); formerly referred to as intrauterine growth retardation.

intrauterine insemination – the introduction of semen into the vagina or uterus by mechanical or instrumental means rather than by sexual intercourse.

intravenous injection – a hypodermic injection into a vein for the purpose of injecting a contrast medium.

intravenous urography – procedure used in radiography wherein contrast is administered intravenously to help visualize the urinary system.

intussusception – bowel prolapses into distal bowel (telescoping) and is then propelled in an antegrade fashion.

invasive mole – tumor that penetrates into and through the uterine wall.

in vitro fertilization (IVF) – a method of fertilizing the human ova outside the body by collecting the mature ova and placing them in a dish with a sample of spermatozoa.

ischemic rest pain – critical ischemia (lack of blood) of the distal limb when the patient is at rest.

islets of Langerhans – portion of the pancreas that has an endocrine function and produces insulin, glucagon, and somatostatin.

isoechoic – echo texture that resembles the surrounding tissue. Isoechoic masses can be difficult to identify.

isthmus – small piece of thyroid tissue that connects the lower lobes of the gland.

IUP – intrauterine pregnancy.

jaundice – excessive bilirubin accumulation causes yellow pigmentation of the skin; first seen in the whites of the eyes.

jejunoileal atresia – blockage of the jejunum and ileal bowel segments that appears as multiple cystic structures within the fetal abdomen.

junctional fold – small septum within the gallbladder, usually arising from the posterior wall.

juxtathoracic – near the chest wall (thorax).

kilohertz (kHz) – 1000 Hz.

Klatskin's tumor – cancer at the bifurcation of the hepatic ducts; may cause asymmetric obstruction of the biliary tree.

Kupffer cells – special hepatic cells that remove bile pigment, old blood cells, and the by-products of phagocytosis from the blood and deposit them into the bile ducts.

large for gestational age (LGA) – fetus measures larger than would be expected for dates (diabetic fetus).

lateral arcuate ligament – thickened upper margin of the fascia covering the anterior surface of the quadratus lumborum muscle.

left atrium – filling chamber of the heart.

left crus of the diaphragm – tendinous connection of the diaphragm that arises from the sides of the bodies of the first two lumbar vertebrae.

left gastric artery – artery that arises from the celiac axis to supply the stomach and lower third of the esophagus.

left hypochondrium – left upper quadrant of the abdomen that contains the left lobe of the liver, spleen, and stomach.

left lobe of the liver – lobe that lies in the epigastrium and left hypochondrium.

left portal vein – the main portal vein branches into the left and right portal veins to supply the liver.

left renal artery – artery that arises from the posterolateral wall of the aorta directly into the hilus of the kidney.

left renal vein – leaves the renal hilum, travels anterior to the aorta and posterior to the superior mesenteric artery to enter the lateral wall of the inferior vena cava.

left ventricle – pumping chamber of the heart.

leiomyoma – most common benign gynecologic tumor in women during their reproductive years.

lemon sign – seen on sonography, sign of frontal bones collapsing inward; occurs with spina bifida.

lesser omentum – membranous extension of the peritoneum that suspends the stomach and duodenum from the liver; helps to support the lesser curvature of the stomach.

lesser sac – peritoneal pouch located behind the lesser omentum and stomach.

lesser saphenous vein – vein that originates on the dorsum of the foot and ascends posterior to the lateral malleolus and runs along the midline of the posterior calf; vein terminates as it joins the popliteal vein.

leucopoiesis – white blood cell formation stimulated by presence of bacteria.

leukocyte – white blood cell; primary function is to defend the body against infection.

leukocytosis – increase in the number of leukocytes.

leukopenia – abnormal decrease of white blood corpuscles; may be drug induced.

levator ani muscles – a pair of muscles that form the floor of the pelvis.

lienorenal ligament – ligament between the spleen and kidney that helps hold the spleen in place and supports the greater curvature of the stomach.

ligament – fibrous band of tissue connecting bone or cartilage to bone that aids in stabilizing a joint.

ligamentum teres – termination of the falciform ligament; seen in the left lobe of the liver.

ligamentum venosum – transformation of the ductus venosus in fetal life to closure in neonatal life. It separates left lobe from caudate lobe; shown as echogenic line on the transverse and sagittal images.

limb–body wall complex – anomaly with large cranial defects, facial cleft, large body wall defects, and limb abnormalities.

linea alba – fibrous band of tissue that stretches from the xiphoid to the symphysis pubis.

linea semilunaris – line that extends from the ninth costal cartilage to the pubic tubercle.

lipase – pancreatic enzyme that acts on fats; enzyme is elevated in pancreatitis and remains increased longer than amylase.

lipoma – common benign tumor composed of fat cells.

liver function tests – specific laboratory tests that look at liver function (aspartate or alanine aminotransferase, lactic acid dehydrogenase, alkaline phosphatase, and bilirubin).

lobular carcinoma in situ (LCIS) – see lobular neoplasia.

lobular neoplasia – term preferred by many authors to replace LCIS (not considered a true cancer nor treated as such) and atypical hyperplasia.

long axis – plane that transects heart perpendicular to dorsal and ventral surfaces of body and parallel with long axis of heart.

loop of Henle – portion of a renal tubule lying between the proximal and distal convoluted portions; reabsorption of fluid, sodium, and chloride occurs in the proximal convoluted tubule and the loop of Henle.

lower uterine segment – thin expanded lower portion of the uterus at the junction of the internal os and sacrum that forms in the last trimester of pregnancy.

lymph – alkaline fluid found in the lymphatic vessels.

lymphangiectasia – dilation of a lymph node.

lymphoma – malignancy that primarily affects the lymph nodes, spleen, or liver.

macrocephaly – enlargement of the fetal cranium as a result of ventriculomegaly.

macroglossia – hypertrophied tongue.

macrosomia – birth weight greater than 4000 g or above the 90th percentile for the estimated gestational age; these infants have fat deposition in the subcutaneous tissues.

main lobar fissure – boundary between the right and left lobes of the liver; seen as hyperechoic line on the sagittal image extending from the portal vein to the neck of the gallbladder.

main portal vein – vein formed by union of the splenic vein and superior mesenteric vein; enters the liver at the porta hepatis.

main pulmonary artery – main artery that carries blood from the right ventricle to the lungs.

major calyces (also known as the **infundibulum**) – area of the kidneys that receives urine from the minor calyces to convey to the renal pelvis.

malpighian corpuscles – small, round, deep red bodies in the cortex of the kidney, each communicating with a renal tubule.

mammary layer – middle layer of the breast tissue (one of three layers recognized on breast ultrasound between the skin and the chest wall) that contains the ductal, glandular, and stromal portions of the breast.

Marfan's syndrome – hereditary disorder of connective tissue, bones, muscles, ligaments, and skeletal structures.

maternal serum alpha-fetoprotein (MSAFP) – antigen present in the fetus; the maternal serum is tested between 16 and 18 weeks of gestation to detect abnormal levels; can also be tested directly from the amniotic fluid from amniocentesis.

maternal serum quad screen – a blood test conducted during the second trimester (15 to 22 weeks) to identify pregnancies at a higher risk for chromosomal anomalies (trisomy 21 and trisomy 18) and neural tube defects.

maximum or **deep vertical pocket** – method to determine the amount of amniotic fluid; pocket less than 2 cm may indicate oligohydramnios; greater than 8 cm indicates polyhydramnios. This method is used more often in multiple gestation pregnancy.

McBurney's point – site of maximum tenderness in the right lower quadrant; usually with appendicitis.

mean velocity – velocity based on the time average of the outline velocity (maximum velocity envelope).

mechanical index – an index that defines the low acoustic output power that can be used to minimize the destruction of microbubbles by energy in the acoustic field; when the microbubbles in microbubble-based ultrasound contrast agents are destroyed, contrast enhancement is lost.

Meckel's diverticulum – congenital sac or blind pouch found in the lower portion of the ileum; a remnant of the proximal part of the yolk stalk.

meconium ileus – small-bowel disorder marked by the presence of thick echogenic meconium in the distal ileum.

medial arcuate ligament – thickened upper margin of the fascia covering the anterior surface of the psoas muscle. It connects the medial borders of the two diaphragmatic crura as they cross anterior to the aorta.

mediastinum testis – linear structure within the midline of the testes.

medulla of the adrenal – central tissue of the adrenal gland that secrets epinephrine and norepinephrine.

medulla of the kidney (also known as the **pyramid**) – inner portion of the renal parenchyma that contains the loop of Henle.

medullary carcinoma – neoplastic growth that accounts for 10% of thyroid malignancies.

medullary pyramids – large and hypoechoic in the neonate.

megahertz (MHz) – 1,000,000 Hz.

Meigs' syndrome – benign tumor of the ovary associated with ascites and pleural effusion.

membranous or velamentous insertion of the cord – insertion of the cord into the membranes before it enters the placenta.

menarche – onset of menstruation; state after reaching puberty in which menses occur normally every 27 to 28 days.

meninges – linings of the brain.

meningocele – open spinal defect characterized by protrusion of the spinal meninges.

meningomyelocele – open spinal defect characterized by protrusion of meninges and spinal cord through the defect, usually within a meningeal sac.

menopause – cessation of menstruation.

menses – monthly flow of blood from the endometrium.

menstrual age – gestational age of the fetus determined from the first day of the last normal menstrual period (LMP) to the point at which the pregnancy is being assessed.

mesentery – a fold from the parietal peritoneum that attaches to the small intestine anchoring it to the posterior abdominal wall.

mesosalpinx – free margin of the upper portion of the broad ligament where the oviduct is found.

mesothelium – tissue that lines the body cavities of the embryo, part of which develops into the peritoneum.

meta- – change.

metabolism – physical and chemical changes that occur within the body.

metastatic disease – tumor that develops away from the site of the organ; most common form of neoplasm of the liver; most common primary sites are colon, breast, and lung.

microcephaly – head smaller than the body.

micrognathia – abnormally small chin; commonly associated with other fetal anomalies.

microphthalmos – small eyes.

middle cerebral artery (MCA) – large terminal branch of the internal carotid artery.

midline echo complex (the falx) – widest transverse diameter of the skull; proper level to measure the biparietal diameter.

minor calyces – area of the kidneys that receives urine from the renal pyramids; form the border of the renal sinus.

mitral atresia – thickened, underdeveloped mitral apparatus.

mitral regurgitation – failure of the leaflets to close completely, allowing blood to leak backward into the left atrium.

mitral valve – atrioventricular valve between the left atrium and left ventricle.

molar pregnancy – also known as gestational trophoblastic disease; abnormal proliferation of trophoblastic cells in the first trimester.

molecular imaging agents – agents include Optison, Definity, Imagent, Levbovist, and Sono Vue.

monoamniotic – multiple pregnancy with one amniotic sac.

monochorionic – multiple pregnancy with one chorionic sac.

monozygotic – twins that arise from a single fertilized egg that divides to produce two identical fetuses.

Morison's pouch – right posterior subphrenic space that lies between the right lobe of the liver, anterior to the kidney and right colic flexure, where fluid may lie or an abscess may develop.

MSD – mean sac diameter.

mucinous cystadenocarcinoma – malignant tumor of the ovary with multilocular cysts.

mucinous cystadenoma – benign tumor of the ovary that contains thin-walled, multilocular cysts.

mucosa – mucous membrane; thin sheet of tissue that lines cavities of the body that open to the outside; it is the first layer of bowel.

multicentric breast cancer – breast cancers occurring in different quadrants of the breast that are at least 5 cm or more apart; multicentric cancers are more likely to be of different histologic types than is a multifocal cancer.

multicystic dysplastic kidney disease (MCDK) – multiple cysts replace normal renal tissue throughout the kidney; usually causes renal obstruction; most common cause of renal cystic disease in the neonate; may have contralateral ureteral pelvic junction obstruction.

multifocal breast cancer – breast cancer occurring in more than one site within the same quadrant or the same ductal system of the breast.

multinodular goiter – nodular enlargement of the thyroid associated with hyperthyroidism.

multiplanar imaging – ability to collect data from axial, coronal, and sagittal planes for reconstruction into 3-D format.

Murphy's sign – positive sign implies exquisite tenderness over the area of the gallbladder upon palpation.

muscle – a type of tissue consisting of contractile cells or fibers that affects movement of an organ or part of the body.

muscularis – third layer of bowel.

myelin – substance forming the sheath of Schwann cells.

myeloschisis – cleft spinal cord resulting from failure of the neural tube to close.

myocardium – thickest muscle in the heart wall.

myometritis – infection within the myometrium of the uterus.

myometrium – middle layer of the uterine cavity that appears very homogeneous with sonography.

nabothian cyst – benign tiny cyst within the cervix.

naked tuberosity sign – the deltoid muscle is on the humeral head; seen with a full-thickness tear of the rotator cuff.

neck of the pancreas – small area of the pancreas between the head and the body; anterior to the superior mesenteric vein.

neonate – infant during the early newborn period.

neoplasm – refers to any new growth (benign or malignant).

nephroblastomatosis – abnormal persistence of fetal renal blastema (potential to develop into Wilms' tumor).

nephron – functional unit of the kidney; includes a renal corpuscle and a renal tubule.

neuroblastoma – malignant adrenal mass that is seen in pediatric patients.

nonimmune hydrops (NIH) – group of conditions in which hydrops is present in the fetus but not a result of fetomaternal blood group incompatibility.

nonmaleficence – refrain from harming oneself or others.

nonpalpable – cannot be felt on clinical examination; nonpalpable breast mass is one that is usually identified on screening mammogram and is too small to be felt as a breast lump on BSE or CBE.

nonresistive – vessels that have high diastolic component and supply organs that need constant perfusion (internal carotid artery, hepatic artery, and renal artery).

Non-Stress Test (NST) – test that utilizes Doptone (a brand of Doppler instrumentation used in obstetric examinations) to record the fetal heart rate and its reactivity to the stress of uterine contraction.

normal situs – indicates normal position of the abdominal organs (liver on right, stomach on left, heart apex to the left).

nuchal cord – condition that occurs when the cord is wrapped around the fetal neck.

nuchal lucency – increased thickness in the nuchal fold area in the back of the neck associated with trisomy 21.

obstructive disease – blockage of bile excretion within the liver or biliary system.

obturator internus muscle – arises from the anterolateral pelvic wall surrounding the obturator foramen to insert on the greater trochanter of the femur.

oculodentodigital dysplasia – underdevelopment of the eyes, fingers, and mouth.

oligohydramnios – insufficient amount of amniotic fluid.

-ology – study of; *physiology*: study of body functions.

omphalocele – anterior abdominal wall defect in which abdominal organs (liver, bowel, stomach) are atypically located within the umbilical cord and protrude outside the wall; highly associated with cardiac, central nervous system, renal, and chromosomal anomalies. It develops when there is a midline defect of the abdominal muscles, fascia, and skin.

omphalomesenteric cyst – cystic lesion of the umbilical cord.

oophoritis – infection within the ovary.

ophthalmic artery – first branch of the internal carotid artery.

Ortolani maneuver – patient lies in the supine position. The examiner's hand is placed around the hip to be examined with the fingers over the femoral head. The hip is flexed 90 degrees and the thigh is abducted.

osteogenesis imperfecta – metabolic disorder affecting the fetal collagen system that leads to varying forms of bone disease; intrauterine bone fractures, shortened long bones, poorly mineralized calvaria, and compression of the chest found in type II forms.

otocephaly – underdevelopment of the jaw that causes the ears to be located close together toward the front of the neck.

ovarian carcinoma – malignant tumor of the ovary that may spread beyond the ovary and metastasize to other organs via the peritoneal channels.

ovarian cyst – cyst of the ovary that may be found in the fetus; results from maternal hormone stimulation and is usually benign.

ovarian hyperstimulation syndrome (OHS) – a syndrome that presents sonographically as enlarged ovaries with multiple cysts, abdominal ascites, and pleural effusions. Often seen in patients who have undergone ovulation induction post administration of follicle-stimulating hormone or a GnRH analogue followed by hCG.

ovulation induction therapy – controlled ovarian stimulation with clomiphene citrate or parenterally administered gonadotropins.

ovarian torsion – partial or complete rotation of the ovarian pedicle on its axis.

Paget's disease of the breast – surface erosion of the nipple that results from direct invasion of the skin of the nipple from underlying breast cancer.

palpable – can be felt on clinical examination; palpable breast lump is one that is identified on CBE or BSE.

pampiniform plexus – multiple veins that drain the testicles; when a varicocele is present, dilation and tortuosity may develop.

pancreatic ascites – fluid accumulation caused by a rupture of a pancreatic pseudocyst into the abdomen; free-floating pancreatic enzymes are very dangerous to surrounding structures.

pancreatic duct – duct that travels horizontally through the pancreas to join the common bile duct at the ampulla of Vater.

pancreatic pseudocyst – "sterile abscess" collection of pancreatitis enzymes that accumulate in the available space in the abdomen (usually in or near the pancreas).

pancreaticoduodenal arteries – arteries that help supply blood to the pancreas along with the splenic artery.

pancreatitis – inflammation of the pancreas; may be acute or chronic.

papillary carcinoma – most common form of thyroid malignancy.

paralytic ileus – dilated, fluid-filled loops of bowel without peristalsis secondary to obstruction, decreased vascularity, or abnormal metabolic state.

parametritis – infection within the uterine serosa and broad ligaments.

paraovarian cyst – cystic structure that lies adjacent to the ovary.

parasternal – transducer placement over the area bounded superiorly by left clavicle, medially by sternum, and inferiorly by apical region.

pariet- – wall; *parietal membrane*: membrane that lines the wall of a cavity.

parietal peritoneum – layer of the peritoneum that lines the abdominal wall.

parity – number of live births.

partial mole – condition that develops when two sperm fertilize an egg.

partial situs inversus – reversal of the heart or the abdominal organs (dextrocardia or liver on the left, stomach on the right).

partial thromboplastin time – laboratory test that can be used to evaluate the effects of heparin, aspirin, and antihistamines on the blood clotting process; PTT detects clotting abnormalities of the intrinsic and common pathways.

patent ductus arteriosus – open communication between the pulmonary artery and descending aorta that does not constrict after birth.

peau d'orange – French term that means "skin of the orange"; descriptive term for skin thickening of one breast that, on clinical breast examination, resembles the skin of an orange. Such an appearance can result from an inflammatory breast condition (mastitis), simple edema, or skin involvement from underlying breast cancer.

pelv- – basin; *pelvic cavity*: basin-shaped cavity enclosed by the pelvic bones.

pelvic girdle – formation of the hip bones by the ilium, ischium, and pubis.

pelvic inflammatory disease (PID) – all-inclusive term that refers to all pelvic infections (endometritis, salpingitis, hydrosalpinx, pyosalpinx, and tuboovarian abscess).

pelvic kidney – location of the kidney when the kidney does not migrate upward into the retroperitoneal space.

pelviectasis – dilated renal pelvis measuring 5 to 9 mm in the anteroposterior direction.

pennate – featherlike pattern of muscle growth.

pentalogy of Cantrell – rare anomaly with five defects: omphalocele, ectopic heart, lower sternum, anterior diaphragm, and diaphragmatic pericardium.

perforating veins – veins that connect the superficial and deep venous systems.

pericardium – sac surrounding the heart, reflecting off the great arteries.

perineurium – the surrounding connective tissue of muscle.

period – duration of a single cycle of a periodic wave or event.

peripheral occlusive arterial disease – narrowing or stenosis of the peripheral arteries.

peripheral zone – posterior and lateral aspect of the prostate.

perirenal space – located directly around the kidney; completely enclosed by renal fascia.

peristalsis – rhythmic dilatation and contraction of the gastrointestinal tract as food is propelled through it.

peritoneal cavity – potential space between the parietal and visceral peritoneal layers.

peritoneal lavage – invasive procedure that is used to sample the intraperitoneal space for evidence of damage to viscera and blood vessels.

peritoneal recess – slitlike spaces near the liver; potential space for fluid to accumulate.

peritonitis – inflammation of the peritoneum.

periventricular leukomalacia – echogenic white matter necrosis best seen in the posterior aspect of the brain or adjacent to the ventricular structures.

peroneal veins – veins that drain blood from the lateral lower leg.

phagocytosis – process by which cells engulf and destroy microorganisms and cellular debris; "cell-eating"; for example, the red pulp destroys the degenerating red blood cells.

Phalen's sign (Phalen's test, Phalen's maneuver, or Phalen's position) – an increase in wrist compression due to hyperflexion of the wrist for 60 seconds; this test is done with the patient holding the forearms upright and pressing the ventral side of the hands together.

phenylketonuria (PKU) – hereditary disease caused by failure to oxidize an amino acid (phenylalanine) to tyrosine, because of a defective enzyme; if PKU is not treated early, mental retardation can develop.

pheochromocytoma – benign adrenal tumor that secretes hormones that produce hypertension.

phlegmasia alba dolens – swollen, painful white leg.

phlegmasia cerulea dolens – swollen, painful cyanotic leg.

phrenocolic ligament – one of the ligaments between the spleen and splenic flexure of the colon.

phrygian cap – gallbladder variant in which part of the fundus is bent back on itself.

Pierre Robin syndrome – micrognathia and abnormal smallness of the tongue usually with a cleft palate.

piezoelectric effect – generation of electric signals as a result of an incident sound beam on a material that has piezoelectric properties; in the converse (or reverse) piezoelectric effect, the material expands or contracts when an electric signal is applied.

piriformis muscle – muscle that arises from the sacrum between the pelvic sacral foramina and the gluteal surface of the ilium.

pitting – process by which the spleen removes abnormal red blood cells.

placenta – organ of communication (nutrition and products of metabolism) between the fetus and the mother; forms from the chorion frondosum with a maternal decidual contribution.

placenta accreta – growth of the chorionic villi superficially into the myometrium.

placenta increta – growth of the chorionic villi deep into the myometrium.

placenta percreta – growth of the chorionic villi through the myometrium.

placenta previa – placental implantation that encroaches upon the lower uterine segment; the placenta comes first and bleeding is inevitable.

placental grade – technique of grading the placenta for maturity.

placental grading – arbitrary method of classifying the maturity of the placenta with a grading scale of 0 to 3.

placental insufficiency – abnormal condition of pregnancy manifested by a restricted rate of fetal and uterine growth. One or more placental abnormalities cause dysfunction of maternal-placental or fetal-placental circulation.

placental migration – movement of the placenta as the uterus enlarges the placenta; a low-lying placenta may move out of the uterine segment in the second trimester.

planar reconstruction – movement of the intersection point (point of rotation) of the three orthogonal image planes throughout the 3-D volume and rotating the image planes; the sonographer or physician has the liberty to generate anatomic views from an infinite number of perspectives.

plantar flexion – pointing of the toes toward the plantar surface of the foot.

pleur – rib; *pleural membrane*: membrane that encloses the lungs within the rib cage.

pleural effusion (hydrothorax) – accumulation of fluid within the thoracic cavity.

pneumothorax – a collection of air or gas in the pleural cavity.

polycystic kidney disease – poorly functioning enlarged kidneys.

polycystic ovarian disease – endocrine disorder associated with chronic anovulation.

polycythemia – excess of red blood cells.

polycythemia vera – chronic, life-shortening condition of unknown etiology involving bone marrow elements; characterized by an increase in red blood cell mass and hemoglobin concentration.

polydactyly – anomalies of the hands or feet in which there is an addition of a digit; may be found in association with certain skeletal dysplasias.

polyhydramnios – excessive amount of amniotic fluid.

polyp of gallbladder – small, well-defined soft tissue projection from the gallbladder wall.

polysplenia – condition where there is more than one spleen; associated with cardiac malformations.

popliteal artery – artery that begins at the opening of the adductor magnus muscle and travels behind the knee in the popliteal fossa.

popliteal vein – vein that originates from the confluence of the anterior tibial veins and posterior and peroneal veins.

porta hepatis – central area of the liver where the portal vein, common duct, and hepatic artery enter.

portal confluence – see confluence of the splenic and portal veins.

portal vein – vein formed by the union of the superior mesenteric vein and splenic vein near the porta hepatis of the liver.

portal venous hypertension – results from intrinsic liver disease; may cause flow reversal to the liver, thrombosis of the portal system, or cavernous transformation of the portal vein.

portal-splenic confluence – junction of the splenic and main portal vein; posterior border of the body of the pancreas.

postcoital test (PCT) – a clinical test done within 24 hours after intercourse to assess sperm motility in cervical mucus.

posterior arch vein – main tributary of the greater saphenous vein.

posterior cerebral artery (PCA) – artery that originates from the terminal basilar artery and courses anteriorly and laterally.

posterior communicating artery (PCoA) – courses posteriorly and medially from the internal carotid artery to join the posterior cerebral artery.

posterior pararenal space – space found between the posterior renal fascia and the muscles of the posterior abdominal wall.

posterior tibial veins – veins that originate from the plantar veins of the foot and drain blood from the posterior lower leg.

posterior urethral valve – the presence of a valve in the posterior urethra; occurs only in male fetuses; most common cause of bladder outlet obstruction in the male neonate.

postterm – fetus born later than the 42-week gestational period.

Potter's syndrome – condition characterized by renal agenesis, oligohydramnios, pulmonary hypoplasia, abnormal facies, and malformed hands and feet.

Pourcelot resistive index – Doppler measurement that takes the highest systolic peak minus the highest diastolic peak divided by the highest systolic peak.

preeclampsia – also known as *pregnancy-induced hypertension (PIH)*. A complication of pregnancy characterized by increasing hypertension, proteinuria, and edema.

premature atrial and ventricular contractions – fetal cardiac arrhythmia resulting from extra systoles and ectopic beats.

premature rupture of the membranes (PROM) – leaking or breaking of the amniotic membranes causing the loss of amniotic fluid, which may lead to premature delivery or infection.

premenarche – time period in young girls before the onset of menstruation.

preterm – fetus born earlier than the normal 38- to 42-week gestational period.

primary yolk sac – first site of formation of red blood cells that will nourish the embryo.

proboscis – a cylindrical protuberance of the face that in cyclopia or ethmocephaly represents the nose.

profunda femoris artery – artery posterior and lateral to the superficial femoral artery.

projectile vomiting – condition found in pyloric stenosis in the neonatal period; after drinking, the infant experiences projectile vomiting secondary to the obstruction.

proliferative phase – days 5 to 9 of the menstrual cycle; endometrium appears as a single thin stripe with a hypoechoic halo encompassing it; creates the "three-line sign."

prostate specific antigen – laboratory test that measures levels of the protein prostate specific antigen in the body; elevated levels could indicate prostate cancer.

prothrombin time – laboratory test used to detect clotting abnormalities of the extrinsic pathway; measured against a control sample, PT tests the time it takes for a blood sample to coagulate after thromboplastin and calcium are added to it.

prune-belly syndrome – dilation of the fetal abdomen secondary to severe bilateral hydronephrosis and fetal ascites; fetus also has oligohydramnios and pulmonary hypoplasia.

pseudoaneurysm – perivascular collection (hematoma) that communicates with an artery or a graft and has the presence of pulsating blood entering the collection.

pseudoascites – sonolucent band near the fetal anterior abdominal wall seen in the fetus over 18 weeks (does not outline the falciform ligament or bowel as ascites will).

pseudo-dissection – condition seen in a patient with aortic dissection; there is no intimal flap seen, only hypoechoic thrombus near the outer margin of the aorta with echogenic laminated clot.

pseudogestational sac – decidual reaction that occurs within the uterus in a patient with an ectopic pregnancy.

psoas major muscle – begins at the level of hilum of the kidneys and extends inferiorly along both sides of the spine into the pelvis.

pudendal artery – the internal and external pudendal arteries partially supply the scrotal wall and epididymis and occasionally the lower pole of the testis.

pulmonary embolism – blockage of the pulmonary circulation by a thrombus or other matter; may lead to death if blockage of pulmonary blood flow is significant.

pulmonary hypoplasia – small, underdeveloped lungs with resultant reduction in lung volume; secondary to prolonged oligohydramnios or as a consequence of a small thoracic cavity.

pulmonary stenosis – thickening and narrowing of the pulmonic cusps; causes blood to back up into the right ventricle and atrium.

pulmonary veins – four pulmonary veins bring blood from the lungs back into the posterior wall of the left atrium; there are two upper (right and left) and two lower (right and left) pulmonary veins.

pulsatility index (PI) – Doppler measurement that uses peak systole minus peak diastole divided by the mean.

pulse duration – measure of the ring-down (an artifact that occurs when the ultrasound transducer strikes the ribs) time of a transducer after excitation.

pulsed wave transducer – single crystal that sends and receives sound intermittently; a pulse of sound is emitted from the transducer, which also receives the returning signal.

pyloric canal – canal located between the stomach and duodenum.

pyocele – pus located between the visceral and parietal layers of the tunica vaginalis.

pyogenic – pus producing.

pyogenic abscess – pus-forming collection of fluid.

pyosalpinx – retained pus within the inflamed fallopian tube.

pyramidal lobe – lobe of the thyroid gland that is present in small percentage of patients; extends superiorly from the isthmus.

pyramids – area of the kidneys that convey urine to the minor calyces.

radial – descriptive term used to denote area of the breast relative to a clock.

radial artery – artery that begins at the brachial artery bifurcation.

reactive hyperemia – alternative method to stress the peripheral arterial circulation.

real-time – ultrasound instrumentation that allows the image to be displayed many times per second to achieve a "real-time" image of anatomic structures and their motion patterns.

rectouterine pouch (pouch of Douglas) – area in the pelvic cavity between the rectum and the uterus that is likely to accumulate free fluid.

rectus abdominis muscle – muscle of the anterior abdominal wall.

rectus sheath hematoma – hemorrhage within the anterior rectus sheath muscle usually secondary to trauma.

recurrent rami – terminal ends of the centripetal (intratesticular) arteries that curve backward toward the capsule.

red pulp – tissue composed of reticular cells and fibers (cords of Billroth); surrounds the splenic sinuses.

reducible hernia – capable of being replaced in a normal position; the visceral contents can be returned to normal intraabdominal location.

refractile shadowing (edge artifact) – the bending of the sound beam at the edge of a circular structure, resulting in the absence of posterior echoes.

refraction – change in the direction of propagation of a sound wave transmitted across an interface where the speed of sound varies.

renal agenesis – interruption in the normal development of the kidney resulting in absence of the kidney; may be unilateral or bilateral.

renal artery – artery that arises from the posterolateral wall of the aorta, travels posterior to the inferior vena cava to supply the kidney.

renal artery stenosis – narrowing of the renal artery; historically, this has been very difficult to evaluate sonographically.

renal capsule – first layer adjacent to the kidney that forms a tough, fibrous covering.

renal corpuscle – part of the nephron that consists of Bowman's capsule and the glomerulus.

renal hilum – area in the midportion of the kidney where the renal vessels and ureter enter and exit.

renal pelvis – area in the midportion of the kidney that collects urine before entering the ureter.

renal sinus – central area of the kidney that includes the calyces, renal pelvis, renal vessels, fat, nerves, and lymphatics.

renal vein thrombosis – obstruction of the renal vein resulting in kidney becoming enlarged and edematous.

resistive index – peak systole minus peak diastole divided by peak systole (S-D/S 5 RI); an RI of 0.7 or less indicates good perfusion; an RI of 0.7 or higher indicates decreased perfusion.

resolution – ability of the transducer to distinguish between two structures adjacent to one another.

respect for persons – incorporates both respect for the autonomy of individuals and the requirement to protect those with diminished autonomy.

respiratory phasicity – change in blood flow velocity with respiration.

rete testis – network of the channels formed by the convergence of the straight seminiferous tubules in the mediastinum testis; these channels drain into the head of the epididymis.

reticuloendothelial cells – certain phagocytic cells (found mainly in the liver and spleen) make up the reticuloendothelial system (RES), which plays a role in the defense against infection and synthesis of blood proteins and hematopoiesis.

retromammary layer – deepest of the three layers of the breast noted on breast ultrasound. The retromammary layer is predominantly fatty and can be thin. The retromammary layer separates the active breast glandular tissue from the pectoralis fascia overlying the chest wall muscles.

retroperitoneum – space behind the peritoneal lining of the abdominal cavity.

retroverted – refers to the position of the uterus when the fundus is tipped posteriorly.

Rh blood group – system of antigens that may be found on the surface of red blood cells. When the Rh factor is present, the blood type is Rh positive; when the Rh antigen is absent, the blood type is Rh negative. A pregnant woman who is Rh negative may become sensitized by the blood of an Rh positive fetus. In subsequent pregnancies, if the fetus is Rh positive, the Rh antibodies produced in maternal blood may cross over the placenta and destroy fetal cells, causing erythroblastosis fetalis.

rhabdomyoma – benign cardiac tumor of the heart that is associated with tuberous sclerosis.

right atrium – filling chamber of the heart.

right crus of the diaphragm – arises from the sides of the bodies of the first three lumbar vertebrae.

right gastric artery – artery that supplies the stomach.

right hepatic artery – artery that supplies the gallbladder via the cystic artery.

right hypochondrium – right upper quadrant of the abdomen that contains the liver and gallbladder.

right lobe of the liver – largest of the lobes of the liver.

right portal vein – the main portal vein branches into the right and left portal veins to supply the lobes of the liver.

right renal artery – artery that arises from the posterolateral wall of the aorta and travels posterior to the inferior vena cava to enter the hilum of the kidney.

right renal vein – vein that leaves the renal hilum to enter the lateral wall of the inferior vena cava.

right ventricle – pumping chamber of the heart that sends blood into the pulmonary artery.

ROI – region of interest.

rugae – inner folds of the stomach wall.

saccular aneurysm – localized dilatation of the vessel.

sagittal plane – vertical plane through the longitudinal axis of the body that divides it into two portions.

salpingitis – infection within the fallopian tubes.

saphenous opening – gap in the fascia lata, which is found 4 cm inferior and lateral to the pubic tubercle.

sciatic nerve – largest nerve in the upper thigh.

scoliosis – abnormal curvature of the spine.

scrotum – dependent sac containing the testes and epididymis.

S/D ratio – difference between peak systole and peak diastole.

secondary yolk sac – sac formed at 23 days when the primary yolk sac is pinched off by the extra embryonic coelom.

second generation agents – agents containing heavy gasses (i.e., Optison).

secretin – hormone released from small bowel as antacid; stimulates secretion of bicarbonate.

secretory (early) phase – days 10 to 14 of the menstrual cycle; ovulation occurs; the endometrium increases in thickness and echogenicity.

secretory (luteal) phase – days 14 to 28 of the menstrual cycle; the endometrium is at its greatest thickness and echogenicity with posterior enhancement.

semilunar valve – valve located in the aortic or pulmonic artery.

seminal vesicles – reservoirs for sperm located posterior to the bladder.

sentinel node – represents the first lymph node along the axillary node chain. This is the node chain the surgeon identifies for evidence of metastasis.

sepsis – spread of an infection from its initial site to the bloodstream.

septa testis – multiple septa formed from the tunica albuginea that course toward the mediastinum testis and separate the testicle into lobules.

septicemia – infection in the blood.

septum primum – first part of the atrial septum to grow from the dorsal wall of the primitive atrium; fuses with the endocardial cushions.

septum secundum – part of the atrial septum that grows into the atrium to the right of the septum primum.

seroma – accumulation of serous fluid within tissue.

serosa – fourth layer of bowel; thin, loose layer of connective tissue, surrounded by mesothelium covering the intraperitoneal bowel loops.

serous cystadenocarcinoma – most common type of ovarian carcinoma; may be bilateral with multilocular cysts.

serous cystadenoma – second most common benign tumor of the ovary; unilocular or multilocular.

serum amylase – pancreatic enzyme that is elevated during pancreatitis.

short axis – plane that transects heart perpendicular to dorsal and ventral surfaces of body and perpendicular to long axis of heart.

sickle cell anemia – inherited disorder transmitted as an autosomal recessive trait that causes an abnormality of the globin genes in hemoglobin.

sickle cell crisis – condition in sickle cell anemia in which the malformed red cells interfere with oxygen transport, obstruct capillary blood flow, and cause fever and severe pain in the joints and abdomen.

simple ovarian cyst – smooth, well-defined cystic structure that is filled completely with fluid.

single umbilical artery – condition of one umbilical cord instead of two; it has a high association with congenital anomalies.

single ventricle – condition in which there are two atria with one ventricle.

sinoatrial node – forms in the wall of the sinus venosus near its opening into the right atrium.

situs inversus – heart and abdominal organs are completely reversed.

sludge – low-level echoes found along the posterior margin of the gallbladder; move with change in position.

small for gestational age (SGA) – fetus measures smaller than would be expected for dates.

soleal sinuses – large venous reservoirs that lie in the soleus muscle and empty into the posterior tibial or peroneal veins.

sonohysterography – technique that uses a catheter inserted into the endometrial cavity with the insertion of saline solution or contrast medium to fill the endometrial cavity for the purpose of demonstrating abnormalities within the cavity or uterine tubes.

spatial pulse length – spatial extent of an ultrasound pulse burst.

Spaulding's sign – overlapping of the skull bones; occurs in fetal death.

specific gravity – laboratory tests that measure how much dissolved material is present in the urine.

spectral analysis waveform – graphic display of the flow velocity over period of time.

spectral broadening – change in the spectral width that increases with flow disturbance.

spermatic cord – structure made up of vas deferens, testicular artery, cremasteric artery, and pampiniform plexus that suspends the testis in the scrotum.

spermatocele – cyst within the vas deferens containing sperm.

spherocytosis – condition in which erythrocytes assume a spheroid shape; hereditary.

sphincter of Oddi – small muscle that guards the ampulla of Vater.

sphygmomanometer – device used to measure blood pressure.

spiculation – fingerlike extension of a malignant tumor; usually appears as a small line that radiates outward from the margin of a mass.

spina bifida – neural tube defect of the spine in which the dorsal vertebrae (vertebral arches) fail to fuse together, allowing the protrusion of meninges and/or spinal cord through the defect; two types exist: spina bifida occulta (skin-covered defect of the spine without protrusion of meninges or cord) and spina bifida cystica (open spinal defect marked by sac containing protruding meninges and/or cord).

spina bifida aperta – open (non–skin-covered lesions) neural tube defects, such as myelomeningocele and meningocele.

spina bifida occulta – closed defect of the spine without protrusion of meninges or spinal cord; alpha-fetoprotein analysis will not detect these lesions.

splaying – widening.

splenic agenesis – complete absence of the spleen.

splenic artery – one of the three vessels that arise from the celiac axis to supply the spleen, pancreas, stomach, and greater omentum; forms the superior border of the pancreas.

splenic flexure – the transverse colon travels horizontally across the abdomen and bends at this point to form the descending colon.

splenic hilum – site where vessels and lymph nodes enter and exit the spleen; located in the middle of the spleen.

splenic sinuses – long, irregular channels lined by endothelial cells or flattened reticular cells.

splenic vein – vein that drains the spleen; travels horizontally across the abdomen (posterior to the pancreas) to join the superior mesenteric vein to form the portal vein; serves as the posterior medial border of the pancreas.

splenomegaly – enlargement of the spleen.

spontaneous – flow is present without augmentation.

-stasis – standing still; *homeostasis*: maintenance of a relatively stable internal environment.

strabismus – eye disorder in which optic axes cannot be directed to the same object.

strangulated hernia – an incarcerated hernia with vascular compromise.

subclavian artery – artery that originates at the inner border of the scalenus anterior and travels beneath the clavicle to the outer border of the first rib to become the axillary artery.

subclavian steal syndrome – symptoms of brain stem ischemia associated with a stenosis or occlusion of the left subclavian, innominate, or right subclavian artery proximal to the origin of the vertebral artery.

subclavian vein – continuation of the axillary vein.

subcostal – placement of the transducer located near body midline and beneath costal margin.

subcutaneous layer – most superficial of the three layers of the breast identified on breast ultrasound, the subcutaneous layer is mainly fatty; it is located immediately beneath the skin and superficial to the mammary layer. The subcutaneous layer can be very thin and difficult to recognize.

subependyma – fragile area beneath the ependyma that is subject to bleed in the premature infant.

subhepatic – inferior to the liver.

subjective assessment of fluid – sonographer surveys uterine cavity to determine visual assessment of amniotic fluid present.

subluxed – occurs when the femoral head moves posteriorly and remains in contact with the posterior aspect of the acetabulum.

submandibular window – window formed when transducer is placed at the angle of the mandible and angled slightly medially and cephalad toward the carotid canal.

submucosa – one of the layers of the bowel, under the mucosal layer; contains blood vessels and lymph channels.

submucosal leiomyoma – type of leiomyoma found to deform the endometrial cavity and cause heavy or irregular menses.

suboccipital window – window formed when the transducer is placed on the posterior aspect of the neck inferior to the nuchal crest.

subphrenic – below the diaphragm.

subserosal – type of leiomyoma that may become pedunculated and appear as an extrauterine mass.

subvalvular aortic stenosis – formation of a membrane beneath the aortic leaflets causes left ventricular outflow obstruction.

succenturiate placenta – one or more accessory lobes connected to the body of the placenta by blood vessels.

sulcus – groove on the surface of the brain that separates the gyri.

superficial femoral artery – artery that courses the length of the thigh through Hunter's canal and terminates at the opening of the adductor magnus muscle.

superficial femoral vein – vein that originates at the hiatus of the adductor magnus muscle in the distal thigh and ascends through the adductor (Hunter's) canal.

superficial inguinal ring – triangular opening in the external oblique aponeurosis.

superior mesenteric artery – artery that arises inferior to the celiac axis to supply the proximal half of the colon and the small intestine.

superior mesenteric vein – vein that drains the proximal half of the colon and small intestine, travels vertically (anterior to the inferior vena cava) to join the splenic vein to form the portal veins.

superior vena cava – vessel receiving venous return from the head and upper extremities into the upper posterior medial wall of the right atrium.

superior vesical arteries – after birth the umbilical arteries become the superior vesical arteries.

supracristal septal defect – high membranous septal defect just beneath the pulmonary orifice.

suprapubic – above the symphysis pubis.

suprasternal – transducer placement in the suprasternal notch.

supraventricular tachyarrhythmias – abnormal rhythms above 200 beats per minute with a normal sinus conduction rate of 1:1.

surface mode – in the surface-light mode there are brighter image intensity values to structures that are closer to the viewer and darker image intensity values to structures that are further from the viewer.

synovial sheath – membrane surrounding a joint, tendon, or bursa that secretes a viscous fluid called synovia.

systemic lupus erythematosus (SLE) – inflammatory disease involving multiple organ systems; fetus of a mother with SLE may develop heart block and pericardial effusion.

systole – part of the cardiac cycle in which the ventricles are pumping blood through the outflow tract into the pulmonary artery or the aorta.

systolic to diastolic (S/D) ratio – Doppler determination of the peak systolic velocity divided by the peak diastolic velocity.

tachycardia – heart rate more than 100 beats per minute.

tail of Spence – a normal extension of breast tissue into the axillary or arm pit region.

tail of the pancreas – tapered end of the pancreas that lies in the left hypochondrium near the hilus of the spleen and upper pole of the left kidney.

target (donut) sign – characteristic of gastrointestinal wall thickening consisting of an echogenic center and a hypoechoic rim; frequently associated with sectional areas of the gastrointestinal tract; the muscle is hyperechoic, and the inner core is hypoechoic.

tendinitis (tendinopathy, tendinosis, or tenosynovitis) – inflammation of a tendon.

tendon – fibrous tissue connecting muscle to bone.

tentorium – "tent" structure in the posterior fossa that separates the cerebellum from the cerebrum.

teratoma – solid tumor.

terminal ductal-lobular unit (TDLU) – smallest functional portion of the breast involving the terminal duct and its associated lobule containing at least one acinus (tiny milk-producing gland). The TDLU undergoes significant monthly hormone-induced changes and radical changes during pregnancy and lactation. The TDLU is the site of origin of nearly all significant pathological processes involving the breast, including all elements of fibrocystic condition, fibroadenomas, and in situ and invasive breast cancer (both lobular and ductal).

testicle – male gonad that produces hormones that induce masculine features and production of spermatozoa.

testicular artery – artery arising from the aorta just distal to each renal artery; it divides into two major branches supplying the testis medially and laterally.

testicular vein – the pampiniform plexus forms each testicular vein; the right testicular vein drains directly into the inferior vena cava, whereas the left testicular vein drains into the left renal vein.

tethered spinal cord – fixed spinal cord that is positioned in an abnormal position.

tetralogy of Fallot – a congenital anomaly consisting of four defects: membranous ventricular septal defect, overriding of the aorta, right ventricular hypertrophy, and pulmonary stenosis.

thalamus – portion of the midbrain that serves as two landmarks for the sonographer that abut both sides of the third ventricle.

thalassemia – group of hereditary anemias occurring in Asian and Mediterranean populations.

thanatophoric dysplasia – lethal short-limb dwarfism characterized by a marked reduction in the length of the long bones, pear-shaped chest, soft-tissue redundancy, and frequently clover-leaf skull deformity and ventriculomegaly.

theca-lutein cysts – multilocular cysts that occur in patients with hyperstimulation (hydatidiform mole and infertility patients); appear as multiple cysts within each ovary; complication of hyperstimulation.

Thompson's test – a test used to evaluate the integrity of the Achilles' tendon that involves plantar flexion with squeezing of the calf.

thoracentesis – surgical puncture of the chest wall for removal of fluids; usually done by using a large-bore needle.

thoracic outlet syndrome – changes in arterial blood flow to the arms related to intermittent compression of the proximal arteries.

three-dimensional (3-D) ultrasound – permits collection and review of data obtained from a volume of tissue in multiple imaging planes and rendering of surface features.

thrombocytes – platelets in blood.

thyroglossal duct cyst – congenital anomaly that presents in the midline of the neck anterior to the trachea.

thyroiditis – inflammation of the thyroid.

thyroid-stimulating hormone (TSH) – hormone secreted by the pituitary gland that stimulates the thyroid gland to secrete thyroxine and triiodothyronine.

tibial-peroneal trunk – arterial branch that exits after the anterior tibial artery and bifurcates into the posterior tibial artery and the peroneal artery.

time gain compensation (TGC) – also referred to as *depth gain compensation*; ability to compensate for attenuation of the transmitted beam as the sound wave travels through tissues in the body; usually, individual pod controls allow the operator to manually change the amount of compensation necessary for each patient to produce a quality image.

Tinel's sign (Hoffmann-Tinel sign, Tinel's symptom, or Tinel-Hoffmann sign) – pins-and-needles type tingling felt distally to a percussion site. Sensation can be either an abnormal or a normal occurrence (i.e., hitting the elbow creates a tingling in the distal arm).

TIPS – transjugular intrahepatic portosystemic shunt.

tissue specific ultrasound contrast agent – a type of contrast agent whose microbubbles are removed from the blood and are taken up by specific tissues in the body; one example is the agent Sonozoid

-tomy – cutting; *anatomy*: study of structure, which often involves cutting or removing body parts.

transducer – any device that converts signals from one form to another.

transitional zone – prostate area that is located on both sides of the proximal urethra and ends at the level of the verumontanum.

transorbital window – transducer placement on the closed eyelid.

transparent mode – sometimes called x-ray mode, is best for viewing a relatively low-contrast block of soft tissue.

transposition of the great arteries – failure of the truncus arteriosus to complete its rotation during the first trimester; causes the pulmonary artery to arise from the left ventricle and the aorta to arise from the pulmonary artery (blue baby at birth).

transpyloric plane – horizontal plane that passes through the pylorus, the duodenal junction, the neck of the pancreas, and the hilum of the kidneys.

transtemporal window – transducer placement on the temporal bone cephalad to the zygomatic arch anterior to the ear.

transvaginal transducer – high-frequency transducer that is inserted into the vaginal canal to obtain better definition of first-trimester pregnancy.

transverse lie – description of the fetus lying transversely (horizontally) across the abdomen.

Treacher Collins syndrome – underdevelopment of the jaw and cheek bone and abnormal ears.

tricuspid atresia – underdevelopment of the tricuspid valve (usually associated with hypoplasia of the right ventricle and pulmonary stenosis).

tricuspid valve – atrioventricular valve found between the right atrium and right ventricle.

trigonocephaly – premature closure of the metopic suture.

trimester – pregnancy is divided into three 13-week segments called trimesters.

true knots of the umbilical cord – knots formed when a loop of cord is slipped over the fetal head or shoulders during delivery.

true (minor) pelvis – found below the brim of the pelvis; the cavity of the minor pelvis is continuous at the pelvic brim with the cavity of the major pelvis.

truncus arteriosus – common arterial trunk that divides into the aorta and pulmonary artery.

tuboovarian abscess (TOA) – infection that involves the fallopian tube and the ovary.

tunica adventitia – outer layer of the vascular system.

tunica albuginea – inner fibrous membrane surrounding the testicle.

tunica intima – inner layer of the vascular system.

tunica media – middle layer of the vascular system; veins have thinner tunica media than arteries.

tunica vaginalis – membrane consisting of a visceral layer (adherent to the testis) and a parietal layer (adherent to the scrotum) lining the inner wall of the scrotum; a potential space between these layers is where hydroceles may develop.

Turner's syndrome – congenital endocrine disorder caused by failure of the ovaries to respond to pituitary hormone stimulation; cystic hygroma often seen.

twin-to-twin transfusion – monozygotic twin pregnancy with single placenta and arteriovenous shunt within the placenta; the donor twin becomes anemic and growth restricted with oligohydramnios; the recipient twin may develop hydrops and polyhydramnios.

tympany – predominant sound heard over hollow organs (stomach, intestines, bladder, aorta, gallbladder).

ultrasound contrast agents – agents that can be administered intravenously to evaluate blood vessels, blood flow, and solid organs.

umbilical – around the navel.

umbilical cord – connecting lifeline between the fetus and placenta; it contains two umbilical arteries and one umbilical vein encased in Wharton's jelly.

umbilical herniation – failure of the anterior abdominal wall to close completely at the level of the umbilicus.

uncinate process – small, curved tip of the pancreatic head that lies posterior to the superior mesenteric vein.

unicornuate uterus – anomaly of the uterus in which only one horn and tube develop.

ureteropelvic junction – junction of the ureter entering the renal pelvis; most common site of obstruction.

ureteropelvic junction obstruction – most common neonatal obstruction of the urinary tract; results from intrinsic narrowing or extrinsic vascular compression.

ureterovesical junction – junction where the ureter enters the bladder.

ureters – retroperitoneal structures that exit the kidney to carry urine to the urinary bladder.

urethra – small, membranous canal that excretes urine from the urinary bladder.

urethral atresia – lack of development of the urethra; condition causing a massively distended bladder (prune belly).

urinary amylase – pancreatic enzyme that remains elevated longer than serum amylase in patients with acute pancreatitis.

urinary bladder – muscular retroperitoneal organ that serves as a reservoir for urine.

urinary incontinence – the uncontrollable passage of urine.

urinoma – cyst containing urine.

uterine synechiae – scars within the uterus secondary to previous gynecological surgery.

uterovesical space – anterior pouch between the uterus and bladder.

uterus didelphys – complete duplication of the uterus, cervix, and vagina.

VACTERL – **v**ertebral abnormalities, **a**nal atresia, **c**ardiac abnormalities, **t**racheo**e**sophageal fistula, and **r**enal and **l**imb abnormalities.

vagina atresia – failure of the vagina to develop.

valvulae conniventes – normal segmentation of the small bowel.

varicocele – dilated veins caused by obstruction of the venous return from the testicle.

varicose veins – dilated, elongated, tortuous superficial veins.

vas deferens – tube that connects the epididymis to the seminal vesicle.

vasa previa – condition that occurs when the umbilical cord vessels cross the internal os of the cervix.

vascular ultrasound contrast agents – a type of ultrasound contrast agent whose microbubbles are contained in the body's vascular spaces; examples of this type of agent include Optison, Definity, Imagent, Levovist, SonoVue.

vasovagal – concerning the action of stimuli from the vagus nerve on blood vessels.

veins – collapsible vascular structures that carry blood back to the heart.

velocity – speed of the ultrasound wave; determined by tissue density.

velocity envelope – trace of the peak velocities as a function of time.

ventricular septal defect – communication between the right and left ventricles.

ventriculitis – inflammation or infection of the ventricles that appears as echogenic linear structures along the gyri; may also appear as focal echogenic structures within the white matter.

ventriculomegaly – abnormal accumulation of cerebrospinal fluid within the cerebral ventricles resulting in dilation of the ventricles; compression of developing brain tissue and brain damage may result; commonly associated with additional fetal anomalies.

veracity – truthfulness, honesty.

vertebral artery – branches of the subclavian artery that merge to form the basilar artery.

vertex – position of fetus with head down in the uterus.

vertigo – sensation of having objects move about the person or sensation of moving around in space.

verumontanum – junction of the ejaculatory ducts with the urethra.

villi – inner folds of the small intestine.

visceral peritoneum – layer of peritoneum that covers the abdominal organs.

vital signs – medical measurements used to ascertain how the body is functioning.

volar – the anterior portion of the body when in the anatomical position.

volume rendering – the volume is evaluated by rotating the volume data to a standard orientation and then scrolling through parallel planes. The data may be rotated to assess oblique planes.

wall echo shadow (WES) sign – sonographic pattern found when the gallbladder is packed with stones.

wandering spleen – spleen that has migrated from its normal location in the left upper quadrant.

wave – propagation of energy that moves back and forth or vibrates at a steady rate.

wavelength – distance over which a wave repeats itself during one period of oscillation.

Wharton's jelly – myxomatous connective tissue that surrounds the umbilical vessels and varies in size.

white blood cells – cells that defend the body by destroying invading microorganisms and their toxins.

white pulp – tissue composed of lymphatic tissue and lymphatic follicles.

Wilms' tumor – most frequent malignant tumor in the neonate and infant.

yolk sac – circular structure seen between 4 and 10 weeks that supplies nutrition to the fetal pole (the developing embryo); it lies within the chorion outside the amnion.

yolk stalk – the umbilical duct connecting the yolk sac with the embryo.

zygote – fertilized ovum resulting from union of male and female gametes.

zygote intrafallopian transfer (ZIFT) – a human fertilization technique in which the zygotes are injected through a laparoscope into the fimbriated ends of the fallopian tubes. Recently, this has been performed under ultrasound guidance.

Index

Page numbers followed by *f, t,* or *b* indicate figures, tables, or boxes, respectively. Numbers in **boldface** type are in Volume Two.